Forensic Medicine and Toxicology
for Medical Students

Get free online access to author's video lectures/demonstration of important forensic topics/procedures

List of videos with QR code placement

Topic of video	Chapter number	Page number
Do's and don'ts for a doctor in court	1	18
Identification of male vs female skull	5	87
Development of latent fingerprints	6	108
Evisceration methods	7	135
Brain death demonstration	8	147
Coup and contrecoup injury	13	271
Bloodstains and blood group examination	29	486
Demonstration of gastric lavage	35	538
Examination of drunkenness	47	625

Steps to access free videos:
1. *Scan the QR code at the page number pertaining to topic mentioned above.*
2. *Play and start watching.*

Forensic Medicine and Toxicology
for Medical Students

Including Clinical and Pathological Aspects

As per the Competency Based Medical Education Curriculum (NMC)

Sixth Edition

Gautam Biswas MD (UCMS)
Professor and Head
Department of Forensic Medicine and Toxicology
Dayanand Medical College and Hospital
Ludhiana, Punjab, India

Forewords
Ponni Arunkumar
Ashok Moondra

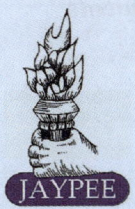

JAYPEE BROTHERS MEDICAL PUBLISHERS
The Health Sciences Publisher
New Delhi | London

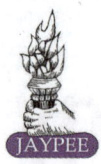
Jaypee Brothers Medical Publishers (P) Ltd

Headquarters
Jaypee Brothers Medical Publishers (P) Ltd
EMCA House, 23/23-B
Ansari Road, Daryaganj
New Delhi 110 002, India
Landline: +91-11-23272143, +91-11-23272703
+91-11-23282021, +91-11-23245672
Email: jaypee@jaypeebrothers.com

Corporate Office
Jaypee Brothers Medical Publishers (P) Ltd
4838/24, Ansari Road, Daryaganj
New Delhi 110 002, India
Phone: +91-11-43574357
Fax: +91-11-43574314
Email: jaypee@jaypeebrothers.com

Overseas Office
J.P. Medical Ltd
83 Victoria Street, London
SW1H 0HW (UK)
Phone: +44 20 3170 8910
Fax: +44 (0)20 3008 6180
Email: info@jpmedpub.com

Website: www.jaypeebrothers.com
Website: www.jaypeedigital.com

© 2024, Jaypee Brothers Medical Publishers

The views and opinions expressed in this book are solely those of the original contributor(s)/author(s) and do not necessarily represent those of editor(s) of the book.

All rights reserved. No part of this publication may be reproduced, stored or transmitted in any form or by any means, electronic, mechanical, photocopying, recording or otherwise, without the prior permission in writing of the publishers.

All brand names and product names used in this book are trade names, service marks, trademarks or registered trademarks of their respective owners. The publisher is not associated with any product or vendor mentioned in this book.

Medical knowledge and practice change constantly. This book is designed to provide accurate, authoritative information about the subject matter in question. However, readers are advised to check the most current information available on procedures included and check information from the manufacturer of each product to be administered, to verify the recommended dose, formula, method and duration of administration, adverse effects and contraindications. It is the responsibility of the practitioner to take all appropriate safety precautions. Neither the publisher nor the author(s)/editor(s) assume any liability for any injury and/or damage to persons or property arising from or related to use of material in this book.

This book is sold on the understanding that the publisher is not engaged in providing professional medical services. If such advice or services are required, the services of a competent medical professional should be sought.

Every effort has been made where necessary to contact holders of copyright to obtain permission to reproduce copyright material. If any have been inadvertently overlooked, the publisher will be pleased to make the necessary arrangements at the first opportunity.

Inquiries for bulk sales may be solicited at: jaypee@jaypeebrothers.com

Forensic Medicine and Toxicology for Medical Students

First Edition: 2010
Second Edition: 2012
Third Edition: 2015
Fourth Edition: 2019
Fifth Edition: 2021
  Reprint Edition: 2022
Sixth Edition: **2024**

ISBN: 978-93-5696-962-9

Printed at: Samrat Offset Pvt. Ltd.

Anupama and Gaurav...
With lots of love...

Contributors
(for Images)

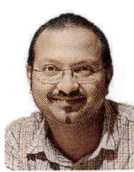
Abhishek Das
Associate Professor and Head
Department of Forensic Medicine and Toxicology
Calcutta National Medical College
Kolkata, West Bengal, India

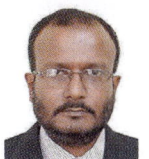
Amarjyoti Patowary
Professor and Head
Department of Forensic Medicine and Toxicology
North Eastern Indira Gandhi Regional Institute of
Health and Medical Sciences
Shillong, Meghalaya, India

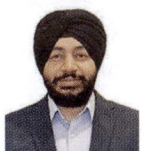
Aminder Singh
Associate Professor
Department of Pathology
Dayanand Medical College and Hospital
Punjab, India

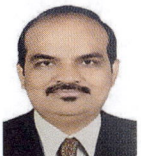
Amit Parmar
Additional Dean and Professor
Department of Forensic Medicine and Toxicology
Govt Medical College
Gujarat, India

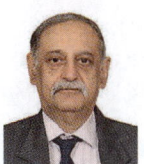
Anil Kohli
Director-Professor
Department of Forensic Medicine and Toxicology
University College of Medical Sciences and
Guru Teg Bahadur Hospital
Dilshad Garden, Delhi, India

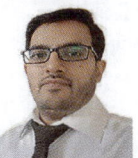
Chandresh I Tailor
Associate Professor and I/C Head
Department of Forensic Medicine and Toxicology
Government Medical College and New Civil Hospital
Gujarat, India

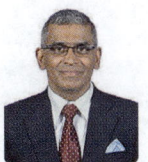
Dinesh MG Fernando
Head
Department of Forensic Medicine
Faculty of Medicine
University of Peradeniya
Sri Lanka

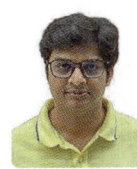
Dipak Harjivan Vora
Associate Professor
Department of Forensic Medicine and Toxicology
Govt Medical College and SSG Hospital
Gujarat, India

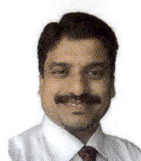
Hareesh Kumar
Additional Dean and Professor
Department of Forensic Medicine and Toxicology
Government Medical College
Rajasthan, India

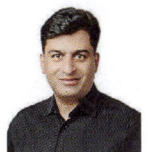
Hitesh Chawla
Professor
Department of Forensic Medicine and Toxicology
SHKM Govt. Medical College
Haryana, India

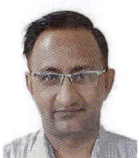
Jitender Kumar Jakhar
Professor
Department of Forensic Medicine and Toxicology
Post Graduate Institute of Medical Sciences
Rohtak, Haryana, India

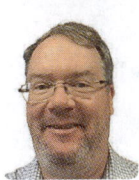
Joseph A Prahlow
Forensic Pathologist, Deputy Medical Examiner
Professor and Vice Chair
Department of Pathology
Western Michigan University Homer Stryker
MD School of Medicine
Kalamazoo, Michigan, USA

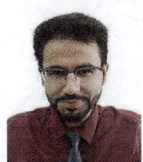
Karan Pramod
Senior Resident
Department of Forensic Medicine and Toxicology
GGS Medical College
Punjab, India

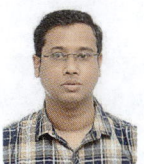
Lishu Chaure
Demonstrator
Department of Forensic Medicine and Toxicology
Bharat Ratna Late Shri Atal Bihari Vajpayee
Memorial Medical College
Chhattisgarh, India

Contributors

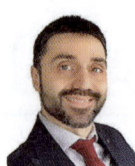
Lorenzo Gitto
Assistant Medical Examiner-Forensic Pathologist
Cook County Medical Examiner's Office
Chicago, Illinois, United States

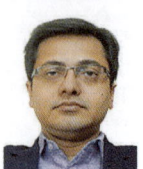
Mohit Gupta
Professor
Department of Forensic Medicine and Toxicology
Vardhman Mahavir Medical College and
Safdarjung Hospital
New Delhi, India

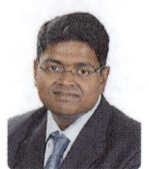
O Murugesa Bharathi
Associate Professor
Department of Forensic Medicine and Toxicology
Indira Gandhi Medial College and Research Institute
Puducherry, India

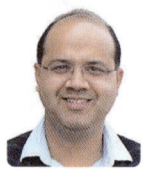
Parmod Goyal
Principal, Professor and Head
Department of Forensic Medicine and Toxicology
Adesh Institute of Medical Sciences and Research
Bathinda, Punjab, India

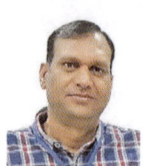
Rajendra Singh Kulhari
Assistant Professor
Department of Forensic Medicine and Toxicology
Sardar Patel Medical College
Bikaner, Rajasthan, India

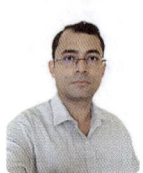
Sandip Mukhopadhyay
Associate Professor
Department of Forensic Medicine and Toxicology
Nil Ratan Sircar Medical College
Kolkata, West Bengal, India

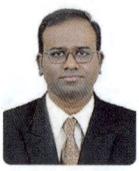
Senthil Kumaran M
Associate Professor and In-Charge Head
Department of Forensic Medicine and Toxicology
All India Institute of Medical Sciences
Tamil Nadu, India

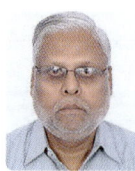
Shashidhar Mestri
Professor and Head (*Retired*)
Department of Forensic Medicine and Toxicology
Karpaga Vinayaga Institute of Medical Sciences
Tamil Nadu, India

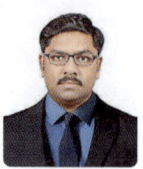
Siddesh RC
Associate Professor
Department of Forensic Medicine and Toxicology
SS Institute of Medical Sciences and Research Center
Karnataka, India

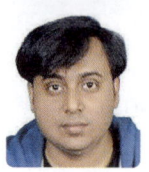
Soumeek Chowdhuri
Assistant Professor
Department of Forensic Medicine and Toxicology
Calcutta National Medical College and Hospital
Kolkata, West Bengal, India

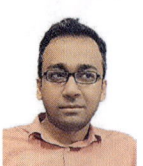
Sujash Biswas
Associate Professor
Department of Forensic Medicine and Toxicology
Rampurhat Govt Medical College and Hospital
Birbhum, West Bengal, India

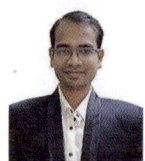
Tikendra Dewangan
Forensic Expert
District Hospital, Dantewada
Chhattisgarh, India

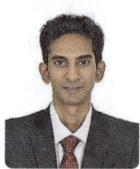
Viswakanth B
Professor
Department of Forensic Medicine and Toxicology
Kanachur Institute of Medical Sciences and Hospital
Mangaluru, Karnataka, India

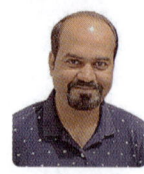
Vivek Kumar
Associate Professor
Department of Forensic Medicine and Toxicology
Jalpaiguri Government Medical College & Hospital
West Bengal, India

Foreword

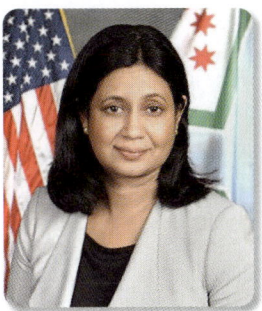

Forensic pathology presents a unique challenge—an intricate blend of medical expertise and legal scrutiny. It navigates the complexities of investigating deaths, often facing the weight of unraveling mysteries while adhering to rigorous scientific protocols and legal requisites. The practitioner's role in deciphering truth from evidence is pivotal, standing as a testament to the demanding yet profoundly rewarding nature of this field.

"*Forensic Medicine and Toxicology for Medical Students*" stands as a testament to the richness and complexity of this discipline, encapsulating a wide array of chapters that unveil the multifaceted nature of forensic practice. Written by Gautam Biswas, an experienced expert deeply involved in the field, this compendium goes beyond being just a set of chapters. It guides the reader through the complex pathways of forensic medicine. It embodies the dedication, responsibility, and unwavering commitment to truth embraced by those devoted to this fascinating discipline.

From the very outset, this compendium sets a robust foundation, touching upon legal procedures and the ethical considerations inherent in medical practice. The initial chapters serve as an anchor, grounding the reader in the fundamental principles that underpin the intricate intersection between medicine and the legal system.

What distinguishes this anthology is its in-depth investigation into injuries and their legal-medical implications. From deaths related to asphyxia to firearm injuries and transportation incidents, the chapters offer a thorough view of various trauma encountered in forensic practice. Accompanied by high-definition color photos and diagrams, these sections guide the reader through the complex landscape of traumatic injuries within forensic investigations.

The compendium fearlessly delves into the intricate and sensitive realms of human behavior. It discusses critical subjects such as neglect, criminal abortions, abuse, and sexual violence, shedding light on the challenging realities faced by forensic experts. These sections deftly blend scientific rigor with a relentless pursuit of factual truths, presenting raw realities in an objective manner.

Moreover, the inclusion of chapters exploring toxicology in such depth is commendable. From basic toxicology principles to common drugs of abuse, from corrosive poisons to organic and inorganic irritants, the compendium offers a comprehensive exploration of toxic substances and their impact on human physiology. This comprehensive exploration of toxicology deepens the understanding of forensic investigations, particularly their wide-ranging legal implications.

"*Forensic Medicine and Toxicology for Medical Students*" is a commendable resource that not only educates but also inspires a deeper appreciation for the profound complexities inherent in forensic practice, representing a guide for students, residents, forensic professionals, educators, and forensic enthusiasts.

Ponni Arunkumar MD
Chief Medical Examiner
Cook County Medical Examiner's Office
Chicago, Illinois, United States

Foreword

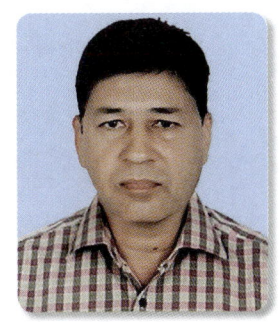

It gives me immense pleasure and pride to write Foreword for the 6th edition of the *"Forensic Medicine and Toxicology for Medical Students"*. Gautam Biswas is sincere, hardworking, and great academician. Nowadays, writing a book is a difficult task as the taste of students has changed; they are reading only the PDF contents that are available online. An author has to work very hard to get into the psyche of the students and make it part of their bookshelf. Dr Biswas keeps the book updated and makes continuous efforts to improve it. In furtherance to that, this modernized and revised edition of the textbook will be useful for both UG and PG students.

The textbook is structured in such a way that recent changes prescribed by the National Medical Commission (NMC) are incorporated in the book. It is a competency-based book covering the whole course in a systematic manner. Online Multiple Choice Questions (MCQs) and contents are included to help students during NEET PG and UG examinations and various competitive examinations. This book includes an interesting case study along with every chapter to arouse interest of the student so that they can understand the chapter in better way. Not only the content of the book is meticulous but language is also very simple; colored photographs are included as well as diagrams and charts to make it understandable and interesting. The original photographs taken by various faculty members throughout the country are included in the book—this is a great thought and students can learn in a better way.

I felt proud to see the medical students following this book even in Mauritius (where I visited as an examiner) and procure this book from India. It gives a proud feeling that Indian authors are also popular outside the country. In true sense, it is an example of "Make in India". I hope that the 6th edition of this book will be loved by students and faculty alike, and many more editions will be coming in the future.

Ashok Moondra MBBS MD
Senior Professor and Head
Department of Forensic Medicine and Toxicology
Government Medical College
Kota, Rajasthan, India

Preface to the Sixth Edition

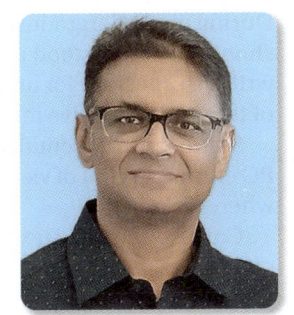

It gives me an immense pleasure to introduce the 6th edition of my textbook *Review of Forensic Medicine and Toxicology*. The book has been retitled as *"Forensic Medicine and Toxicology for Medical Students"*. This book is being revised regularly to incorporate new research, new technology, new laws, and new regulations so as to provide up-to-date information to the readers. The book conforms to the National Medical Commission (NMC's) "Competency Based Undergraduate Curriculum for the Indian Medical Graduate". The previous edition was a move toward this direction making it more learner-centric, patient-centric, gender-sensitive, outcome-oriented, and environment-appropriate. The current edition adds up to this direction.

This edition of *"Forensic Medicine and Toxicology for Medical Students"* has been thoroughly updated with extensive modifications in its look and content, although the format and layout remain the same. Similar to the last edition, this edition too comes in full colored text incorporating the competencies listed in the NMC document. At the beginning of each chapter, there are learning objectives featuring brief statements as to what the students are expected to learn after completion of the topic. It will be useful for preparing for professional examinations also.

Like previous editions, this text is presented in a concise and lucid form with line diagrams, boxes, tables, differentiations, and flowcharts are colored and designed to make the book interesting to read, easy to comprehend, recollect, and reproduce. Colored images from several clinical case studies have been added to make the concept clearer. Additionally, colored boxes in the form of "Pearls" have been added to highlight salient features/points. "Mnemonics" have been included wherever possible. Interesting anecdotes and facts, concepts, theories, recent advances, and topic-related information have been added wherever needed. Older terminologies have been discarded and newer ones introduced.

There are some new innovative ideas which will help the reader in understanding the topic in a better way—colored images featuring clinical cases/postmortem have been incorporated after completion of the topic along with thought-provoking questions that the readers can deal with confidently when they actually come across similar cases. There is a separate table of "High Yield" at the end of each chapter which gives a summary of important definitions and points—take-away messages from the chapter. Additionally, a case report is given at the end (after "high yield") pertaining to some topic already discussed in the chapter (as suggested by few students). This will create more interest and will help in retaining the information in the long run. Another innovative approach is the addition of "QR codes" to select topics which the reader can utilize to watch the video for better understanding of the concept.

The Multiple Choice Questions (MCQs) from recent PG entrance examinations are included as online content for the students which they can access with the unique code provided along with each book. This will help the reader to get an insight into that topic and prepare for viva-voce and subsequent postgraduate entrance examinations (INCET/NEET/NEXT).

It is my hope that this edition will find favorable response from medical students (both undergraduate and postgraduate) like the previous editions and also offer significant help to medical practitioners, in-service doctors, and forensic pathologists.

Any mistakes or misinterpretations inadvertently done may be brought to my notice. It will be rectified and duly acknowledged in the next edition.

Gautam Biswas

Preface to the First Edition

During my undergraduate days, I felt that textbooks should contain necessary information, not have too many details and should be understood easily, i.e., they should be comprehensive, clear and concise. Keeping this in mind, this book is written, especially for undergraduates and for those preparing for the postgraduate (PG) entrance test. The entire concept of this book is to give information in as few words as possible without omitting necessary details.

Some topics (Identification, Injuries, Sexual Offences, Forensic Psychiatry and Toxicology) which are important from PG entrance point of view, are in more detail. All topics are updated and recent advances/changes have been incorporated wherever needed.

Concise and lucid text (bullet's format), line-diagrams, boxes, tables, differentiations and flowcharts given at appropriate places, are designed to make the book interesting-to-read, easy-to-comprehend, recollect and reproduce.

The information given in boxes is 'desirable to know', that a student may skip if there is shortage of time or if preparing for the professional examination. Rest of the information is 'must know', i.e., one should go through it definitely.

In section two (Toxicology), all the poisons are given in the same format throughout so that the student is able to understand and reproduce them during the examination. The section is up-to-date and some additional topics have been added for the PG entrance test.

Topic-wise MCQs are given at the end of most of the chapters. They are based on the recall of students who appeared in these examinations, and will help the reader to get insight of that topic and prepare for the PG entrance. It will also make preparation for viva voce easy and interesting for the student.

Appendices I and II give a list of important questions, which the students should prepare for the professional examination and are based on the latest MBBS curriculum prepared by Directorate General of Health Services and National Medical Council. There are two categories—must know and desirable to know, the student may prepare according to the time and can devote to the subject.

It is my hope that this new book will find favorable response from medical students and also offer significant help to medical practitioners, in-service doctors and forensic scientists.

It has been my endeavor to keep the book error-free, however, there may be some typographical errors. If the reader comes across any such error or wants to send any comment/suggestion, please do write or send an e-mail. It will be duly acknowledged in the subsequent edition.

Gautam Biswas

Acknowledgments

I am thankful for the blessings of my mentors and teachers, who taught me to inquire, think, and persevere. I deeply appreciate the invaluable suggestions of Dr Anil Kohli, Director-Professor, Forensic Medicine, UCMS and GTB Hospital, whose immeasurable suggestions and wisdom can never be appropriately or adequately acknowledged. Dr Dasari Harish, Professor and Head, GMCH, Chandigarh, gave useful suggestions for improvement of this book for which I am grateful to him. I am so very thankful to Dr Viswakanth B, Dr O Murugesa Bharathi, and Dr Lishu Chaure for being my troubleshooters/problem solvers/fixers, whenever I got stuck; they were always available with the solutions! Dr Viswakanth has provided valuable inputs for the chapter on Medical Jurisprudence, ART Acts, Surrogacy Acts, Sexual Offences, and Homosexuality for which I am highly indebted to him. Dr Kulhari, Dr O Murugesa Bharathi, and Dr Lishu Chure have been instrumental for getting some of the exceptional images that are part of this book.

Faculty from all over India and outside India have contributed many amazing images. I am indebted to them for their contributions. I sincerely acknowledge the encouragement given by Dr Anil Aggrawal (Maulana Azad Medical College, New Delhi), Dr Suresh Kumar Dhattarwal (PGIMS, Rohtak), Dr Parmod Goyal (Adesh Institute of Medical Science and Research, Bathinda), and Jitender Kumar Jakhar (PGIMS, Rohtak). Dr Virendar Pal Singh, my friend and colleague, deserves special appreciation for providing constant support in this venture.

I also express my thanks to Dr Aminder Singh (Professor, Department of Pathology, DMCH) and Dr Ajay Kumar (Professor, Department of Anatomy, DMCH) for their valuable contribution in updating the text. I thank some of my students, notably Abhay, Harjas, Prisha, Ritvik, Siddhant, Simran and Yukta for reviewing some of the chapters and providing valuable suggestions. I am thankful to Depositphotos, Wikipedia, various newspapers, journals, and blogs for the case reports and some photos. I have taken permissions for some of the images and case reports and acknowledged the same wherever possible. If missed inadvertently, kindly let me know so that I can acknowledge the same in the next edition.

I would like to express my sincere gratitude to Shri Bipin Gupta, Secretary, Managing Society, DMCH; Dr Sandeep Puri, Principal, DMCH; Dr Gurpreet Singh Wander, Vice-Principal, DMCH; and Dr Sandeep Kaushal, Dean Academics, DMCH, for their continuous support, motivation, encouragement, and invaluable suggestions.

I am indebted and obliged to the following faculty for their wholehearted support, valuable suggestions, and blessings (*in random order*):

1. Dr Mukul Chopra (CMC, Ludhiana, Punjab)
2. Dr Jayesh Dudhe (GMCH, Nagpur)
3. Dr Baljit Singh Khurana and Dr Rajiv Chaudhary (SGRD Medical College, Amritsar, Punjab)
4. Dr Rajiv Joshi (GMC, Faridkot, Punjab)
5. Dr Anju Gupta (PIMS, Jalandhar, Punjab)
6. Dr Aakashdeep Aggarwal (GMC, Patiala, Punjab)
7. Dr Hitesh Chawla (GMC, Mewat)
8. Dr CS Gupta (ASCOMS, Jammu)
9. Dr Aditya Sharma (IGMC, Shimla)
10. Dr Farida Noor (GMCH, Srinagar, Jammu and Kashmir)
11. Dr Sandhya Arora (GMCH, Jammu)
12. Dr SK Verma and Dr Arvind Kumar (UCMS and GTB Hospital, Delhi)
13. Dr Mukta Rani (LHMC, New Delhi)
14. Dr Sunil Kumar Naggar (MAMC, New Delhi)
15. Dr Anil Mittal and Dr Gaurav Jain (VMMC, New Delhi)
16. Dr Upender Kishore (BSAM College and Hospital, Rohini, New Delhi)
17. Dr Vijay Arora (RPGMC, Tanda, Himachal Pradesh)
18. Dr Sangeet Dhillon (Dr YS Parmar Medical College, Nahan, Himachal Pradesh)
19. Dr Sanjay Chandel (Dr Radhakrishnan GMC, Hamirpur)
20. Dr Prabh Sharan Singh (MMU Medical College, Solan, Himachal Pradesh)

21. Dr Sanjoy Das (HIMS, Dehradun, Uttarakhand)
22. Dr CP Bhaisora (GMCH, Haldwani, Uttarakhand)
23. Dr Lalit Kumar Varshney and Dr Shah Alam (SGRRI, Dehradun, Uttarakhand)
24. Dr Vijay Pal Khanagwal (KCGMC, Karnal, Haryana)
25. Dr Dildar Singh (Maharaja Agrasen Medical College, Agroha, Haryana)
26. Dr Gaurav Sharma and Dr Anil Garg (BPSGMC, Sonipat, Haryana)
27. Dr Gaurav Aggarwal (MSY Medical College, Meerut, UP)
28. Dr Mukesh Yadav (GMC, Banda, UP)
29. Dr Pooja Rastogi (SIMS, Greater Noida, UP)
30. Dr Arbind Kumar (Nalanda Medical College, Patna, Bihar)
31. Dr Binay Kumar (AIIMS, Patna, Bihar)
32. Dr Gunajit Das (Dhubri Medical College, Dhubri, Assam)
33. Dr Amar Jyoti Patowary (NEIGRIHMS, Shillong, Meghalaya)
34. Dr Satyakam Jena (Hi-Tech Medical College, Cuttack, Orissa)
35. Dr Swapnil Agarwal (PMC and Shree Krishna Hospital, Gujarat)
36. Dr Lavlesh Kumar (SBKS Medical Institute and Research Center, Vadodara, Gujarat)
37. Dr Tanuj Kanchan (All India Institute of Medical Sciences, Jodhpur, Rajasthan)
38. Dr PK Tiwari (GMC, Kota, Rajasthan)
39. Dr Sanjeev Choudhary (Geetanjali Medical College, Udaipur, Rajasthan)
40. Dr Jagadeesh Narayanareddy (VIMS and Research Center, Bengaluru, Karnataka)
41. Dr Prateek Rastogi (KMC, Mangaluru, Karnataka)
42. Dr Pradeep Kumar MV (HIMS, Haveri, Karnataka)
43. Dr Pramod Kumar GN (KIMS, Karwar, Karnataka)
44. Dr Prakash Babladi (MR Medical College, Gulbarga, Karnataka)
45. Dr Sudha R (Osmania Medical College, Hyderabad, Telangana)
46. Dr Avishek Kumar (CU Shah Medical College and Hospital, Surendranagar, Gujarat)
47. Dr Sandeep Singh (LN Medical College, Bhopal, MP)
48. Dr Sarthak Juglan (GR Medical College, Gwalior, MP)
49. Dr Seema Sutay (Index Medical College, Indore, MP)
50. Dr Raghavendra Vidua (AIIMS, Bhopal)
51. Dr Krishnadutt Chavali (AIIMS, Raipur, Chhattisgarh)
52. Dr Freminston Marak (IGMC and RI, Puducherry)
53. Dr Pannag P Kumar (Goa Medical College, Goa)
54. Dr Shailesh Mohite (TNMC and Nair Hospital, Mumbai, Maharashtra)
55. Dr Indrajit Khandekar (MGIMS, Sevagram, Maharashtra)
56. Dr Harish Pathak and Dr Ravindra Deokar (KEM Hospital, Mumbai, Maharashtra)
57. Dr Sudhir Ninave (JNMC, Wardha, Maharashtra)
58. Dr Tapas Kumar Bose (JIMSH, Kolkata, West Bengal)
59. Dr Uday Basu (ESIC Medical College & Hospital, Joka, Kolkata, West Bengal)
60. Dr P Mukhopadhyay (Malda Medical College, Malda, West Bengal)

I express my appreciation to the whole team of M/s Jaypee Brothers Medical Publishers (P) Ltd., for their patience, encouragement, and professionalism during the entire process. I am especially indebted to Shri Jitendar P Vij (Group Chairman), Mr Ankit Vij (Managing Director), Mr MS Mani (Group President), Dr Madhu Choudhary (Director-Educational Publishing), Ms Pooja Bhandari [Director-Production (Books and Journals)], Ms Sunita Katla (Executive Assistant to Group Chairman and Publishing Manager), Ms Samina Khan (Executive Assistant to Director-Content Strategy), and Dr Aditya Tayal (Team Lead-UG Publishing). I also thank production team comprising Mr Ajay Kumar Sharma [DGM-Production (Books and Journals)], Mr Rajesh Sharma (Production Coordinator), Mr Sumit Kumar (Cover Visualizer), Ms Neelam (Proofreader), Mr Dinesh Bhardwaj and Mr Kulwant Singh (Typesetters), and Mr Nitesh Jain (Graphic Designer) for shaping up this book and making all the changes without any complaints.

This work would not have been possible without the blessings of my family. I would like to thank my parents for their unconditional love, support, and blessings. I would like to express my earnest gratitude and love for my wife Anupama and son Gaurav for their constant support and encouragement. Last but not least, I wish to offer my apologies to all my colleagues, friends, and students, whose names I have omitted inadvertently, for without their constant support, encouragement, and well wishes, the book would not have been completed.

Contents

Section 1: Jurisprudence and Forensic Medicine

Chapter 1: Legal Procedure   3

- History of Forensic Medicine   3
- Inquest   6
- Police Inquest   7
- Magistrate Inquest   7
- Courts of Law   9
- Subpoena/Summons   11
- Conduct Money   12
- Medical Evidence   12
- Types of Witness   15
- Recording of Evidence   16
- Conduct and Duties of a Doctor in the Witness Box   18

Chapter 2: Medical Practitioner—Duties and Malpractices   20

- National Medical Commission   20
- Powers and Functions   21
- State Medical Council (SMC)   22
- Duties of a Doctor   24
- Professional Secrecy   27
- Privileged Communication   28
- Medical Malpractice   29
- Professional Misconduct (Infamous Conduct)   29
- Erasure of Name   31
- Types of Physician–Patient Relationship   32
- Professional Negligence   32
- Safeguards Against Litigation   35
- Defenses Against Negligence   36
- Doctrine of Res Ipsa Loquitur   36
- Calculated Risk Doctrine   37
- Doctrine of Common Knowledge   37
- Contributory Negligence   37
- Corporate Negligence   38
- Products Liability   38
- Medical Maloccurrence   38
- Therapeutic Misadventure/Hazard   39
- Vicarious Liability/Respondeat Superior   39
- Consent   40

Chapter 3: Ethical and Social Aspects of Medical Practice   45

- Medical Ethics   45
- Euthanasia (Mercy Killing)   47
- Stem Cell Research   48
- Human Experimentation   49
- Malingering (Shamming)   51
- Oath   51
- Declaration of Geneva   52
- Doctors and Media   54
- Press Conference   54
- Challenges in Medico-legal cases   54
- Communication Skills   55
- Conflict   56

Chapter 4: Acts Related to Medical Practice   60

- The Transplantation of Human Organs Act, 1994   60
- The Consumer Protection Act, 2019   63
- Medical Indemnity Insurance   64
- The Workmen's Compensation Act, 1923   65
- Employees' State Insurance (ESI) Act, 1948   65
- The Protection of Children from Sexual Offenses (POCSO) Act, 2012   66
- The Transgender Persons (Protection of Rights) Act, 2019   67
- The Assisted Reproductive Technology (Regulation) Act, 2021   68
- The Medical Termination of Pregnancy (Amendment) Act, 2021   69
- The Preconception and Prenatal Diagnostic Techniques Act, 1994   71
- The Protection of Women from Domestic Violence Act, 2005   73
- The Mental Healthcare Act, 2017   73

Chapter 5: Identification I   79

- Corpus Delicti   79
- Race and Religion   80
- Sex   81
- Disorders of Sexual Development   83
- Sex from Skeletal Remains   86
- Age   90
- Age from Ossification of Bones   94
- Bone Age Estimation   97
- Age Determination in Adults Over 25 years   97
- Medico-legal Importance of Age   100
- Stature   100
- Scars   102
- Tattoo Marks   102

Chapter 6: Identification II   106

- Anthropometry (Bertillon System)   106
- Dactylography   106
- Poroscopy   110
- Lip Prints (Cheiloscopy)   110
- Hair   111
- Medico-legal Questions   111
- Superimposition   115
- Forensic Odontology   115
- Miscellaneous Methods of Identification   117

Chapter 7: Medico-legal Autopsy — 120

- Purpose/Objectives of Autopsy 121
- Procedure for Medico-legal Autopsies 121
- Instruments for Autopsy Examination 122
- External Examination 123
- Internal Examination (Evisceration) 125
- Skin Incisions 125
- Evisceration Methods 125
- Abdomen and Pelvis 126
- Chest 127
- Heart 128
- Neck 130
- Skull and Brain 130
- Description of an Organ 132
- Report 133
- Demonstration of Pneumothorax 133
- Demonstration of Air Embolus 133
- Collection of Samples 134
- Preservation of Viscera 135
- Preservation of Samples 136
- Samples for Laboratory Investigations 137
- Obscure and Negative Autopsy 138
- Digital Autopsy 139
- Examination of Decomposed, Mutilated and Skeletonized Remains 140
- Medico-legal Questions 140
- Exhumation 143

Chapter 8: Thanatology — 146

- Death 146
- Brain/Brainstem Death 147
- Cause, Mechanism and Manner of Death 149
- Cause of Death 150
- Modes of Death (Proximate Causes of Death) 152
- Anoxia 153
- Sudden Death 153
- Coronary Atherosclerosis 154

Chapter 9: Signs of Death — 158

- Immediate Changes (Somatic Death) 158
- Suspended Animation (Apparent Death) 159
- Early Changes (Molecular Death) 159
- Postmortem Staining (Livor Mortis) 160
- Algor Mortis (Cooling of the Dead Body) 163
- Rigor Mortis 165
- Cadaveric Spasm (Instantaneous Rigor) 167
- Heat Stiffening 167
- Cold Stiffening 169
- Putrefaction/Decomposition 169
- Decomposition of Submerged Body 173
- Floatation of a Dead Body on Water 174
- Entomology 174
- Adipocere (Saponification) 175
- Mummification 175
- Estimation of Time Since Death (TSD)/Postmortem Interval (PMI) 176
- Preservation of Dead Bodies 180
- Presumption of Survivorship 180
- Presumption of Death 181

Chapter 10: Asphyxial Deaths — 183

- Etiology of Asphyxia 183
- Clinical Effects of Asphyxia 184
- Hanging 184
- Autopsy of Neck (Asphyxial Deaths) 186
- Postmortem Findings in Hanging 187
- Medico-legal Questions 189
- Strangulation 190
- Ligature Strangulation 191
- Postmortem Examination 191
- Medico-legal Questions 192
- Throttling (Manual Strangulation) 194
- Postmortem Examination 194
- Medico-legal Questions 196
- Hyoid Bone Fractures 196
- Suffocation 197
- Drowning 201
- Postmortem Examination 203
- Medico-legal Questions 208
- Autoerotic Asphyxia (Sexual Asphyxia) 209

Chapter 11: Injuries — 213

- Classification of Wounds/Injuries 213
- Abrasion 214
- Bruise/Contusion 217
- Lacerated Wound 221
- Incised Wound (Cut/Slash/Slice) 223
- Chop Wounds 226
- Stab Wound/Punctured Wound 227
- Defense Wounds 231
- Fabricated/Fictitious/Forged Wounds 232

Chapter 12: Firearm Injuries — 235

- Classification of Firearms 236
- Rifled Firearms 236
- Smooth Bore Firearms/Shotguns 237
- Caliber (Gauge/Bore) 238
- Bullet 238
- Cartridge 240
- Gunpowders (Propellant Charge) 241
- Mechanism of Discharge of Projectile 242
- Wound Ballistics and Mechanism of Injury 242
- Firearm Wounds 243
- Characteristics of Shotgun Wounds 245
- Characteristics of Rifled Firearms Wounds 246
- Firearm Wounds on Skull 249
- Exit Wounds 249
- Peculiar Effects of Firearms 252
- Postmortem Examination 253
- Preservation and Marking of Exhibits 254
- Medico-legal Questions 255
- Detection of Gunshot Residues 258

Chapter 13: Regional Injuries — 262

- Craniocerebral Injuries 262
- Biomechanics of Head Injury 263
- Soft Tissue Injury 263

- Skull Fractures 264
- Brain Injury 268
- Cerebral Concussion 268
- Diffuse Axonal Injury 269
- Cerebral Contusion and Laceration 270
- Coup and Contrecoup Injury 271
- Intracranial Hematoma 273
- Epidural/Extradural Hematoma 273
- Subdural Hematoma 275
- Subarachnoid Hematoma 277
- Intracerebral Hematoma 279
- Diffuse Injury to the Brain 282
- Facial Injuries 283
- Spinal Cord 284
- Neck 285
- Vertebral Column 285
- Chest 285
- Lungs 286
- Heart 286
- Abdomen 287
- Kidneys 288
- Bones and Joints 289

Chapter 14: Thermal Injuries 293

- Cold Injury 293
- Heat Injury 295
- Heat Stroke/Heat Hyperpyrexia 296
- Burns 298
- Postmortem Examination 301
- Medico-legal Questions 305
- Scalds 307
- Electrical Injuries (Electrocution) 308
- Judicial Electrocution 311
- Lightning Stroke 311

Chapter 15: Transportation Injuries 314

- Pedestrian Injuries 314
- Injuries Sustained by Vehicle Occupants 318
- Role of Seat Belts and Air Bags 320
- Motorcycle and Cycle Injuries 320
- Postmortem Examination 321
- Alcohol, Drugs and Trauma 322
- Railway Injuries 322

Chapter 16: Explosion Injuries and Fall from Height 324

- Explosion Injuries 324
- Classification of Injuries 325
- Fall from Height 327
- Injury Patterns 328

Chapter 17: Medico-legal Aspects of Injuries 332

- Grievous Hurt 333
- Punishments 337
- Causes of Death from Wounds 338
- Medico-legal Questions 342
- Injury Report 345
- Mode of Starvation 349

Chapter 18: Neglect and Starvation Deaths 349

- Pathophysiology 350
- Signs and Symptoms 350
- Postmortem Findings 351
- Medico-legal Questions 351

Chapter 19: Radiation Sickness, Anesthetic and Operative Deaths 353

- Ionizing Radiation Reactions 353
- Anesthetic and Operative Deaths 354
- Postmortem Examination 355

Chapter 20: Infanticide and Child Abuse 358

- Postmortem Examination of Infants 359
- Age of Fetus 361
- Rule of Hasse 361
- Demonstration of Centers of Ossification 363
- Viability of Fetus/Infant 364
- Live-Born/Dead-Born/Stillborn 364
- Postmortem Findings 365
- Signs of Dead-born Fetus 368
- Signs of Stillborn Fetus 369
- Infant Death 370
- Battered Baby Syndrome 373
- Child Abuse 375
- Sudden Infant Death Syndrome 376
- Munchausen Syndrome by Proxy 377

Chapter 21: Criminal Abortion 380

- Classification of Abortion 380
- Criminal Abortion 381
- Complications of Criminal Abortion 384
- Duties of a Doctor in Suspected Case of Criminal Abortion 385
- Examination of a Woman with Alleged History of Abortion 385
- Trauma and Abortion 387

Chapter 22: Erectile Dysfunction and Sterility 389

- Causes of Erectile Dysfunction and Sterility in Males 389
- Causes of Impotence and Sterility in Females 392
- Examination of a Person in an Alleged Case of Erectile Dysfunction and Sterility 393
- Nullity of Marriage and Divorce 394
- Sterilization 395
- Artificial Insemination (AI) 397
- Surrogate Mother 399
- Normal Female genitalia 401

Chapter 23: Virginity, Pregnancy and Delivery 401

- Medico-Legal Aspects 403
- Pregnancy 404
- Presumptive Signs/Symptoms 404
- Probable Signs of Pregnancy 405
- Positive/Conclusive Signs of Pregnancy 407
- Pseudocyesis (Spurious/False/Phantom Pregnancy) 409
- Superfecundation 409

- Superfetation *409*
- Legitimacy and Paternity *410*
- Signs and Symptoms of Recent Delivery in Living *411*
- Signs of Remote Delivery in Living *412*
- Medico-legal Aspects of Pregnancy and Delivery *412*

Chapter 24: Sexual Offenses 416

- Rape *417*
- Duties of a Doctor in Case of a Survivor of Sexual Assault (Rape) *420*
- Examination of Sexual Assault Survivor *421*
- Examination *425*
- Specimens for Laboratory Examination *429*
- Opinion *430*
- Corroborative Signs of Sexual assault *431*
- Rape on Deflorate/Sexually Active Woman *432*
- Rape on Children *433*
- Medico-legal Questions *433*
- Indicators of Sexual Abuse *434*
- Examination of Rape Accused *435*
- Incest *436*
- Adultery *437*

Chapter 25: Homosexuality 439

- Sodomy *439*
- Examination of Passive Partner of Sodomy *440*
- Opinion *441*
- Examination of Active Partner of Sodomy *442*
- Legal Aspects *442*
- Lesbianism/Tribadism *443*
- Bestiality/Zoophilia *444*
- Buccal Coitus *444*

Chapter 26: Paraphilia 446

- Sadism (Algolagnia) *446*
- Masochism (Passive Algolagnia) *447*
- Transvestic Fetishism (Eonism) *448*
- Voyeurism (Scoptophilia) *449*
- Exhibitionism *449*
- Fetishism *449*
- Frotteurism (Toucherism) *450*
- Pedophilia *450*
- Masturbation (Onanism) *450*
- Insertion of Foreign Objects/Fingers *451*
- Indecent Assault *452*

Chapter 27: Postmortem Artifacts 455

- Artifacts due to Postmortem changes *455*
- Third Party Artifacts *457*
- Environmental Artifacts *459*
- Miscellaneous Artifacts *459*

Chapter 28: Forensic Psychiatry 461

- Delusion *461*
- Hallucination *462*
- Illusion *464*
- Impulse *465*
- Obsession–Compulsion *465*
- Lucid Interval *466*
- Role of Forensic Psychiatrist *467*
- Psychiatric Assessment *468*
- Classification of Mental, Behavioral or Neurodevelopmental Disorders (ICD-11) *469*
- Neurodevelopmental Disorders *469*
- Schizophrenia *470*
- Catatonia *472*
- Mood Disorders *473*
- Anxiety or Fear-related Disorders *474*
- Obsessive-Compulsive or Related Disorders *475*
- Stress Disorders *476*
- Dissociative Disorders *477*
- Feeding or Eating Disorders *477*
- Bodily Distress or Bodily Experience Disorders *478*
- Substance use or Addictive Behaviors Disorders *478*
- Impulse Control Disorders *478*
- Disruptive Behavior or Dissocial Disorders *479*
- Personality Disorders and Related Traits *479*
- Factitious Disorders *479*
- Neurocognitive Disorders *479*
- Sleep-Wake Disorders *480*
- Mental Disorder and Responsibility *481*

Chapter 29: Bloodstain Analysis 486

- Bloodstain Pattern Analysis *486*
- Presumptive Tests for Blood *487*
- Confirmatory Tests for Blood *488*
- Species Identification *488*
- Genetic Markers in Blood *490*
- Medico-legal Application of Blood (Groups) *491*
- Medico-legal Questions *493*

Chapter 30: Seminal Stains and Other Biological Samples 496

- Purpose of Seminal Identification *497*
- Examination of Seminal Stains *497*
- Confirmatory Tests *498*
- Individualization of Seminal Stains *500*
- Medico-legal Questions *501*
- Identification of Biological Samples and Body Fluids *501*

Chapter 31: DNA Fingerprinting 504

- Restriction Fragment Length Polymorphism *504*
- Polymerase Chain Reaction *506*
- Specimen Selection and Preservation *508*
- Uses of DNA Fingerprinting *509*
- Limitations of DNA Testing *510*

Chapter 32: Torture and Custodial Deaths 512

- Types of Torture *512*
- Medical Practitioner and Torture *514*
- Custodial Deaths *515*

Chapter 33: Medico-legal Aspects of HIV 518

- HIV Testing Policy *518*
- Healthcare Workers and HIV Infection *519*
- Partner Notification (Contact Tracing/Partner Counseling) *519*
- Clinical Trials and HIV *520*
- Blood Donation and HIV *520*

Chapter 34: Newer Techniques and Recent Advances — 522
- Polygraph *522*
- Brain Fingerprinting (Brain Mapping) *523*
- Narco-analysis *523*
- Facial Reconstruction *524*
- Crime Scene Investigation *525*

Section 2: Toxicology

Chapter 35: General Toxicology — 531
- Medico-legal Aspects of Poisons *532*
- Classification of Poisons *533*
- Toxicokinetics and Toxicodynamics of Poisons *534*
- Poisoning in the Living *534*
- Duties of a Doctor in a Case of Suspected Poisoning *535*
- Medical Records *536*
- Suicide/Homicide/Accident *536*
- Management of Poisoning Cases *537*
- Removal of Unabsorbed Poison *538*
- Administration of Antidotes *540*
- Elimination of Poison by Excretion *542*
- Diagnosis of Poisoning in Dead *543*
- Samples Preserved for Toxicological Analysis *545*
- Failure to Detect Poison *545*
- Chromatography *546*

Chapter 36: Corrosive Poisons — 549
- Mineral/Inorganic Acids *549*
- Vitriolage (Vitriol Throwing) *551*
- Chemical Colitis *552*
- Oxalic Acid (Acid of Sugar) *552*
- Carbolic Acid (Phenol) *553*
- Strong Alkalis (Caustic Alkalis) *554*

Chapter 37: Inorganic Metallic Irritants—Arsenic — 557
- Signs and Symptoms (Acute Poisoning) *558*
- Treatment *559*
- Postmortem Findings *559*
- Chronic Arsenic Poisoning *560*
- Postmortem Findings *561*
- Postmortem Imbibition of Arsenic *561*

Chapter 38: Inorganic Metallic Irritants—Mercury — 563
- Signs and Symptoms (Acute Poisoning) *564*
- Treatment *565*
- Postmortem Findings *565*
- Chronic Mercury Poisoning (Hydrargyrism) *565*
- Specific Features/Diseases *566*

Chapter 39: Inorganic Metallic Irritants—Lead — 568
- Chronic Lead Poisoning (Plumbism/Saturnism) *569*
- Signs and Symptoms *570*
- Treatment *572*
- Postmortem Findings *573*

Chapter 40: Inorganic Metallic Irritants—Copper — 575
- Signs and Symptoms *576*
- Treatment *576*
- Postmortem Findings *577*
- Chronic Copper Poisoning *577*

Chapter 41: Inorganic Metallic Irritants—Thallium — 579
- Signs and Symptoms *579*
- Treatment *580*
- Postmortem Findings *580*

Chapter 42: Other Inorganic Metallic Irritants — 582
- Cadmium *582*
- Barium *583*
- Zinc *584*
- Metal Fume Fever *585*

Chapter 43: Non-metallic Irritants — 587
- Phosphorus *587*
- Signs and Symptoms *587*
- Postmortem Findings *589*
- Chronic Phosphorus Poisoning *590*
- Iodine Poisoning *590*

Chapter 44: Organic Irritants—Plant — 592
- Ricinus Communis (Castor) *592*
- Croton Tiglium (Jamalgota) *593*
- Abrus Precatorius (Rati/Rosary Pea/Gunchi/Jequirity) *594*
- Suis *595*
- Semecarpus Anacardium *595*
- Capsicum Annuum *596*
- Calotropis (Rubber Bush) *597*

Chapter 45: Organic Irritants—Animal — 599
- Snakes *599*
- Signs and Symptoms of Ophitoxemia *602*
- Management *605*
- Postmortem Findings *608*
- Scorpions *609*
- Bees and Wasps *610*
- Spiders *610*

Chapter 46: Somniferous Poisons (Narcotic Poisons) — 613
- Opium *613*
- Signs and Symptoms *614*
- Treatment *615*
- Postmortem Findings *616*
- Chronic Morphine Poisoning (Morphinism) *618*

Chapter 47: Inebriants—Alcohol — 620
- Signs and Symptoms (Acute Poisoning) *622*
- Treatment *623*
- Drunkenness *625*
- Laboratory Diagnosis *628*
- Collection of Samples in the Living *629*
- Alcoholism *629*
- Delirium Tremens *630*
- Wernicke's Encephalopathy *631*
- Korsakoff's Psychosis *631*
- Methyl Alcohol (Methanol) *632*
- Ethylene Glycol *634*

Chapter 48: Sedative-hypnotic—Barbiturates — 637
- Signs and Symptoms 637
- Treatment 638
- Postmortem Findings 639
- Barbiturate Automatism (Self-poisoning) 639
- Dhatura/Datura 641

Chapter 49: Deliriants—Dhatura/Datura — 641
- Signs and Symptoms 642
- Treatment 643
- Postmortem Findings 644

Chapter 50: Deliriants—Cannabis — 646
- Signs and Symptoms 647
- Treatment 648
- Run-amok 648

Chapter 51: Deliriants—Cocaine — 650
- Signs and Symptoms 651
- Treatment 651

Chapter 52: Spinal Poisons — 654
- Strychnos Nux-vomica 654
- Signs and Symptoms 655
- Treatment 656
- Aconite 658

Chapter 53: Cardiac Poisons — 658
- Nicotiana Tabacum (Tobacco) 660
- Digitalis Purpurea (Foxglove) 660
- Oleander (Kaner) 661
- Nerium Odorum 662
- Cascabela Thevetia 662
- Cerbera Odollam 663

Chapter 54: Hydrocyanic Acid — 666
- Signs and Symptoms 667
- Treatment 667
- Postmortem Findings 668
- Judicial Execution 669

Chapter 55: Asphyxiants — 671
- Carbon Monoxide (CO) 671
- Treatment 672
- Postmortem Findings 673
- Tear Gases 674
- Methyl Isocyanate (MIC) 675

Chapter 56: Agricultural Poisons — 677
- Organophosphorus Compounds (OPCs) 677
- Signs and Symptoms 678
- Treatment 680
- Postmortem Findings 682
- Endrin 683
- Paraquat 684
- Pyrethrins and Pyrethroids 685

Chapter 57: Alphos (Aluminum Phosphide) — 687
- Signs and Symptoms 688
- Treatment 688
- Postmortem Findings 690
- Paracetamol (Acetaminophen) 692

Chapter 58: Medicinal Poisons — 692
- Iron 693
- Phenytoin 694
- Lithium 694
- Antipsychotic Drugs (Tranquilizers) 695
- Tricyclic Antidepressants 696
- Benzodiazepines 696
- Acetylsalicylic Acid (Aspirin) 697
- Antibiotics 699
- Muscle Relaxants 699
- Local Anesthetics 699
- Propofol 700
- Insulin 700

Chapter 59: Drug Dependence and Date Rape Drugs — 703
- Patterns of Drug use Disorders 703
- Psychoactive Substances 704
- Hallucinogens 707
- Date Rape Drugs 709
- Complications of Drug Abuse 710
- Postmortem Findings 710
- Medical Jurisprudence 712

Chapter 60: Supplement — 712
- Medical Acts 713
- Decompression Sickness 717
- Altitude Illness 717
- Toxicology 718
- Boric Acid (Hydrogen Borate/Orthoboric Acid) 718
- Hydrofluoric Acid 719
- Methemoglobinemia Inducing Agents 720
- Ergot 720
- Cantharides (Spanish Fly) 721
- Isopropyl Alcohol 722
- Peripheral Nerve Poisons 722
- Cardiac Poisons 724
- Carbon Dioxide 725
- Hydrogen Sulfide 726
- Biological Weapons 728
- Naphthalene 729
- Kerosene Oil Poisoning 730
- Food Poisoning 732
- Poisonous Foods 734

Answer Key 737

Index 739

Synopsis

SUMMARY I

Summary of some important sections of IPC, CrPC and IEA

Section	Issue/Offence (with punishment)
Criminal responsibility	
82	Act of a child under 7 years of age (age of criminal responsibility in India)
83	Act of a child 7–12 years of age of immature understanding
84	Act of a person of unsound mind (criminal responsibility of mentally ill)
85	Act of a person intoxicated involuntarily (not responsible)
86	Act of a voluntarily intoxicated person
Consent	
87	Act not intended to cause death or grievous hurt done with consent
88	Act done in good faith for benefit of the person, with consent, not intended to cause death
89	Act done in good faith for benefit of minor or insane person
90	Conditions of valid consent
92	Act done in good faith for benefit of a person without consent to save life (emergency treatment)
166B	Punishment for non-treatment of victim (up to 1 year with/without fine)
Summons	
174	Punishment for non-attendance of court after receiving summons (up to 6 months with/without fine up to ₹ 1000)
176	Omission to give notice to public servant by person legally bound to give it
177	Furnishing false information (up to 6 months with/without fine up to ₹ 1000; if it is related to commission of an offence: up to 2 years with/without fine)
Evidence	
191	Giving false evidence (perjury)
192	Fabricating false evidence
193	Punishment for false evidence (for perjury—up to 7 years and fine; and in any other case—up to 3 years and fine)
197	Punishment for issuing or signing false certificate (up to 7 years and fine)
201	Punishment for causing disappearance of evidence of offence or giving false information to screen offender (up to 7 years)
202	Punishment for intentional omission to give information of offence by person bound to inform (up to 6 months with/without fine)
204	Destruction of document or electronic record to prevent its production as evidence (up to 2 years with/without fine)
228A	Punishment for disclosure of identity of rape victim (up to 2 years and fine)
284	Punishment for negligent conduct with respect to poisonous substance (up to 6 months with/without fine up to ₹ 1000)
Homicide	
299	Defines culpable homicide not amounting to murder
300	Defines murder
302	Punishment for murder (death or life imprisonment)
303	Punishment for murder by a person already undergoing life imprisonment (death)
304	Punishment for culpable homicide not amounting to murder (up to 10 years in prison to life imprisonment)
304A	Punishment for causing death by rash and negligent act (up to 2 years with/without fine)
304B	Punishment for dowry death (7 years to life imprisonment)
305	Abetment to suicide of child or insane person (up to 10 years and fine)

306	Punishment for abetment of suicide (up to 10 years and fine)	
307	Attempt to commit murder (up to 10 years and fine)	
309	Punishment for attempt to commit suicide (not punishable)*	
Abortion		
312	Punishment for causing miscarriage (3 years, may extend to 7 years if the woman was quick with child, with/without fine)	
313	Punishment for causing miscarriage without woman's consent (10 years to life imprisonment and fine)	
314	Punishment for death caused by an act done with intent to cause miscarriage [10 years to life imprisonment (if without consent) and fine]	
315	Punishment for any act done with intent to prevent a child from being born alive, or to cause it to die after its birth (up to 10 years with/without fine)	
316	Punishment for causing death of a quick unborn child by an act amounting to culpable homicide (up to 10 years and fine)	
317	Punishment for exposure and abandonment of child <12 years by parent or guardian (up to 7 years with/without fine)	
318	Punishment for concealment of birth by secret disposal of dead body (up to 2 years with/without fine)	
Injuries		
319	Defines hurt	
320	Defines grievous hurt	
323	Punishment for voluntarily causing hurt (1 year with/without fine up to ₹ 1000)	
324	Punishment for voluntarily causing hurt by dangerous weapons or means (up to 3 years with/without fine)	
325	Punishment for voluntarily causing grievous hurt (up to 7 years and fine)	
326	Punishment for voluntarily causing grievous hurt by dangerous weapons or means (up to 10 years and fine)	
326A	Punishment for voluntarily causing grievous hurt by acids (10 years to life imprisonment and fine paid to victim)	
326B	Punishment for voluntarily throwing or attempting to throw acid (5–7 years and fine)	
328	Punishment for causing hurt by means of poison with intent to commit an offence (10 years and fine)	
337	Causing hurt by rash and negligent act endangering life or personal safety of others (up to 6 months with/without fine of ₹ 500)	
338	Causing grievous hurt by rash and negligent act endangering life or personal safety of other (up to 2 years with/without fine of ₹ 1000)	
351	Defines assault	
352	Punishment for assault (3 months with/without fine)	
Kidnapping		
361	Defines kidnapping (<16 in males, <18 for females) from lawful guardianship	
362	Defines abduction	
363	Punishment for kidnapping (up to 7 years and fine)	
364	Kidnapping or abducting in order to murder (10 years to life imprisonment and fine)	
364A	Kidnapping for ransom, etc. (life imprisonment/death and fine)	
366	Kidnapping or abducting a woman to compel her for marriage, etc. (up to 10 years and fine)	
366A	Procuration of minor girl (<18 years) for illicit intercourse (up to 10 years and fine)	
366B	Importation of girl from foreign country (<21 years) for illicit intercourse (up to 10 years and fine)	
Sexual offences		
375	Defines rape	
376(1)	Punishment for rape (10 years to life imprisonment and fine)	
376(2)	Punishment for custodial rape (10 years to life imprisonment and fine)	
376(3)	Punishment for raping a girl <16 years (20 years to life imprisonment and fine)	
376A	Punishment for causing death or persistent vegetative state of victim (20 years to life imprisonment/death)	
376AB	Punishment for raping a girl <12 years (20 years to life imprisonment and fine/death)	
376B	Punishment for sexual intercourse by husband upon his wife during separation (2–7 years and fine)	
376C	Punishment for sexual intercourse not amounting to rape (5–10 years and fine)	

* As per the Mental Healthcare Act, 2017, attempted suicide has been decriminalized and no punishment is to be given.

376D	Punishment for gang rape (20 years to life imprisonment)
376 DA	Punishment for gang raping a girl <16 years (life imprisonment and fine)
376 DB	Punishment for gang raping a girl <12 years (life imprisonment and fine/death)
376E	Punishment for repeat offenders of rape (life imprisonment/death)
377	Punishment unnatural offences (up to 10 years or life imprisonment and fine)
498	Punishment for enticing/taking away/detaining a married woman with criminal intent (up to 2 years with/without fine)
498A	Punishment for husband or relative of husband of a woman subjecting her to cruelty (up to 3 years and fine)
509	Punishment for word, gesture or act intended to insult the modesty of a woman (up to 3 years and fine)
510	Punishment for misconduct in public by a drunken person (up to 24 h with/without fine)
290	Punishment for public nuisance, e.g., frotteurism (fine of ₹ 200)
294	Punishment for obscene acts and songs, e.g., exhibitionism (up to 3 months with/without fine)
297	Trespassing on burial places, e.g., necrophilia and necrophagia (up to 1 year with/without fine)

Section	CrPC
2C	Cognizable offence
8C	Punishment of narcotic or substance abuse
39	Public to give information of certain offences under the IPC
53(1)	Examination of accused by doctor at the request of a police officer
53(2)	Examination of female accused only by or under the supervision of female doctor
53A	Examination of rape accused by a medical practitioner
54	Examination of arrested person by doctor at the request of the arrested person
61–69	Summons
164A	Medical examination of victim of rape
174(1)	Inquiry by police officer into cause of death
174(3)	Compulsory autopsy of dowry death
176	Inquiry by Magistrate into cause of death
291	Deposition of medical witness
327	Examination of a survivor of sexual assault must be conducted in camera
350	Summary procedure for punishment for non-attendance by a witness in obedience to summons
357C	Treatment of rape victims free of cost and information to the police
416	Postponement of capital sentence on pregnant woman

Section	IEA
3	Evidence
32(1)	Dying declaration
45	Opinion of experts
107	Presumption of being alive (burden of proving death of person known to have been alive within 30 years)
108	Presumption of death (burden of proving that person is alive who has not been heard of for 7 years)
114A	Presumption as to absence of consent in certain cases of rape
137	Procedures in examining witness in a court of law (examination-in-chief)
138	Order of examinations
141	Leading questions
142	When leading questions must not be asked
143	When leading questions may be asked
146	Questions lawful in cross-examination
148	Court to decide when a witness is compelled to answer
151	Indecent and scandalous questions
154	Question by party to his own witness (hostile witness)
159	Refreshing memory
162	Production of documents

Time scale of postmortem changes

Time scale	Significant changes
Few min to 1 h	Segmented blood within retinal blood vessels (Kervorkian sign)
30 min to 1 h	Retina pale, dull patches of postmortem (PM) staining develop, no fall in rectal temperature
2 h	Opacity of cornea, rigor mortis start developing
3–4 h	Tache noire develop in eyes, confluence of PM staining, body cold to touch
4 h	Well-developed PM staining
4–8 h	Intraocular tension falls to zero
5–6 h	Complete PM staining, optic disk outline is hazy
7–10	Blurred optic disk outline, flies lay eggs
8–12 h	Fixed PM staining, cornea permanently hazy, rigor mortis fully developed, architecture of kidney maintained
16–20 h	Body temperature attains environmental temperature (temperate countries)
12–24 h	Cornea white and flattened, rigor mortis present in the body, greenish discoloration in right iliac fossa (in summers), liver soft and flabby, distension of abdomen, postmortem purge, larvae or maggots of flies appear in body, disturbed architecture of kidneys
24–36 h	Rigor mortis pass off, blisters appear on surface of liver, marbling of veins seen, marked changes in kidneys
36–48 h	Tongue protrude out, prominent marbling of veins and distention of abdomen, greenish discoloration in right iliac fossa (in winters), blisters on lower surface of trunk and thighs, putrefactive odor is noticeable
48–72 h	Postmortem staining gets displaced, eyes protrude, fish-mouth like appearance of face, hair and nails become loose, brain is soft, pinkish-gray, autolytic changes in kidneys, steady increase in vitreous potassium (till 100 h)
3–5 days	Teeth become loose, skin of hands and feet come off, innumerous maggots, pupa seen, body lice die
5–10 days	Abdomen burst open, puffiness of body pass off, brain and other tissues liquefy, complete life cycle of fly
7–15 days	Adipocere
3–12 months	Mummification
>12 months	Skeletonization (in soil buried bodies)

SUMMARY II

Signs associated with poisons

System	Signs	Poisons suspected
Eyes	Miosis	Opioids, phenol, organophosphorus (OPC), carbamates, muscarinic type mushrooms, physostigmine, neostigmine, pilocarpine, ethanol, nicotine, barbiturates, benzodiazepines, caffeine, clonidine
	Mydriasis	Dhatura, atropine, belladonna, cannabis, ergot, endrin, strychnine, botulism, oleanders, hydrogen cyanide (HCN), anticholinergics, antihistamines, amphetamine, cocaine, methanol, lysergic acid diethylamide (LSD)
	Lacrimation	OPC, irritant gas or vapors
	Retinal hyperemia	Methanol
	Poor vision	Methanol, botulism, CO
	Nystagmus	Sedatives, hypnotics, CO, barbiturates, ethanol
Skin	Bullae	CO, barbiturates
	Cyanosis	Central nervous system (CNS) depressants
	Erythema	Boric acid, mercury, cyanide, anticholinergics
	Dry hot skin	Anticholinergics, dhatura, botulism
	Diaphoresis	OPC, cocaine, muscarinic mushrooms, nitrates
	Needle tracks	Heroin, amphetamine, phencyclidine
GIT	Salivation	OPC, salicylates, corrosives, strychnine
	Dry mouth	Anticholinergics, dathura, amphetamines, antihistamine
	Gum lines	Lead, mercury, arsenic
	Burns	Corrosives, oxalate-containing plants
	Cramps	Arsenic, lead, thallium, OPC
	Epigastric tenderness	Nonsteroidal anti-inflammatory drugs (NSAIDs), salicylates
	Diarrhea	Arsenic, boric acid, iron
	Constipation	Lead, opioids, botulism
	Hematemesis	Corrosives, salicylates, iron
CVS	Bradycardia	Digoxin, narcotics, OPC, petroleum products, mushrooms, cyanide
	Tachycardia	Alcohol, amphetamine, sympathomimetics, substances containing atropine, tricyclic antidepressants, salicylates, cocaine
	Arrhythmias	Chlorinated solvents, chloral hydrate, digitalis glycosides, OPC, opioids, sedative-hypnotics, tricyclic antidepressants, amphetamines, anticholinergics, caffeine, cocaine, phenothiazine, arsenic, methadone
	Cyanosis	Aniline dyes, nitrites, phenacetin—causing methemoglobinemia
	Hypotension	Narcotics, barbiturates, iron, antidepressants, phenothiazines, disulfiram, cyanide, CO, H_2S, arsenic, certain mushrooms, nitrites, nitrates
	Hypertension	Antihistaminics, anticholinergics (atropine), amphetamines, phenylpropanolamine, LSD, cocaine, monoamine oxidase (MAO) inhibitors
Respiration	Slow and depressed	Alcohol, barbiturates (late), narcotics, botulinum toxin, carbamates, elapid venom, strychnine, sedatives, hypnotics
	Tachypnea	Barbiturates (early), methanol, paraldehyde, cocaine, salicylates, CO, cyanide, ethylene glycol, amphetamines
Temperature	Hypothermia	Ethanol, opioids, barbiturates, sedatives, hypnotics, phenothiazines, hypoglycemic agents, benzodiazepines, tricyclic antidepressants, CO
	Hyperpyrexia	Amphetamines, atropine, quinine, cocaine, dinitrophenol, phencyclidine (PCP), salicylates, strychnine, tricyclic antidepressants, marking nut, dhatura, cocaine, aspirin, strychnine, antihistaminic, pethidine, nicotine

CNS	Altered consciousness	Narcotics, sedatives, hypnotics, alcohol, ethylene glycol, CO, OPC, insecticides
	Restless, delirious	Dhatura, alcohol, marijuana, cocaine, heroin, methaqualone, sympathomimetics, anticholinergics, heavy metals
	Ataxia	Alcohol, barbiturates, sedatives, narcotics, benzodiazepines, CO, insulin
	Paralysis	Botulin, heavy metals, poison hemlock
	Coma	Antihistamines, barbiturates, benzodiazepines, ethanol, opioids, phenothiazines, CO, cyanide, OPC, lead, antidepressants
	Seizures	Amphetamines, antidepressants (especially tricyclic antidepressants), cocaine, PCP, withdrawal from alcohol or sedative-hypnotics

Antidotes at a glance

S.No.	Toxic agent	Specific antidote	S.No.	Toxic agent	Specific antidote
1.	Acetaminophen	N-acetyl cysteine	9.	CO	Oxygen, hyperbaric oxygen
2.	Anticholinergics (e.g., dhatura, atropine)	Physostigmine	10.	Cyanide	Amyl nitrite pearls, sodium nitrite, sodium thiosulfate
3.	Benzodiazepines	Flumazenil	11.	Methemoglobinemia	Methylene blue
4.	OPC	Atropine and pralidoxime (2-PAM)	12.	Arsenic	British anti-Lewisite (BAL)
5.	Carbamate	Atropine	13.	Mercury	2,3-dimercaptopropanesulfonate (DMPS), dimercaptosuccinic acid (DMSA), BAL
6.	Methanol, ethylene glycol	Ethanol, fomepizole	14.	Lead	CaEDTA, BAL
7.	Opioids	Naloxone	15.	Copper	Penicillamine, BAL, calcium disodium ethylenediamine tetraacetate (CaEDTA)
8.	Snake venom	Anti-snake venom (ASV) serum	16.	Iron	Desferrioxamine

Classification of poisons based on their effect/outcome

S.No.	Category	Poisons
1.	Stupefying poisons	Alcohol, dhatura, cannabis, chloral hydrate
2.	Abortifacients	Calotropis, aconite, lead, arsenic, mercury, KMnO$_4$, croton, marking nut, cantharides
3.	Cattle poisons	Rati, oleander, calotropis, aconite, arsenic, OPC, strychnine
4.	Arrow poisons	Rati, croton, calotropis, aconite, strychnine, curare, snake venom
5.	Aphrodisiacs*	Cantharidin, ginseng, lead, mandrake, nutmeg, puncturevine, yohimbine, belladonna, henbane
6.	Priapism	Cantharidin, cocaine, spider envenomation (black widow)
7.	Decreases libido	Benzodiazepines, barbiturates, ethanol
8.	Poisons resisting putrefaction	Arsenic, antimony, mercury, thallium, cyanide, phosphorus, fluoride, alphos, ZnP, barbiturates, OPC, strychnine, yellow oleander, dhatura, hyoscine, nicotine, CO
9.	Poisons rapidly destroyed in body	Chloral hydrate, sodium nitrite, volatile poisons, thiopental sodium, cocaine, aconite
10.	Knock-out agents	Potassium bromide, chloral hydrate, dhatura, cannabis (*bhang*)
11.	Froth producing	Barbiturates, opium, Tik-20, endrin, copper sulfate, kerosene, OPC
12.	Hallucinogens	LSD, mescaline, alcohol, cannabis, cocaine, amphetamine
13.	Artificial bruise producing	Calotropis, marking nut, plumbago
14.	Blister forming	Barbiturates, meprobamate, marking nut, plumbago, calotropis, croton, CO, tricyclic antidepressants
15.	Curiosity poisons	Castor, borax paste, iodine, rati, poisonous mushrooms
16.	Formication (as if ants creeping under skin)	Cocaine, phosphorus, ergot
17.	Acidic drugs secreted into the stomach	Salicylic acid, probenecid, phenylbutazone, thiopental, barbital
18.	Basic drugs secreted into the stomach	Theophylline, quinine, aniline, antipyrine, phencyclidine, dextromorphan, tolazoline

*Aphrodisiacs heighten sexual desire, pleasure or performance.

Competencies Covered

No.	Competency The student should be able to	Page No.
FM 1.1	Demonstrate knowledge of basics of Forensic Medicine like definitions of forensic medicine, Clinical Forensic Medicine, Forensic Pathology, State Medicine, Legal Medicine and Medical Jurisprudence.	3
FM 1.2	Describe history of forensic medicine.	3
FM 1.3	**LEGAL PROCEDURE** Describe legal procedures including Criminal Procedure Code, Indian Penal Code, Indian Evidence Act, Civil and Criminal Cases, Inquest (Police Inquest and Magistrate's Inquest), cognizable and non-cognizable offences.	4, 6, 9
FM 1.4	**LEGAL PROCEDURE** Describe Courts in India and their powers: Supreme Court, High Court, Sessions Court, Magistrate's Court, Labor Court, Family Court, Executive Magistrate Court and Juvenile Justice Board.	9
FM 1.5	**LEGAL PROCEDURE** Describe court procedures including issue of summons, conduct money, types of witnesses, recording of evidence oath, affirmation, examination in chief, cross examination, re-examination and court questions, recording of evidence and conduct of doctor in witness box.	11, 15, 16, 18
FM 1.6	Describe offenses in court including perjury; court strictures vis-a-vis medical officer.	16
FM 1.7	Describe dying declaration and dying deposition.	12
FM 1.9	Describe the importance of documentation in medical practice in regard to medico-legal examinations, medical certificates and medico-legal reports especially: ♦ Maintenance of patient case records, discharge summary, prescribed registers to be maintained in health centers. ♦ Maintenance of medico-legal register like accident register. ♦ Documents of issuance of wound certificate. ♦ Documents of issuance of drunkenness certificate. ♦ Documents of issuance of sickness and fitness certificate. ♦ Documents for issuance of death certificate. ♦ Documents of Medical Certification of Cause of Death—form number 4 and 4A. ♦ Documents for estimation of age by physical, dental and radiological examination and issuance of certificate.	12, 345, 535, 625
FM 1.10	Select appropriate cause of death in a particular scenario by referring ICD 10 code.	150
FM 1.11	Write the correct cause of death certificate as per ICD 10 code.	150
FM 2.1	**THANATOLOGY** Define, describe and discuss death and its types including somatic/clinical/cellular, molecular and brain-death, cortical death and brainstem death.	146
FM 2.2	Describe and discuss natural and unnatural deaths.	149
FM 2.3	Describe and discuss issues related to sudden natural deaths.	153
FM 2.4	Describe salient features of the Organ Transplantation and The Human Organ Transplant (Amendment) Act, 2011 and discuss ethical issues regarding organ donation.	60
FM 2.5	Discuss moment of death, modes of death—coma, asphyxia and syncope.	146, 152
FM 2.6	Discuss presumption of death and survivorship.	180
FM 2.7	Describe and discuss suspended animation.	158
FM 2.8	Describe and discuss postmortem changes including signs of death, cooling of body, postmortem lividity, rigor mortis, cadaveric spasm, cold stiffening and heat stiffening.	158, 160, 163, 165
FM 2.9	Describe putrefaction, mummification, adipocere and maceration.	169, 175
FM 2.10	Discuss estimation of time since death.	176

Competencies Covered

FM 2.11	**AUTOPSY** Describe and discuss autopsy procedures including postmortem examination, different types of autopsies, aims and objectives of postmortem examination.	120, 121
FM 2.12	Describe the legal requirements to conduct postmortem examination and procedures to conduct medico-legal postmortem examination.	121
FM 2.13	Describe and discuss obscure autopsy.	138
FM 2.14	Describe and discuss examination of clothing, preservation of viscera on postmortem examination for chemical analysis and other medico-legal purposes, postmortem artifacts.	135, 455
FM 2.15	Describe special protocols for conduction of medico-legal autopsies in cases of death in custody or following violation of human rights as per National Human Rights Commission Guidelines.	515
FM 2.16	Describe and discuss examination of mutilated bodies or fragments, charred bones and bundle of bones.	140
FM 2.17	Describe and discuss exhumation.	143
FM 2.18	**CRIME SCENE INVESTIGATION** Describe and discuss the objectives of crime scene visit, the duties and responsibilities of doctors on crime scene and the reconstruction of sequence of events after crime scene investigation.	525
FM 2.19	**INVESTIGATION OF ANESTHETIC, OPERATIVE DEATHS** Describe and discuss special protocols for conduction of autopsy and for collection, preservation and dispatch of related material evidences.	354
FM 2.20	**MECHANICAL ASPHYXIA** Define, classify and describe asphyxia and medico-legal interpretation of postmortem findings in asphyxial deaths.	183
FM 2.21	**MECHANICAL ASPHYXIA** Describe and discuss different types of hanging and strangulation including clinical findings, causes of death, postmortem findings and medico-legal aspects of death due to hanging and strangulation including examination, preservation and dispatch of ligature material.	184, 190
FM 2.22	**MECHANICAL ASPHYXIA** Describe and discuss pathophysiology, clinical features, postmortem findings and medico-legal aspects of traumatic asphyxia, obstruction of nose and mouth, suffocation and sexual asphyxia.	197, 209
FM 2.23	Describe and discuss types, pathophysiology, clinical features, postmortem findings and medico-legal aspects of drowning, diatom test and, Gettler test.	201
FM 2.24	**THERMAL DEATHS** Describe the clinical features, postmortem finding and medico-legal aspects of injuries due to physical agents like heat [heat-hyper-pyrexia, heat stroke, sun stroke, heat exhaustion/prostration, heat cramps (miner's cramp)] or cold (systemic and localized hypothermia, frostbite, trench foot, immersion foot).	293, 295
FM 2.25	Describe types of injuries, clinical features, pathophysiology, postmortem findings and medico-legal aspects in cases of burns, scalds, lightening, electrocution and radiations.	298, 307, 308, 311, 353
FM 2.26	**STARVATION DEATHS** Describe and discuss clinical features, postmortem findings and medico-legal aspects of death due to starvation and neglect.	349
FM 2.27	**INFANTICIDE** Define and discuss infanticide, feticide and stillbirth,	358, 364, 369
FM 2.28	**INFANTICIDE** Describe and discuss signs of intrauterine death, signs of live birth, viability of fetus, age determination of fetus, DOAP session of ossification centers, hydrostatic test, sudden infants death syndrome and Munchausen's syndrome by proxy.	361, 363, 364, 368, 376
FM 3.1	**IDENTIFICATION** Define and describe corpus delicti, establishment of identity of living persons including race, sex, religion, complexion, stature, age determination using morphology, teeth—eruption, decay, bite marks, bones—ossification centers, medico-legal aspects of age.	79, 80, 90, 100, 115
FM 3.2	**IDENTIFICATION** Describe and discuss identification of criminals, unknown persons, dead bodies from the remains—hairs, fibers, teeth, anthropometry, dactylography, foot prints, scars, tattoos, poroscopy and superimposition.	102, 106, 111, 115
FM 3.3	**MECHANICAL INJURIES AND WOUNDS** Define, describe and classify different types of mechanical injuries, abrasion, bruise, laceration, stab wound, incised wound, chop wound, defense wound, self-inflicted/fabricated wounds and their medico-legal aspects.	213, 214, 217, 221, 223, 226, 227, 231
FM 3.4	**MECHANICAL INJURIES AND WOUNDS** Define injury, assault and hurt. Describe IPC pertaining to injuries.	213, 332

FM 3.5	**MECHANICAL INJURIES AND WOUNDS** Describe accidental, suicidal and homicidal injuries. Describe simple, grievous and dangerous injuries. Describe antemortem and postmortem injuries.	333, 342
FM 3.6	**MECHANICAL INJURIES AND WOUNDS** Describe healing of injury and fracture of bones with its medico-legal importance.	214, 217, 221, 223, 289
FM 3.7	Describe factors influencing infliction of injuries and healing, examination and certification of wounds and wound as a cause of death—primary and secondary.	149, 217, 338, 345
FM 3.8	**MECHANICAL INJURIES AND WOUNDS** Describe and discuss different types of weapons including dangerous weapons and their examination.	333, 345
FM 3.9	**FIREARM INJURIES** Describe different types of firearms including structure and components. Along with description of ammunition propellant charge and mechanism of firearms, different types of cartridges and bullets and various terminology in relation of firearm—caliber, range, choking.	236, 238, 241
FM 3.10	**FIREARM INJURIES** Describe and discuss wound ballistics—different types of firearm injuries, blast injuries and their interpretation, preservation and dispatch of trace evidences in cases of firearm and blast injuries, various tests related to confirmation of use of firearms.	243, 253, 258, 324
FM 3.11	**REGIONAL INJURIES** Describe and discuss regional injuries to head (scalp wounds, fracture skull, intracranial hemorrhages, coup and contrecoup injuries), neck, chest, abdomen, limbs, genital organs, spinal cord and skeleton.	263, 271, 273, 284, 285, 287, 288, 289
FM 3.12	**REGIONAL INJURIES** Describe and discuss injuries related to fall from height and vehicular injuries—primary and secondary impact, secondary injuries, Crush syndrome, railway spine.	284, 314, 327, 338
FM 3.13	**SEXUAL OFFENCES** Describe various sections of IPC and CrPC related to definition of rape and sexual assault, medical examination of rape victim and accused of rape, police information by the doctors and medical care with recent amendments notified till date (i.e., Section 375 IPC, 166B IPC, 357C and 164A, 53A of CrPC). Describe the relevant provisions of POCSO Act related to medical care and police information.	66, 417
FM 3.14	**SEXUAL OFFENCES** Describe and discuss the examination of the victim of an alleged case of rape, and the preparation of report, framing the opinion and preservation and dispatch of trace evidences in such cases.	421
FM 3.15	**SEXUAL OFFENCES** Describe and discuss examination of accused and victim of sodomy, preparation of report, framing of opinion, preservation and dispatch of trace evidences in such cases.	439
FM 3.16	**SEXUAL OFFENCES** Describe and discuss informed consent in sexual intercourse. Describe and discuss histories of gender and sexuality-based (sexual orientation) identities and rights in India. Describe history of decriminalization of 'adultery' and consensual adult homosexual sexual behavior. Describe sexual offences with its medicolegal significance— ◆ Forced/non-consensual penetrative anal sex ◆ Forced/non-consensual oral sex ◆ Sexual acts with animals/bestiality/zoophilia ◆ Forced/non-consensual insertion of fingers or objects ◆ Forced/non-consensual touching or groping or disrobing ('indecent assault').	67, 417, 437, 439, 442, 444, 451, 452
FM 3.17	**PARAPHILIAS** Describe the difference between paraphilia and paraphilic disorder. Describe paraphilic disorder as per the latest guidelines of DSM and ICD and describe medico-legal implications of paraphilic disorder by referring scientific literature and legal justification (if any). Describe and discuss the various paraphilias in the context of informed consent during any sexual interaction.	446
FM 3.18	**VIRGINITY** Describe legitimacy and its medicolegal importance. Describe and discuss how 'signs' of virginity (so called 'virginity test', including finger tests on female genitalia) are unscientific, inhuman and discriminatory. Describe and discuss how to appraise the courts about unscientific basis of these tests if court orders it.	401, 409, 496
FM 3.19	**PREGNANCY AND DELIVERY** Discuss the medico-legal aspects of pregnancy and delivery, signs of pregnancy, precipitate labor superfetation, superfecundation and signs of recent and remote delivery in living and dead.	370, 404, 409, 411, 412

FM 3.20	Discuss disputed paternity and maternity.	409
FM 3.21	Discuss Pre-conception and Pre-natal Diagnostic Techniques (PC&PNDT)—Prohibition of Sex Selection Act, 2003 and Domestic Violence Act, 2005.	71, 73
FM 3.22	**IMPOTENCE AND STERILITY** Define and discuss impotence, sterility, frigidity, sexual dysfunction, premature ejaculation. Discuss the causes of impotence and sterility in male and female.	389
FM 3.23	Discuss sterilization of male and female, artificial insemination, test tube baby, surrogate mother, hormonal replacement therapy with respect to appropriate national and state laws.	395, 397
FM 3.24	Discuss the relative importance of surgical methods of contraception (vasectomy and tubectomy) as methods of contraception in the National Family Planning Programme.	395
FM 3.26	Discuss the national guidelines for accreditation, supervision and regulation of assisted reproductive technology (ART) clinics in India.	68
FM 3.27	**ABORTION** Define, classify and discuss abortion, methods of procuring medical termination of pregnancy (MTP) and criminal abortion and complication of abortion—MTP Act, 1971.	69, 380, 381, 384
FM 3.28	Describe evidences of abortion—living and dead, duties of doctor in cases of abortion, investigations of death due to criminal abortion.	385
FM 3.29	**CHILD ABUSE** Describe and discuss child abuse and battered baby syndrome.	373
FM 3.30	**TORTURE** Describe and discuss issues relating to torture, identification of injuries caused by torture and its sequelae, management of torture survivors.	512
FM 3.31	**TORTURE AND HUMAN RIGHTS** Describe and discuss guidelines and protocols of National Human Rights Commission regarding torture.	515
FM 4.1	**MEDICAL JURISPRUDENCE** Describe medical ethics and explain its historical emergence.	45
FM 4.2	Describe the Code of Medical Ethics 2002 conduct, Etiquette and Ethics in medical practice and unethical practices and the dichotomy.	29
FM 4.3	Describe the functions and role of Medical Council of India (now NMC) and State Medical Councils.	20
FM 4.4	Describe the Indian Medical Register.	20, 31
FM 4.5	Rights/privileges of a medical practitioner, penal erasure, infamous conduct, disciplinary committee, disciplinary procedures, warning notice and penal erasure.	29, 31
FM 4.6	Describe the laws in relation to medical practice and the duties of a medical practitioner towards patients and society.	24
FM 4.7	Describe and discuss the ethics related to HIV patients.	518
FM 4.8	Describe the Consumer Protection Act, 2019 (Medical Indemnity Insurance, Civil Litigations Compensations), Workman's Compensation Act and ESI Act.	63, 65
FM 4.9	Describe the medico-legal issues in relation to family violence, violation of human rights, National Human Rights Commission (NHRC) and doctors.	58
FM 4.10	Describe communication between doctors, public and media.	54
FM 4.11	Describe and discuss euthanasia.	47
FM 4.12	Discuss legal and ethical issues in relation to stem cell research.	48
FM 4.14	Describe and discuss the challenges in managing medico-legal cases including development of skills in relationship management—human behavior, communication skills, conflict resolution techniques.	54
FM 4.16	Describe and discuss bioethics.	46
FM 4.17	Describe and discuss ethical principles: Respect for autonomy, non-malfeasance, beneficence and justice.	46
FM 4.18	Describe and discuss medical negligence including civil and criminal negligence, contributory negligence, corporate negligence, vicarious liability, res ipsa loquitur, prevention of medical negligence and defenses in medical negligence litigations.	32, 35, 36, 37, 38, 39
FM 4.19	Define consent. Describe different types of consent and ingredients of informed consent. Describe the rules of consent and importance of consent in relation to age, emergency situation, mental illness and alcohol intoxication.	40
FM 4.20	Describe therapeutic privilege, malingering, therapeutic misadventure, professional secrecy, human experimentation.	27, 39, 40, 49, 51
FM 4.21	Describe products liability and Medical Indemnity Insurance.	38, 64

FM 4.22	Explain oath—Hippocrates, Charaka and Sushruta and procedure for administration of oath.	51
FM 4.23	Describe the modified declaration of Geneva and its relevance.	51
FM 4.24	Enumerate rights, privileges and duties of a registered medical practitioner. Discuss doctor-patient relationship—professional secrecy and privileged communication.	24, 27, 31
FM 4.25	**CLINICAL RESEARCH AND ETHICS** Discuss human experimentation including clinical trials.	49
FM 4.27	Describe and discuss ethical guidelines for biomedical research on human subjects and animals.	49
FM 5.1	**FORENSIC PSYCHIATRY** Classify common mental illnesses including post-traumatic stress disorder (PTSD).	469
FM 5.2	**FORENSIC PSYCHIATRY** Define, classify and describe delusions, hallucinations, illusion, lucid interval and obsessions with exemplification.	461
FM 5.3	Describe civil and criminal responsibilities of a mentally ill person.	481
FM 5.4	Differentiate between true insanity from feigned insanity.	467
FM 5.5	Describe and discuss delirium tremens.	630
FM 5.6	Describe the Indian Mental Health Act, 2017 with special reference to admission, care and discharge of a mentally ill person.	73
FM 6.1	Describe different types of specimen and tissues to be collected both in the living and dead: Body fluids (blood, urine, semen, feces saliva), skin, nails, tooth pulp, vaginal smear, viscera, skull, specimen for histopathological examination, blood grouping, human leukocyte antigen (HLA) typing and deoxyribonucleic acid (DNA) fingerprinting. Describe Locard's exchange principle.	106, 134, 508
FM 6.2	Describe the methods of sample collection, preservation, labeling, dispatch, and interpretation of reports.	134, 508
FM 7.1	Enumerate the indications and describe the principles and appropriate use for: ♦ DNA profiling ♦ Facial reconstruction ♦ Polygraph (lie detector) ♦ Narcoanalysis ♦ Brain mapping ♦ Digital autopsy ♦ Virtual autopsy ♦ Imaging technologies.	139, 504, 510, 522, 524
FM 8.1	**FORENSIC TOXICOLOGY** Describe the history of toxicology.	531
FM 8.2	Define the terms toxicology, forensic toxicology, clinical toxicology and poison.	531
FM 8.3	Describe the various types of poisons, toxicokinetics, and toxicodynamics and diagnosis of poisoning in living and dead.	533, 543
FM 8.4	Describe the laws in relations to poisons including Narcotic Drugs and Psychotropic Substances (NDPS) Act, medico-legal aspects of poisons.	533
FM 8.5	Describe medico-legal autopsy in cases of poisoning including preservation and dispatch of viscera for chemical analysis.	545
FM 8.6	Describe the general symptoms, principles of diagnosis and management of common poisons encountered in India.	537
FM 8.7	Describe simple bedside clinic tests to detect poison/drug in a patient's body fluids.	545
FM 8.8	Describe basic methodologies in treatment of poisoning: Decontamination, supportive therapy, antidote therapy, procedures of enhanced elimination.	537
FM 8.9	Describe the procedure of intimation of suspicious cases or actual cases of foul play to the police, maintenance of records, preservation and dispatch of relevant samples for laboratory analysis.	535, 545
FM 8.10	Describe the general principles of analytical toxicology and give a brief description of analytical methods available for toxicological analysis: Chromatography—thin layer chromatography, gas chromatography, liquid chromatography and atomic absorption spectroscopy.	546
FM 9.1	Describe general principles and basic methodologies in treatment of poisoning: Decontamination, supportive therapy, antidote therapy, procedures of enhanced elimination with regard to caustics Inorganic—sulfuric, nitric, and hydrochloric acids; organic—carboloic acid (phenol), oxalic and acetylsalicylic acids.	549, 552, 697
FM 9.2	Describe general principles and basic methodologies in treatment of poisoning: Decontamination, supportive therapy, antidote therapy, procedures of enhanced elimination with regard to phosphorus, iodine, barium.	583, 587, 590

Competencies Covered

FM 9.3	Describe general principles and basic methodologies in treatment of poisoning: Decontamination, supportive therapy, antidote therapy, procedures of enhanced elimination with regard to arsenic, lead, mercury, copper, iron, cadmium and thallium.	557, 563, 568, 575, 579, 582, 693
FM 9.4	Describe general principles and basic methodologies in treatment of poisoning: Decontamination, supportive therapy, antidote therapy, procedures of enhanced elimination with regard to ethanol, methanol, ethylene glycol.	620, 632, 634
FM 9.5	Describe general principles and basic methodologies in treatment of poisoning: Decontamination, supportive therapy, antidote therapy, procedures of enhanced elimination with regard to organophosphates, carbamates, organochlorines, pyrethroids, paraquat, aluminium and zinc phosphide.	584, 677, 683, 684, 685, 687
FM 9.6	Describe general principles and basic methodologies in treatment of poisoning: Decontamination, supportive therapy, antidote therapy, procedures of enhanced elimination with regard to ammonia, carbon monoxide, hydrogen cyanide and derivatives, methyl isocyanate, tear (riot control) gases.	555, 666, 671, 674
FM 10.1	Describe general principles and basic methodologies in treatment of poisoning: Decontamination, supportive therapy, antidote therapy, procedures of enhanced elimination with regard to: ♦ Antipyretics—paracetamol, salicylates ♦ Anti-infectives (common antibiotics—an overview) ♦ Neuropsychotoxicology—barbiturates, benzodiazepines phenytoin, lithium, haloperidol, neuroleptics, tricyclics ♦ Narcotic analgesics, anesthetics, and muscle relaxants ♦ Cardiovascular toxicology: Cardiotoxic plants—oleander, odollam, aconite, digitalis ♦ Gastrointestinal and endocrine drugs—insulin.	613, 637, 658, 660, 661, 663, 692, 694, 696, 697, 699, 700
FM 11.1	Describe features and management of snake bite, scorpion sting, bee and wasp sting and spider bite.	599, 609, 610
FM 12.1	Describe features and management of abuse/poisoning with following chemicals: Tobacco, cannabis, amphetamines, cocaine, hallucinogens, designer drugs and solvent.	646, 650, 660, 706, 707
FM 13.2	Describe medico-legal aspects of poisoning in Workman's Compensation Act.	65
FM 14.6	**EXAMINATION OF HAIR AND SEMEN** Demonstrate and interpret medico-legal aspects from examination of hair, fiber, semen and other biological fluids.	491, 497
FM 14.7	**EXAMINATION OF BLOOD** Demonstrate and identify particular stain in blood and identify the species of its origin.	487
FM 14.8	Demonstrate the correct technique to perform and identify ABO and Rh blood group of a person.	490
FM 14.16	To examine and prepare medico-legal report of drunk person in a simulated/supervised environment.	625
FM 14.17	To identify and draw medico-legal inference from common poisons, e.g., dhatura, nux vomica.	592, 641, 654

Source: Medical Council of India, Competency Based Undergraduate Curriculum for the Indian Medical Graduate. 2018; Vol. 1: 228-48.

SECTION 1: Jurisprudence and Forensic Medicine

Section Outline

1. Legal Procedure 3
2. Medical Practitioner—Duties and Malpractices 20
3. Ethical and Social Aspects of Medical Practice 45
4. Acts Related to Medical Practice 60
5. Identification I 79
6. Identification II 106
7. Medico-legal Autopsy 120
8. Thanatology 146
9. Signs of Death 158
10. Asphyxial Deaths 183
11. Injuries 213
12. Firearm Injuries 235
13. Regional Injuries 262
14. Thermal Injuries 293
15. Transportation Injuries 314
16. Explosion Injuries and Fall from Height 324
17. Medico-legal Aspects of Injuries 332
18. Neglect and Starvation Deaths 349
19. Radiation Sickness, Anesthetic and Operative Deaths 353
20. Infanticide and Child Abuse 358
21. Criminal Abortion 380
22. Erectile Dysfunction and Sterility 389
23. Virginity, Pregnancy and Delivery 401
24. Sexual Offenses 416
25. Homosexuality 439
26. Paraphilia 446
27. Postmortem Artifacts 455
28. Forensic Psychiatry 461
29. Bloodstain Analysis 486
30. Seminal Stains and Other Biological Samples 496
31. DNA Fingerprinting 504
32. Torture and Custodial Deaths 512
33. Medico-legal Aspects of HIV 518
34. Newer Techniques and Recent Advances 522

CHAPTER 1

Legal Procedure

LEARNING OBJECTIVES

Must know
1. Inquest, Police and Magistrate inquest
2. Courts in India and their powers
3. Offenses (bailable and non-bailable; cognizable and non-cognizable)
4. Subpoena/summons
5. Conduct money
6. Recording of evidence: Oath, examination-in-chief, leading question, cross-examination, perjury
7. Documentary evidence, dying declaration
8. Types of witness: Expert, common, hostile
9. Police and Magistrate inquest (Diff.)
10. Dying declaration and dying deposition (Diff.)

Desirable to know
1. Medical examiner system, coroner's inquest
2. Common and expert witness (Diff.)
3. Conduct of a doctor in the witness box

FM 1.1
Demonstrate knowledge of basics of forensic medicine like definitions of forensic medicine, clinical forensic medicine, forensic pathology, state medicine, legal medicine and medical jurisprudence.

NOTA BENE

Forensic science refers to a group of scientific disciplines which are concerned with the application of their particular scientific area of expertise to law enforcement, criminal, civil, legal and judicial matters. Forensic scientists examine objects, substances (including blood/drug samples), chemicals (paints/explosives/toxins), tissue traces (hair/skin) or impressions (fingerprints/tyremarks) left at the scene of crime—*a multidisciplinary subject*.

Definitions

- **Forensic medicine*** (Legal medicine or State medicine): It is the *application of principle and knowledge of medical sciences* to legal purposes and legal proceedings so as to aid in the administration of justice.
- **Clinical forensic medicine:** It is the branch of medicine that deals with both the *provision of clinical services* (i.e., diagnosis, treatment and management) to patients and the *medico-legal aspects* of patient care.
- **Forensic pathology**: Investigation of sudden, unexpected and/or violent deaths that includes determining *the cause of death and the circumstances of how the death occurred*.
- **Medical jurisprudence**: It is the *application of knowledge of law* in relation to practice of medicine. It includes:
  - Doctor-patient relationship
  - Doctor-doctor relationship
  - Doctor-State relationship.

FM 1.2
Describe history of forensic medicine.

HISTORY OF FORENSIC MEDICINE

Forensic medicine has humble and ancient origins.
- Law-medicine problems were found written in records in Egypt, Sumer, Babylon, India and China dating 4000–3000 BC.
- Manu (3102 BC) was the first traditional king and lawgiver in India. Manusmriti, a famous treatise where rules for marriage, punishment for adultery, incest and sexual offenses were formulated.

---

*Latin *forensis*: of or before the forum. In Rome, 'forum' was the meeting place, where civic and legal matters used to be discussed by those with public responsibility.

SECTION 1: Jurisprudence and Forensic Medicine

- Code of Hammurabi specified by King of Babylon (about 1754 BC) is the oldest known medico-legal code.
- Hippocrates (460–377 BC), Father of Western medicine discussed the lethality of wounds and contributed to the field of ethics.
- First descriptions of examination of injuries were found carved on pieces of bamboo dating back to the Qin dynasty in China, from about 220 BC.
- First medico-legal autopsy in history was conducted by the Roman physician Antistius who examined the body of Julius Caesar after his assassination in 44 BC.
- Charaka Samhita, the first treatise on Indian medicine which dates back to 100–200 BC.
- Sushruta, father of Indian surgery gave the Sushruta Samhita in 200–300 AD.
- During the 6th century, Justinian law called medico-legal experts to testify in cases of rape, criminal abortion and murder.
- Chinese publication in the 13th century titled 'Hsi Yuan Lu' or 'Instructions to the Coroner' dealt with findings in cases of infanticide, drowning, hanging, poisoning and assault.
- In Germany, during the 16th century, the code of Bamburg brought about a requirement for medical testimony in forensic cases. This code also allowed the opening of bodies to examine the depth of and damage caused by wounds.
- Ambroise Pare (1510–1590), a French surgeon is considered the father of modern forensic pathology. He studied the effects of violent death on internal organs, and wrote *Reports in Court*, a procedure on writing of legal report in relation to medicine.
- In 1602, first book on forensic medicine was published by Italian physician, Fortunato Fedele.
- Paolo Zacchia published *Questiones Medicolegales* (1621–1651) in three volumes and is considered the father of forensic psychiatry and father of legal medicine.
- The first recorded medico-legal autopsy performed in India was by Edward Bulkley in 1693 at Madras (now Chennai) on a suspected case of arsenic poisoning.
- The first publication on forensic medicine in UK was by William Hunter in the 18th century. His essays were on injuries found on murdered illegitimate children.
- In the 18th century, Italian anatomist Giovanni Morgagni (1682–1771) dissected the bodies of the dead and compared the alterations in their organs with the symptoms of the diseases that had caused death. He published a book in 1761 on 640 postmortem he had conducted.
- The three great pioneers of forensic medicine born in the 18th century were Johann Casper (1796–1864), Mathieu Orfila (1787–1853) and Marie Devergie (1798–1879). They devoted their life in the study and development of forensic medicine as we understand it today.
- In 1807, Andrew Duncan became the first professor in forensic medicine at Edinburgh.
- In 1858, Sir William Herchel advocated the use of fingerprint in identification of a person.
- Alfred Swaine Taylor published the '*Principles and practice of Medical Jurisprudence*' in 1865.
- In 1879, Alphonse Bertillon was the first to utilize anthropometry in law enforcement.
- In 1890, Sir Francis Galton systemized the use of fingerprints and its use for identification.
- The first chair in medical jurisprudence was instituted in Calcutta Medical College in 1845 and Dr CTO Woodford was the first Professor.
- Dr Jaising Modi was the first to handle cases of medico-legal nature and published the first book in India 'Forensic Medicine'.
- Prof Alec Jeffreys pioneered the use of DNA profiling for identification in 1984.

> **FM 1.3**
> Describe legal procedures including Criminal Procedure Code, Indian Penal Code, Indian Evidence Act, Cognizable and non-cognizable offenses.

Law is a set of rules that are created and enforced by a particular country or community through social or governmental institutions to regulate the actions of its members. It can be:

a. **Substantive law:** It deals with those areas of law which establish the rights and obligations of individuals, what individuals may or may not do. For example, the Indian Penal Code.
b. **Procedural law:** It deals with and lays down the ways and means by which substantive law can be enforced. For example, Criminal Procedure Code and Indian Evidence Act.

Types of Law

In Indian judicial system, there are four types of law:

1. **Criminal law** deals with criminal offenses, regulates the apprehension, charging and trial of suspected individuals, and fixes penalties and modes of punishments applicable to convicted persons. Punishment can be imprisonment with/without fine or death sentence. For example, rape, assault, murder, robbery, kidnapping, etc. are considered offenses under criminal law.
2. **Civil law** deals rules, procedures, regulations and judicial precedents that help in resolving the various disputes which are non-criminal. These disputes are either between individuals or organizations. For example, cases of defamation, custody of children, property disputes, copyright, insurance claims, etc.
3. **Common law** is case law or judicial precedent which is derived from judicial decision of courts and similar tribunals.
4. **Statutory law** is established by an Act of the legislature that is signed by the executive (President/Governor) or legislative body.

Indian Penal Code (IPC)

IPC is the official criminal code of India intended to cover all aspects of criminal law. The IPC defines specific crimes and provides punishment for them. Some examples are:

a. **Crimes against the human body**
   - These offenses are provided for in Chapter XVI of the Code from Sec. 299 which deals with culpable homicide to Sec. 377 which deals with unnatural offenses.
   - The chapter deals with all kinds of offenses which can be committed against the human body, from the very lowest degree i.e., simple hurt or assault to the gravest ones which include murder, kidnapping and rape.

b. **Crimes against property**
   - These crimes are defined and punished under Chapter XVII from Sec. 378 which defines theft, to Sec. 462 which prescribes punishment for the offense of breaking upon an entrusted property.
   - The offenses dealt under this chapter include theft, extortion, robbery, cheating, forgery etc.

c. **Offenses against the State**
   - These crimes are defined and punished under Chapter VI from Secs. 121 to 130 and are some of the most rigorous penal provisions of the entire code.
   - This includes the offense of waging war against the State under Sec. 121 and sedition under Sec. 124A.

d. **General exceptions**
   - Secs. 76–106 (Chapter IV) represent the general exceptions which are basically exceptional circumstances where the offender can escape criminal liability.
   - Concepts that are elaborated upon in this chapter include insanity, consent and acts of children below a certain age.

Criminal Procedure Code (CrPC)

- CrPC deals with procedures of investigation and the mechanism for punishment of offenses against the substantive criminal law.
- It is a comprehensive document designed to provide due process to the accused by laying down a procedure for cognizance, arrest, bail, collection of evidence, trial and determination of innocence or guilt.
- The procedure ensures that the rights of individuals are protected against the strong State machinery.
- **Offense** is 'any act or omission made punishable by law for the time being in force'. The offenses can be:
  a. **Bailable offenses*** are those in which bail can be granted by the law. The court cannot refuse bail, and the police have no right to keep the person in custody. For example, causing death by rash or negligent act (Sec. 304-A IPC), causing miscarriage (Sec. 312 IPC), or voluntarily causing hurt (Sec. 323 IPC) and grievous hurt (Sec. 325 IPC).
  b. **Nonbailable offenses** are those in which bail cannot be granted. These are serious offenses and the decision for bail is taken by a Judicial Magistrate only. For example, cases of murder (Sec. 302 IPC), attempt to murder (Sec. 307 IPC), dowry death (Sec. 304-B IPC), causing miscarriage without woman's consent (Sec. 313 IPC) or voluntarily causing grievous hurt by dangerous weapons (Sec. 326 IPC).
- According to Sec. 2(h) of the code, an *investigation* is the process of collecting evidence by either a police officer or any other person that is authorized by a Magistrate to do so.
- The process of investigation is thorough and full of intricate procedures—any irregularities in the procedure may result in the acquittal of the accused.
- For the purposes of investigation, cases under CrPC have been divided into cognizable and non-cognizable cases **(Diff 1.1)**.
- **FIR ('First Information Report'):** It is the written document prepared by the police officer regarding the commission of a 'cognizable offense' (Sec. 154 CrPC).
- For the purposes of trials, the cases under CrPC can be classified into four categories:
  1. **Sessions case:** These are cases where the punishment for the offenses involved is death, life imprisonment or imprisonment for a period of ≥7 years. In such cases, the trial is to be handled by a Sessions Court.

DIFFERENTIATION 1.1: Cognizable and non-cognizable offense

S. No.	Feature	Cognizable offense	Non-cognizable offense
1.	Nature of crime	Serious	Not much serious
2.	FIR	Can be registered without Magistrate's permission	Cannot be registered without Magistrate's permission
3.	Arrest by police	May arrest without warrant from the Magistrate	Cannot arrest without warrant
4.	Sec. of CrPC	2(c)	2(l)
5.	Examples of cases	Rape, murder, dowry death	Causing miscarriage, voluntarily causing hurt, cheating, public nuisance

---

* Bail means the temporary release of an accused; it is not only the essence of criminal procedure but also a safeguard of individual liberty.

2. **Summons case:** Case relating to an offense punishable with imprisonment for a term <2 years, e.g., voluntarily causing hurt, and is tried by a Magistrate. These are relatively less serious offenses and the procedure involved is also simpler.
3. **Warrant case:** Case related to an offense punishable with death, life imprisonment or imprisonment for ≥2 years, e.g., murder, dowry deaths, attempt to murder cases, etc.
4. **Summary case:** Summary trials are those kinds of trials where speedy justice has to be given, which means those cases which are to be disposed of speedily and the process of these cases is quite simplified.

Trial Procedure

- The procedure for trials is interwoven with detailed procedures; they are in place so that the guilty may be punished but also the innocent persons get every possible opportunity to prove their innocence.
- Once the innocence or guilt of an accused is determined, the aggrieved party has the option to go in appeal and challenge the decision within the stipulated statutory time.
- The appeals generally lie from a Magistrates Court to the Sessions Court, from the Sessions Court to the High Court and from the High Court to the Supreme Court.

Indian Evidence Act (IEA)

- IEA relates to evidence on which the court come to conclusion regarding facts of the case. It is common to both the criminal and civil procedure.
- IEA defines evidence in court and states its admissibility.
- **Objectives:** Aid the courts in ascertaining the truth, to prevent inquiries from becoming prolonged and delay the judicial process, and to ensure that judges do not grow confused or muddled due to irrelevant or inconsequential evidence.
- **Purpose:** Define the sources of evidence for Indian courts.
- Evidence which does not fall under the IEA is not admissible in court, even if it is the key to determining the truth of the matter.
- Evidence law is supported by three main pillars:
  i. Evidence should only consist of matters in issue
  ii. Hearsay evidence does not have evidentiary value
  iii. There should be an effort to provide the best evidence in all cases.
- Sec. 3 of IEA is an important clause that provides the definition of important terms that appear throughout the Act. It defines:
  a. What constitutes a court, i.e., who is authorized by this Act to collect evidence and reach a decision
  b. Different types of evidence, documents
  c. What is a fact?
  d. What is relevant?
  e. How a fact is proved, disproved and not proved?
  f. How it sets up the reading of the rest of the Act, and the interpretation of evidence law according to it?
- **Court:** 'Court' consists of all Judges and Magistrates, and any person who is legally authorized to take evidence, with the exception of arbitrators and tribunals.
- **Fact:** 'Fact' may be defined as "anything, state of things, relation of things that can be sensed (external fact)".
- **Facts in issue:** Facts in issue are those facts that are sought to be proved and are also called "principal facts" or *factum probandum*. When the rights and liabilities of the parties are dependent on a fact that is in dispute or controversy, that fact is in issue.
- **Relevant facts:** Relevant facts are those which are needed to prove or disprove a fact in issue. Relevant facts are also called evidentiary facts (*factum probans*).
- **Document:** A document within the meaning of this Act is any writing, marks, figures inscribed on a surface for the purpose of recording a matter.
- **Evidence** means to discover, determine or arrive at the truth.

> **NOTA BENE**
>
> The government introduced three Bills—the Bharatiya Nyaya Sanhita (BNS) Bill, 2023, Bharatiya Nagarik Suraksha Sanhita (BNSS) Bill, 2023 and Bharatiya Sakshya (BS) Bill, 2023 to repeal the British-era IPC, IEA and CrPC respectively.

FM 1.3

Describe Inquest, Police inquest and Magistrate inquest

■ INQUEST

Definition: An inquest is an inquiry or investigation into the cause of death where death is apparently *not due to natural causes.**

It is done in cases of:
i. Sudden death.
ii. Suicide, homicide and infanticide.
iii. Death from accident, drowning, poisoning, drug mishap or machinery.
iv. Unexplained death or death from burns or fall from height.
v. Death under anesthesia or on operation table or from postoperative shock.
vi. Death due to alleged medical negligence or within 24 hours (h) of admission in a hospital.
vii. Death of a convict in jail, police custody, mental hospital or correctional school.
viii. Dowry deaths (in India).
ix. Death due to any industrial disease (not held in India).

---

* If death is due to natural causes, e.g., old age, brain hemorrhage, tuberculosis, myocardial infarction etc, the body is handed over to the relatives for cremation/burial without any further investigations.

Types of Inquest

Two types of inquests are held in India **(Diff. 1.2)**:
  i. Police inquest *(most common)*
  ii. Magistrate inquest

Other types of inquests *(not held in India)*:
  i. Coroner's inquest
  ii. Medical examiner system
  iii. Procurator fiscal

■ POLICE INQUEST

- The provision for holding of inquest is outlined in **Sec. 174 CrPC**.
- Police inquest is held by a police officer (known as the Investigation Officer—IO) not below the rank of senior head constable in all cases of unnatural deaths with the exceptions mentioned under Magistrate inquest.
- An inquest is a fact finding inquiry, to establish reliable answers to four important questions. The *first* relates to the identity of the deceased, the *second* to the place of his death, the *third* to the time of death, and the *fourth* question is related to his apparent cause of death (whether accidental, suicidal, homicidal or caused by animal).
- The rules of procedure forbid any expression of opinion on any other matter.
- It is not the requirement of law to mention the name of the accused, the weapon carried by them and who were the witnesses of the assault in the inquest report.
- Even if there is some discrepancy between the inquest report and the postmortem report, the list of injuries mentioned in the postmortem report will prevail over the details of the inquest report.

Procedure

- Police officer, on receipt of information of death, gives intimation to the nearest Executive Magistrate empowered to hold inquests.
- He then proceeds to the place of occurrence and holds an inquiry into the matter, in the presence of two or more respectable inhabitants of the locality (witnesses). The witnesses are called *panchas*.
- The inquest report so prepared is known as *panchnama*.
- If no foul play is suspected, the dead body is handed over to the relatives for disposal.
- In suspicious cases, the body is sent for postmortem examination to the nearest authorized doctor with a requisition and a copy of the inquest.
- The report is then forwarded to the District Magistrate or Sub-Divisional Magistrate (SDM).

The police officer may summon persons who appear to know the facts of the case, and the person is bound to attend and answer questions put to him **(Sec. 175 CrPC)**.

Refusal to answer questions is punishable under **Sec. 179 IPC** with imprisonment up to 6 months and/or fine of ₹ 1000.

■ MAGISTRATE INQUEST

Inquest is conducted by District Magistrate, Judicial Magistrate, SDM or any Executive Magistrate empowered

DIFFERENTIATION 1.2: Magistrate and police inquest

S.No.	Feature	Magistrate inquest	Police inquest
1.	Investigating officer	Inquest conducted by DM, SDM or Magistrate who is qualified and experienced	Conducted by police officer who is not qualified in law or medicine
2.	Section under which conducted	Sec. 176 CrPC	Sec. 174 CrPC
3.	Informing Magistrate	Need not inform anyone	Needs to inform the Magistrate of the area
4.	Types of cases handled	Can hold inquest in all cases of suspicious deaths	Cannot hold inquest in cases of death in custody, jail, police encounter or dowry deaths
5.	Witnesses	Police helps the Magistrate. Does not require signature of the witnesses	*Panchas* help, who are chosen at random to sign the report
6.	Value of statements made by witness	Valuable and admissible in court	No value, not admissible in court
7.	Warrant for arrest	Can issue arrest warrant of the accused	Cannot issue warrant, but can arrest an accused in cognizable offense
8.	Exhumation	Can order a body to be exhumed	Cannot order
9.	Autopsy	Does not send dead bodies for autopsy indiscriminately	Sends dead bodies for autopsy indiscriminately
10.	Analysis of viscera	Can order chemical analysis of viscera	Cannot order
11.	Quality of investigation	Superior to police inquest	Inferior to Magistrate inquest

by State Government, such as the Sub-Collector or Tehsildar.
- **Sec. 176 CrPC** deals with inquiry by Magistrate into cause of death.
- It is practiced all over India.
- It is not held routinely, but only when especially indicated.

Indications for Magistrate Inquest

1. Death in police encounter.
2. Disappearance or death of a person in police custody or during police interrogation.
3. Death of a convict in jail or a patient in psychiatric hospital.
4. Exhumation (where the body is dug out of a grave).
5. Rape alleged to have been committed on any woman in the custody of the police.
6. Dowry death (suicide/death of a woman within 7 years of marriage).
7. Admission of a mentally ill person in a psychiatric hospital under certain provisions of Mental Health Care Act, 2017.
- In addition to the above, the Magistrate reserves the right to hold an inquest in any other case of death which he deems fit.
- Inquiry by Judicial Magistrate or Metropolitan Magistrate is *mandatory* in cases of custodial death/disappearance or custodial rape. In all other cases, an Executive Magistrate can hold an inquiry.
- When such an inquiry is to be held, the Magistrate should inform the relatives, i.e., parents, children, brothers, sisters or spouse of the deceased and allow them to remain present at the inquiry.

- The Judicial Magistrate holding the inquest should forward the body for examination by the Civil Surgeon or any other doctor appointed by the State Government within 24 h of the death of a person.

Purpose

The main intention behind the Magistrate inquest is to ensure that:
a. No person is unjustly deprived of his liberty and his rights as citizen.
b. No person, who is deprived of his liberty, can die as a result of neglect or brutality of the people who are in-charge of him.
c. In case of a buried body, there is no doubt with regards to identity, cause of death or manner of death.
d. The death is not a 'dowry death'.

> **NOTA BENE**
> **Investigation vs. Inquiry (Diff. 1.3)**
> - *Investigation* includes all proceedings under the CrPC for the collection of evidence conducted by a police officer or any person, other than a Magistrate, who is authorized by the Magistrate.
> - *Inquiry* is a judicial proceed which is conducted by the Magistrate or court to determine whether the further proceedings of the cases moves to trial.

Coroner's Inquest (Diff. 1.4)

- **Coroner** is usually an advocate, attorney or 1st class Magistrate with 5 years experience or a Metropolitan Magistrate.
- Appointed by state Government to inquire into causes of unnatural or suspicious deaths.

DIFFERENTIATION 1.3: Investigation and inquiry

S.No.	Feature	Investigation	Inquiry
1.	Official involved	Police officer or someone authorized by Magistrate	Magistrate
2.	Objective	Collect evidence for the prosecution	Determine the truth or falseness of certain facts with a view to take certain actions
3.	Section defining	Sec. 2(h) CrPC	Sec. 2(g) CrPC
4.	Stage	First stage of a criminal case	Second stage
5.	Action	Not a judicial proceeding	Judicial proceeding

DIFFERENTIATION 1.4: Coroner's and Magistrate's court

S.No.	Feature	Coroner's court	Magistrate's court
1.	Type of court	Court of inquiry	Court of trial
2.	Accused	Need not be present during trial	Should be present during the trial
3.	Punishment	No power to impose fine/punish	Can impose fine and punishment
4.	Contempt of court	Can punish a person for contempt, if committed within the premises of his court	Can punish whether offense is committed within or outside the premises of court
5.	Status in India	Not followed	Followed

- Coroner's inquest is currently held in some states of US, Australia, Canada, UK, New Zealand, Hong Kong and some other countries, **but not in India**.
- The coroners have quasi-judicial power—powers resembling those of a court of law or judge, and can enquire death caused by accident, homicide, suicide, or by an unknown cause.

Open verdict means an announcement of the commission of crime without naming the criminal (when the perpetrator of crime is not identified).

Medical Examiner System

- This type of inquest is conducted in most of the states of the US. A medical man (Board Certified or Board eligible forensic pathologist) is appointed to hold an inquest.
- He visits the scene of crime/accident to gather first hand evidence and interview people to obtain as much information as possible regarding circumstances of death.
- After that, he performs autopsy and correlates autopsy findings with evidence, and determines the cause and manner of death.
- The system is superior to other inquest where non-medical men/coroner conducts the inquiry.
- But the medical examiner does not have any judicial powers, such as, he cannot examine the witness under oath and cannot authorize the arrest of any person.

NOTA BENE

- In India, the coroner system was introduced by the British in 1902 in Kolkata and Mumbai. Later on, the system was removed from Kolkata, and still later from Mumbai (since 26th July, 1999).
- **Procurator fiscal** is a public prosecutor in Scotland and has powers in the investigation of criminal matters (similar to coroner system). Amongst his roles is the investigation of sudden, unexplained or suspicious deaths including fatal accidents. He can request an autopsy to be performed by a forensic pathologist and presents cases for the prosecution in the courts.

A 35-year-old married woman died in unnatural conditions within 5 years of her marriage. Her parents complained of frequent demand of dowry by her in-laws.

a. Her autopsy will be conducted under Sec._____
b. Dowry deaths are punishable under Sec._____

FM 1.3, 1.4
- Civil and Criminal cases.
- Describe Courts in India and their powers: Supreme Court, High Court, Sessions Court, Magistrate's Court, Labor Court, Family Court, Executive Magistrate Court and Juvenile Justice Board.

COURTS OF LAW

A court of law is a place where legal matters are decided by a judge or a magistrate to adjudicate legal disputes between parties and carry out the administration of justice in civil, criminal and administrative matters in accordance with the rule of law.

In India, the courts of law are of two types **(Flowchart 1.1)**:

1. **Civil court**
   - A court of law that tries and determines civil cases, usually disagreements between individual people or private organizations, rather than with criminal activity.
   - Judge can order payment of money/fine or make decisions about family/home/land.
   - The court of the District Judges is the highest civil court in a district. Most of the civil cases are filed in the court of the *Munsiff*.
   - The court of the District Judge has both original and appellate jurisdiction. Against the decision of the District judge, an appeal is made in the High Court.

2. **Criminal court**
   - A court that has jurisdiction and authority to try and punish individuals accused of committing a crime as per criminal law.

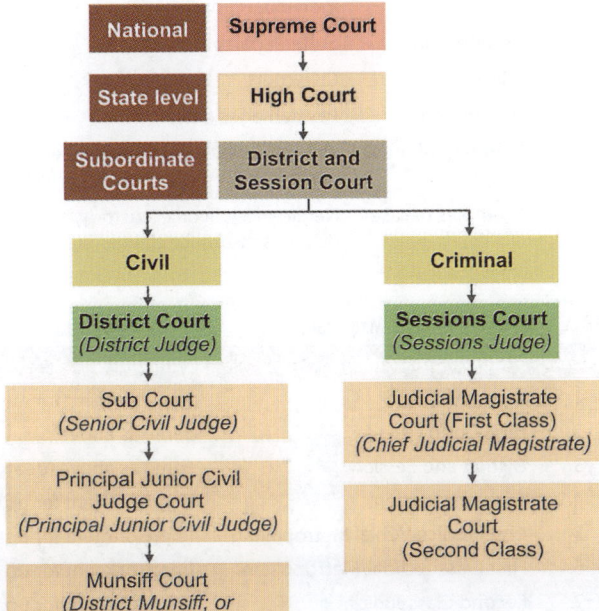

Flowchart 1.1: Civil and criminal courts in India

- Judge can punish by imprisonment with/without fine or pronounce death sentence.
- The government files a case against someone for committing a crime in the criminal court since it is considered an act against a state and not only the victim. Therefore, state becomes operative when a crime is committed. The person accused of committing the crime is called the defendant.

Difference between civil and criminal cases is highlighted in **Diff. 1.5**.

Criminal Courts and its Powers

Criminal courts are of four types **(Flowchart 1.1 and Table 1.1)**:

1. **Supreme Court** is the highest judicial tribunal and the highest court of appeal; located in New Delhi. It has the power of supervision over all courts in India. The law declared by it is binding on all courts.
2. **High Court** is usually located in the capital of every State (with few exceptions) and is the highest court in the state. Judges in a High Court are appointed by the President of India in consultation with the Chief Justice of India and the Governor of the State. It deals with appeals from lower courts and writ petitions. It may try any offense and pass any sentence authorized by law (Sec. 28 CrPC).
3. **Sessions Court** is usually located at the district headquarters and is also known as *District Session Court,* and presided over by a 'District and Sessions Judge'.
   - He is known as a District Judge when he presides over a civil case, and a Sessions Judge when he presides over a criminal case.
   - Appointment of District Judge is done either by the state Government in consultation with the High Court or by way of elevation of Judges from courts subordinate to district courts.
   - It can try cases which have been committed to it by a Magistrate.
   - It can pass any sentence authorized by law including death sentence which is subject to confirmation by the High Court (Sec. 28 CrPC).
4. **Magistrates' Courts** are of three types:
   i. Chief Judicial Magistrate (CJM): CJM is the senior most Judicial Magistrate First Class.
   ii. Judicial Magistrate First Class.
   iii. Judicial Magistrate Second Class.

- In metropolitan cities with more than 1 million population, the Chief Judicial Magistrate and First Class Judicial Magistrate are designated as Chief Metropolitan Magistrate and Metropolitan Magistrate respectively.
- The High Court appoints the Judicial Magistrate of first class to the CJM (Sec. 12 CrPC).
- Powers of Magistrate court is given in Sec. 29 CrPC. Higher court can enhance the sentence awarded by it.

DIFFERENTIATION 1.5: Civil and criminal case

S.No.	Feature	Civil case	Criminal case
1.	Definition	Dispute between two or more parties in their individual capacities	Prosecution by the State against a person/organization, for committing a public wrong (offense against the State)
2.	Complainant	Sufferer party	Public prosecutor on behalf of the State
3.	Trial by	Civil court	Criminal court
4.	Punishment	Pay damages (fine)	Fine, community service, probation, imprisonment, death
5.	Standard of proof	'Preponderance of the evidence'—the winner's side of the story is more probably true than not true	'Beyond a reasonable doubt'—party needs to prove that his version of the facts is highly likely
6.	Examples of cases	Negligence, divorce, custody, of child consumer disputes insurance claims, etc.	Assault, robbery, murder, arson, rape, etc.

TABLE 1.1: Powers of Judge/Magistrate

S.No.	Judge/Magistrate	Punishment	Amount of fine
1.	Supreme Court	Imprisonment for any period including death sentence	Any amount
2.	High Court	Same as above	Any amount
3.	District and Session	Same as above (death sentence needs confirmation by High Court)	Any amount
4.	Assistant Session	Imprisonment for up to 10 years	Any amount
5.	Chief Judicial/Chief Metropolitan	Imprisonment for up to 7 years	Any amount
6.	First Class Judicial/Metropolitan	Imprisonment for up to 3 years	Up to ₹ 10,000
7.	Second Class Judicial	Imprisonment for up to 1 year	Up to ₹ 5,000

Labor Courts

- Labor court is a governmental judiciary body which deals with disputes between an employee and employer (e.g., wrongful termination, unpaid salary, sexual harassment, denied maternity benefit etc.) during the course of employment.
- Case has to be filed within a year from the date of dispute.
- Proceedings are governed by the Industrial Dispute Act.

Family Courts

- Family courts were established to hear all cases that relate to familial and domestic relationships, such as marriage, divorce, domestic violence, alimony, child custody, etc.
- In India, the Family Courts Act, 1984 was implemented for the welfare of women.
- *Main purpose:* Try the cases away from the intimidating atmosphere of regular courts and reduce the backlog of cases.

Executive Magistrates

- Executive Magistrates (including DM, SDMs, Tehsildars) are officers of the Executive branch.
- State government appoints these Executive Magistrates.
- Judicial Magistrate can handle all cases including criminal cases, whereas Executive Magistrate can handle cases relating to public peace, maintenance of law and order, etc.
- These officers cannot try any accused nor pass verdicts.
- Usually, they are officers of the Revenue Department who are invested with specific powers under both CrPC and IPC.

Juvenile Justice Board

- Under the Juvenile Justice (Care and Protection of Children) Act, 2015, the State Government constitutes the Juvenile Justice Boards for each district.
- The Board consists of a Metropolitan Magistrate/Judicial Magistrate First Class (Principal Magistrate) and two social workers, out of which at least one should be a female.

Functions

1. To adjudicate cases of juvenile offenders and monitor institutions for juvenile offenders.
2. Ensure that the children's rights are protected in the process of inquiry, arrest and rehabilitation.
3. Maintain liaison with the Child Welfare Committee.

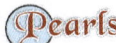

Sentences authorized by the law (Sec. 53 IPC)
i. Death
ii. Imprisonment for life
iii. Imprisonment—rigorous (hard labor) or simple
iv. Forfeiture of property
v. Monetary fine
vi. Treatment, training and rehabilitation of juvenile offenders

Capital Punishment

- **Capital punishment** or **death penalty** is the killing of a person by judicial process as a punishment for an offense.
- Various methods of carrying out death sentence are: hanging, electrocution, shooting, cyanide poisoning, lethal injection, garroting and guillotine.
- Sec. 354(5) CrPC, 1973 states that 'When any person is sentenced to death, the sentence shall direct that he be hanged by the neck till he is dead.'* This is also provided under Air Force, Army and Navy, and the execution has to be carried out *either by hanging by neck till death or by being shot to death.*
- The power of amnesty for capital punishment in India is vested with the President of India.

NOTA BENE

- Lethal injection is usually the method of execution in the US.
- **Guillotine:** Device used for carrying out executions by decapitation. It consists of a tall upright frame from which a heavy blade is suspended. The blade is raised with a rope and then allowed to drop, severing the victim's head from his body. The device was used for execution in France and, more particularly, during the French Revolution.

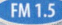 **FM 1.5**

Describe summons, conduct money, types of witnesses.

SUBPOENA/SUMMONS

Definition: *Subpoena* (Latin, under punishment) is a document compelling the attendance of a witness in a court of law, under penalty, on a particular day, time and place for the purpose of giving evidence.

- **Sec. 61–69 CrPC** deals with summons.
- It is issued by the court in writing, in duplicate and signed by the presiding officer of the court and bears the seal of the court (Sec. 61 CrPC).
- It is served on the witness by a police officer, by an officer of the court or any other public servant.
- The witness retains one copy and returns the other duly signed by him on the back, in acknowledgment of its receipt (Sec. 62 CrPC).

---

* Capital punishment in IPC: 302 (murder); 354A (kidnapping for ransom); 376A (rape and injury which caused death or PVS); 376DB (gang rape of a child <12 years) etc.

- Summon must be obeyed, and if the witness fails to attend the court, then:
  i. In civil cases, he is liable to pay damages.
  ii. In criminal cases, the court may issue notice under Sec. 350 CrPC. If it finds that the witness neglected to attend the court without justification, may sentence him to imprisonment and/or fine, or may issue bailable or non-bailable warrant to secure the presence of witness (Sec. 172–174 IPC and Sec. 87 CrPC).
- It may also require the witness to bring with him any books, documents or other things under his control, which he is bound by law to produce in evidence.
- The witness may be excused from attending the court, if he has valid and urgent reason.
- If a witness is summoned by two courts on the same day, one criminal and other civil, he should attend the criminal court (criminal courts have priority over civil courts).
- Higher court has priority over the lower. If summoned to two courts on the same day, either civil or criminal, he must first attend the higher court.
- If a witness receives two summons on the same date from the same type of court, he should attend the court from which he received the summon first, and inform the other court.

NOTA BENE

- Subpoena can be of two types:
  i. *Subpoena duces tecum:* Person is required to bring certain documents or other evidence to the court (usually the postmortem or the medico-legal report) specified in the subpoena.
  ii. *Subpoena ad testificandum:* Requires the individual to testify before the court.

CONDUCT MONEY

Definition: It is the fee offered or paid to a witness (e.g., doctor) in *civil cases* at the time of serving the summons to meet the expenses towards attending the court.
- If fee is not paid or if he feels that the amount is less, the witness can bring this fact to the notice of the Judge before giving evidence in the court. The Judge will decide the amount to be paid.
- In criminal cases, no fee is paid to the witness at the time of serving the summons. He must attend the court and give evidence because of the interest of the State in securing justice; otherwise he will be charged with contempt of court. However, conveyance charges and daily allowance are paid according to the Government rules.

FM 1.7, 1.9
- Describe dying declaration and dying deposition.
- Describe the importance of documentation in medical practice.

MEDICAL EVIDENCE

Definition: It is defined as legal means to prove or disprove any medico-legal issue in question. It is of two types:
  i. Documentary evidence
  ii. Oral evidence.

Documentary Evidence

Definition: It comprises of all documents (including electronic records), to be produced before the court for inspection during the course of trial **(Fig. 1.1)**. It can be:
1. **Primary:** The document itself produced for the inspection of the court.
2. **Secondary:** Certified copies of the original documents issued by authorized person.

It includes:
  i. **Medical certificates**
   - Issued by a qualified registered medical practitioner (RMP) in relation to ill health, death, insanity, age or sex.
   - No fee is to be charged for issuing death certificates. Death certificate should not be issued without inspecting the body, and if the doctor is not sure of the cause of death, the matter should be reported to the police.
   - Issuance of false certificate is treated as forgery or making false document under Secs. 463 and 464 IPC which is punishable with imprisonment up to 2 years with/without fine (Sec 465 IPC).
   - Issuance of false certificate is a professional misconduct and punishable with *penal erasure*.
  ii. **Medico-legal reports**
   - Reports prepared by a doctor at the request of the IO for his guidance, usually in criminal cases, e.g., injury, postmortem, sexual assault, pregnancy, abortion or delivery.
   - Injury report is prepared when there is a requisition from the person himself or the police/Magistrate.
   - Postmortem reports are made only when there is a requisition from the police officer or Magistrate.
   - Reports are *not* admitted as evidence, unless the doctor attends the court and testifies to the facts under oath.*
   - Report should show competence, lack of bias and offer concrete professional advice. The doctor should avoid technical terms as far as possible.

---

* Recently, Orissa High Court held that a postmortem report, if its genuineness is uncontested by the accused can be treated a substantive evidence without the need for formal proof (no need to examine the doctor).

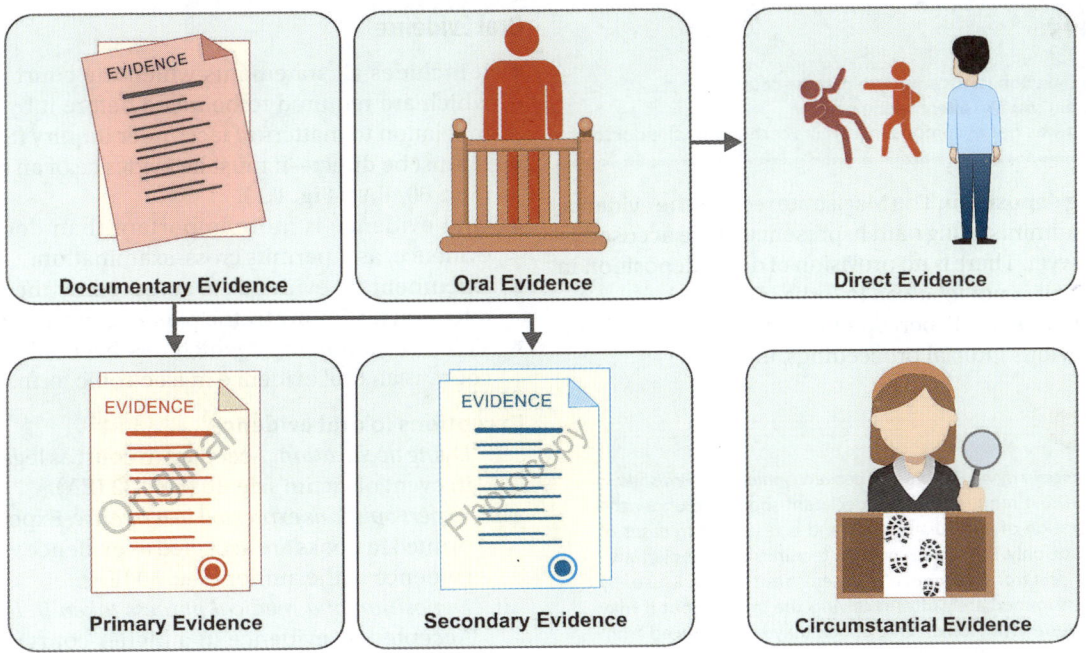

Fig. 1.1: Types of evidence

> **NOTA BENE**
>
> Medical certificates (sickness/fitness/vaccination/disability certificate) issued by doctors are not certificates required by law and hence not covered under Sec. 197 IPC (issuing false certificate). However, if such documents are submitted in the court as evidence, and proved to be false then it is equivalent to giving false evidence (Sec. 197 IPC) and punishable with imprisonment up to 7 years and fine (Sec. 193 IPC).

iii. **Dying declaration**

Definition: It is a written or oral statement of a person, who knows that his death is imminent, concerning what he believes to be the cause or circumstances of his death.*

- A dying declaration is called as '*leterm mortem*' which means 'words said before death'.
- The law does not provide who can record a dying declaration, nor is there any prescribed form, format or procedure for the same.
- The dying declaration has been incorporated in **Sec. 32 IEA**. It must have corroborative evidence to support it before it can be accepted (**Sec. 157 IEA**).

Procedure and features of dying declaration

- The doctor should certify that the person is conscious and his mental faculties are normal, i.e., he is in *compos mentis*.
- Oath is not administered because of the belief that a dying person tells the truth. This is based on the maxim '*nemo moriturus praesumitur mentire*' which means 'no one at the point of death is presumed to lie'—a man will not make his creator with a lie in his mouth.†
- *No leading questions* are asked.
- Ideally, a Magistrate should be called to record the declaration—gives more strength and reliability.
- When death is imminent, the statement may be recorded in the presence of two witnesses by the doctor or the police officer without losing time in waiting for the Magistrate.
- Statement of the declarant should be recorded in the form of a simple narrative, in the same vernacular the declarant speaks and understands, without any alteration or phrases.
- If the person is unable to speak, he can make the declaration by signs and gestures in response to the question.
- While recording the statement, if the declarant becomes unconscious, the person recording it must record as much information as he has obtained and sign it himself.
- Fitness of the declarant to make statement is certified again at the conclusion of the statement.
- Declaration is sent to the Magistrate in a sealed cover.
- If the declarant survives, the person is called to give oral evidence. It may be used to corroborate or contradict his statement in the court.

---

* Although, dying declaration is documentary in nature, legally it is considered as oral and hearsay evidence too.

† A dying declaration is admissible as evidence even though it has not been made on oath and the person making it cannot be cross examined. It is an exception to the rule of hearsay evidence.

Pearls

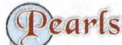

Dying declaration is not admissible in the court if:
1. Declarant survives after making it.
2. Patient was not in compos mentis (as certified by the doctor).

Dying deposition: The Magistrate records the evidence after administering oath in presence of the accused or his lawyer. There is no provision of dying deposition in IEA, so it is not followed in India **(Diff. 1.6)**.

iv. **Miscellaneous:** Expert opinion from books, deposition in previous judicial proceedings, etc.

NOTA BENE

- *Difference in dying declaration between Indian and British law:* In the UK, it requires that the declarant should be under the expectation of immediate death and is restricted in cases of homicide only. But there is no such requirement in Indian law.
- *Dying declaration made in a state of shock:* Shock usually appears immediately after receiving the injuries, but it may supervene after some time. Shock may be produced from exhaustion resulting from several injuries combined, though each one of them separately may be very slight. After receiving mortal injuries involving a vital organ, a very guarded reply is required to be given by a medical witness as to whether a person is capable of speaking, walking or performing any other volitional act.
- The declaration can be made to a police officer, public servant, village headman or any member of public, but its evidential value will be less. The only requirement in such cases is that the person recording it must be sure that the statement was made in a proper mental condition. A doctor's certificate about the dying man's mental condition is not necessary to make the declaration acceptable as evidence. The judgment can be made by the individual recording the statement.
- FIR lodged by dying person is valid dying declaration.

Oral Evidence

- It includes all statements which the court permits or which are required to be made before it by a witness, in relation to matters of fact under inquiry (Sec. 3 IEA).
- It must be direct—it must be evidence of an eyewitness (Sec. 60 IEA) **(Fig. 1.1)**.
- Oral evidence is more important than documentary evidence, as it permits cross-examination.
- Documentary evidence is accepted by the court only after oral testimony by the person concerned.
- Video conferencing** which has been allowed by the court, is an oral evidence in electronic form.

Exceptions to oral evidence

i. *Dying declaration:* Accepted in court as legal evidence in event of victim's death (Sec. 32 IEA).
ii. *Expert opinions expressed in a treatise:* Expert opinions printed in books are accepted as evidence without oral evidence of the author (Sec. 60 IEA).
iii. *Deposition of a medical witness taken in lower court:* Accepted as evidence in a higher court when it has been recorded and attested by a magistrate in presence of the accused who had an opportunity to cross-examine the witness (Sec. 291 CrPC).
iv. *Report of certain government scientific experts:* Admitted as evidence without their oral examination, e.g., reports of Chemical Examiner or Director of Fingerprint Bureau/Haffkine Institute/CFSL (Sec. 293 CrPC).
v. *Evidence given by a witness in a previous judicial proceeding:* Admitted in a subsequent judicial proceeding when the witness is dead or cannot be found or is incapable of giving evidence, or cannot be called without unreasonable delay or expense to the court (Sec. 33 IEA).

DIFFERENTIATION 1.6: Dying declaration and dying deposition

S.No.	Feature	Dying declaration	Dying deposition
1.	Statement	Recorded by anyone—Magistrate/doctor/village headman/police/any member of public	Always recorded by a Magistrate*
2.	Oath	Not required	Must
3.	Accused or his counsel	Not present	Always present
4.	Cross-examination	Not done	Done
5.	Legal value	Comparatively less	Much more
6.	Admissibility, if declarant survives	Not admitted, but has corroborative value	Fully admitted
7.	Nature	Merely recording of statement	Complete court procedure
8.	Type of evidence	Documentary	Oral
9.	Role of doctor	Assess compos mentis Record the statement in absence of Magistrate, but in presence of witnesses	Assess compos mentis Statement always recorded by the Magistrate
10.	Status in India	Followed	Not followed

* Or Reader of court or before the lawyers of two parties.
** Video conferencing is live visual connection between the court and the medical witness located at different sites to facilitate recording of the evidence using computer network.

vi. *Public records:* Birth and death certificates, and certificates of marriage.
vii. *Hospital records:* Routine entries, such as date of admission, discharge, pulse, temperature, etc., are admissible without oral evidence.

- **Circumstantial evidence or indirect evidence** is the evidence consisting of collateral facts from which an inference may be drawn and are consistent with the direct evidence, such as finding blood on the clothes of the accused or footprint that matches a shoe of the accused.
- **Hearsay evidence:** Any evidence that is offered by a witness of which he does not have direct knowledge, but his testimony is based on what others have said. For example, Anil heard from Sunil about an accident that Sunil witnessed but that he had not, and Anil repeated in the court Sunil's story as evidence of the accident.

> Another type of evidence used in criminal law is **real or physical evidence** which consists of material items involved in a case, objects and things, such as fingerprints, DNA, weapon, tape recording, computer printout, photographs etc. In order to be used at trial, real evidence must be relevant, material and authentic. The court will hear evidence from an expert witness explaining the significance or the relevance of the real evidence before it is admitted.

FM 1.5
Describe types of witnesses.

TYPES OF WITNESS

Definition: A witness is a person who gives sworn testimony (evidence) in a court of law as regards facts and/or inferences that can be drawn from these.

Types (Diff. 1.7)
i. Common, percipient, ordinary or lay witness
ii. Expert or skilled witness

- **Expert witness** is a person who has been trained or skilled in a technical or scientific subject. He can volunteer a statement, if he feels that justice is likely to be miscarried owing to the court having failed to elicit an important point.
- Doctors are not necessarily expert witnesses. Medical practitioners are considered '*professional witnesses*' akin to *witnesses of fact* when he is providing factual medical evidence, e.g., the doctor may confirm the physical examination findings in case of an accident or a diagnosis made after investigation or may report the findings of an X-ray or treatment given to the patient. The medical practitioner is not giving comment or opinion on any report based on the medical facts.
- The difference between a 'professional witness' and an 'expert witness' is that, experts can offer opinions beyond the facts of what they have personally witnessed and can respond to questions about hypothetical situations posed to them. In most cases, medical evidence is expert evidence.
- When a doctor describes the dimensions of an injury, e.g., stab wound, he acts like an ordinary witness, but when opines the cause of death as hemorrhage due to antemortem injury to the femoral artery, he acts as an expert witness.

Hostile witness is a person who willfully or with motive (bribe/intimidation) conceals part of the truth or tells a lie or gives completely false evidence in a court.
- It is contradictory to the statement the witness made in the previous deposition (e.g., statement recorded by the police).
- Any witness—common or expert can be declared hostile witness.

DIFFERENTIATION 1.7: Common and expert witness

S.No.	Feature	Common witness	Expert witness
1.	Definition	Gives evidence about the facts observed or perceived by him (**Sec. 118 IEA**)	Person especially skilled in foreign law, science or art (**Sec. 45 IEA**)
2.	Volunteering a statement	Not allowed	Can volunteer
3.	Drawing inference from observations	Not allowed	Can draw
4.	Expressing opinion on observations made by others	Not allowed	Can express
5.	Responsibility	Less	Highly responsible
6.	Punishment for giving false evidence	Less punishment	Severely punished in some countries
7.	Conduct money	Cannot claim	Can claim
8.	Examples	Any person	Handwriting or fingerprint expert, doctor, chemical examiner

SECTION 1 : Jurisprudence and Forensic Medicine

> **NOTA BENE**
> - A witness who has seen the event first-hand is known as an eyewitness.
> - **Testimony:** Testimony is a solemn attestation as to the truth of a matter.
> - The Supreme Court has defined a **hostile witness** as 'one who is not desirous of telling the truth at the instance of the party calling him', and an **unfavorable witness** is 'one called by a party to prove a particular fact, who fails to prove such a fact or proves an opposite fact' (Sat Pal vs Delhi Administration).
> - Supreme Court held that the deposition of a hostile witness can be taken into consideration to the extent that the same is in consonance with the case of the prosecution and found to be reliable under careful judicial scrutiny. Evidence tendered by a prosecution witness would not get entirely erased merely because the prosecution has chosen to treat him as hostile.

FM 1.5, 1.6
- Describe court procedures including recording of evidence, oath, affirmation, examination in chief, cross examination, re-examination and court questions, and conduct of doctor in witness box.
- Describe offenses in court including perjury; court strictures vis-a-vis medical officer.

RECORDING OF EVIDENCE

Testifying

- A deposition is testimony of a witness.
- A deposition is a discovery device—lawyers gather information on what factual and expert witnesses says orally and assess the relative effectiveness of their testimony.
- The purpose of discovery is to identify all the facts related to the case.
- All persons are competent to testify in the court, unless they fail to understand the questions or give rational answers due to (a) tender years [child], (b) extreme old age or (c) disease (physical/mental) **[Sec. 118 IEA]**.

Presentation of Evidence

After receiving subpoena, the witness must appear before the court at the appointed time with the relevant documents. The evidence is probed for areas of uncertainty, inconsistency or any factors which may make it appear unreliable. Evidence is presented in a systematic order (Sec. 138 IEA):
1. Oath (Sec. 51 IPC)
2. Examination-in-chief (Sec. 137 IEA)
3. Cross-examination (Sec. 141–146 IEA)
4. Re-examination (Sec. 137–138 IEA)
5. Court questions (Sec. 165 IEA, Sec. 311 CrPC).

Oath/Affirmation

- An oath is a verbal promise to tell the truth in the name of God.
- Oath is taken holding the Gita, Bible or New/Old Testament.
- It is compulsory for the witness to take an oath in the witness box before he gives his evidence. He is required to swear by Almighty God that he will tell the truth, the whole truth and nothing but the truth.
- A child of <12 years of age need not take oath.
- **Affirmation** is a verbal, solemn and formal declaration, which is made in place of an oath, if the witness is an atheist. An affirmation has the same effect as an oath.
- **Refusing oath/affirmation** is punishable with imprisonment up to 6 months with/without fine of ₹ 1000 (Sec. 178 IPC).

Perjury (false evidence): A witness who after taking oath or making a solemn affirmation, willfully makes a false statement which he knows or believes to be the false (Sec. 191 IPC and Sec. 344 CrPC) is liable to be prosecuted for perjury under **Sec. 193 IPC** with imprisonment up to 7 years and fine.

Reasons behind perjury:
a. Witness may have taken bribe
b. He may be under threat
c. He may have personal bias towards one party

> **NOTA BENE**
> - In the US, punishment for perjury is imprisonment up to 5 years, while in the UK it is up to 7 years.
> - In some countries, such as France, Italy and Germany, suspect's evidence is not taken under oath or affirmation and thus cannot commit perjury, regardless of what they say during their trial.

Examination-in-Chief (Direct Examination)

- It is the examination of a witness by the party who calls him.
- In criminal cases, the public prosecutor commences this examination.
- **Objectives** are to place before the court all the facts that bear on the case, and if the witness is an expert, his interpretation of these facts.
- *No leading questions are allowed* except in those cases in which the Judge permits or the witness is declared 'hostile'.

> **NOTA BENE**
> - **Leading question (suggestive interrogation):** Any question suggesting the answer which the person putting it wished or expects to receive (Sec. 141 IEA). It includes a material fact and admits of a conclusive answer by a simple 'Yes' or 'No'. For example, "Was the length of the knife 15 cm?" Instead the question should be "What was the length of the knife?"
> - Leading questions must not be asked, if objected to by the adverse party, in an examination-in-chief or in re-examination, except with the permission of the court (Sec. 142 IEA).
> - **Loaded questions:** They contain false or unproven assumptions that make it difficult to answer and are objectionable. For example, "Have you stopped taking a bribe for medico-legal reports?" indirectly asserting that the person used to take bribes.

Cross-examination

It is the examination of a witness by the adverse party (defense lawyer).

Objectives

i. To elicit facts favorable to his case.
ii. To test the accuracy of the statements made by the witness.
iii. To modify or explain what has been said.
iv. To develop new or old facts.
v. To discredit the witness.
vi. To remove any overemphasis which may have been given to any of fact in direct examination.

♦ The lawyer tries to weaken the evidence of the witness by showing that his details are inaccurate, conflicting, contradictory and untrustworthy.
♦ *Leading questions are allowed* (Sec. 143 IEA) to test the accuracy, credibility and reliability of the witness.
♦ Cross-examination has no time limit, may last for hours or even days.
♦ The court has the power to disallow questions which are indecent or scandalous (Sec. 151 IEA) or intended to insult or annoy, or offensive in form (Sec. 152 IEA).

During cross-examination, if any question is not understood, the witness should ask the lawyer to explain it better. Moreover, he should not volunteer any unrelated information.

> **NOTA BENE**
>
> Cross-examination is considered as one of the most reliable methods to extract the truth from the witnesses. A cross-examination is like a:
> ♦ *Legal lie-detector*—used by the lawyer to test the veracity of evidence tendered by the opposite side.
> ♦ *Legal surgery*—blade of questions is used to dissect the body of evidence adduced by the other side. Like a surgeon, a cross-examiner has to attack only limited areas of evidence only which are troubling the client.
> ♦ *Double-edged sword*. It is said "if you know how to wield, it helps to cut enemy's neck, otherwise, it cuts own hands", i.e., it may end up harming the defendant more than that to the other side.
> ♦ *Mental duel*—it is a dignified fight between a cross-examiner and the witness.

Re-examination (Re-direct Examination)

It is the examination of a witness subsequent to the cross-examination by the party who called him.

Objectives

i. To clear any doubts that may have arisen during cross-examination.
ii. To explain some matter in its proper perspective, so that underemphasis or possible misinterpretation may be avoided.

Leading questions are not allowed. Opposing lawyer has the right of re-cross-examination on any new point which has been raised.

Court Questions/Questions by the Judge

A judge may ask any question to the witness at any stage of the trial to clear any doubtful points.

The deposition of the witness is handed over to him. The witness after carefully going through it, is required to sign at the bottom of each page and on the last page immediately below the last paragraph, and to initial any corrections (Sec. 278 CrPC). The witness should not leave the court without the permission of the Judge.

Judicial stricture: An adverse comment or a signature of disapproval; it is a criticism from a court of law to any person or administrative authority.
♦ It is figured as considered judgments and acts as a warning without convicting the person/authority.
♦ There are multiple instances where judiciary has passed strictures against doctors for poor quality of medico-legal work or illegible handwriting of doctors in MLRs.

Some of the important sections of IPC, CrPC and IEA are given in the Synopsis (beginning of the Unit).

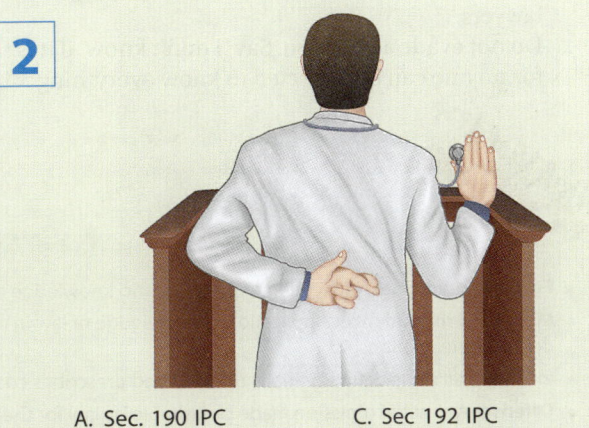

A witness, who after taking oath, willfully makes a statement which he knows or believes to be false is guilty of offense under:

A. Sec. 190 IPC　　C. Sec 192 IPC
B. Sec. 191 IPC　　D. Sec. 193 IPC

> **NOTA BENE**
>
> **Evidence through video conferencing**
> Supreme Court has held that the recording of evidence through video conferencing is legal [Sec. 273 and 275(1) CrPC]. Most of the courts have allowed the medical witness to depose through video conferencing, since personal appearance in the court would be expensive, inconvenient and time consuming. Punjab and Haryana High court has directed the State Governments to set up video conferencing rooms in the Civil Hospitals to facilitate recording of evidence of medical experts. However, the court must satisfy itself regarding the identity of the witness.

> **FM 1.5**
> Describe conduct of doctor in witness box.

CONDUCT AND DUTIES OF A DOCTOR IN THE WITNESS BOX

When summons is served, he must attend the court punctually. As a rule, his evidence is taken at the appointed time. Following are the do's and don'ts in the witness box:
  i. Take all records and relevant reports that may have to be quoted in the box.
  ii. Be well dressed and modest.
  iii. Do not discuss the case with anyone in the court except the lawyer by whom you were asked to testify.
  iv. Stand up straight, be relaxed, calm and not be frightened or nervous. Look people in the eye when you speak, for it gives the impression of honesty.
  v. Never attempt to memorize. The law allows refreshing your memory from copies of reports.
  vi. Speak slowly, distinctly and audibly so that the typist can record your evidence.
  vii. Use simple language, avoiding technical terms to the best of your ability.
  viii. Address the Judge by his proper title such as 'Sir' or 'Your honor'.
  ix. Be polite, pleasant and courteous to the lawyer. Do not underestimate the medical knowledge of the lawyers.
  x. Do not evade a question. Say 'I don't know' if it is so, for no one can be expected to know everything.
  xi. Do not loose your temper. An angry witness is often a poor witness.
  xii. Retain independence of your mind. A biased expert is a useless expert.
  xiii. Listen carefully to the questions. Do not hesitate to ask the questions to be repeated, if you do not understand it. Avoid long discussions.
  xiv. If you believe the question is unfair, look at your lawyer before answering. If he fails to object, turn to Judge and ask whether you should answer the question.
  xv. Do not overemphasize replies to questions from cross-examining lawyers.
  xvi. Watch for *double barreled/double direct* questions (asking on two different issues within one question). The answer to each part of the question may be different.
  xvii. When asked to comment upon the competence of a colleague, avoid any insulting remarks. If you do not wish to make any statement, say that you have 'no opinion' or 'no comments'.
  xviii. Say 'In my opinion…', do not use phrase such as 'I think…' or 'I imagine…' Be prepared to give reasons for your opinion, if asked.
  xix. Do not be drawn outside your particular field of competence. Avoid speaking on a subject in which you have little or no practical experience.
  xx. Do not refuse to answer any question—a medical witness has no professional privilege.
  xxi. Do not volunteer any information beyond that is asked for in the question.

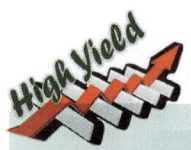

- **Forensic medicine:** Application of principle and knowledge of medical sciences to aid in administration of justice.
- **Medical jurisprudence:** Application of knowledge of law in relation to practice of medicine such as doctor-patient/doctor-doctor/doctor-State relationship.
- Indian Penal Code defines various offenses and prescribes code for punishment in the court of law.
- **Offense:** Any act of omission made punishable by law for the time being in force.
- **Cognizable offense:** Police officer can arrest a person without warrant from the Magistrate [Sec. 2 (c) CrPC].
- **Non-cognizable offense:** Police officer cannot arrest without a warrant.
- **Warrant case:** Offense is punishable with death, imprisonment for life or for a term ≥2 years.
- **Summons case:** Offense is punishable with imprisonment for a term <2 years.
- Inquest is an inquiry/investigation into the cause of unnatural death.
- Two types of inquest are held in India—police *(most common)* and magistrate inquest.
- Inquest not held in India—coroner inquest and medical examiner system.
- Police inquest is done by a person not below the rank of sub-inspector/senior head constable.
- Sec. 176 CrPC deals with Magistrate inquest.
- Magistrate inquest is held in police firing/interrogation deaths, death of convicts in jail, dowry deaths, rape in police custody, exhumation.
- Supreme Court and High Court are the courts of appeal.
- Judicial execution is practiced in India by hanging.
- Death sentence issued by Session's Court has to be confirmed by High Court.

CHAPTER 1 : Legal Procedure

- Lowest court to give imprisonment up to 10 years is Assistant Session court.
- Chief Judicial Magistrate can give imprisonment up to 7 years and unlimited fine.
- **Summons:** Document compelling the attendance of a witness in a court, under penalty, on a particular day, time and place for giving evidence.
- Issuing a false certificate (e.g., medical certificate) to be used in court as evidence is like giving false evidence (Sec. 197 IPC) and punished under Sec. 193 IPC (perjury).
- **Conduct money:** Fee paid to a witness in *civil case* (not in criminal case). It is paid by the party who has called him as a witness and decided by the Judge.
- Types of medical evidence—documentary and oral.
- Documentary evidence should be supported by oral evidence who issued it.
- Death certificate is issued free of charge.
- **Dying declaration:** No oath is taken; no cross-examination is done (Sec 32 IEA).
- If a person survives after giving dying declaration, it is used as corroborative evidence.
- Dying deposition is *not* followed in India.
- Oral evidence is more important than documentary evidence; *permits cross-examination*.
- Documentary evidence along with oral evidence is required in postmortem reports.
- Expert witness can volunteer a statement in the court of law.
- **Hostile witness:** Person who willfully tells a lie or gives completely false evidence in court.
- **Perjury:** Willfully making a false statement by a witness under oath. Punishment under Sec. 193 IPC with imprisonment up to 7 years and fine.
- Leading questions are *not* allowed in examination-in-chief and re-examination.
- Leading questions are allowed in cross-examination, dying deposition, and to a hostile witness.
- Oath is compulsory in a deposition. Child <12 years is not required to take an oath.
- Deposition is a statement on oath made by a witness in a judicial proceeding.
- During trial, the Judge can ask questions during any part of the trial.
- No time limit for examination-in-chief or cross-examination.

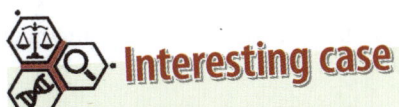

Perjury (Jessica Lal Case, 1999)

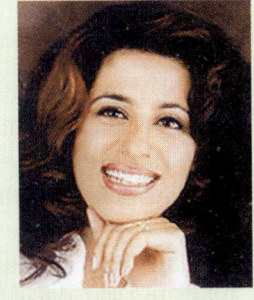

Jessica Lal was shot dead in April 1999 by Manu Sharma after she had refused to serve him liquor at a restaurant in south Delhi. He was convicted and sentenced to life imprisonment by the High Court in 2006. The trial court had acquitted him earlier, but the Delhi High Court had reversed the order and the Supreme Court (SC) had upheld his life sentence in 2010.

Two cartridge cases recovered from the crime spot was the lone evidence to link the accused to the crime as the weapon of offense could not be recovered. The ballistic expert thus became a crucial witness in the case. The Delhi police had asked for his opinion on whether the bullets fired at Jessica were from the same firearm. In a written statement, he had stated that a conclusive opinion on the question was not possible in the absence of the firearm for testing in the laboratory. Later on, in his oral deposition before the trial court he said that the bullets appear to have been fired from different firearms. The Delhi high court declared him 'hostile' and initiated perjury proceedings against him as the court believed that his opinion was 'calculated to let the accused off the hooks' as the defense had formed its definite plan about a 'two weapon theory'.

But the SC observed that 'scientifically it is not possible for an expert to give a definite opinion by only examining the cartridges as to whether they have been fired from the same firearm. It is significant to note that his opinion that the cartridges appeared to have been fired from different firearms was based on the trail court's insistence to give the opinion without examining the firearm. In other words, it was not even his voluntary, let alone deliberate deposition before the court. Therefore, it is unjust, if not unfair, to attribute any motive to the appellant that there was a somersault from his original stand in the written opinion.' The court held that a forensic expert being a professional gives an 'opinion on facts' during the trial unlike any other 'witness of facts' who must present facts as put forth by the prosecution. The ballistic expert charged for perjury by the Delhi high court was cleared of the charge by the SC.

CHAPTER 2: Medical Practitioner—Duties and Malpractices

LEARNING OBJECTIVES

Must know
1. Constitution, powers and functions of National Medical Commission
2. Functions of State Medical Council
3. Professional misconduct, penal erasure, warning notice
4. Professional secrecy
5. Privileged communication
6. Unethical acts
7. Duties, rights and privileges of a registered medical practitioner
8. Prevention of medical negligence
9. Defenses in medical negligence suits
10. Medical maloccurrence, therapeutic misadventure
11. Professional negligence, Res ipsa loquitur
12. Examples of medical negligence
13. Contributory negligence
14. Consent, types, informed consent, rules
15. Vicarious liability
16. Civil and criminal negligence (Diff.)
17. Professional misconduct and negligence (Diff.)

Desirable to know
1. Types of physician-patient relationship
2. Corporate negligence
3. Products liability
4. Calculated risk doctrine
5. Doctrine of common knowledge

FM 4.3, 4.4
- Describe the functions and role of National Medical Commission.
- Describe the Indian Medical Register.

NATIONAL MEDICAL COMMISSION

Introduction
- The National Medical Commission (NMC) Act, 2019 has repealed the Indian Medical Council Act, 1956 (IMC Act). This Act provides for setting up of National Medical Commission (NMC) in place of Medical Council of India (MCI).
- The MCI was established in 1934 under the IMC Act, 1933. In 1956, the old Act was repealed and a new one was enacted. This was further modified in 1964, 1993 and 2001.
- The MCI, a statutory body, responsible for establishing and maintaining uniform standards of medical education, and recognition of medical qualifications was superseded by the government.
- NMC became operational from 25th September 2020.
- Currently, the NMC is the umbrella regulatory body with certain other bodies under it which regulates medical education and practice in India.

Constitution
- NMC is comprised of 33 members, including one Chairman, ten *ex officio* members and 22 part-time members. Out of the 22 part-time members, 19 will be nominated by States and Union Territories.
- The Chairperson, certain part-time members and the Secretary are appointed by the Central Government on the recommendation of a Search Committee (*a seven member committee*).

Autonomous Boards
The Act provides for constitution by the Central Government of the following autonomous boards under the supervision of the NMC:
- Undergraduate Medical Education Board (UGMEB)
- Postgraduate Medical Education Board (PGMEB)
- Medical Assessment and Rating Board (MARB)
- Ethics and Medical Registration Board (EMRB)

CHAPTER 2 : Medical Practitioner—Duties and Malpractices

Medical Advisory Council

- The Act also provides for the constitution of an advisory body, known as the Medical Advisory Council (MAC) by the Central Government.
- **Composition:** The MAC would be comprised of the Chairperson and all members of the NMC (*as ex-officio members*), the Chairman of the University Grants Commission, the Director of the National Assessment and Accreditation Council, and various other members to be nominated by the State Governments, Ministry of Home Affairs in the Government of India, State Medical Council, and the Central Government.
- **Function:** The MAC shall act as the primary platform through which the States and Union Territories may put forth their views and concerns before the NMC and help in shaping the overall agenda, policy and action relating to medical education and training. Further, the MAC shall advise the NMC on measures to determine and maintain, and to coordinate maintenance of the minimum standards in all matters relating to medical education, training and research, and measures to enhance equitable access to medical education.

POWERS AND FUNCTIONS

National Medical Commission

1. Lay down policies for maintaining a high quality and high standards in medical education.
2. Lay down policies for regulating medical institutions, medical researches and medical professionals.
3. Assess the requirements in healthcare, including human resources for health and healthcare infrastructure and develop a road map for meeting such requirements.
4. Promote, co-ordinate and frame guidelines and lay down policies by making necessary regulations for the proper functioning of the Commission, the Autonomous Boards and the State Medical Councils (SMCs).
5. Ensure co-ordination among the Autonomous Boards.
6. Ensure compliance by the SMCs of the guidelines framed and regulations made under this Act for their effective functioning.
7. Exercise appellate jurisdiction with respect to the decisions of the Autonomous Boards.
8. Lay down policies and codes to ensure observance of professional ethics and to promote ethical conduct by medical practitioners.
9. Frame guidelines for determination of fees and all other charges in respect of 50% of seats in private medical institutions and deemed to be universities.
10. **Entrance and exit tests**
    - NMC conducts a National Eligibility-cum-Entrance Test (NEET) for admission to the UG and PG superspecialty in all medical institutions governed by the Act, as well as common counseling so that there is transparency in admissions.
    - Subsequently, a common final year UG medical examination [National Exit Test (NEXT)] will held for granting licenses to practice medicine and for enrolment in the State Register/National Register, for admission to PG courses and screening test for foreign medical graduates.
11. **Recognition of medical qualifications granted by statutory or other body:** The medical qualifications granted by statutory or other bodies including Diplomate of National Board (DNB), which are covered by the categories listed in the Schedule shall be recognized medical qualifications.
12. **Withdrawal of recognition of qualification granted by medical institutions**
    On receiving a report from the MARB, if the Commission is of the opinion that:
    - The courses of study and examination do not conform to the standards specified by the UGMEB or PGMEB, or
    - The standards and norms for infrastructure, faculty and quality of education are not adhered to and the medical institution has failed to take necessary corrective action to maintain specified minimum standards, it may withdraw recognition granted to such medical qualification.
13. **Recognition of medical qualifications granted by medical institutions outside India**
    - The Commission may either grant or refuse recognition (after due verification) to such medical qualification on receiving application from an authority in any country outside India.
    - All medical qualifications which have been recognized before the date of commencement of this Act and are included in the Second Schedule and Part II of the Third Schedule to the IMC Act, shall also be recognized medical qualifications under this Act.
14. **Derecognition of medical qualifications granted by medical institutions outside India:** If the Commission is of the opinion that a recognized medical qualification which is included in the list is to be derecognized, it may order derecognition and remove it from the list (after verification with the authority of that country).
15. **Issuing good standing certificate:** The certificate ensures that the medical practitioner has a good track record and there is no ethical breech or disciplinary proceedings against him. It is valid for 6 months from the date of issue.
16. **Community health providers:** The NMC may grant a limited licence to practise medicine at mid-level as a community health provider (CHP). CHPs can independently prescribe specified medicine in primary and preventive healthcare. Beyond that, the CHP can prescribe medicine only under the supervision of duly registered medical practitioners (RMP).

Undergraduate and Postgraduate Medical Education Boards

1. Regulation of the standards of medical education at the undergraduate (UG), postgraduate (PG) and super-speciality level.
2. Develop competency-based dynamic curriculum at all levels.
3. Develop competency-based dynamic curriculum for addressing the needs of primary health services, community medicine and family medicine (by UG Board).
4. Develop competency-based dynamic curriculum at PG and superspeciality level so as to develop appropriate skill, knowledge, attitude, values and ethics to provide healthcare, impart medical education and conduct medical research (by PG Board).
5. Frame guidelines for setting up of medical institutions, having regard to the needs of the country and the global norms.
6. Determine the minimum requirements and standards for conducting courses and examinations.
7. Determine standards and norms for infrastructure, faculty and quality of education in medical institutions.
8. Facilitate development and training of medical institute faculty members in Medical Education Technologies.
9. Facilitate research and the international student and faculty exchange programs.
10. Specify norms for compulsory annual disclosures (electronically or otherwise) by medical institutions, in respect of their functions that has a bearing on the interest of all stakeholders including students, faculty, the Commission and the Central Government.
11. Recognition of medical qualifications granted by universities or medical institutions in India. Moreover, all medical qualifications which have been recognized before the date of commencement of this Act and are included in the First Schedule and Part I of the Third Schedule to the IMC Act, shall also be recognized qualifications and shall be listed and maintained by the respective boards.
12. Promote and facilitate PG courses in family medicine (by PG board only).

Medical Assessment and Rating Board

1. **Assessment and rating of medical colleges:** Determine the procedure for assessing and rating the medical institutions for their compliance with the standards laid down by UGMEB or PGMEB.
2. **Rating of institutions:** Conduct or empanel independent rating agencies to conduct, assess and rate all medical institutions.
3. **Permission for establishment of a new medical college/starting PG course/increase in seats:** Conduct evaluation and assessment of any medical institution at any time, and assess and evaluate the performance, standards and benchmarks of such medical institution. Criteria for approving or disapproving scheme will be based on adequacy of financial resources, academic faculty and hospital facilities.
4. **Inspections of medical colleges:** Carry out inspections of medical institutions for assessing and rating such institutions. It may hire and authorize any third party agency or persons for assessing and rating such institutions.
5. **Punitive measures:** It may issue warning, impose fine, reduce intake, stop admissions or withdraw recognition of a medical institution for failure to maintain the minimum standards.

Ethics and Medical Registration Board

1. **National Register:** Maintain National Registers (including in electronic form) of all licensed medical practitioners containing the name, address and all recognized qualifications possessed. It should also ensure electronic synchronization of the National Register and the State Register.
2. **Professional conduct and medical ethics:** It shall ensure compliance of the code of professional and ethical conduct through the SMC.
3. **Interaction with SMCs:** Continuous interaction with SMCs to effectively promote and regulate the conduct of medical practitioners and professionals.
4. **Appellate powers:** Exercise appellate jurisdiction with respect to the actions taken by a SMC.

Schedules under MCI (IMC Act)
- **First Schedule:** Recognized medical qualifications granted by Universities in India.
- **Second Schedule:** Recognized medical qualifications granted outside India.
- **Part I of the 3rd Schedule:** Qualification granted by medical institutions not included in 1st schedule.
- **Part II of the 3rd Schedule:** Qualification granted outside India, but not included in 2nd schedule.

NOTA BENE

MCI has asked the Health Ministry to make it mandatory for all doctors to re-register with the SMCs and MCI every 5 years. SMCs of certain States, such as Punjab, Delhi, Odisha, Rajasthan and Maharashtra have provision for re-registration of doctors under their respective statutes.

STATE MEDICAL COUNCIL (SMC)

Composition of the State Medical Council
- Medical teachers from different Universities of the State elected by the teachers of different medical institutions.

- Members elected by registered medical practitioners of the State.
- Some members are nominated by the State Government. They elect a President and a Vice-President from amongst themselves.

Functions of SMC

i. **Maintenance of Medical Register**
   - As per the NMC Act, the SMC should maintain and regularly update the State Register in a electronic format.
   - On payment of prescribed fees, the name, address and qualifications are entered in the register.
   - A provisional registration is granted to a student who has passed the qualifying examination, but has to undergo a certain period of training (internship for 1 year) in an approved institution, and permanent registration is granted after that training period.
   - Additional qualification obtained subsequent to registration or for any alteration may be done after payment of requisite fees to the SMC.

ii. **Renewal of registration:** Medical practitioners need to participate in CME programmes for at least 30 hours (h) to renew their registrations every 5 years. Several States are planning to bring legislation in order to make the process of re-registration mandatory for doctors.

iii. **Disciplinary control:** The Council is entrusted with disciplinary control over the registered medical practitioner **(Flowchart 2.1)**. SMC can issue warning, suspension or penal erasure of the name of medical practitioner found indulging in unethical practice*. It can act against doctors for professional negligence too. The SMC takes cognizance of any misconduct (professional) in case:
   - The medical practitioner has been convicted by court for any criminal offense.
   - A complaint has been lodged against him by some person or body (within 2 years of the cause of action).
   - Upon receipt of any complaint, the SMC would hold an enquiry and give opportunity to the registered medical practitioner to be heard.
   - If the doctor is found to be guilty of committing professional misconduct, the Council may punish as deemed necessary or may direct the removal of the name of the delinquent practitioner from the register, altogether or for a specified period.
   - Decision on complaint against delinquent physician is taken within a time limit of 6 months.
   - An inquiry against a doctor should be initiated by SMC with which he/she is registered. The role of the NMC/EMRB is only as an appellate authority to the Central Health Ministry to decide on an appeal against the decision of the SMC on disciplinary matters.

iv. **Removal of name of medical practitioner:** SMC is empowered to erase from the register the name of any registered medical practitioner with whom it is unable to establish communication.

v. **Restoration of name of medical practitioner:** It can direct restoration of any name of registered medical practitioner so removed.

Pearls
- Warning is a cautionary notice given by the NMC/SMC after enquiry on finding a doctor guilty of infamous conduct.
- Warning notice is a list of offenses which are considered as infamous conduct.

NOTA BENE
NMC is now considering bringing uniformity across the country in the assessment of liability and award of disciplinary action in case of professional misconduct. The disciplinary action may be graded at 5 levels (depending on the severity of offense):

1. **Level 1:** Reformation in the form of advisory, instruction or warning.
2. **Level 2:** Role of the RMP in causing harm was not proved conclusively but breached relevant regulations. Maximum punishment is suspension of registration up to 1 month.
3. **Level 3:** Role of the RMP in causing harm was proved conclusively and breached relevant regulations. Maximum punishment is suspension of registration up to 3 months.
4. **Level 4:** Role of the RMP in causing harm was proved conclusively and breached relevant regulations. Maximum punishment is suspension of registration from 3 months to 3 years.
5. **Level 5:** Role of the RMP in causing wilful, intentional harm or unlawful prohibited was proved conclusively after a detailed enquiry. This will be taken as a unique case and no precedent needs to be cited. The punishment is to debar a member from practice permanently (permanent suspension of registration).

As per the NMC Act, 2019, a RMP aggrieved by the decision taken by a SMC may appeal to the Ethics and Medical Registration Board (EMRB) against such action, and if further aggrieved by the decision of the EMRB may appeal to the Commission within 60 days.

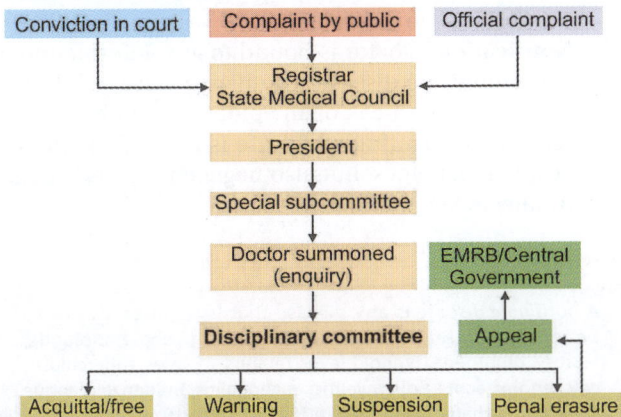

Flowchart 2.1: Disciplinary functions of State Medical Council

---

* Imposition of monetary penalty has been added under the NMC Act.

DUTIES OF A DOCTOR (FLOWCHART 2.2)

Duties of a Doctor in General

i. **Character of physician:** A physician should uphold the dignity and honor of his profession and render service to humanity; reward or financial gain is a subordinate consideration.

ii. **Maintaining good medical practice**
- The physician should try to improve medical knowledge and skills, and should practice methods having scientific basis. He should participate in CME programmes for *at least 30 h every 5 years*.
- *Membership in medical society:* He should affiliate with associations and societies for the advancement of his profession.

iii. **Maintenance of medical records**
- Physician should maintain the medical records (which should be fully digitize) of his indoor patients for a period of *3 years* from the date of last contact with the patient for treatment. In a case where medical records and consent obtained from a patient were not produced, negligence was established.
- On request for medical records, either by the patients or legal authorities, the same should be issued within the period of 72 h (it is planned to extend it to 5 working days). This applies to a doctor in his private capacity, in case of indoor patients whom he might have treated/operated in hospital/nursing home.
- He should maintain a register of medical certificates issued. He should record the signature and/or thumb mark, address and at least one identification mark of the patient and keep a copy of the certificate.

iv. **Display of registration numbers**
- Physician should display the unique registration number accorded to him by the EMRB/SMC in his clinic and in all his prescriptions, certificates, money receipts given to his patients. A doctor was held guilty for printing incorrect information about his qualification on the prescription paper.
- Physicians should display as suffix to their names only recognized medical degrees or such certificates/diplomas and memberships/honors which confer professional knowledge.

v. **Use of generic names of drugs:** Physician should prescribe drugs with generic names (and not brand names), and ensure that there is a rational prescription and use of drugs.

vi. **Highest quality assurance in patient care:** He should not employ in connection with his professional practice any attendant who is not registered, or permit such persons to attend, treat or perform operations upon patients wherever professional discretion or skill is required.

vii. **Exposure of unethical conduct:** Physician should expose, without fear or favor, incompetent or corrupt, dishonest or unethical conduct on the part of members of the profession.

viii. **Payment of professional services**
- Physician should clearly display his fees in his chamber and/or hospitals he is visiting.
- He should announce his fees before rendering service and not after the operation or treatment is underway.

ix. **Evasion of legal restrictions:** Physician should observe the laws of the country in regulating the practice of medicine and should not assist others to evade such laws.

Duties of a Doctor towards the State

i. **Poisoning cases**
- He should assist the police in determining whether the poisoning is accidental, suicidal or homicidal.
- In case of death, certificate should mention about the poisoning with recommendation for postmortem examination.

ii. **Notification:** Doctor is bound to give information of communicable diseases (notifiable diseases), births, deaths and outbreak of an epidemic to public health authorities. Failing which he is not only liable for criminal penalties, but also negligence suits brought by affected persons.

> **NOTA BENE**
>
> A *notifiable disease* is any disease that is required by law to be reported to government authorities, e.g., cholera, plague, leprosy, diphtheria, typhoid fever, tetanus, measles, tuberculosis, chickenpox, acute poliomyelitis, encephalitis, influenza, dengue fever, hemorrhagic fevers, hepatitis, HIV, COVID-19, etc.

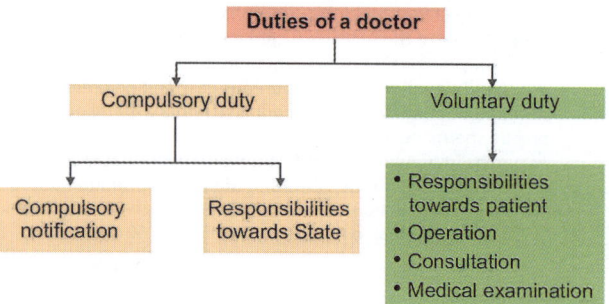

Flowchart 2.2: Duties of a medical practitioner

iii. **Geneva convention**
- In 1949, in Geneva, four conventions were agreed upon. Each convention lays down the persons it protects.
- The wounded or sick of the armed forces (*1st convention*), ship-wrecked (*2nd convention*), prisoners of war (*3rd convention*) or civilians of enemy nationality (*4th convention*) are to be treated by the physician without any adverse distinction based on gender, race and nationality.

iv. **Responding to emergency military service as and when required.**

Duties of a Doctor towards Patients

i. **Exercise reasonable degree of skill and knowledge**
- It begins the moment the physician–patient relationship is established (i.e., when the physician agrees to treat the patient).
- He owes this duty even when the patient is treated free of charge.
- It neither guarantees cure nor an assured improvement.
- A practitioner (e.g., MBBS) is not liable because some other doctors of greater skill and knowledge (e.g., MD/MS) would have prescribed a better treatment or operated better in the same circumstances.

ii. **Attendance and examination**
- When a doctor agrees to attend a patient, he is under an obligation to attend to the case, as long it requires attention.
- He can withdraw after giving reasonable notice or when he is asked by the patient to withdraw.
- If the doctor is called by police to attend a case of road side accident, he may give first aid and advice, but no doctor–patient relationship is established.

iii. **Furnish proper and suitable medicines**
- He should give a legible prescription. He should write the prescribed drugs in capital letters—mistakes arising out of illegibly written names of medicines as opposed to other kinds of indecipherable documents—can be very dangerous.
- Doctor is held responsible for any temporary or permanent damage in health, caused to the patient due to wrong prescription.

iv. **Instructions:** Doctor should give full instructions to his patients or their attendants regarding use of medicines (quantities and timings), injections (whether to be given intramuscularly or intravenously) and diet.

v. **Prognosis:** The patient or his relatives should have such knowledge of the patient's condition as will serve the best interests of the patient and the family (*truth telling/veracity*).

vi. **Control and warn**
- Doctor should warn patients of the side-effects involved in the use of prescribed drug, otherwise it might amount to negligence.
- If the doctor fails to inform the known dangerous effects of a drug/device, he becomes liable not only for the harm suffered by the patient but also for injuries his patient may cause to third parties.

vii. **Third parties:** If a patient suffers from an infectious disease, the doctor should warn not only the patient, but also third parties who are close to the patient.

viii. **Children and disabled persons** being incapable of taking care of themselves, the doctor should arrange for their proper care, e.g., supervised application of hot water bottles.

ix. **Consent:** A mentally sound adult (≥18 years) must be told of all the relevant facts in nonmedical terms and in a language he understands, and then obtain consent.

x. **Operations**
- Doctor should explain the nature and extent of operation, and take consent of patient.
- He should take proper care to avoid mistakes, such as operating on the wrong patient or on wrong limb, or leave any instrument or swab inside a body cavity.
- He should not delegate his duty to operate a patient to another doctor.
- He should not experiment without valid reason or valid consent from the patient.
- He should avail the assistance of qualified and experienced anesthetists.
- Death on operation table should be followed by postmortem examination.

xi. **Investigations**
- All cases of accident, unless they are minor, should be X-rayed.
- For proper diagnosis and to know the progress, the doctor should advise investigations, like biopsy, X-rays, CT scan, etc.
- Wrong interpretation of X-ray is liable to be held as negligent.

xii. **Emergency cases**
- He has moral, ethical and humanitarian duty to help the patient in saving his life.
- In medico-legal injury cases, a doctor is obliged to give medical aid and to save life of the patient.

xiii. **Professional secrecy/Confidentiality:** The doctor should keep secret all information regarding the patient that he comes to know in course of professional work.

Duties of a Doctor in Consultation

i. **Consultation for patient's benefit** is of foremost importance. Unnecessary consultations should be avoided.

ii. **Statement to patient after consultation** should take place in the presence of the consulting physician, except if otherwise agreed. Differences of opinion should not be divulged unnecessarily.
iii. **Treatment after consultation:** The attending physician should make subsequent variations in the treatment, if any unexpected change occurs. The attending physician may prescribe medicine at any time for the patient, whereas the consultant may prescribe only in case of emergency or as an expert when called for.
iv. **Patients referred to specialists:** When a patient is referred to a specialist by the attending physician, a case summary of the patient should be given to the specialist, who should communicate his opinion in writing to the attending physician.

> *Consultation is advised with a specialist in the following conditions:*
> i. In case of emergency.
> ii. If the patient requests consultation.
> iii. If quality of care or management can be considerably enhanced.
> iv. In cases where diagnosis remains obscure.
> v. In case of homicidal poisoning.
> vi. In connection with organ transplantation.
> vii. When treatment or operation involves risk of life.
> viii. When operation affecting vitality, intellectual or generative functions is to be performed.
> ix. When an operation involves mutilation or destruction of an unborn child.
> x. When an operation is to be performed on a patient who has received injuries in a criminal assault.
> xi. To take decision about termination of pregnancy beyond 20 weeks of pregnancy.
> xii. While dealing with a criminal abortion or an attempted criminal abortion case.

- A referring physician is relieved of further responsibility when he completely transfers the patient to another physician.
- The referring physician may be held liable under the *doctrine of negligent choice,* if it can be proved that the consultant was incompetent or had a reputation as an errant physician.

Consultation through Telemedicine

- Recently, in the wake of COVID-19 outbreak, guidelines for consultation through telemedicine were issued to enhance health services and access to patients **(Box 2.1)**.
- The guidelines place the onus on the doctor to decide whether a teleconsultation will suffice, or if an in-person consultation is needed.
- If a physical examination is critical for consultation, the doctor should not proceed until a physical examination can be arranged.

> **Box 2.1** Basic guidelines for telemedicine
> a. Only registered medical practitioners (RMPs) are entitled to provide telemedicine consultation from any part of India.
> b. *Modes:* Three primary modes—video, audio or text (chat, messaging, email, fax, etc.) for consultations.
> c. *Identification:* Consultations should not be anonymous, both patient and doctor should know each other's identity.
>   - The doctor should ensure that there is a mechanism for the patient to verify his credentials and contact details. He should display the registration number on prescriptions, website, electronic communication (WhatsApp/email, etc.) and receipts, etc. given to his patients.
>   - Doctor should verify the patient's identity by name, age, address, email ID, phone number, etc.
> d. *Age verification:* Doctors need to be sure about the patient's age before prescribing any medication. He can ask for the patient's age proof if in doubt. Teleconsultation for minors will be allowed only with an identified adult family member.
> e. Consent is necessary for any telemedicine consultation. If patients initiate the consultation, then their consent is implied. If the doctor initiates the consultation, the patient's explicit consent is needed via email, text, audio/video message.
> f. *Prescribing medicines:* Doctors should provide the patient a copy of the prescription. There are certain restrictions on the type of medications that can be prescribed based on the type of consultations.
>   - Doctors can prescribe over-the-counter drugs (e.g., paracetamol, ORS, zinc, iron, etc.) ('List O') through any mode of consultation.
>   - 'List A' drugs (e.g., hypertension, skin ailments, eye/ear drops etc.) can be prescribed over video-consultations only and in a follow-up consultation for a refill, while 'List B' medicines can be prescribed after follow-up consultation ('add-on'), after an initial in-person consultation.
>   - Drugs that cannot be prescribed includes drugs in Schedule X of Drugs and Cosmetics Act and Rules and any drugs listed in the NDPS Act, 1985 (anticancer drugs, morphine, etc.).
> g. *Consultation fees:* The same fees will be charged for a telemedicine consultation as for an in-person consultation.
> h. *Right to stop consultation:* Both the patient and the doctor have the right to discontinue the teleconsultation at any stage.

- Telemedicine cannot replace physical examination that may require palpation, percussion or auscultation; that requires physical touch and feel.
- It is not applicable to conduct surgical or invasive procedure remotely nor can provide for consultations outside the jurisdiction of India.
- Apart from direct doctor–patient consultation, telemedicine consultations can be held between a caregiver and doctor; doctor to doctor; and health worker to doctor.

Ethics, data privacy, and confidentiality

- Privacy and confidentiality to be maintained as per NMC guidelines for professional conduct, ethics, etc., while using telemedicine.
- It will be considered as 'misconduct' if doctors misuse patient images and data, especially private and sensitive in nature, prescribe medicines from the specific restricted list, insist on a teleconsultation when the patient is willing to travel to a facility, and solicit patients via any advertisements.

- The doctor will not be held responsible for any privacy or confidentiality breach, if it was a technology breach or if somebody else was responsible for it.

Records: It is the doctor's responsibility to maintain the records of the telemedicine interaction and other documents 'for the period as prescribed from time to time'. This includes patient records, diagnostics, data used in the consultation, and prescriptions.

Responsibility of Doctors towards Each Other

i. **Conduct in consultation:** No insincerity, rivalry or envy should be indulged in. All due respect should be observed towards the physician in-charge of the case, and no statement or remark be made, which would impair the confidence the patient has reposed in him.

ii. **Consultant not to take charge of the case:** Consultant should normally not take charge of the case, especially on the solicitation of the patient or friends.

iii. **Appointment of substitute:** A physician should accept to attend another physician's patients during his temporary absence from his practice, only when he has the capacity to discharge the additional responsibility along with his other duties.

> **FM 4.20, 4.24**
> - Describe professional secrecy.
> - Discuss doctor–patient relationship: professional secrecy and privileged communication.

■ PROFESSIONAL SECRECY

Definition: The doctor is obliged to maintain the secrets that he comes to know concerning the patient in the course of a professional relationship, *except* when he is required by the law to divulge the secrets or when the patient has consented for its disclosure.

It is a fundamental tenet that whatever a doctor sees or hears in the life of his patient must be treated as totally confidential. Disclosure would be failure of trust and confidence.

Following principles should be followed:

i. Physician should not answer any query by third parties, even when enquired by close relatives, either with regard to the nature of illness or any subsequent effect of such illness on the patient, without his consent.

ii. If the patient is *major* (≥18 years), physician should not disclose any facts about the illness without his consent to parents or relatives even though they may be paying the doctor's fees. In case of minor or insane person, guardians or parents should be informed of the nature of illness.

iii. A doctor should not disclose the illness of his patient without his consent, even when requested by a public or statutory body, *except* in case of notifiable diseases.

iv. In case of a patient who happens to be a celebrity, press conference regarding patient's condition should not be held without his consent. There may be improper access and snooping to the medical information of celebrities by hospital workers, so a doctor needs to be extra careful in securing the records.

v. Even in case of husband and wife, the facts relating to the nature of illness of one must not be disclosed to the other, without the consent of the concerned person. Particular caution is required over the disclosure of sexual matters, such as pregnancy, abortion or venereal disease, as disclosure might cause conflict between them.

vi. In divorce and nullity cases, no information should be given without the consent of the concerned person.

vii. When a domestic servant is examined at the request of the master, the physician should not disclose any facts about the illness to the master without the consent of servant, even though the master is paying the fees. Similarly, the medical officer of firm or factory should not disclose without the patient's consent.

viii. Medical officers in government service are also bound by code of professional secrecy, even when the patient is treated free.

ix. A person in police custody as an undertrial prisoner has the right not to permit the doctor who has examined him to disclose the nature of his illness to any person. If convicted, he has no such right and physician can disclose the findings to the authorities.

x. Postmortem findings should not be revealed to the relatives, and the report should be given to the police only. However, if an application is filed under the Right to Information Act, 2005, the condition may have to be revealed and entire PM report has to be given to the relatives.

xi. Any information regarding a dead person may be given only after obtaining the consent from a relative.

xii. In examination of a dead body, certain facts may be found, the disclosure of which may affect the reputation of the deceased or cause mental torture to his relatives, and as such, the autopsy surgeon should maintain secrecy.

xiii. The medical examination for *life insurance policy* is a voluntary act by the examinee, and consent to the disclosure of findings may be taken as implied.

Punishment for breaching professional secrecy: The patient can bring forth a:

i. Criminal action in the form of defamation under Sec. 499 IPC (imprisonment for up to 2 years and/or fine under Sec. 500 IPC).

ii. Civil action for damages.

iii. Complain to SMC/NMC, who can initiate disciplinary action.

PRIVILEGED COMMUNICATION

Definition: It is a statement, made bonafide upon any subject matter by a doctor to the concerned authority having corresponding interest, due to his legal, social or moral duty to protect the interests of the community or of the State.

- It is an exchange of information between two individuals in a confidential relationship, and *an exception to professional secrecy*.
- To be privileged, it must be made to the person who has a duty towards it. If made to more than one person or to a person who has not got a direct interest in it, the plea of privilege fails.
- Doctor should first persuade the patient to obtain his consent, before notifying the proper authority. However, disclosure can be done without consent (if consent is not forthcoming).

Types

Privilege can be two types:
i. *Absolute privilege:* Any statement made in the court of law.
ii. *Qualified privilege:* Notification or births, deaths, reporting of color blindness of bus driver, notifiable diseases to municipal authorities.

Examples

i. **Civic benefit**: If there is a potential threat of 'grave harm' to the safety or health of the patient and the public, the doctor must decide whether to inform the authority about the condition.
   - For example, engine or bus driver, pilot or ship navigator may be suffering from epilepsy, hypertension, alcoholism, drug addiction, poor visual acuity or color blindness; or a teacher with tuberculosis or a person with infectious diseases (e.g., enteric infection) working as a cook. In all these cases, the proper course is for the doctor to explain the risks to the patient and to persuade him to allow the doctor to report the problem to his employers. If the patient refuses, then it is always wise to seek the advice of senior colleagues before making any disclosure.
   - A syphilitic taking bath in public pool or a patient with sexually transmitted disease is about to get married is a privileged communication, but an impotent person getting married is not.
ii. **Notifiable clauses:** Doctor has a statutory duty to notify births, deaths, stillbirths, infectious diseases, therapeutic abortions, drug addictions, epidemic and food poisoning to public health authorities.
iii. **Suspected crime:** If the physician learns of a crime, such as assault, terrorist activity, traffic offense or homicidal poisoning by treating the victim or assailant, he is bound to report it to the nearest Magistrate or police officer **(Sec. 39 CrPC)**.
   - But sometimes, the issue of confidentiality clashes with the need to protect some individual or the public from possible further danger (e.g., a below-age of consent girl came to a doctor with STD). The doctor is usually required to obtain a list of the patient's sexual contacts to inform them that they need treatment. However, the patient may be reluctant to divulge the names of her older sexual partners, for fear that they will be charged with *statutory rape*. The same issue may arise where a doctor suspects a child or an elderly person, disabled or incompetent person is being abused, but here the overriding consideration is the safety of these individuals.
   - It has been made mandatory to report to the police any case of sexual abuse in children (≤18 years) as per the Protection of Children from Sexual Offenses Act, 2012.
   - At times, assault may occur within a family, e.g., between spouses or close relatives, the victim may not wish to bring criminal charges, and so the doctor must not assume that consent for disclosure has been given.
   - The doctor knowing or having reason to believe that an offense has been committed by a patient when he is treating, intentionally omits to inform the police, can be punished with imprisonment up to 6 months with/without fine **(Sec. 202 IPC)**.
iv. **Patient's own interest:** Doctor may disclose patient's condition to his relatives so that he may be properly treated, e.g., to warn parents/guardians of patient's melancholia or suicidal tendencies.
v. **Self-interest:** In case of civil and criminal suits by the patient against the doctor, evidence about patient's condition may be given.
vi. **Negligence suits:** When doctor is employed by opposite party to examine a patient who has filed a suit for negligence, the information thus acquired is not a professional secret (no physician–patient relationship), and the doctor may testify to such information.
vii. **Court ordered examination:** If a court orders an examination for the purposes of reporting back to the court about the physical or mental condition of the person, then he should be told that examination findings is not confidential. The report becomes part of the court record.
viii. **Court of law:** Doctor cannot claim professional secrecy concerning the facts about illness of his patient in court of law. He has to answer the questions about patient's confidential matters to avoid risk penalties for contempt of court.

A doctor can disclose and discuss the medical facts of a case with other doctors and paramedical staff, such as nurses, radiologist and physiotherapist to provide better service to the patient.

CHAPTER 2 : Medical Practitioner—Duties and Malpractices

FM 4.2, 4.5
- Describe the Code of Medical Ethics 2002 Conduct, Etiquette and Ethics in medical practice and unethical practices and dichotomy.
- Discuss infamous conduct.

MEDICAL MALPRACTICE

The term '*medical malpractice*' covers all failures in the conduct of doctors, where it impinges upon their professional skills, ability and relationships.

It can be divided into two broad types (Diff. 2.1):
 i. **Professional misconduct**—where the personal or professional behavior falls below that which is expected of a doctor.
 ii. **Medical negligence**—where the standard of medical care given to a patient is considered to be inadequate.

Under the Indian Medical Council Act, 1956, the MCI made the following regulations which are called the **Indian Medical Council (Professional Conduct, Etiquette and Ethics) Regulations, 2002** (amended in 2009 and 2020).

Code of Medical Ethics: At the time of registration, all the doctors are self-warned about certain unethical practices (infamous conduct) and the disciplinary action by the SMC (also called as *warning notice*). The applicant should certify that he/she has read and agreed to abide by the same, and submit a declaration duly signed.

PROFESSIONAL MISCONDUCT (INFAMOUS CONDUCT)

Definition: Any conduct of the doctor which might reasonably be regarded as disgraceful or dishonorable and unethical behavior as judged by professional men of good repute and competence.

It involves abuse of professional position and noncompliance with applicable laws and regulations.

The following acts (unethical) of commission or omission on the part of a physician constitutes professional misconduct:
 i. **Advertising:** *He should not:*
    a. Solicit patients directly or indirectly, through social media, by a physician or a group of physicians or by institutions.
    b. Make use his name for any advertising through any mode (such as using an unusually large signboard), so as to invite attention to his professional position.
    c. Give any recommendation, endorsement or statement with respect of any drug, surgical, therapeutic appliance or software/platforms with his name, signature or photograph (**no association with manufacturing firms**) nor shall he boast of cases, operations or cures or permit the publication of report thereof through any mode.
    d. Print self-photograph or any such material of publicity in the letterhead or on sign board of the consulting room.
    e. Breach social/electronic media guidelines or contribute to the lay press articles and give interviews regarding diseases and treatments which may have the effect of advertising himself. He is allowed to do public education through media without soliciting patients for himself or the institution.
    f. Affix a signboard on a chemist's shop or in places where he does not reside or work.

    A medical practitioner is, however, permitted to make a formal announcement in press regarding the following:
    - Starting or resumption or change of type of practice.
    - Change of address.
    - Temporary absence from duty.
    - Public declaration of charges.
    - Acquiring new equipment or starting a new procedure or operation (as per Punjab Medical Council).
 ii. **Patent and copyrights:** He may patent surgical instruments, appliances, procedures and medicine. However, it is unethical, if the benefits of such patents are not made available in situations where the interest of large population is involved.
 iii. He should not **run an open shop for dispensing of drugs and appliances** prescribed by other physicians, but can sell medication to his own patients..
 iv. **Rebates and commission (dichotomy/fee splitting/ 'cut practice'):** He should not give or receive any gift or commission in consideration of referring, recommending or procuring of patient for medical, surgical or other treatment, or for getting specimen or material for diagnostic purposes.

DIFFERENTIATION 2.1: Professional negligence and professional misconduct

S.No.	Feature	Professional negligence	Professional misconduct
1.	Offense	Absence of care and skill or willful negligence	Violation of code of Medical Ethics
2.	Duty of care	Should be present	Need not be present
3.	Damage to person	Should be present	Need not be present
4.	Trial by	Courts—civil or criminal	State Medical Council
5.	Punishment	Fine, imprisonment or both	Erasure of name or warning
6.	Appeal	Higher court	EMRB and Central Government

v. **Secret remedies:** He should not prescribe or dispense secret remedial agents of which he does not know the composition.
vi. **Torture and human rights:** He should not aid or abet torture or be a party to either infliction of psychological or physical trauma.
vii. **Euthanasia:** He should not practice euthanasia. However, withdrawal of life-supporting measures after brain death can be done as per provisions of Transplantation of Human Organs Act, 1994.
viii. **Pharmaceutical and allied health sector industry:** A medical practitioner should not receive any gift, cash or monetary grants, travel facility or accept any hospitality, like hotel accommodation from any pharmaceutical industry for vacation or for attending conferences, seminars, workshops or CME program as a delegate.
ix. **Prescribing drugs in brand names:** The medical practitioner should not write illegibly and write the generic names, and there should not be an irrational prescription and use of drugs.
x. If he **does not maintain the medical records** of his indoor patients for a period of 3 years and refuses to provide the same within 72 h (planning to extend to 5 working days) when the patient requests for it.
xi. If he **does not display the unique registration number** accorded to him by the EMRB/SMC in his clinic, prescriptions and certificates issued by him.
xii. Physician posted in **rural area is found absent on more than two occasions** during inspection by the Head of the District Health Authority or the Chairman, Zila Parishad.
xiii. Physician posted in a **medical college** as teaching faculty or otherwise is **found absent on more than two occasions**, if it is certified by the Principal/Medical Superintendent.
xiv. Providing **falsified and misleading information** to the NMC via Form A. The form is filled by the doctor during inspection of the medical college.
xv. Prescribing medicines through telemedicine without an appropriate diagnosis/provisional diagnosis.
xvi. Conducting the unscientific 'two-finger test' (also known as 'virginity test') to test the laxity of the vagina in rape survivor/victim.
xvii. Offering conversion therapy to any individual belonging to the LGBTQIA+ community.

Further, he should NOT:
i. **Commit adultery or misbehave** with a patient. He should respect the boundaries of the doctor-patient relationship.
ii. Be **drunk and disorderly** so as to interfere with proper practice of medicine.
iii. Get **convicted by court of law** for offenses involving moral turpitude/criminal acts.
iv. Do **sex determination tests** with the intent to terminate the life of a female fetus.
v. **Issue false, misleading or improper certificates** for subsequent use in the courts or for administrative purposes.

vi. **Violate the provisions of Drugs and Cosmetics Act.** He should not:
 - Sell Schedule 'H' and 'L' drugs and poisons to the public, except to his patient.
 - Prescribe steroids/psychotropic drugs when there is no medical indication.
vii. **Supply or sell addiction forming drugs** to a patient other than medical grounds.
viii. **Give cover,** i.e., assist someone who has no medical qualification to attend, treat or perform an operation, in cases requiring professional discretion or skill.
ix. **Perform an illegal abortion/operation** for which there is no medical, surgical or psychological indication.
x. **Issue certificates of proficiency in modern medicine** to unqualified or nonmedical person.
xi. **Disclose professional secrets.**
xii. **Refuse on religious grounds** such as sterilization, birth control, circumcision and medical termination of pregnancy when it is indicated.
xiii. **Publish photographs/case reports** of his patients **without their consent** in any medical or other journal or social media in a manner by which their identity could be revealed.
xiv. **Use touts or agents or social media** to entice patients.
xv. **Claim to be specialist** when he has no special qualification in that branch.
xvi. **Undertake in vitro fertilization or artificial insemination** without the informed consent of the female patient and her spouse, as well as the donor.
xvii. Do clinical **drug trials** or other **research** involving patients or volunteers without proper consent and not abiding by the guidelines of ICMR and New Drugs and Clinical Trials Rules, 2018.

The instances of offenses and professional misconduct which are given above *do not constitute a complete list of the infamous acts* which calls for disciplinary action. Circumstances may arise from time to time in relation to which there may occur questions of professional misconduct that do not come within any of these categories.

A patient was referred for a CT scan to a nearby diagnostic center. The doctor received commission from the center for sending the patient. Name the term to describe it. Is this ethical?

1

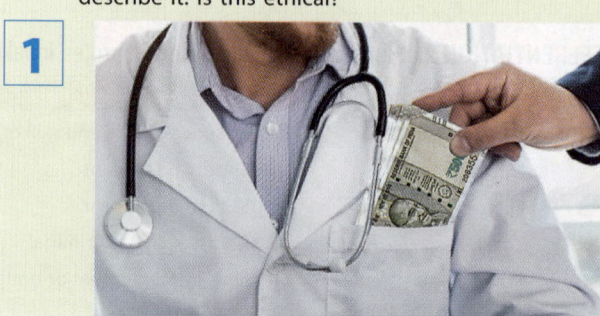

CHAPTER 2 : Medical Practitioner—Duties and Malpractices

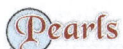earls

Important offenses can be described as 6 A's (Fig. 2.1)
1. Association with unqualified persons
2. Advertising
3. Abortion (criminal)
4. Adultery
5. Addiction
6. Alcohol

NOTA BENE

Conduct of RMPs on Social/Electronic and Print Media
NMC is planning to provide guidelines for RMPs on social media in the forthcoming regulations:
- RMPs can provide educative information and make announcement on social media—should be factual and can be verified.
- He should avoid discussing the treatment or prescribing medicine to patients. He should not post patient's photographs or scans.
- He should not indulge in purchasing 'likes', 'followers' or pay money for search algorithms' for higher ratings or soliciting patients.
- He should refrain from sharing images of cured patients, surgery/procedure videos displaying exceptional results.

FM 4.5
Discuss penal erasure.

ERASURE OF NAME

The name of the doctor is removed from the SMC register:
- After the death of registered medical practitioner.
- When entries of the medical practitioner are erroneous or fraudulent.
- In case of professional misconduct, which is known as *penal erasure*. When the name is permanently removed, it is termed as **professional death sentence**.
- When the registered medical practitioner is not traceable at the address recorded with the Council.

NOTA BENE

Sometimes, professional incompetence, professional misconduct and professional incapacitation are used interchangeably which needs to be distinguished:
- **Professional incompetence:** Failure to exercise due care and diligence in professional responsibilities due to lack of knowledge or skill.
- **Professional incapacity:** Inability to carry out professional activities and responsibilities/obligations due to a physical or mental condition/illness that may limit the capacity to fulfill his professional responsibilities/obligations temporarily or permanently.

FM 4.4, 4.24
- Rights/privileges of a medical practitioner.
- Enumerate rights, privileges of a registered medical practitioner.

Rights and Privileges of Registered Medical Practitioners

i. Right to choose his patient—he may refuse any patient without reason, but he should not refuse emergency treatment required by the patient.
ii. Right to use title and description of the qualification to his name.
iii. Right to practice medicine.
iv. Right to dispense medicine to his patient.
v. Right to possess and supply dangerous drugs to his patients.

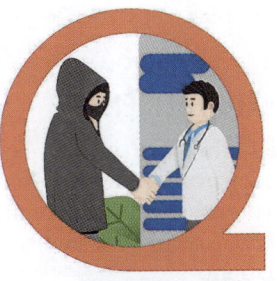
Association with unqualified persons

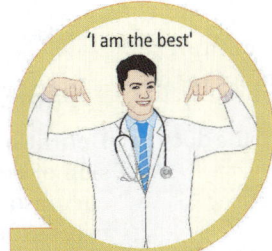
Advertising

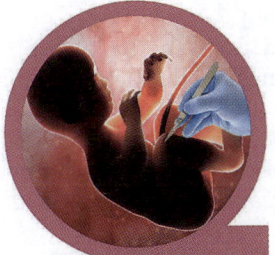
Abortion (criminal)

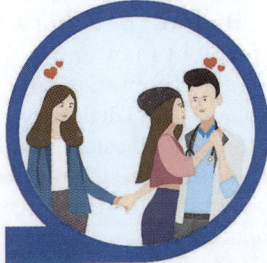
Adultery

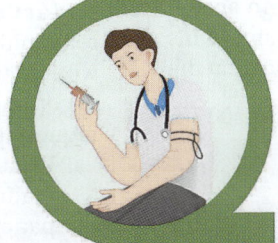
Addiction

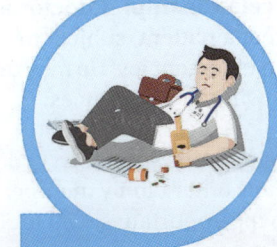
Alcohol

Fig. 2.1: 6 A's of professional misconduct

vi. Right to give evidence at any inquest or in the court of law, as an expert witness.
vii. Right to issue medical/fitness certificates and medico-legal reports.
viii. Right to recovery of fees—if the patient does not pay the justified fees, help of court can be taken.
ix. Right to hold office as a physician or surgeon meant to be held by a physician or surgeon.
x. Right to be exempted from acting as a juror in course of holding an inquest (not applicable in India).

Privileges and Rights of Patients

i. **Access** to healthcare facilities and emergency services regardless of age, sex, religion, social or economic status.
ii. **Choice:** To choose his own doctor freely.
iii. **Continuity:** To receive continuous care for his illness from doctor/institution.
iv. **Comfort:** To be treated in comfort during illness and follow-up.
v. **Complaint:** Right to complain and redressal of grievances.
vi. **Confidentiality:** All information about his illness should be kept confidential.
vii. **Dignity:** To be treated with care, compassion, respect without any discrimination.
viii. **Information:** Should receive full information about his diagnosis, investigations, treatment plans, alternative therapy, procedures, diagnosis, complications and side-effects.
ix. **Privacy:** To be treated in privacy.
x. **Refusal:** Can refuse any specific or all measures.
xi. **Records:** Can have access to his records and demand summary or other details.

Duties of a patient

i. He should furnish the doctor with complete information about the facts and circumstances of his illness.
ii. He should strictly follow the instructions of the doctor as regards diet, medicine and lifestyle.
iii. He should pay a reasonable fee to the doctor.

TYPES OF PHYSICIAN–PATIENT RELATIONSHIP

It is of two types:
1. **Therapeutic relationship:** A doctor is free to accept or refuse to treat a patient, subject to constraint of his work, except in emergencies. He may refuse to treat the patient in following circumstances:
    i. Beyond his practicing hours.
    ii. Not belonging to his speciality.
    iii. Doctor or any other family member is ill.
    iv. Doctor having important social function in family.
    v. Illness beyond the competence and qualification of the doctor or beyond the facilities available in his setup.
    vi. Doctor is having alcohol.
    vii. Patient is malingering.
    viii. Patient has been defaulting in payment.
    ix. Patient or his relatives are abusive/uncooperative/violent (NMC has proposed the same in their recent guidelines. RMP should document and report the behavior).
    x. Patient refuses to give consent.
    xi. Patient demanding specific drugs, such as amphetamine, steroids, etc.
    xii. Patient rejecting low-cost remedies in favor of high cost alternatives.
    xiii. At night, on grounds of security, if patient is not brought to him.
    xiv. An unaccompanied minor or female patient (in case of male doctor).
    xv. When doctor remains engaged with an emergency or more serious case.
    xvi. Any new patient, if he is not the only doctor available.
2. **Formal relationship:** It pertains to the situation where the third party has referred the person/patient for impartial medical examination, e.g.:
    i. Pre-employment
    ii. Insurance policy
    iii. Yearly medical checkups
    iv. Cases of sexual assault or victims of crimes
    v. Intimate body searches and other medico-legal cases
    vi. In certain psychiatric illnesses referred by court/police

Doctor has to comply with the directive of the party demanding such examination.

> **FM 4.18**
> Describe and discuss medical negligence including civil and criminal negligence.

PROFESSIONAL NEGLIGENCE

Definition: The failure to exercise reasonable care and skill of an ordinary prudent medical practitioner in the circumstances; a breach of duty to act with care appropriate to the situation, which resulted in bodily injury (harm/loss) or death of the patient.

- *Negligence consists of two acts:* Not doing something that a reasonable man, under the circumstances would do **(act of omission)**; or doing something which a reasonable prudent man under the circumstances would not do **(act of commission)**.
- According to Black's Law Dictionary, medical negligence requires that the plaintiff establish the following **(4 Ds)**:
    i. Existence of the physician's *duty* of care* to the plaintiff, based on the existence of the physician–patient relationship.

---
* Duty of care in deciding to undertake the case, what treatment to give and in administration of that treatment.

ii. Applicable standard of care and its violation (*dereliction of duty*), i.e., a breach in the duty caused by the defendant's negligent act or omission.
iii. *Damage* (a compensable injury), i.e., pain and suffering, disability and disfigurement, past and future medical bills, lost wages, wrongful death, etc.
iv. Causal connection between the violation of care and the harm complained of (*direct causation*), i.e., a direct link between the defendant's negligent act or omission and an injury suffered by the plaintiff.

♦ In a lawsuit for malpractice or negligence (civil), the 'patient' is known as the *plaintiff* and the 'physician' becomes the *defendant*.

♦ Malpractice requires the demonstration of negligence or substandard practice that caused harm. To successfully sue a physician for malpractice, the plaintiff must prove damage has been caused by the doctor's conduct **(Flowchart 2.3)**.

Flowchart 2.3: Basic principle of negligence (example)

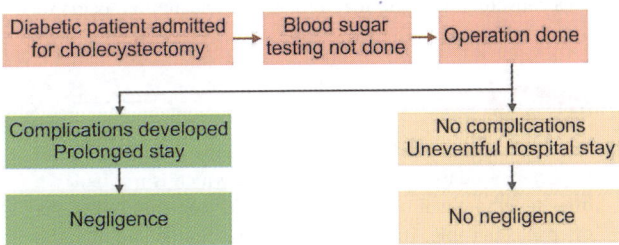

> **NOTA BENE**
>
> ♦ **Tort:** A wrong or harm other than breach of contract; breach of a noncontractual duty towards another person which caused harm or loss. The same action may be both a tort, for which a person may seek compensation, and a crime, punishable by the State.
> ♦ **Degree of care:** The level of caution, prudence or forethought legally required to avoid causing harm or loss to another person. In determining liability, a person may be required to exercise degrees of care variously described as 'ordinary', 'due', 'reasonable', 'great', or 'utmost'.
> ♦ **Gross negligence:** Negligence beyond the ordinary; a reckless or wanton disregard of the duty of care toward others.
> ♦ **Active negligence:** An action that is the result of negligence as opposed to a passive inaction or failure to act which is the cause of negligence.
> ♦ **Liability:** An actual or potential legal obligation, duty or responsibility to another person; the obligation to compensate, in whole or in part, a person harmed by one's acts or omissions.
> ♦ **Chain of causation:** In claims in tort, or prosecutions in criminal law, the causal relationship between the defendant's wrong doing and the victim's loss or injury should be obvious for successful outcome. For example, if A hits B over the head, and B sustains a concussion, A is responsible.
> ♦ **Bolam test:** The test judged by the medical professional's peers is used to assess standard of care when deciding medical negligence. 'If a doctor reaches the standard of a responsible body of medical opinion, he is not negligent'.
> ♦ **Bolitho test:** Another test for assessment of medical negligence. 'Experts should direct their minds to the question of comparative risks and benefits in order to reach a defensible conclusion on the matter in question. A clinical conclusion which does not have *risk analysis* at its heart is not likely to be deemed a responsible conclusion.'
> ♦ **Damages:** Money awarded in a suit or legal settlement as compensation for an injury or loss caused by a wrongful or negligent act or a breach of contract.
> 'Damage' should be distinguished from 'damages'. *Damage* (injury or harm) to the patient may be physical, mental or financial. *Damages* are assessed by the court based on parameters, such as loss of earning, medical and surgical costs, or reduction of quality of life.

Types (Diff. 2.2)

Professional negligence is of two types:
i. Civil
ii. Criminal

Civil Negligence

Question of civil negligence arises:
a. When a patient, or in case of his death, any relative brings suit in a civil court for realization of compensation from his doctor, if he has suffered injury due to negligence.
b. When doctor brings a civil suit for the realization of his fees from patient or his relatives, who refuse to pay the same, alleging professional negligence.

Civil negligence involves:
♦ Such act on the part of the treating physician which causes some suffering, harm, damage or death to the patient
♦ Damage is such, which can be compensated by paying money
♦ Does not come under the purview of CrPC and IPC
♦ Does not demand legal punishment.

Criminal Negligence

♦ Criminal negligence is more serious than civil negligence.
♦ Practically limited to cases in which the patient has died.
♦ Mostly associated with drunkenness or impaired efficiency due to the use of drugs by doctors.
♦ Doctor shows gross incompetency and inattention in the selection and application of remedies, undue interference by him or criminal indifference to the patient's safety.
♦ **Sec. 304-A IPC** deals with criminal negligence; 'whoever causes the death of any person by doing any rash or negligent act not amounting to culpable homicide is punished with imprisonment up to 2 years with/without fine'.

DIFFERENTIATION 2.2: Civil and criminal negligence

S.No.	Feature	Civil negligence	Criminal negligence
1.	Offense	No specific and clear violation of law	Must have specifically violated a particular criminal law in question
2.	Negligence	Simple absence of care and skill	Gross negligence, inattention or lack of competence
3.	Conduct of physician	Compared to a generally accepted simple standard of professional conduct	Not compared to a single test
4.	Consent for act	Good defense, cannot recover damages	Not a defense, can be prosecuted
5.	Trial by	Civil court	Criminal court
6.	Evidence	Strong evidence is sufficient	Guilt should be proved beyond reasonable doubt
7.	Punishment	Liable to pay damages	Imprisonment, fine or both
8.	Contributory negligence	Defense for doctor	Not a defense
9.	Double jeopardy*	Can be tried twice for crime	Cannot be tried twice for the same crime
10.	Damage	Repairable damage or harm to patient	Irreparable damage to the patient
11.	Dispute	Between two parties in their individual capacities	Between the State and the offending doctor
12.	Complainant	Sufferer party is the complainant	Public prosecutor on behalf of the State is the complainant

Double jeopardy is a procedural defense (in India, US, Canada, Mexico and Japan—a constitutional right) that forbids a defendant from being tried a second time for the same crime.

- If death is not caused to the patient, then the doctor can be charged under **Sec. 337 IPC** (causing hurt by rash or negligent act to endanger life for which punishment is imprisonment up to 6 months and/or fine ₹ 500/-), or **Sec. 338 IPC** (causing grievous hurt by rash or negligent act to endanger life for which punishment is imprisonment up to 2 years and/or fine ₹ 1,000/-).
- The concept of negligence differs in civil and criminal law. What may be negligence in civil law may not necessarily be negligence in criminal law. For an act to amount to criminal negligence, the degree of negligence should be much higher, i.e., gross or of a very high degree. Negligence which is neither gross nor of a higher degree may provide a ground for action in civil law but cannot form the basis for prosecution.
- The Supreme Court has held that to prosecute a doctor for criminal negligence, it must be shown that the accused did something or failed to do something which in the given facts and circumstances no doctor in his ordinary senses and prudence would have done or failed to do. The expression 'rash or negligent act' as occurring in Sec. 304-A IPC has to be read as 'grossly'.

Examples of Medical Negligence

It is impossible to give a complete list of negligent situations in medical practice. However, some situations that frequently give rise to allegations of negligence are given in **Table 2.1**.

A physician may be liable to both civil and criminal negligence by a single act, e.g., if he performs an unauthorized operation on a patient, he may be sued in civil court for damages and prosecuted in criminal court for assault.

NOTA BENE

The police sometime register the cases of professional negligence deaths under Sec. 304 IPC which is nonbailable offense, whereas if it is registered under Sec. 304-A IPC, the offense is bailable. The basic difference is that in Sec. 304, the act is intentional, while in 304-A, the act is never done with the intention to cause death.

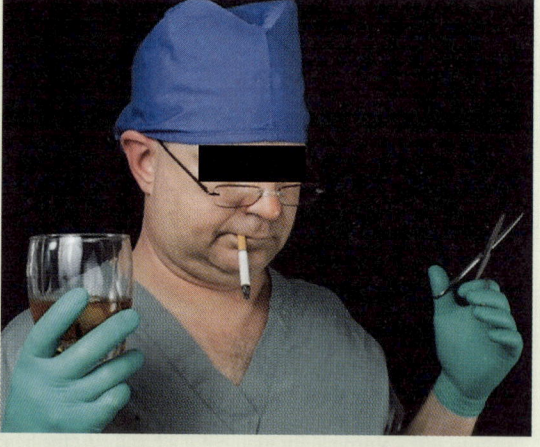

A patient was operated upon by this doctor resulting in death. The doctor will be charged under:

A. Sec. 299 IPC C. Sec. 304-A IPC
B. Sec. 300 IPC D. Sec. 304-B IPC

Burden of Proof

The accused (doctor) is innocent until proven guilty, and the prosecution must prove the case against him. The plaintiff

TABLE 2.1: Examples of medical negligence

General Errors
- Inadequate medical records and failure to examine the patient himself/herself or follow protocol
- Failure to attend a patient with consequent damage
- Failure to admit to hospital when necessary
- Failure to obtain informed consent for any procedure
- Making a wrong diagnosis in the absence of skill and knowledge
- Administration of incorrect type/quantity of drugs, especially by injection
- Failure to immunize and perform sensitivity tests
- Failure to act on radiological or laboratory reports

Medicine
- Failure to diagnose myocardial infarcts and other medical conditions
- Failure to refer a patient to hospital or for specialist opinion
- Toxic results of drug administration/administration of contraindicated drug

Surgery
- Delayed diagnosis of acute abdominal lesions
- Retention of instruments, tubes, towels, sponges and swabs in operation sites
- Operating on the wrong patient, wrong side of the body, wrong limb, digit or even organ
- Failed vasectomy, without warning of lack of total certainty of consequent sterility
- Diathermy burns

Obstetrics and Gynecology
- Unwanted pregnancy due to failed tubal ligation
- Complications of hysterectomy—ureteric ligation and vesicovaginal fistulae
- Brain damage in the newborn due to hypoxia from prolonged labor
- Mismanagement of delivery, especially under the influence of alcohol/drug
- Performing abortion without indication (criminal abortion)

Orthopedics and Emergency Medicine
- Missed fractures, especially of the scaphoid, skull, femoral neck and cervical spine
- Over-tight or prolonged use of plaster casts resulting in tissue and nerve damage
- Undiagnosed intracranial hemorrhage
- Missed foreign bodies in eyes and wounds, especially glass
- Inadequately treated hand injuries, particularly tendons

Anesthesiology
- Hypoxia resulting in brain damage
- Neurological damage from spinal or epidural injections
- Peripheral nerve damage from splinting during infusion
- Incompatible blood transfusion
- Incorrect or excessive use of anesthetic agents

(patient) bears the burden of proof and must convince the judge by a preponderance of the evidence that its case is more plausible.

- In civil cases, a preponderance of the evidence is at least 51%. It means that Judges in a medical negligence case must be persuaded that the evidence presented by the plaintiff is more plausible as the proximate cause of the injury than any counterargument offered by the defendant.
- In criminal cases, the prosecution must prove their case 'beyond reasonable doubt' akin to a 98% or 99% certainty.

> **FM 4.18**
> Describe and discuss prevention of medical negligence and defenses in medical negligence litigations.

SAFEGUARDS AGAINST LITIGATION

Some ways/methods to minimize litigation are sited below:

- **Awareness of potential areas of litigation and medico-legal problems:** Doctor should be aware of the risks involved in certain procedures and should have clear knowledge of the changes in legislation which might influence his practice.
- **Good 'doctor–patient' relationship:** Sympathy, good rapport and taking keen interest in the patient's apprehensions and complaints are hallmarks in gaining the patient's confidence. A suspicious patient who has no faith in the physician is a potential litigant.
- **Appropriate training and maintenance of authorized protocol:** Up-to-date and adequate training of medical and nursing staff is needed. It is dangerous to venture beyond one's capability and qualifications. Maintaining a time-tested, well accepted protocol is necessary. It is wise to seek a second opinion.
- **Maintaining standard medical service:** Limited work load and adequate infrastructure are needed to maintain good quality service. Minimum standard for nursing homes or hospitals, whether public or private, must be maintained.
- **Proper counseling and informed consent:** Counseling and informed consent is mandatory before each medical/investigative/operative procedure.
- **Proper investigation:** Any noninvasive/invasive procedures should be done, provided the risks and benefits are duly informed, and written consent has been taken.
- **Adequate supervision and timely referral:** Adequate supervision by a well organized graded system is recommended. Early detection of complications by resident doctors and timely notification of the consultant, especially in emergency cases, may prevent mishaps.
- **Surgical intervention:** Surgical procedures should always be performed in places where there is sufficient

equipment and qualified staff. Junior doctors should be trained well, and supervised in surgical care of the patient.
- **Meticulous record keeping:** Often proper record keeping can prove the doctor innocent in the court. However, fabrication of records after any mishap is dangerous.
- **Morbidity and mortality audits:** Discussions, analysis and constructive criticism of errors and omissions help in improving and maintaining standard of patient care.
- **Medical indemnity insurance:** The doctor must cover himself with indemnity insurance.
- **Medical defense procedure:** Efficient defense lawyer is important to defend one against a malpractice and negligence suit. The lawyer must be aware of the expected standard of patient care.

DEFENSES AGAINST NEGLIGENCE

In case of alleged negligence, following may be helpful for defense:
- No duty owed to patient, i.e., no doctor–patient relationship was established.
- Duty discharged according to prevailing standards.
- **Informed consent for the act:** The patient was duly informed of the consequences (patient had actual, subjective knowledge of the risk involved in the treatment/procedure).
- Patient was guilty of contributory negligence—patient most likely would have avoided injuries had he/she not also been negligent.
- Therapeutic misadventure.
- Medical maloccurrence.
- **Error of judgment:** The court has held that the error of judgment is not negligence. If, e.g., one of the risks inherent in an operation takes place or some complication ensues which lessens the benefit that was hoped for, he makes an error of judgment. Moreover, doctor is not responsible if patient does not respond to the treatment.
- **Mistake of fact** is a situation where a person not intending to do unlawful act, does so because of wrong conclusion or understanding of fact. The guilty mind was never there while doing the act. It can be a factor in reducing civil liability but not criminal liability.
- **Res judicata** means 'the things have been decided'. According to this principle, once the case is completed between two parties, it cannot be tried again between the same parties. Suppose a patient sues a hospital for any malpractice and the things are decided in the District Commission and looses the case, he can appeal to higher court, i.e., State Commission, National Commission and Supreme Court. But after getting decision from the higher court, he cannot lodge a fresh complaint for the same negligence in the lower court.
- **Limitation:** The case against the doctor should be filed within 2 years from the date of alleged negligence.

No fee was charged for the treatment cannot be a defense in cases of negligence.

> **FM 4.18**
> Discuss Res Ipsa Loquitur.

DOCTRINE OF RES IPSA LOQUITUR

- Generally, professional negligence of a doctor must be proved in the court by expert evidence of another physician.
- The patient need not prove negligence in case where the rule of *res ipsa loquitur* applies, which means '*the thing or fact speaks for itself.*'
- Applies to civil negligence only.
- Error is so self-evident that the patient's lawyer need not prove the doctor's guilt with medical evidence. The doctor has to prove his innocence.
- Rule is applied when the following three conditions are satisfied:
  i. In the absence of negligence, the injury would not have occurred, i.e., its occurrence ordinarily bespeaks negligence.
  ii. Doctor had exclusive control over the injury producing instrument/treatment.
  iii. Patient was not guilty of contributory negligence, i.e., injury was not the result of his own voluntary act or neglect.

Examples

  i. Blood transfusion misadventure (e.g., infected blood, blood group mismatch).
  ii. Failure to give tetanus toxoid vaccine in cases of injury.
  iii. Prescribing an overdose of medicine producing ill effects.
  iv. Wrong-site surgery (surgery on the wrong person, wrong organ or limb, or wrong vertebral level), or wrong-procedure.
  v. Leaving a pair of scissors/instruments in abdomen.
  vi. Failure to remove swabs during operation, causing complications/death.
  vii. Loss of use of hand due to prolonged splinting.

In such situations, the breach of duty is obvious, so the strategy of the defense generally must be to show that the patient was not harmed by the breach.

> **NOTA BENE**
>
> **Gossypiboma** or **textiloma** denotes complications resulting from foreign materials accidentally left inside a patient's body. The list of implements includes sponges (most common), swabs, towels, needles, instruments, catheters, metal clips, contraceptive coils, and retractors.

CALCULATED RISK DOCTRINE

- The doctrine is that, *res ipsa loquitur* should not be applied when the injury complained is of type that may occur even though reasonable care has been taken.
- It is an important defense to any doctor.
- Doctor has to produce evidence/statistics that the accepted method of treatment he employed had unavoidable risks.
- For example, when a patient undergoing coronary bypass dies during the surgery, it becomes a case of professional accident as there is already an inherent risk of 2–5% associated with it.

DOCTRINE OF COMMON KNOWLEDGE

- It is based on the assumption that the issue of negligence in the particular case is not related to specialized knowledge or technical matters of the medical profession, but an act involving application of common knowledge.
- Experts may not provide evidence regarding matters of 'common knowledge'.
- It is a variant of *res ipsa loquitur*.
- Here, the patient must prove the act of commission or omission, but he need not produce evidence to establish the standard of care.

FM 4.18 Discuss contributory negligence.

CONTRIBUTORY NEGLIGENCE

Definition: Any unreasonable conduct, or absence of ordinary care on part of the patient or his attendant, which combined with doctor's negligence contributed to the injury complained of, as a direct cause and without which the injury would not have occurred.

- Good defense (called as '*affirmative defense*') for the doctor in civil cases, but not in criminal cases.
- Doctor has to prove patient's negligence. But, doctor is expected to foresee that the patient may harm himself and to warn accordingly.
- For example, patient did not give proper history, failure to follow doctor's instructions regarding drugs, tests and diet.
- Damages awarded by the court may be reduced.

The doctrine of contributory negligence is subject to following exceptions:

1. **Last clear chance doctrine:** A negligent patient can still recover damages if he is able to show that the doctor had the last opportunity to avoid the accident. For example, if the patient complains of visual disturbance which is due to side effects of the drug prescribed in the follow-up visit and the doctor do not take remedial action that result in subsequent blindness, then plea of contributory negligence fails.
2. **Avoidable consequences doctrine.**

Doctrine of Avoidable Consequence

- Once plaintiff (patient) has been injured, he must take reasonable steps to lessen the consequences of his original injury. A defendant (accused) will not be liable of any further injury that the plaintiff could have reasonably avoided.
- The doctrine is different from contributory negligence, which is unreasonable conduct by plaintiff. It occurs before or simultaneously with the wrong committed by the defendant.
- The doctrine refers to unreasonable conduct by the plaintiff after the defendant has wronged the plaintiff. The amount of recovery is reduced.
- Thus, if the plaintiff, after injury, unreasonably refuses to accept medical attention for a foot injury and as a result ultimately suffers amputation of the foot that otherwise would have healed, then the avoidable consequences rule would deny recovery for loss of foot but would not affect other damages.

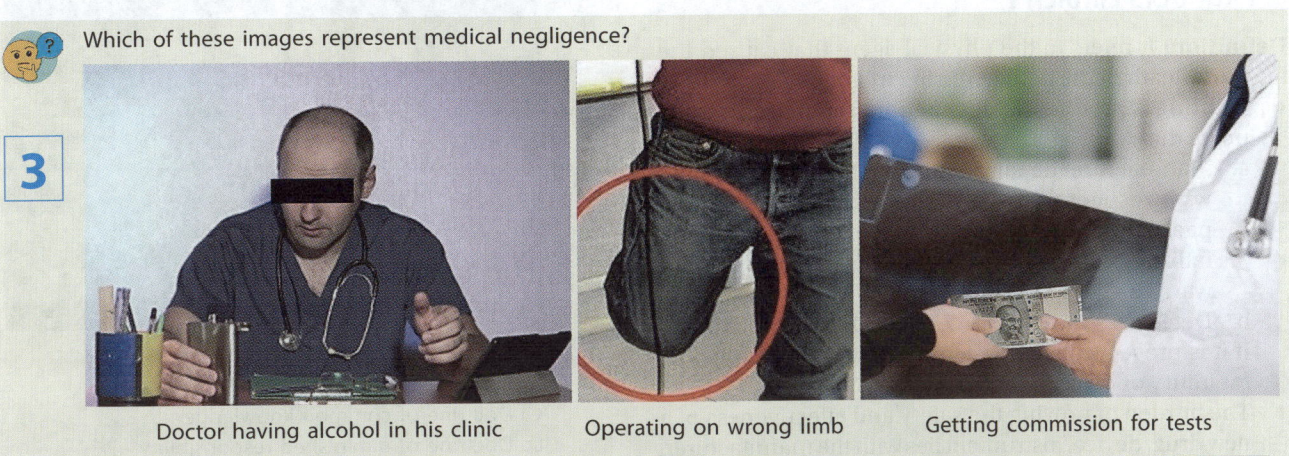

3. Which of these images represent medical negligence?

Doctor having alcohol in his clinic | Operating on wrong limb | Getting commission for tests

SECTION 1 : Jurisprudence and Forensic Medicine

> **NOTA BENE**
> - **Composite negligence:** Injury is caused to the person without any negligence on his part, but as a result of the combined effect of the negligence of some other persons (two or more). In such a case, each wrong doer is jointly and severally liable to the injured for payment of the entire damages, and the injured person has the choice of proceeding against all or any of them.
> - **Concurrent negligence:** The presence of negligence by both the plaintiff and defendant with regard to a case.
> - **Collateral negligence:** Negligence by an employee as a result of a careless or negligent act or omission.
> - **Comparative negligence:** Tort law distribution of liability which reduces the amount of compensation given to a plaintiff in proportion to the damages that may have been caused by the plaintiff's own negligent actions.

Discuss corporate negligence.

CORPORATE NEGLIGENCE

Definition: It is the failure of those in hospital administration/management who are responsible for providing the treatment, accommodation and facilities necessary to carry out the purpose of the institution, to follow the established standard of conduct.

It occurs when the hospital:
- Provides defective equipment or drugs.
- Selects or retains incompetent employees including doctors.
- Fails in some other manner to meet the accepted standard of care, and such failure results in injury to a patient to whom the hospital owes a duty.

Describe products liability.

PRODUCTS LIABILITY

Definition: It refers to the physical agent that caused the injury or death of the patient during treatment.
- To bring a product liability action, the plaintiff must prove that:
  a. Manufacturer departed from standards of due care, with respect to design, manufacture, assembly, packaging, not conforming to the express warranty, failure to test and inspect for defects or failure to warn or give adequate instructions.
  b. Defect was the proximate cause of injury/death.
  If it is proved, the manufacturer becomes responsible for injury or death.
- The burden of proving the safety and effectiveness of a new drug/device/instrument lies with the manufacturer.

- A product liability action cannot be brought, if at the time of harm:
  a. The product was misused, altered, or modified.
  b. The personnel while using such product was under the influence of alcohol or any non-prescription drug.

MEDICAL MALOCCURRENCE

- Medical maloccurrence is a legal term which defines a less than ideal outcome that is unrelated to the quality of medical care delivered by the healthcare team. This includes:
  - Medical and surgical complications that can be anticipated, and represent unavoidable risks of appropriate medical care.
  - Complications that arise unpredictably and are unavoidable.
  - Complications that arise as a result of decisions made by patient and doctor with fully informed consent but appear, in retrospect, to have been a less appropriate choice.
- Maloccurrence is often unrelated to the reasonable risks of quality of care that was provided.
- In some cases, in spite of good medical attention and care, an individual fails to respond properly.

Examples
i. Idiosyncratic response to drugs in some patients.
ii. Damage to recurrent laryngeal nerve during thyroidectomy leading to vocal cord paralysis.
iii. Rupture of the posterior capsule is a well-known complication of cataract surgery. The surgeon is not necessarily negligent if this occurs during the procedure.

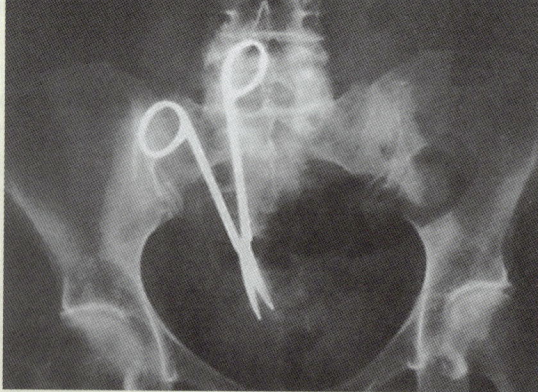

Which of the following options best describe the image?

A. Doctrine of avoidable consequence
B. Doctrine of res ipsa loquitur
C. Doctrine of common knowledge
D. Doctrine of diminished responsibility

Describe therapeutic misadventure.

THERAPEUTIC MISADVENTURE/HAZARD

Definition: It is a case in which a patient has been injured (results in measurable disability, prolonged hospitalization or both) or had died due to some unintentional/inadvertent/unintended act by doctor or his agent or hospital (somewhat similar to medical maloccurrence).
- The injury or an 'adverse event' is caused by medical management rather than by an underlying disease.
- It includes medication errors, medical and surgical errors, surgical complications, iatrogenic or nosocomial infections, or postoperative complications.
- Such mishap does not provide ground for negligence, for example:
    a. Hypersensitivity reactions caused by penicillin, tetracycline or aspirin.
    b. Radiological procedures for diagnostic purposes, e.g., poisoning by barium enema, traumatic rupture of rectum or chemical peritonitis during barium enema.
    c. Thyroid cancer with I^{131} therapy.
    d. Fatal complications from hemolytic reactions with blood transfusion.
    e. Prolonged use of diethylstilbestrol, a synthetic form of estrogen, may cause breast cancer.

NOTA BENE
- **Medical error:** Failure of a planned action to be completed as intended or use of a wrong, inappropriate or incorrect plan to achieve an aim.
- **Misadventure** is mischance, accident or disaster. It is of three types:
    i. **Therapeutic:** When treatment is being given.
    ii. **Diagnostic:** When diagnosis is the only objective at that time, e.g., injection of radiopaque dye in radiological investigation, bronchoscopy and angiography.
    iii. **Experimental:** Where patient has agreed to serve as a subject in an experimental study (drug/operative procedure).

Describe and discuss vicarious liability.

VICARIOUS LIABILITY/RESPONDEAT SUPERIOR

Definition: An employer is responsible not only for his own negligent act, but also for the negligent act of his employees by the principle of *'respondeat superior'* (Latin, 'let the master answer'), if three conditions are satisfied:
   i. There must be an employer-employee relationship.
   ii. The employee's conduct must occur within the scope of his employment.
   iii. Incident must occur while on the job.

- It also called the *'Master-Servant Rule'* or *'Captain of the Ship Doctrine'*.
- In medical practice, usually, the principal doctor becomes responsible for any negligence of his assistants (both medical and paramedical). Both may be sued by the patient, even though the principal has no part in the negligent act.
- A doctor may be associated temporarily with another doctor with the establishment of an employee–employer relationship between them. Thus, if one surgeon assists another in the operating room for a fee, the assistant is considered as an employee of the principal surgeon.
- When two doctors practice as partners, each is liable for negligence of the other, even though one may have no part in the negligent act.
- If a swab, sponge or instrument is left in the patient's body after the operation, the surgeon is liable for damage. A surgeon is not liable for the negligence of anesthetist, and the anesthetist is not liable for the negligence of the operating surgeon.
- **'Borrowed servant doctrine':** An employee may serve more than one employer, e.g., the nurse employed by a hospital to assist in operations will be the 'borrowed servant' of the operating surgeon during the operation, and the servant of the hospital for all other purposes.
- Physicians and surgeons are not responsible for the negligent acts of competent nurse or other hospital personnel, unless such acts are carried out under their direct supervision and control.
- A hospital, as an employer, is responsible for negligence of its employees who are acting under its supervision and control.
- Hospital management cannot be held responsible for the negligent acts of members of the senior medical staff in the treatment of patients, if it can be proved that the management exercised due care and skill, in selecting properly qualified and experienced staff.
- Hospital management is held responsible for the mistakes of resident physicians and interns in training, who are considered employees when performing their normal duties. A physician is responsible for the acts of the interns and residents carried out under his direct supervision and control.
- Both the employer and employee are sued by the patient, because the employee may lack funds for paying the damages. Usually, liability will be fixed upon those actually at fault and those whose control over the negligence is demonstrable.
- To avoid vicarious liability, an employer must demonstrate either that the employee was not negligent or the employee was reasonably careful or that the employee had gone on a *'detour'*, wherein the employee was acting in his own right, rather than on the employer's business.

NOTA BENE

In a case, Mr. Y was referred by the surgeon for preoperative assessment to a cardiologist who declared him fit for surgery. He developed cardiorespiratory arrest during surgery and died. The court observed that the cardiologist, in preoperative check, found BP 150/100 mm Hg and ST changes in anterolateral lead in ECG. The anesthetist was also duty bound to assess the patient's condition for anesthesia. The court found the surgeon vicariously liable in selecting the cardiologist and anesthetist of his choice. The sharing of the liability of the surgeon was 30%, cardiologist 60% and anesthetist 10% of the total compensation granted by the court. The hospital was acquitted.

FM 4.19, 4.20

- Define consent. Describe different types of consent and ingredients of informed consent. Describe the rules of consent and importance of consent in relation to age, emergency situation, mental illness and alcohol intoxication.
- Describe therapeutic privilege.

CONSENT

Definition: Consent (Latin, 'to feel or sense with') means voluntary agreement, compliance or permission.

As per the **Sec. 13 of the Indian Contract Act, 1872**: 'two or more persons are said to consent when they agree upon the same thing in the same sense (meeting of the minds).'

Types (Flowchart 2.4)

Broadly, consent is of two types:
1. **Implied:** When the patient presents himself at the doctor's clinic or outpatient, it is held to imply that he is agreeable to be examined. This does not imply to procedures more complex than *inspection, palpation, percussion* and *auscultation*. For other examinations, such as rectal and vaginal examination, or withdrawal of blood for diagnostic purposes, expressed permission should be obtained.
2. **Expressed:** Specifically stated by the patient in distinct and explicit language. It can be:
   i. *Oral/verbal consent* is obtained for relatively minor examinations or therapeutic procedures, preferably in presence of disinterested party, such as patient's attendant or nurse.

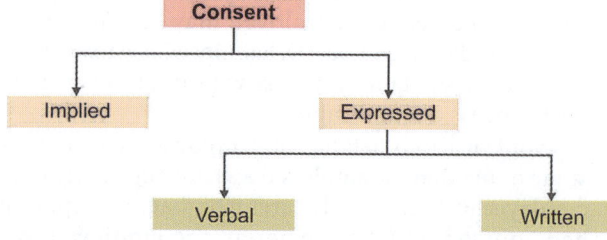

Flowchart 2.4: Types of consent.

ii. *Written consent* is to be obtained for:
   - All minor and major diagnostic procedures
   - General anesthesia
   - Operations

Doctrine of Informed Consent

Definition: Consent of the patient for any procedure or treatment that is taken after fully informing him about the nature of his condition.

This doctrine implies an understanding by the patient of:
i. His/her condition or nature of illness
ii. Purpose or necessity for further testing
iii. Natural course of condition and possible complications
iv. Nature of procedure or treatment proposed
v. Risks and benefits of treatment or procedure
vi. Risks and benefits of alternative treatment or procedure
vii. Prognosis in the absence of intervention
viii. Duration and approximate cost of treatment
ix. Expected outcome and follow-up.

- The information provided to patients should be simple, easy to understand language and list any possible major complications to enable the patient to determine whether to undergo or decline a procedure (*informed refusal*) **(Box 2.2)**.
- There is no need to explain remote or theoretical risks involved which may frighten or confuse the patient and result in refusal to take treatment.
- There are no clear parameters laid down regarding the quantum of information to be given for informed consent. Therefore, it is reasonable information which a doctor deems fit considering best practices.
- The standard to which physicians are held in negligence suits is that of a 'reasonable physician' dealing with a 'reasonable patient.'**

Box 2.2 Disclosure of information during informed consent

Name of the procedure: PCNL*
Benefits: Removal of stone, amelioration of symptoms, such as pain, vomiting and blood in urine, small incision, shorter hospital stay, faster recovery.
Risks and undesirable consequences: Infection and bleeding, retained stone, recurrence of stone, failure to remove the stone, need of ESWL,¥ injury to surrounding organs, gut and blood vessels, risk of anesthesia.
Alternatives:
a. *ESWL*: May need multiple sessions, failure to adequately clear stone, pain and discomfort, blocked ureter, need for ancillary procedures.
b. *Open surgery*: Large incision, severe bleeding, infection, risk of anesthesia, prolonged hospital stay, longer recovery.

* Percutaneous nephrolithotomy (PCNL) is a surgical procedure to remove stones from the kidney by a small puncture wound through the skin.
¥ Extracorporeal shock wave lithotripsy (ESWL) uses sound waves or shock waves to break stones into small fragments that can pass spontaneously in urine.

** **Montgomery test** requires a doctor to take reasonable care to ensure that the patient is aware of 'any material or significant risks' involved in any recommended treatment and give the fullest possible information or all possible options. There is a shift towards a 'prudent patient test' or 'reasonable patient' rather than 'reasonable doctor'.

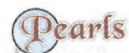

Exceptions to informed consent
- Emergencies
- Medical examination requested by a police officer of an arrested accused under Sec. 53 (1) CrPC
- Therapeutic privilege
- Therapeutic waiver
- Medico-legal postmortems (Sec. 174 CrPC)
- Psychiatric examination or treatment by court order
- Use of placebos
- Prisoners
- Person suffering from disease under 'notified' category (to notify the authorities only)
- Treatment of notifiable diseases for greater community interest.

Emergency cases: If a patient is unconscious and there is an imminent danger to the life of the patient and there is no designated surrogate or the surrogate is unavailable, then the law presumes that consent has been deemed to be given (*implied consent*, **Sec. 92 IPC**). For implied consent to apply, the injured must require emergency treatment to save life or limb, and the treatment rendered must be so limited. Once the emergency treatment is no longer required, the doctrine of implied consent does not govern.

Therapeutic privilege: In patients prone to anxiety, full disclosure (e.g., presence of malignancy or unavoidable total results) may inflict harm/suffering to the patient. The doctor should use therapeutic privilege in the interest of the patient and may withhold information. However, he should disclose full information to the competent relative of the patient.

Therapeutic waiver: A competent person who is aware of being entitled to informed consent may give up his right by waiving it.

Placebo: The doctor may use placebos in certain self-limiting conditions or in patients with high psychological overlay or in those who insist for some particular medication (e.g., addiction forming drugs). Informed consent may be withheld, since there are high chances of benefit to the patient with negligible risk.

Prisoners: Prisoners and persons released on bail can be treated without their consent in the interest of the society.

Consenting Ages for Treatment

Purpose	Required age
Medical examination and treatment	≥12 years*
Medico-legal examination	≥12 years (parent/guardian if <12 years)
Inmates of hostel	≥12 years (Warden if <12 years)
Invasive/diagnostic procedures, general anesthesia and surgical operations	≥18 years

---
* Child <12 years of age, or unsound mind: Parent/guardian

- In accordance to the Indian Contract Act, a person is generally competent to contract (i) if he has attained the age majority (18 years in India), (ii) is of sound mind, and (iii) is not disqualified by any law to which he is subject to.
- Impairments to reasoning and judgment which may make it impossible for someone to give informed consent include basic intellectual or emotional immaturity, high levels of stress, such as PTSD, severe mental retardation or illness, senility, delirious intoxication, severe sleep deprivation, Alzheimer's disease and coma.

Reasons for Obtaining Consent

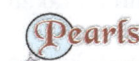

To examine, treat or operate without consent is considered:
a. Assault in law
b. Doctor may be charged for negligence
c. Deficiency in medical services

Rules of Consent

i. Consent should be free, voluntary, clear, intelligent, informed, direct and personal. There should be no undue influence, fraud, misrepresentation of facts, compulsion, coercion or other consequences.
ii. Informed consent for any minor/major surgical or diagnostic procedure should be in written format. It provides evidence that consent was in fact obtained, if necessity arises.
   - It should be in a proper form and suitably drafted for the circumstances. The more specific the consent, the less likely it will be construed against the doctor or hospital in the court.
   - The written consent should be witnessed by another person, present at the signing to prevent any allegation that the consent was forged or obtained under pressure. Hence, it has to be signed by the patient (unless minor, unconscious or insane wherein a legal guardian/next of kin should sign—*substituted consent*), doctor and an independent witness.
   - Video recording of consent, particularly for clinical trials has also been proposed.
iii. Any procedure beyond routine physical examination, such as operation, blood transfusion or collection of blood requires expressed consent.
iv. The doctor should explain the object of examination to the patient, and patient should be informed that the findings would be included in the report.
v. Patient should be informed that he has right to refuse to submit to examination. If he refuses, he cannot be examined.

vi. A person ≥18 years of age can give valid consent to suffer any harm, which may result from an act not intended or not known to cause death or grievous hurt **(Sec. 87 IPC)**. This section is not meant for doctors as the act is not done for benefit of the opposite party.

vii. A person can give valid consent to suffer any harm which may result from an act not intended or not known to cause death, done in good faith and for his benefit **(Sec. 88 IPC)**. This section is meant for doctors as the act is done in good faith for the benefit of the opposite party.

viii. A child <12 years of age and an insane person cannot give valid consent to suffer any harm which may result from an act done in good faith and for his benefit. The consent of the parent or guardian should be taken **(Sec. 89 IPC)**.

Loco parentis (Latin, 'in place of a parent'): In an emergency involving children, when their parents or guardians are not available, consent is taken from the person-in-charge of the child, e.g., a school teacher can give consent for treating a child who becomes sick during a picnic away from home, or the consent of the principal of a residential school.

ix. The consent given by an insane or intoxicated person, who is unable to understand the nature and consequences of that to which he gives his consent is invalid **(Sec. 90 IPC)**.

x. **Sec. 92 IPC** deals with cases of emergency, e.g., head injury requiring urgent decompression. It states that any harm caused to a person in good faith, even without the person's consent, is not an offense, if the circumstances are such that it is impossible for that person to signify consent and has no guardian or other person in lawful charge of him from whom it is possible to obtain consent in time for the thing to be done in benefit. *In an emergency, the law implies consent.*

xi. Even in emergency, unless patient is unconscious, the consent offered by the parents of major (≥ 18 years) is void and amount to negligence.

xii. Nothing is said to done in good faith which is done without due care and attention **(Sec. 52 IPC)**.

xiii. Consent of the inmates of the hostel is necessary, if they are ≥ 12 years of age. Within 12 years, the principal or warden can give consent.

xiv. In civil cases, examination should not be done without the consent of the person.

xv. In criminal cases, the victim cannot be examined without her consent. The court cannot force a person to get medically examined.
- In sexual assault cases, victim should not be examined without her written consent.
- In medico-legal cases of pregnancy, delivery and abortion, the woman should not be examined without her consent.

xvi. Under **Sec. 53 (1) CrPC**, an accused can be examined by a doctor by using reasonable force, if requested by a police officer (not below S.I.), if examination* may provide evidence to the commission of the offense.
- Whenever an accused female is to be examined, the examination *shall be made only by, or under the supervision of a female medical practitioner.* Such an examination by a male doctor must not be carried out even in the presence of a female nurse **[Sec. 53 (2) CrPC]**.

xvii. Under **Sec. 54 CrPC**, an arrested person may be examined by a doctor at his request to detect evidence in his favor, a copy of the report is to be furnished by the doctor to the arrested person.

xviii. Consent of one's spouse is not necessary for the treatment of other. Husband or wife has no right to refuse consent to any operation, which is required to safeguard the health of the partner.

xix. For receiving artificial insemination and donation of ovum or sperm, consent of spouse is legally required, since gametes may be construed as belonging to spouse also. Consent of spouse is legally not required, but preferable/desirable to avoid marital conflict for:
  a. Medical termination of pregnancy
  b. Sterilization [consent of the spouse is not required (as per the Ministry of Health and Family Welfare guidelines)]
  c. Any operation that may affect the sexual life (breast reduction, penectomy, etc.)

xx. Consent given for a diagnostic procedure cannot be considered as consent for therapeutic treatment. Consent given for a specific treatment/procedure is not valid for conducting some other treatment/procedure. The Supreme Court has held that the unauthorized additional surgery however beneficial to the patient, in saving time, expenses, pain and suffering are not grounds of defense in an action for negligence. The only exception to this rule is if the unauthorized procedure was done to save the life or preserve the health of the patient.

xxi. There can be a common consent for:
- Diagnostic and operative procedures where they are contemplated
- Particular surgical procedure and an additional/further procedure that may become necessary during the course of surgery.

xxii. The law provides the consent in any procedure made compulsory by State, e.g., mass immunization.

---

*This includes examination of blood, bloodstains, semen, swabs in cases of sexual offenses, sputum and sweat, hair samples and fingernail clippings using modern and scientific techniques including DNA profiling.

xxiii. In case of consent for donation of organ after death, the will of the deceased is enough.
xxiv. In prenatal diagnostic procedures, informed written consent of pregnant woman is obtained and a copy of the consent is given to the woman.
xxv. Pathological autopsy should not be carried out without the consent of next of kin of the deceased.
xxvi. Medico-legal autopsy does not require any consent from the relatives of the deceased.

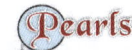

Consent is invalid if:
- It is not an informed consent.
- Given for committing a crime or an illegal act, such as criminal abortion.
- Obtained by misrepresentation or fraud.
- Given by one who had no legal capacity to give it, e.g., a minor or an insane person.

NOTA BENE

- **Paternalism:** The interference with a person's liberty of action, justified by reason referring exclusively to the welfare, good, happiness, needs, interest or values of the person being coerced.
- **Substituted consent:** If a person in need of treatment is incapable of giving informed consent, consent (proxy consent) must be obtained from next of kin. The order of succession is generally spouse, adult child, parent, sibling, lawful guardian and then relatives.
- **Blanket (open) consent:** The consent taken at the time of admission, and practiced in most hospitals that cover almost everything a doctor might do to a patient without mentioning anything specific. It is of questionable legal validity.
- **Presumed consent** assumes that an individual agrees in principle to the said procedure; if not, he must withdraw his consent, i.e., 'opt out'.
- The National Consumer Disputes Redressal Commission has held that the fixed format for consent form for medical procedures as an *'unfair trade practice'* as the pre-printed from fits in for any procedure and is a case of *'administrative arbitrariness'*.

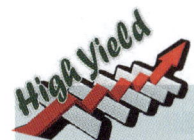

- The National Medical Commission Act, 2019 has repealed the Indian Medical Council Act, 1956.
- NMC will maintain a national register, recognize medical qualifications granted by medical institutions and statutory bodies, hold NEET for admission to UG and PG courses and common EXIT examination for medical graduates to pass before practicing or pursuing PG courses.
- If the patient is major (≥18 years), the facts relating to the nature of illness *must not be disclosed to anyone else without his consent* **(professional secrecy).**
- Privileged communication is an exception to professional secrecy.
- Doctor is bound to report any suspected crime to the Magistrate/police officer **(Sec. 39 CrPC).**
- It is mandatory to report any sexual abuse in children (≤18 years) **[POCSO Act, 2012].**
- If the doctor intentionally omits to inform the police, then imprisonment is up to 6 months with/without fine **(Sec. 202 IPC).**
- **Professional misconduct:** Conduct of doctor that is regarded disgraceful/ dishonorable as judged by professional men of good repute and competence.
- Dichotomy is splitting of fees and is an unethical act.
- Repeated intentional advertisement by a doctor in newspaper is professional misconduct.
- **Warning notice** is a list of offenses which are considered as infamous conduct.
- **Warning** is a cautionary notice given by the MCI/SMC after enquiry on finding a doctor guilty of infamous conduct.
- **6 A's of professional misconduct—A**lcohol, **A**ddiction, **A**dultery, **A**dvertisement, **A**bortion (criminal), **A**ssociation with unqualified persons
- **Penal erasure:** Name of RMP is removed from SMC in case of *professional misconduct*. When the name is permanently removed— *professional death sentence.*
- **Professional negligence:** Inadequate standard of medical care given to a patient leading to injury/death. Negligence consists of two acts—*act of omission or act of commission*.
- **4 D's of medical negligence—D**uty of care, **D**erelict in duty, **D**amage, **D**irect causation.
- **Damages:** Money awarded as compensation for an injury or loss caused by a negligent act.
- Trial of professional misconduct is by State Medical Council; trial of professional negligence is by court.
- In a lawsuit for malpractice/negligence (civil), 'patient' is known as *plaintiff* and 'physician' becomes *defendant*.
- Case should be filed ≤2 years from the date of negligence *(limitation period)*.
- The patient was treated free of charge is not a defense in cases of negligence.
- **Res ipsa loquitur** means the evidence speaks for itself.
- In negligence cases, the burden of proof lies on the plaintiff.
- **Burden of proof lies on the doctor:** Res ipsa loquitur and contributory negligence cases.

- ◆ **Expert evidence is not needed in:** Res ipsa loquitur and doctrine of common knowledge.
- ◆ **Burden of proof lies on manufacturer:** Product liability.
- ◆ **Sec. 304-A IPC** deals with death due to *criminal negligence*; punishment is imprisonment up to 2 years with/without fine'.
- ◆ **Therapeutic misadventure:** Death of a patient due to an unintentional act by the doctor.
- ◆ **Contributory negligence:** Unreasonable conduct or absence of ordinary care on part of the patient/his attendant, which along with doctor's negligence resulted in the injury.
- ◆ **Vicarious liability:** Employer is responsible not only for his own negligent act, but also for the negligent act of his employees by the principle of **'respondeat superior'**.
- ◆ Vicarious liability is also called the *Master-Servant Rule* or *Captain of the Ship Doctrine*.
- ◆ The surgeon is responsible for the negligent action of his team members by respondent superior.
- ◆ **Consent:** Two or more persons are said to consent when they agree upon same thing in same sense.
- ◆ **Consent is invalid** if obtained from a person who is minor, intoxicated, insane or under threat.
- ◆ In sexual assault cases, victim should not be examined without her written consent.
- ◆ Accused can be examined by a doctor by using reasonable force, if requested by a police officer **[Sec. 53 (1) CrPC]**.
- ◆ Accused female has to be examined only by a female doctor. Examination by a male doctor must not be carried out even in the presence of a female nurse **[Sec. 53 (2) CrPC]**.
- ◆ **Loco parentis:** The school principal can give consent for treatment of children, when the legal guardian is unavailable.
- ◆ **Sec. 92 IPC** deals with cases of emergency (law implies consent).
- ◆ Law provides consent in any procedure made compulsory by State, e.g., mass immunization.
- ◆ *Organ donation after death:* Consent of legal guardian/Will of deceased.
- ◆ *Pathological autopsy:* Consent is required from next of kin of deceased.
- ◆ *Medico-legal autopsy:* Consent is not required from relatives.
- ◆ *Treatment/operation of spouse:* Consent of one's spouse is not required.
- ◆ *Artificial insemination, donation of ovum/sperm:* Consent of spouse is required.
- ◆ *Prenatal diagnostic procedures:* Informed written consent of pregnant woman.
- ◆ Consent of spouse is legally *not* required, but preferable to avoid marital conflict for: MTP, sterilization and operation affecting sexual life (breast reduction, penectomy, etc.).

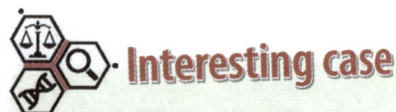

Negligence (Case of Bob East, 1985)

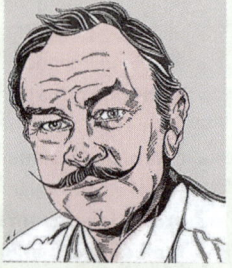

In 1985, Bob East a 64-year-old prize-winning Miami Herald newspaper photographer was admitted at Jackson Memorial Hospital for removal of a malignant tumor that involved his cheekbone and his right eye **(Fig. A)**. He decided to have his eye donated to the medical school for research.

After East was anesthetized, the Chief Surgeon instructed attending anesthetist to remove 50 cc of cerebrospinal fluid (CSF) from the base of his spine. This was to reduce pressure on the brain's surface to facilitate movement at the rear of the cancerous eye. The CSF was to be re-injected 'to check for leaks' in the covering of the brain which is exposed during surgery—a routine procedure. The anesthetist left the task to a resident and left the operating room (OR) to attend another case. The resident drained the fluid and left it in a capped, labeled syringe.

In the meantime, an ophthalmology resident from the eye institute came and left a small, unmarked vial of glutaraldehyde (toxic substance used to sterilize instruments and to preserve tissue removed during surgery) on a tray in the OR to preserve the eye after its removal. As the operation progressed, a nurse spotted the vial and asked what it was. One of the members of the surgical team said 'CSF', she marked it placed the vial next to the syringe containing the CSF.

As the surgeons completed their work, the surgeon ordered the CSF to be re-injected and the anesthetist was summoned. The anesthetist came and injected the syringe containing the CSF into his spinal column. Then he picked up the vial of glutaraldehyde marked 'CSF', drew it into a syringe and injected it too. *No one has explained why both portions were injected when only one had originally been withdrawn.*

The patient's pulse slowed and his blood pressure sank immediately. Emergency measures were taken to keep him breathing. No one could figure out what had gone wrong. But when the ophthalmology resident returned and asked for the vial, the anesthetist realized his mistake. An hour earlier he had injected the lethal glutaraldehyde into the spine of East. After the error was discovered, doctors tried to drain as much of the glutaraldehyde as possible, but it was too late. The injection left East brain dead. Brain scans disclosed no signs of life. Five days later his ventilator was withdrawn and he was declared dead. An autopsy showed the solution had hardened up organs like stone. This negligent act resulted in policy changes requiring no unmarked vials to ever be brought into an OR.

CHAPTER 3: Ethical and Social Aspects of Medical Practice

Learning Objectives

Must know
1. Medical ethics and etiquette
2. Bioethics and medical ethics (Diff.)
3. Euthanasia, types (Diff.)
4. Malingering
5. Ethical guidelines for biomedical research
6. Oath
7. Declaration of Geneva
8. Addressing a press conference
9. Communication skills
10. Conflict management
11. NHRC guidelines regarding human rights violation

Desirable to know
1. Stem cell research
2. Clinical trials
3. Hippocratic oath
4. Various declarations of World Medical Association
5. Social aspects of assault, rape, attempted suicide, homicide, domestic violence, dowry-related cases

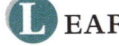

Describe medical ethics and explain its historical emergence.

MEDICAL ETHICS

Definitions

- **Medical ethics:** It is concerned with *moral principles* for the members of the medical profession in their dealings with each other, their patients and the State. It is a self-imposed code of conduct assumed voluntarily by medical professionals.
- **Medical etiquette:** These are the *conventional laws and customs of courtesy* which are followed between members of same profession. A doctor should behave with his colleagues, as he would like to have them behave with him, for e.g., he should not charge another doctor or members of his family for professional service.

Historical Emergence of Medical Ethics

- By the 18th and 19th centuries, medical ethics emerged as a more self-conscious discourse.
- In 1803, the English physician Thomas Percival published *Medical Ethics* and reportedly coined the phrase 'medical ethics'.
- In 1847, the American Medical Association adopted its first code of ethics, adapted from the ethical code of conduct published by Thomas Percival.
- The Nuremberg Code was the first international code laying ethical principles for clinical research. This was the outcome of inhuman experiments by the Nazi doctors in their concentration camps.
- In 1964, the World Medical Association (WMA) developed the Declaration of Helsinki for clinical research. It contains 32 principles, which stress on informed consent, confidentiality of data, vulnerable population and requirement of a protocol, including the scientific reasons of the study, to be reviewed by the ethics committee.
- In 1979, the US laid down its guidelines for ethical principles in the Belmont Report after discovery of the Tuskegee's syphilis study in which treatment was withheld from African American men with syphilis so that scientists could study the course of the disease. The National Commission for the Protection of Human Subjects of Biomedical and Behavioral Research in the US, for the first time enunciated the three basic ethical principles for research involving human subjects: respect for persons, beneficence and justice.
- In 1982, the Council for International Organizations of Medical Sciences (CIOMS) developed 'International

Ethical Guidelines for Biomedical Research Involving Human Subjects'. They especially stressed upon ethical issues in less developed countries, such as investigator's duties regarding consent, appropriate inducements, special/vulnerable populations, therapeutic misconceptions and post-trial access.
- In 1980, Indian Council of Medical Research (ICMR) issued a Policy Statement related to ethical aspects of human research. In line with the advances in medical research, ICMR updated the ethical guidelines in 2000 and then in 2006. Although not a law, these guidelines have been put into force through Schedule Y.
- In 2002, the Medical Council of India (MCI) brought out the code of ethics for all medical professionals 'Indian Medical Council (Professional Conduct, Etiquette and Ethics) Regulation.
- In 2017, the ICMR issued the National Ethical Guidelines for Biomedical and Health Research Involving Human Participants. The purpose of these guidelines is to safeguard the dignity, rights, safety and well-being of the human participants involved in biomedical and health research.
- Some of the influential codes of ethics and regulations that developed through the years are given below:

Code of ethics and regulations	Year
Hammurabi code of medical ethics	1754 BC
Charaka code of medical ethics	100-200 BC
Hippocratic code of ethics	400 BC
Boston Medical Society (self-regulation)	1808
American Medical Association code of ethics	1847
British General Medical Council's code of ethics	1858
German code of science and medicine	1898
Nuremberg code of ethics	1947
Code of medical ethics—MCI	1956
WMA declaration of Helsinki	1964
ICMR Policy statement on ethical considerations involved in research on human subjects	1980
Revised code of ethics—MCI	2002
ICMR Biomedical and Health Research involving Human Participants	2017

FM 4.16, 4.17
- Describe and discuss bioethics.
- Describe and discuss ethical principles: respect for autonomy, nonmaleficence, beneficence and justice.

Bioethics and Medical Ethics

- *Ethics* is the set of philosophical beliefs and practices concerned with distinction between right and wrong.
- *Bioethics*, a subfield of ethics, is an area of philosophy which concerns ethical issues in applied and practical biomedical scientific technologies.
- In 1970, the term 'bioethics' was used for the first time by Potter.
- Bioethics is based on the principle of solidarity, as well as freedom, tolerance, equal opportunity, social justice and human dignity.
- Bioethics and medical ethics are closely related to each other since both are concerned with humans **(Diff. 3.1.)**.
- Bioethics is generally more to do with theoretical ethical issues and concepts, and follows the four basic principles when evaluating the merits and demerits surrounding all biomedical technologies.
- The four basic principles are:
  1. **Autonomy** refers to the right of the patient to retain control over his body. It requires that patients should have autonomy of thought, intention and action when making decisions regarding health care procedures, i.e., the decision-making process must be free of coercion or coaxing. This principle is the basis for the practice of 'informed consent' in the doctor–patient relationship.
  2. **Beneficence:** The doctor should act in the 'best interest' of the patient—the procedure and treatment is provided with the intent of doing benefit to the patient. The goal of providing benefit can be applied both to individual patient and society as a whole.
  3. **Nonmaleficence:** Requires that the doctor should not intentionally create a harm or injury to the patient (*primum non nocere*—first do no harm), either through acts of commission or omission.

DIFFERENTIATION 3.1: Bioethics and medical ethics

S.No.	Feature	Bioethics	Medical ethics
1.	Basic difference	Refers to the philosophical study of ethics of medical and biological research	Moral principles which concern the practice of medicine
2.	Focus	Utilitarian, concepts surrounding all biomedical technologies	Doctor's duty to the individual patient
3.	Scope	More extensive, societal-oriented	Applied narrowly, mainly patient-oriented
4.	Application	Guides for public policy, stem cell research, xenotransplantation, use of animals in research	Clinical obligations, patient autonomy and interest, telling errors

This principle affirms the need for medical competence.

4. **Justice** is usually defined as a form of fairness—a fair distribution of goods in society. The burdens and benefits of treatments must be distributed equally among all groups in society regardless of their gender, race or religion.

> **NOTA BENE**
> - **Mnemonic for basic principles ABCDE**—A: Autonomy; B: Beneficence; C: Confidentiality; D: Do no harm (non-maleficence); E: Equity/Justice.
> - **Doctrine of double effect:** Some interventions may bring an intended positive effect along with an unintended negative outcome (serious harm, such as the death). This principle is commonly referred to in euthanasia to justify the case where a doctor gives drugs (e.g., morphine) to a patient to relieve distressing symptoms even though he knows doing this may shorten the patient's life.
> - **Collusion** is a secret agreement made between the doctor and a patient or between patients and caregivers to hide the diagnosis of a serious or life-threatening illness from the patient, particularly seen in relation to patients with cancer. Collusion is generally an act of love or a need to protect another from pain.
>   - But principles of informed consent and patient autonomy mandate clear ethical obligations to provide patients with as much information as they desire about their illness and its treatment.
>   - It has been found that collusion isolate the patient, cause family disruption, incurs tremendous psychosocial stress on patient and relatives and leads to poor standard of healthcare.

FM 4.11
Describe and discuss euthanasia.

EUTHANASIA (MERCY KILLING)

Definition: Euthanasia (Greek, good death) denotes producing painless death of a person suffering from hopelessly incurable and painful disease.

Types: It can be of two types **(Diff. 3.2)**
i. Active euthanasia
ii. Passive euthanasia

It can also be classified into:
i. **Voluntary euthanasia:** Wherein the individual requests euthanasia, either during illness or before, if complete incapacitation is expected.
ii. **Nonvoluntary euthanasia:** Where an individual is incapable of perception and feeling, and hence cannot decide or distinguish between life and death, such a person cannot give informed consent, for e.g., when resuscitation is not expected after severe brain damage as in coma patients or severely defective infants.
iii. **Involuntary euthanasia:** Where an individual may distinguish between life and death, and any medical killing is involuntary, i.e., against the will of the person. It is ethically, morally and legally considered as murder. This is not to be confused with medical killing in cases of capital punishment.

Arguments against Euthanasia

i. It is against medical ethics.
ii. Medical science is making rapid progress; a disease which is incurable today may became curable tomorrow.
iii. It would not only be for people who are 'terminally ill', but may be used to commit murder. It could be misused by doctors coming hand in glove with relatives.
iv. It can become a means of health care cost containment.
v. It may become involuntary.
vi. It is a rejection of the importance and value of human life.
vii. It is a crime against society and equivalent to legalizing murder and suicide. It will encourage people to commit suicide.

Reasons for Euthanasia

i. **Unbearable pain:** Patient should be allowed a dignified painless death, instead of prolonging the same through the torture of pain and disease.
ii. **High cost of medical treatment:** It may pose economic and psychological burden to the patient's relative.
iii. Right to commit suicide.
iv. **Patient should not be forced to stay alive:** Medical science too has its limitation and cannot cure all diseases.

DIFFERENTIATION 3.2: Active and passive euthanasia

S.No.	Feature	Active euthanasia	Passive euthanasia
1.	Definition	Positive merciful act, to end useless suffering or a meaningless existence	Discontinuing or not using extraordinary life-sustaining measures to prolong life
2.	Principle	It is an act of commission	It is an act of omission
3.	Procedure	Administration of lethal doses of opium/barbiturate/sodium thiopental and then a muscle relaxant	Allowing death by not resuscitating a terminally ill or incapacitated patient or defective newborn infant
4.	Characteristic feature	Using measures that would hasten death	Not using measures that would delay death
5.	Followed in	Netherlands, Belgium and Luxembourg	India, Mexico and in some States of the US (e.g., with holding tube-feeding)

NOTA BENE

- Supreme Court had allowed passive euthanasia in patients with permanent vegetative state but rejected active euthanasia.
- Currently, the Supreme Court has allowed an individual to draft a *'living will'*. A 'living will' is made by a person, in his normal state of mind, seeking voluntary euthanasia in case of terminal illness, if he reaches an irreversible vegetative state. The 'advance directives' can be issued and executed by 'next friend and relatives' of terminally ill people, but a medical board to take a final call.
- A family member or friend of the terminally ill person who has not written a 'living will' can go to the High Court, which will constitute a medical board to decide if passive euthanasia is needed.
- **Physician-assisted suicide (PAS)** is the physician prescribing a drug or other action to facilitate a patient taking his own life, with the committed action taken by the patient. The terms 'PAS' and 'euthanasia' are often used interchangeably.
- Belgium, Netherlands, Luxembourg, Switzerland and the US States of Oregon, Washington, Montana, Vermont permit some forms of euthanasia.
- By far, most reported cases of euthanasia concern cancer patients.
- **Palliative care:** The provision of reasonable medical and nursing procedures for the relief of physical pain, discomfort or emotional and psychological suffering, as well as providing food and water in terminally ill patients.

FM 4.12 Discuss legal and ethical issues in relation to stem cell research.

STEM CELL RESEARCH

Introduction

- Stem cell research (SRC) offers understanding basic mechanisms of human development and differentiation, and hold potential for therapies and cures for diseases, such as diabetes, heart disease, spinal cord injuries, Parkinson's, Alzheimer's, etc.
- Rapid progress in SRC has introduced a host of ethical and policy issues.
- In India, there is no law to regulate the SRC.
- ICMR and Department of Biotechnology has issued guidelines on SRC, the National Guidelines for Stem Cell Research, 2017 to ensure that all researches with human stem cells are conducted in an ethical and scientifically responsible manner.
- The underlying philosophy is to prevent the commercialization of unproven stem-cell therapies and generation of new knowledge based on the sound scientific rationale while addressing all ethical concerns.
- An important aspect of the guideline is that it clarifies the ambiguity over who has legal jurisdiction over the uses of stem cell.

Salient Features

- Stem cells and their derivatives are defined as 'drug' as per the Drugs and Cosmetics Act, 1940.
- Any stem cell use in patients, other than that for hematopoietic stem cell reconstitution for approved indications, is investigational at present.
- The guidelines do not apply to research using (i) nonhuman stem cells and their derivatives; (ii) hematopoietic stem cells, and (iii) platelet-rich plasma and autologous chondrocyte/osteocytes implantation.
- Clinical trials using stem cells should be in compliance with Schedule Y (Drugs and Cosmetic Act), Good Clinical Practice (GCP) guidelines and ICMR's ethical guidelines for biomedical research.
- Mandatory registration of the Institutional Committee for Stem Cell Research.
- All clinical trial must have a NMC registered postgraduate medical specialist in the subject domain of the trial.

Ethical and Scientific Issues

Health, safety and rights of the donor are of the utmost importance:

1. Human participants enrolled for clinical trials are not liable to pay any charges toward procedures, investigations and/or hospitalization related to the trial. Identity of the donor shall be kept confidential at all times.
2. Mandatory video consent is necessary.
3. Mandatory screening for six major transmittable diseases (HIV-1 and 2, hepatitis B virus, hepatitis C virus, *Treponema pallidum*, human T-lymphotropic virus and cytomegalovirus) or any other risk factors for genetic disorders.
4. Intellectual property rights of donated material will not vest with donor, but may be shared (to be mentioned in informed consent form). If commercialization brings any financial benefit, it may be passed on to donor/community.
5. 'Permissible' research includes establishment of embryonic stem cell (ESC) and induced pluripotent stem cells; 'restrictive' research involve human preimplantation embryos processed by in vitro fertilization (IVF)/intracytoplasmic sperm injection (ICSI)/somatic cell nuclear transfer to derive ESC lines; and 'prohibited' research involve human germline gene therapy and reproductive cloning.
6. **Genome modification** is restricted only to in vitro studies. In vitro studies on preimplantation human embryos must be carried out within 14 days of fertilization or formation of primitive streak, whichever is earlier. Uterine implantation (human/animal) of manipulated cells with the intent of developing a whole organism is prohibited.
7. **Banking** of umbilical cord blood or ESC/induced pluripotent stem cell (iPSC) lines is permitted only

in licensed institutions. Commercial banking of all other biological materials is not permitted.

8. **Procurement:** If cells/tissues have been developed utilizing IVF method, permission is mandatory. Archival period for stem-cell lines and related information is 10 years. For procurement of fetal or placental tissue, processes must comply with all obligations under the MTP Act, 1971 (Amendment Act 2021). The medical person responsible for patient careof and the investigator using the fetal material shall not be the same. The consent for fetal tissue donation should be obtained in advance and not just before or at the time of the procedure. If there is disagreement between parents, the mother's wish shall prevail. Consent for donation of blastocysts for establishment of human ESC lines should be obtained from the donor at least 24 hours (h) in advance. Donors retain the right to withdraw consent until the blastocysts are actually used in cell line derivation.
9. Import of stem cell lines for basic research will not require "no objection certificate" but those required for clinical trials and originating oversees require import clearance. For export of indigenously developed cell lines, clearances must be obtained.
10. **Publicity:** The advertising and publicity of probable benefits of stem cell therapy through any mode by clinicians are not permitted.

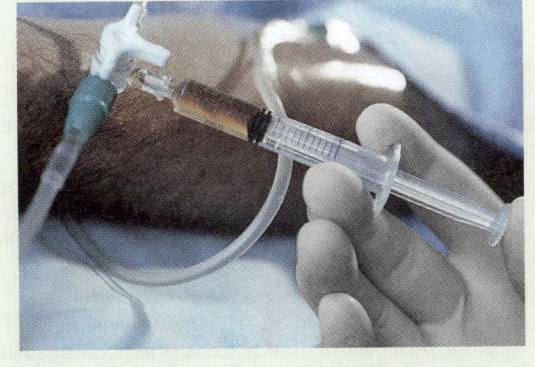

Type of euthanasia represented by the image:
1

FM 4.20, 4.25, 4.27

- Describe human experimentation.
- Discuss human experimentation including clinical trials.
- Describe and discuss ethical guidelines for biomedical research on human subjects and animals.

HUMAN EXPERIMENTATION

Introduction

- The Nuremberg Code consisting of 10 ethical principles (formulated in 1947) is one of the most influential documents in the history of clinical research.
- WMA's Declaration of Helsinki in 1964 is regarded as the basic document on medical research involving human subjects.
- The ICMR issued the Policy Statement on Ethical Considerations Involved in Research on Human Subjects in 1980.
- The revised ICMR guidelines 'National Ethical Guidelines for Biomedical and Health Research Involving Human Participants, 2017' have adapted important guidance points from various international guidelines keeping in mind the diverse sociocultural milieu of our country.
- These guidelines are applicable to all biomedical, social and behavioral science research for health conducted in India involving human participants, their biological material and data.

Constitution of Ethics Committee

- The number of persons in an ethics committee (EC) should be between 7 and 15 (preferably 8–12 members). A minimum of five persons is required to form the quorum without which a decision regarding the research should not be taken.
- The Institutional Ethics Committee should appoint from among its members a Chairman who should be from outside the Institution to maintain the independence of the Committee.
- The Member Secretary should be from the same Institution and should conduct the business of the Committee.
- Other members should be a mix of medical/nonmedical, scientific and non-scientific persons including lay persons to represent the differed points of view.

The composition of ethics committee is given in **Box 3.1**.

Box 3.1 Composition of ethics committee (EC)

Chairperson	One-two clinicians from various institutes
Member Secretary	One lay person from the community
One legal expert or retired judge	One-two persons from basic medical science area
One philosopher/ethicist/theologian	One social scientist/representative of nongovernmental voluntary agency

Ethical Guidelines for Biomedical Research

a. The four basic principles—autonomy, beneficence, nonmaleficence and justice must be adhered to in any biomedical research in order to protect the dignity, rights, safety and well-being of participants.
b. ECs must ensure that the research is conducted in accordance with the basic principles given in **Box 3.2**.

There are some general issues that must be kept in focus during the conduct of biomedical and health research involving human participants **(Table 3.1)**.

> **Box 3.2** General principles
>
> *Principle of essentiality:* Human participation should be considered only if essential for the research.
>
> *Principle of voluntariness:* It's the right of the participant to agree or not to agree to participate in research.
>
> *Principle of non-exploitation:* Benefits and burdens of the research are distributed fairly and without any discrimination.
>
> *Principle of social responsibility:* Research should not create social and historic divisions or disturb social harmony.
>
> *Principle of privacy and confidentiality:* Privacy of participant is maintained, her/his identity and records are kept confidential.
>
> *Principle of risk minimization:* Ensure minimization of risks, and care and compensation is given if any harm occurs.
>
> *Principle of professional competence:* Persons conducting research should be competent, qualified and experienced.
>
> *Principle of maximization of benefit:* Research should maximize the benefits to the participants/society.
>
> *Principle of institutional arrangements:* Institutes should facilitate research by providing infrastructure, manpower, funds and training.
>
> *Principle of transparency and accountability:* Conducted in a fair, honest, impartial and transparent manner to guarantee accountability.
>
> *Principle of totality of responsibility:* Researchers are responsible for their actions.
>
> *Principle of environmental protection:* Research should be in compliance with existing guidelines and regulations.

TABLE 3.1: General ethical issues

Ethical issues	Explanation
Benefit-risk assessment	Every research has some inherent probabilities of harm or risk; so maximize benefits and minimize risks to participants. Risks can be physical (death, disability, infection), psychological (depression, anxiety), economic (job loss) or social (discrimination or stigma from participating in a certain trial).
Informed consent	Informed consent from the participant/legally acceptable/authorized representative in writing is mandatory and should carry the specified elements in simple, layman's language. They should make their own decision about whether they want to participate or continue participating in research.
Privacy and confidentiality	Researcher should safeguard the privacy and confidentiality of participants and research-related data from unauthorized access and keep the information confidential.
Distributive justice	Benefits and burdens of research should be equitably distributed among the participating individuals or communities.
Payment for participation	Participants should not be made to pay for research-related expenses incurred beyond routine clinical care. Participants may also be paid for inconvenience incurred, time spent and other incidental expenses in either cash or kind or both as deemed necessary.
Compensation for research related harm	Research participants who suffer direct physical, psychological, social, legal or economic harm are entitled to financial compensation or other forms of assistance. Investigator/ institution or insurance company should compensate for research related harm.
Ancillary care	Free medical care may be offered as ancillary care for non-research-related conditions or incidental findings.
Conflict of interest	Policies for declaration and management of financial or nonfinancial (personal, academic or political) conflict of interest for researchers, EC, institution and sponsor must be implemented by research institutes. To minimize potential conflicts of interest, an independent review panel with no vested interest in the study should review the proposal.
Selection of vulnerable groups as participants	Primary basis for recruiting and enrolling participants should be the scientific goals of the study—not vulnerability, privilege, or other factors. The selection of vulnerable and special groups (incapable of protecting their own interests because of personal disability, environmental burdens, social injustice, lack of power, understanding or ability to communicate), with provisions for additional safeguards and close monitoring.
Community engagement	Engaging with the community from the beginning of research till after its completion helps to improve design and conduct of research and ensures greater responsiveness to health needs. However, every individual participant's consent is essential.
Post-research access and benefit sharing	Post-research access and benefit-sharing may be done with individuals, communities and populations, wherever applicable after completion of study.

Research Involving Animals

- As per NMC guidelines, animal experiments should be designed and done only if absolutely necessary and meaningful.
- Proper care and compassion should be there, and minimize pain and suffering during the experiments.

Clinical Trials

Clinical trials must be conducted in accordance with the Indian Good Clinical Practice guidelines, Declaration of Helsinki, National Ethical Guidelines for Biomedical and Health Research Involving Human Participants (2017) and revised Schedule Y of the Drugs and

CHAPTER 3 : Ethical and Social Aspects of Medical Practice

Cosmetics Act, 1940 and other applicable regulations and guidelines.
- Clinical trial interventions could be of drugs, vaccines, biosimilars, biologics, phytopharmaceuticals, radiopharmaceuticals, diagnostic agents, public health or sociobehavioral interventions, technologies, devices, surgical techniques or traditional systems of medicine.
- An investigator should determine if the clinical trial is within the regulatory ambit and if so, all Central Drug Standards and Control Organization (CDSCO) requirements should be followed.
- If students are conducting clinical trials as part of their thesis, guides/and institutions should take the responsibilities of sponsor.
- Clinical trials must be prospectively registered which is mandatory for trials under the purview of CDSCO.
- Patients should not be charged for trial interventions that are added on as part of research.
- Ancillary care may be provided to clinical trial participants for non-study/trial related illnesses arising during the period of the trial.
- Adverse effects of drugs should be reported in a timely manner.
- Institutions must obtain grants, insurance coverage or set up corpus funds to meet the costs related to treatment/management and payment of compensation.
- Clinical trials should be scientifically and ethically sound and preclinical studies should precede trials on humans.
- Bioavailability/Bioequivalence studies involving healthy volunteers may pose risks due to adverse effects of drugs and require safeguards.
- Precautions should be taken to protect participants from harm when a placebo is used.
- Trials on devices should follow the same requirements as for new drugs. Similarly, surgical interventions must also follow the ethical guidelines.
- If a study involves biosimilars, the product quality, preclinical data and bioassay must demonstrate similarity with a reference biologic.
- Clinical trials with stem cells should follow the National Guidelines for Stem Cell Research, 2017.
- Community trials may be conducted to evaluate preventive strategies, such as mass drug administration.
- Research that involves sexual minorities or intravenous drug users should ensure community engagement.
- Trials using diagnostic agents should follow the same protocols as for trials on new drugs.
- Radioactive materials and X-rays should be used with more precaution in persons who have not completed family.
- Clinical trials among women for contraceptives or if they are pregnant or lactating should involve abundant precautions and care.
- Therapeutic misconception should be addressed to in oncology trials.

FM 4.20
Describe malingering.

MALINGERING (SHAMMING)

Definition: It is a conscious planned feigning or pretence to having a disease in order to achieve a specific goal.

Reasons

i. By soldiers or policemen to evade their duties
ii. By prisoners to avoid hard work
iii. By businessmen to avoid business contracts
iv. By workmen to claim compensation
v. By beggars to attract public sympathy
vi. By criminals to avoid legal responsibility

Diseases feigned: Ophthalmia, neurasthenia, dyspepsia, aphasia, intestinal colic, sciatica, diabetes, vertigo, spitting of blood, epilepsy, ulcers, insanity, burns, paralysis of limbs, rheumatism, artificial bruise, lumbago, etc.

- Usually the signs and symptoms do not conform to any known disease.
- Patients can distort or exaggerate their symptoms, but true simulation is very rare.
- History of the case should be taken from the person himself and his relatives or friends, and any inconsistencies in this description of the symptoms are noted.
- A complete examination is essential after removing the bandages, if any, and washing the part.
- It can be diagnosed by keeping the patient under observation, and watching him without his knowledge.

Medico-legal importance: If a patient gets a medical certificate by narrating false symptoms and uses for any purpose, he may be sued under **Sec. 198 IPC** for false evidence (punishment is 7 years and fine under **Sec. 193 IPC**) or sued for cheating under **Sec. 415 IPC** (punishment is 1 year and/or fine under **Sec. 417 IPC**).

FM 4.22, 4.23
- Explain oath—Hippocrates, Charaka and Sushruta and procedure for administration of oath.
- Describe the modified Declaration of Geneva and its relevance.

OATH

- Oath is a solemn promise, often invoking a divine witness, regarding one's future action or behavior.
- Oaths are neither a universal endeavor nor a legal obligation, and they cannot guarantee morality.
- Affirmation strengthens a doctor's resolve to behave with integrity in extreme circumstances.
- Medical colleges incorporate medical ethics into the core curriculum, and all medical graduates make a

commitment, by means of affirmation, to observe an ethical code.

Charaka's Oath

The Charaka's oath of initiation is an Indian oath for medical students which appear in the *Charaka Samhita*, a medical text written around 100–200 BC by the Indian physician Charaka.

- The oath contains several unique elements, including the requirements to lead the life of a celibate, eat no meat and carry no arms.
- It mandates that the physician must seek consent before entering a patient's quarters, must be accompanied by a male member of the family if he is attending a woman or minor, must inform and gain consent from patient or the guardians if the patient is a minor, must never resort to extortion for his service, never involve himself in any other activities with the patient or patient's family (such as negotiating loans, arranging marriage, buying or selling property), speak with soft words and never use cruel words, only do "what is calculated to do good to the patient", and maintain the patient's privacy.
- In it, physicians can refuse to treat people who were not favored by the king. This shows that oaths were a product of the sociocultural factors of the times they were created.

Sushruta Oath

- **Sushruta** (200–300 AD) was a physician in ancient India known as the "Father of Indian Medicine" and "Father of Plastic Surgery" for inventing and developing surgical procedures.
- Before beginning the training during that time, the students were required to take a solemn oath.

'*Thou shalt renounce all evil desires, anger, greed, passion, pride, egotism, envy, harshness, meanness, untruth, indolence and other qualities that bring infamy upon oneself.*'

'*Thou shalt clip thy nails and hair close, observe cleanliness . . . and dedicate thyself to the observance of truth, celibacy and the salutation of elders . . . '*

'*The preceptor, the poor, the friendly, the travellers, the lowly, the good and the destitute—those thou shalt treat when they come to thee like thy own kith and kin and relieve their ailments . . .*'

a. Sushruta emphasized the fact that knowledge was not an individual monopoly and that medical remuneration was secondary to service.
b. The doctors should serve the patient with the motto 'service to man is service to God.'

Hippocratic Oath

- Hippocrates, the Father of Medicine, constructed the groundwork for the principles of ethics in 400 BC in his establishment of the Hippocratic Oath.
- The oath sets the standards of conduct at a time when healers were considered near divine and no laws or litigations existed. The oath became universal only towards the early 19th century.
- In its original form, it requires a new physician to swear, by the Gods of healing of Greek pantheon, to uphold specific ethical standards. This was to help them understand the gravity of their situation and what is expected from their conduct as healers.
- The oath exhorts to treat the ill to the best of one's ability, to preserve a patient's privacy, to teach the secrets of medicine to the next generation, and so on. It embodies the principles of beneficence, confidentiality and non-maleficence.
- It is said that the exact phrase 'first do no harm' (*primum non nocere*) is a part of the original Hippocratic oath.
- The changing cultural and social environment of modern society, accompanied by the advancement in scientific knowledge and therapeutic tools, has surfaced the need to reframe ethical perspective in modern medicine.
- In 1960s, the oath was changed to require 'utmost respect for human life from its beginning,' making it a more secular obligation, not to be taken in the presence of God or any Gods, but before only other people.
- In 2019, the oath was changed again to include 'protection of the environment which sustains us.' This further widened the focus of care from the individual, to the community and to the ecosystem.

DECLARATION OF GENEVA

- The Declaration of Geneva was adopted by WMA at Geneva in 1948 and has been amended many times, the last being in 2017.
- The Declaration is one of the core documents of medical ethics and was intended as a revision of the Hippocratic oath to a formulation that could be comprehended and acknowledged in a modern way.
- It is a standard practice for policy review of the declaration by WMA every 10 years so as to maintain its accuracy, essentiality and relevance.

Declaration

The current declaration which is also known as the *Physician's Pledge*, states:

As a member of the medical profession:
- I solemnly pledge to dedicate my life to the service of humanity.
- The health and well-being of my patient will be my first consideration.
- I will respect the autonomy and dignity of my patient.
- I will maintain the utmost respect for human life.

- I will not permit considerations of age, disease or disability, creed, ethnic origin, gender, nationality, political affiliation, race, sexual orientation, social standing or any other factor to intervene between my duty and my patient.
- I will respect the secrets that are confided in me, even after the patient has died.
- I will practice my profession with conscience and dignity and in accordance with good medical practice.
- I will foster the honor and noble traditions of the medical profession.
- I will give to my teachers, colleagues and students the respect and gratitude that is their due.
- I will share my medical knowledge for the benefit of the patient and the advancement of healthcare.
- I will attend to my own health, well-being, and abilities in order to provide care of the highest standard.
- I will not use my medical knowledge to violate human rights and civil liberties, even under threat.

I make these promises solemnly, freely and upon my honor.

Salient Features

- The important difference between the Declaration of Geneva and other key ethical documents is the lack of overt recognition of patient autonomy. The following clause '*I will respect the autonomy and dignity of my patient*' highlights the importance of patient self-determination.
- To more explicitly invoke the standards of ethical and professional conduct expected of physicians by their patients and peers, the clause '*I will practise my profession with conscience and dignity*' was augmented to include the wording '*and in accordance with good medical practice.*'
- The revisions also included a physician-centric line about maintaining health and awareness to provide proper care. It incorporated the clause of physician well-being '*I will attend to my own health, well-being, and abilities in order to provide care of the highest standard.*' This reflects not only the humanity of physicians, but also the role physician self-care can play in improving patient care.
- With regard to professional relationships the clause '*I will give to my teachers, colleagues, and students the respect and gratitude that is their due*' replaced the line 'My colleagues will be my sisters and brothers,' because the tone was considered outdated. To complement this principle, it added a clause referring more explicitly to the obligation to teach and forward knowledge to the next generation of physicians.
- Age, disability, gender, and sexual orientation have been added as factors that must not interfere with a doctor's duty to a patient. Secrets are to remain confidential '*even after the patient has died.*' The violation of 'human rights and civil liberties' replaces 'the laws of humanity' as a forbidden use of medical knowledge.
- Furthermore, the revised text is meant to be used by all active physicians (*as member of the medical profession*); earlier the text was used by beginners only ('At the time of being admitted as a member of the medical profession').

Administration of Oath

- Medical students usually take an oath when they graduate but there is no standard approach.
- Over the years, it has become an emotional rite of passage in medical school graduations across the world.
- Usually, the Dean of medical college administers the oath to the graduates, he invites the fresh graduates present to stand and recommit themselves to the oath's principles by raising their right hands.

Medico-legal Issues

- There is no direct punishment for breaking the Hippocratic Oath, although it may construed as medical malpractice which carries a wide range of punishments, from legal action to civil penalties.
- In ancient times, the punishment for breaking the oath could range from a penalty to losing the right to practice medicine.

NOTA BENE

- **Declaration of Tokyo:** This was adopted in 1975 which refers to the guidelines for doctors concerning *torture, degradation* or *cruel treatment of prisoners.*
- **Declaration of Helsinki:** The WMA developed this declaration in 1964. It refers to the *ethical principles for medical research involving human subjects,* including research on identifiable human material and data.
- **Declaration of Oslo:** It was a statement by the WMA in 1970 on *therapeutic abortion.*
- **Declaration of Malta:** This was adopted by the WMA in 1991 for *hunger strikers.* The principle of beneficence urges physicians to resuscitate them, but respect for individual autonomy restrains physicians from intervening when a valid and informed refusal has been made.
- **Declaration of Lisbon:** This was adopted by the WMA in 1981. The declaration represents some of the principal *rights of the patient* that the medical profession endorses and promotes.
- **Declaration of Ottawa:** This declaration on *child health* was adopted by the WMA in 1998. Physicians along with parents advocate for healthy children.
- **Declaration of Sydney:** This declaration was adopted in 1968 on the *determination of death and the recovery of organs.*
- **Declaration of Venice:** This declaration on *terminal illness* was adopted in 1983, which considers both euthanasia and physician-assisted suicide as unethical.
- **Declaration of Taipei:** WMA adopted this in 2002 on *ethical considerations regarding health databases and biobanks.*
- **Declaration of Chicago:** The declaration on *quality assurance in medical education* was adopted in 2017.

Describe communication between doctors, public and media.

DOCTORS AND MEDIA

- The ubiquitous nature of the news media makes it a powerful tool for directing attention to specific issues.
- Public engagement for doctor can include everything from discussions with the mainstream media to the creation of own media.
- Doctors should effectively use media to communicate with the healthcare professionals, as well as the public.
- Use of public networks and the mainstream media to advance healthcare issues needs to be identified as part of our work.
- However, the doctors do not see public engagement as part of their job. Fear of being misrepresented or misunderstood is a common concern for doctors in such media interactions.
- But, effective media communication is key responsibility of health professionals. Every conversation with the media is an opportunity to reach and influence innumerable people.
- Self-monitoring, accountability, having a good communication strategy can go a long way in improving the medical related news coverage.

Usefulness of Media

- Many people receive their health information from the media. It is essential to get the right information across and to control the story.
- Sensitize the media and public towards science and the process of discovery.
- Doctors should communicate medical information in a way that the public can understand and provide clear information about the concepts of risk and how to apply them.
- Effective communication is particularly critical during crises. Well-constructed and properly delivered media messages can inform and calm a worried public, reduce misinformation, and focus attention on what is most important.
- Media raise awareness and level of debate in society and gain public feedback on controversial issues.
- Doctor should pitch a story and not a research topic. Care should be taken to educate the public and desist from promoting self.
- Maintain a good relationship with journalists/editors and try to establish yourself as a media source.
- The media should have a social and ethical responsibility to ensure accuracy and balance of information and selection of reliable sources when communicating with the people.

PRESS CONFERENCE

- While addressing a press conference, one should prepare three to five key messages on what one wish to say but do not be derailed.
- It is all too easy to be caught unprepared, especially on short-notice or demanding media interviews, and preparation is vital.
- Communicate badly and one may be perceived as incompetent, uncaring or dishonest. Communicate well and one can reach more people with a clear and credible public health message.
- If someone from the media puts a question which is irrelevant to the immediate issue, the response should be 'it is a very important issue and we will discuss it in detail at a later sitting but today we wish to concentrate on the topic….'.
- However, one should be prepared to take provocative questions. It is always better to provide some extra reading material to the media personnel.

Do's

- Be attentive during conversation.
- Maintain distance between speakers during a conversation.
- Before speaking up one should consider what is humorous and what is inappropriate/taboo.
- Should take turns during conversations—loudness, speed of delivery, length of delivery, silence, and time to respond to another's point.
- Should consider when to enter into and exit from conversations.

Don'ts

- Do not demand to 'approve' the story before it goes to print or on air.
- Do not be defensive or hostile when questioned about risks, side effects or contradicting opinions.
- Do not become overexposed to the media, positioning yourself as the only expert or try to market your own work.
- Desist from passing on some sensational story or viewpoint which is neither research nor news so as to get publicity and remain in the news.

Describe and discuss the challenges in managing medico-legal cases including development of skills in relationship management—human behavior, communication skills, conflict resolution techniques.

CHALLENGES IN MEDICO-LEGAL CASES

Doctors come across medico-legal cases (MLC) during their practice.

The challenges faced while dealing with a MLC can be:

Unable to decide or differentiate between a MLC and a non-MLC case	Incomplete documentation and answering the court as witness
Incorrect/improper history	Improper/inadequate sampling
Patients/attendants refusing MLC	Patient absconded
Delayed treatment due to the confusion	Giving opinion for 'fit for statement'
Delay in intimation to police	Handling the police and the violent public
Financial issues especially in an insured patient	Cases referred from other hospital

A proper counseling session can be arranged for patients for all MLCs, so that they can have a better understanding and knowledge regarding the case.

Key Skills for Doctors doing Medico-legal Work

- Ability to work any time of day or night, often under pressure
- Good practical skills
- Communication skills, compassion and a courteous manner
- Ability to solve problems
- Effective decision-making skills
- Leadership and management skills
- Continue learning throughout career
- Analytical ability
- Time management

Relationship Management

- Relationship management is basically interpersonal communication skills. It is the ability to inspire and influence patients, coworkers and teammates, ability to communicate and build bonds with patient, and the ability to resolve conflict.
- Interpersonal skills are built on basic communication skill. Appropriate communication integrates both patient- and doctor-centered approaches.

COMMUNICATION SKILLS

- Good communications skills are vital for good doctor–patient relationship.
- Currently, doctor–patient relationship is undergoing severe strain and leading to conflicts, communication skills become all the more important.
- Better communication saves more time and more lives in the long run and also lead to less litigation.
- Better understanding between parties—and a doctor's willingness to admit to errors, show concern, and apologize—can help prevent patients from seeking retribution through lawsuits.

Effective communication has three basic components:
1. Verbal component deals with the content of the message including selection of the words.
2. Nonverbal component includes body language, such as posture, gesture, facial expression and spatial distance.
3. Paraverbal component includes tone, pitch, pacing and volume of the voice.

Verbal component is important and it includes information about the nature, course and prognosis of the patient; investigations, risks/benefits of treatment/invasive procedures and cost.

Although most of us focus on the verbal component; non-verbal and paraverbal components are equally important.

Benefits of Good Communication Skills

The main goals of doctor–patient communication are creating a good interpersonal relationship, facilitating exchange of information and including patients in decision making **(Box 3.3)**.

Patients sue because of a feeling that they were not heard, that their needs were not attended to, and that nobody seemed to care, and as a result, a bad outcome resulted due to a mistake or negligence.

Communication Strategies

First interaction is extremely important to win patient's confidence.

Prerequisites

- Put the patient at ease and make him feel comfortable.
- The patient's confidentiality and privacy should be maintained. He should not be made to state the reason for his visit when other people are present. The discussions should not be done while walking in the corridors.
- While talking, tone of voice should be agreeable, not critical.
- Time of consultation should neither be too little nor too long.

Box 3.3 Goals of good communication skills

- Manage and interact effectively with a 'difficult' patient
- Adjust for language barriers, such as accents or colloquial expressions
- Clearly present diagnosis and/or treatment options
- Increase patient's compliance to doctor's advices
- Exhibit empathy for patient/patient care
- Gain a clear understanding of patient needs or medical issues
- Influence a patient to adopt healthy living or lifestyle changes
- Initiate and grow a trusting relationship
- Understand and work with cultural distinctions or attitudes
- Decrease work stress and increase job satisfaction

Listen to the Patients

Doctors should spend more time listening effectively during the appointment.

- Greet the patient first. It is desirable to address the patient by his name.
- Establish eye contact and maintain it at reasonable intervals.
- Some patients may be nervous, a general nonmedical inquiry may be started in order to develop a comfortable environment for the patient.
- Do not interrupt the patient when he is expressing something.
- Encourage request for information.
- The doctor should show a genuine interest in what the patient is saying with his mannerism, body language and active involvement.
- Inattentive listening can distract the patient from telling his history effectively.
- Doctors should acknowledge what the patient is saying and encourage them to continue, and even removing physical barriers between the two (i.e., not talking from behind a computer or while using mobile phone).
- While concluding, one must ask the patient if he has got any further queries.

Communicating with the Attendants

- Attendants are apprehensive and at times full of doubts and queries.
- Important especially when patient is in critical condition.
- The communication should be formal and conducted once or twice daily.
- Discuss and appreciate the efforts made by them.
- Most of the attendants surf internet for information, their queries should be satisfied by giving better references.
- Always explain the dynamic nature of the condition—especially important for critically injured patients. They are more convinced and ready to accept bad outcome if the same fact is explained beforehand.
- Try to convince that all efforts are being made to bring situation under control or will be controlled.
- Presenting the information in the right manner is important. A life-threatening condition should not be conveyed in a frightening way.
- If something goes wrong, taking the patient and his relatives into confidence helps.

> **NOTA BENE**
>
> **Breaking bad news**
> - If a junior doctor is on duty, it is better to call a senior doctor for breaking bad news. The patient's relatives should be taken to a separate room or place and make them sit before breaking the news. The communication should be made as reassuring as possible. Often the caregivers may become angry or emotional. Both the extremes of situation should be dealt calmly and with empathy. A second opinion is recommended in such situations.

> - A 6-step guide known as **SPIKES protocol** for holding family meetings is advised in which difficult decisions need to be made.
> S—**S**etting up the interview; P—Assessment of the patient's or family's **p**erception of the situation; I—**I**nvitation; K—**K**nowledge or information sharing; E—**E**motions addressed with **e**mpathy; S—**S**ummarize and **s**trategize

Communicating with Colleagues

Postgraduate students, fellows, residents and interns along with nursing and supportive staffs are part of the team.

- They will be united and motivated if they are not put down or scolded in front of patients or attendants. If doubts arise in the minds of patients, insecurity will be created in absence of consultants.
- Greatest courtesy should be displayed for all staffs including nurses, paramedical staffs and other supporting staffs.
- Appreciate the hard work and ability of the doctors and supporting staff.
- Audit and regular feedback improves in professional practice. Never delay to give appreciation and dare to give positive criticism.

CONFLICT

Definition: Disagreement within oneself or between people that cause harm or have the potential to cause harm. Disagreement can be of ideas, perspectives, priorities, preferences, beliefs, values and goals.

- It is widely recognized that human interactions have the potential to develop conflict and health arena is no exception.
- Conflicts can be between doctors and patients/families/attending physicians/residents.
- Conflicts between doctors and patients/family members may arise in case of forceful role in decision-making (e.g., the use of persuasion), suppressing key information, family's inadequate understanding of the patient's medical condition or the risks and benefits of therapies, or physicians' inability to communicate information effectively.
- Physicians must acknowledge that these cognitive distortions are not personal shortcomings of family members but rather their behavioral adaptations to stress. Failure to do so creates opposition between those advocating for the patient, resulting in conflict.
- Mitigating such conflict is a key skill that doctors should possess to maintain appropriate focus on care that will maximize patients' well-being, improve family members' outcomes and decrease the frequency of moral distress and burnout among physicians.
- Helpful behaviors include the use of supportive skills, such as acknowledging family members' emotions and expressing nonabandonment.

- Physicians' emotions matter in how they approach, manage, and respond to potential or actual conflicts with family members that arise during high-stakes decision-making. Their behavioral attributes are likely to influence how they prognosticate, communicate, and provide recommendations to surrogate decision-makers.

Classification of Conflict

1. **Intrapersonal:** Conflict takes place within an individual; it is psychological involving the individual's thoughts, values, principles and emotions.
2. **Interpersonal:** Conflict between two individuals due to incompatible choices and opinions.
3. **Intragroup:** Conflict occurs among individuals within team members.
4. **Intergroup:** Conflict due to misunderstanding among different teams within an organization.

Conflict Management

Conflict theorists suggest that conflict is a positive force in society and that human groups must handle conflicts in productive ways. Conflict management is the process of limiting the negative (destructive) aspects of conflict while increasing its positive (constructive) aspects.

Strategies of conflict management for managing stressful situations:

- **Collaboration** (win/win): Collaborating means working together by integrating ideas set out by multiple people so as to find a creative solution acceptable to everyone. Common grounds for agreement and common interests are pursued. Most time consuming strategy.
- **Negotiation/compromise** (win some/lose some): Adjusting with each other's opinions and ideas, and thinking of a solution where some points of both the parties can be entertained. The parties attempt to strike some sort of a bargain so as to minimize losses and maximize gains.
- **Accommodation** (lose/win): Accommodation means giving up of one's own ideas and thoughts so that the other party achieve its desired outcome. Accession is unlikely to result in a successful strategy in the long term.
- **Competing** (win/lose): Competing means when there is a dispute a person or a group is not willing to collaborate, work or adjust but it simply wants the opposite party to lose. This technique can further escalate conflict or losers may retaliate.
- **Avoidance** (no winners/no losers): It involves no declaration or statement for one of the parties to the other and no cooperation from the other party is sought or gained. The ideas suggested by both the parties are rejected and a third person (mediator) is involved who takes a decision without favoring any of the parties. A mediator in the healthcare setting would be either the head of department, CEO of the hospital or some high-level administrator. This technique may lead to postponing the conflict but may make matters worse.
- **Domination and intimidation:** The use of authority to impose one's will over another. This requires the greatest amount of assertiveness, and may backfire as some negotiators are by nature submissive individuals who may sound inauthentic when trying to dominate another.

The use of each technique had its advantages and disadvantages and no one technique is best for all situations. When a disagreement arises, often the *best course of action is negotiation to resolve the disagreement.*

Process of Negotiation

Preparation

- Set realistic goals and be flexible
- Revisit the circumstances behind the conflict
- Schedule specific start and finish times for the meetings
- Find a neutral ground for holding the meeting
- Minimize distractions
- Ensure break-out spaces for all

Exploration of Shared Interests

- Each party shares what they hope to achieve from the negotiation and satisfy them.
- Conducted in a nonadversarial manner.
- Listen carefully to what is being expressed.
- All the relevant issues should be laid on the table and both the parties should acknowledge it.

Enlarging of Shared Interests

- Highlight points of agreement and disagreement.
- Define common ground for agreement, for e.g., good patient care. Often, the points of agreement outweigh the points of disagreement.
- Delineate disagreement, for e.g., unresolved differences, clarify lingering ambiguities. The points of disagreement need to be reframed as points of lesser value.
- Identify and try to expand on small agreements.
- Avoid communication freezers, for e.g., negative personal comments or interjections.
- Develop and agree on a work plan for working on issues. Clarify rules and tasks for participants.
- This stage concludes when the parties are ready to share the investment of energy in finding solutions to the remaining problems.
- Work at reframing continuing issues in a more palatable way.

Enlightened Interests

- This is essentially a brainstorming session where the parties are encouraged to come up with creative solutions to the remaining points of disagreement.

- A zone of "no obligation" is set up, and creativity can flourish without either side needing to commit to anything.

Aligned Interests

- With multiple solutions available, each party can now debate what combination of solutions results in maximal recognizable gain for the parties.
- Whatever disagreement remains after this process can be deferred until a future round of negotiations, thus separating persistent points of argument from the agreement which has already been reached.
- The negotiation over solutions will require each party to make some concessions.

> **FM 4.9**
> Describe the medico-legal issues in relation to family violence, violation of human rights, NHRC and doctors.

Family Violence

Definition: Family and domestic violence represents any use of force, threats or other forms of coercion sufficient to injure or endanger the physical and/or psychological integrity of the victim, which is committed by one family member against other person(s) with whom he/she lives or has lived with, or with whom is/was in an intimate relationship.

Risk factors associated with violence include husbands being unemployed, associated with younger women who are in short-term relationships, belonging to a lower socioeconomic group, poor educational status, and alcohol and substance abuse.

- Family violence is a common problem in India and victims may suffer physical, psychological and emotional abuse.
- The National Human Rights Commission (NHRC) has considered domestic violence as violation of human rights as majority of the victims is female with male being the abusers.

Site of injuries: Head and neck and musculoskeletal injuries along with sexual abuse.

Responsibility of doctors: Doctors should be able to identify family violence victims and potential abusers in their clinical setting. The NHRC has also observed that doctors are always expected to maintain high standards of professionalism and should consider it their duty to report domestic violence.

- Emergency physicians are often the first to evaluate and identify family violence victims. They must be able to assess and identify the signs and symptoms of injury and provide initial treatment of victims. Injuries often require immediate evaluation and treatment after an assault.
- When healthcare professionals identify family violence, they should have a plan that includes providing community resource information related to shelter, counseling, advocacy groups, child protection and legal aid.
- Forensic experts can be of great help not only for court proceedings, but also in the designing appropriate standards for conducting clinical medico-legal examination, prevention programs and strategies in fighting family violence.
- Family violence including marital rape is associated with a high degree of secondary victimization that occurs during the medical procedures, pre-investigation and court proceedings, and additionally discourages victims in reporting the offence.
- Documentation (characteristics of injury on the victim's body and sampling of biological material as physical evidence) and reporting by forensic expert plays significant role in getting justice for the victim of family violence.

Rights of children: A child <14 years of age cannot be engaged as domestic servants. National Commission of Protection of Child Rights (NCPCR) and Child Welfare Committees refer the cases with suspected violation of child rights for forensic evaluation.

> **NOTA BENE**
> **Legal sections:** Laws to criminalize domestic violence in India were enacted, such as the Dowry Prohibition Act, 1986 and the Protection of Women from Domestic Violence Act, 2005. Even after the enactment of many laws and many women NGOs, the incidence of domestic and intimate partner violence in India is still on the rise.

Violation of Human Rights and NHRC

- Torture and other human rights abuses have been common throughout history.
- Doctors may participate in torture either by act of commission (certifying someone fit for interrogation or intentionally inflicting severe pain or suffering) or by act of omission (falsifying medical certificate or withholding treatment).
- Human Rights Watch has reported on a wide range of abuses against individuals under medical supervision, including the practice of forcible anal and vaginal examination, female genital mutilation and the failure to provide life-saving abortion, palliative care and treatment for drug dependency.
- Ethical guidelines uniformly prohibit doctors from any form of participation in torture.
- Doctors have an important role in detecting, documenting and prosecuting those involved in torture. Doctors working in places where systematized abuse is common, such as prisons and interrogation centers are likely to observe and link patterns of injury. Doctors may come across sequelae of physical abuse during autopsy.
- In India, NHRC has issued guidelines for doctors to deal with cases involving human right violation which emphasizes on right of prisoners regarding prompt medical assistance whenever felt necessary.

- This includes prevention of torture while in custody, and therefore, provisions have been made for mandatory medical examination by doctors every 48 h during his detention in custody and at the time of his release from the police custody.
- In cases of death in custody, it is mandatory for the DMs and SPs of every district to report to the Secretary General of the Commission about such incidents of death in police or judicial custody within 24 h of occurrence or having come to know about such incidents.
- Postmortem examination is to be conducted by board/panel of doctors including forensic expert and video-recording of examination in such cases is mandatory.

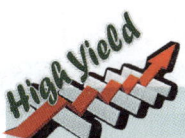

- **Medical ethics:** Moral principles for doctors in their dealings with each other, patients and the State.
- **Medical etiquette:** Conventional laws and customs of courtesy followed between members of same profession.
- **Bioethics:** Discipline dealing with the ethical implications emerging from medical and biological research.
- **Four basic principles' of bioethics:** Autonomy, non-maleficence, beneficence and justice.
- **Malingering:** Conscious planned feigning of a disease to achieve a specific goal.
- **Euthanasia:** Producing painless death of a person suffering from hopelessly incurable and painful disease.
- Passive euthanasia is legal in India, Mexico and in some States of US.
- **Conflict:** An active disagreement and argument between people with opposing opinions or principles.
- **Main cause of conflict:** Poor communication skill with patient.
- **Best course of action to resolve conflict:** Negotiation.
- Relationship management is basically interpersonal communication skills.

Interesting case

Euthanasia (Case of Aruna Shanbaug, 1973)

Aruna Shanbaug was working as a nurse at KEM Hospital, Mumbai. In 1973, she was sexually assaulted by a ward boy in the hospital basement. He sodomized and strangulated her with a dog chain. She was found next morning with the chain round her neck. Aruna suffered brainstem and cervical cord injury, and went into in a vegetative state **(Figs. A and B)**. The ward boy was caught and convicted for theft and assault but not for rape and unnatural sex. He served two concurrent seven year terms and was released in 1980.

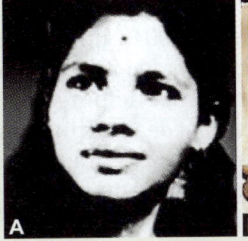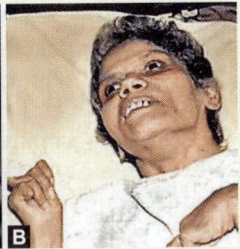

In 2010, the Supreme Court (SC) admitted the petition made by activist-journalist Pinki Virani to withdraw her life support. It sought a report on her medical condition from the hospital. In 2011, a three-member medical board concluded that the patient was not brain dead but met 'most of the criteria of being in a permanent vegetative state'. In March 2011, the SC in a landmark judgement issued a set of broad guidelines legalizing passive euthanasia. It permitted withdrawal of life-sustaining treatment from patients not in a position to make an informed decision. These guidelines stated that the decision to discontinue life support must be taken by parents, spouse or other close relatives, or in the absence of them, by a 'next friend'. The decision also requires court approval. In its judgment, the court rejected Virani's petition as they declined to recognize Virani as the 'next friend' of Aruna, and instead treated the KEM Hospital staff as the 'next friend' (nurses taking care of her opposed the plea). In 2015, Aruna died of pneumonia after being in a persistent vegetative state for nearly 42 years.

In 2014, SC cited inconsistencies in earlier verdicts on passive euthanasia including the one given in Aruna's case and referred the PIL of NGO 'Common Cause' seeking nod to allow terminally-ill persons to execute a living will for passive euthanasia to a Constitution bench. In 2018, SC recognized 'living will' (advance directive)* and laid down guidelines on procedures to be adopted for it. The court said that the 'living will' should be permitted since a person cannot be allowed to continue suffering in a comatose state when he does not wish to live. The SC said that directions and guidelines and its directive shall remain in force till legislation is brought on the issue.

---

* A living will is a written document by way of which a patient can give his explicit instructions in advance about the medical treatment to be administered when he is terminally ill or no longer able to express informed consent.

CHAPTER 4

Acts Related to Medical Practice

LEARNING OBJECTIVES

Must know
1. The Transplantation of Human Organs Act, 1994
2. The Consumer Protection Act, 2019
3. The POCSO Act, 2012
4. The MTP (Amendment) Act, 2021
5. The PCPNDT Act, 1994
6. The Assisted Reproductive Technology Act, 2021
7. The Mental Healthcare Act, 2017

Desirable to know
1. The Workman's Compensation Act, 1923
2. The ESI Act, 1948
3. The Protection of Women from Domestic Violence Act, 2005
4. The Transgender Persons (Protection of Rights) Act, 2019
5. The Surrogacy Act, 2021

Describe salient features of the Transplantation of Human Organs Act, 1994 and discuss ethical issues regarding organ donation.

THE TRANSPLANTATION OF HUMAN ORGANS ACT, 1994

- This Act was enacted in 1994 (amended in 2011 and 2014) for the removal, storage and transplantation of human organs for therapeutic purposes and for the prevention of commercial dealings in human organs.
- Under this Act 'human organ' means any part of a human body consisting of a structured arrangement of tissues which, if wholly removed, cannot be replicated by the body.

Salient Features

Authority for removal of human organs
1. Any donor (>18 years of age) may authorize the removal before his death of any organ of his body for therapeutic purposes.
2. If any donor had in writing (in presence of 2 or more witnesses) or in documents like driving license authorized the removal of any organ after his death for therapeutic purposes, the person lawfully in possession of dead body should allow the doctor all reasonable facilities for removal.
3. When no such authority is there, person lawfully in possession of dead body can authorize the removal of any organ including eye/cornea of the deceased person.
4. When human organ is to be removed, the medical practitioner should satisfy himself that life is extinct in such body or in case of brainstem death, it has been certified by:
    i. The doctor in-charge of hospital in which the brainstem death has occurred.
    ii. An independent doctor, being a specialist nominated by the above in-charge from the panel of names approved by Appropriate Authority.
    iii. A neurologist or a neurosurgeon, nominated by the in-charge from the panel.
    iv. The doctor treating the person whose brainstem death has occurred.

Under any circumstances, *brainstem death tests should not be performed by transplant surgeons or any doctor in the transplant team or a member of the Authorization Committee.*

After next of the kin (NOK) or person in lawful possession of the body authorizes removal and gives consent for donation of human organ(s) or tissue(s) or both, the registered medical practitioner (RMP) of the hospital through Transplant Coordinator should inform the registered Human Organ Retrieval Center by telephone/fax/electronic mail for removal, storage or transportation.

Removal of human organs cannot be authorized wherein:
i. An inquest may be required to be held in relation to such body.
ii. A person who has been entrusted the body solely for the purpose of cremation.

Authority for removal of human organs in case of unclaimed bodies in hospital or prison
- If not claimed by any near-relatives within 48 hours (h) from time of death, the authority lies with the management of hospital or prison or by employee of the hospital or prison authorized by management.
- If there is reason to believe that any near-relative of the deceased person is likely to claim the body even beyond 48 h, no authority should be given.

Authority for removal of organs from bodies sent for postmortem or pathological examination: Person competent under this Act can give authorization, if such organ is not required for the purpose for which the body has been sent.

Donation in Medico-legal Cases
- After the authority for removal of organs and/or tissues, and consent to donate from a brainstem dead are obtained, the RMP should make a request to the SHO of the area, either directly or through the police post located in the hospital to agree for retrieval of organs from the donor. It has to be ensured that, by retrieving organs, the determination of the cause of death is not jeopardized.
- In cases where the definite cause of death is established clinically by the RMP, the postmortem may be waived off by the competent officer on the request of the RMP and Investigating Officer (IO) of the case.
- The RMP who is designated to do the postmortem can do the organ retrieval also. Otherwise, he should be present at the time of retrieval of organs/tissues by the retrieval team. The postmortem report in respect of the organs/tissues being retrieved should be prepared at the time of retrieval. Rest of the postmortem procedure should take place at the autopsy room.
- For the purpose of organ(s)/tissue(s) retrieval, request for postmortem beyond specified timings, can be made by the RMP and IO of the case.

Restriction on Removal and Transplantation of Human Organs (Table 4.1)
i. Human organ should not be removed from the body of donor *before his death* and transplanted into recipient, unless the donor is a *near-relative**.

TABLE 4.1: Characteristics of recipients of human organs

Donor	Recipient	Organs transplanted
Living	Near-relative	Bone marrow, kidney, part of liver and pancreas
Living	Not a near-relative but with approval of Authorization Committee	–do–
Cadaver/brain dead	Any recipient	Most organs

ii. When donor authorizes the removal of his organs *after his death*, the organs may be transplanted into the body of *any recipient*. However, such a consent becomes invalid if the next of kin (NOK) refuses to allow removal of organs for transplantation since the legal heir (NOK) is the owner of the body.
iii. If any donor authorizes the removal of his organs *before his death* to such recipient not being near-relative *by reason of affection or attachment towards the recipient*, the organs should not be removed and transplanted without prior approval of Authorization Committee.

The law made it legal:
- Not-so-close relatives who have stayed with the patient can donate organs, provided there is no commercial dealing.
- Swapping of organs between two unrelated families, if the organs of the respective willing 'near relative' donors are found medically incompatible for the intended recipients.

Regulation of hospitals conducting the removal, storage or transplantation of human organs
i. Hospital not registered under this Act should not be engaged in transplantation activities.
ii. Medical practitioner should not conduct transplantation at any unregistered place under this Act.
iii. The eyes and the ears may be removed at any place from dead body of any donor for therapeutic purposes by a doctor. Removal of eye can be done by a trained technician to facilitate eye donation.

The doctor is also prohibited from removal or transplantation of human organs for any purpose other than *therapeutic purposes*.

Offenses and Penalties

Punishment for doctor on removal of human organs without authority
i. Punishable with imprisonment for 10 years and fine up to ₹ 25 lakh.
ii. Removal of his name from the register of State Medical Council for a period of 3 years for the 1st offense and permanently for the subsequent offense.

Punishment for commercial dealings in human organs: Punishable with imprisonment for a term from 5 to 10 years and fine of ₹ 20 lakh to 1 crore.

---
* Spouse, son, daughter, father, mother, brother or sister, grandparents, grandchildren, uncles and aunts are considered near-relatives.

Duties of the Medical Practitioner Regarding Organ Transplantation

I. In case of *live donation*, the doctor should satisfy himself before removing an organ from the donor that:
   i. Donor has given his authorization.
   ii. Donor is in proper state of health and fit to donate the organ.
   iii. Donor is a near-relative of the recipient and sign a certificate after carrying out HLA and/or DNA testing on donor and recipient.
   iv. In case recipient is a spouse of donor, record the statements of both and sign a certificate.
   v. In case of a donor not being a near-relative, the permission from the Authorization Committee has been obtained.
   vi. If a donor and/or recipient is/are foreign nationals, the approval of the Authorization Committee has been obtained.

II. In case of *cadaveric donation*, the doctor should satisfy himself that:
   i. Donor has authorized before his death, the removal of his organ for therapeutic purpose, in presence of two or more witnesses, at least one of whom is a near-relative.
   ii. Person lawfully in possession of dead body has signed a certificate as specified under the Act.

III. A doctor, before removing organ from a *brainstem dead* person, should satisfy that:
   i. Certificate regarding the brainstem dead from the board of medical experts is present. In case of non-availability of a neurosurgeon or a neurologist to certify brain death, an intensivist or anesthetist can be included on the medical board. It is mandatory for the ICU/treating medical staff to request relatives of a brain dead patient for organ donation.
   ii. In case of a person <18 years, a certificate has been signed by either of the parents of such person. Living organ/tissue donation by minors is not permitted, except on exceptional medical grounds and with prior approval of the Appropriate Authority and the Government concerned.

Authorization Committee

i. The medical practitioner involved in organ transplantation team should not be a member of the Authorization Committee.
ii. In case of foreigners, where the transplant is between a married couple, the Committee must evaluate the factum and duration of marriage and verify documents such as marriage certificate, or marriage photograph.
iii. Transplantation is not permitted if the recipient is a foreign national and donor is an Indian national, unless they are near-relatives.
iv. When the proposed donor and the recipient are not 'near-relatives', the Committee should evaluate that:
   a. there is no commercial transaction between the recipient and the donor.
   b. there is no middleman or tout involved.
   c. financial status of the donor and the recipient, evidence of their vocation and income for the previous three financial years.
   d. donor is not a drug addict.
   e. next of the kin of unrelated donor is interviewed regarding awareness about his/her intention to donate an organ and/or tissue, the authenticity of the link between the donor and the recipient and the reasons for donation.

Ethical Issues in Organ Donation

Justice for both the donor and the recipient must the grounding principle guiding transplant doctors.

1. **Setting safety standards:** The most prominent of concern is the potential harm to the donor. In living donations, the doctor is risking the life of a healthy person to save or improve the life of patient. There should not be any manipulation, coercion, significant pain, emotional suffering or morbidity. Complying with the principle of justice requires more attention to the vulnerable donor.
2. **Faith and personal values:** There should not be any breach of religious (Christianity supports donation whereas Jehovah's witnesses and Jews do not support donation) or personal values to satisfy organ demand.
3. **Transparency of rules for allocation of organs:** The recipient is also a vulnerable human component. Justice for the recipient relates to just allocation of the organ which is medically appropriate and ethically fair and acceptable. It should be based on time of waiting, immunological matching, medical urgency and age of the patient.
4. **Equality of access in transplant service:** Characteristics of recipients such as race, religion, gender and socioeconomic status or cognitive impairment should not have a primary place in the selection of recipients.
5. **Checking commercialization:** The gap between demand and supply of organs for transplant has yielded to organ trafficking, transplant tourism* and commercialism. It essential to prevent commercialization of organs and exploitation of the healthy poor.

> **NOTA BENE**
>
> ◆ Organ donation is considered in case of brain death (37 different tissues and organs can be donated including 6 life saving organs—kidneys, liver, heart, lungs, pancreas and intestine), since ventilator supplies necessary oxygen to these organs functioning, whereas tissues like cornea, heart valves, bone and skin can be harvested after cardiac death as well.

*** Transplant tourism** refers to patients traveling across the borders to be transplanted elsewhere, and it is widely condemned on ethical grounds.

- One set of corneas are given to two people needing sight. Heart valves are used in valve replacement surgery (common in children), skin grafts are used in burn patients, and bone, tendons and ligaments can be used in reconstructive surgeries.
- Organs and tissues that can be transplanted: liver, kidney, pancreas, pancreatic islet cells, small intestine, lung, heart, corneas, skin graft, blood vessels, bone and hand. Living donors can donate one kidney, portion of pancreas and part of liver.
- Maximum time an organ can be stored before transplant: heart: 3 h; liver and pancreas: 12 h; kidneys: 24 h; cornea: 2 weeks; middle ear, skin, bone marrow: 5 years; heart valve: 10 years.
- Maximum time for organ retrieval in case of normal death: skin: 3 h; cornea: 6 h.
- In Spain, England, Sweden, Luxembourg, Bulgaria, Austria and Singapore, every dead person can provide organs, unless the deceased person expressly rejected it (presumed consent). Nonetheless, doctors ask the family for permission.

FM 4.8
Describe the Consumer Protection Act, 2019; Medical Indemnity Insurance, Civil Litigations and Compensations.

■ THE CONSUMER PROTECTION ACT, 2019

Purpose: The Consumer Protection Act (CPA) was brought into existence for the protection of interests of the consumer and for settlement of consumer disputes within a limited time frame and with fewer expenses. This enables a patient to make a complaint to a redressal forum in respect of a defective (negligent) service, if the service has been paid for.

- The Consumer Protection Act, 2019 replaced the more than three decades old Consumer Protection Act, 1986.
- This Act is applicable on all the products and services, until or unless any product or service is especially debarred out of the scope of this Act by the Central Government.
- In the Act of 1986, medical service was not included within the ambit of services. However, in 1995, healthcare was included as 'service' in Sec. 2(1) (o) of CPA by the Supreme Court (IMA vs. VP Shanta & Ors). In the new Act too, 'healthcare' has not been included in the list of services enlisted under its definition [Sec. 2(42) of the 2019 Act]. This issue has also been clarified by the Bombay High court too.
- The legislators have taken 'healthcare' out of inclusion list, but has not included in the exclusion list. The CPA 2019 defines services as '*but not limited to*' before listing the categories of services which means that healthcare can be included under this definition.

Salient Features

Central Consumer Protection Authority (CCPA): The Act proposes the establishment of CCPA to address issues related to consumer rights, unfair trade practices, misleading advertisements and impose penalties for selling faulty and fake products.

- **Unfair trade practices:** Sharing of personal information given by the consumer in confidence is considered unfair trade practices, unless such disclosure is made in accordance with the provisions of any other law or in public interest.

E-filing of complaints: The consumer can file complaints with the jurisdictional consumer forum located at the place of residence/work of the consumer. It also enables the consumer to file complaints electronically and for hearing and/or examining parties through video-conferencing.

Mediation: There is a provision for settlement of disputes by way of mediation at the stage of complaint or at any later stage, if acceptable to both parties. In the event of failure to settle the dispute, the respective commissions shall continue to adjudicate the dispute.

Redressal Agencies (Flowchart 4.1)

It is established at three different levels:
i. **District Commission** consisting of President and not less than 2 members appointed by the State government in consultation with the Central government, situated in each district of the State.
ii. **State Commission** consisting of President and not less than 2 members appointed by the State government in consultation with the Central government, situated in the capital of each State.
iii. **National Commission** is the apex consumer body consisting of President and not less than 4 members appointed by Central government, situated in New Delhi and run by the Central Government.

Experts to assist National Commission or State Commission: Provision has been made for experts in case there is an application by a complainant for an opinion that involves the larger interest of consumers.

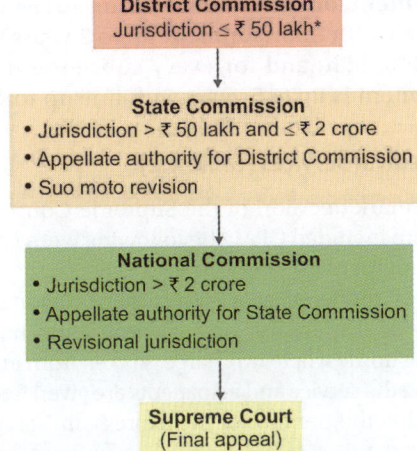

Flowchart 4.1: Structure of consumer commissions

*The pecuniary jurisdiction is determined based on the value of goods and services paid and not on the basis of compensation sought for.

Limitation Period

The District, State, and National Commissions will not admit a complaint, unless it is filed within 2 years from the date of occurrence of the cause of action.

> **NOTA BENE**
>
> - **Discover rule (discovery of harm)** states that the statute of limitations starts to run when the patient discovers or reasonably should discover the injury. The purpose of this rule is to give patients the right to file a lawsuit after the standard statute of limitations expired, when they might not have known (or might not have had reason to suspect) that they were harmed by a doctor's medical negligence.
> - In *VN Shrikhande vs. Anita Sena Fernandes (ASF)*: ASF, a nurse by profession underwent open cholecystectomy. She continued experiencing pain for 9 years since a gauge was left in her abdomen. She underwent a second surgery to remove the gauge. Charges for negligence and compensation of ₹50 lakhs was demanded by the petitioner. The Supreme Court rejected the case on limitation grounds while highlighting the Discovery Rule is not applicable in this case due to the reason that she should have consulted the doctor after the surgery if she was experiencing pain and cannot claim the compensation after a period of 9 years (SC/0868/2010).

Appeals

- Any appeal against the order of the District Commission or the State Commission under this Act must be filed within 45 days of the order.
- Any person who is aggrieved by an order of the National Commission has a right to appeal to the Supreme Court (appellate authority) within a period of 30 days from date of the order.

Offenses and Penalties

- **Penalty for noncompliance of direction of Central Authority:** Punished with imprisonment up to 6 months with/with fine up to ₹20 lakh.
- **Punishment for false or misleading advertisement:** Punished with imprisonment up to 2 years with fine up to ₹10 lakh; and for every subsequent offense, punishment is up to 5 years with fine up to ₹50 lakh.

CPA and Medical Services (Table 4.2)

In the landmark decision of the Supreme Court, medical services were included CPA. The following were concluded from the judgment:
i. Services rendered at a government hospital, health center or dispensary, non-governmental hospital or nursing home where no charge is taken from any person availing the service and all patients are given free service, is outside the purview of the expression 'service'.

TABLE 4.2: Arguments against/for CPA

Arguments against CPA	Arguments for CPA
There are Civil Courts, hence, no need of Consumer Courts	Civil courts have failed in delivery of justice at fewer expenses
The cases are hurried through because of time limits	Cases are disposed of speedily (within 90 days). Frivolous adjournments are not allowed to prevent the delay
As there is no court fee, any one can appeal, increasing the litigation and wasting valuable time and energy of the physician	Complainant is not required to pay court fee. So, even a poor victim of professional negligence can get compensation
No doctor would take risky cases for fear of litigation	All principles of natural justice are followed, like in Civil Courts
As there is no scope for testimony by medical experts, there is very likelihood of the justice being miscarried (in District Commission)	Both parties can produce their own evidence, lawyer and expert
Deterioration of the doctor-patient relationship. Doctors would resort to defensive medicine, leading to increase in the cost of healthcare	It is the consumer's choice to go to Consumer or Civil Court; once case is decided by consumer court, doctor cannot be punished for the same offense by a Civil Court

ii. The medical services delivered on payment basis fall within 'service' as defined in Sec. 2 (1) (o) of the Act of 1986.*
iii. Similarly, hospital and nursing homes, which provide free service to some patients who cannot afford to pay, and charges are required to be paid by persons who are in a position to pay, are covered under this Act.
iv. When a person has an insurance policy for medical treatment and all charges are borne by insurance company, the service rendered by a doctor would not be free of charge.

Further, this judgment concedes that the summary procedure prescribed by the CPA would suit only glaring cases of negligence, and in complaints involving complicated issues requiring recording of the evidence of experts, the complainant can be asked to approach the civil courts.

FM 4.21

Describe Medical Indemnity Insurance.

MEDICAL INDEMNITY INSURANCE

Professional indemnity is a contract under which the insurance company agrees, in return for the payment of premiums, to indemnify (cover) the insured doctor as a result of his claimed professional negligence.

---

* The Bombay High Court held that mere repeal of the 1986 Act by 2019 Act would not result in exclusion of 'healthcare' services from the definition of the term 'service'. Services rendered by doctors in lieu of fees/charges are under the purview of the 2019 Act.

Objectives of Medical Indemnity Insurance
  i. To look after and protect the professional interests of the insured doctor.
  ii. To arrange, conduct and pay for the defense of such doctor.
  iii. To arrange all other professional assistance including pre-litigation advice.

This insurance covers doctors against civil liabilities arising out of wrong treatments, mishaps or mistakes. It pays the cost of litigation, court fees, settlements, loss of documents, breach of confidentiality, defamation, etc.

> **FM 4.8, 13.2**
> - Describe the Workman's Compensation Act & ESI Act.
> - Describe medico-legal aspects of poisoning in Workman's Compensation Act.

■ THE WORKMEN'S COMPENSATION ACT, 1923

This Act provides for the payment of compensation to workmen for injuries sustained by them in an accident, arising out of and in the course of employment.
- This Act is applicable to establishments with ≤20 workers.
- This Act has been amended and called the **Employee's Compensation (Amendment) Act, 2017.**
- If a workman is killed, his dependants will be entitled to compensation for his death.
- The amount of compensation depends upon whether the injury has caused death, permanent total disablement or permanent partial disablement.
- The employer is liable to compensate the employee if:
  a. The injury is caused due to an accident in the course of employment.
  b. The employee contracts any occupational disease during the course of employment.
- The employer is not liable to pay compensation:
  a. If an injury does not cause total or partial disability for a period of >3 days.
  b. If any injury results in death or permanent total disablement caused by an accident, when at the time of sustaining the injury, the workman was under the influence of drink or drugs or willfully disregarded or removed any safety guard or other device provided for his safety.

Disablement is loss of earning capacity of an employee due to an injury.
The Act classifies disablement into two categories: Partial (loss of thumb/fingers, partial loss of vision, etc.) and total disablement (loss or amputation of hand and foot, permanent loss of vision or hearing, etc.).

Occupational diseases occurring during the course of employment due to exposure which includes occupational poisoning, bronchiectasis, asbestosis, asthma, cataract, and infectious diseases.

Duties of a Doctor
1. Assess the degree of disablement of the employee, whether partial or total.
2. Estimate the percentage in case of permanent partial disablement.
3. Regular checkups for the diagnosis and prevention of occupational diseases.
4. Establishing a causal relationship between injury and malignancy according to Ewing's postulates.
5. Maintenance of records for any future litigation against the employer.

Workman's Compensation Act and Poisoning
- Those who suffer from poisoning that were a result of their job is covered by the Act. If it is proven that the poisoning resulted from working, several benefits may be available. These benefits may include compensation for medical expenses, vocational and physical rehabilitation, wage losses, and more.
- The following poisons/toxins are implicated as causative agents under this Act—heavy metals like mercury, lead, arsenic, cadmium and manganese; benzene, bichromates, carbon disulfide, chromic acid, halogenated hydrocarbons, nitrous fumes, organophosphates and phosphorous.

■ EMPLOYEES' STATE INSURANCE (ESI) ACT, 1948

An autonomous corporation, Employees' State Insurance Corporation (ESIC) was established by ESI Act by the government. Employees' State Insurance (ESI) is a self-financing social security and health insurance scheme for Indian workers.
- The Act provides for medical, cash, maternity, disability and dependent benefits to the insured persons funded by the contributions made by the employers and the employees.
- This is applicable to establishment employing ≥10 employees.
- The Act covers employees with salary up to ₹ 21,000 (from Jan 2017).

Objectives: Its main aim is to provide economic security to people who work in certain factories and establishments in contingency such as illness, maternity, sickness or other health hazards due to exposure to employment injury or occupational hazard.
- The employees registered under it are entitled to medical treatment for themselves and their dependents, unemployment cash benefit and maternity benefit in case of women employees.
- In case of employment-related disablement or death, there is provision for a disablement benefit and a family pension respectively.

ESIC also runs medical and nursing colleges in some ESI hospitals across India. These colleges admit students on the basis of marks obtained in the competitive examinations conducted at the central level (NEET-UG).

> **FM 3.13**
> Describe the relevant provisions of POCSO Act related to medical care and police information.

THE PROTECTION OF CHILDREN FROM SEXUAL OFFENSES (POCSO) ACT, 2012

- The POCSO Act, 2012 (amended in 2019) has been drafted to strengthen the legal provisions for the protection of children from offenses, such as sexual assault, sexual harassment and child pornography.
- The POCSO Act defines a child as any person below the age of 18 years and provides protection to all children (both males and females—*the Act is gender neutral*, unlike the IPCs) under the age of 18 years from sexual abuse.
- The crimes and cases under this Act are nonbailable.

Offenses and Punishments (Flowchart 4.2)

1. **Penetrative sexual assault:** A person is said to commit 'penetrative sexual assault' if he:
   a. Penetrates his penis to any extent, into the vagina, mouth, urethra or anus of a child or makes the child to do so with him or any other person; or
   b. Inserts any object or a part of the body (not being his penis) to any extent, into the vagina, urethra or anus of a child or makes the child to do so with him or any other person; or
   c. Manipulates any part of the body of the child so as to cause penetration into the vagina, urethra, anus or any part of body of the child or makes the child to do so with him or any other person; or
   d. Applies his mouth to the penis, vagina, anus, urethra of the child or makes the child to do so to him or any other person.

   Punishment

Offense	Punishment
For penetrative sexual assault on a child <16 years of age	Imprisonment for 20 years which may extend for the remainder of natural life + fine
For penetrative sexual assault on a child between 16 and 18 years of age	Imprisonment for 10 years which may extend for the remainder of natural life + fine
For aggravated penetrative sexual assault	Rigorous imprisonment for 20 years which may extend to a life sentence + fine or death sentence

2. **Sexual assault:** Any physical contact with sexual intent but without penetration like touching the vagina, penis, anus or breast of the child or making the child touch the vagina, penis, anus or breast of such person or any other person.
   Punishment: Imprisonment for ≥3–5 years and fine.
   For aggravated sexual assault: Imprisonment for ≥5–7 years and fine.

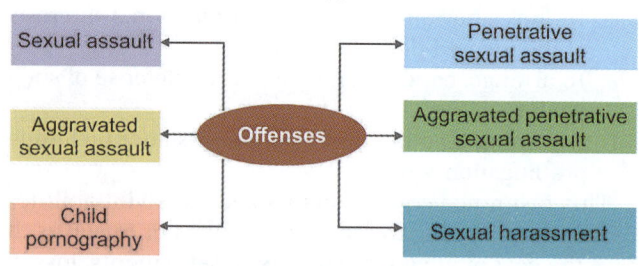

Flowchart 4.2: Types of offenses

3. **Sexual harassment of the child:** It is considered sexual harassment when a person with sexual intent:
   a. Utters any word/sound, or makes any gesture or exhibits any object or part of body with the intention to be heard or seen by the child; or
   b. Makes a child exhibit her body or any part of her body, so as it is seen by the person or any other person; or
   c. Shows any object to a child in any form or media for pornographic purposes; or
   d. Repeatedly or constantly follows or watches or contacts a child either directly or through electronic, digital or any other means; or
   e. Threatens to use, in any form of media, a real or fabricated depiction through electronic, film or digital or any other mode, of involvement of the child in a sexual act; or
   f. Entices a child for pornographic purposes.
   Punishment: Imprisonment for up to 3 years and fine.

4. **Use of child for pornographic purposes:** A person is guilty of the offense if he uses a child in any form of media, for the purposes of sexual gratification, which includes:
   a. Representation of the sexual organs of a child; or
   b. Usage of a child engaged in real or simulated sexual acts (with or without penetration); or
   c. Indecent or obscene representation of a child.
   Punishment: Imprisonment for 5 years and fine, and in subsequent conviction: 7 years and fine.

Salient Features (Flowchart 4.3)

- An offense is treated as "aggravated" when the abused child is mentally ill, below 12 years, or committed by a person in a position of trust or authority of child, such as a family member, member of security forces, police officer, public servant, etc.
- There is provision for punishment even in abetment or an attempt to commit the offenses defined in the Act.

CHAPTER 4: Acts Related to Medical Practice

Flowchart 4.3: Features of POCSO Act

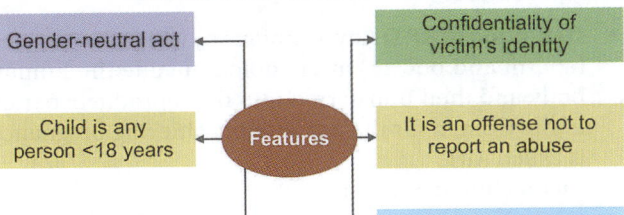

- The punishment for the attempt to commit is up to half the punishment prescribed for the commission of the offense.
- It is mandatory for healthcare providers to report to the police about the offense. Failure to report attracts punishment with imprisonment of up to 6 months with/without fine.
- It is also mandatory for police to register an FIR in all cases of child abuse.
- A child's statement can be recorded even at the child's residence or a place of her choice and should be preferably done by a female police officer not below the rank of Sub-Inspector (if the victim is a female).
- The child's medical examination can be conducted even prior to registration of an FIR. This discretion is left up to the Investigation Officer (IO). The IO has to get the child medically examined in a government or local hospital within 24 h of receiving information about the offense. This is done with the consent of the child or parent or a competent person whom the child trusts and in their presence.
- The police are also required to bring the matter to the attention of the Child Welfare Committee (CWC) within 24 h of receiving the report and should also indicate if the child is in need of care and protection; and steps taken by them in this regard.
- For speedy trial, the evidence of the child has to be recorded within a period of 30 days. The Special Court has to complete the trial within 1 year.
- There is provision for relief and rehabilitation of a child. The child must be compensated for physical and psychological trauma, and financial loss.
- The burden of proof is shifted on the accused, keeping in view the vulnerability and innocence of children, and following the principle of "guilty until proven innocent".
- To prevent misuse of the law, punishment is given for false complaints or false information with malicious intent.
- The media is barred from disclosing the identity of the child without the permission of the Special Court. The punishment for breaching this provision is imprisonment from 6 months to 1 year.

FM 3.16
Describe and discuss histories of gender and sexuality-based (sexual orientation) identities and rights in India.

THE TRANSGENDER PERSONS (PROTECTION OF RIGHTS) ACT, 2019

This Act has been implemented with the objective to provide for protection of rights of transgender people, their welfare, and other related matters. This Act was passed after years of struggle put by these deprived people **(Table 4.3)**.

Definitions

- **Transgender:** A person whose gender does not match with the gender assigned to that person at birth. It includes trans-person with intersex variations, gender-queer and person having such socio-cultural identities as *kinnar, hijra, aaravani* and *jogta*.
    - It is irrespective of whether they had undergone sex reassignment surgery or hormone therapy or any other such therapy.
    - This Act *does not cover gay, lesbians, or bisexuals*.
- **Intersex:** A person who at birth shows variation in his or her primary sexual characteristics, chromosomes or hormones from normal standard of male or female body.

TABLE 4.3: Timeline of various developments concerning gender and sexual identities

Year	Developments
1226-1526	Hijra community evolved and gained recognition in the society
1861	The British Raj brought in the IPC and introduced Sec 377 IPC banning homosexual practices
1871	Hijras were declared 'Criminal tribe' for not complying with British Raj and homosexuality was one of the reasons under Criminal Tribes Act 1871
1981	All-India Hijra Conference brought together 50,000 Hijras who traveled to Agra to fight for their rights
1990	Ashok Row Kavi, founded India's first magazine for queer men 'Bombay Dost'
2006	Raj Rao founded the Queer Studies Circle at Pune University and proposed to offer courses on LGBTQ+ literature at university level
2009	Election Commission instructed that the format of the registration forms to include an option of "others" for the transsexual people
2014	SC recognized hijras, eunuchs, and intersex people as a "third gender" (National Legal Services Authority vs. Union of India)
2015	The Rights of Transgender Persons Bill passed by the Rajya Sabha
2019	The Transgender Persons Act 2019 was enacted for protection of rights of transgender persons

- **Trans-male:** By birth female → by puberty time → starts showing male characteristics (ambiguous primary sexual characteristics + secondary sexual characters) → so transformed in to male (like) → trans-male.
- **Trans-female:** By birth male → by puberty time → starts showing female characteristics (ambiguous primary sexual characteristics + secondary sexual characters) → so transformed in to female (like) → trans-female.

Rights of Transgender Persons

- **Prohibition against discrimination** in relation to opportunities for education, job, healthcare services, and access to services, etc. It further reinforces transgender persons' right of movement, right to property and holding of public or private office.
- **Right to be recognized as transgender:** Every person has a right to be recognized as a transgender.
    - **Certificate of identity:** Right to self-perceived gender identity from the District Magistrate, without the requirement of any medical or physical examination. It further provides that a person undergoing surgery for change of gender to either male or female may make an application for issuance of a revised certificate indicating change in gender.
- **Right of residence:** No transgender person shall be separated from parents or immediate family on the ground of being a transgender.
- **Healthcare:** The Act also seeks to provide rights of health facilities to transgender persons including separate HIV surveillance centers, and sex reassignment surgeries.
    - It also states that the government shall review medical curriculum to address health issues of transgender persons, facilitate access to hospitals and other healthcare centers; and provide comprehensive medical insurance schemes for them.
- **Offenses and penalties:** Offenses, such as indulging transgender persons in forced or bonded labor or denial of access to public places; physical, emotional or sexual abuse; or other offenses committed under the provisions the Act are punishable with imprisonment for 6 months to 2 years along with fine.

FM 3.26
Discuss the national guidelines for accreditation, supervision and regulation of ART clinics in India.

THE ASSISTED REPRODUCTIVE TECHNOLOGY (REGULATION) ACT, 2021

The Assisted Reproductive Technology (ART) Act was enacted in 2021 to regulate the ART clinics, to provide ethical guidelines to ART clinics and to prevent misuse of ART services by ART clinics.

Salient Features

- **Definition of ART:** Any technique by which the gametes (sperm and oocyte) are handled outside the human body and then transferred into the reproductive tract of the women for the purpose of achieving pregnancy is called ART.
- ART techniques include:
    a. Artificial insemination
    b. IVF-ET (in vitro fertilization and embryo transfer)—zygote intrafallopian transfer (ZIFT) and gamete intrafallopian transfer (GIFT)
    c. Intracytoplasmic sperm injection (ICSI)
    d. Surrogacy
- **Qualifications of doctor:** The doctor performing ART services should have MD or DNB degree in Obs & Gyne. An MBBS doctor working in an ART clinic should have at least performed 50 oocyte retrieval procedures independently.
- **Commissioning couple** (intending couple): An infertile married couple opting for ART services.
- **Intending woman:** A divorcee who is currently not married or a widow opting for ART services.
- **Age limit of intending couple/woman**
    - The husband should be between 21-55 years.
    - The wife/intending woman should be between 21-50 years.
- **Donors and age limit of donors**
    - Any healthy married or unmarried male Indian can donate sperms. His age limit should be 21-55 years.
    - Any healthy married or unmarried female Indian can donate oocytes. Her age limit should be 23-35 years.
- **Number of donation:** Oocyte donor can donate only once in her lifetime. There is no restriction for the sperm donors. However, the semen of one donor can be used only to one intending couple or intending woman.
- The semen of one donor can be used for 1 couple or woman until that ART cycle gets completed. Mixing of semen of 2 donors is not allowed. Mixing of husband's semen with donor's semen is allowed. Donor's blood group must be same as husband's blood group.
- **Confidentiality:** The couple/woman should not know who the donor is and vice versa. This responsibility of maintaining confidentiality is the duty of ART clinic. Disclosure of the donor's identity is to be made only when the court asks for it.
- **Legitimacy of the child:** A child born through ART is considered legitimate and can inherit all rights like that of a naturally born child.
- **Consent:** In artificial insemination by husband (AIH), consent should be taken from both husband and wife. In artificial insemination by donor (AID), consent should be taken from:
    a. Husband, wife and the donor (if single) or
    b. Husband, wife, the donor and the donor's wife.

CHAPTER 4 : Acts Related to Medical Practice

c. Intending woman and donor (if the donor is single)
d. Intending woman, donor and donor's wife
- **Storage of gametes:** They can be stored only upto a period of 10 years. After that, they must be discarded.
- **Commercial dealings outside India:** Gametes of Indian donors should not be supplied outside India for any purpose by ART clinics or banks.
- Sex selection should not be done while handling gametes (except for those clauses mentioned as exceptions in PCPNDT Act).
- ART clinics should not make advertisements to attract couples/women for ART services or use agents to procure donors.
- **Maintenance of records:** Should maintain the registers for a period of 10 years and send data of the couples/women and donors details to the national registry.
- **Punishments:** Contravening any rules of this Act will lead to imprisonment up to 7 years with fine of ₹ 10-25 lakh.

THE SURROGACY ACT 2021
The Surrogacy Act 2021 was enacted to regulate and lay down rules for the practice of surrogacy by surrogacy clinics in India.

Definitions
- *Surrogacy* is a practice in which a woman agrees to carry and give birth to a child for a married couple or intending woman with the intention of giving up the child after its birth.
- *Surrogate mother* is a woman who agrees to carry and give birth to a child for a married couple or intending woman with the intention of giving up the child after its birth.

Types of Surrogacy
a. **Gestational surrogacy:** The gametes of an intending couple are fertilized in vitro and then transferred into the uterus of the surrogate mother.
b. **Biological surrogacy:** The oocyte of the surrogate mother is fertilized with the spermatozoa of the husband of the intending couple.
c. **Commercial surrogacy:** The surrogate mother is paid separate money for agreeing to carry a child along with the money for all the medical expenses during her pregnancy.
d. **Altruistic surrogacy:** The surrogate is not paid any separate money for agreeing to carry a child. Instead, she is paid money only for her medical expenses during her pregnancy. She is also given a medical insurance cover for a period of pregnancy and 3 years postdelivery.
  - In India, only gestational altruistic surrogacy is allowed. Biological or commercial surrogacy is not allowed.
- **Age limit of intending couple/woman**
  a. Husband should be between 26-55 years.
  b. Wife should be above between 23-50 years.
  c. Age limit of intending woman should be between 35-45 years to avail surrogacy service.
  - Only Indian intending couples and intending women can be allowed to avail surrogacy. The surrogate mother should also be of Indian origin.
- **Characteristics of surrogate:** A woman can offer her service to become a surrogate only once in her life. A surrogate mother should preferably be a married woman having a child of her own and she should be between 25 to 35 years. In some cases, even an unmarried woman of 25 to 35 years who is willing to offer her service as a surrogate, can be allowed if approved by the Board (the woman is referred to as 'willing woman'). The surrogate mother can or need not be genetically related to the intending couple or intending woman. Once a woman becomes a surrogate mother, then in future she cannot donate oocytes.
- The intending couple should not have any surviving child before availing surrogacy (either by natural birth or adoption).
- **Consent:** A written informed consent must be obtained from the surrogate mother, intending couple and intending woman. The surrogate mother is not allowed to withdraw her consent for surrogacy once she is pregnant.
- In some cases, if there is any need to terminate the pregnancy then it should fall under the ambit of MTP Act.
- A maximum of 3 attempts to achieve pregnancy in a surrogate mother is allowed.
- No sex selection is permitted during the process of in vitro fertilization prior to transferring the embryo into the uterus of the surrogate mother (except for those clauses mentioned as exceptions in PCPNDT Act).
- Unmarried Indian and foreign couples, LGBTQ and other third gender are not allowed to avail surrogacy services in India. Married foreign couples, foreign women or a foreign woman who never married in her life are not allowed to avail surrogacy services from Indian woman.
- **Confidentiality** not applicable since it is gestational surrogacy. Surrogate woman should give up all parental right over the child and should handover the child to the intending couple or intending woman.
- **Legitimacy of the child:** A child born through surrogacy is considered legitimate and can inherit all rights like that of a naturally born child.
- **Adultery or rape:** It does not amount to adultery or rape when done with consent as there is no sexual intercourse.
- **Qualification of the doctor:** The doctor should be having an MD or DNB degree in Obs & Gyne. An MBBS doctor working in any surrogacy clinic should have at least performed 50 oocyte retrieval procedures independently.
- Surrogacy clinics should not make advertisements to attract couples/women for surrogacy services and neither arrange for a surrogate woman nor should use agents to procure volunteers for surrogacy. The intending couples or intending women should arrange for their own surrogate woman.
- **Maintenance of records:** Surrogacy clinics should maintain the registers for a period of 25 years.
- **Punishments:** Whoever contravenes any rules of this Act will be punished with imprisonment up to 7 years with fine of ₹10-25 lakh.

FM 3.27
Discuss MTP (Amendment) Act, 2021 and methods of procuring MTP.

THE MEDICAL TERMINATION OF PREGNANCY (AMENDMENT) ACT, 2021

The Medical Termination of Pregnancy (MTP) Act, 1971 came into force on 1st April 1972, and amended in 2002 and recently in 2021 to provide for the termination of certain pregnancies by the registered medical practitioners (RMP) for protection and preservation of the lives of women.

Indications for Termination of Pregnancy (Fig. 4.1)

i. **Therapeutic:** In order to prevent injury to the physical health of pregnant woman. Indications are:
   - Cardiac disease (Grades III and IV)
   - Chronic glomerulonephritis

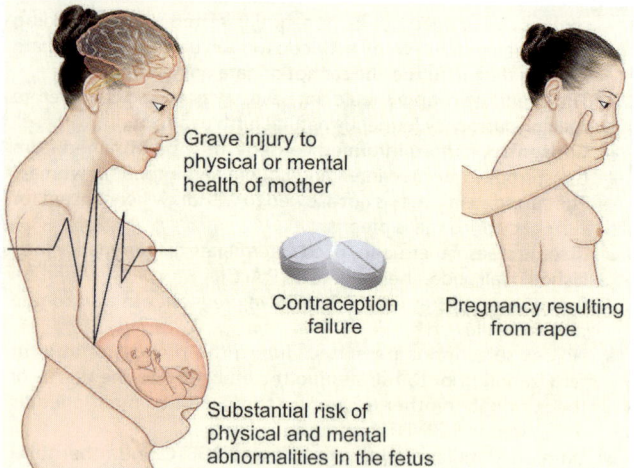

Fig. 4.1: Indications for MTP

- Intractable hyperemesis gravidarum
- Malignant hypertension
- Epilepsy/Insanity
- Cervical or breast carcinoma
- Diabetes with retinopathy
- Toxemia of pregnancy.

ii. **Eugenic:** Risk of the child being born with serious physical or mental abnormalities. Indications are:
- Mother exposed to teratogenic drugs (warfarin) or radiation exposure (>10 rads) in early pregnancy.
- German measles (Rubella), chickenpox, viral hepatitis or other viral infections, if contacted within 1st trimester.
- Structural (anencephaly), chromosomal (Down's syndrome) or genetic abnormalities of the fetus.
- Parents have inheritable mental condition or chromosomal abnormalities.

iii. **Socioeconomic:** Almost the sole indication, to prevent grave injury to the physical and mental health of the pregnant lady. Conditions include:
- Unplanned pregnancy with low socioeconomic status (80% of cases).
- Pregnancy as a result of failure of contraception used by the woman (married or unmarried) or her partner. All the pregnancies can be terminated using this criterion.

iv. **Humanitarian:** Pregnancy caused by rape.

MTP Act Rules (Flowchart 4.4)

Emergency cases: Pregnancy can be terminated by any RMP, even without required experience at any place, irrespective of duration of pregnancy, if it is necessary to save the life of pregnant woman.

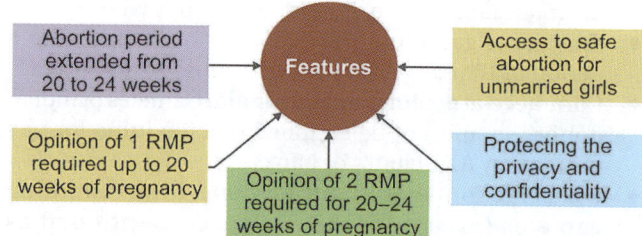

Flowchart 4.4: Features of MTP (Amendment Act) 2021

TABLE 4.4: Requirement of doctors as per the MTP (Amendment) Act 2021

Time since conception	MTP (Amendment) Act 2021
Up to 20 weeks	1 doctor¥
20–24 weeks	2 doctors for special categories of pregnant women
More than 24 weeks	Medical board, in case of substantial fetal abnormality
Anytime during the pregnancy	1 doctor, if necessary to save the pregnant woman's life

¥Doctor refers to RMP with experience/training in Obs & Gyne.

Length of pregnancy: Under MTP Act, pregnancy cannot be terminated after 20 weeks of pregnancy. However, there are some exceptions [as per the recent MTP (Amendment) Act 2021] **(Table 4.4):**
- The upper gestation limit of termination is up to 24 weeks for special categories of women. These include survivors of rape, victims of incest and other vulnerable women (like differently-abled women, minors), etc.
- Termination can be done beyond 24 weeks in cases of substantial fetal abnormalities diagnosed by a Medical Board*.

Opinion of only one doctor will be required up to 20 weeks of gestation and two doctors for termination of pregnancy of 20-24 weeks.

Consent: Consent of woman is mandatory, except when she is minor (<18 years) or mentally ill, where consent of the guardian is obtained. Consent of husband is not necessary.

Maintenance of register: The register with details of the patient is maintained for a period of 5 years, and professional secrecy should be maintained.

Place where MTP can be performed

MTPs can only be conducted at:
i. A hospital established or maintained by Government, or
ii. A place approved by Government or a District level Committee with the Chief Medical Officer or District Health Officer as the Chairperson of the said Committee.

---

* Medical board will comprise of (i) A gynecologist (ii) A pediatrician (iii) A radiologist (iv) Other members as may be specified by the State government.

Qualification and Experience of RMP using Medical and Surgical Methods

For RMP conducting MTP up to 12 weeks

The doctor should have the experience of assisting an RMP in conducting 25 cases of MTP, out of which at least 5 cases should have been performed independently, in an approved hospital by the Government.

For RMP conducting MTP beyond 12 weeks

The doctor should have either:
- Post-graduate degree/diploma in Obs & Gyne
- Six months of house surgery in Obs & Gyne, or
- One year or more in the practice of Obs & Gyne at any hospital.

Special provision for RMP conducting MTP up to 9 weeks using only medical methods [as per MTP (Amendment) Rules 2021)]
- Experience at any hospital for a period of not less than 3 months in the practice of Obs & Gyne; or
- Independently performed 10 cases of MTP by medical methods under the supervision of a RMP in a hospital/institution approved by the Government.

Offenses and Penalties

- **Contravention of the rules by the doctor:** Liable to be punished with rigorous imprisonment of 2–7 years. A person who willfully contravenes or fails to comply with the requirements of any regulation under this Act is punished with fine of ₹ 1000.
- It is a cognizable offense for which a police officer can arrest a doctor for violations without warrant.
- if he is a government servant, he will be liable to face disciplinary action including dismissal from service.
- The doctor may only reveal the details of a woman whose pregnancy has been terminated to a person authorized by the law. Violation is punishable with imprisonment up to 1 year with/without fine.

Methods to bring about abortion are given in Table 4.5.

TABLE 4.5: Methods of inducing abortion under MTP Act

1st trimester (up to 12 weeks)	2nd trimester (up to 20 weeks)
Medical	• **Dilatation and evacuation** (13–14 weeks)
• Mifepristone (RU-486)	• **Intrauterine instillation of hyperosmotic solution**
• Mifepristone and misoprostol (PGE$_1$)	i. Intra-amniotic hypertonic urea (40%), saline (20%)
• Methotrexate and misoprostol	ii. Extra-amniotic: Ethacrydine lactate, prostaglandins (PGE$_2$, PGF$_{2\alpha}$)
• Tamoxifen and misoprostol	• **Prostaglandins** (PGE$_1$, PGE$_2$, PGF$_{2\alpha}$): Intravaginally, intramuscularly or intra-amniotically
Surgical	• **Oxytocin infusion**
• Manual vacuum aspiration (MVA)	• **Hysterotomy**
• Dilatation and evacuation (D & E)	
• Suction evacuation and/or curettage	

NOTA BENE

- It is unrealistic to produce a definitive list of conditions that constitute 'serious physical or mental abnormalities' since accurate diagnostic techniques are as yet unavailable. Likewise, the consequences of abnormality are difficult to predict.
- In a landmark judgment, the Supreme Court struck down a high court order directing the MTP of an adult woman without her consent on grounds of 'mental retardation' (*parens patriae* jurisdiction). The MTP Act states that a guardian can make decisions on behalf of a 'mentally ill person', but this cannot be done on behalf of a person who is in a condition of 'mental retardation'. The SC observed that the State must respect the personal autonomy of a mentally retarded woman with regard to decisions about MTP.
- Complications are much less in legal abortions done before 8 weeks (5%), but it is about five times more in mid-trimester termination, irrespective of the method employed.
- Deaths during legal abortions are rare. Such deaths are due to:
   i. Hemorrhage and shock due to trauma, atonic uterus or incomplete abortion
   ii. Infection
   iii. Emboli (thrombotic, amniotic, or air)
   iv. Complications of anesthesia.
- Deaths by *method of abortion* in developed countries (in decreasing rate of occurrence):
   i. Hysterectomy/hysterotomy
   ii. Instillation methods (including saline)
   iii. Dilatation and evacuation
   iv. Dilatation and curettage.
- Curettage is the most common method of abortion used and results in the most deaths because of this, even though it has the lowest rate of death by type of procedure.
- Deaths due to hemorrhage and sepsis are complications of perforation of the uterus. While perforation is a recognized complication of any procedure involving instrumentation of the uterus, death due to sepsis/hemorrhage should not occur and strongly suggest the possibility of medical negligence.
- In India, contrary to the western countries, the mortality from saline method has been found be much higher as compared to termination by abdominal hysterectomy.

FM 3.21

Discuss Pre-conception and Prenatal Diagnostic Techniques (PCPNDT)-Prohibition of Sex Selection Act, 1994.

THE PRECONCEPTION AND PRENATAL DIAGNOSTIC TECHNIQUES ACT, 1994

The Government enacted the Prenatal Diagnostic Techniques (Regulation and Prevention of Misuse) Act,

1994 and renamed it after amendment in 2003 as 'The Pre-conception and Prenatal Diagnostic Techniques (Prohibition of Sex Selection) Act" [PCPNDT Act] in order to check female feticide.

- The Act provides for the **prohibition of sex selection**, before or after conception.
- 'Prenatal diagnostic procedures' means any gynecological, obstetrical or medical procedures, such as ultrasonography, fetoscopy, samples of amniotic fluid, chorionic villi, embryo, blood or any other tissue or fluid of a man, or of a woman before or after conception, for conducting any type of analysis or prenatal diagnostic tests for selection of sex before or after conception.
- 'Prenatal diagnostic test' means ultrasonography or any analysis of amniotic fluid (amniocentesis), fetal biopsy, chorionic villi, blood or any tissue or fluid of a pregnant woman or conceptus conducted to detect any abnormalities or diseases as given in clause 2.
- 'Prenatal diagnostic techniques' includes all prenatal diagnostic procedures and prenatal diagnostic tests.

Any medical practitioner or any other person should not conduct or aid in conducting any prenatal diagnostic techniques at a place other than a place registered under this Act.

An amendment in the Act allows medical practitioners (MBBS doctors) to conduct sonography tests on pregnant women, provided they undergo 6 months training imparted within the well-defined syllabus prescribed by the Act at accredited institutions.

Regulation of Prenatal Diagnostic Techniques

Clause 1: Any place including a registered genetic counseling center, laboratory or clinic should not be used for conducting prenatal diagnostic techniques except for the purpose given in clause 2 and after satisfying any of the conditions in clause 3.

Clause 2: Prenatal diagnostic techniques should be used for the detection of any of the following abnormalities:
  i. Chromosomal abnormalities
  ii. Genetic metabolic diseases
  iii. Hemoglobinopathies
  iv. Sex linked genetic diseases
  v. Congenital anomalies
  vi. Single gene disorder
  vii. Mental disability.

Clause 3: Prenatal diagnostic techniques should be used in pregnant women, if any of the following conditions are satisfied:
  i. Age ≥35 years.
  ii. Undergone two or more spontaneous abortions or fetal loss.
  iii. Has been exposed to potentially teratogenic agents, such as drugs, radiations, infections or chemicals.
  iv. The pregnant woman or her spouse has a family history of mental retardation or physical deformities, such as spasticity or any other genetic disease.

Written consent of pregnant woman and prohibition of communicating the sex of fetus

1. Prenatal diagnostic procedures should not be conducted unless:
   a. The doctor has explained all known side-effects and after-effects of such procedures to the patient.
   b. He has obtained her written consent in a language which she understands.
   c. A copy of her written consent obtained above is given to the pregnant woman.
2. The person conducting prenatal diagnostic procedures including ultrasonography *should not communicate* to the pregnant woman or her relative, the sex of the fetus by words, signs or in any other manner. The person should give a declaration on each report on ultrasonography/image scanning that he has neither detected nor disclosed the sex of fetus of the pregnant woman to anybody.*
3. The pregnant woman before undergoing ultrasonography/image scanning should declare that she does not want to know the sex of her fetus.

Maintenance and Preservation of Records

- All such registered genetic/ultrasound/imaging centers should maintain a register showing, in serial order, the names and addresses of the men or women given counseling, subjected to prenatal diagnostic procedures or tests, the names of their spouses or fathers and the date on which they first reported.
- All case related records, forms of consent, laboratory results, microscopic pictures, sonographic plates or slides should be preserved for a period of 2 years. In the event of any legal proceedings, the records are to be preserved till the final disposal of the case.
- In case the records are maintained on computer or other electronic equipment, a printed copy of the record should be taken and preserved after authentication by a person responsible for such record.

Offenses and Penalties

- Any person, organization, genetic counseling center/laboratory/clinic should not issue any advertisement in any manner regarding facilities of prenatal determination of sex.
- Any medical person who contravenes the provisions of this Act is punished with imprisonment up to 3 years and fine up to ₹ 10,000, and on any subsequent

---

* However, sex can be disclosed in sex-linked disorders found at ultrasound and in metabolic disorders found in amniocentesis or chorionic villus sampling, e.g., Alport syndrome or Fabry's disease (which affects only males).

conviction with imprisonment up to 5 years and fine up to ₹ 50,000. His name is removed from the register of the Council for a period of 5 years for the first offense and permanently for the subsequent offense.
- Any person who seeks the aid of genetic counseling laboratory/clinic or medical practitioner for purposes other than specified above, is punished with imprisonment up to 3 years and fine up to ₹ 50,000, and on any subsequent conviction with imprisonment up to 5 years and fine up to ₹ 1 lakh.
- Every offense under this Act is cognizable, non-bailable and non-compoundable.

Medico-legal Implications

1. Every incomplete/error in paperwork and sex determination has same punishment. There is equal punishment for any offense under the Act. Thus, incomplete/errors in paperwork and sex determination is treated at par.
2. Irregularities in record keeping are offenses under this Act.
3. It is a legal mandate to submit PCPNDT Form F along with ultrasound report, ultrasound images, gynecologist's OPD consultation sheet and identification documents of each patient as a 'physical printed hard copy' duly signed by a radiologist/sonologist. Form F has to be filled by the doctor and not by any clerk.
4. There is multiplication of records in form of patient register, form F and declaration copy to be given to patient.
5. Under the Act, the equipment found in unregistered centers is simply sealed and seized, and offense is registered. The machine becomes property of the government and can be de-sealed only by the court order.
6. Referral slip needs to be preserved under the Act.

> **NOTA BENE**
> - **Non-bailable:** The Magistrate has the power to refuse bail and remand a person to judicial or police custody.
> - **Non-compoundable:** Case (e.g., rape, 498-A) which cannot be withdrawn by the petitioner.

FM 3.21
Discuss Domestic Violence Act, 2005.

THE PROTECTION OF WOMEN FROM DOMESTIC VIOLENCE ACT, 2005

Salient Features

- The term 'domestic violence' covers all forms of physical, sexual, verbal, emotional and economic abuse that can harm, cause injury, endanger the health, safety, life, limb or well-being, either mental or physical of the aggrieved person.
- Aggrieved person is not just the wife, but a woman who is the sexual partner of the male irrespective of whether she is his legal wife or not. It also includes daughter, mother, sister, child (male or female), widowed relative, or any woman residing in the household who is related in some way to the respondent.
- 'Respondent' is any male, adult person who is, or has been, in a domestic relationship with the aggrieved person, that includes his mother, sister and other relatives; the case can also be filed against relatives of the husband or male partner.
- *Information to Protection Officer*: The information regarding any acts of domestic violence does not necessarily have to be lodged by the aggrieved party but by any person who has reason to believe that such an act has been or is being committed. Any medical officer, neighbors, social workers or relatives can all take initiative on behalf of the victim.
- *Duties of medical facilities*: If an aggrieved person or a Protection Officer or a service provider requests the medical practitioner to provide any medical aid to the victim, the doctor should provide medical aid to the aggrieved person in the medical facility.
- *Penalties*: The Magistrate can impose a penalty of up to 1 year of imprisonment with/without a fine of up to ₹ 20,000/- for an offense under this Act. The offense is also considered cognizable and nonbailable. The decision can be taken under the sole testimony of the aggrieved person; the court may conclude that an offense has been committed by the accused.
- The Act also allows the Magistrate to make the respondent pay compensation and damages for injuries including mental torture and emotional distress caused by acts of domestic violence.
- The Magistrate can impose monetary relief and monthly payments of maintenance. The respondent can also be made to meet the expenses incurred and losses suffered by the aggrieved person and can also cover loss of earnings, medical expenses, loss or damage to property.

FM 5.6
Describe the Mental Health Act, 2017 with special reference to admission, care and discharge of a mentally ill person.

THE MENTAL HEALTHCARE ACT, 2017

- This Act was passed in April 2017 and superseded the previous Mental Health Act, 1987.
- It provides for mental healthcare and services for persons with mental illness and to protect, promote and fulfill the rights of such persons during their mental healthcare (**Flowchart 4.5**).

Flowchart 4.5: Salient features of Mental Healthcare Act

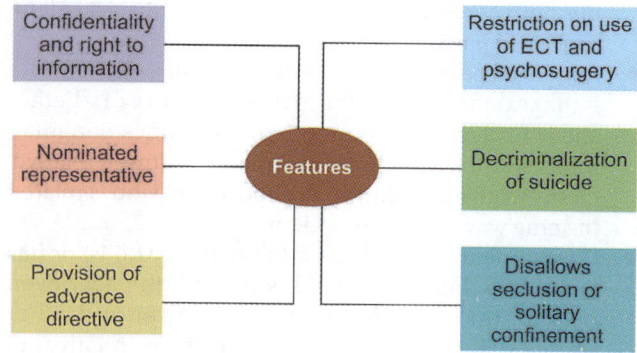

Definitions

- **Mental illness:** Disorder of thinking, mood, perception, orientation or memory that grossly impairs judgment, behavior, capacity to recognize reality or ability to meet the ordinary demands of life; mental conditions associated with the abuse of alcohol and drugs, but *does not include mental retardation*.
- **Mental healthcare:** Analysis and diagnosis of a person's mental condition and treatment, as well as care and rehabilitation for his mental illness.
- **Mental health establishment:** Any establishment (government, local authority, trust, private or public, corporation, organization, etc.) for care, treatment, convalescence and rehabilitation of persons with mental illness.
- **Independent patient admission:** Admission of person with mental illness to a mental health establishment, who has the capacity to make decisions or requires minimal support in making decisions.

Decriminalizing Attempt to Commit Suicide

- The Act decriminalized the attempt to commit suicide with the presumption that such persons to be under severe stress, and ensures that they are offered opportunities for treatment and rehabilitation from the government to reduce the risk of recurrence.
- Previously, under **Sec. 309 IPC**, it was punishable with up to 1 year simple imprisonment with/without fine.

Advance Directive

- Under this Act, any major person (legal guardian in case of minor) has the right to make an advance directive in writing, specifying the way the person wishes to be/not to be cared for and treated for a mental illness, and to appoint as his nominated representative to take decisions on his behalf when a medical practitioner deems him to lack capacity to decide.
- Every medical officer/psychiatrist should propose or give treatment in accordance to this valid advance directive.
- It can be overruled if an application is made in that behalf to the mental healthcare Board. In addition, advance directives do not apply in the case of emergency treatment.

Capacity to Make Mental Healthcare and Treatment Decisions

- The Act allows persons suffering from mental illness to make decisions regarding their health, given that they have the appropriate knowledge to do so.
- Every person, including a person with mental illness is supposed to have capacity to make decisions regarding his mental healthcare or treatment if he has ability to understand the information, appreciate the consequences of a decision on the treatment or admission, and communicate his decision by means of speech, expression or gesture.

Rights of Persons with Mental Illness

The Act aims to safeguard the rights of the people with mental illness, along with access to healthcare without discrimination from the government. Moreover, insurers are now bound to make provisions for medical insurance for the treatment of mental illness on the same basis as is available for the treatment of physical ailments.

- The person should be treated confidentially and have the rights to information about his illness, treatment and side effects.
- Any photograph or any other information relating to his mental illness should not be released to the media without his consent.
- A child <3 years of a woman receiving treatment should not be separated from her during her stay in such hospital.

Informed Consent

Any person with mental illness admitted under this Act should be provided treatment, after taking into account (as the case may be):

a. Informed consent of the patient
b. Advance directive (if any)
c. Informed consent of the person with the support from his nominated representative (capacity to consent reviewed every 7 days).

Voluntary Admission of Independent Patient (Flowchart 4.6)

- Any major person who considers having a mental illness and desires to be admitted may request the medical officer in-charge of the psychiatric hospital to be admitted as an independent patient for treatment.

CHAPTER 4 : Acts Related to Medical Practice

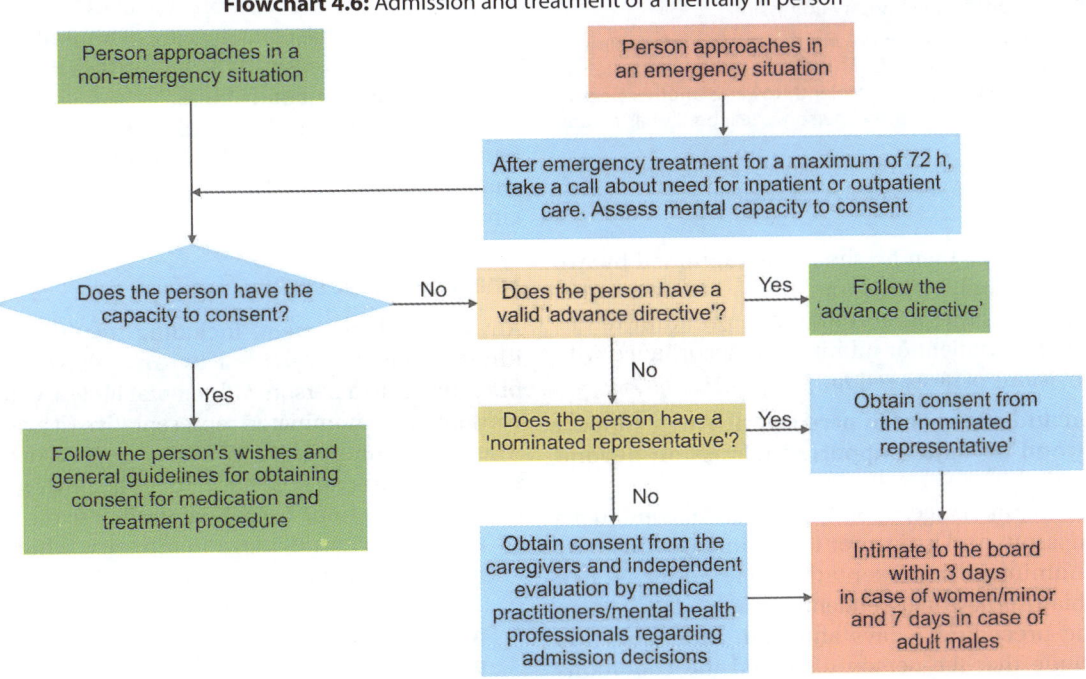

Flowchart 4.6: Admission and treatment of a mentally ill person

- The doctor should make an inquiry as deem fit, and if satisfied that the person requires treatment as an in-patient, he may admit such patient.

Admission of Minor

- In case of a minor, the nominated representative may make such request to the medical officer in-charge of a mental health establishment for admission.
- The doctor may admit such a minor, if two psychiatrists, or one psychiatrist and one mental health professional or one psychiatrist and one medical practitioner, have independently examined the minor on the day of admission or in the preceding 7 days and both independently conclude that he requires treatment as an in-patient.
- When a minor attains the age of 18 years, the doctor in-charge should classify him as an independent patient.
- In the case of minor girls, where the guardian is male, a female attendant is to be appointed by him to stay with her in the hospital for the entire duration of her admission.
- If the guardian requests discharge of the minor, then he should be discharged.
- Any admission of a minor to be informed by the in-charge to the concerned Board within a period of 72 h. Any admission of a minor beyond a period of 30 days should be immediately informed to the Board. The Board will review within a period of 7 days of being informed, of all admissions of beyond 30 days and subsequent 30 days.

Discharge of Voluntarily Independent Patient

- The medical officer in-charge should immediately discharge any person admitted voluntarily as independent patient on his request.
- The doctor may not discharge such a patient for 24 h for assessment if he is of the opinion that the patient is unable to understand the nature and purpose of his decisions and requires substantial support from his guardian, or for such conditions mentioned in the **Box 4.1**.
- After assessment, the person is either admitted as a supported patient or discharged from the establishment within 24 h.

Involuntary Institutionalization

This involuntary admission can be for a period of 30 days. It is only when this period is to be extended beyond the 30 days that the Board must confirm the admission.

Admission and treatment of persons with mental illness with high support needs up to 30 days (supported admission)

- The medical officer in-charge upon application by the nominated representative may admit such person, if the person has been independently examined on the day of admission or in the preceding 7 days, by a psychiatrist and a mental health professional/medical practitioner, and both independently conclude that the patient displayed the conditions mentioned in **Box 4.1**.
- The admission is for 30 days. If the doctor in-charge is of the opinion that the patient requires further treatment

> **Box 4.1** Provisions for involuntary admission
> a. Recently threatened/attempted or is threatening/attempting to cause bodily harm to himself; or
> b. Recently behaved/is behaving violently towards another person or has caused/is causing another person to fear bodily harm from him; or
> c. Recently shown/is showing an inability to care for himself to a degree that places the individual at risk of harm.

beyond 30 days, then he should be examined by two psychiatrists for his admission.
- After 30 days, the person may remain admitted as independent patient or admitted in accordance with the provisions of next section.

Admission and treatment of persons with high support needs beyond 30 days (supported admission beyond 30 days)
i. The doctor in-charge, upon application for continuous admission and treatment beyond 30 days by the nominated representative may admit, if two psychiatrists have independently examined the person in the preceding 7 days and both independently conclude that the person displayed the conditions mentioned **Box 4.1**; and
ii. Both psychiatrists, after taking into account an advance directive, if any, certify that admission is the least restrictive care option possible under the circumstances; and
iii. The person continues to remain ineligible to receive care and treatment as an independent patient.
- The doctor in-charge should report all admissions/readmission within 7 days to the concerned Board.
- The Board will within 21 days from the date of last admission/readmission permit such admission/readmission or order discharge.

Admitting Person with Mental Illness by Magistrate

a. When any person with mental illness or who may have a mental illness is brought before a Magistrate, he may order:
  - that the person is taken to a mental health establishment for assessment and treatment.
  - admission in a mental health establishment for ≤10 days to enable the doctor in-charge to carry out an assessment and plan for treatment, if any.
b. On completion of the period of assessment, the doctor in-charge is required to submit a report to the Magistrate, and dealt with in accordance with the provisions of this Act.

Duties of Police Officers in Respect of Persons with Mental Illness

The officer in-charge of a police station has a duty to take under protection any person (within the limits of the police station):

a. found wandering whom he believes has mental illness and is incapable of taking care of himself; or
b. whom he has reason to believe to be a risk to himself or others due to mental illness.

Such person should be taken to the nearest public health establishment within 24 h for assessment, and should not be detained in the police lock up/prison in any circumstances.

Emergency Treatment

Any medical treatment, including treatment for mental illness, may be provided by any registered medical practitioner to a person with mental illness, with informed consent of the nominated representative (if available), and where it is immediately necessary to prevent:
a. death or irreversible harm to his health; or
b. inflicting serious harm to himself or to others; or
c. causing serious damage to property, which is directly related to his mental illness
- This Act does not allow any medical officer or psychiatrist to use electroconvulsive therapy (ECT) as emergency treatment.
- The emergency treatment should be limited to 72 h (may extend up to 7 days in case of emergency/disaster declared by Government) or he has been assessed at a mental health establishment, whichever is earlier.

Prohibited Procedures

The Act has restricted the following procedures on any person with mental illness:
a. ECT without the use of muscle relaxants and anesthesia
b. ECT for minors (if necessary, only with informed consent of guardian and prior permission of the Board)
c. Sterilization of men or women, when such sterilization is intended as a treatment for mental illness
d. Chained in any manner or form whatsoever.

Restraints and Seclusion

a. A person with mental illness should not be subjected to seclusion or solitary confinement, and physical restraint may only be used when:
  - it is the only means available to prevent imminent and immediate harm to himself/others
  - it is authorized by the psychiatrist in-charge of the person's treatment.
b. Physical restraint should not to be used for a prolonged period than it is absolutely necessary.
c. The doctor in-charge is responsible for ensuring the method, nature of restraint, justification for its imposition and the duration, which is recorded in his medical notes.
d. The restraint should not be used as a form of punishment or merely on the ground of shortage of staff in such establishment.

e. The guardian should be informed of restraint within 24 h, and concerned Board monthly.
f. The patient under restraint should be kept in a place where he can cause no harm to himself/others and under regular supervision of the medical personnel.

Registration of Mental Health Establishment

Any person or organization should not establish or run a mental health establishment without being registered with the Authority under the provisions of this Act.

Offenses and Penalties

- Penalties for establishing mental health establishment without registration—fine ₹ 5000–50,000 for first contravention; fine ₹ 50,000 to ₹ 2 lakh for a second contravention, and fine ₹ 2–5 lakh for every subsequent contravention.
- Any health professional knowingly serves in mental health establishment not registered under this Act—fine of ₹ 25,000.
- Anyone contravening any of the provisions/rule/regulation is punished with imprisonment for up to 6 months with/without fine (up to ₹ 10,000) [first contravention]; and for any subsequent contravention—imprisonment for up to 2 years with/without fine (₹ 50,000 to ₹ 5 lakh).

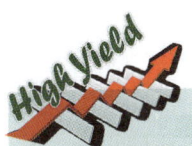

- **Human organ:** Any part of a human body consisting of a structured arrangement of tissues which, if wholly removed, cannot be replicated by the body.
- Transplantation of human Organs Act (THOA) is meant for using human organs for *therapeutic purposes*.
- Person ≥18 years of age may authorize in writing removal of organs for transplant before his death.
- Transplantation of bone marrow is outside the purview of THOA.
- The eyes and ears may be removed at any place from dead body of any donor for therapeutic purposes by a doctor.
- Brainstem death tests *should not* be performed by transplant surgeons, any doctor in the transplant team or a member of the Authorization Committee.
- In case of bodies sent for PM/pathological examination, competent person can give authorization, if such organ is not required for knowing the cause of death.
- Organs and tissues that can be transplanted: liver, kidney, pancreas, pancreatic islet cells, small intestine, lung, heart, corneas, skin graft, blood vessels, bone and hand.
- **Maximum time for cornea retrieval for transplantation:** 6 hours.
- **Punishment for doctor contravening the provisions of TOHA:** Imprisonment for 10 years and fine up to ₹ 25 lakh and penal erasure from SMC register for 3 years.
- **Apex body dealing with medical negligence cases:** National Consumer Commission.
- **Limitation period for filing a complaint under CPA:** 2 years.
- **Indications for termination of pregnancy under MTP Act:** Therapeutic, eugenic, humanitarian and socio-economic.
- The POCSO Act defines a child as any person below the age of 18 years and provides protection to all children (both males and females) under the age of 18 years from sexual abuse.
- There is no maternal age limit wherein MTP is not allowed.
- For MTP up to 20 weeks: single doctor opinion; 20–24 weeks: two doctors opinion is required.
- Pregnancy cannot be terminated beyond 20 weeks of pregnancy. Above 20 weeks, MTP only on therapeutic considerations, i.e., to save her life, special categories of women (victims of rape, incest etc) and substantial fetal abnormality.
- Consent of woman is mandatory, except when she is minor (<18 years) or mentally ill, where consent of the guardian is obtained. Consent of husband is not necessary.
- PCPNDT Act was enacted in order to check female feticide.
- Under the PCPNDT Act, there is prohibition of sex selection, before or after conception.

SECTION 1 : Jurisprudence and Forensic Medicine

- Prenatal diagnostic techniques include all prenatal diagnostic procedures and prenatal diagnostic tests (USG, fetoscopy or analysis of amniotic fluid, chorionic villi, blood).
- Written informed consent of pregnant woman is taken for any prenatal diagnostic techniques/procedures under the PCPNDT Act.
- Under the PCPNDT Act, doctor should not communicate the sex of fetus.
- **Punishment for doctor contravening the provisions of PCPNDT Act:** Imprisonment up to 3 years and fine up to ₹10,000 (offense is cognizable, non-bailable and non-compoundable).
- The Mental Healthcare Act 2017 decriminalized the attempt to commit suicide.
- Any independent voluntarily admitted patient in psychiatric hospital should be immediately discharged on his request.
- **Maximum period of stay under involuntary institutionalization:** 30 days.
- **Supported admission ≥30 days:** Doctor in-charge may admit such person (requested by nominated representative), if admission is advised by two psychiatrists independently.
- Magistrate can order admission in a mental health establishment for ≤10 days to enable the doctor in-charge to carry out an assessment and plan for treatment, if any.
- The doctor should not use ECT as emergency treatment.

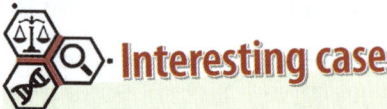

Interesting case

Negligence and Compensation (Case of Anuradha Saha, 1998)

Anuradha Saha, a US-based NRI consulted the doctor after developing skin rashes, which was not considered significant and was advised rest. When the rashes increased, the doctor prescribed Depomedrol injection (80 mg twice daily), a step which was later faulted by medical experts at the apex court. Instead of improving, her condition worsened rapidly after the administration of the steroids. She was admitted to the AMRI Hospital, Kolkata. As her condition did not improve, she was taken to a hospital in Mumbai in an air ambulance. There diagnosis of toxic epidermal necrolysis (TEN)* was made. She died of complications from steroid overdose after a month in May 1998.

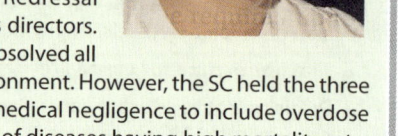

Kunal Saha, her husband filed criminal and civil cases against doctors and both hospitals for gross negligence. In March 1999, he filed a petition before the National Consumer Disputes Redressal Commission (NCDRC) demanding ₹ 77 crore from the three treating doctors, hospital and its directors. The case was dismissed by the NCDRC, but he moved the Supreme Court (SC). In 2009, the SC absolved all the doctors and the hospitals of criminal negligence in treatment, which spared them of imprisonment. However, the SC held the three doctors and the Kolkata hospital culpable to civil liability for medical negligence. It redefined medical negligence to include overdose of medicines, not informing patients about side-effects of drugs, not taking extra care in case of diseases having high mortality rate, and hospitals not providing amenities fundamental for patients.

In 2013, the SC held the hospital vicariously liable and directed the hospital and the three doctors to pay an amount of ₹ 5.96 crore as compensation. It was calculated to be ₹ 11.41 crore, as the court ordered that he was entitled to 6% interest on the compensation amount from 1999. The court directed that out of the total compensation amount, ₹ 10 lakh each to be paid by two doctors and ₹ 5 lakh by the other doctor. The rest of the amount along with the interest is to be paid by the hospital. It is called the 'Jackpot Judgment', as it is the highest penalty paid by any hospital in India till date.

---

* TEN is a rare life-threatening exfoliative skin disease characterized by widespread blistering detachment (necrolysis) leaving a tender glistening raw surface, mostly caused by reactions to drugs.

CHAPTER 5

Identification I

LEARNING OBJECTIVES

Must know
1. Identification, types, medico-legal importance
2. Corpus delicti
3. Cephalic index
4. Nuclear sexing, Barr body, Davidson body
5. Disorders of sexual development with examples
6. Klinefelter and Turner syndrome
7. Eruption of temporary and permanent teeth
8. Gustafson's method
9. Spacing of jaw, superadded and successional teeth, period of mixed dentition
10. Age estimation: Ossification of long bones
11. Fusion of skull sutures
12. Estimation of stature
13. Tattoo marks, scars, medico-legal importance
14. Medico-legal importance of age
15. Male and female—skull, pelvis and mandible (Diff.)
16. Age changes in mandible (Diff.)

Desirable to know
1. Stack, Boyde and Miles' method of age estimation
2. Age changes in symphysis pubis
3. Sexual development in adolescents

Definitions

- **Identification:** *Determination of the individuality of a person* based on certain physical characteristics.
- **Identity:** Set of characteristics that individualize a person.

It can be:
i. **Complete (absolute):** Absolute fixation of the individuality of a person.
ii. **Partial (incomplete):** Ascertainment of only some facts (e.g., race, sex, age or stature) about the identity, while the others remain unknown.

Identification is necessary in:
1. *Living persons* pertaining to:

Criminal cases	Civil cases
♦ Persons accused of assault, murder or rape	♦ Marriage
♦ Interchange of newborn babies in hospitals	♦ Passport/license
	♦ Inheritance
♦ Impersonation	♦ Insurance claim
♦ Absconding soldiers and criminals	♦ Missing persons
	♦ Disputed sex

2. *Dead people*
   i. In cases of fire, explosion and accidents.
   ii. When an unknown dead body is found on the road, fields, railway compartment or water.
   iii. In cases of decomposed body.
   iv. In cases of mutilated body.
   v. Skeleton.

Before identifying the patient in the court, the doctor should verify the identification marks noted by him.

FM 3.1
Define and describe corpus delicti.

CORPUS DELICTI

Corpus delicti ('body of offense') refers to the principle that it must be proven that a crime has actually occurred before a person can be convicted of committing the crime. In a charge of homicide, it includes:
i. Positive identification of the dead body (victim).
ii. Proof of its death by criminal act of accused.
- The term includes body of the victim, bullet or clothing showing marks of the weapon, spilled blood or photographs showing fatal injuries.
- The main part of corpus delicti is the establishment of identity of the body and infliction of violence in a particular way, at a particular time and place by the person or persons charged with crime and none other.

- The identification of a dead body and proof of corpus delicti is essential before a sentence is passed in murder trials, as unclaimed, decomposed bodies or portions of a dead body (such as a forearm or a leg) or bones are sometimes produced to support a false charge.

Identification Data

In living and dead both
1. Race and religion
2. Sex
3. Age
4. Teeth
5. General development and stature
6. Anthropometric measurements
7. Fingerprints, lip prints and footprints
8. External peculiarities, like scar or tattoo
9. Hair, blood, DNA
10. Personal effects: Clothes, pocket contents

In living only
1. Handwriting
2. Speech and voice
3. Gait, manner and habit
4. Memory and education

- Sex, age, ancestry and stature are primary characteristics of identification—they are unaltered even after death.
- Method of identification using biometric features includes fingerprints, hand geometry, face, voice, iris or retina scan, etc.
- Biochemical method of identification can be DNA analysis, bomb curve analysis, stable isotope analysis.

FM 3.1

Define and describe establishment of identity of living persons including race, religion, complexion, sex.

RACE AND RELIGION

Important in cases of mass disasters, e.g., in case of railway accidents or air crashes, when persons of different races are traveling together.

Race: Biological grouping within the human population classified according to genetically transmitted differences.

It is determined by:
i. **Clothing:** Traditional Indian dress is different from Western dress.
ii. **Complexion:** Skin is black in Negroes, brown in Indians and fair in Europeans (Caucasian).
iii. **Eye:** Indians have dark or brown iris, while Negroes have dark brown, and Europeans have blue or gray iris.
iv. **Hair:** Ethnic variations are discussed in Chapter 6. Indians have black, long and fine hair, which is rounder and thicker than Caucasians or Negroes.
v. **Skull: Cephalic Index** (identified by Swedish anatomist Anders Rezitus) *or index of breadth or cranial index* is the percentage of breadth to length in any skull.

$$CI = \frac{\text{Maximum transverse breadth of skull}}{\text{Maximum anteroposterior length of skull}} \times 100$$

Length and breadth are measured by calipers.
- It is useful anthropologically to find out racial difference from skull shape. Skull can be classified into three types based on cephalic index (CI)—dolichocephalic, mesaticephalic brachycephalic, **(Table 5.1)**. Another variant *hyperbrachycephalic* with very round or broad head (CI 85–89.9) can be seen among Kyushu of Japan and in Apert syndrome.
- Since, the Indian skull is Caucasian with few Negroid characters, we take the value for Europeans, i.e., 75–79.9 (mesaticephalic skull).
- CI is also useful in estimating the age of fetuses for legal and obstetrical reasons.

Difference between Caucasian, Mongolian and Negroid skull is given in **Diff. 5.1**.

vi. **The indices of long bones** may also help in identifying races, e.g., brachial index (radiohumeral index), intermembral index, humerofemoral index and the crural index (tibiofemoral index).

TABLE 5.1: Different types of skull based on cephalic index **(Figs. 5.1A and B)**

Type of skull	Cephalic index	Race
Dolichocephalic (long-headed)	70–74.9	Negroid (Aryans, Aborigines, Negroes)
Mesaticephalic (medium-headed)	75–79.9	Caucasoids (Europeans, Chinese, Indians)
Brachycephalic (short-headed)	80–84.9	Mongoloids (Mongolians, Native Americans)

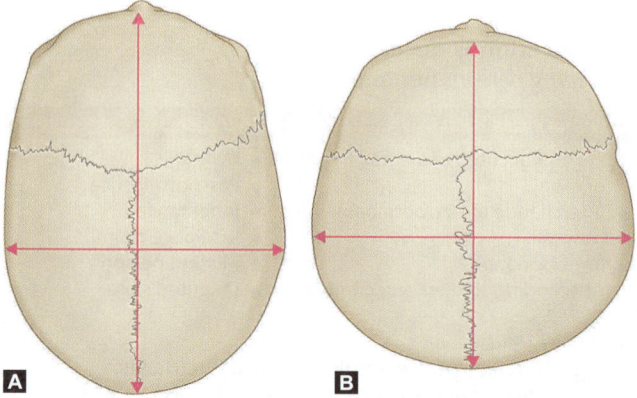

Figs. 5.1A and B: Cephalic index: (A) Dolichocephalic skull; (B) Brachycephalic skull

CHAPTER 5 : Identification I

DIFFERENTIATION 5.1: Caucasian, Mongolian and Negroid skull

S.No.	Feature	Caucasians	Mongols	Negroes
1.	Skull	Rounded	Square	Narrow and elongated
2.	Forehead	Raised	Inclined	Small and compressed
3.	Face	Straight lower face—orthognathism	Large and flattened, malar bones prominent	Jaw projecting—prognathism, malar bones prominent
4.	Orbits	Triangular	Small, round	Square
5.	Nasal opening	Narrow and elongated	Rounded	Broad
6.	Palate	Triangular	Rounded or horseshoe shaped	Rectangular
7.	Nasal index	<0.48	0.48–0.53	>0.53

> **NOTA BENE**
> - **Brachial index** = (Length of Radius/Length of Humerus) × 100
>   For Europeans: 74.5, Negroes: 78.5
> - **Crural index** = (Length of Tibia/Length of Femur) × 100
>   For Indians: 86.5, Negroes: 86.2, Europeans: 83.3
> - **Humerofemoral index** = (Length of Humerus/Length of Femur) × 100
>   For Europeans: 69, Negroes: 72.4
> - **Intermembral index** = (Length of Humerus + Radius/Length of Femur + Tibia) × 100
>   For Europeans: > 70, Negroes: < 70.5

> **NOTA BENE**
> **'Mongolian spots'**: These hyperpigmented spots or patches are most often found over the lumbosacral region of infants, and occur in people of different races (90% of Native Americans, 80% of Asians and 10% of whites) which help in racial identification.

 Identify this instrument. Mention its uses.

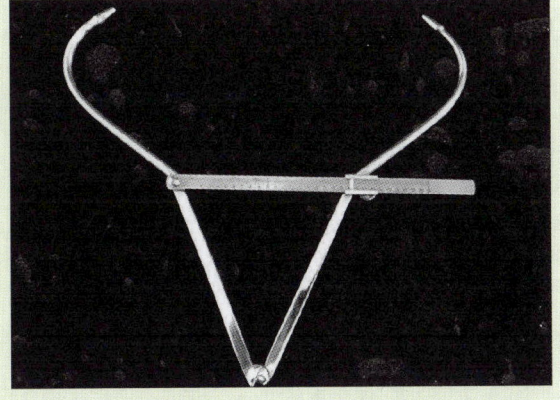

Religion

- *Hindu males* are not circumcised, may have sacred thread, necklace of wooden beads, caste marks on forehead, tuft of hair on back of the head and piercing of ear lobes.
- *Muslim males* are normally circumcised, have marks of corns and callosities on lateral aspect of knees and feet due to their posture during prayer.
- *Hindu females* put on saris, vermilion on head, silver toe ornaments, tattoo marks, nose ring aperture in left nostril and few openings for ear rings along the helix.
- *Muslim females* put on trousers, no vermilion mark, nose ring in the septum, several openings on the helix for ear rings and no tattoo marks.

SEX

- **Sex:** Biological term denoting the genetic, physiologic and anatomical characteristics of an individual, based on which we can identify ourselves into 'males' and 'females'.
- **Gender:** Sociological construct that denotes how an individual identifies according to social norms (social roles, position and behavior), based on which an individual exhibits 'masculine' or 'feminine' qualities. It is the sexual identity of an individual from birth to puberty and adulthood.*
- **Intersex:** Intermingling of sexual characters of either sex in one individual to a varying degree including the physical form, reproductive organs and sexual behavior.

> In normal cases, in the living:
> - **Most certain evidence of sex:** Possession of ovaries in females, and testes in males.
> - **Highly probable evidence of sex:** Possession of sexual structures, e.g., developed breasts and vagina in females, and male distribution of hair and penis in males.
> - **Presumptive evidence of sex:** Outward appearance of individual features, contours of face, clothes, voice and figure.

Reasons for Sex Determination

- *Identification in living*: Sex is important in any chain of identity data and determination of the individuality of a person.

---

*To identify whether an individual is 'male' or 'female', the correct terminology is 'sex verification tests' and not 'gender verification tests' or 'femininity testing'.

- *Participation in sports*: Sex segregation in sports is based on the long-term endogenous androgen exposure of men at puberty that lead to the physiological gap with women.
- For deciding whether an individual can *exercise certain civil rights* extended to one sex only.
- For deciding questions relating to legitimacy, divorce, paternity, marriage, impotence, rape and affiliation.

At present, there are three frequent circumstances wherein determination of sex has become necessary—sports, pre-employment and sex specific crimes. Routinely at birth, identifying biological sex of an individual is based on 'external genitalia' (*phenotype sex*), i.e., whether it is penis and scrotum (in males) or vulva and vagina (in females).

Identification of 'sex' of an individual may become problematic in:
  i. **Intersex:** They can be natural or acquired ('hijras' are castrated before puberty and 'zenanas' are castrated after puberty). They may have features resembling one sex and the internal gonads could be of other sex or of both sexes (true hermaphrodite).
  ii. **Transvestism:** It is the practice of wearing the clothes of the opposite gender.
  iii. **Transgender:** It is denoting or relating to an individual whose self-identity does not conform unambiguously to conventional notions of male or female gender. It is a state of one's gender identity or gender expression not matching one's assigned sex which may result in gender dysphoria.
  iv. **Transsexuals:** Individuals who have undergone sex change surgeries or sex reassignment (male-to-female or female-to-male) **(Figs. 5.2A and B)**.*
  v. **Concealed sex:** Individuals who hide their real sex for a motive by cross dressing.
  vi. **Advanced decomposition and skeleton:** Sex can be determined in decomposed body by identifying uterus or prostate, which resist putrefaction.

Identification of biological sex in concealed sex and transvestism can be easily done by physical examination, but difficulty arises in cases of ambiguous genitalia wherein the external genitalia are a combination of both sexes.

Sex Verification Tests

  i. *Physical morphology*: External examination is done to determine the sex **(Diff. 5.2)**.
  ii. *Nuclear sexing or sex chromatin or microscopic test*: Buccal epithelial cells or hair follicle cells are examined microscopically to detect the presence of 'Barr body'.
  iii. *Gonadal biopsy*: Detection of 'internal gonads and sex chromosomes' (*genotype sex*), i.e., the identification of testes and XY sex chromosomes (in males), or ovary and XX sex chromosomes (in females) is a *confirmatory method* of determining sex.
  iv. *Gene-based test*: Polymerase chain reaction (PCR) is used to detect SRY gene (sex-determining region of the Y-chromosome) and/or the DYZ1 region of Y chromosome which is diagnostic. SRY gene is expressed in a small group of somatic cells of the developing gonads, and it is responsible for the expression of a male-specific cell membrane component (the H-Y antigen) and induces them to become Sertoli cells.
  v. *Assay of testosterone levels* also helps in differentiating the sex of an individual. For females, they should have levels <10 nmol/l (lower than the lower limit of normal for male).

Usually, combinations of all these tests are carried out to determine the 'sex' of the individual.

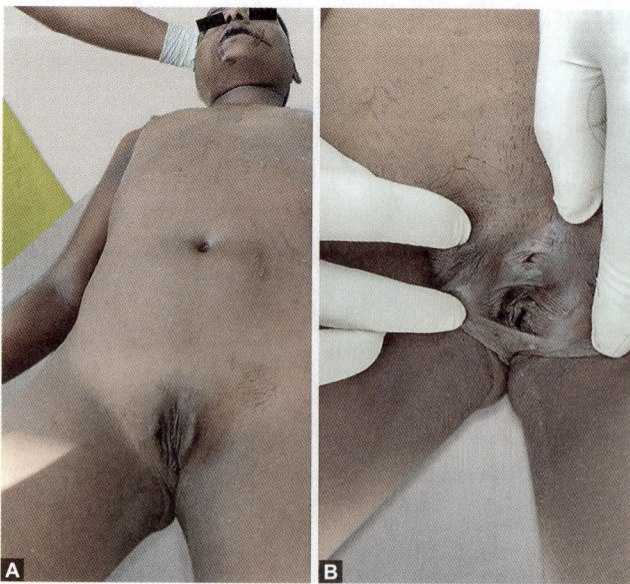

Figs. 5.2A and B: (A) Transexual/transgender; (B) Vaginal reconstruction

Nuclear Sexing

Definition: It is a method of sexing cells which may help in determining sex in doubtful cases, decomposed and mutilated bodies and fragmentary remains **(Table 5.2)**.

Histological Examination

  i. **Barr body (sex chromatin):** It is the condensed, inactive, single X-chromosome found in the nuclei of somatic cells of most females and whose presence is the basis of sex determination tests **(Fig. 5.3)**. In XO (Turner's syndrome) there will be none, and in XXX there will be two Barr bodies. It is seen during mitosis in the interphase nucleus as dark staining,

---

* As per ICD-11, transsexuals and transgender are considered under **gender incongruence** which is characterized by a marked and persistent incongruence between an individual's experienced gender and the assigned sex.

DIFFERENTIATION 5.2: Determination of sex from physical/morphological feature

S.No.	Feature	Male	Female
1.	General built	Muscular, strong, stout	Less muscular, delicate, slender
2.	Scalp hair	Short, thick, coarse	Long, fine, thin
3.	Facial hair	Present	Absent
4.	Pubic hair	Thick, coarse, extends upwards with apex at umbilicus (rhomboidal)	Thin, fine, horizontal, covers mons veneris (triangular)
5.	Adam's apple	Prominent	Less prominent
6.	Shoulders	Broader than hip	Narrower than hip
7.	Waist	Not well-defined	Well-defined
8.	Trunk	Abdominal segment smaller	Abdominal segment larger
9.	Thorax	Dimensions more	Dimensions less
10.	Thighs	Cylindrical	Conical due to short femur and greater fat
11.	Breasts	Not developed	Developed after puberty
12.	Uterus and vagina	Absent	Present
13.	Penis	Present	Absent
14.	Gonads	Testes	Ovaries

TABLE 5.2: Chromatin positivity in males and females

Test	Male (%)	Female (%)
Barr body	0–4	20–80
Davidson body	0	3
Fluorescent feulgen	0–2	50–70
Quinacrine dihydrochloride	45–80	0–4

small planoconvex mass of chromatin lying near the nuclear membrane. Buccal smear is usually used.

> **NOTA BENE**
> *Murray Barr* and *Edward Bertran* while working on stained sections of nerve cells in cats noticed a tiny, dark staining blob that was always present only in the nucleus of the female cats and never in the males. It was subsequently determined to be inactive X-chromosome, and came to be known as **Barr body**.

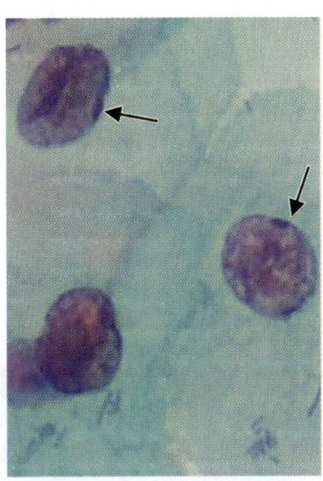

Fig. 5.3: Barr body (arrows)

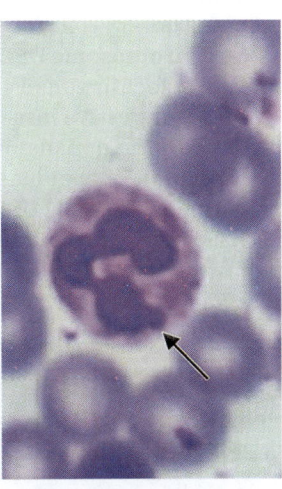

Fig. 5.4: Davidson body in neutrophil (arrow)

ii. **Davidson-Smith body:** In females, neutrophil leukocytes contain an attachment of drumstick form (**Fig. 5.4**). A drumstick consists of a small nuclear mass of about 1.5 μ in diameter, attached to the body of the nucleus by means of a thin filament.
- Sex chromosomes (XX or XY) can be determined in the cells that are dividing, e.g., bloodstains, cartilage, bone marrow, teeth pulp and hair root.
- In decomposed bodies, sex chromatin is difficult to make out.
- Hair follicles are important for cell sexing since they resist putrefaction, and both Barr body and Y-chromosome can be demonstrated.
- **Quinacrine dihydrochloride** is used for staining Y-chromosome that is seen as bright fluorescent body (commonly referred to as f–body).
- **Fluorescent Feulgen reaction** using Acriflavin Schiff reagent is used for staining X-chromosome that is seen as bright yellow spot in nuclei.

DISORDERS OF SEXUAL DEVELOPMENT

Disorder of sexual development (DSD) is a broad term encompassing any condition where external genitalia are atypical in relation to chromosome and gonads. It results from some defect in embryonic development. Earlier, Davidson divided 'intersex' into four groups:
  i. Gonadal agenesis
 ii. Gonadal dysgenesis
iii. True hermaphroditism
iv. Pseudohermaphroditism

- Currently, the term DSD is used to substitute the obsolete nomenclature of 'intersex', 'hermaphrodite' and 'pseudohermaphrodite', since they are based only on identifying the gonads and they fail to take into consideration whether those gonads are functioning or not.
- Moreover, the nomenclature was perceived to be pejorative or stigmatizing by some affected families.
- The karyotype is used as a prefix to define the category of DSD, replacing the earlier terminology of male or female pseudohermaphroditism (now known as XY DSD or XX DSD, respectively).

The new terms and possible diagnosis in such cases are given in **Table 5.3** and **Flowchart 5.1**. Some of these are briefly described below:

1. **Ovotesticular DSD (true hermaphroditism):** It is a rare condition; also known as double-sex or bisexual. Both ovarian and testicular tissues are present. External genitalia of both sexes exist in one individual, but sex chromatin may be either male or female pattern (46XX or 46XY or mosaics). True hermaphroditism is very similar to mixed gonadal dysgenesis. The karyotype could be 46XX/46XY or 46XX/47XXY.
2. **Sex chromosome DSD (gonadal dysgenesis):** It refers to a defect in gonad formation that is characterized by a progressive loss of primordial germ cells in the developing gonads of an embryo with consequent formation of hypoplastic and dysfunctioning gonads composed mainly of fibrous tissue—**streak gonads**. External sexual characters are present, but testes or ovaries fail to develop at puberty. Some examples are:

    i. **Klinefelter syndrome:** It is the most common sex chromosome disorder associated with male hypogonadism, most common presentation being 47XXY karyotype (**Box 5.1 and Fig. 5.5A**).
       - Prevalence is 1:500 to 1:1000 males, chances are more with increasing maternal age.
       - These individuals are anatomically male, but fail in external genitalia examination, and have false positive Barr body testing.
    ii. **Turner syndrome (congenital ovarian hypoplasia syndrome):** First described by Henry Turner (1938), it is the most common sex chromosome disorder associated with female hypogonadism with 45XO karyotype (prevalence 1:2000 to 2500 newborns females) (**Box 5.2 and Fig. 5.5B**).
       - These individuals are anatomically female, pass in external genitalia examination, but have false negative Barr body testing.
    iii. **Swyer syndrome:** The individuals with pure gonadal dysplasia and a 46XY karyotype will display variable degrees of undermasculinization, dependent upon the amount of testicular dysplasia. Both XX and XY gonadal dysgenesis are due to mutation or deletion of part of the sequence of the SRY gene.
    iv. **Mosaicism:** It is a genetic abnormality with mixture of cells with XX and XY, or X and XY sex chromosomes. Accordingly, there may be false positive or false negative Barr body tests depending on number of X chromosomes.

TABLE 5.3: Classification of disorders of sexual development (DSD)

Old name	New name	Possible diagnosis
True hermaphrodite	Ovotesticular DSD	46XX/46XY or 45X/46XY
Male pseudohermaphrodite	46XY DSD	Androgen insensitivity syndrome 5-α-reductase deficiency
Female pseudohermaphrodite	46XX DSD	Congenital adrenal hyperplasia
XX male or XX sex reversal	46XX testicular DSD	
XY sex reversal	46XY complete gonadal dysgenesis	
Gonadal dysgenesis	Sex chromosome DSD	45XO Turner 47XXY Klinefelter

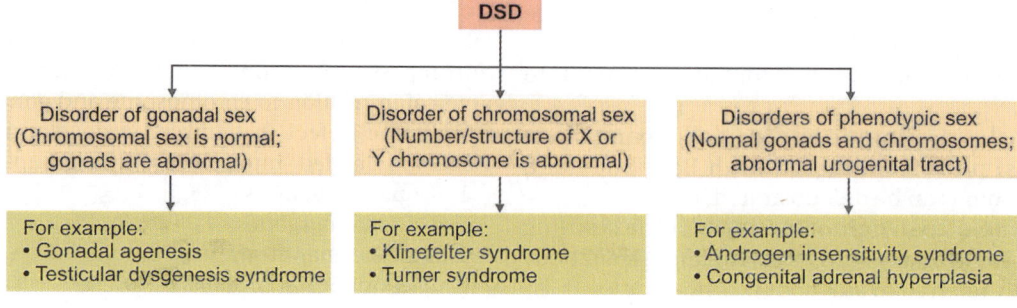

Flowchart 5.1: Classification of disorders of sexual development (DSD)

CHAPTER 5: Identification I

Box 5.1 Klinefelter syndrome

Clinical features
- Delay in onset of puberty, gynecomastia at puberty.
- Axillary and pubic hair are absent, hair on chest and chin are reduced.
- Signs of eunuchoidism, tall stature and abnormal body proportions (decreased upper to lower segment ratio).
- Firm, fibrotic, small testes and non-tender to palpation. Erectile dysfunction, loss of libido and azoospermia.
- Mental deficiency and other abnormalities, such as clinodactyly or synostosis.
- Problems with coordination and behavioral difficulties including immaturity, poor judgment, shyness, etc.

Diagnosis: Karyotyping using lymphocytes or fibroblasts or prenatally from aminocytes or chorionic villi, or by determining the presence of RNA for X-inactive-specific transcriptase (XIST) in peripheral blood leukocytes by PCR. Serum testosterone is low, and FSH, LH and estradiol are elevated.

Histological features: Testicular dysgenesis with hyalinization and fibrosis of seminiferous tubules.

Box 5.2 Turner syndrome

Clinical features
- Short stature *(most common feature)*.
- Micrognathia, high-arched palate, webbed neck, low hairline.
- Ptosis with low-set ears, widely spaced nipples.
- Cubitus valgus (wide carrying angle), short fourth and fifth metacarpals and metatarsals, hyperconvex nails.
- Lymphedema of hands and feet, pigmented nevi and keloid formation.
- Learning disability, often involving visual-spatial skills without typical mental retardation.
- *Cardiovascular* anomalies: Coarctation of the aorta and aortic stenosis.
- *Renal* abnormalities: Hydronephrosis, horseshoe kidney, hypertension.
- Increased urinary gonadotropin excretion.
- *Sexual* infantilism due to gonadal dysgenesis with primary amenorrhea.
- High incidence of osteoporosis, type II diabetes.

Diagnosis: Evaluation for childhood short stature often leads to the diagnosis. Hypogonadism is confirmed in girls who have high serum levels of FSH and LH. A karyotype showing 45XO establishes the diagnosis.

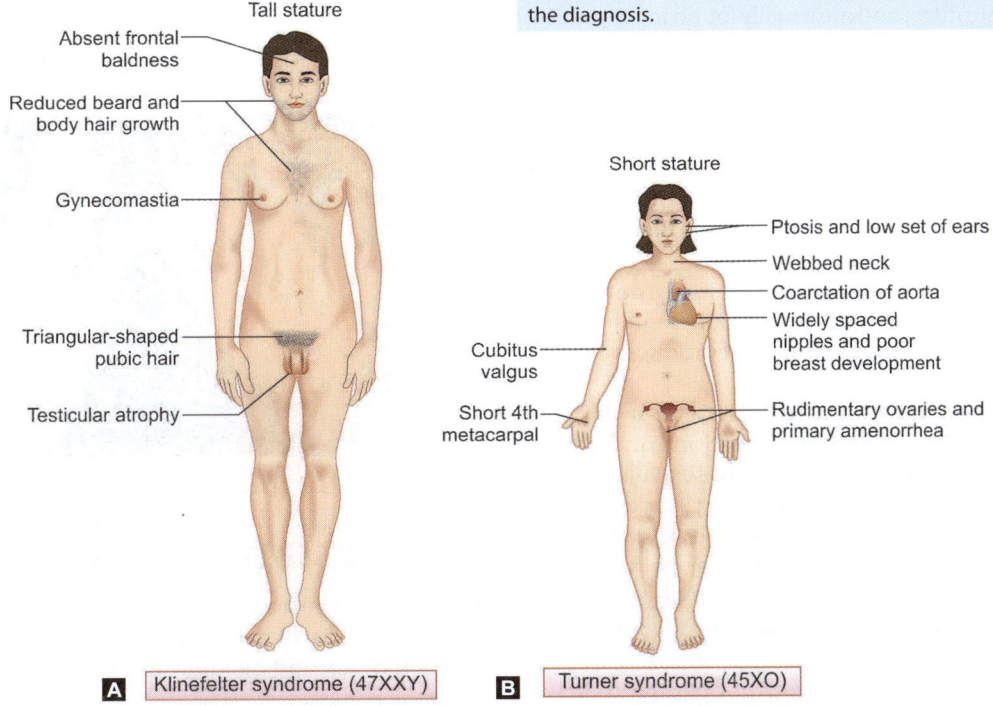

Figs. 5.5A and B: Features seen: (A) Klinefelter; (B) Turner syndrome

3. **Androgen receptor deficiency:** Androgen insensitivity is caused by receptors that are insensitive to androgens, particularly testosterone. As a result, even though they are genetically male (46 XY DSD) and possess testes, but fail to develop male characteristics. These individuals are born and raised as girls and have female gender identity. They would fail the Barr body test as they have only one X chromosome. It can be:
   i. **Complete androgen insensitivity syndrome** (cAIS), previously known as *testicular feminization syndrome* (most common form).

- It is an X-linked recessive condition resulting in failure of normal masculinization of the external genitalia.
- They have female external genitalia with normal labia, clitoris and vaginal introitus with normal size breasts but with primary amenorrhea and scanty or absent axillary and pubic hair.
- Internally, there is a short blind-pouch vagina with absence of uterus, fallopian tubes and ovaries.

   ii. **Incomplete androgen insensitivity:** The phenotype may range from mildly virilized female external genitalia (clitoromegaly without other external anomalies) to mildly undervirilized male external genitalia (hypospadias and/or diminished penile size) with gynecomastia. They tend to be tall.

In both cases, affected individuals have normal testes with normal production of testosterone and normal conversion to dihydrotestosterone (DHT), which differentiates this condition from 5-α reductase deficiency.

4. **5-α reductase deficiency (5-ARD):** This is an autosomal recessive sex-limited condition resulting in the inability to convert testosterone to DHT. Since, DHT is required for the normal masculinization of the external genitalia in utero, genetic males with 5-ARD deficiency are born with ambiguous genitalia.
    - The individual presents with a clitoral-like phallus, markedly bifid scrotum, pseudovaginal blind-ending introitus with perineoscrotal hypospadias and a rudimentary prostate.
    - Uterus and fallopian tubes are absent.
    - Testes are intact and are usually found in the inguinal canal or scrotum or occasionally in the abdomen.
    - At puberty, musculature, body and facial hair develop owing to normal levels of testosterone.
    - These individuals fail in external examination of genitals and fail in Barr body testing.

5. **Congenital adrenal hyperplasia (CAH):** It is a condition wherein adrenal glands produce excessive amounts of testosterone in females.
    - These individuals develop secondary male characteristics but are genetically female (46XX, DSD), lacking testes and male reproductive organs (masculinized females).
    - Among the various forms of CAH, the 21-hydroxylase deficiency resulting from mutations or deletions of CYP21A is most common, but sexual ambiguity can also be seen in defects in 17-hydroxylase, 3b-hydroxysteroid dehydrogenase, 17-ketosteroid reductase and 11b-hydroxylase.
    - Phenotypically female at birth, but do not develop breasts or menstruate in adolescence; they may present with hypertension.
    - Genital anomalies range from complete fusion of the labioscrotal folds and a phallic urethra to clitoromegaly, partial fusion of the labioscrotal folds, or both. These individuals fail in external examination of genitals but would have positive Barr body testing.

Recently, the Supreme Court directed that all documents (including voter/Aadhar card) should have a third category marked '*transgender or third gender*'. It would only apply to transgender people but not to gays, lesbians or bisexuals.

NOTA BENE

- Men with Klinefelter syndrome are at a higher risk of autoimmune diseases, diabetes mellitus, leg ulcers, osteopenia and osteoporosis, tumors (breast and germ cells), gonadotroph adenoma and gonadotroph hyperplasia liver adenoma, systemic lupus erythematosus (SLE), rheumatoid arthritis and Sjögren syndrome.
- **Hypergonadotropic hypogonadism** (defective development of testes or ovaries and associated with excess pituitary gonadotropin secretion) is seen in Klinefelter syndrome, Noonan syndrome, viral orchitis (mumps), cytotoxic drugs and testicular syndrome, viral orchitis (mumps), cytotoxic drugs and testicular irradiation. In women with hypergonadotropic hypogonadism, the most common cause is Turner syndrome.
- Cardiovascular disease is the most common cause of death in adult women with Turner syndrome. Most common heart defects are bicuspid aortic valve (30% of children), coarctation of the aorta (5–10%) and aortic dissection. Other anomalies seen are hypoplasic left-heart syndrome, partial anomalous pulmonary venous drainage and atrial septal defects.

A 15-year-old female patient presented with complaint of primary amenorrhea. Clinically, she was short with prominent epicanthal folds, low hairline, mutliple facial nevi and a small fourth finger of both hands. Previous images of USG pelvis revealed a steaky uterus with non-visualized ovaries. What is your diagnosis?

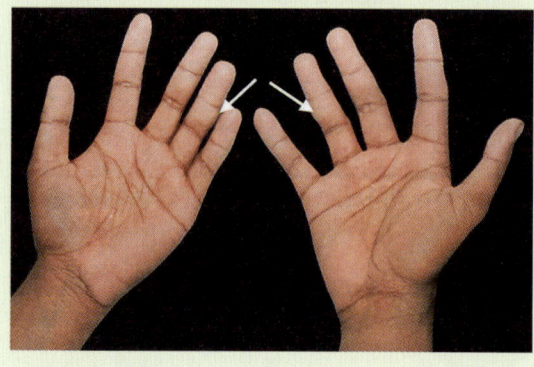

SEX FROM SKELETAL REMAINS

- Recognizable sex differences appear after puberty *except* in the pelvis. In pelvis, sex features are independent of each other, and one may even contradict the other in same pelvis.
- Among the long bones, *femur is most useful for sex determination* [larger and higher neck-shaft angle (collo-diaphyseal angle) in males, femur head diameter (males >45 mm; females <41 mm), oblique length (447-459 mm in males; females 409-426 mm), and bicondylar width (males >78 mm; females <72 mm)].
- The sex of long bones can be determined on the basis of medullary index from tibia, humerus, ulna and radius. Sternum is least useful.

The accuracy in sexing from adult skeletal remains is given in **Table 5.4** (as reported by Wilton M Krogman).

Traits diagnostic of sex from skeleton are given in **Diff. 5.3 to 5.6** *and* **Table 5.5**.

Summary of various indices is given in **Table 5.6**.

CHAPTER 5 : Identification I

TABLE 5.4: Accuracy of sexing based on skeletal remains

Skeletal remains	Accuracy in sexing (%)
Entire skeleton	100
Skull + pelvis	98
Pelvis alone (best single bone)	95
Skull alone	92
Long bones	80–85
Long bones + pelvis	98

NOTA BENE

- The **preauricular sulcus** is characteristic of the *female pelvis*. The pelvic portion of the anterior sacroiliac ligament is attached to it. Its prominence results from obstetrical trauma during the course of delivery which allows for differentiation between nulliparous women and males vs females who have given birth.
- **Ashley's rule:** It is used to know the *sex of the sternum* for Europeans. Also known as '149 rule'—male sternum is >149 mm and female sternum is <149.

DIFFERENTIATION 5.3: Male and female skull (Fig. 5.6)

S.No.	Feature	Male skull	Female skull
1.	General appearance	Larger, heavier, rugged, marked muscular ridges	Smaller, lighter, walls thinner, smoother
2.	Cranial capacity	More capacious (1450–1550 cc)	Less capacious (1300–1350 cc)
3.	**Forehead**	Receding, irregular, rough, less rounded	Vertical, round, full, infantile, smooth
4.	Glabella	Prominent	Less prominent
5.	Supraorbital/supraciliary margin	Thick and rounded	Sharp
6.	**Supraorbital ridge**	Pronounced, 'loaf shaped' ridge	Smooth, little or no projection
7.	**Frontonasal junction (Nasion)**	Distinct angulation	Smoothly curved
8.	Orbits	Square, small	Rounded, large
9.	**Mastoid process**	Large, round, blunt	Small, smooth, pointed
10.	**Nuchal crest**	Well-defined ledge or hook of bone (rugged)	Absent or slight (smooth)
11.	Frontal and parietal eminence	Less prominent	Prominent
12.	Zygomatic arch	Prominent	Not prominent
13.	Occipital area (muscle markings and protuberance)	Prominent	Not prominent
14.	Digastric groove	Deep	Shallow
15.	Condylar facet	Long, narrow	Short, broad
16.	**Palate**	Large, U-shaped, broad	Small, parabolic
17.	Foramen magnum	Relatively large, long	Small, round
18.	Mental eminence	Large projection	Little or no projection
19.	Nasal aperture	High, thin sharp margins	Lower, wider, rounded margins
20.	Suprameatal crest	Present (extends)	Absent (no extension)

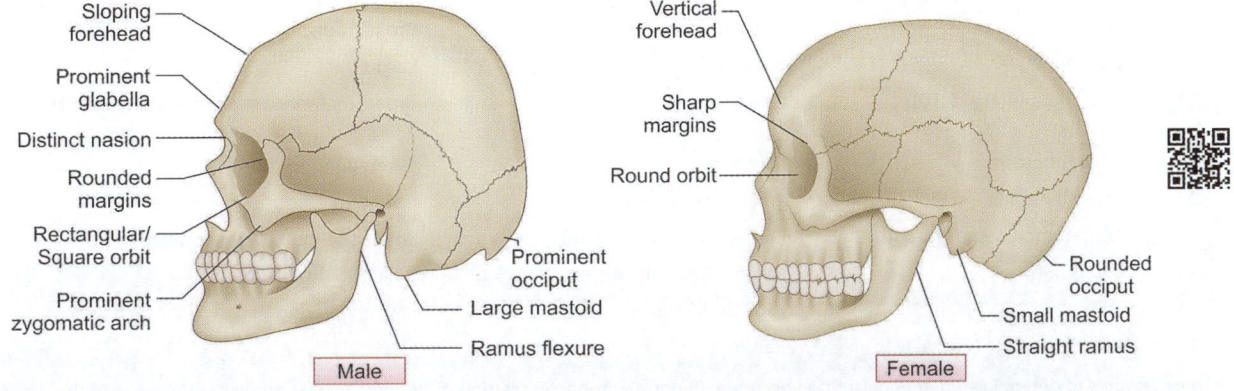

Fig. 5.6: Male and female skull

DIFFERENTIATION 5.4: Male and female mandible (Fig. 5.7)

S.No.	Feature	Male mandible	Female mandible
1.	General appearance	Larger, thicker	Smaller, thinner
2.	**Chin** (symphysis menti)	Square or U-shaped	Rounded
3.	**Angle of body with ramus** (gonial angle)	Less obtuse (<125°), prominent	More obtuse (>125°), not prominent
4.	**Ramus flexure**	Rearward angulation of the posterior border of ramus	Straight ramus
5.	Angle of mandible	Everted	Inverted
6.	Body height at symphysis	Greater	Smaller
7.	Ascending ramus	Greater breadth	Smaller breadth
8.	Muscular markings	Prominent	Not prominent

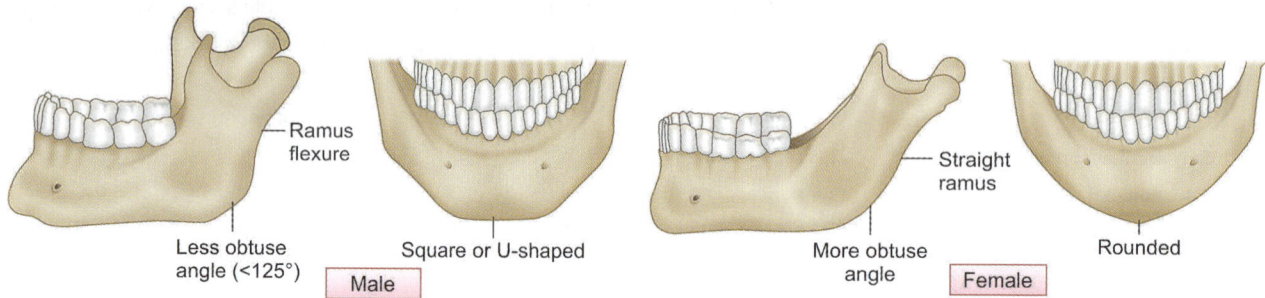

Fig. 5.7: Male and female mandible

DIFFERENTIATION 5.5: Male and female pelvis (Figs. 5.8 and 5.9)

S.No.	Feature	Male pelvis	Female pelvis
1.	General appearance	Massive, rougher, prominent muscular markings	Less massive, slender, smoother, muscular markings not prominent
2.	**Shape**	Deep funnel with heart shaped inlet	Flat bowl shaped with elliptical/circular inlet
3.	**Preauricular sulcus** (attachment of anterior sacroiliac ligament)	Not frequent, narrow, shallow	More frequent, broad, deep
4.	**Subpubic angle**	V-shaped, sharp angle, 70–75°	U-shaped, rounded, broader angle, 90–100°
5.	**Greater sciatic notch (Fig. 5.11)**	Narrow, deep, small	Broad, shallow, large
6.	Ventral arc	Absent	Present
7.	Subpubic contour	Straight	Concave
8.	Medial aspect of ischiopubic ramus	Broad and flat	Sharp, ridged
9.	Pelvic cavity	Conical, funnel shaped	Broad, round
10.	Pelvic outlet	Smaller	Larger
11.	Body of pubis (Fig. 5.10)	Narrow, triangular	Broad, rectangular, pits on posterior surface, if borne children*
12.	Ischial tuberosity	Inverted	Everted
13.	Iliopectineal line	Well-marked, rough	Rounded, smooth
14.	Obturator foramen (Fig. 5.10)	Large, oval, base upwards	Small, triangular, apex forwards
15.	Acetabulum	Large, 52 mm diameter	Small, 46 mm diameter
16.	Ilium	High and vertical	Low and flaring
17.	Auricular surface (Fig. 5.11)	Raised	Flat

*Three features to determine whether parturition occurred: (i) dorsal pitting, (ii) scarring of the preauricular groove, (iii) scarring of the groove for the interosseous ligament (interosseous groove).

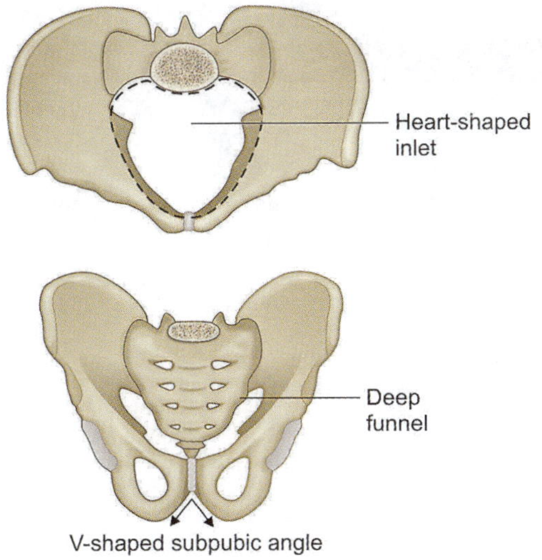

Fig. 5.8: Male pelvis

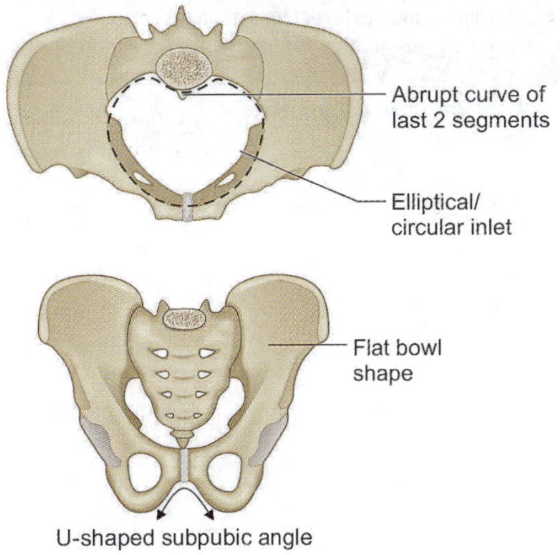

Fig. 5.9: Female pelvis

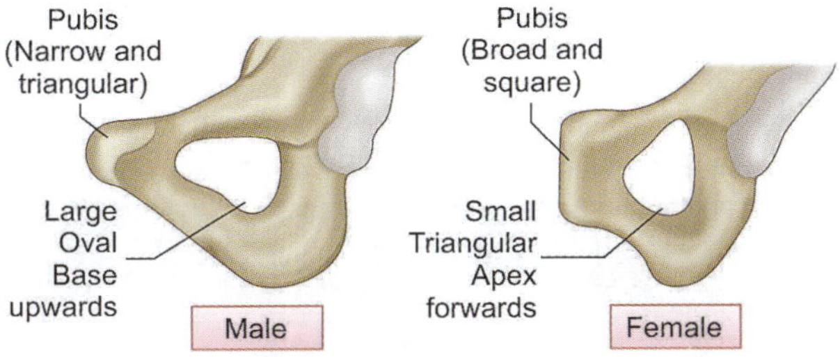

Fig. 5.10: Pelvis: Obturator foramen

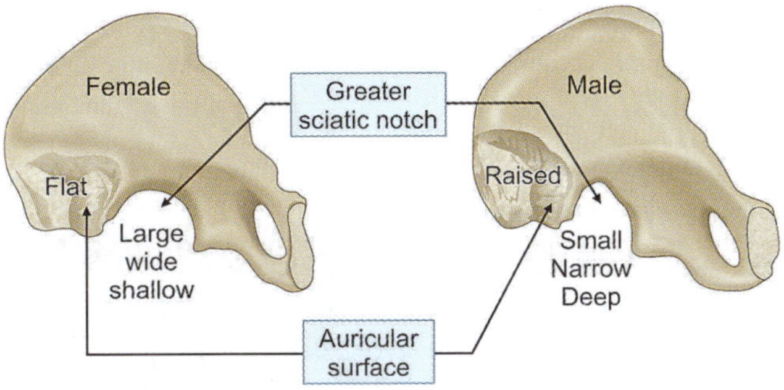

Fig. 5.11: Pelvis: Greater sciatic notch and auricular surface

DIFFERENTIATION 5.6: Male and female sacrum (Fig. 5.12)

S.No.	Feature	Male sacrum	Female sacrum
1.	General appearance	Long, heavier, rough, narrow	Short, lighter, smooth, broad
2.	Breadth of body of 1st sacral vertebra	More than breadth of one side ala	Less than breadth of one side ala
3.	Inner curvature (Fig. 5.7)	Uniformly curved anteriorly	Abruptly curved at the last two segments
4.	Sacroiliac articulation	Large, extends up to 3rd segment	Small, extends up to 2–2½ segment
5.	Sacroiliac joint surface	Large, less sharply angulated	L-shaped, elevated anteriorly

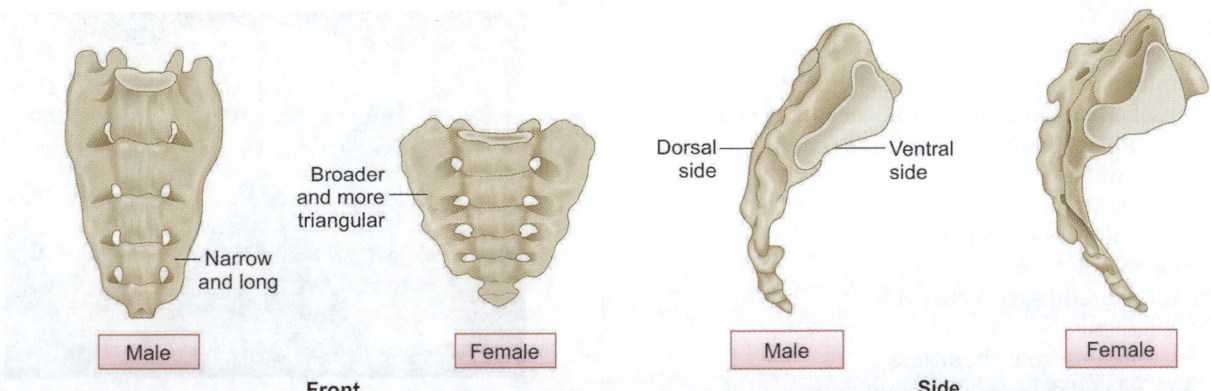

Fig. 5.12: Sacrum

TABLE 5.5: Diagnostic indexes for determination of sex

S.No.	Index	Formula	Male	Female
1.	Washburn/Ischiopubic index (Best index)	$\dfrac{\text{Length of pubis}}{\text{Length of ischium}} \times 100$	73–94 (average 75)	91–115 (average 100)
2.	Sciatic notch index	$\dfrac{\text{Width of sciatic notch}}{\text{Depth of sciatic notch}} \times 100$	145	166
3.	Sternal index	$\dfrac{\text{Length of manubrium}}{\text{Length of body}} \times 100$	46.2	54.3
4.	Corporobasal index	$\dfrac{\text{Breadth of body of 1st sacral vertebra}}{\text{Breadth of base of sacrum}} \times 100$	>42	<42
5.	Sacral index	$\dfrac{\text{Transverse diameter of base of sacrum}}{\text{Anterior length of sacrum}} \times 100$	<114	>114
6.	Chilotic line index	$\dfrac{\text{Sacral part of chilotic line}}{\text{Pelvic part of the chilotic line}} \times 100$	>100	<100
7.	Kimura's base-wing index (Alar index)	$\dfrac{\text{Width of wing (ala of sacrum)}}{\text{Width of base (transverse diameter of body of S1)}} \times 100$	65	80

TABLE 5.6: Indices useful for identification

Race	Sex	Species
Cephalic index	Ischiopubic index	Medullary index
Nasal index	Sciatic notch index	
Brachial index	Chilotic line index	
Crural index	Ilium index	
Intermembral index	Sacral index	
Humerofemoral index	Kimura's base-wing index	
	Corporobasal index	
	Sternal index	

Define and describe age determination using morphology, teeth-eruption, decay, bones-ossification centers.

AGE

Age determination can be done through many means, and an analysis of all possible age-related attributes is best for an overall estimate. Some of the utilized features include:
i. Dental eruption
ii. Epiphyseal unions
iii. Pubic symphyseal morphology
iv. Cranial suture closures
v. Mandibular and sacral changes
vi. Miscellaneous
   a. Secondary sexual characters
   b. Age-related degenerative conditions.

Is this a male or female skull? Give reasons.

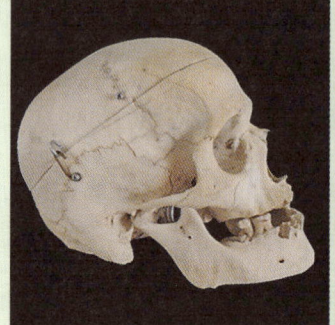
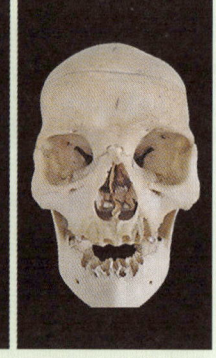

3

Which one of these statements is true?

4

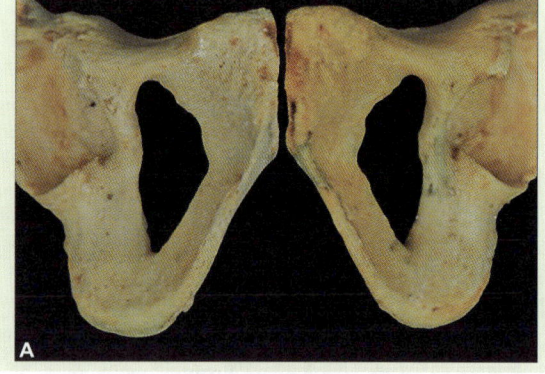

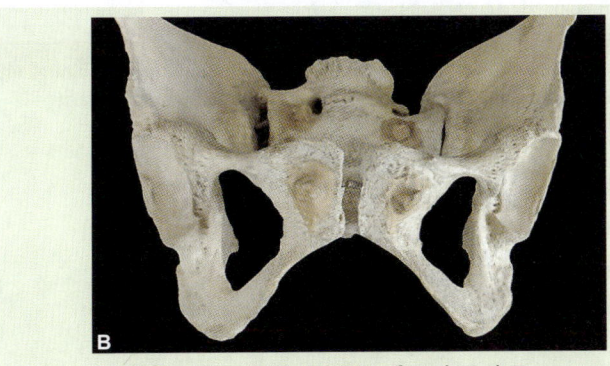

1. (A) is male pelvis and (B) is female pelvis
2. (A) is female pelvis and (B) is male pelvis
3. Both (A) and (B) are female pelvis
4. Both (A) and (B) are male pelvis

Dentition in Determining Age

Age can be determined by using the criteria like eruption and calcification of teeth, Demirjian method, Stack's method, Miles method, Boyde's method and Gustafson's method.

- Teeth are especially useful to determine age in children and adolescents since the developmental stages are well known and characterized. Radiological analysis of dental development is preferred over morphological analysis.
- Alveolar cavities which contain teeth are formed around the 3–4th month of intrauterine life (IUL).
- At birth, rudiments of all the temporary teeth and the 1st permanent molars may be found in jaw.
- Each tooth has a crown, neck and a root embedded in jaw bone (**Fig. 5.13**).
- Teeth are composed of *dentin* covered on the crown by enamel and on the root by cementum which is attached to the alveolar bone by periodontal membrane. Tooth enamel is the hardest substance in the body containing primarily hydroxypatite (crystalline calcium phosphate).

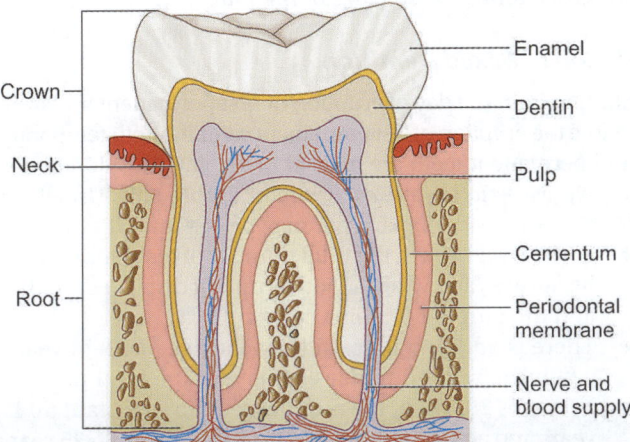

Fig. 5.13: Parts of a tooth

- Mineralization proceeds from crown tips down the sides of the tooth.
- Root mineralization does not begin until crown formation is complete and root formation ceases with the reduction of apical foramen. As the root becomes longer, the crown erupts through the bone.
- Mineralization of deciduous dentition begins in utero, early in 2nd trimester, and root formation of third molar may not be complete until 20 years of age.
- During eruption of a permanent tooth, the overlying root of its deciduous predecessor simultaneously undergoes absorption, until only the crown remains. The unsupported crown then falls off.
- Age of eruption of teeth depends upon:
  i. Heredity
  ii. Environment
  iii. Nutrition
  iv. Endocrine factors.

Each individual has two sets of teeth (Diff. 5.7)
  i. Temporary/deciduous/milk teeth
  ii. Permanent teeth

Temporary teeth

- *20 in number*: 4 incisors, 2 canines and 4 molars in each jaw (**Table 5.7** and **Fig. 5.14**).
- The eruption of the deciduous teeth commences at about 6–7 months after birth and is completed about 2nd–3rd year. the lower central incisors anteceding those of the upper. However, upper lateral incisor erupts earlier than its lower quadrant counterpart.
- In ill-nourished children, especially in rickets, dentition may be delayed.
- In congenital syphilis, teeth may be premature or even present at birth.

Permanent teeth: 32 in number—4 incisors, 4 pre-molars, 2 canines and 6 molars in each jaw (**Table 5.7** and **Fig. 5.15**).

Developmentally teeth are divided into two sets:
  a. **Super-added permanent teeth:** These teeth do not have deciduous predecessors. All permanent molars belong to this category (6 in each jaw).
  b. **Successional permanent teeth:** These teeth erupt in place of deciduous teeth, e.g., permanent premolars erupt in place of deciduous molars (10 in each jaw).
- Usually permanent tooth erupts first in lower jaw.
- Permanent teeth appear few months earlier in girls than in boys.
- Eruption of teeth is useful in estimating age up to 15 years. The third molar (wisdom tooth) erupts after this time, but is so variable in eruption that it is not a reliable age indicator.
- However, the developmental characteristics of eruption and mineralization of 3rd molars are useful for age estimation. The assessment distinguishes between the stages of alveolar eruption, gingival eruption, and having reached the occlusal plane. The latter two stages can be

DIFFERENTIATION 5.7: Temporary and permanent teeth

S.No.	Feature	Temporary teeth	Permanent teeth
1.	Size	Smaller, lighter, narrower, except temporary molars which are longer than permanent premolars	Heavier, stronger, broader, except permanent premolars
2.	Direction of anterior teeth	Vertical	Inclined forward
3.	Crown color	China-white	Ivory-white
4.	Neck	More constricted	Less constricted
5.	Ridge	Present at the junction of the crown and the root	Not present
6.	Root	Roots of molars are smaller, more divergent	Roots of molars are larger, less divergent
7.	Incisors	Smooth incisal edge	Ridged, especially on incisal surface
8.	Radiology	Presence of tooth germ beneath tooth will suggest that tooth is temporary	No such thing visible in case of permanent teeth

TABLE 5.7: Eruption of deciduous and permanent teeth

Tooth	Deciduous teeth (months)	Permanent teeth (years)
Central incisor	6–8 (lower, 1st to erupt) 7–9 (upper)	6–8
Lateral incisor	7–9 (upper) 10–12 (lower)	7–9
First premolar	Absent	9-11
Second premolar	Absent	10–12
First molar	12–14	6–7 (1st to erupt)
Canine	17–18	11–12
Second molar	20–30 (2–2½ years)	12–14
Third molar	Absent	17–25

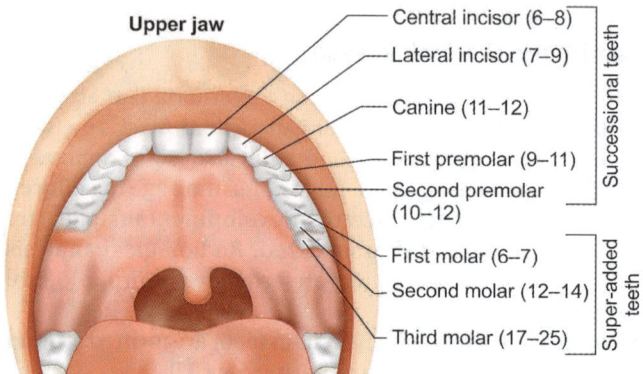

Fig. 5.15: Eruption of permanent teeth (in years)

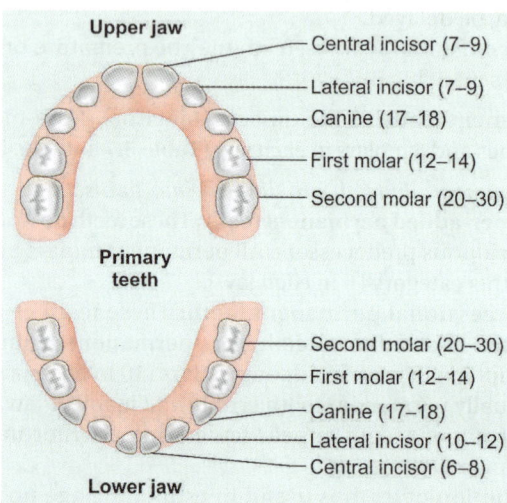

Fig. 5.14: Eruption of deciduous teeth (in months)

determined by oral visual inspection and do not require an X-ray. The mineralization of third molars is assessed with an orthopantomogram.
- The mandibular third molar is the most commonly impacted tooth in the mouth and is closely followed by maxillary third molar, maxillary canine and mandibular canine respectively.
- If, in the jaw all 3rd molars are present, then the age is over 18 years, but their absence gives no certain idea about age.

Spacing of Jaw

After eruption of 2nd molars, the ramus of mandible grows behind to make room for the eruption of 3rd molar teeth which is known as *spacing of the jaw*.

Period of Mixed Dentition

Starting from the day of eruption of first permanent molar till before the eruption of last permanent canine—both temporary and permanent teeth are present in the jaw. This duration is known as *period of mixed dentition* **(Table 5.8)**. Usually, it is between 6 and 11 years, but may persist until 12–13 years.
- From 6 to 11 years, the total number of teeth remains 24 because as and when a tooth erupts, it displaces another and the number remains constant.
- There is addition of teeth from the age of 12–14 years, when the second molar erupts and the total number becomes 28. Then, the number remains constant till 17 years and again 4 more teeth are added from 17–25 years and the number becomes 32.

CHAPTER 5: Identification I

TABLE 5.8: Number of teeth with age*

Age (years)	Number of teeth	
2.5–5	20	(All deciduous)
6	21–24	(Eruption of 1st permanent molars)
7–9	24	(12 permanent—8 incisors, 4 molars) (12 deciduous—4 canines, 8 molars)
10	24	(16 permanent—8 incisors, 4 molars, 4 premolars) (8 deciduous—second molars and canines)
11	24	(20 permanent—8 incisors, 4 molars, 8 premolars) (4 deciduous—canines)
12–14	25–28	(Eruption of 2nd permanent molars)
14–17	28	(All permanent)
17–25	29–32	(Eruption of 3rd molars)

* Total number of permanent teeth = (Age in years–5) × 4

NOTA BENE

- **Stack's method:** Method to estimate the age from sum of the weight of the erupting teeth of *fetus and infant* (from 5 months in utero to postnatal age of 7 months).
- **Boyde's method:** Estimate age of dead infants, based on counting the number of cross striations in the enamel of teeth (incremental lines) from *neonatal line* (darkest band) onwards. Neonatal line is formed soon after birth.
- **Open apices method:** Cameriere proposed this radiological method of estimation of age in children based on relationship between age and measurement of open apices and length of the tooth axis major. This method uses the seven left mandibular teeth; simple, non-destructive and reliable.
- **Demirjian method:** Dental age estimation in children based on assessment of maturity score of lower left permanent mandibular teeth (except 3rd molar) using an orthopantomogram.
- **Lamendin method:** Periodontosis and translucency of root are taken into consideration for estimation of age at death for adults by analyzing single-rooted teeth—considered better than Gustafson's method.
- **Miles' method:** Amount of wear on all three permanent molars is assessed for age estimation. Miles also developed a formula to determine age at death by measuring the thickness of enamel and dentin from neonatal line and divided it by daily rate of formation.
- **Histological technique:** The amount of dentin laid down after the formation of the neonatal line (incremental lines) in deciduous dentition, and counting of cross-striations and striae of Retzius in primary and secondary enamel may help in finding the chronological age. Once enamel depositions are complete, the use of cemental annulations rings can be used.
- **Aspartic acid racemization:** During the course of aging, L-forms of amino acids (in crown dentin) are transformed by racemization to D-forms. Thus, the extent of racemization of amino acids may be used to estimate the age. Of all amino acids, aspartic acid racemization is most commonly used for age estimation.
- **Radiocarbon analysis of tooth enamel:** Method to determine the year of tooth formation based on levels of radiocarbon present in tooth enamel.

Estimation of age from teeth beyond 25 years
The various methods that can be used to determine age from teeth are:
- Gustafson's method
- Aspartic acid racemization
- **Chemical method:** Estimation of nitrogen content of enamel (increases with age), carbonate content (decreases with age) and concentration of ions—Cu, Se and Fe (increases with age).
- Miles' method
- Radiocarbon dating of tooth enamel

- Of the non-destructive methods (where tooth is not required to be taken out), assessing stages of development of mineralization of the teeth using radiographs are more reliable than those using tooth counts.
- *Amino acid racemization* is considered to be most reliable destructive method of dental age estimation.

Gustafson's Method

- Age estimation consists of microscopic examination of longitudinal section of central part of the tooth to assess changes in teeth as a result of wear and tear with advancing age.
- Estimate age between 25 and 60 years.
- Useful only while examining a *dead body or skeletal remains,* as teeth need to be extracted for examination.
- It is based on criteria given in **Table 5.9 and Figure 5.15**.
- Anterior teeth are more suitable than posterior teeth. Merit decreases from incisors to premolars, molars are quite unsuitable.
- All changes are absent at 15 years. Error is ± 10–15 years. Limit of error increases above 50 years of age.

Other Information from Teeth

- **Sex determination**
  i. *Visual and microscopic*: Mandibular canines show the greatest dimensional differences with larger teeth in males than in females. Optical scanner and radiogrammetric measurements of root length and crown diameter of mandibular permanent teeth help in sex determination.
     - Identifying Y-chromosome in dental pulp tissue using quinacrine and fluorescent microscopy.
     - Isolation of sex-specific banding patterns in DNA profiles of X and Y-chromosomes.
  ii. *Sex determination from enamel protein*: Amelogenin (AMEL) is a major protein found in human enamel. It has a different signature in male and female.
- **Race**
  i. *'Shovel-shaped'* upper central incisors can be found in most Mongoloids and Americans. In white races,

TABLE 5.9: Gustafson's criteria **(Fig. 5.16)**

S.No.	Changes	Description
1.	Attrition	Wearing down of occlusal surface due to mastication, first involving enamel, then dentin and lastly pulp
2.	Periodontosis	Retraction of gum margin and loosening of tooth exposing the neck and adjacent parts of roots
3.	Secondary dentin	Progressive infilling of the dental pulp cavity decreases the size of cavity and may completely obliterate it
4.	Cementum apposition	Cementum increase in thickness around the root due to changes in tooth position; continuously deposited throughout life and forms incremental lines
5.	Root resorption	Involves both cementum and dentin. Starts at apex and extends upwards. *Least reliable of all criteria*
6.	Root transparency	Occurs in root from below upwards in lower jaw and above downwards in upper jaw due to rarefaction of the dentin tissue. *Most reliable of all criteria.*

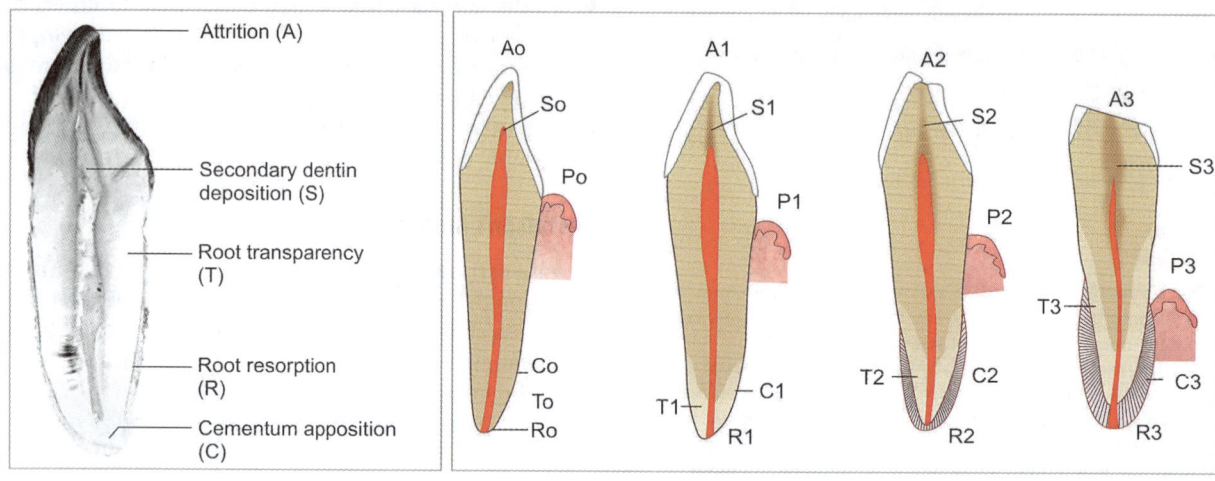

Fig. 5.16: Gustafson's method and its criteria

lateral incisor in upper jaw is smaller than the central, especially in females.
  ii. *Carabelli's cusp* (seen in whites), *taurodontism* (bull tooth) and *enamel pearls* (common in Mongoloids) have been listed as racial determinants.

> **NOTA BENE**
> - **Carabelli's tubercle** is an anomalous cusp on the lingual surface of maxillary first permanent molars, most commonly seen among Europeans (75–85%) (50% of American whites and 34% of Afro-Americans).
> - **Taurodontism** is an aberration of teeth that lacks the constriction at the level of the cementoenamel junction characterized by elongated pulp chambers and apical displacement of bifurcation or trifurcation of the roots, giving it a rectangular shape.
> - **Enamel pearls** are small nodules of enamel on the root surface of permanent maxillary molar.
> - Taurodontism, especially in maxillary molars, enamel pearls on premolars and congenital lack of upper 3rd molars are commonly seen in *Mongoloids*.

- **Occupation and habits**
  i. Cobblers or tailors usually show notched upper incisors from wear and tear.
  ii. Dark brown stains on the back of incisors are seen in 'cigarette smokers'.
- **Social status:** From general cleanliness, dentures and dental fillings by gold, silver or other metal.

AGE FROM OSSIFICATION OF BONES

- The clavicle is the first bone to ossify in the body from two membranous primary ossification centers during the 5–6th postovulatory week. A secondary center forms in the sternal end between 15–17 years and fuses by 20–22 years. In majority of the bones, primary centers of ossification appear between 7th and 12th weeks of IUL. By the age of 11–12th week of IUL, there are 806 centers of ossification.
- The process of appearance and union has a sequence and time (approximate age ranges) **(Table 5.10 and Fig. 5.17)**.
- Ossification begins centrally in an epiphysis and spreads peripherally as it gets bigger.
- Process of union of epiphysis and diaphysis is called *fusion*. Union is a process not an event.
- Some researchers have used five grades of epiphyseal union: unobservable (0), beginning (1), active (2), recent (3) and complete (4), and these offer a possibly more accurate estimate of age.

TABLE 5.10: Appearance of ossification centers (in males)

S.No.	Bone	Centers of ossification	Age of appearance	Age of union	
1.	Sternum	Manubrium	5th month IUL	60–70 years	(Manubriosternal joint)
		1st sternebrae	5th month IUL		(From below upwards; 3rd and
		2nd and 3rd sternebrae	7th month IUL	14–25 years	4th–15 years; 2nd and 3rd–20 years;
		4th sternebrae	10th month IUL		1st and 2nd–25 years)
		Xiphisternum	3rd year postnatal	40–45 years	(With body)
2.	Clavicle	Medial end	15–17 years	20–22 years	
3.	Scapula	Coracoid base	10–11 years	14–15 years	
		Acromion process	14–15 years	17–18 years	
Upper Limb					
4.	Humerus	Head	1 year	At 5–6 years, the three fuses	
		Greater tubercle	3 years	together (conjoint epiphysis) and at	
		Lesser tubercle	5 years	17–18 years, fuses with the shaft	
		Capitulum	1 year		
		Trochlea	9–10 years	At 14–15 years, all three	
		Lateral epicondyle	10–11 years	fuses with the shaft*	
		Medial epicondyle	5–6 years¥	16 years	
5.	Radius	Upper end	5–6 years	15–17 years	
		Lower end	1–2 years	17–19 years	
6.	Ulna	Upper end (olecranon)	8–9 years	15–17 years	
		Lower end	5–6 years	17–19 years	
7.	Carpals	Pisiform	9–12 years	—	
Lower Limb					
8.	Hip bone	Ischiopubic rami	—	7 years	
		Triradiate cartilage	—	12–14 years	
		Iliac crest$	15–16 years	19–21 years	
		Ischial tuberosity	16–17 years	20–22 years	
9.	Femur	Head	1 year	17–18 years	
		Greater trochanter	4 years	14–15 years	
		Lesser trochanter	14 years (puberty)	15–17 years	
		Lower end	9 months IUL	17–18 years	
10.	Tibia	Upper end	At birth	17–18 years	
		Lower end	1 year	16–17 years	
11.	Fibula	Upper end	4 years	17–18 years	
		Lower end	2 years	16–17 years	
12.	Tarsals	Calcaneum	5th month IUL		
		Talus	7th month IUL		
		Cuboid	9th month IUL		

* Ossification centers of lateral epicondyle, capitulum and trochlea fuse with each other at about 13–14 years to form a conjoint epiphysis which fuses with shaft at about 14–15 years.
¥ Sequence of appearance of elbow ossification centers: CRITOE: Capitulum → Radial head → Internal (medial) epicondyle → Trochlea → Olecranon → External (lateral) epicondyle.
$ Radiographically, Risser classification is used to grade skeletal maturity of ossification and fusion of iliac crest on a scale of 0-5. Risser 0 indicates that there is significant amount of growth remaining, while Risser 5 indicates skeletal maturity.

- Capitate and hamate ossifies during infancy (1 year), the former preceding the later. Between 2 and 6 years, the number of carpal bones present on X-ray represents the approximate age in years, e.g., three carpal bones—3 years (**Fig. 5.18**).
- X-rays of elbow, wrist, clavicle and shoulder joints (upper extremity) and pelvis, knee and ankle joints (lower extremity) are usually recommended to determine the age before 25 years of age.
- Radiography of the hand and wrist is the commonest modality used to calculate bone age of a child.
- Following the wrist skeletal development, the assessment of the ossification stage of the medial clavicular epiphysis is quite helpful, as the clavicles are the last long bones to ossify in the skeleton. Ossification stage of the medial clavicular epiphysis is done using thin-slice CT (method of choice) and evaluated according to a 5-stage classification system.
- Determination of age based on the union of epiphyses with a range of ± 6 months is given in **Table 5.11**. In females, epiphyseal union occurs 1–2 years earlier than males.

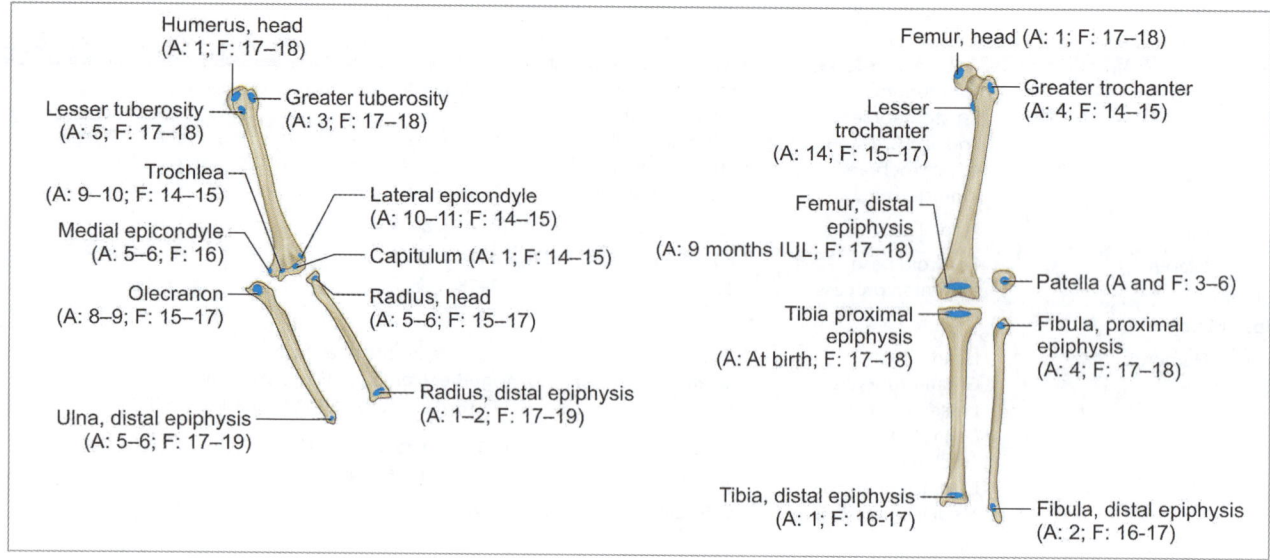

Fig. 5.17: Appearance (A) and fusion (F) of ossification centers of upper and lower limbs (in years).

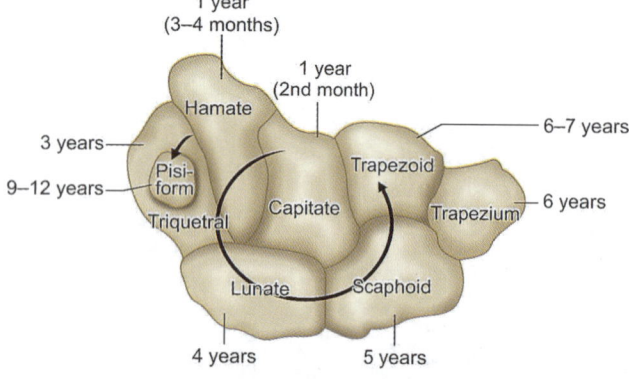

Fig. 5.18: Sequence of (left wrist dorsal aspect) ossification of carpal bones (simplified)

- If all the epiphyses of all the long bones are united, the person is most probably over 25 years of age.

TABLE 5.11: Radiological age determination (before 25 years)

S.No.	Site for X-ray (region)	Age (years)	
		Female	Male
1.	Elbow	13–14	15–16
2.	Wrist	16–17	18–19
3.	Shoulder	17–18	18–19
4.	Iliac crest	18–19	19–21
5.	Ischial tuberosity and inner end of clavicle	21–22	21–23

A. Estimate the age of this person from the given radiograph.
B. Observe the pelvic bone. What could be the age of this person? Give reasons.

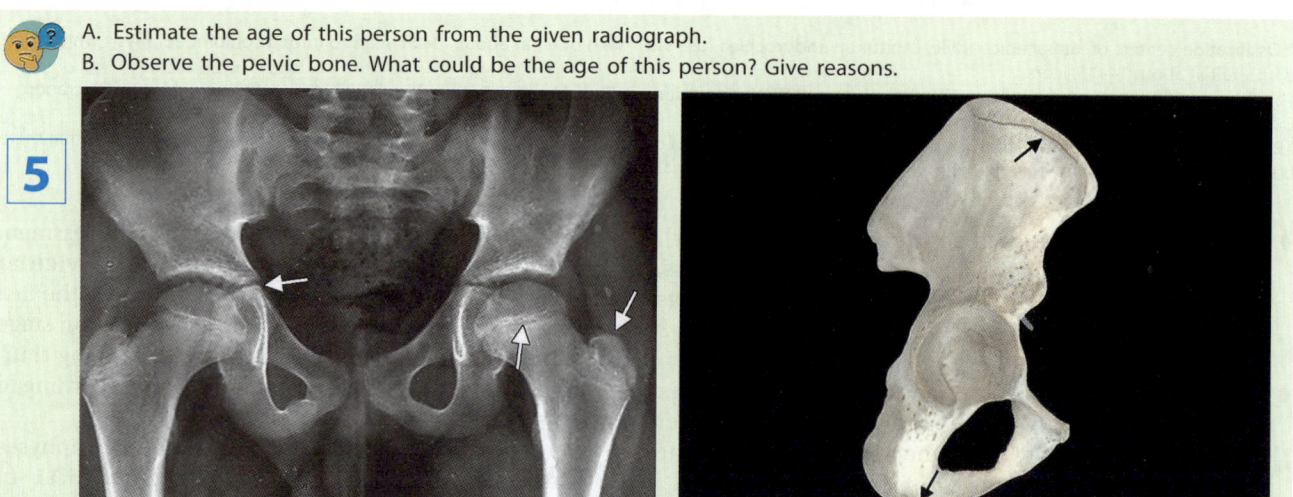

A. _____
B. _____

BONE AGE ESTIMATION

- Age estimation is mainly done by a board of forensic physicians, radiologists, dentists and pediatricians.
- Currently, the essential components of age estimation is given in **Box 5.3**.
- Bone development is influenced by a number of factors, including nutrition, hormonal secretions, genetics, differences in ethnicity, socioeconomic status and accelerated development or developmental disorders. Other factors include: variability among methods, degree of variability in the estimation of skeletal maturation, and dispersion of the values of skeletal maturation.
- Pre-existing illnesses can lead to a developmental delay and thus to an underestimation of age.
- Endocrine disorders that lead to accelerated skeletal maturity include: precocious puberty, adrenogenital syndrome and hyperthyroidism. Physical examinations should specifically look for gigantism, acromegaly, dwarfism, virilization in girls, dissociated virilism in boys, goiter and exophthalmos.

Box 5.3 Age assessment protocol
- Medical history and physical examination to assess the physical development and to rule out development-related illnesses and medications.
- Dental examination with orthopantomogram.
- X-ray examination of the hand and wrist joint.
- Thin-slice CT of the medial end of clavicle (indicated if there is complete ossification of wrist).

Recent advances in skeletal age assessment
- *Radiographic methods* remain the gold standards. A correct positioning is essential because poor positioning can change the appearance of some bones. It is also preferable to employ scoring methods to these techniques and percentiles rather than bone age in years and months.
- *CT visualization* of the clavicle has been extensively studied but requires a high dose of radiation.
- *Magnetic resonance imaging (MRI)* based methods are being developed but require more research to evaluate the reliability and validity.
- *Ultrasound imaging* has some limitations that include operator dependence, lower intra-rater and inter-rater reliability of assessment and difficulties with standardization of documentation and imaging transfer.
- The iliac bone and femoral head have also been studied for computation of bone age, but no standardized methods have yet been generated.
- *Computerized bone age estimation system:* The use of automated bone age determination system in Europe (BoneXpert) has been validated for various ethnicities and children with endocrine disorders.

AGE DETERMINATION IN ADULTS OVER 25 YEARS

After the age of 25 years, estimation of age becomes more uncertain.

Symphyseal Surface of Pubis

- The pubic symphyseal face in the young is characterized by an undulating surface, such as the crenulated surface of a typical non-fused epiphyseal plate.
- This surface undergoes a regular progressive change from 18 years onwards.
- It is the *best single criterion* for determining age-at-death for individuals from third to fifth decade.
- Morphologic changes seen in males with increasing age are given in **Table 5.12 and Figure 5.19**.

Skull Suture Closure

- This method estimates age utilizing the degree of closure, union or ossification of the cranial sutures (**Table 5.13** and **Fig. 5.20**).
- The closure of the skull sutures is considered to be a reasonably reliable index of age estimation between 25–40 years of age (useful in living also).
- Closure of skull sutures begins on the inner side (endocranially) 5–10 years earlier than on the outer side (ectocranially). The closure of ectocranial suture is variable and it may not close at all (lapsed union). It is more commonly seen in sagittal suture.
- *The most successful estimate* of age is done from sagittal suture, followed by lambdoid and then coronal. The sutures start closing on the inner side at about 25 years of age. On the outer side, posterior one-third of sagittal

TABLE 5.12: Age determination from pubic symphysis (in males)

Age	Features
<20 years	Compact bone near its surface
About 20 years	• Surface markedly irregular/uneven • Ridges runs transversely across articular surface
25–40 years	• Ridges gradually disappear • Surface has granular appearance • Outer and inner margins completely defined
40+(Early 5th decade)	Oval smooth surface with raised upper and lower ends
Late 5th decade	Narrow beaded rim develops on margin
50+(6th decade)	Erosion of surface and breakdown of ventral margins
60+(7th decade)	Surface becomes irregularly eroded

Note: If male criteria are used for females, the age would be underestimated by about 10 years.

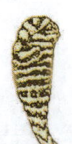 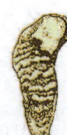 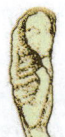 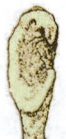 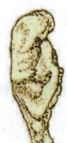

About 20 years   25–30 years   30–35 years   35–45 years   50+

Fig. 5.19: Changes in pubic symphyseal surface with age

suture closes at about 30–40 years; anterior one-third of sagittal and lower half of coronal at about 40–50 years; and middle of sagittal and upper half of the coronal at about 50–60 years **(Fig. 5.21)**.

- Lambdoid suture starts closing between 25 and 30 years and complete closure occurs between 65 and 70 years.
- Last skull suture to close is the *temporoparietal suture* (70–80 years)
- A *lateral head skiagram* is preferable for observing the sutures.

TABLE 5.13: Age determination from skull suture closure

S.No.	Suture closure	Age
1.	Posterior fontanelle (occipital)	At birth to 6 months
2.	Anterior fontanelle (bregma)	1½–2 years
3.	Two halves of mandible	1–2 years
4.	Metopic suture (between frontal bones)	1 year (3–9 months), may remain unfused
5.	Basiocciput and basisphenoid	18–20 years (females) 20–22 (males)
6.	Lambdoid suture	45–50 years
7.	Parieto-temporal	60–70 years

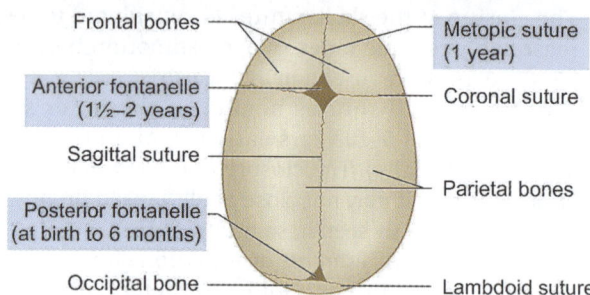

Fig. 5.20: Normal skull of the newborn

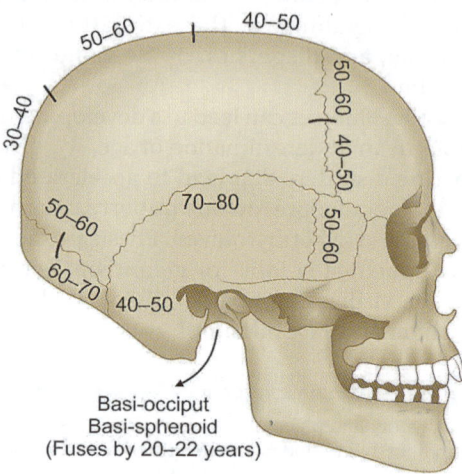

Fig. 5.21: Age (in years) of skull suture closure

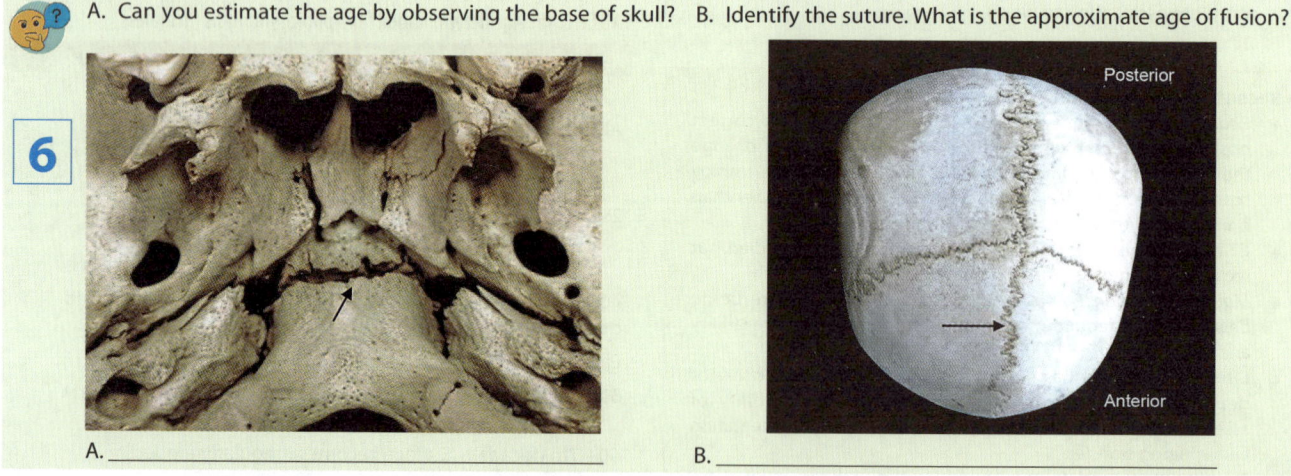

A. Can you estimate the age by observing the base of skull?
B. Identify the suture. What is the approximate age of fusion?

A. _____
B. _____

Age Estimation from Mandible

It is given in **Diff. 5.8** and **Figure 5.22**.

Sacrum

The five sacral vertebrae remain separated by cartilage until puberty, and with the onset of puberty, ossification of intervertebral discs starts from below upwards and fusion becomes complete by 20–25 years.

General Features in Estimation of Age

It includes secondary sexual characters, baldness or graying of hair, arcus senilis and skeletal changes.

Secondary Sexual Characters

- The secondary changes for estimation of age are not very helpful, but give an estimate of prepubertal and pubertal ages.

DIFFERENTIATION 5.8: Mandibles of infancy, adult and old age (Fig. 5.22)

S.No.	Feature	Infancy	Adult	Old age
1.	Body	Shallow	Thick and long	Shallow
2.	Ramus (medico-legal angle)	Short, oblique, forms obtuse angle with body	Less obtuse angle (almost right angle)	Obtuse angle with body (about 140°)
3.	Mental foramen	Opens near the lower margin and directed forwards	Opens midway between upper and lower margins and directed horizontally backwards	Opens near the alveolar margin
4.	Condyloid process	At a lower level than coronoid process	Elongated and projects above coronoid process	Neck is bent backwards

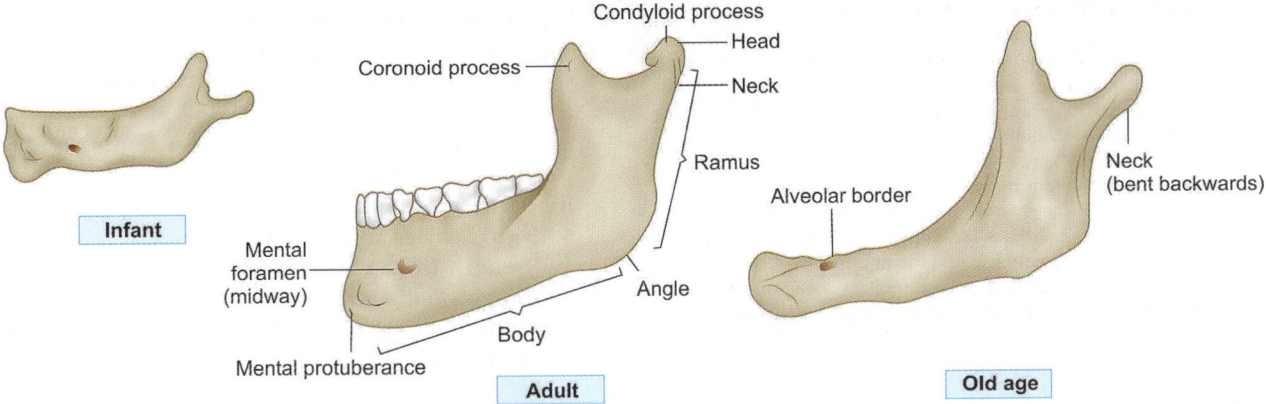

Fig. 5.22: Mandible at different ages

- Best known is the **Tanner staging**, which give sequential physical and physiological changes during puberty. A summary of important findings is given in **Diff. 5.9**.

Older Years

Many non-pathogenic conditions, such as arthritis and osteoporosis become more prevalent and pronounced in old age and can be used as corroborative evidence in the determination of age.

i. Baldness or graying of hair does not carry much value in calculating age. But, pubic hair does not turn gray before 50–55 years.
ii. **Arcus senilis:** Opaque zone around periphery of cornea may be noticed as a result of lipoid degeneration after 50 years, but is not complete before 60 years.
iii. **Pterygia:** Localized, elevated yellow-white areas that develop on the conjunctiva and cornea. Located most often nasally but sometimes temporally, and are usually bilateral. Pterygia are generally found in middle-aged or elderly individuals.
iv. **Skeletal changes**
  - Thyroid and cricoid cartilage (1st tracheal ring) tend to ossify by about 45–50 years.
  - Greater cornu fuse with the body of hyoid by 40–45 years.
  - Xiphisternum and manubrium unite with the body of sternum around 40 years and above 50 years respectively.
  - Lipping of lumbar vertebrae occurs around 40–50 years (osteophytosis) and atrophic changes occur in intervertebral disc with diminution of joint space at about 50–60 years.
  - Radiological thinning of the cortex and progressive rarefaction of apex of medullary cavity of head of humerus and femur are helpful in determination of the age.

DIFFERENTIATION 5.9: Summary of sexual development

S.No.	Feature	Girls	Boys
1.	Onset	10–12 years	12–14 years
2.	First sign	Breast development (thelarche)	Testicular enlargement (gonadarche)
3.	Growth spurt	Early (10–11 years)	Late (12–13 years)
4.	Sexual maturity	Menarche: 13–14 years	Spermarche: 15 years
5	Order of maturity	Thelarche → pubarche → peak growth velocity → menarche	Testicular development → pubarche → axillary hair → beard

- Skull bones with advancing age tend to become lighter and thinner.

X-rays of skull, vertebrae and sterum are used to determine age in old people.

> **NOTA BENE**
> - **Phase changes in the sternal rib:** Age estimation based on sequential morphological changes at the sternal end (costochondral joint) between the rib and sternum of the 4th rib. These changes are similar to those that occur on the pubic symphyseal face.
> - **Cortical bone histology:** Age estimation based on calculating the rate of osteon turnover or replacement osteon from midshaft of long bone sections. Best correlation come from the fibula, then femur and tibia.
> - **Harris lines:** These are the small growth lines within the bones. No two individuals have the same pattern, i.e., they are unique. Identification of a person is possible from these lines.
> - **Age estimation from bone marrow:** The normal cellularity varies with age. The marrow is approximately 100% cellular during the first 3 months of life, slowly declining in cellularity until 30 years of age, then it remains at about 50%. This can give an estimation of different age groups (newborn, child, adults and elderly) but not the exact age of the person.

FM 3.1
Describe medico-legal aspects of age.

MEDICO-LEGAL IMPORTANCE OF AGE

Age estimation is important for issues pertaining to illegal trafficking (child labor), legal medicine (kidnapping/human trafficking/illegal migration), sexual exploitation, criminal cases, adoption of individuals without birth certificates, and natural or mass disasters. Medico-legal importance of various age groups is given in **Table 5.14**.

- **Evidence:** Competency for giving evidence depends upon understanding, but not on age. A child of any age can give evidence, if the court is satisfied that the child is truthful **(Sec. 118 IEA)**.
- **Criminal abortion:** A woman who has passed the childbearing age cannot be charged of procuring criminal abortion.
- **Identification:** An approximate age is important in any chain of identity data.
- **Impotence and sterility:** A boy is sterile though not impotent before puberty; woman becomes sterile after menopause.

FM 3.1
Define and describe stature.

STATURE

- Stature estimation from skeletal remains is a common parameter in forensics used to aid in the identification of dead bodies.
- Stature varies at different times of day by 1.5–2 cm. It is less in the afternoon and evening due to reduced elasticity of intervertebral discs and the longitudinal vertebral muscles.
- After the age of 30, the natural process of senile degeneration causes gradual decrease in stature by 0.6 mm/year on average.
- On an average, the body lengthens after death by about 2 cm, due to complete loss of muscle tone, relaxation of large joints and loss of tensioning effect of paraspinal muscles on intervertebral discs.
- If the body has been dismembered or skeletonized, the approximate stature may be determined by:
  i. Length of entire skeleton and 2.5–4 cm for thickness of soft parts.
  ii. Length from tip of middle finger to the tip of the opposite finger when arms are fully extended.
  iii. Twice the length of one arm with 30 cm added for two clavicles and 4 cm for sternum.
  iv. Length from vertex to the symphysis pubis is roughly half of stature.
  v. Length from sternal notch to symphysis pubis multiplied by 3.3.

Stature from Bones

The methods in use to determine the stature can be divided into:
a. Least squares regression equation and other regression principles.
b. Stature: bone length ratios.
c. Skeleton height and adjustment for missing soft tissue.

Sex and race of the individual should be taken into account while applying these methods:

- When whole skeleton is not available, but one or the other long bones are available, then regression equations are used.
- **Karl Pearson's regression formula** (first reported in 1899) is the most commonly used method to determine the stature based on long bones. The formula for femur being: Stature = $81.306 + 1.88 \times F$ (length of femur in males).
- Several authors have offered regression equations, viz. Breitinger, Telkkä, Dupertius and Hadden, Trotter and Gleser, and Muñoz. They are derived for one population (usually Europeans and North Americans) and as such not suitable for Indians. Moreover, these formulae are not valid for children.
- Combination of bones is more reliable than a single bone, and long bones of lower limb (femur and tibia) give better estimate than upper limbs (humerus and radius).
- *Multiplication factors to calculate stature* for femur: 3.6–3.8; tibia and fibula: 4.48; humerus: 5.30; radius 6.7–6.9 and ulna: 6.0–6.3 (approximately).
- In taking measurements of bones, their lengths are measured using Hepburn type osteometric board **(Fig. 5.23)**.

TABLE 5.14: Medico-legal importance of various age groups

Age	Medico-legal importance
5 years	Custody of a minor who is below 5 years is with the mother
7 years	Below this age, child is not responsible for his criminal act, as he does not understand the nature and consequences of his act **(Sec. 82 IPC)**
7–12 years	A child may or may not be held responsible for his act by the court, depending upon whether the child has attained sufficient maturity to understand the nature and consequence of the act **(Sec. 83 IPC)**
10 years	If a child below this age is removed from his lawful guardian for purpose of robbing movable property from his possession, it will amount to **kidnapping (Sec. 369 IPC)**
12 years	• Age of consent for general physical examination including medico-legal examination • A child under this age need not take oath • A child under 12 years cannot give valid consent to suffer any harm which may occur from any act done in good faith and for his benefit **(Sec. 89 IPC)**. • If a child under 12 years is guilty under the Indian Railways Act, 1889 for his willful negligent act or omission, then his father or guardian has to execute a bond for such amount and such period for the good conduct of the child (no punishment is awarded to child)
14 years	**Employment:** Prohibition of child below this age in any employment even as a domestic help (except in non-hazardous family business or as an artist, actor, singer, sports) and is a cognizable offense (CLPR Act 2016)
14–18 years	Adolescents are not allowed in hazardous occupation (mining, inflammable substances, explosives etc) but can work in non-hazardous industries.
16 years	• Taking away a *male* under this age without consent of guardian amounts to **kidnapping (Sec. 361 IPC)** • Learner license to drive a vehicle of 50 cc engine and without any gear
17 years	Admission in a medical college
18 years	• **Statutory rape:** Intercourse with a girl below this age, irrespective of whether with or without her consent amounts to rape • **Judicial punishment:** Below this age, an offender is child and is tried in a Juvenile court, and if convicted, sent to reformatory school (no imprisonment or death sentence)* • Age of **majority** except when the individual is under guardianship of the court • Age of **marriage for females** • Can **cast vote** (in India, UK, US, Australia and most of the countries) • Mentally sound person can make a valid will **(testamentary capacity)** • Age for permanent license to drive a private motor vehicle • Taking out or enticement of a *girl* below this age from custody of her guardian amounts to **kidnapping** • Kidnapping a girl below this age for purpose of begging is punishable (imprisonment of 10 years with/without fine) • Can be **employed** in any authorized job in a factory • Can give valid consent to suffer any harm which may result from an act not intended or not known to cause death or grievous hurt **(Sec. 87 IPC)** • Minimum age for entering a government service • A pregnant female can give valid consent for termination of pregnancy (MTP Act) • A person can authorize the removal of organ from his body for therapeutic purposes (Transplantation of Human Organs Act) • Abetment to suicide of a person below this age is severely punishable (imprisonment up to 10 years to life imprisonment and fine) • Procurement of girl under this age for illicit intercourse is punishable [10 years imprisonment and fine **(Sec. 366A IPC)**]
21 years	• Age of **marriage for males** • If a girl below this age is 'imported' to India from foreign country for the purpose of illicit intercourse, the act amounts to **kidnapping (Sec. 366 B IPC)** • Person under the guardianship of the Court of Wards attains **majority**
25 years	• Age for contesting membership of Parliament and other legislative bodies • Age limit for entering in some government services • According to Punjab Excise Act, a person below this age cannot buy and consume liquor
35 years	• Minimum age for appointment as President, Vice-President and Governor of States in India • Prenatal diagnostic tests/procedures cannot be conducted if the pregnant female is below this age (PCPNDT Act)
55–65 years	Age of retirement from services under the government, statutory bodies, autonomous bodies/institutes or from judiciary services

* Child offenders (16–18 years) committing heinous offenses (e.g. rape, murder) can be tried in Children's court after preliminary assessment.

♦ A simple rule of thumb is that humerus is 20%, tibia 22%, femur 27% and the spine 35% of an individual's height in life.

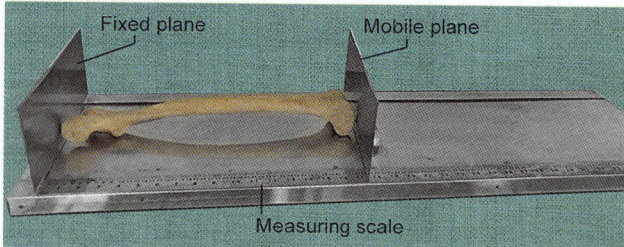

Fig. 5.23: Osteometric board

Describe and discuss identification of criminals, unknown persons, dead bodies from scars and tattoos.

SCARS

Definition: It is a fibrous tissue covered by epithelium without hair follicles, sweat glands or pigment, produced from the healing of a wound.
♦ Scar is formed, if injury is at the level of dermis and below.
♦ The most superficial wounds which involve the epidermis, e.g., superficial burns or abrasions will heal by epithelialization alone without scar formation.

Examination: Good lighting is essential. Description of scars should include number, site, size and shape, level it bears to the body surface, fixed or free, smoothness or irregularity of the surface, color, presence or absence of glistening, tenderness, condition of the ends—whether tapering or not, and the probable direction of the original wound.

Characteristic of Scars

Wound/injury	Features
Lacerated and infected wounds	Firm, irregular and attached to deeper tissues
Incised wounds	Linear scars
Stab wound (knife)	Oval, elliptical, depressed, triangular, irregular scar
Bullet wound	Circular depressed scar
Burns and corrosive acids	Irregular scar
Scalds	Spotted appearance
Vaccination scars	Circular or oval, flat or slightly depressed

Growth: Scars produced in childhood grow in size, especially if situated on chest or limbs.

Age of scars: Refer to **Table 5.15**.

Erasure: Scar can be erased by excision and skin grafting.

TABLE 5.15: Age determination of scars

Features	Duration
Firm union, reddish/bluish scar	5–6 days
Pale, soft and sensitive (tender)	2 weeks–2 months
Tough, brownish, glistening, wrinkled and little tender	2–6 months
Tough, white, glistening, corrugated and non-tender	>6 months

Medico-legal Importance

i. Identification of the individual.
ii. Shape of scar may indicate the nature of weapon or agent that caused injury.
iii. Age of scar indicates time of infliction of injury which may have value as circumstantial evidence.
iv. If a person is disfigured by scar due to assault, it constitutes grievous hurt (**Sec. 320 IPC**).
v. Striae gravidarum and linea albicantes may indicate previous pregnancy in females.
vi. To charge an enemy with assault, a person may attribute scar due to disease as those of wound.
vii. Scars on wrist or throat may indicate previous attempts at suicide.
viii. Linear needle scars indicate an IV drug abuser, and depressed scars a skin popper.

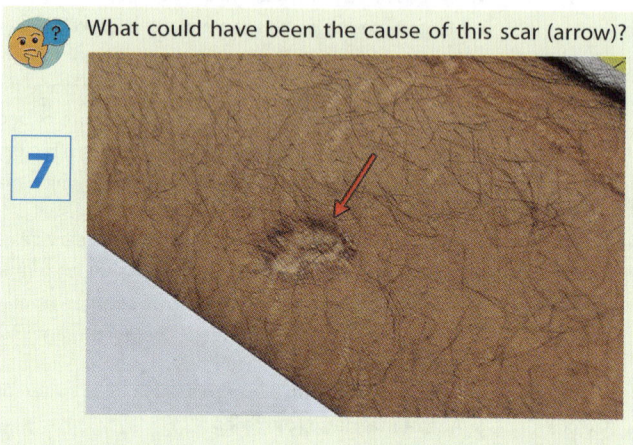

What could have been the cause of this scar (arrow)?

TATTOO MARKS

Definition: Tattoos (Tahitian or Polynesian *tatau*: to mark or strike) are designs made in the skin by multiple small puncture wounds with needles dipped in coloring matter which is attached to an oscillating unit.

Dyes used: Indigo, cobalt, carbon, vermilion, cadmium, selenium, Prussian blue and India ink.
♦ Color, design, size and situation should be noted.
♦ The permanency of tattoo marks depends upon the type of dye used, the depth of its penetration and the

part of body tattooed. Permanent tattoos are obtained if:
  i. Black, blue and red dyes are employed.
  ii. The dye penetrates the dermis.
  iii. The part of body is protected by clothing.
- A latent (faded) tattoo mark becomes visible by rubbing that part and examining with magnifying lens. The use of high contrast photography, computer image enhancement, UV lamp or infra-red photography is also helpful for identifying faded tattoos.
- Tattoos are recognized even in decomposed bodies and bodies recovered from water when the epidermis is removed **(Fig. 5.24)**.
- Since some pigment migrates from the tattoo site to the body's lymph nodes, pigmentations of the axillary lymph nodes in upper extremities tattoos could be identified with the naked eye during autopsy.

Complications: Septic inflammation, abscess, gangrene, syphilis, hepatitis B, AIDS, leprosy and tuberculosis.

Classification of Tattoos

The American Academy of Dermatology distinguishes five types of tattoos:
  i. **Traumatic tattoos** (*'natural tattoos'*) resulting from injuries (road traffic injuries) or close range firearm (unburnt gunpowder) or pencil lead; these are *unintentional* and *unwanted* tattoos.
  ii. **Amateur tattoos** are applied by anyone at home, using a needle and a single color carbon based ink, e.g., India ink applied at varying depths.
  iii. **Professional tattoos** (using both traditional methods and modern tattoo machines) are created by a trained tattoo artist at a salon or tattoo parlor which contains several colors and applied uniformly beneath the skin.
  iv. **Cosmetic tattoos** (also known as *'permanent makeup'*) camouflage skin discolorations, such as birthmarks (hemangiomas) or scars, tattooing 'hair follicles' into bald areas or corneal tattooing (using India Ink) in perforating injury. Two other methods exist: chemical dyeing with gold or platinum chloride and carbon impregnation.
  v. **Medical tattoos** are used for indicating a medically relevant condition or body location, e.g., medical alert tattoos (like insulin-dependent diabetes mellitus or drug allergy), blood group tattoo, reconstructive surgery (nipple-areola complex in mastectomy), delineating the radiation field, and endoscopic tattoos for directing endoscopic procedures.

Erasure of Tattoo

  i. **Surgical methods**
     - **Dermabrasion** using dermabraders [e.g., tannic acid, silver nitrate (*Variot's method*) or trichloroacetic acid (chemical peels)] or '*salt abrasion*' wherein salts like zinc chloride are applied or *Q-switched Nd:YAG laser*. Laser beam vaporizes the particles of the dye and are expelled from tissues in gaseous form.
     - Complete excision and skin grafting.
     - Production of burns by means of red hot iron.
     - Scarification.
     - Using carbon dioxide snow.
  ii. Electrolysis.
  iii. Caustic or corrosive substances remove pigment by producing inflammatory reaction and superficial scar, e.g., mixture of papain in glycerin.

Chronic eczema may cause the tattoo designs to disappear.

Medico-legal Importance

It helps in knowing the:
  i. **Identity** of a person, particularly the dead or decomposed individual—his name or spouse's or friend's; date of birth or joining of service.
  ii. **Religion and nationality:** Designs of Cross or Christ (in Christians), and Hanuman or Lord Krishna (in Hindus).
  iii. **Political affiliations**, e.g., hammer and sickle, lotus or right hand.
  iv. **Race:** Tattooing on the chest and limbs is common amongst the Japanese.
  v. **Profession/occupation:** Some gangs have certain specific emblems of tattoo marks. Some occupations, e.g., coal miners leave visible tattoo marks on the hands and face.
  vi. **Behavioral characteristics:** Tattoos have been associated with high-risk behaviors including alcohol and drug use, violence, carrying weapons, sexual activity, eating disorders and suicide.
     - Erotic tattoos of the sexual fanatic, blue bird design on the extensor surface of the web of thumb of homosexuals, number 13 inside the lower lip of drug pushers, addict type of tattoo marks to conceal injection sites.
  vii. It may also represent **social status** of that individual.

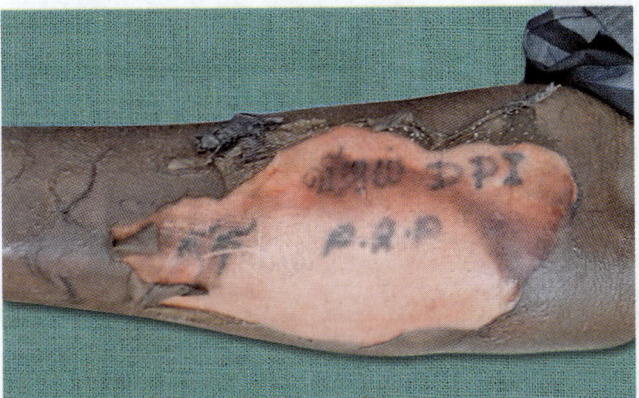

Fig. 5.24: Tattoos seen when epidermis is removed

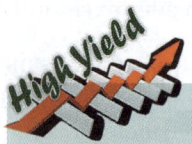

- Sex, age and stature are primary characteristics of identification.
- **Determination of race of individual:** Cephalic index.
- Indian skull is Caucasian with few Negroid characters, CI—75-79.9 (mesaticephalic skull).
- **Disorder of sexual development:** External genitalia atypical in relation to chromosome and gonads.
- **Most certain evidence of sex:** Possession of ovaries in females and testes in males.
- **Confirmatory method of sex determination:** Gonadal biopsy (identification of sex chromosomes).
- In females, Barr body (sex chromatin) is the inactive, condensed X-chromosome found in the cells.
- In XO (Turner's syndrome) there will be no Barr body, and in XXX there will be two Barr bodies.
- XX or XY can be determined in the cells that are dividing, e.g., bloodstains, cartilage, bone marrow, tooth pulp and hair root.
- *Davidson body* can be seen in the neutrophils of females.
- Quinacrine dihydrochloride is used to stain Y-chromosome (referred to as f-body).
- Fluorescent Feulgen reaction using Acriflavin Schiff reagent is used for staining X-chromosome.
- *Streak gonads* are seen in gonadal dysgenesis.
- **Most common DSD associated with male hypogonadism:** Klinefelter syndrome (47XXY).
- **Most common DSD associated with female hypogonadism:** Turner syndrome (45XO).
- **Complete androgen insensitivity syndrome** *(testicular feminization syndrome):* X-linked recessive condition; failure of normal masculinization in genetically male (46XY DSY) individual. Negative Barr body testing.
- **Most common cause of congenital adrenal hyperplasia:** 21-hydroxylase deficiency.
- **Accuracy of sexing based on skeletal remains:** Entire skeleton: 100%; Skull + Pelvis –98%; Pelvis alone (*best single bone*): 95%.
- **Important features to differentiate sex in skull:** Supraorbital margin and ridge, nasion and nuchal crest.
- **Important features to differentiate sex in pelvis:** Pre-auricular sulcus, sub-pubic angle and greater sciatic notch.
- Pre-auricular sulcus is prominent in females.
- Males have more corporobasal index and chilotic line index.
- Females have more sternal index, ischiopubic index, alar index and sciatic notch index.
- **Ashley's rule** *(149 rule):* Determination of sex from sternum for Europeans.
- **First temporary tooth to appear:** Lower central incisor (6–8 months).
- **First permanent tooth to appear:** First molar (6–7 years).
- **Last temporary tooth to fall:** Canine.
- Eruption of temporary teeth is completed by 2½ years.
- Mixed dentition is seen in: 6–11 years of age.
- Total number of teeth between 6 and 12 years: 24.
- Number of permanent teeth present at 8 years: 12.
- Permanent molars are super-added permanent teeth.
- Permanent premolars are successional permanent teeth.
- *Stack method* of dental age estimation is used for infants.
- **Gustafson's method:** Age estimation (beyond 25 years) based on microscopic examination of wear and tear tooth in dead body/skeletal remains.
- **Most reliable criteria of Gustafson's method:** Root transparency.
- **Most reliable non-destructive method of estimation of age from tooth:** Mineralization of teeth to assess stages of development using radiographs.
- **Most reliable destructive method:** Amino acid racemization.
- 'Shovel-shaped' upper central incisors, taurodontism, enamel pearls and congenital lack of upper 3rd molars seen in Mongoloids.
- 'Carabelli's cusp' is seen in Europeans (Caucasian).
- Clavicle—first bone to ossify during the 5–6th postovulatory week.
- The first bone to ossify in the wrist is capitate (1 year).
- Between 2–6 years, the number of carpal bones present on X-ray represents the age in years, e.g., three carpal bones—3 years.
- Pisiform gets ossified by 9-12 years of age.

- **Commonest modality to determine bone age of a child:** X-ray of hand and wrist.
- **Last long bone to ossify in the skeleton** (helps in age estimation): Medial clavicular epiphysis.
- **Best bone to determine age-at-death from third to fifth decade:** Symphyseal surface of pubis.
- **Most successful age estimation from skull suture closure:** Sagittal suture.
- **Last fontanelle to close:** Anterior fontanelle (1½–2 years).
- **Last skull suture to close:** Temporoparietal suture.
- **Best method to estimate age based on secondary sexual characters:** Tanner staging.
- **First pubertal change:** Breast development (in females) and testicular enlargement (in males).
- Child <7 years is not held criminally responsible (Sec. 82 IPC).
- Child below 12 years is not required to take oath.
- Child <14 years cannot be employed for any type of work (not even domestic help).
- Person attains majority at 18 years (21 years if under guardianship of Court of Wards).
- Juvenile offender is a person who has committed a crime and is <18 years of age.
- Female <18 years and male <21 years cannot marry.
- A person can cast vote at 18 years.
- **Consent:** Can give valid consent for general physical and medico-legal examination at ≥12 years; any major diagnostic or operative procedure, donating organs and consent for sexual intercourse is ≥18 years.
- **Kidnapping:** Taking away a person (boy <16 years, girl <18 years) by illegal means.
- Child of any age can give evidence, if the court is satisfied that the child is truthful.
- **Most common method to determine the stature from long bones:** Karl Pearson's regression formula.
- *Hepburn's osteometric board* is used to measure the length of long bones.
- For estimation of stature, femur is more reliable among the long bones.
- **Multiplication factors to calculate stature:** *Femur:* 3.6–3.8; *tibia and fibula:* 4.48; *humerus:* 5.30; *radius:* 6.7–6.9; *ulna:* 6.0–6.3.
- Corneal tattooing can be done with gold chloride.
- Tattoos can be identified from pigmentations of regional lymph nodes.

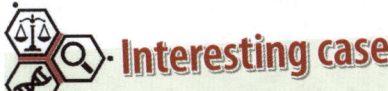 **Interesting case**

Tattoo Mark in Identification (The Shark Arm Case, 1935)

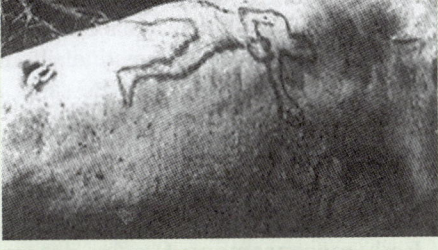

In 1935, a shark on display in an aquarium in Sydney, Australia vomited up a human arm. The arm was well preserved and it had a tattoo of two boxers. It had a rope tied around its wrist. A medical examination showed it had not been bitten off—there were no tooth marks and the limb had been cleanly removed at the shoulder with a blade. The police started a homicide investigation.

A man recognized the description of the tattoo in the news paper and told police the arm might belong to his brother James Smith. He had gone missing weeks before. The police were able to obtain fingerprints from the hand and matched with Smith.

Police found out that Smith had last been seen drinking with person called Patrick Brady. Then, they went to a cottage hired by Brady. The owner of the cottage said that a mattress and a tin trunk had gone missing. The police also found evidence that Smith had worked for a man named Reginald Holmes. He was a wealthy boat builder but was also involved in drug smuggling. He admitted Smith had worked for him. However the two men had fallen out and, the police believed, Smith had been blackmailing Holmes. He was killed to silence him. The police arrested Patrick Brady and Reginald Holmes. He told police that Brady killed Smith. He said Brady brought the severed arm to his house and tried to blackmail him with it, threatening to kill him too if he did not pay him money.

CHAPTER 6

Identification II

LEARNING OBJECTIVES

Must know
1. Dactylography, types, medico-legal importance
2. Examination of hair, medico-legal importance
3. Human and animal hair (Diff.)
4. Cheiloscopy
5. Superimposition

Desirable to know
1. Anthropometry
2. Poroscopy
3. Forensic odontology, charting of teeth
4. Palatoscopy

FM 3.2, 6.1
- Describe and discuss identification of criminals, unknown persons, dead bodies from anthropometry, dactylography, poroscopy and footprints.
- Describe Locard's Exchange Principle.

ANTHROPOMETRY (BERTILLON SYSTEM)

The first scientific method of criminal identification, called anthropometry, is attributable to *Alphonse Bertillon* (regarded as first forensic expert). He developed this system based on principle that the measurements of various parts of the human body do not alter after adult age (21 years). Bertillonage was ultimately replaced by fingerprints system as a scientific method of personal identification, since different individuals can have the same anthropometric measurements.

Anthropometry includes:
- **Descriptive data:** Color of hair, eyes, complexion, shape of nose, ears and chin ('*portrait parle*').
- **Body measurement:** Height, anteroposterior (AP) diameter of head and trunk, span of outstretched arms, length of middle finger, left little finger, left forearm and left foot, length and breadth of right ear, and color of left iris (11 such measurements).
- **Body marks,** such as moles, scars and tattoo marks.
- **Photographs** of front view and right profile of the head are also taken.

DACTYLOGRAPHY

Dactylography (**dermatoglyphics, Galton system**) is the study of fingerprints as a method of identification. A fingerprint match is widely accepted as *most reliable evidence of identification*. This system was first used by Sir William Herschel in 1858. Sir Francis Galton systematized this method in 1892.

What are fingerprints?
- The fingers, palms of the hands and soles of the feet of humans (and some other primates)* bear friction ridge skin **(Fig. 6.1)**. On the tip of the fingers, the friction ridge skin forms a number of basic patterns. Within each basic pattern are numerous possible variations.
- Dermal carvings or ridges appear first time from the 12th–16th week of intrauterine life (IUL) and their formation gets completed by 24th week, i.e., 6th month IUL, and remain constant throughout embryonic life, birth and the life of the individual.
- The arrangement and distribution of the patterns are unique to an individual, and no two hands resemble each other.
- An individual's genetic makeup plays a part in determining the basic shapes of the patterns and ridges, but it is not the only factor as identical twins have identical genetic makeup, but distinguishably different fingerprints (fingerprints are influenced by both genetic and environmental factors during development in the

---

* Fingerprints are not unique to humans. Chimpanzee and gorillas also have fine ridges on their fingertips.

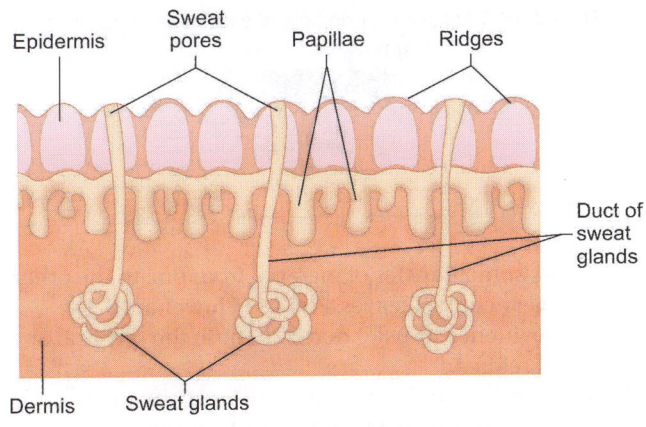

Fig. 6.1: Cross section of friction skin

TABLE 6.1: Types of fingerprint ridges

S.No.	Type	Percentage (%)
1.	Loop (ulnar/radial)	60–70
2.	Whorl	30–35
3.	Arch	5–10
4.	Composite	2–3

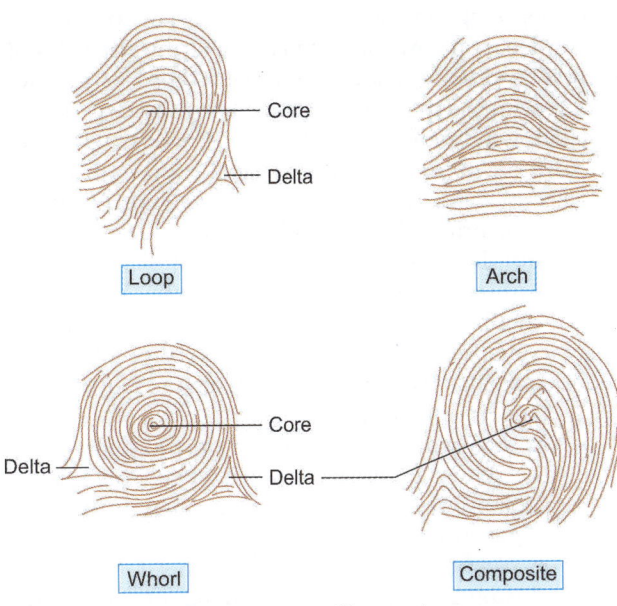

Fig. 6.2: Types of fingerprints

womb). The probability that two individuals will have the same conventional fingerprint is about one in 1 billion.
- Fingerprints do not change throughout life, unless damage has occurred to the dermal skin layer.
- *Temporary loss* of fingerprints may be seen when there is swelling of the fingers, e.g., when stung by bee, but returns when the swelling recedes.
- *Permanent loss* of fingerprint pattern occurs in leprosy, electric injury and after exposure to radiation (injury should involve 1–2 mm beneath the skin surface).
- Fingerprints can be erased permanently and deliberately by criminals to reduce their chance of conviction. Erasure can be achieved in a variety of ways including burns, acids and plastic surgery.

NOTA BENE
- Ridge atrophy with alteration of ridge pattern is seen in celiac disease, dermatitis, eczema, psoriasis, acanthosis nigricans, scleroderma, and dry and atrophic skin. Anticancer drug *capecitabine* may cause the loss of fingerprints. Elderly persons may have fingerprints that are difficult to capture, since the elasticity of skin decreases with age.
- People with certain genetic disorders, such as Baird syndrome (congenital milia), Zinsser–Cole–Engman syndrome (dyskeratosis congenita), Naegeli–Franceschetti–Jadassohn syndrome, dermatopathia pigmentosa reticularis and adermatoglyphia are seen *without* fingerprints.

Fingerprint Patterns

There are four basic ridge patterns depending on presence of core and delta as given in **Table 6.1 and Figure 6.2**. A ridge curving on itself is called the *core*. Convergence of ridges from three directions is called a *delta* (or triradius).
- In **loops**, ridges enter from one side, recurve and exit from same side they entered (there is one core and one delta). Loops can be subdivided into (a) radial: ridges enter and exit from radial side; (b) ulnar: ridges enter and exit from ulnar side.
- In **whorls**, ridges make a complete 360° circuit around the center of the print (there are two deltas).
- **Arches** show no core or deltas, and are subdivided into:
  a. *Plain arch:* Ridges enter from one side, rise to a slight bump and exit out from the opposite side;
  b. *Tented:* Similar to plain arch, but the ridges stand at an angle of 45° or more.
- **Composite** contains at least two different patterns, other than the basic arch. Sometimes, it is also referred to as 'accidental'.

If a scar is formed, it will constitute a valuable addition to the identification process.

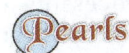 **Pearls**

If a pattern contains neither core nor delta, it is an arch; if it contains one core and one delta, it is a loop; and if it contains one core and two deltas, it is a whorl.

Recording of Fingerprints

Hands are washed, cleaned and dried to ensure clear prints. Print is taken using printer's ink on an unglazed white paper.
  i. **Plain or dab impression** is obtained by gently pressing the inked surface of the tip of finger on paper.

ii. **Rolled impression** is taken by rolling the inked finger from side to side.
- In case of criminals, impressions of all the ten digits of both hands are taken.*
- It is customary and conventional to take the *left thumb impression of male* and *right thumb impression of female* in lieu of signature for illiterate person and on legal and other documents. The reason cited is that in earlier days, males being working class (and as most people are right handed) may have some injury/scar on their right thumb.
- In a dead body, if fingertips are dried up or shrivelled, the prints can be taken after soaking the fingers in an alkaline solution (e.g., KOH). The surface of the fingers can be rounded out and smoothened by injecting glycerin, melted paraffin, hot water or air into the tissues.
    - If the prints obtained by the above methods are not found decipherable, then the palmer skin of the terminal phalanx of each finger may be removed from both the hands and placed in a labeled bottle containing 10% formalin or a solution of glycerin and alcohol for preservation, and transported to the Fingerprint Bureau.
    - In case of advanced putrefaction and in drowning, the skin may come out like a glove which can be preserved in formalin for the development of fingerprints.
- Prints can be obtained from the dermis if epidermis is lost, histological section up to a depth of 0.6 mm from finger pad surface can give satisfactory results.

Types of Evidentiary Fingerprints

Three types of fingerprint may be encountered:
i. **Patent (visible) print** needs no processing to be clearly recognizable as a fingerprint. It is often made from grease, dark oil, dirt or blood, rendering it visible and recognizable, and even suitable for comparison without additional processing.
ii. **Plastic (impression/indentation) print** is a recognizable fingerprint indentation in a soft surface, such as butter, soap, cheese, paint, putty or tar. Such prints have a distinct three-dimensional character, immediately recognizable and require no further processing.
iii. **Latent print** requires additional processing to be rendered visible and suitable for comparison. Processing of latent prints is called *development, enhancement* or *visualization*.

Locard's Principle of Exchange

- Edmond Locard who was a pioneer in forensic science in France formulated the *Locard's principle*. 'When two objects come into contact with each other, there is

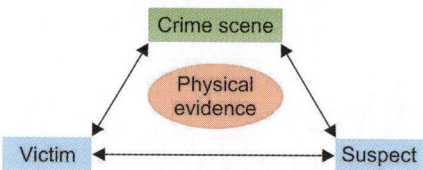

Flowchart 6.1: Locard's principle of exchange: Transfer of physical evidence

always some transfer of material from one to the other, i.e., every contact leaves a trace' **(Flowchart 6.1)**.
- Such evidence transfer occurs in both the physical and digital realms.
- Once this transfer is detected and the substance classified and/or individualized, the forensic specialist will have a clue as to what may have occurred at the scene. The forensic scientist's job is to uncover and reconstruct how the evidence fits into the investigation of a crime.
- For example, fingerprints left behind on a knife, semen deposited in vagina or shoe prints left under a window at a crime scene. An analysis of the impression and wear pattern of the shoes might reveal the make, model and individualization of the shoes which will provide stronger link to the suspect.

Development/Enhancement of Latent Prints

Latent prints are the most prominent example of Locard's Principle of Exchange.

Composition of latent print residue: Palmer and planter surface is completely free from hair and sebaceous glands, but there is profusion of sweat glands (called eccrines), the composition of which forms the basis for latent fingerprint residue; contamination by sebaceous secretions is also quite common from people touching their faces **(Fig. 6.1)**.
- The salts predominant in perspiration are sodium and potassium chlorides, with the organic fraction containing mainly amino acids, urea and lactic acid. Free fatty acids, triglycerides and wax esters prevail in sebaceous secretions.
- Fingerprints are stable compounds and unless they are exposed to extremes of heat or humidity and/or friction, they may persist indefinitely.
- Most methods for the development of latent prints were developed on the basis of knowledge about the latent print residue composition.

Fingerprint Development

Various developments methods are summarized in **Table 6.2**.

---
* **Exemplar/known prints** are fingerprints deliberately collected from a subject, whether for purposes of enrollment in a system or when under arrest for a suspected criminal offense.

CHAPTER 6: Identification II

TABLE 6.2: Development techniques for fingerprints

Nonporous surface (e.g., glass, gloss-painted surfaces, metal and plastic)	*Porous surface* (e.g., paper, wallpaper, cardboard and matt emulsion painted surfaces)*
Vacuum metal deposition (most sensitive, use gold and zinc)	Desferrioxamine (most sensitive)
Fingerprint powders (milled aluminum or brass, or molybdenum disulfide)	Ninhydrin (produces purple color—*Ruhemann's purple*)
Superglue fuming (methyl or ethyl cyanoacrylate)	Physical developer (aqueous solution of silver nitrate + 2 detergents)
Small particle reagent (molybdenum disulfide)	Powders (black or magnetic powder)
Iodine fuming	Superglue fuming

> **NOTA BENE**
> **Other methods for detecting latent prints**
> - *Radioactive sulfur dioxide:* Useful for fabrics and adhesive tapes.
> - *Sudan black:* Useful for surfaces contaminated by grease or foodstuffs.
> - *Osmium tetraoxide:* Useful for both porous and nonporous surfaces.
> - *Electronography:* This technique involve dusting the skin surface with lead (or iron) and then exposure to long wave X-rays (**Grenz rays**). Emission of radiation from the lead powder can be captured on a photographic film. The silver halides present in the film are darkened by the radiation and can produce an image of ridge detail present on the skin surface.
> - *Scanning electron microscopy with an energy dispersive X-ray spectrometer* can be used for imaging of latent fingerprints.

Identification Protocol

- The unknown impression is examined, and all minutiae are analyzed and then compared to the known, to determine if a relationship exists. An acronym ACE-V for four stages for the examination process is given—Analysis, Comparison, Evaluation and Verification.
- Weight is assigned in a comparison, not only to the number of minutiae in agreement, but also the rarity and clarity of those characteristics. Differences in appearance due to recording technique, pressure and other factors must be anticipated.
- The comparison can result in one of *three possible conclusions*: insufficient ridge detail to form a conclusion, exclusion or identification, i.e., that they were made by the same finger.

Fingerprint Classification

- The modified Henry system followed in the US is used for the classification of 10-print sets or a fingerprint card, for one individual.
- The development of computerized fingerprint storage and retrieval systems has made searching larger files for single and partial prints routine. It has also rendered classification largely unnecessary.
- By convention, 12 points of fine comparison were accepted as proof of identity (suggested by Locard). For quite a few decades, a 'minimum number of minutiae (points)' rule is being followed. A fingerprint expert or digital systems need 4-5 points as a minimum for a match—although the more points matched, the better.

Medico-legal Application

i. Identification of criminals whose fingerprints were found at scene.
ii. Identification of fugitive through fingerprint comparison.
iii. Exchange of criminal identifying information with identification bureau of foreign countries in cases of mutual interest.
iv. Identification of unknown deceased person, persons suffering from amnesia, missing persons and unconscious patient.
v. Identification in disaster work.
vi. Identification in case of accidental exchange of newborn infants.
vii. Identification of licensing procedure for automobile, firearm, aircrafts, etc., and for issuance of passport and visa.
viii. Problems of mistaken identity and detection of bank forgeries.
ix. *Biometric system for health workers:* Fingerprint scanners wirelessly sync with a health worker's smartphone to link patient's fingerprint to their health record.
x. *Biometric attendance:* NMC has directed the faculty and residents to mark their attendance by Aadhar Enabled Biometric Attendance System (AEBAS) so as to check absenteeism in all private and government medical institutions.
xi. Electronic fingerprint readers have been introduced for security applications, such as log-in authentication for the identification of computer users. Fingerprint sensors gained popularity in the mobile/notebook PC market.
xii. *Electronic registration and library access*: Fingerprints can be used to validate electronic registration, cashless catering and library access.
xiii. *Sex determination:* The amino acid content in fingerprints can be used to determine sex of the individual. In this method, ninhydrin is combined with an optimized extraction protocol.
xiv. *Identification of recently handled materials:* Extrinsic materials that are left in a fingerprint after recent handling of such materials can be demonstrated using infrared spectromicroscopy which can link as to who

---

* The reagents used for these surfaces react either with amino acids, fats and lipids or chlorides absorbed into the surface.

was handling key materials (including explosives)—can be a powerful investigative tool.

xv. *Detection of drug use:* The secretions in fingerprint contain residues of various chemicals and their metabolites—tobacco, marijuana, cocaine and methadone, which can be detected.

xvi. The police department in Canada has advised parents to fingerprint their children, if they apprehend kidnapping.

> **NOTA BENE**
>
> ♦ Sir Francis Galton published his book in 1892, *'Finger Prints'* and is regarded as a classic work.
> ♦ The first 'Fingerprint Bureau' in the world was officially established in Kolkata on 12th June 1897 at Writers' Building.
> ♦ Sir Edward Henry devised a fingerprint-classification system that was adopted in British India. He presented it in the UK in 1899.
> ♦ **Automated Fingerprint Identification System (AFIS)** is a storage, search, retrieval and exchange system for finger and palm print electronic images and demographic data (biometric data). AFIS utilizes specialized computer software configurations to create unique algorithms based upon relationships between the characteristics present within the finger or palm friction ridge.* To match a print, a fingerprint technician scans the print in question, and computer algorithms are utilized to mark all minutiae points, cores and deltas detected on the print. This enables a fingerprint to be compared with millions of file prints within a matter of seconds.

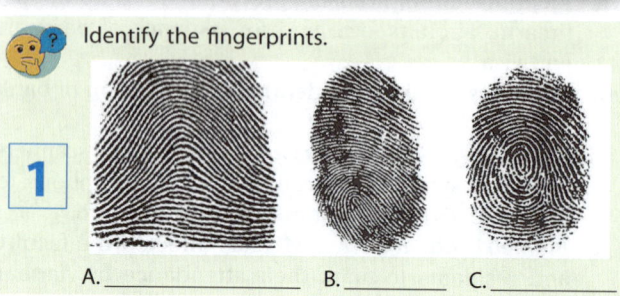

Identify the fingerprints.

A. _____ B. _____ C. _____

POROSCOPY

Poroscopy is the term applied to a specialized study of pore structure found on the papillary ridges of the fingers as a means of identification.

♦ Ridges on fingers and hands are studded with microscopic pores formed by mouths of ducts of subepidermal sweat glands. Each millimeter of ridge contains 9–18 pores. There are about 550–950 sweat pores per square centimeter in finger ridges, and less (400) in the palms and soles **(Fig. 6.3)**.

♦ Poroscopy is the further study of fingerprints, discovered and developed by Edmond Locard in 1912. He observed that like the ridge characteristics, the pores are also permanent, immutable and individual, and these are useful to establish the identity of individuals when available ridges do not provide sufficient ridge characteristics.

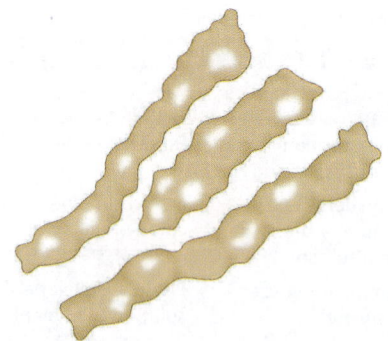

Fig. 6.3: Sweat pores as they appear on ridges

Podography (Footprints)

Skin patterns of toes and heels are as distinct and permanent as those of fingers. Footprints of newborn infants are used in maternity hospitals to prevent exchange or substitution of infants. Records are also kept for air force flying personnel.

> **NOTA BENE**
>
> ♦ **Ridgeology** refers to friction ridge identification that is associated with all the ridges on the volar areas and not just on the fingertips.
> ♦ **Edgeoscopy** (term coined by Salil K Chatterjee in 1962) is the study of the characteristics formed by the sides or edges of papillary ridges as a means of identification.
> ♦ **Forensic podiatry:** Specialty using clinical podiatric knowledge for the purpose of person identification. Techniques of forensic podiatry include identification from podiatry records, the human footprint, footwear, and the analysis of gait forms captured on CCTV cameras. The most valuable techniques relate to the comparison of the foot impressions seen inside the shoes.

LIP PRINTS (CHEILOSCOPY)

♦ The study of lip prints is called *cheiloscopy*.
♦ It is said that a person's lip prints are unique and can be useful for personal identification (currently lip print identification is not accepted as evidence in court of law).
♦ Lip prints are revealed at the point of direct, physical contact of the individual's lips with an object at the scene of crime, e.g., cutlery and crockery items, particularly if a meal was eaten, or on the surface of windows, plastic bags and cigarette ends.
♦ Suzuki has divided lip prints into five main types **(Fig. 6.4)**. Type I represents grooves running vertically over the lips. Type I' has partial length grooves of Type I variety. They do not cover the entire breadth of the lips. Type II represents the branched grooves and Type III

---

* To create a digital fingerprint, a person places his finger on the scanner and holds it there for a few seconds. Ink-free digital imprints of ten fingers are taken. The main ways of scanning fingers may be optical, ultrasonic, capacitive or thermal.

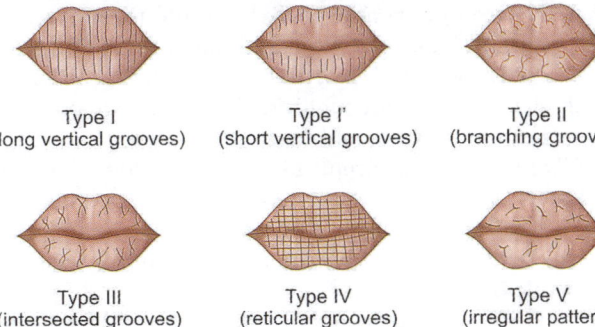

Fig. 6.4: Types of lip prints

 A. Study of lip prints left behind in crime scene is called _____.
B. Predominant pattern (type) which can be seen in lower lip is _____.

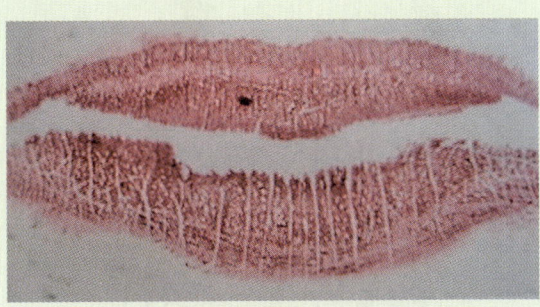

represents the intersected grooves. Type IV represents the reticular pattern, much like a wire mesh. Type V represents all other patterns. These are irregular non-classified patterns.

Recent Advances in Identification

Retina and iris scanning
- Eye-based biometrics is considered the most secure of all biometrics.
- Useful in high-security applications, such as prisons, governmental agencies and schools.
- Eye scanning consists of 2 forms—iris scanning and retina scanning.
- First biometric eye-scanning was the retina recognition.
- Retinal scanners examine the patterns of retinal blood vessels by casting either natural or infrared light onto them. It is an extremely accurate process as the retinal patterns are stable over time and unique to individuals. However, the equipment for retina scanning is bulky, complex and costly and the procedures tend to be uncomfortable for users.
- Iris scanning is a newer technology. An iris scan is a high-quality photograph taken under near-infrared illumination. Iris patterns are complex, containing more raw information than a fingerprint. Irises are unique and even identical twins exhibit different iris patterns. Iris recognition involves standard imaging cameras that are not specialized or expensive.

Facial recognition
- Major advantage of facial recognition over other biometric technologies is that it is nonintrusive. It does not require individuals to provide fingerprint or eyes scanned.
- However, facial recognition is affected by time. The appearance and shape of a face change with one's aging process and alterations to face (surgery, accidents, shaving or burns).
- Several methods have been devised—one technique analyzes the bone structure and the eyes, nose and cheeks. Another technology recognizes a neural-network pattern in a face and scans for 'hot spots' using infrared technology. The infrared creates a so-called 'facial thermogram'.

Voice recognition
- Voice recognition differs from other biometric as it uses acoustic information instead of images. Each individual has a unique set of voice characteristics that are difficult to imitate.
- Its advantage over other biometrics is that voice data can be transmitted over phone lines which can be used in security, fraud prevention and monitoring.
- Voice recognition use three types of speaker verification—text dependent, text prompted and text independent.

FM 3.2
Describe and discuss identification of criminals, unknown persons, dead bodies from the remains—hairs and fibers.

HAIR

- Examination of hair **(tricology)** can provide crime investigators with important clues.
- Apart from burning, hair is virtually indestructible.
- It remains identifiable even on bodies in an advanced state of decomposition, or attached to the weapon of offense after a crime has been committed.

When a sample of hair is submitted for examination, the following questions need to be answered.

MEDICO-LEGAL QUESTIONS

Q. Is the material hair or some other fiber?

Hair consists of bulb or root, shaft and a tip **(Fig. 6.5)**.
- *Root* is the portion of hair at the base of skin. It has a base known as bulb, embedded inside the hair follicle.
- *Shaft* is the portion of hair lying above the skin and tapers to terminate at the free end as *tip*.

On sectioning, hair can be divided into three zones **(Fig. 6.6)**:
i. **Cuticle:** Outermost layer, consists of thin non-pigmented microscopic scales.
ii. **Cortex:** Middle layer, consists of longitudinally arranged elongated cells. Within these cells are fibrils on which there may be granules of pigment. It has keratin that is responsible for the charring and acrid odor when the hair is burned.
iii. **Medulla:** Innermost layer, composed of keratinized remains of cells.

These three zones are also seen in the root or bulb, but the tip is usually nonmedullated.

Fibers
- Fibers can be classified into two groups: natural and artificial (manmade).

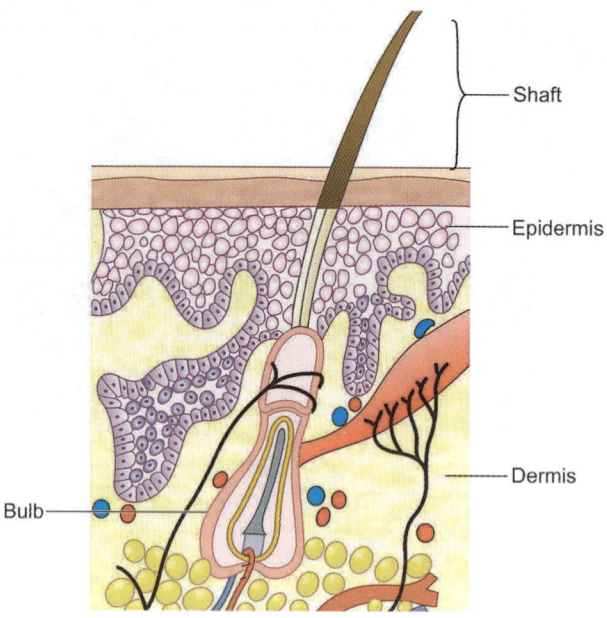

Fig. 6.5: Parts of hair

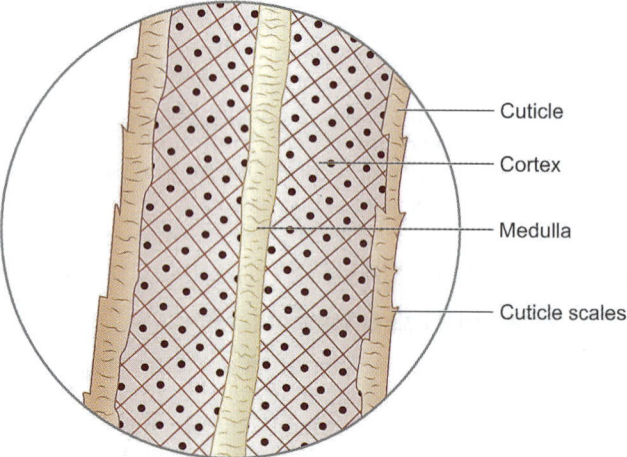

Fig. 6.6: Longitudinal section of human hair

i. *Natural fibers* are subdivided into three classes: animal (e.g., silk, wool and hair), vegetable (e.g., cotton, jute and coir) and mineral (e.g., asbestos).
ii. *Artificial fibers* are subdivided into synthetic-polymer, natural-polymer and other fibers.

- All animal fibers, except silk can be considered as hair fibers.
- Most natural fibers have distinctive appearances that can be detected under the comparison microscope **(Table 6.3)**.
- Synthetic fiber that cannot easily be identified with the microscope can be subjected to infrared spectrophotometry.

Q. If hair, is it human or animal hair?

Difference between human and animal hair is given in **Diff. 6.1 (Figs. 6.7 and 6.8)**.

> The **medullary index (MI)** is defined as the ratio of the diameter of the medulla to the diameter of shaft of whole hair.
> $$MI = \frac{\text{Diameter of medulla}}{\text{Diameter of hair}}$$

Q. What could be the racial profile of the person?

- Important differences are given in **Diff. 6.2** and **Figure 6.9A**.
- These features become somewhat less useful for identifying people of mixed ancestry.

TABLE 6.3: Microscopic features of different fibers

Fiber	Features
Cotton	Flattened and twisted tubes consisting of long tubular cells with thickened edges and blunt pointed ends
Silk	Consists of long clear threads without any cells. They have smooth surface and are finely striated
Wool	Being an animal hair, it shows an outer layer of flattened cells and overlapping margins. Interior is composed of fibrous tissue, but sometimes medulla is present

DIFFERENTIATION 6.1: Human and animal hair

S.No.	Feature	Human hair	Animal hair
1.	External	Delicate, fine and thin	Coarse and thick
2.	Color	Black, gray, reddish or reddish-brown	Any color, can have banded appearance
3.	**Cortex**	Thick, well striated, 4–10 times as broad as medulla	Thin, rarely twice as broad as medulla
4.	**Medulla**	Narrow, may be continuous, interrupted, fragmented or even absent	Broad, continuous and always present
5.	**Medullary index**	<1/3	>1/3
6.	Shaft diameter	50–150 μ	25 μ or >3000 μ
7.	Root	Bulb or ribbon-shaped	Brush-like
8.	Tip	Cut or frayed (scalp hair)	Tapered
9.	Cuticular scales	Short, broad, thin and irregularly annular	Large and have step-like or wavy projections
10.	Pigment granules	Uniformly distributed	Mostly clumped near the medulla
11.	Precipitin test (with intact root)	Specific for human	Specific for animal

CHAPTER 6 : Identification II

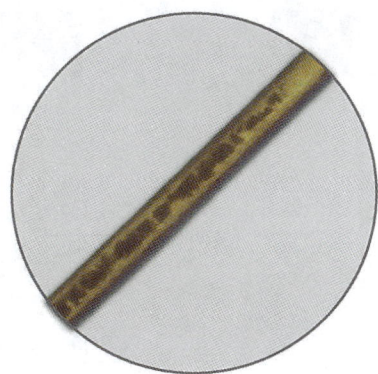

Fig. 6.7: Human hair

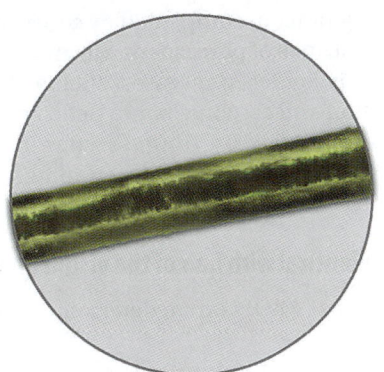

Fig. 6.8: Animal hair

DIFFERENTIATION 6.2: Ethnic differences in human hair

S.No.	Feature	Caucasians	Mongolians	Negroes
1.	Color	Light brown	Black or dark brown	Black or dark brown
2.	Consistency	Fine to medium	Coarse	Short, curly, finest
3.	Shape	Oval	Round	Flat
4.	Shaft diameter	Slight variation	Constant diameter	Wide variation
5.	Pigmentation	Uniform	Coarse granules	Irregular
6.	Cuticle	Thin	Thick	Medium
7.	Medulla	Fragmented or absent	Unbroken	Fragmented or absent

Q. From what part of body has the hair originated?

- *Scalp hair:* Long, soft, taper from root to tip, split ends, and circular on cross section **(Fig. 6.9B)**.
- *Beard and moustache*: Thicker, straight, blunted tip, and triangular on cross section.
- *Axillary and pubic hair*: Stout, short, lack of uniformity, and curly with frayed or split ends.
- *Eyebrow, eyelashes and nostril hair*: Short and stiff, thick, tapering abruptly, and triangular on cross section **(Fig. 6.9B)**.
- *Body hair*: Soft, fine and flexible, lack of uniformity of medulla, milder pigmentation, and narrow tip.

Q. Is it male or female hair?

- Beard and moustache are specific for males. Male hair is usually thicker, coarser and darker as compared to females.
- Barr bodies can be detected in the hair follicles in about 20–80% of females and only about 0–4% of the males.
- Sexing can be done if root sheath is present, using DNA analysis.

Q. What could be the age of the person?

Whether the hair is that of an infant or adult can be said.
- *Lanugo hair* of the newborn are fine, downy, soft, non-pigmented, nonmedullated, and cuticular scales have smooth edges.
- Adult hair are coarser, pigmented and medullated having a complex cuticular pattern.
- Gray hair are apparent after the age of 40, and are devoid of any pigment.

Q. Has the hair being altered by dyeing, bleaching or diseased?

- Bleached or colored hair are dry, brittle, lusterless and rough. Abrupt color change to a very light color indicates bleaching.
- Color in cuticle indicates dyeing. Microscopical examination with incident fluorescence illumination may show whether hair is dyed or not.

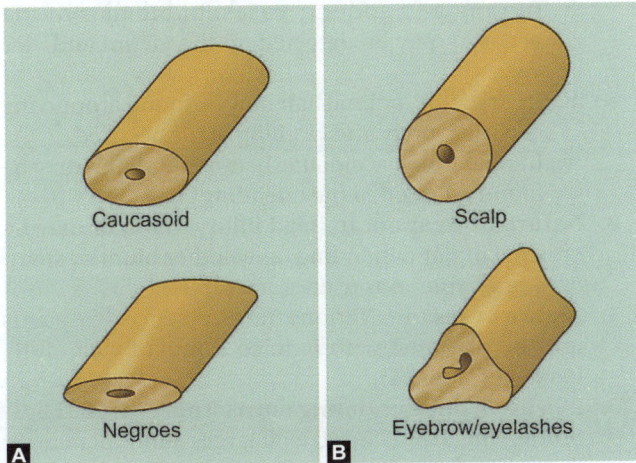

Figs. 6.9A and B: Cross section of hair

- Curly appearance accompanied by constrictions in the shaft is indicative of permanent waving.
- Hair color is lighter in diseases, such as kwashiorkor, malnutrition and certain vitamin deficiencies.
- Tunneling of hair by fungal hypae can produce distinctive transverse lines—seen in hair exposed to fungi, and occur in buried bodies.

Q. Is the hair identical with hair of the victim or the suspect?

- Blood groups (ABO) can be determined from a single hair bulb.
- Microscopic examination of scalp hair may provide information of pediatric conditions, such as Menkes disease, Netherton's syndrome, monilethrix, etc.
- If some root structure is present, standard DNA profiling can be used.
- Even if the shaft is there, mitochondrial DNA (mtDNA) testing can be tried.

Q. Did the hair fall naturally or was it forcibly removed?

- The bulb of naturally fallen hair is distorted, atrophied and the hair sheath is absent (**Fig. 6.10A**).
- In forcibly plucked hair, the hair sheath is ruptured, bulb is swollen, larger and irregular (**Fig. 6.10B**).
- If the root is not present, an even break with regular edges indicates that it was cut off, and an irregular break indicates the hair was broken off.

Q. What is the cause of injury?

- In uncut hair, the tip is pointed and nonmedullated (**Fig. 6.11**).
- Sharp weapon produces a clean uniform cut surface (**Fig. 6.11**).
- Blunt force injury result in flattening and splitting of hair shaft.

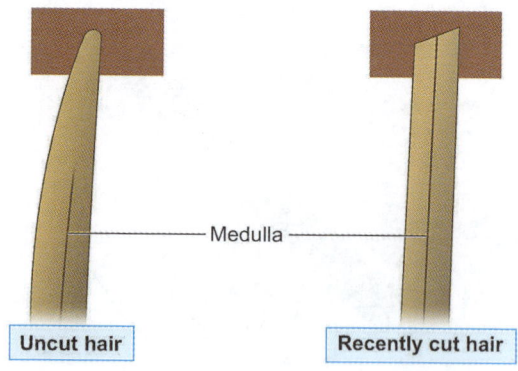

Fig. 6.11: Tip of hair

- Singed hair due to burns or firearm injury are swollen, fragile, curled, twisted and have a peculiar odor.

> **NOTA BENE**
>
> **Postmortem root banding** may be seen in decomposed body, wherein an opaque band about 0.5 mm above the root bulb can be observed with transmitted light microscope.

Medico-legal Application

1. **Identification:** Hair remains identifiable long after the commission of crime and provides valuable physical evidence. In homicidal cases, presence of hair in the grip of the hand of the deceased in cadaveric spasm may help in identification of the assailant.
2. **Establish relationship between offense, offender and the victim.** Suitable hair can be compared microscopically with known hair samples to determine if they could have come from the same source. This is augmented by mtDNA sequencing.
    i. It is an important clue when similar hair may be detected on the alleged weapon and on the body of the assailant.
    ii. In rape and sodomy cases, pubic hair of the accused may be detected on the victim and vice versa.
    iii. In bestiality, animal hair may be found around the genitalia, body and clothing of the accused.
    iv. In road traffic accidents, hair of the victim may be found adhered to the offending car.
3. **Nature of weapon:** In head injury, the hair may be crushed or cut depending on whether blunt or sharp cutting weapon was used.
4. **Nature of assault:** Various trace evidence, like stains may be attached with hair, so it must be carefully looked (**Table 6.4**).
5. It helps in **differentiating burns from scalds**. Hair is brittle, singed or charred with large round vacuoles at the point of burning which is absent in scalds.

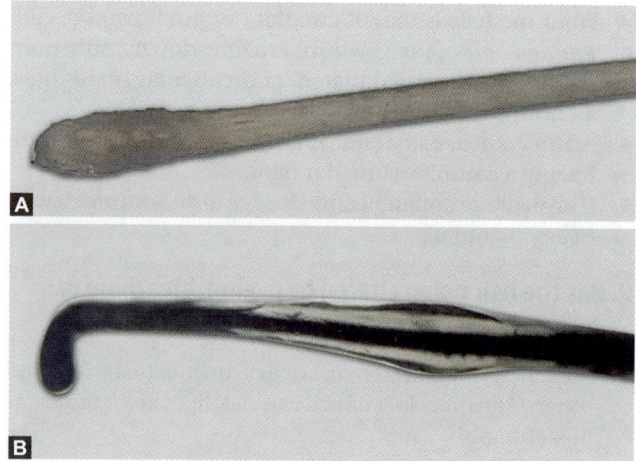

Figs. 6.10A and B: (A) Root of a naturally fallen hair; (B) Healthy hair bulb (plucked)

CHAPTER 6 : Identification II

TABLE 6.4: Stains attached on the hair

Type of stains	Suggestive information
Seminal	Sexual offense
Blood	Injury
Salivary	Asphyxial deaths
Mud	Struggle/road traffic accident
Carbon particles	Burns/firearm injury
Dyes	Concealment of natural color

6. Singeing of hair indicates **burns** or close range **firearm injury**.
7. **Alcohol testing:** Hair alcohol testing is used to know whether or not a person has consumed alcohol at a frequent and excessive rate over a period of time. The concentration of ethyl glucuronide and fatty acid ethyl esters found in a hair sample reflects the consumption of alcohol over the period covered by the sample.
8. **Time since death** can be estimated from growth of scalp hair or beard (growth rate: 2.5 mm/week or 0.4 mm/day) *if the date of last shave is known*. It is possible to calculate for what period the deceased survived after his last shave.
9. **Age and sex** can be determined.
10. **Cause of death:** Poisons, such as *arsenic, thallium or lead* can be determined from hair. Sometimes, accidental poisoning may occur with compounds like aniline derivatives including paraphenylene diamine (PPD) and resorcinol found in hair dye.

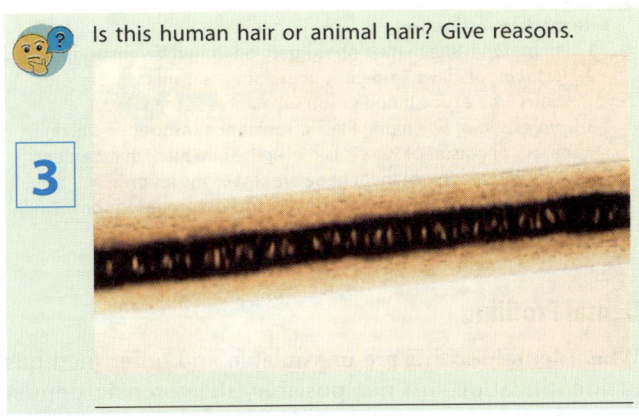

Is this human hair or animal hair? Give reasons.

FM 3.2
Describe and discuss superimposition.

SUPERIMPOSITION

- Technique applied to determine whether the recovered skull is that of the person in the photograph.
- Technologically, skull-photo superimposition have passed through three phases—the photographic, video, and computer-assisted superimposition techniques.

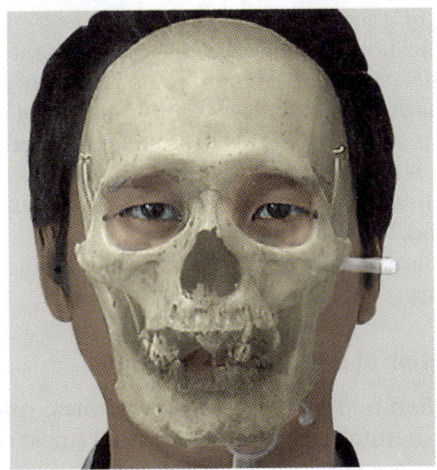

Fig. 6.12: Computer-assisted superimposition technique

- While performing photographic superimposition, the comparison photograph is enlarged to the size of the unknown skull and then the skull is positioned in the same orientation as the facial photograph.
- Recently, computer-assisted superimposition has become a popular method which digitize the skull and facial photograph using a video computer with appropriate software, and then compare the two images morphologically by image processing **(Fig. 6.12)**.
- The complete skull is required to obtain positive identification. Without the mandible, it cannot be positively be identified as the presumed person, even if a good match is seen in skull-superimposition image.
- The coincidence of dentition between the skull and facial photograph (if incisors and canines are seen) could lead to positive identification.
- When evaluating anatomical consistency between the parts, special attention should be paid to their outline, the facial tissue thickness at various anthropometric points, and the positional relationships between skull and face-eyebrow to supraorbital margin, eye to orbit, nose to nasal aperture, lips to teeth and ear to external auditory meatus.
- If they are well matched with each other, it can only be stated that the skull could be that of the photographed person.
- Test is of a more negative value, because it can be *definitely be stated* that the skull and photograph are not those of the same person.

FM 3.1, 3.2
- Define and describe—establishment of identity of living persons: Bite marks.
- Describe and discuss identification of criminals, unknown persons, dead bodies from the remains—teeth.

FORENSIC ODONTOLOGY

Definition: It deals with the application of dentistry to aid in the administration of justice.

The work of a forensic odontologist includes:
- Identification of unknown bodies through dental records.
- Identification of bite marks on the victims of attack.
- Comparison of bite marks with the teeth of a suspect and presentation of this evidence in the court as an expert witness.
- Identification of bite marks on other substances, such as wood, leather and foodstuffs.
- Age estimation of living individuals, cadavers and skeletal remains.

Identification of Human Remains

Unidentified bodies due to violent crimes, road traffic accidents, natural and manmade disaster (mass casualties normally associated with aviation disasters), drowning, burns, murder, suicide or dead from natural causes rely on dental evidence to positively identify the body.
- Postmortem dental remains can be compared with antemortem dental records, including written notes, study casts, radiographs, etc. to confirm identity.
- Individuals with numerous and complex dental treatments are often easier to identify than those individuals with little or no restorative treatment.
- Once the postmortem record is complete, a comparison with antemortem dental records can be carried out. A range of conclusions can be reached when reporting a dental identification.
- Even if only a few teeth are available, odontologists can determine age, smoking habit, state of oral hygiene, and identify individual features which may match with antemortem records.
- In cases where the subject has no teeth, useful information can still be obtained from the study of any dentures and by X-ray of mouth and skull.

Recent Advances in Dental Identification
In problem cases, a variety of techniques are used to assist in the identification issue. These include:
- Incremental line and other histology studies (*Maples* noted that 2nd molar was best for histological ageing techniques).
- Scanning electron microscopy with/without energy-dispersive X-ray analysis.
- Metal ratio analysis in bone and teeth, especially magnesium/zinc ratio.
- Serology studies for blood groups, serum proteins and polymorphic enzymes.
- DNA analyses: Dental pulp material is a good source for DNA analysis; two vital teeth (preferably molars, canines/premolars) are extracted and sent for examination.

Bite Marks

Bites are commonly seen in cases of:
i. *Sexual assault*: Marks are usually seen on breasts, neck, shoulders, thighs, abdomen, pubis or vulva.
ii. *Child abuse*: Marks are seen anywhere on the body, such as arms, hands, shoulders, cheeks, buttocks and trunk.
iii. Bite marks on foodstuffs (apples, cheese or chocolate), leather (key rings or belts) and wood (pencils) in cases where a perpetrator might have taken a bite out of something in the victim's home and left it behind.
iv. Police officers may be bitten by the resisting offenders.
v. In sporting events, such as football, rugby or wrestling.
vi. In assaults, where marks may be found anywhere on the body.

Nature of bite marks: Comprise of a crop of punctate hemorrhages varying from small petechiae to large ecchymoses merging into a confluent central bruise. Human bite is semicircular or crescentic caused by the front teeth (incisors and canines) with a gap on either side due to separation of upper and lower jaw, whereas deep parabolic arch or U-shaped is characteristic of an animal bite. There may be abrasions, bruises and lacerations or a combination of all these.
- *Self-inflicted bite marks* are present on accessible parts of the body, e.g., shoulders or arms, usually seen in psychiatric patients or teenage girls.
- *Accidental marks* resulting from falls on to the face and during fits, biting of tongue and lips may also be there.
- *In sexual assault*, sucking action during bites reduces the air pressure in the center, and produces multiple petechial hemorrhages due to rupture of small capillaries and venules.

Identification from bite marks is possible, if incisors and canines have some characteristic features.

NOTA BENE

Bite mark investigation
1. *Photograph:* Bite mark is photographed from different angles.
2. *Swabbing of saliva:* To identify or exclude assailant from 'secretor' status who exude blood group substances in the saliva.
3. *Impression of bite mark:* Plastic substance (rubber or silicone based) or plaster of Paris is laid over the bite mark that hardens and produces permanent negative cast of the lesion.
4. Skin carrying the bite is removed and preserved in formalin during autopsy.

Dental Profiling

When dental records are unavailable and other methods of identification are not possible, the forensic dentist often produces a 'picture' of the general features of the individual known as *dental profiling*. It will typically provide information of the deceased's age, ancestral background, sex, and socioeconomic status. In some instances, it is possible to provide additional information regarding occupation, dietary habits, habitual behaviors, and occasionally, on dental or systemic diseases.

Charting of Teeth

On the charts, following peculiarities are recorded:
i. Any extractions, recent or old
ii. Any fillings, number, position and composition

iii. Artificial teeth, whether of gold, porcelain or stainless steel
iv. Prosthetic work in mouth, such as bridge work or braces
v. Any crowned teeth
vi. Any broken teeth
vii. Pathological conditions in teeth, jaws or gums
viii. Congenital defects, such as Hutchinson's teeth or ectopic teeth
ix. Malpositioned teeth that are rotated or tilted
x. General state of hygiene, such as caries, plaque, tobacco staining, or gingivitis
xi. Racial pointers, such as shovel-shaped upper central incisors, enamel pearls, Carabelli's cusps or multi-cusped molars.

Most widely used systems are:
1. **FDI** (*Federation Dentaire Internationale*)—**two-digit system**: A two-digit notation indicating tooth and quadrant is the *most commonly used method* (quadrant number before teeth number). The first digit indicates the quadrant (1 to 4; 1 for upper right quadrant and continues clockwise till lower right quadrant) and second digit indicates tooth type (1 to 8, starting from mid-line to third molar which is similar to Palmer system). Thus, lower right canine will be numbered 43.*

   A. **Permanent teeth**

	Upper right-1	Upper left-2	
Patient's right	18 17 16 15 14 13 12 11	21 22 23 24 25 26 27 28	Patient's left
	48 47 46 45 44 43 42 41	31 32 33 34 35 36 37 38	
	Lower right-4	Lower left-3	

   B. **Deciduous teeth**

	Upper right-5	Upper left-6	
Patient's right	55 54 53 52 51	61 62 63 64 65	Patient's left
	85 84 83 82 81	71 72 73 74 75	
	Lower right-8	Lower left-7	

2. **Universal (Cunningham) system:** Follows the plan advocated by American and International Society of Forensic Odontology. The permanent teeth are numbered from 1 to 32, and lettering the deciduous teeth A to T, starting at the posterior upper right and continuing in a clockwise direction. The 'Army system', 'Navy system' and 'Bosworth system' are variations of this system.

Right	1 2 3 4 5 6 7 8	9 10 11 12 13 14 15 16	Left
	32 31 30 29 27 27 26 25	24 23 22 21 20 18 18 17	

3. **Palmer's notation:** Adult teeth are numbered 1 to 8, with deciduous teeth indicated by a letter A to E. The Palmer notation⁺ consists of a symbol (⌐ ⌐ ¬ ¬) designating in which quadrant the tooth is found and a number indicating the position from the midline. For example, the left and right maxillary lateral incisor has the same number, i.e., '2', but the right one would have symbol, '⌐', underneath it, while the left one would have, '⌐'.

Right	8 7 6 5 4 3 2 1	1 2 3 4 5 6 7 8	Left
	8 7 6 5 4 3 2 1	1 2 3 4 5 6 7 8	

4. **Haderup system:** It is similar to Palmer notation, except it uses a plus sign (+) to designate upper teeth and a minus sign (-) for lower. For the deciduous teeth, a zero was additionally placed in front of the number. This notation was adopted by the Scandinavian countries.

Right	8+ 7+ 6+ 5+ 4+ 3+ 2+ 1+	+1 +2 +3 +4 +5 +6 +7 +8	Left
	8- 7- 6- 5- 4- 3- 2- 1-	-1 -2 -3 -4 -5 -6 -7 -8	

5. **Diagrammatic or anatomical chart:** In this, each tooth is represented by a pictorial symbol that gives the same number of tooth surfaces as those on that particular tooth in mouth. Incisors and canines are represented by four surfaces, premolars and molars by five.

Medico-legal Application

1. **Identification:** Dental identification is the most useful method of identification after dactylography (not much use in developing countries, as dentists often do not keep records).
   - Identification of unknown dead bodies.
   - Identification of burnt, mutilated or decomposing remains, as the teeth are very resistant to decomposition, incineration, trauma or destruction, particularly in mass disasters.
2. **Age** estimation of an individual.
3. Identification of race, sex, occupation or habits (betel nut chewing or smoking) of an individual.
   Microscopic examination of teeth can confirm sex by the presence or absence of Y-chromatin, and DNA analysis can also reveal sex.
4. **Grievous hurt:** Fracture/dislocation of tooth amounts to grievous hurt according to **Sec. 320 IPC**.
5. **Cause of death:** Since teeth resist putrefaction, deposition of metals can be detected after considerable time after death, e.g., lead poisoning, or phossy jaw.
6. Dentures (partial or complete) are useful in identification, if they have the patient's name or code number in them.
7. Criminals can be identified through bite marks left either on human tissues or foodstuffs. However, a number of DNA exonerations have occurred in recent years for individuals convicted based on erroneous bite mark identifications.

MISCELLANEOUS METHODS OF IDENTIFICATION

Clothes and Personal Effects

They are helpful in establishing identity in case of mass disasters. It is necessary to preserve the clothes along with

---

* There is no modified FDI system as given in most of the books. It is a misnomer.
⁺ It was originally named **Zsigmondy system** (oldest method, introduced in 1861). Permanent teeth were numbered 1 to 8, and the deciduous teeth were depicted using Roman numerals I, II, III, IV, V from the midline. Palmer changed this to A, B, C, D, E.

any articles, such as driving license, cell phone, watch, spectacles, ornaments and wallet found on a dead body for the purpose of future identification. The clothes are examined for mark of the tailor, foreign material or any tear.

Occupational Marks

These are helpful in identifying unknown dead bodies, as certain occupation leave marks by which persons engaged in them may be identified, e.g., clerks may have callosity on the proximal part of right middle finger where the pen usually rests, or dyers/photographers may have there fingers stained with dyes or chemicals.

Handwriting

Opinion regarding the handwriting (graphology) is usually given by the expert in this field, and doctors are seldom asked to testify. But, sometimes, the doctor may have to examine a person so as to acertain whether he is able to write when a plea of paralysis or mental incapacity is put forward.

Speech, Voice, Ticks, Manner and Habit

Sometime, it is possible to identify a living person from certain peculiarities, like stammering, nasal twang and jerky movement of muscle of the face or shoulder.

> **NOTA BENE**
>
> *Other methods of identification*
> 1. **Palatoscopy/palato-print/rugoscopy:** It is the study of palatal rugae in order to establish identity. Rugae ('*plica palatine*') are anatomical fold or wrinkles formed 12–14th week of IUL in the maxillary portion of the oral cavity. This irregular fibrous connective tissue is located on the anterior third of the palate, each side of the median palatal raphe and behind the incisive papilla. Palatine rugae are unique and can be used for identification in circumstances when it is difficult to identify a dead person through dental records or fingerprints (even in advanced decomposition).
>
>   This method is useful since:
>   - Rugae pattern remain stable throughout life and does not change during growth.
>   - It is protected from trauma and heat due to its situation and by buccal pad of fat and tongue.
>   - Even in twins, the pattern of rugae may be similar but not identical.
> 2. **Ameloglyphics** (amelo: enamel; glyphics: carvings): The study of pattern of enamel rods is a recent technique in identification as the enamel of teeth is highly calcified structure that resists putrefaction; tooth print is composed of combination of basic subpatterns and are unique to single tooth, exhibiting dissimilarity both between teeth of same individual, as well as different individuals. This method can be recommended for those individuals working in dangerous occupations, such as fire fighters, soldiers, jet pilots, divers, and people who live or travel to politically unstable areas.
> 3. **Fronal sinus print:** It is unique to a particular individual, and these are permanent and fixed (after 15 years of age), and rarely alter following infection or injury. For comparison, antemortem X-ray of skull taken on occipitomental plane is compared with postmortem X-rays.
> 4. **Vascular grooves and sutural pattern:** The sutural pattern on the skull bone, particularly of sagittal and lambdoid sutures are complex and are individualistic. Similarly, the vascular grooves over skull bone, particularly of middle meningeal vessels are individualistic. Rather, vascular grooves over skull are more helpful for identification as compared to suture lines, because these are well demonstrable in X-rays.
> 5. **Ear print:** It is the study of shapes of the ear lobules and tips of ears, as well as the hardness or softness of the helix and lobules, and hairiness of the helix and tragus. These characters of the ears are considered to be individualistic.
> 6. **Nose print:** The lines on the nose and shape of the tip of nose are considered to be individualistic. Chance impressions may be found over door, wall and mirror at the scene of crime or even on the body of the victim or accused.
> 7. **Nail print:** It is the study of the depressions and elevations (striations), numbers, distribution and dimensions of the ridges on the surface of the nails, which are considered to be individualistic. They remain unchanged throughout life, and with advancement of age the striations become more prominent. The longitudinal striations are present over both convex and concave surfaces of finger and toe nails.
> 8. **EV method of identification:** The electrocardiogram (ECG or EKG) and vector cardiogram (VCG) trace expresses cardiac features that are unique to an individual. As a biometric, heartbeat data are difficult to disguise, reducing the likelihood of successfully applying falsified credentials into an authentication system.
> 9. **'Barium meal' X-ray of stomach:** It is also considered to be individualistic and may be helpful in identification, if previous record is available.

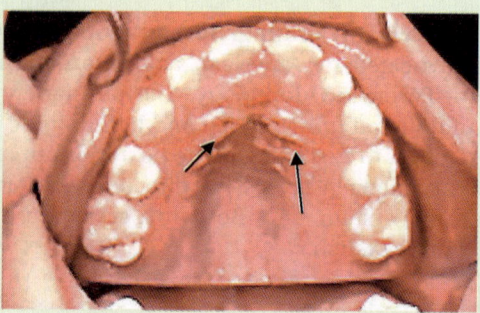

Study of transverse palatal rugae inside the mouth (arrows) is called:

CHAPTER 6 : Identification II

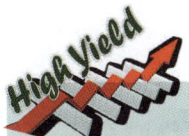

- **First scientific method of criminal identification:** Bertillon system/anthropometry.
- **Most reliable method of identification:** Fingerprints (Galton system/dactylography)
- Identical twins have identical genetic makeup, but different fingerprints.
- Fingerprints are not inherited and paternity cannot be proved by fingerprints (paternity testing only by DNA fingerprint).
- Fingerprinting was first used by Sir William Herschel. Sir Francis Galton systematized this method.
- World's first *'Fingerprint Bureau'* was established in Kolkata in 1897 at Writers' Building.
- **Permanent impairment of fingerprint:** Leprosy, electric injury, exposure to radiation, anticancer drug *capecitabine*.
- **Most common ridge pattern:** Loop.
- *Locard's Principle of Exchange* states that every contact leaves a trace.
- No minimum number of features required for making fingerprint identification.
- **Poroscopy:** Study of pore structure on papillary ridges of fingers.
- **Cheiloscopy:** Study of lip prints.
- The order of effectiveness of biometric systems are palm scans, hand geometry, iris scan, retina scan and fingerprint.
- **Medullary index (MI):** Ratio of diameter of medulla to diameter of shaft of whole hair—determine species.
- Determination of *human* hair is based on the relative size and appearance of the *medulla*, the appearance of the scales, and the diameter of the *hair* shaft.
- Most *animal hairs* have a smaller diameter and larger medullary index than human.
- In human, medulla is generally amorphous, often broken or fragmented and occupies <1/3 the width of hair shaft.
- In animals, medulla is sharply defined, always present, continuous and occupies >1/3 the width of hair shaft.
- **Superimposition** technique is most useful for identification from skull.
- **Most commonly used method for charting of teeth:** FDI system (two-digit notation indicating tooth and quadrant).
- For identification, palatoprints are taken from anterior third of the palate.

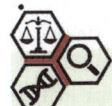 **Interesting case**

Superimposition Technique (Sheena Bora Case, 2012)

Sheena Bora, an executive working in Mumbai, went missing in April 2012. After a month, the police in Raigad found a body after villagers complained of a foul odor. No identification was made and the remains were sent to a hospital in Mumbai. No link was made with the Sheena Bora case. She was allegedly administered a sedative, strangulated inside a car and then burnt and dumped in Raigad by her mother (co-founder of INX Media) with help from her ex-husband and driver. The murder came to light three years later in 2015 after the driver spilled the beans. The skeletal remains were exhumed and the police found bones, including a skull, from the spot. Digital superimposition was carried out to match the skull and mandible recovered.

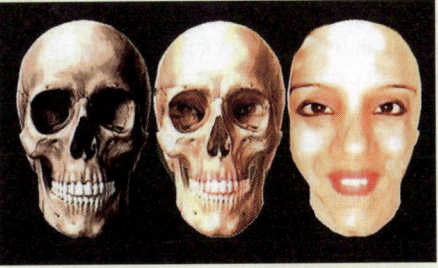

Four sets of live photographs of Sheena with different facial profiles and respective corresponding profiles' skull photographs were used. The computerized superimposition was done using software which involved cropping and additional preparing. It also compared the exactness over visible teeth of the victim in live photographs (with smile and visible front teeth) and the corresponding teeth in the skull. The forensic medicine expert opined that all the landmarks and facial characteristics along with teeth superimposition were found correctly matching, and identified the remains as hers. A DNA test has also confirmed the bones were Sheena's remains.

CHAPTER 7

Medico-legal Autopsy

LEARNING OBJECTIVES

Must know
1. Autopsy, types, objectives/purpose
2. Evisceration techniques
3. Instruments used in postmortem examination
4. Procedures, formalities of medico-legal autopsies
5. Types of skin incisions
6. Antemortem and postmortem thrombus (Diff.)
7. Collection and preservation of samples
8. Preservation of viscera and preservatives used
9. Digital autopsy
10. Exhumation

Desirable to know
1. Dissection of the heart
2. Subendocardial hemorrhage
3. Delivery of the brain
4. Posterior approach to spinal cord dissection
5. Demonstration of pneumothorax and air embolus
6. Obscure and negative autopsy
7. Second autopsy
8. Chain of evidence
9. Autopsy room hazards
10. Examination of bundle of bones

Describe and discuss different types of autopsies, aims and objectives of postmortem examination.

Definitions

Autopsy*: Systematic examination of a dead person for medical, legal and/or scientific purposes.
- The examination of a dead body involves external and internal examination and incorporating the results of special tests (including radiology).
- The internal examination involves, but is not limited to, examining the contents of the cranium, chest and abdomen. Further dissection may occur in particular circumstances.

It is of three types **(Diff. 7.1)**:
i. **Academic autopsy:** Dissection carried by students of anatomy.
ii. **Pathological, hospital or clinical autopsy:** Done by pathologists to diagnose the cause of death or to confirm a diagnosis. Consent signed by the next of kin is required for these autopsies.
iii. **Medico-legal or forensic autopsy:** Scientific examination of a dead body carried out under the laws of the State for the protection of rights of citizens in cases of sudden, suspicious, obscure, unnatural, litigious or criminal deaths. The basic purpose of this autopsy is to establish the cause and manner of death.

- It is said '*the only thing worse than no autopsy is a partial autopsy.*' In every case, the autopsy must be complete, i.e., all the body cavities should be opened, and every organ must be examined.
- The autopsy should be carried out by the registered medical practitioner, preferably with training in forensic medicine. The doctor should remove the organs himself. The attendant should prepare the body and help the doctor where required, such as sawing the skull cap, reconstructing the body, etc. As the autopsy is proceeded with, details of the examination should be taken down verbatim by an assistant.
- The person responsible for handling, moving and cleaning the body is often called a *diener* (German, servant).

---
* Autopsy (Greek *autos*—self, *opis*—view)—to see for oneself; also called necropsy (Greek *necros*—dead, *opis*—view) or postmortem examination (post—after, mortem—death).

DIFFERENTIATION 7.1: Medico-legal autopsy and pathological autopsy

S.No.	Feature	Medico-legal autopsy	Pathological/Clinical autopsy
1.	Done in	Unnatural deaths	Natural deaths
2.	Purpose/Indication	To determine cause of death and time since death	To know pathophysiology of disease causing death
3.	Done by	Forensic medicine experts	Pathologists
4.	Consent	From State	From next of kin
5.	Body handed over to	Investigating Officer/Constable	Relatives

NOTA BENE

- **Endoscopic autopsy (keyhole autopsy):** In this, internal organs are seen through endoscopes or laparoscopes. It is done in cases where the family of the deceased objects to the performance of a conventional autopsy for religious or other reasons. The technique has proven to be accurate, more rapid than conventional autopsy and left the body virtually intact.
- **Needle autopsy:** A biopsy needle is used to take the samples of tissues and examined microscopically only.
  Virtopsy (digital autopsy), endoscopic autopsy and needle autopsy are examples of limited autopsy (anything less than a complete autopsy).
- **Verbal autopsy:** A protocolized procedure that allows the classification of causes of death through analysis of data derived from structured interviews with family, friends, and caregivers.
- **Psychological autopsy** is an investigative procedure of reconstructing a person's state of mind prior to death. This is based upon information gathered from personal documents, police and medical records and interviews with survivors of the deceased-families, friends and others who had contact with the person. The typical case is one in which there is some doubt as to whether death was accidental, self-inflicted or malicious, and whether the deceased played an active role in his own demise. Such matters can be especially important in life insurance claims that are void if death was suicidal.

PURPOSE/OBJECTIVES OF AUTOPSY

Who, when, where, why, what and how are the questions that the autopsy assists in answering. The objectives of medico-legal autopsy are to determine:

i. Identification of the deceased in case of decomposed, burnt, mutilated or an unidentified body.
ii. Cause of death, whether natural or unnatural, and to interpret the significance and effect of the disease present in case of natural death.
iii. Approximate time of death, mode of death, age of injuries, and place of death.
iv. Manner of death, whether accidental, suicidal or homicidal.
v. Poison or weapon responsible for death in case of homicide.
vi. Volitional activity possible after receiving the trauma, and survival time.
vii. Extent of external and internal injuries present.
viii. Whether the injury present is expected to cause death in ordinary course of nature.
ix. Whether deceased received any treatment before death.
x. In case of homicide, whether:
   - One or more person(s) was/were involved.
   - Any trace evidence was left behind on the body that may help in identification of the assailant.
   - Any other offense was related with the death, e.g., strangulation along with sexual assault.
   - More than one method or weapon was involved in the crime, e.g., firearm along with knife.
   - The body has been displaced from the original place of disposal.
   - The relative positions of victim and the assailant(s) can be deciphered.
xi. In case of newborns, to determine the question of live birth and viability of the baby.
xii. In case of mutilated or skeletal remains, to determine if they are human, and if human, whether they belong to one or more than one person, the probable cause of death and approximate time since death.

FM 2.11, 2.12
- Describe and discuss autopsy procedures including postmortem examination.
- Describe the legal requirements to conduct postmortem examination and procedures to conduct medico-legal postmortem examination.

PROCEDURE FOR MEDICO-LEGAL AUTOPSIES (FLOWCHART 7.1)

i. **Visit to the scene of crime:** It is useful in certain cases, such as homicide, poisoning, road traffic accidents, firearm injuries and sexual offenses. In many cases, crime can be excluded in favor of accident, suicide or even natural causes.
ii. **Authorization:** It should be conducted only when there is an official order authorizing the autopsy, from the police or Magistrate.
iii. All registered medical practitioners (RMP) in government service can conduct the examination. Autopsy is conducted by two doctors where death of a female due to burns or other suspicious reasons has occurred within 7 years of her marriage. A panel of doctors is also constituted in case of custodial deaths, death in operation table and second autopsy. Ideally, a board should have odd number of members so that in case of differences of opinion, a conclusion can be reached.

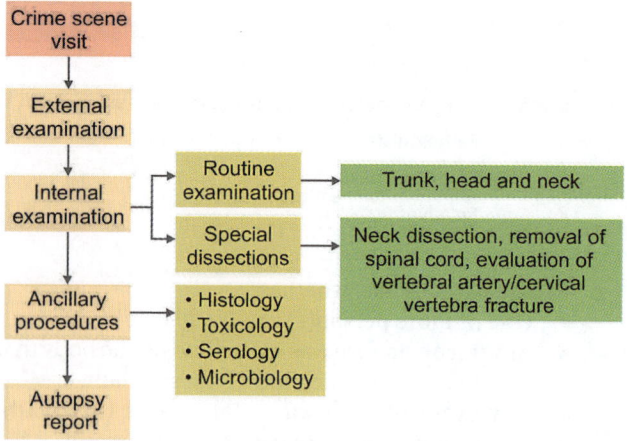

Flowchart 7.1: Components of a medico-legal autopsy

iv. No unauthorized person should be present at the autopsy (although, there are no written rules for the same).* However, the Investigating Officer (IO) may be shown certain findings found during autopsy contrary to the inquest report.

v. The medico-legal autopsy should be conducted in an authorized center. The *body should never be embalmed before autopsy*, since histopathological examination will be impossible. It may be necessary to do an autopsy at the site, when the body is in an advanced state of putrefaction.

vi. Even if the body is decomposed, autopsy should be performed, as certain important lesions may still be found. Help from a forensic entomologist can provide accurate estimation of victim's death and other valuable information in such cases.

vii. It should be performed, as soon as possible after receiving the requisition, without undue delay. The requisition is accompanied with a copy of the inquest report, a dead-body challan which includes the name, age, sex, identification marks and religion of the deceased, apparent cause of death and any other paper of importance. Before starting the autopsy, the doctor should go through the inquest report and the requisition thoroughly, and put his signature on all the papers after marking them serially. However, it should be kept in mind that the inquest report may have scanty, misleading or incorrect history.

viii. The autopsy should be conducted in daylight, since it is said that color changes, such as jaundice, changes in bruises and postmortem staining cannot be appreciated in the artificial light. Moreover, postmortem is not an emergency, and unless there is serious threat to law and order situation or instruction comes from District Magistrate, it should not be done after 5 PM. However, the government has allowed postmortem at night (which should be video recorded) in some special circumstances and availability of lighting and infrastructure. Postmortem for organ donation should be done on priority and can be conducted even after sunset if adequate infrastructure is available.

ix. If the body is received in the mortuary at night, it is preserved at 4°C after noting the date and exact time.¥ A preliminary examination is done to note external appearances, body (rectal) temperature, extent of postmortem staining and rigor mortis. The actual postmortem is conducted on the next day.

x. **Identification:** A police officer or any other authorized person and two relatives should identify the dead body in front of the autopsy surgeon. The names of those who identified the body must be recorded. In unidentified bodies, the marks of identification, race, religion, sex, age, dental formula, photographs and fingerprints should be taken.

xi. Medico-legal autopsy does not require any consent from the relatives of the deceased.

xii. Both positive and negative findings should be recorded.

xiii. Nothing should be erased, and all alterations should be initialed in the report.

xiv. **Chain of evidence:** It is absolutely essential to preserve the chain of evidence by identifying the body and maintaining absolute control of specimens removed at autopsy.

xv. **List of articles:** A list is made of all the articles removed from the body, e.g., clothes, jewelry, bullets, etc. They are labeled, sealed, mentioned in the report and handed over to the police constable after obtaining a receipt.

xvi. After completion of autopsy, the body is stitched, washed and restored to the best possible cosmetic appearance, and then handed over to the police constable/IO.

> **NOTA BENE**
>
> **Chain of evidence/custody** requires that from the moment the evidence is collected, every transfer of evidence from person to person be documented and be provable that nobody else could have accessed or tampered that evidence which can compromise the case of the prosecution.

INSTRUMENTS FOR AUTOPSY EXAMINATION

A list of instruments and equipments useful in various postmortem procedures is given in **Box 7.1** and **Figure 7.1**.

---

* In UK and US, there is nothing that specifically forbids the relatives attending the autopsy. At some places, the accused is represented by a lawyer or a doctor acting on his behalf.
¥ It is the job of the technician to ensure that this temperature is maintained. If it falls below 0°C, ice will form within the tissues, and any subsequent histopathological examination of the tissues that may be required after the autopsy will be of little value.

Box 7.1 Essential instruments for postmortem examinations

- **Scalpel** and **disposable blades** of 22 size.
- **Toothed forceps:** Teeth lend strength in gripping the skin and organs.
- **Enterotome:** Large scissors used for opening the intestines.
- **Scissors** used for opening hollow organs and trimming off tissues.
- **Bone cutter:** This is used to cut the ribs and has curved blades.
- **Councilman rib shear/cutter:** Small pruning shears used to cut through the ribs prior to lifting off the sternum.
- **Vibrating saw (Stryker saw):** Instrument of choice for most autopsy surgeons for removing the skull cap.
- **Bone saw:** The hand saw can be used to saw through the skull, but it's very slow-going compared to the vibrating saw. Infections from aerosols being thrown up are other disadvantages.
- **Virchow skull breaker or T-handled chisel:** After scoring the calvarium with the vibrating saw, the chisel is used to separate the top of the calvarium from the lower skull, thus exposing the brain and the meninges.
- **Hammer with hook** is used with the chisel to separate the calvarium from the lower skull.
- **Brain knife:** Long knife used to smoothly cut solid organs into slices for examination.
- **Hagedorn's needle** is used for sewing up the body after autopsy.

Other instruments that should be available: Probe, small ruler and plastic-coated measuring tape, thermometer, hand lens, torch and digital camera.

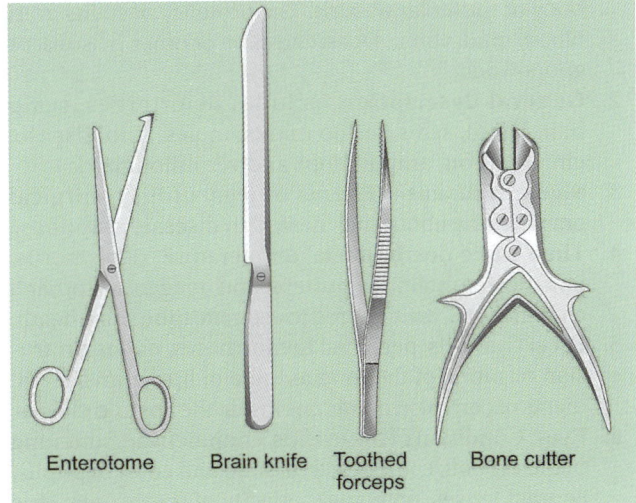
Enterotome Brain knife Toothed forceps Bone cutter

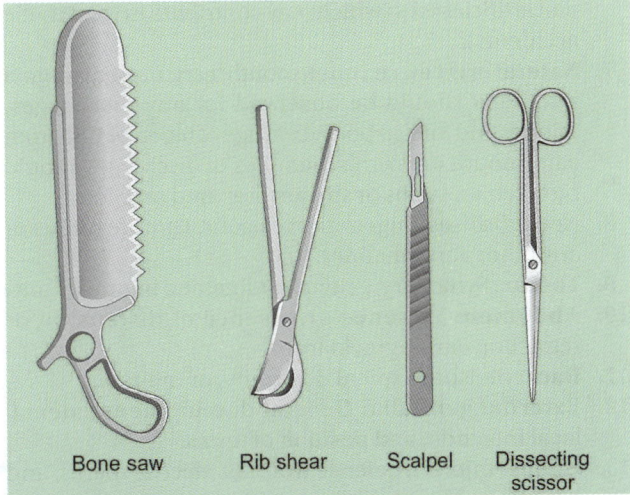
Bone saw Rib shear Scalpel Dissecting scissor

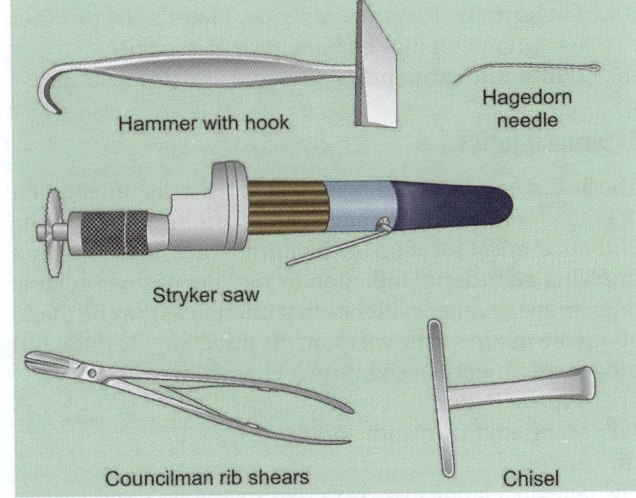
Hammer with hook Hagedorn needle
Stryker saw
Councilman rib shears Chisel

Fig. 7.1: Autopsy instruments

EXTERNAL EXAMINATION

The observation and documentation of various external characteristics of the decedent is the essence of the external examination.

1. **Clothing:** They are listed and their number, labels and laundry marks, design, stains, tears, loss of buttons, cuts, holes or blackening from firearm discharges with their dimensions should be noted.
    - Trace evidence like hair, fibers, paint chips, glass fragments, vegetation and insects are collected, labeled and preserved.
    - Jewelry may provide evidence of identification, pockets may contain medication or drugs of abuse, and personal papers may help in identification and provide medical history.
    - The clothes should be removed carefully without tearing them, to avoid confusion of signs of struggle. If they cannot be removed intact, they should be cut in an area away from any bullet hole or cuts, along the seam of the garment.
    - After autopsy, wet clothing should be air-dried, packed, sealed in paper bags and handed over to the police.
2. The whole surface of the body should be carefully examined before and after washing from head to foot, and back and front, and the details noted.
3. Body length, weight, sex, race, dentition, general state, built, development and nourishment are noted. It should include all surgical procedures, dressings and other diagnostic and therapeutic measures.

Following should be noted in external examination:
1. **Skin:** General condition (rash, petechiae, color, looseness and turgor), asymmetry of any part of the

body or muscular wasting. The presence of stains from blood, mud, vomit, feces, corrosive or other poisons, or gunpowder.
2. **General description** includes deformities, scalp hair, beard, scars, tattoo marks, moles, skin disease, circumcision, amputations and vermilion mark.
3. **Signs of disease:** Edema of legs, dropsy, surgical emphysema about the chest, skin disease, eruptions.
4. **Time since death:** Rectal temperature, rigor mortis, postmortem staining, putrefaction, maggots, stomach contents, etc., are required to estimate time since death.
5. **Face:** Cyanosis, petechial hemorrhages, pallor, protrusion or biting of the tongue, state of lips, gums, teeth, marks of corrosion or injuries inside the lips and cheeks.
6. **Eyes:** Condition of the eyelids, conjunctivae, softening of the eyeball, color of sclera, state and color of pupils, contact lenses, petechiae, opacity of the cornea, lens and artificial eyes (which may contribute in road traffic accidents).
7. **Natural orifices**, i.e., nose, mouth, ears, urethra, vagina and anus should be observed for any discharges, injuries and foreign body. Leakage of blood or CSF from ears, mouth or nostrils. Samples of discharges should be taken on swabs or smears prepared on slides.
8. **Neck:** Bruises, fingernail abrasions, ligature marks or any other abnormalities.
9. **Thorax:** Symmetry, general outline, and injuries, if any.
10. **Abdomen:** Presence or absence of distension or retraction, striae gravidarum.
11. **Back:** Bedsores, spinal deformity, or injuries.
12. **External genitalia:** General development, edema, local infection, and position of testes.
13. **Hands:** Injuries, defense wounds, electric marks, and in clenched hands, if anything is grasped.
14. **Fingernails:** Presence of tissue, blood, dust or other foreign matter may be indicative of struggle.
15. **Limbs and other parts:** Fracture and dislocation.

External Injuries

The final stage of external examination is the documentation of injuries, either by grouping them according to injury type and anatomical location, or by numbering them, without implying an order of infliction or ranking of severity. It is often from the outer evidence that inferences may be made about the nature of the weapon, the direction of attack and other vital aspects. Each injury is characterized by its:
i. Type of injury.
ii. Size (length, breadth and depth).
iii. Shape.
iv. Site (in relation to two external anatomical landmarks).
v. Direction of application of the force.
vi. Margins, edges and base.
vii. Distance of the wound from the heel.
viii. Time of infliction of the injury should be studied from inflammatory and color changes.
ix. Vital reaction.
x. Foreign materials, e.g., hair, grass, fibers, etc.

♦ If the injuries are obscured by hair, it should be shaved.
♦ Deep or penetrating wounds should not be probed until the body is opened.
♦ In burns, their character, position, body surface area involved, and degree should be mentioned.
♦ Concealed punctured wounds, bruising of frenulum of lips, and injection marks should be searched for, if indicated.
♦ The use of printed body sketches is very useful. The position of the injuries should be pictographically depicted on the skeleton diagrams.
♦ Photographic documentation of major injuries is now considered as standard practice. Identifying markers bearing the unique autopsy number, with a measurement scale should be included to ensure that the photographs correspond to the specific case.

NOTA BENE

♦ Special procedures utilized during external examination include photography for the purposes of identification and documentation. *Infrared and UV photography will enhance trace materials, tattoos, bruises and patterned injuries.*
♦ High contrast black-white photography or computer-directed image enhancement can be used to enhance patterned injuries.

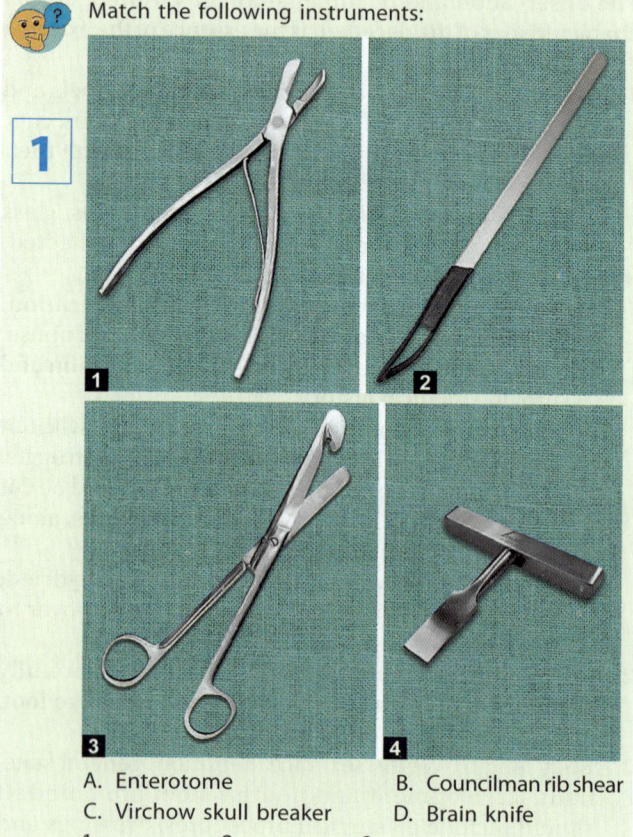

Match the following instruments:

A. Enterotome B. Councilman rib shear
C. Virchow skull breaker D. Brain knife
1._____ 2._____ 3._____ 4._____

INTERNAL EXAMINATION (EVISCERATION)

It is convenient to start the examination with the cavity chiefly affected. All three major cavities of the body, i.e., skull, thorax and abdomen should be opened and examined as a routine. The choice as to which part of body is to be opened first—skull or the body cavities is left to the dissector **(Table 7.1)**.

- In *suspected head injury*, the skull is opened first and then the thorax and the abdomen, but some autopsy surgeons are of the view that it should be opened after blood has been drained out by opening the heart. It is also recommended by some that the brain should be removed first in all autopsies so that abnormal odors can be detected.
- In *suspected asphyxial deaths* due to compression of neck, the skull and abdomen is opened first followed by dissection of the neck. The draining out of blood from neck vessels via the skull provides a comparatively cleaner field for the study of neck structures. The neck incision should not be made until the skull-cap and brain has been removed, to avoid the congestive artifactual hemorrhages in the neck structure.

SKIN INCISIONS

Skin incisions are mostly of four types **(Table 7.2 and Fig. 7.2)**.
- **I-shaped or standard midline incision:** The umbilicus is avoided because the dense fibrous tissue is difficult to penetrate with a needle, when the body is stitched after autopsy.
- **Y-shaped incision:** Some prefer to extend the upper incision in an arc around the inferior portion of the female breasts (*inframammary incision*), but there is a chance of fluids inadvertently leaking from the closed body after autopsy. This is often done in infants and wherever it is desired to avoid disfiguring the front of the neck.

EVISCERATION METHODS (FLOWCHART 7.2)

i. **En masse:** This method, described by *Letulle*, involves removing most of the internal organs in one full

TABLE 7.1: Cavity to be opened in suspected deaths

Suspected death	Cavity dissected
Head injury	Skull first, then thorax and abdomen
Poisoning	Skull (brain) so as to detect abnormal odors
Asphyxial deaths	Skull and abdomen first followed by dissection of neck
All other cases	Thorax and abdomen first, followed by skull

TABLE 7.2: Skin incisions

Types	Incision	Remarks
I-shaped incision	Incision from chin to symphysis pubis	Most commonly used
Y-shaped incision	Straight line of Y corresponding to xiphisternum to pubis and forks of Y runs down medially to chest from acromion process	Commonly followed in US
Modified Y-shaped incision	From suprasternal notch to symphysis pubis and then extends from suprasternal notch over clavicle to its center on both sides and passes upwards over neck behind the ears	For detailed study of neck, like in hanging/strangulation
T-shaped or 'bucket handle' incision	Neck is opened with a transverse incision which runs from acromion to acromion process along the line of clavicles. Midline incision is similar to I-shaped incision.	Also called 'U-shaped' or subclavicular incision

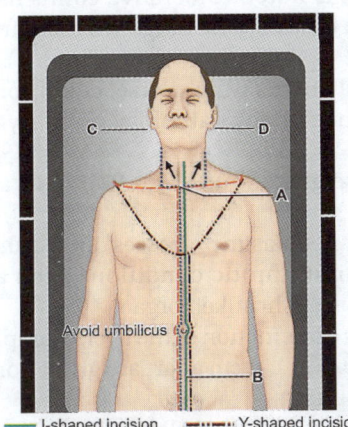 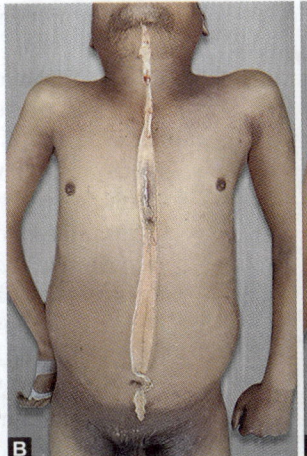 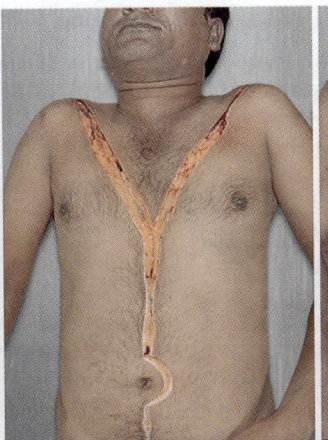 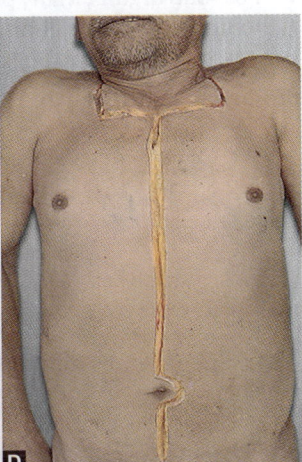

Figs. 7.2A to D: (A) Incision for opening thoracic and abdominal cavities: A. Sternal notch, B. Symphysis pubis, C. Right mastoid process, D. Left mastoid process; (B) I-shaped incision; (C) Y-shaped incision; (D) Modified Y-shaped incision

Flowchart 7.2: Evisceration techniques

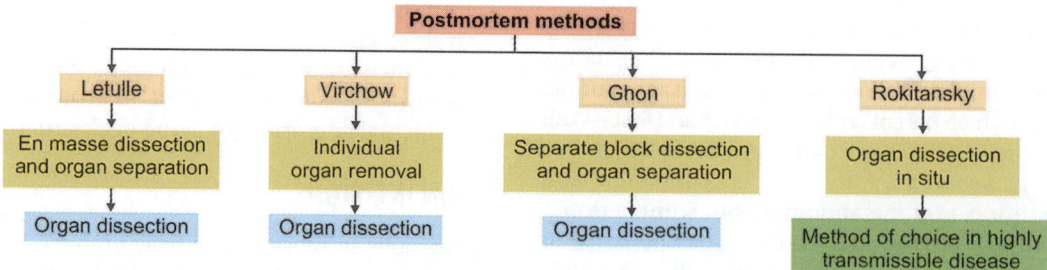

swoop. It is a rapid technique for removing the organs from the body, although the ensuing dissection is the lengthiest. It has the advantage of leaving all attachments intact.

ii. **Virchow's method:** This method of evisceration is simply removal of individual organs one by one with subsequent dissection of that isolated organ. It is useful in assessing individual organ pathology, a quick and effective method, if the pathological interest is in a single organ.

iii. **En bloc removal:** It is a compromise between the above two methods, and most widely used in the UK. *Ghon* developed this method, which is relatively quick, but preserves most of the important inter-organ relationships.

iv. **In situ dissection:** This method, developed by *Rokitansky*, is rarely performed which involves dissecting the organs in situ with little actual evisceration being performed prior to dissection.

No matter which dissection technique is utilized to eviscerate, the autopsy surgeon needs to perform a dissection specific to the organ in question.

- Hollow structures, such as blood vessels and gastrointestinal (GI) tract (esophagus, stomach and intestines) are cut opened in order to reveal the pathology present inside.
- For solid organs, many parallel cuts, in a fashion similar to slicing a loaf of bread ('*bread-loafing*') is done.

Wherever indicated, a small portion of each organ is preserved in formalin for histopathological examination.

Name the skin incision for autopsy shown below:

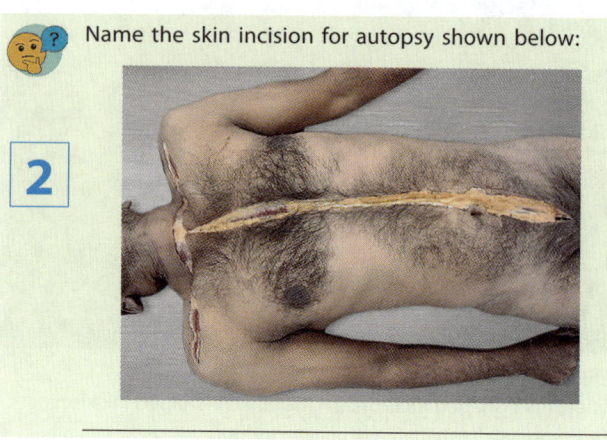

ABDOMEN AND PELVIS

The rectus abdominis muscles are incised up to 5 cm above the symphysis pubis. A small nick is made in the fascia to admit the left index and middle fingers with palmar surfaces up, to protect the underlying structures, and the peritoneum is cut up to the xiphoid. In the abdominal cavity, presence of any blood, pus or fluid, perforation or damage to any organ is looked for. If blood, pus or any other fluid is present, its quantity is measured.

In penetrating wounds of the abdomen, gross injury to liver, kidneys, spleen and intra-abdominal vessels may be seen, and there may be excessive intra-abdominal hemorrhage.

i. **Stomach:** Two ligatures are applied at the cardiac end of the esophagus and two ligatures below the pyloric end of the stomach. The stomach is removed by cutting between the double ligatures at both ends, and is opened along the greater curvature. The mucous membrane is examined for the presence of any stain, congestion, hemorrhage, desquamation, ulceration, sloughing or perforation. The content of the stomach is noted in respect to quantity, nature of material/food, state of digestion, color and smell.

ii. **Intestine:** It is dissected in its entire length. Any injury or reactions due to poison or presence of foreign body, e.g., a bullet, is noted. Ulcerative colitis like lesions is noticed in case of poisoning with mercuric chloride.

iii. **Liver:** It is removed and its weight, size, color, consistency and presence of any pathology or injury is noted.
- Normal liver weighs about 1300–1550 g in an adult.
- Inflammatory or neoplastic processes often cause hepatomegaly, but fibrotic conditions such as cirrhosis will cause a shrunken organ.
- For macroscopic examination of the liver, multiple transverse sections at 1–2 cm apart are given from one side to the other.
- The gallbladder is dissected out along with the liver. Any pathology or stone formation inside it is noted.

iv. **Spleen:** The spleen is removed by cutting through its pedicle; its size, weight, consistency and condition of capsule, and rupture, injuries or disease is noted.

Hilum should be inspected for splenunculi before dissecting the spleen.
- Weight of normal spleen range from 130–170 g.
- It is sectioned in its long axis, and the character of parenchyma, follicles and septa is noted.
- In case of septicemia, the spleen will often be soft and liquefied, and slicing may be impossible.
- With normal spleen or with amyloid deposition or portal hypertension, slicing will be easy.

v. **Pancreas:** The pancreas is removed along with the stomach and duodenum. It is sliced by multiple sections at right angles to the long axis to expose the ductal system.

vi. **Kidneys:** They are removed along with adrenal glands after tying the ureters along with the vessels at least 1 inch away from the hilum.
- The surface of the kidneys along with the covering capsules should be examined for texture, congestion, hemorrhage and injury.
- An adult kidney weighs about 150 g.
- With chronic renal parenchymal disease, such as nephrosclerosis, ischemia or infection, there may be fine or coarse scars associated with capsular fibrosis.
- The kidney is sectioned longitudinally through the convex border into the hilum. The pelvis is examined for calculi and inflammation.
- *Renal infarcts* are pyramidal or wedge-shaped lesions with the base at the cortical surface and the apex pointing to the medullary origin of the arterial supply. Beginning as pale areas of necrosis with hyperemic borders, they progress to yellow-gray lesions that ultimately become depressed V-shaped gray-white furrows.

vii. **Urinary bladder:** It is examined in situ. If bladder contains urine, it is syringed out before opening to avoid any chances of contamination by blood or any other material. The bladder should be examined for any pathology, hemorrhage, congestion or injury. Both the ureters should be opened along their long axes.

viii. **Female genitalia:** The uterus and its appendages should first be examined *in situ* and then removed *en masse* along with the vagina by giving an incision externally on the labia up to the symphysis pubis above and the anus below. Internally, an incision is given around the pelvic brim and continued downwards to the pelvic outlet till it reaches the vaginal incision.

The **uterus** is examined and its dimensions, weight, whether gravid, parous or nulliparous, or any pathology present is noted. In case of gravid uterus, condition of the whole product of conception should be noted. In cases of abortion or attempted abortion, remains of any part of the product of conception inside the cavity, color of endometrial surface, erosion, any injury, ulceration or perforation of vaginal canal (particularly near the fornices) or of the uterine wall is noted. Foreign body may be present inside the uterine cavity. Smell and nature of the fluid present inside the uterine cavity is noted. Evidence of use of instruments may be present in the cervix or in the os.

The **vagina** is examined for any injury, foreign body, condition of hymen, mucous membrane and rugae. Any fluid present in the vagina is aspirated and preserved.

Ovaries should be examined for presence of corpus luteum. Fallopian tubes and ovaries have special medico-legal significance in cases of deaths due to their rupture in ectopic pregnancy.

ix. **Prostate (in males):** It is examined for enlargement or malignancy. In prostatitis, it is firm and in carcinoma, it is hard and granular.

CHEST

The skin and muscles of the chest are dissected sidewise and carried back to the midaxillary line, down to the costal margin and up over the clavicles. The ribs and sternum are examined for fractures, and the chest is opened by cutting the costal cartilages close to the costochondral junctions and starting from the upper border of the second cartilage with a cartilage knife. Then, disarticulation of the sternoclavicular joint is done on each side by inserting the point of knife into the semicircular joint.

The pleural cavity is examined before complete removal of the sternum. *In situ* inspection is done before removal of thoracic organs, which includes observation of the atrium and ventricle for air embolism, distension or collapse of lungs, the chest cavity for fluid, hemorrhage or pus, pleural adhesions, injuries including fracture of ribs.

Lungs

Both the lungs are separated from the mediastinal structures after tying the vessels and the bronchioles.
- The condition of pleura, any sign of pleuritis, petechial hemorrhages, injury, effusion, hemothorax, pneumothorax or pyothorax is noted.
- Normal lungs weigh 250–400 g each in an adult, but may weigh >1 kg in cases of severe cardiac failure or diffuse alveolar damage.
- It is conventional to cut open from large to small airways, from medial to lateral to include all lobes and segments opening along the branches as they are encountered. Impression of the parenchymal appearance and texture is noted, and apical disease like old tuberculous cavities or fungal balls can also be demonstrated.
- The parenchyma is squeezed and any pus or fluid expressed is noted.
- After this, horizontal slicing through each lobe with a brain-knife is made to inspect the rest of the parenchyma.

- It is preferable to make large horizontal slices through the whole lung rather than opening the airways and vessels in cases of large mass lesion (e.g., carcinoma).

Dissection of the Vessels

- The course of pulmonary veins into the lung is traced, and thrombosis and atheroma is looked for, the latter being associated with pulmonary hypertension.
- An antemortem embolus may be coiled, and when straightened resembles a cast of the vessel from which the thrombus originated, usually in the leg.
- Massive pulmonary emboli may block either the main trunk of the pulmonary artery or one of the major pulmonary vessels, more commonly on the right side.
- At autopsy, such large emboli are readily visible and can be easily distinguished from postmortem clot (**Diff. 7.2 and Figs. 7.3A and B**).
- If the postmortem clot is mistaken for a antemortem clot, the cause of death could be determined erroneously.

HEART

- The heart is held at the apex, lifted upwards and separated from other thoracic organs by cutting the inferior and superior vena cava, pulmonary vessels, and ascending aorta as far away as possible from the base of the heart.
- The size and weight of the heart is noted. Adult heart weighs about 250–300 g. Hearts that weigh too much are at risk for sudden, lethal arrhythmias.
- Many approaches can be taken to dissect the heart. The appropriate method is selected on the basis of the age of the patient and any suspected abnormality.
- The overall anatomy of the heart needs to be evaluated for any congenital anomalies. The condition of the valves, presence and degree of atheroma in the valves, and the intima of the large vessels is noted. Any ischemic lesion is searched for. The state of the myocardium, size of the chambers, thickness of right and left ventricle, state of endocardium (subendocardial hemorrhage in the left ventricle), valvular lesions, and condition of the aorta with regards to any aneurysm, atherosclerosis or syphilitic aortitis (*tree bark appearance*) is noted.

Examination of the Heart

Coronary artery disease is seen more commonly than valvular heart disease. The myocardium is examined for fibrosis or recent infarct. The myocardial infarct is easily identifiable when it is of more than 12 hours (h) of age. If an infarct is identified, sections from its central and peripheral zones are useful in dating the onset of ischemic damage and determining any recent extension.

- The extramural coronary arteries are examined by making serial cross-sectional incisions about 3–5 mm apart, in order to evaluate for atherosclerotic narrowing, the common site being 1 cm away from the origin of the left coronary artery (**Fig. 7.4**). The narrowest segments and any areas containing thrombi should be selected for microscopic examination.

  The anterior descending branch of the left coronary artery is cut downwards along the front of the septum, then the circumflex branch on the opposite side of the mitral valve. The right coronary artery is followed from the aorta to the cut near the pulmonary valve and then above the tricuspid valve. The presence of acute coronary lesions, viz. plaque rupture, plaque hemorrhage or thrombus is noted. The extent of

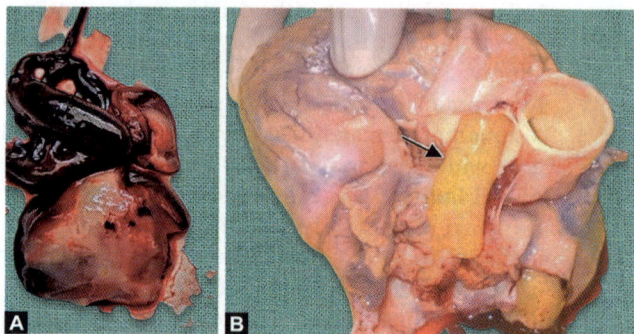

Figs. 7.3A and B: (A) Antemortem clot; (B) Postmortem clot (arrow)

DIFFERENTIATION 7.2: Antemortem clot and postmortem clot (**Figs. 7.3A and B**).

S.No.	Feature	Antemortem clot	Postmortem clot
1.	Origin	As a part of normal hemostasis or pathological derangement of clotting pathway in living	Formed in a dead person due to sedimentation and settling down of blood components
2.	Gross	Dry, granular, firm and friable. Grayish red, lines of Zahn (alternate dark and gray layers of RBCs interspersed with lighter layers of fibrin) are prominent in arterial thrombi	Gelatinous, soft and rubbery. Dark red, dependent portion of clot (called *black currant jelly*) and yellow supernatant, free of red cells (called *chicken fat*)
3.	Shape	Does not form a cast of the vessel	Takes the shape of the vessel or its bifurcation. Forms the cast of the vessel
4.	Attachment to vessel wall	Adheres firmly to the endothelium	Weakly adherent
5.	Location	Anywhere in the body	In dependent parts of the body
6.	Slicing of lung	Clot pour out of cut vessels	Clot does not pour out of cut vessels

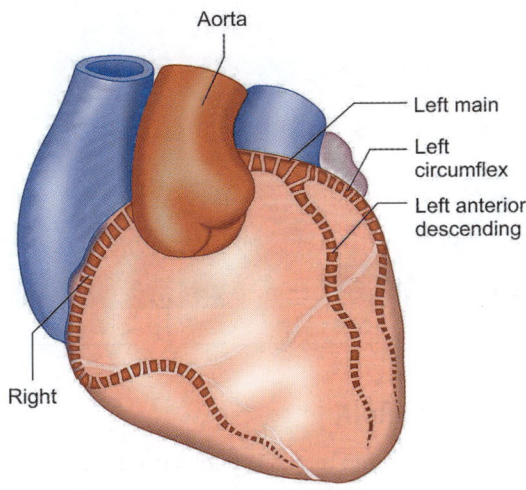

Fig. 7.4: Examination of coronary arteries

coronary artery atherosclerosis is categorized based on the approximate percentage stenosis, caused by the plaque. Anything <50% is considered mild, while 50–75% is considered moderate and >75% is severe.

- Another method to examine the heart is the *inflow-outflow method* or following the direction of blood flow (**Fig. 7.5**). First, the right atrium is opened, followed by the tricuspid valve, and then the pulmonary valve. Next, the left atrium is opened, followed by the mitral valve and the aortic valve. During opening, the valves should be examined before being cut and valve orifice measured. Special sections can be taken at this point to evaluate the conduction (electrical) system of the heart.
- Another lesser used method is the *short axis or ventricular slicing method* (**Fig. 7.6**). With the heart in the anatomical position, the first slice is made through the heart at a point about 3 cm from the apex separating it from the remainder of the heart. Further complete slices are then made in parallel to this slice, 1 cm apart, until reaching below the atrioventricular valves. The remainder is then examined by opening along the path of blood flow. It is useful, if ischemic myocardial disease is suspected, as it clearly demonstrates the distribution of infarction.
- The *intramural or 'sandwich' technique* can be used to cut through the thickness of the left ventricle. The heart is placed open on the cutting board, with the endocardium downwards. A knife is passed into the cut edge of the left ventricle and sliced right through the muscle, keeping equidistant between endocardium and epicardium. The myocardium can then be opened out like a book, showing the interior with any infarcts or fibrotic plaques. *Examination of coronary arteries should precede the examination of heart.*

NOTA BENE

- **Examination of valve:** The circumference of the valve is measured. The circumference of mitral valve is 8–10.5 cm (mean 10 cm) and admits two fingers; tricuspid valve is 10–12.5 cm (12 cm) and admits three fingers; aortic valve is 6–8 cm (7.5 cm) and pulmonary valve is 7–9 cm (8.5 cm). The decrease in circumference is suggestive of stenosis, whereas increased circumference could be due to regurgitation or incompetent valves.
- **Ventricular hypertrophy:** An estimate is made by measuring the thickness of the ventricular walls at a point about 1 cm below the atrioventricular valve. The upper limits of normal are: left ventricle: 1.5 cm, right ventricle: 0.5 cm and atrial muscle: 0.2 cm.

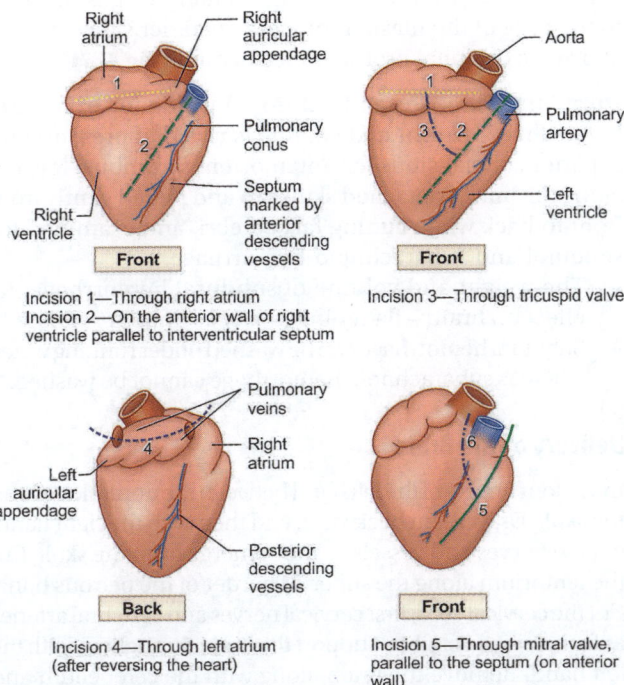

Fig. 7.5: Opening of the heart at autopsy (inflow-outflow method)

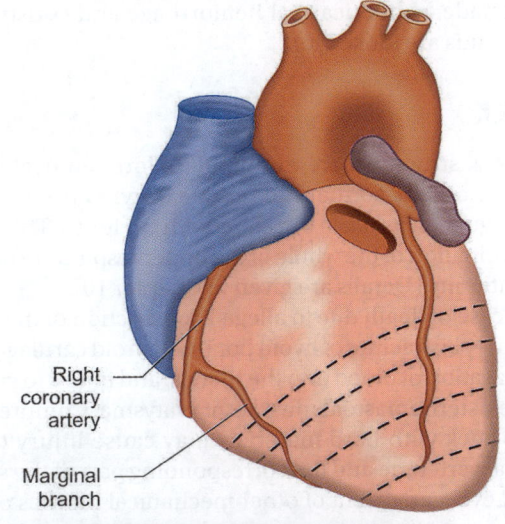

Fig. 7.6: Examination of myocardium (ventricular slicing method)

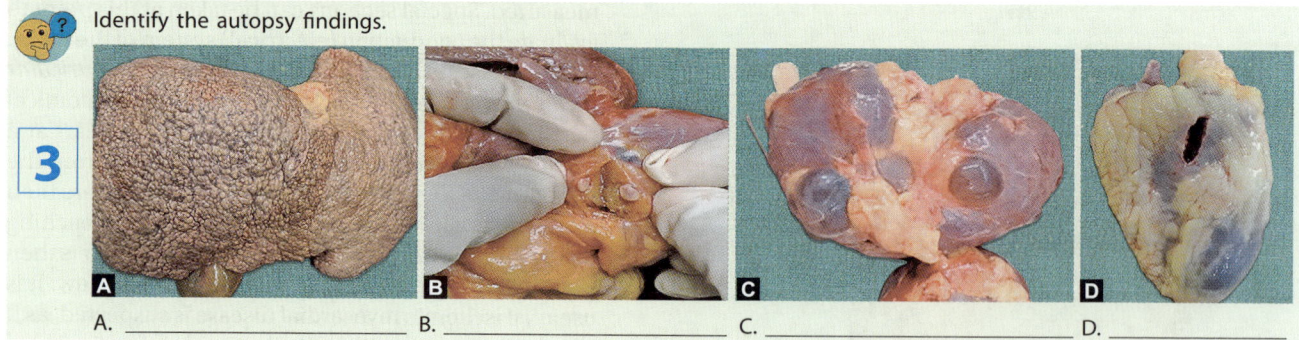

Identify the autopsy findings.

A. _____ B. _____ C. _____ D. _____

Subendocardial or Sheehan's Hemorrhages

These are flame-shaped, confluent hemorrhages and tend to occur in one continuous sheet rather than in patches, seen in the left ventricle, on the left side of the interventricular septum and on the opposing papillary muscles and adjacent columnae carneae.

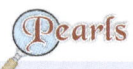

Subendocardial hemorrhages are seen in:
- Severe loss of blood or shock
- Intracranial damage, such as head injury, cerebral edema, surgical craniotomy or tumors
- Death due to ectopic pregnancy, ruptured uterus, abortion, antepartum or postpartum hemorrhage
- Poisoning, e.g., arsenic or oleander

Agonal thrombi: In case of a person dying slowly due to circulatory failure, a firm, stringy, tough, pale-yellow thrombus forms in the cavities, usually on the right side of the heart.

The *pericardium* is examined for presence of any pathology or injury. The contents of the pericardial sac and quantity of fluid is noted. Pericardial effusion, cardiac tamponade, subpericardial hemorrhage and constrictive pericarditis are looked for.

NECK

The neck structures are examined before removal of the thoracic organs so that the tongue, larynx, trachea and esophagus can be taken out along with the lungs. This helps in examination of the whole of the upper respiratory tract in its continuity (Details are given in Chapter 10).

In case of death due to alleged constriction of the neck, there may be fracture of hyoid bone or thyroid cartilage with extravasation of blood into the tissues, and injury to carotid arteries, sternomastoid muscles or platysma. Compression of the neck with hard materials may cause injury to the cervical vertebrae and the corresponding part of the spinal cord. Level and extent of other mechanical injuries on the neck are cautiously examined to know the type of injury, and organs or structures injured resulting in death.

SKULL AND BRAIN

Procedure: A wooden block is placed under the shoulders so that the neck is extended and the head fixed by a headrest. A coronal incision is made in the scalp, which starts from one mastoid to the opposite mastoid process just behind the ear and is continued over the vertex of the scalp. The incision should penetrate upto the periosteum. The scalp is reflected forwards to the superciliary ridges, and backwards to a point just below the occipital protuberance (**Figs. 7.7A and B**). Presence of hematoma, petechial hemorrhage, edema or fracture is noted.

The temporal and masseter muscles are incised on either side for sawing the skull. The saw-line is made in a slightly V-shaped direction (angle of 120°) so that the skull cap can fit back into the correct position on reconstruction of the body. Saw and remove the skull cap, the line of separation is just above the superciliary ridges in front, to the base of the mastoid process on either side, and just above the occipital protuberance behind (**Fig. 7.7C**).

Dura: The dura is examined from outside for extradural hemorrhage (weight and volume is noted, if present) and superior sagittal sinus for antemortem thrombus. It is cut along the line of detached skull cap and pulled gently from front to back while cutting falx cerebri, and examined for subdural and subarachnoid hemorrhage.
- The weight and volume of subdural hemorrhage, its effect on brain—flattening or any asymmetry is noted.
- Subdural hemorrhage can be washed under running water, whereas subarachnoid hemorrhage cannot be washed.

Delivery of the Brain

Insert four fingers of the left hand between the frontal lobes and the skull. Draw them backward, and then with the right hand, cut the nerves and vessels as they emerge from the skull. Cut the tentorium along the superior border of the petrous bone. Cut the cervical cord, first cervical nerves and vertebral arteries as far below as possible. Support the brain throughout with the left hand. Remove the brain along with the cerebellum and brainstem, which is supported by the right hand.
- Examine the remaining venous sinuses and the cranial cavity for antemortem thrombi. Remove the pituitary

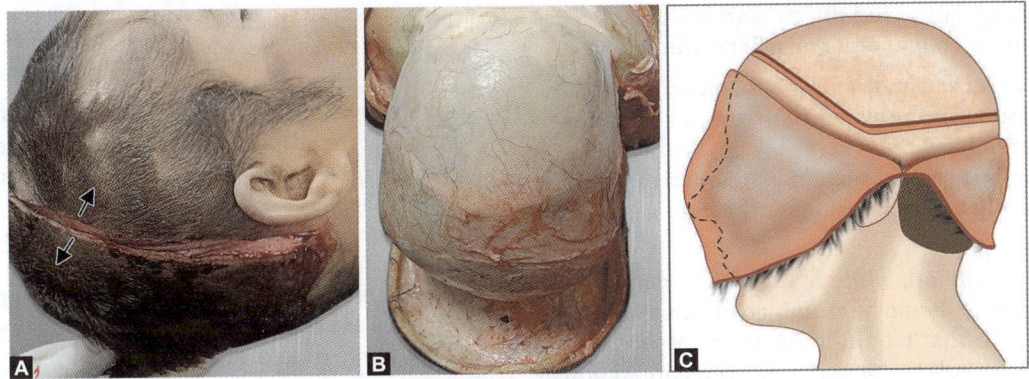

Figs. 7.7A to C: (A and B) Incision for removal and reflection of scalp; (C) Angular saw-line for removal of skull cap to avoid slippage during reconstruction

by chiseling the posterior clinoid processes and incising the diaphragm of the sella turcica around its periphery.
- Pull out the dura, examine the base of the skull and the rest of the cranial cavity for any fracture. Inspect the skull cap for fracture by holding it against the light.
- Remove a wedge-shaped portion of the petrous temporal bone and examine the mastoid for any collection of pus, hemorrhage or fluid in the middle ear.

Examination of the Brain

The brain is weighed, and then examined for any swelling, shrinkage or herniation, upper and lateral surfaces of the brain for asymmetry or flattening of the convolutions. The cerebral vessels is looked at for arteriosclerosis, embolism and aneurysms (especially the circle of Willis).

Berry aneurysms (size varies from few mm to few cm) are usually present at the junction of vessels especially at the junction of the posterior cerebral arteries, the posterior communicating vessels, and the middle cerebral arteries and the anterior communicating arteries. Cerebral infarction may occur due to a thrombus or atheroma.

In most medico-legal autopsies, the brain is examined in the fresh state; however, in select cases, the autopsy surgeon may need the brain 'fixed' prior to further evaluation. Fixation is an important step for proper examination of the brain and spinal cord.

Fixation of the Brain

The best routine fixative is 10% formalin and requires 2–3 weeks for satisfactory fixation. In fetuses and infants, the addition of acetic acid to the fixative solution increases the specific gravity of the fixative and allows the brain to float in the solution; it also makes the tissue firmer without altering its histological characteristics.

Dissection of the Brain

The most utilized and reliable method of brain sectioning is the *coronal cutting method*, whether examination occurs in the fresh state or after formalin fixation. It involves serially sectioning of all parts, including cerebrum, cerebellum and brainstem.

First, the cerebellum and brainstem should be separated from the cerebrum. This is done as high as possible, and cut the surface in a horizontal plane with a brain knife. The brainstem is then separated from the cerebellum at the cerebellar peduncles, as close to the brainstem as possible with a scalpel.

Cerebrum

The cerebrum is then sliced in a coronal plane at 1 cm intervals. If the brain is fresh, it is sliced from the frontal end and from the superior surface. The main aim with the fresh brain is to be as quick as possible, since the brain is so soft that it rapidly collapses.

With fixed brain, the first slice is done through the mammillary bodies (at the basal surface) which divide the brain into half in the exact coronal plane **(Fig. 7.8)**. Thereafter, each half is sliced 1 cm each, in turn, with the flat surface laid downwards. It should be done with a single sweep of a brain knife, to avoid a sawing motion and

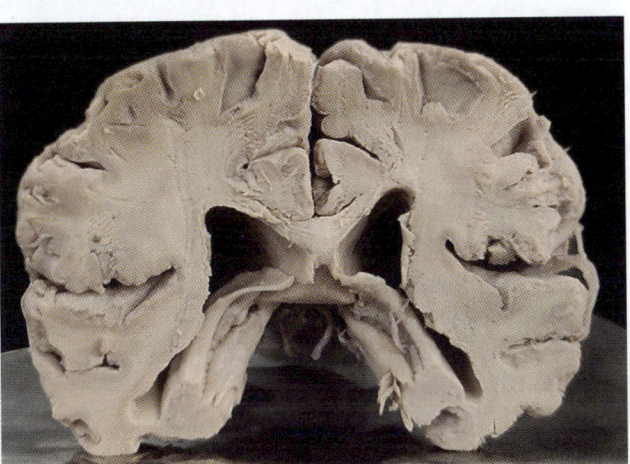

Fig. 7.8: Coronal section through formalin fixed brain

subsequent irregularities on the cut surface. These slices should then be laid out in order on a flat surface.

Other planes that can be used for special cases:
- Cutting the brain in the plane of CT-scans, for comparison with the radiology.
- Single, midline sagittal section, particularly useful if a third or fourth ventricle lesion is expected.

Features to look for:
- The cortical ribbon, white matter, basal ganglia and lateral ventricle should be examined for any asymmetry or brain shift that would indicate space occupying lesion—abscess, large hemorrhage, recent infarction or either metastatic or primary tumors.
- Old infarcts are cystic spaces, which do not produce any brain shift.
- Small focal lesions may not cause any brain shift, e.g., small (lacunar) infarcts associated with hypertension and gray areas of demyelination (plaques) within the white matter.
- Dilatation of lateral ventricle may indicate atrophy.
- Shrinkage of cerebral cortex (gray matter) is common in chronic alcoholics.
- Cerebral fat emboli that have completely obstructed the small vessels of the brain may be visible to the naked eye as punctate hemorrhages in the white matter.
- Petechial hemorrhages in the white matter are commonly found in death from anaphylactic shock.
- In head injury, edema is seen in the white matter around or deep to contusions, lacerations or ischemic lesions. If there is any injury to the brain, successive sections parallel to the wounded surfaces should be made till the whole depth of the wound is revealed.

Cerebellum

The cerebellum is dissected on the horizontal plane with the two lobes being sliced in a 'fan' shape with the middle slice going through the dentate nucleus which gives best histological orientation of the structures.

Brainstem

The brainstem can be sliced at 5 mm intervals perpendicular to its axis, and laid out in order on a flat surface.

In brainstem and cerebellum, any focal lesions must be identified, such as areas of hemorrhage, areas of softening or cystic degeneration that indicate recent or old infarction respectively, and primary or metastatic tumors.

Dissection of head in infants: *Beneke's technique* is used to open the skull in infants (Details in Chapter 20).

Spinal Cord

- The spinal cord can be removed from an anterior or posterior approach, and usually removed separately from the brain.
- If there is no indication, the spinal cord need not be exposed.
- The *anterior approach* is more difficult, but has the advantages of not requiring the body to be turned (messy procedure with evisceration already taken place), and allowing the nerve roots and dorsal ganglia to be dissected.
- The *posterior approach* is both quicker and easier, but best performed before the full postmortem, to avoid the mess. It also allows the spinal cord and the brain to be removed in continuity, but does not allow examination of the nerve roots and basal ganglia.

Posterior Approach to the Spinal Cord

i. A long midline incision is made and the skin, muscle and soft tissues are flapped out sidewise or laterally, 1 inch on either side from the vertebral column.
ii. The posterior arch is cut with the vibrating saw. This dissection can extend superiorly along the cervical vertebrae to the foramen magnum.
iii. The spinal processes and posterior portions of the laminae are removed.
iv. The dura is opened longitudinally to the uppermost part of the incision, where it is cut circumferentially.
v. The nerves are cut and the spinal cord is delivered by steady traction.

DESCRIPTION OF AN ORGAN

- **Size:** Measuring tape is used. A tense capsule indicates enlargement and loose capsule shrinkage.
- **Shape:** Note any deviation from normal.
- **Surface:** Most organs have a delicate, smooth, glistening and transparent capsule of serosa. Any thickening, roughening, dullness or opacity is noted.
- **Consistency:** The softness or firmness is appreciated by application of finger pressure.
- **Cohesion:** It is the strength within the tissue that holds an organ together. It is judged by the resistance of the cut surface to tearing, pressure or pulling.
- **Cut surface:** Note color and structural details.

After completion of autopsy, blood, fluid, etc., are removed from the body cavities. The organs are replaced in the body and any excess space is packed with cotton or cloth, especially in the pelvis and the throat, where blood tends to leak. The dissected flaps are brought close together and sutured by using thin twine and large curved needle. The skull is filled with remaining portion of the brain along with cotton or other absorbent material and the skull cap fitted in place. The scalp is pulled back over the vault, and the scalp stitched with thin strong twine. The body is washed with water, dried and covered with clothes, and then handed over to the police constable accompanying it.

REPORT

After completing the postmortem examination, a complete and concise report should be written in duplicate/triplicate using carbon papers. One copy is given to the IO and another copy is retained for future reference (sometimes a third copy is made for hospital purpose or for the chemical examiner). The report should contain a list of specimens and samples retained for further examination.

- In some States, a computerized report is given to the police.
- The report should be given on the same day, as the details cannot be accurately recorded from memory, if there is too much of delay.
- If laboratory tests have to be carried out, a provisional report is given, and later after obtaining the reports, a supplementary report is given. In suspected cases of poisoning, the opinion should be kept reserved until the Chemical Examiner's report is received. In such cases, viscera should be preserved, and histological and bacteriological examinations may be carried out. The conclusion that death was caused by poison depends on evaluation of clinical, toxicological, circumstantial and autopsy evidence.
- A definite opinion should be given whenever possible, but if the cause of death cannot be ascertained, it should be mentioned in the report. While giving cause of death, the word '*probably*' should be avoided. It must be recognized that the determination of cause and manner of death are opinions, not facts. **The opinion of one autopsy surgeon can differ from another's.**
- A poor opinion is far worse than no opinion at all, as in the latter case, the legal authorities will at least be aware of the deficiency in their evidence, rather than be misled by the assertive factual error of an inexperienced doctor.
- If the cause or manner of death is not found on autopsy, the opinion as to the cause of death should be given as '*undetermined*', and the manner of death as '*unknown*'.

DEMONSTRATION OF PNEUMOTHORAX

Pneumothorax occurs when a leakage through the pleura allows air to enter the pleural cavity, and the communication rapidly closes. It can be demonstrated by three ways during autopsy:

i. The skin and subcutaneous tissues are reflected from the chest wall till the mid-axillary line, being careful not to open the pleural cavity. Care should be taken not to puncture the intercostal soft tissue and penetrate the pleural space, as this releases air from an underlying pneumothorax. Water is poured into the angle between subcutaneous tissue and the chest wall, and the intercostal tissues below the water line are pierced with a blade. If pneumothorax is present, bubbles of air will be seen rising through the water.

ii. Another method is possible before any incision is made. This involves introducing a wide bore needle attached to a 50 mL syringe into the subcutaneous tissue over an intercostal space into the pleural space. The plunger should be removed previously and the syringe filled with water. The water is observed for the presence of any bubbles. A similar procedure is then followed on the other side.

iii. A third method involves postmortem chest X-ray, and assessment in a manner similar to detection of a pneumothorax in the living patient.

DEMONSTRATION OF AIR EMBOLUS

For venous air embolus, a plane chest X-ray before evisceration to demonstrate the pathology may be done. Examination of the retina should be performed with an ophthalmoscope for intravascular bubbles.

During dissection of the neck, the large neck veins should be carefully exposed, but not opened before the heart is dissected *in situ*, to avoid the confusion of introduction of air during evisceration. The abdomen is opened in the usual manner and the contents are moved to inspect the inferior vena cava for bubbles in the lumen through its transparent wall. There are three methods to demonstrate *venous air embolus*:

i. The sternum is removed by dividing the ribs, being careful not to puncture the pericardial sac, and cutting through the sternum distal to the sternoclavicular joint. The internal mammary vessels should be clamped. The anterior pericardial sac is opened and the external epicardial veins inspected for evidence of intraluminal bubbles. Water is introduced to fill the pericardial space. Once completely covered in water, the right atrium and ventricle are incised, and careful inspection is made to identify any air bubbles which may escape.

ii. Another method is by inserting a water-filled syringe (minus plunger) connected to a needle into the right ventricle, the syringe chamber observed for the presence of bubbles.

iii. **Pyrogallol test:** A 2% pyrogallol solution mixed with sodium hydroxide is taken in a syringe. Gas is then aspirated from the right side of the heart and then shaken. The mixture will turn brown, if air is present. In the absence of air, the solution stays clear (indicating gas production by bacteria).

Arterial air emboli are unusual and usually result from traumatic injury involving the pulmonary veins or following introduction of air during cardiopulmonary bypass. Smaller volume of air is associated with such emboli, and as such more difficult to demonstrate.

Systemic emboli may be verified by inspecting the intracranial vessels of the meninges and circle of Willis, and then examining underwater after clamping the internal carotid and basilar arteries.

> **FM 6.1, 6.2**
> - Describe different types of specimen and tissues to be collected both in the living and dead: Body fluids (blood, urine, semen, faeces, saliva), skin, nails, tooth pulp, vaginal smear, viscera, skull, specimen for histopathological examination, blood grouping and HLA typing.
> - Describe the methods of sample collection, preservation, labelling, dispatch, and interpretation of reports.

COLLECTION OF SAMPLES

i. **Blood:** Before autopsy, 10–20 mL of blood can be drawn from the femoral (*best sample*), jugular or subclavian vein by a syringe. Cardiac blood from right chamber of heart is quite useful.
   - Blood should never be collected from the pleural or the abdominal cavities, as it can be contaminated with gastric or intestinal contents, lymph, mucus, urine, pus or serous fluid. Moreover, cellular barrier of mucous and serous membranes breaks down after death, due to which substances (e.g., alcohol and barbiturates) in the stomach and intestine can migrate to the organs in the thorax and abdomen leading to erroneous results.

ii. **Cerebrospinal fluid (CSF):** It is collected by lumbar puncture or from the cisterna magna by inserting a long needle between the atlanto-occipital membrane **(Fig. 7.9A)**. Direct aspiration of CSF can be done from the lateral ventricles or third ventricle after removal of the brain.

iii. **Vitreous humor:** A fine hypodermic needle (20 gauge) attached to a syringe is inserted through the outer canthus into the posterior chamber of the eye, after pulling the eyelid aside, followed by aspiration of 1–2 mL of crystal clear colorless fluid from each eye **(Fig. 7.9B)**. Water/saline is re-introduced through the needle to restore the tension in the globe for cosmetic reasons.

iv. **Lungs:** In solvent abuse ('glue sniffing') and death from gaseous or volatile substances, the lung is mobilized and the main bronchus tied off tightly with a ligature. The hilum is then divided and the lung is put into a glass container immediately and sealed. Plastic (polythene) bags are not suitable, as they are permeable to volatile substances.

v. **Urine:** It can be collected in a suitable sterile or non-sterile 'universal container' for either microbiological or toxicological analysis by suprapubic puncture or when the bladder is opened **(Fig. 7.9C)**. Before dissection, urine can be collected via catheter or abdominal wall puncture.

vi. **Bone:** About 200 g is collected. It is convenient to remove about 10–15 cm of the shaft of the femur.

vii. **Hair:** An adequate sample of head (150-200 hair from the posterior vertex of scalp-region of least growth variation) and pubic hair should be removed by plucking along with roots, and not by cutting, and preserved in separate containers (0.5 g for DNA analysis, upto 10 g for analysis of heavy metals).

viii. **Maggots:** Collect 10 larvae randomly. These are dropped alive into boiling absolute alcohol or 10% hot formalin which kills them in an extended condition (to disclose the internal structure of the larvae). If time of death is an issue, some larvae/maggots should be preserved alive for examination by an entomologist. Maggots may reveal the presence of drugs/poisons in decomposed bodies.

ix. **Nails:** All the nails (fingers and/or toes) should be removed in their entirety and collected in separate envelopes.

x. **Skin:** If there is needle puncture, the whole needle track and surrounding tissue (2–4 cm radius) should be excised. Control specimens should be taken from same area on the opposite side of the body and preserved in a separate container. In firearm cases, a portion of skin around the entrance and exit wounds should be preserved.

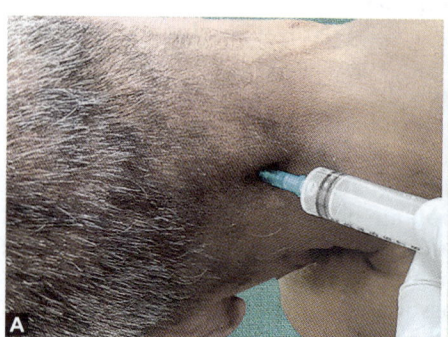 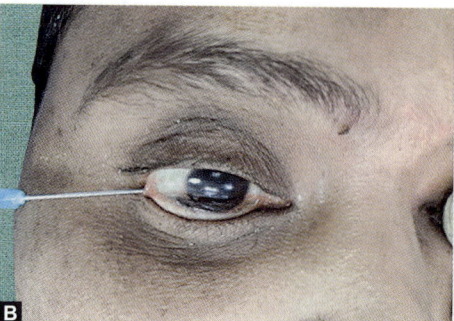 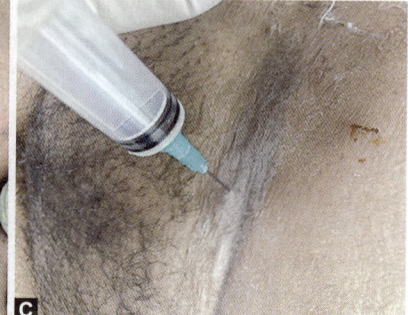

Figs. 7.9A to C: Collection of: (A) Cerebrospinal fluid; (B) Vitreous humor; (C) Urine (suprapubic puncture)
(*Courtesy*: Dr Jatin Bodwal, DDU Hospital, Delhi)

CHAPTER 7 : Medico-legal Autopsy

FM 2.14
Describe and discuss preservation of viscera on postmortem examination for chemical analysis and other medico-legal purposes.

PRESERVATION OF VISCERA

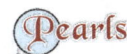

Viscera should be preserved in cases of:
- Suspected death due to poisoning
- Deceased was intoxicated or used to drugs
- Accidental death involving driver of a vehicle or machine operator
- Criminal abortion
- Surgical and anesthetic deaths
- Death due to burns (if needed)
- Advanced decomposition*
- Cause of death could not be found after autopsy
- Any case, if requested by the Magistrate or IO.

The Supreme Court has ruled that in cases of death due to suspected poisoning, the prosecuting agency should send the viscera to a forensic science laboratory immediately after postmortem.

Specimens that must be preserved in cases of suspected poisoning are given in **Tables 7.3 to 7.5 (Fig. 7.10).**

Some practical points that need to be considered:
- The preferred specimens collected at postmortem will depend on the type of case/poison suspected.
- Blood is the most useful sample because toxins present in this can best be related to a physiological effect, and can be used to assess the likelihood of recent exposure to poisons/drugs.
- Urine is the second most important specimen collected. However, the disadvantages are: it is unavailable in half the cases (since it is voided during the dying process), poison may be metabolized so extensively that the

TABLE 7.3: Samples preserved in living persons

Material	Quantity
Vomit	300 mL (whole, if quantity is less)
Stomach washout	500 mL
Blood	10 mL
Urine	100 mL

TABLE 7.4: Viscera preserved during autopsy (routine)

Material	Quantity
Stomach and its contents	Whole
Upper part of small intestine and its contents	About 15–30 cm length (some say 100 cm)
Liver (along with gallbladder)	100 g
Kidney	Longitudinal half of each kidney
Blood	10 mL
Urine	100 mL

TABLE 7.5: Additional viscera and materials required in certain cases

S.No.	Material	Poisoning/circumstances suspected
1.	Heart	Strychnine, digitalis
2.	Brain	Alkaloids, organophosphorus, opiates, strychnine, carbon monoxide, cyanide, barbiturates and volatile organic poisons; hydrophobia/rabies (for negri bodies)
3.	Spinal cord	Strychnine
4.	Cerebrospinal fluid	Alcohol
5.	Vitreous humor	Alcohol, chloroform
6.	Lung	Gaseous poisons, hydrocyanic acid, alcohol, chloroform
7.	Skin	Injected poisons (insulin, morphine, heroin, cocaine and other illicit drugs), firearm injuries
8.	Bone, hair and nails	Heavy metals (arsenic, antimony, thallium)
9.	Fatty tissue	Pesticides and insecticides
10.	Uterus and its appendages	Criminal abortion
11.	Muscle	Decomposition
12.	Spleen	CO, cyanide

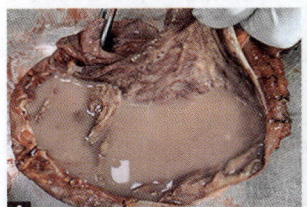 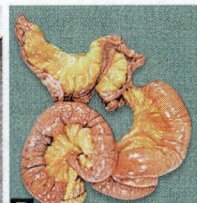 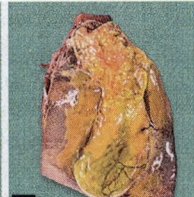 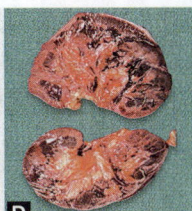 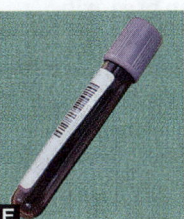 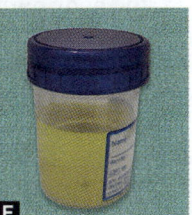

Figs. 7.10A to F: Routine viscera preservation: (A) Stomach along with its contents; (B) Upper part of small intestines; (C) Part of liver along with gallbladder; (D) Half of each kidney; (E) Blood; (F) Urine

---
* When the body is too decomposed to collect any fluids, collect atleast 100 g of muscle from thigh, liver, brain, fat and kidneys.

- parent compound may not detected, and concentration of most poisons are difficult to interpret.
- Vitreous humor is the preferred specimen for postmortem confirmation of alcohol ingestion, since postmortem formation of ethanol does not occur to significant extent in vitreous, and hence useful even in decomposing bodies. It is recommended that this specimen is included routinely in sudden death investigations.
- Stomach content is invaluable in cases of suspected poisoning—establish actual content of poison, determination of route of administration, high concentration of toxins, and analysis is uncomplicated by metabolism. However, detection of poison does not necessarily imply oral ingestion—basic drugs and metabolites in the blood can be secreted through the gastric juice (formed from extracellular fluid) and the juice may be contaminated with bile from retching and vomiting or may be agonal in nature.
- Liver is most important, since large amount of tissue is available, ease of sample collection, high concentration of toxins and availability of large database of liver drug concentrations.
  - A 100 g of tissue is sufficient for most analysis.
  - The right lobe is preferred, since chances of postmortem diffusion of toxins from bowel contents and mesenteric circulation is negligible.
  - With more sensitive analytical methods, the majority of drugs are detected readily in the blood, and it is not necessary to rely on the liver (or any other organ) for their detection.
  - The major disadvantage of the liver as specimen is that it tends to be fatty and putrefy faster than blood.
- Bile has been collected historically, but its usefulness is limited. It may show the presence of number of drugs including morphine/heroin, benzodiazepine, cocaine, methadone, glutathione, many antibiotics and tranquillizers and heavy metals (in chronic poisoning). With the widespread use of sensitive immunoassays and other techniques, the use of bile as a screening specimen is less valuable that it once was.
- Brain, kidney (analysis of heavy metals or ethylene glycol) and spleen are used to determine and interpret the concentration of toxins, i.e., overall assessment of the body burden of a toxin.
- Spleen is useful as a specimen for toxins, such as carbon monoxide (CO) and cyanide that binds to hemoglobin. If septicemia is suspected and the cause of it is not obvious, spleen should be cultured.

PRESERVATION OF SAMPLES

- The ideal samples are the ones in which no preservative has been added and sent to CFSL within few hours. But, practically, it usually gets delayed.
- The specimens and viscera is refrigerated at about 4°C (short-term) or at –20°C or preferably at –80°C (long-term), if not sent to the laboratory.
- In order that putrefaction may not set in and render chemical analysis difficult, certain preservatives are used.

1. Viscera
   - The most commonly used preservative for viscera is **saturated solution of common salt**. It is easily available, cheap and effective preservative. However, the best preservative for preservation of viscera is *rectified spirit*.
   - In cases of suspected alkali or acid poisoning (*except carbolic acid*), only rectified spirit is used. It is *not used* in cases of suspected poisoning with:

♦ Alcohol	♦ Chloroform
♦ Kerosene	♦ Ether
♦ Chloral hydrate	♦ Phosphorus
♦ Formaldehyde	♦ Formic acid
♦ Paraldehyde	♦ Acetic acid

2. Blood for toxicological analysis (for alcohol, cocaine, cyanide and CO) is preserved in sodium or potassium fluoride at the concentration of 10 mg/mL of blood and anticoagulant potassium oxalate, 30 mg/10 mL of blood.
   - Postmortem samples are liable to production of alcohol by microbiological action and higher concentrations of sodium fluoride are required to inhibit this.
   - Heparin and EDTA should not be used as anti-coagulants, since they interfere with detection of methanol.
   - If blood is required only for grouping, no preservative is necessary and small amount of blood is well preserved by soaking in a blotter.
   - In case of suspected CO poisoning, a layer of 1–2 cm of liquid paraffin is added immediately over the blood sample to avoid exposure to atmospheric oxygen. Samples has been found stable with or without refrigeration for up to 4 weeks (if refrigerated, then up to 2 years).
   - If solvent abuse and anesthetic death is suspected, the glass container should have a foil-lined lid to prevent gas from escaping (as gas can permeate rubber) and the container is completely filled to prevent gas from escaping in 'dead' air space.
   - Blood for hematological examination including glycosylated hemoglobin in diabetics should be sent in a clean glass container with anticoagulant (e.g., EDTA).

3. Urine is persevered by adding small amount of phenyl mercuric nitrate or thymol. Fluoride should

be added to urine if alcohol, cyanide or cocaine is suspected.
4. Vitreous humor is preserved using sodium fluoride (10 mg/mL) (for alcohol, diabetes and insulin related deaths).
5. For bones, hair and nails, preservative is not required. It has to be dried in normal temperature and sealed in plastic bag. But, bone marrow is preserved in a test tube containing 4–5 mL of 5% albumin-normal saline solution and stored at 4°C.

- Formalin is *not* used as preservative for chemical analysis because extraction of poison, especially non-volatile organic compounds become difficult.
- All samples should be properly sealed and labeled with the patient's name, hospital number, nature of sample, collection site, preservative used, and date and time of collection. It should be handed over to the IO after obtaining proper receipt.
- The viscera and specimens can be destroyed either after getting the permission from the Magistrate or when the IO informs that the case has been closed.

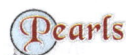

Conditions in which preservative is not necessary:
a. Viscera can be analyzed within 24 h
b. Sample can be kept in refrigerator
c. Hair, nails and bones
d. Lungs (for detecting inhaled poisons)

NOTA BENE
- Sodium fluoride is the most commonly used agent to prevent glycolysis. It inhibits the enzyme enolase and is also effective at inhibiting bacterial growth.
- EDTA can effectively chelate the calcium ion of blood, therefore it can prevent the blood coagulation, does not affect the count and size of the leukocyte and keep erythrocyte invariable. Other anticoagulants are potassium oxalate, citrate or lithium heparin.

Procedure of Preservation

For preservation of viscera, a clean, transparent and preferably sterile glass jar or hard plastic (especially polypropylene) (one liter capacity) with a wide mouth and stoppers should be used. The size of the jar should be such, that at least 1/3rd of the container remains empty after being filled with the preservative to allow for accommodation of the gas, which will evolve out of the organs preserved. However, the preservative should completely immerse the viscera after the contents are well shaken.

- The stomach, small intestine and its contents are preserved in one bottle, part of liver along with gallbladder and kidneys in another bottle and urine in the third bottle **(Table 7.6)**. The stomach and intestines are opened before they are preserved. The liver and kidneys are cut into small pieces to ensure penetration of the preservative. Blood should be sent in a vial(s).
- A sample of the preservative used (sodium chloride or rectified spirit) is separately preserved and sent for analysis *to rule out any poison being present as a contaminant.*
- When additional material is required to be sent, it should be dispatched in separate bottles, like brain in one bottle and vomitus or stomach washout in another bottle. The bottles and vials required for preservation are normally supplied by the office of the Forensic Science Laboratory (FSL).
- The stoppers of the bottles should be well fitting, covered with a piece of cloth and tied by tape or string, and the ends sealed using a departmental seal. Each bottle should be suitably labeled with the autopsy number, name of the deceased, name of the organ, date, time and place of autopsy, followed by signature of the doctor who performed the autopsy.
- The sealed bottles are then put in a viscera box which is sealed. The viscera box along with a specimen of the seal used (put in a separate envelope and sealed) is handed over to the police constable, in return for a receipt. All these precautions are necessary to maintain the chain of evidence.
- Along with the viscera box, the following documents are also sent:
  i. Copy of the inquest papers, brief facts of the case and the case sheet.
  ii. Copy of autopsy report.
  iii. Letter requesting the chemical examiner to examine the viscera and inform the medical officer of its findings.

SAMPLES FOR LABORATORY INVESTIGATIONS

Various samples and their preservation are highlighted in **Table 7.7**.

- **Histopathological examination:** Sections of various internal organs (1.5 × 1.0 × 1.0 cm) in case of suspected abnormality are preserved.
- **Bacteriological/serological examination:** Blood should be kept in sterile container using sterile syringe. It may also be used for biochemical examination.
- **Smears:** In suspected malaria, smears from cerebral cortex, spleen and liver may be taken and examined for malarial parasite.

TABLE 7.6: Contents of viscera bottles

Bottle	Contents
Bottle 1	Stomach, small intestine and its contents
Bottle 2	Part of liver along with gallbladder and kidneys
Bottle 3	Urine
Bottle 4 (vial)	Blood
Bottle 5	Sample of preservative

TABLE 7.7: Sample preservation

Test/Investigation	Sample	Preservative
Histopathology	Sections of internal organs	10% formalin or 95% alcohol
Bacteriology/serology	Blood from right ventricle of heart/femoral vein or artery	No preservatives
Virology	Pieces of tissue	50% sterile glycerin in thermos
Enzymatic studies	Pieces of tissue	Liquid nitrogen
Smears	Vaginal/anal smears (sexual assault)	—
Fibroblasts for tissue culture (karyotyping, metabolic assays, enzyme assays)	Skin, fascia, lung, diaphragm, muscle and cartilage	Phosphate buffer saline Dulbecco's modified Eagle medium (DMEM) RPMI 1640
Tissue for metabolic studies and nucleic acid analysis	Liver, kidney, cardiac and skeletal muscle, and peripheral nerve (inborn errors of metabolism)	Liquid nitrogen or dry ice and stored at −70°C

NOTA BENE

Autopsy Room Hazards

Penetrating injuries are the most common route of transmission for pathogens at autopsy.

1. **Hepatitis B:** *Most transmissible of the blood-borne viruses.*
2. Persons associated with PM examination experiencing needle-stick injuries are at a risk of acquiring **hepatitis C infection** (HCV).
3. Autopsy is an efficient method of transmitting **tuberculosis** from the dead body.
4. Risk of **HIV infection** is considered low when compared with other blood-borne viruses, such as HBV and HCV, but resembles the rates for single contact heterosexual transmission.
   a. First case of documented seroconversion after occupational exposure to HIV: 1984.
   b. Viable HIV can be isolated from cranial bone, brain, cerebrospinal fluid, lymph node, spleen and blood up to 5 days after death, when stored at 6°C.
   c. HIV infection should be suspected, if the body is of:
      i. Male homosexual
      ii. IV drug abuser
      iii. Hemophiliac with repeated blood transfusions
      iv. Female prostitute
      v. Victim of sexual abuse

Risk of transmission from single percutaneous exposure to blood for:
- HBV: 6–30%
- HIV: 0.1–0.36%
- HCV: 2.7–10%

FM 2.13

Describe and discuss obscure autopsy.

OBSCURE AND NEGATIVE AUTOPSY

Obscure Autopsy

In about 20% of all postmortem examination cases, the cause of death may not be clear at the time of dissection of the body, and there are minimal or indeterminate findings or even no positive findings at all. These are a source of confusion to any forensic pathologist.

- In many of these cases, the cause of death can be made out after detailed clinical and laboratory investigations and interview with persons who had observed the deceased before he died.
- These 'obscure autopsies' are more common in the younger age group. An example is the **'obscure syndrome'** seen in Thailand (*'Lai Tai'*), Singapore, China, Japan (*Pokkuri death syndrome*) and Hongkong wherein young workers suddenly die with no demonstrable pathology.
- Before tissue for histology is taken, a full review of the dissection should be undertaken—the coronary system, pulmonary arteries (pulmonary emboli in smaller branches), brain (particularly the basal arteries) and the carotid arteries in the neck.
- When a complete review of the gross pathology has proved unproductive, then a full histological examination is required, especially of the myocardium. Special stains, such as phosphotungstic acid-hematoxylin, dehydrogenase enzyme histochemistry and acridine-orange fluorescence stains may be used.

Causes of Obscure Autopsy

i. **Natural diseases:** Epilepsy, asthma, paroxysmal fibrillation.
ii. **Concealed trauma:** Concussion, blunt injury to the heart, reflex vagal inhibition.
iii. **Poisoning:** Anesthetic overdose, narcotic, neurotoxic, cytotoxic or plant poisoning.
iv. **Biochemical disturbances:** Uremia, diabetes.
v. **Endocrinal disturbances:** Adrenal insufficiency, thyrotoxicosis.
vi. **Miscellaneous:** Allergy, drug idiosyncrasy.

Negative Autopsy

In about 2–5% of all postmortem examination cases, the cause of death remains unknown, even after all laboratory examinations including biochemical, microbiological, virological, microscopic and toxicological examination.

- If at the end of the process, no apparent cause of death is found, then the authorities must be informed that the cause of death cannot be determined and no opinion can be offered in the present state of medical and scientific knowledge.

For example, sudden infant death syndrome (SIDS) could be considered as 'negative autopsy' as by definition, no significant findings are discovered.

- However, negative findings/evidence such as absence of injuries, no evidence of poisoning/lethal infection/well-recognized natural disease may confirm that the deceased did not die of, and in all probability he must have died due to natural causes, rather than some unnatural external event.
- The use of some meaningless terms such as 'heart failure' or 'cardiorespiratory arrest' is pointless and may cause confusion to the police/Magistrate.
- A mode of death is irrelevant in lieu of a cause of death, so is the use of some agonal event such as 'aspiration of vomit'.
- It is also useless to use some unprovable process, such as 'vagal inhibition,' 'reflex cardiac arrest' or 'suffocation,' because these conditions are thought to leave no traces.

Second Autopsy

- Second autopsy or re-postmortem examination is the autopsy conducted on an already autopsied body.
- There is no provision in Indian law for a second autopsy. Instances where second autopsy is requested is given in **Box 7.2**.
- A Committee set up by the Nation Human Rights Commission recommended that the following rules be observed in respect of a second postmortem:
  a. This procedure, ordinarily, should not be undertaken unless either the IO or the concerned authority is of the view that the first postmortem was wrongly done, or done with a view to help the accused to escape punishment.
  b. The second postmortem may also be ordered by the Sub-Divisional Magistrate/Additional District Magistrate of the area concerned, after looking into all the facts.
  c. It should be conducted by a 'Board' of two forensic medicine specialists at a teaching institution where postmortems are being conducted.
  d. The postmortem report of the first doctor should be made available to the Board before conducting the second postmortem.
  e. The doctor who conducted the first postmortem should be informed about the same and be allowed to be present at the second postmortem.

Box 7.2 Indications of second autopsy.
- Relatives are not satisfied with the first autopsy.
- Cause of death cannot be opined in the first instance.
- Expert opinion wherein some question left unanswered or some issues unattended.
- Suspicion of doctor conducting the postmortem coming hand-in-glove with the accused.
- Involvement of the police in concealing the facts.

FM 7.1

Enumerate the indications and describe the principles and appropriate use for: Digital autopsy (virtual autopsy), imaging technologies.

DIGITAL AUTOPSY

Digital autopsy or virtopsy (combination of 'virtual' and 'autopsy') is a bloodless and minimally invasive procedure to examine a body for cause of death.

- It utilizes imaging techniques (MSCT and MRI), photogrammetry and 3-D optical measuring techniques to get a reliable, accurate geometric presentation of all findings (the body surface, as well as the interior).
- Virtopsy is being used in many countries like Switzerland, US, UK, Malaysia, Singapore and Japan.
- Up to 10,000 images can be reconstructed in a typical full-body MSCT virtual autopsy. It is easy to visualize bone, gas and metal fragments (bullets) with MSCT, but discrimination of soft tissue is limited.

Advantages	Disadvantages
Easy accessibility, allows a digital re-examination of the body even decades later (exhumation will become unnecessary)	Touch, feel and smell senses of forensic pathologists are absent
More compatible with religious beliefs held by deceased's family	Visualizing the circulation and possible bleeding is difficult
Take less time than a physical autopsy	No color documentation of body
Decreases the time required for a invasive autopsy as the pathologist is armed with prior information	Soft tissue discrimination is poor with MSCT
Fast localization of foreign objects such as bullets	PM imaging provides no information on macromorphology (i.e., histology, chemistry)
Safer option for pathologists and medical examiners	PM gas formation is difficult to distinguish from bowel gas or gas in wound channels

Uses

1. **Identification** of individuals including dental identification (comparison between postmortem and antemortem data).
2. Determining **time of death** using changes seen in both MSCT and MRI in head injury cases (metabolic information collected in a predefined region of the brain).
3. Determining **cause of death** as it is more effective in identifying vertebral/pelvis fractures (difficult to reach during invasive autopsy), natural death due to cardiac

insufficiency (calcification, cardiac hypertrophy, acute dilatation using MSCT and MRI data). PM coronary angiography can calculate soft and hard plaque volumes. MRCT and MRI can be used to perform perfusion studies of the myocardium.
4. Useful in polytrauma (fractures in RTAs), hanging/strangulation, burns, gunshot injury, drowning and investigation in deaths due to drug abuse.
5. **Age and sex determination** (measurement of bone structures).
6. Image-guided biopsy under CT fluoroscopy for histopathical or microradiological investigation. Gas samples from lungs can be obtained similarly.

Autopsy Radiology

In well-equipped hospital where radiographic facility is available, radiological examination should be done in select cases before starting the autopsy (**Box 7.3**).
- X-ray examination assists in identification, locating foreign objects such as projectiles and documenting old and recent bony injury.
- It is mandatory for X-ray/CT scanning of the body in cases of death in police firing.

FM 2.16
Describe and discuss examination of mutilated bodies or fragments, charred bones and bundle of bones.

EXAMINATION OF DECOMPOSED, MUTILATED AND SKELETONIZED REMAINS

Definitions

- **Forensic anthropology** is that branch of physical anthropology which for forensic purposes deals with identification of skeletonized remains known to be or suspected to be being human.
- **Disaster:** A sudden ecological phenomenon of sufficient magnitude to require external assistance (WHO). As per NDM Act, even a single person dying can be a disaster.
- **Mass disaster:** Death of more than 12 victims in a single event, like fire, air crashes or floods. The number of victims far exceeds the capacity of local death investigation system to handle.
- **Decomposed bodies** show putrefactive changes in varying degree depending upon the time elapsed since death.

Box 7.3	Indications of radiological examination.
Identification and dentistry	Mutilated/charred remains
Sharp force and gunshot wounds	Decomposed body
Air embolism	Barotrauma
Explosives deaths	Child abuse

- **Mutilated bodies** are extensively disfigured, deprived of a limb or a part of the body, but the soft tissues, muscles and skin are still attached to the bones.
- **Fragmentary remains** include only fragments of the body such as head, trunk or limb.
- **Charred bone** is black in color and represents carbonised skeletal material in direct contact with heat and flames; has microscopic residual burned soft tissues adhering to it; more durable than calcined bone.
- **Calcined bone** is thermally altered bone that has lost all of its organic material and moisture and exists as ashen fused bone salts.

In medico-legal practice, many a times, decomposed, mutilated, or even skeletonized bodies are received for autopsy. Careful examination may yield important information in all such cases. In case of mass disaster, the help of the anthropologist is sought for identification, if the remains are skeletonized, charred or largely destroyed.

General description: Decomposed bodies sometimes have earth and clothes stuck to them and/or are infested with maggots. The body may be immersed in a tank of weak carbolic acid (lysol) to soften the earth and get the clothing away without disintegration. Samples of insect eggs or maggots should be obtained for laboratory examination prior to immersing the body in lysol.

In case of skeletal remains, bones are kept in anatomic arrangement and a skeletal chart is drawn, indicating which bones are present. A complete list of all the bones sent for examination should be prepared, and photographs of all the bones are taken. The sand, dust or earth present on the bones is removed with brushes and wooden picks and scrapers. Light applications of acetone help to remove tight dirt.

MEDICO-LEGAL QUESTIONS

Following questions which the autopsy surgeon usually faces in connection with postmortem examination:

Q. Whether the body is of human or animal?

- It is easy to say if the head, trunk or limbs are available, but when pieces of muscles are only available without attached skin or viscera, it is very difficult. In such cases, definite opinion can be given by *precipitin test or antiglobulin inhibition test* (more sensitive than precipitin test) using blood or any other soft tissue, if the tissue is not severely decomposed.
- In case of bones, gross anatomical and microscopic characteristics (Haversian system) and chemical analysis of bone ash may be done. Precipitin test may be useful for confirmation. Serological tests are not useful in case of bones not having extractable plasma proteins or those bones which are burnt or cremated.

Q. Whether it belongs to one or more bodies?

- This is determined by fitting together all separate parts. If there is no disparity or reduplication, and if the color of the skin is same in all parts, they belong to one body.
- For bones, reconstructing the skeleton is done and observed for disproportion in the size of various bones, reduplication and articulation, and if the age, sex and race of all the bones is same.
- If the bones are suspected to be from more than one skeleton, they can be separated by the use of short wave UV light, which emits different color due to fluorescence of organic elements in the bones and inorganic substances on the surface of the bones.

Q. What was the race of the person?

This can be determined from hair and skin, if available, from nasal bridge height, nasal aperture shape, facial prognathism, palate shape, teeth (incisors), the skull (including cephalic index), pelvis and from features and indices of different long bones, particularly the lower extremities (Details in Chapters 5 and 6).

Q. Whether it is male or female?

- Sex can be determined if the head or trunk is available, from the presence and distribution or absence of hair, configuration of the pelvis, skull, mandible, diameter of head of femur and humerus, and measurements of femur, tibia, humerus and radius. Recognizable sex differences are present only after puberty (Details in Chapter 5).
- Sex can also be determined from the recognition of prostate or uterus, which can be identified even in advanced state of putrefaction. Microscopic examination may be done for confirmation. It can also be determined by nuclear sexing or sexing root sheath cells of scalp hair.

Q. What was the age of the individual at the time of death?

- Age can be estimated from general development, color of hair on the scalp, beard, moustache and pubis.
- Closure of the cranial sutures, eruption of teeth, ossification centers of bones, changes in the mandible, symphyseal surface of the pubis, sacrum, and margin of the glenoid cavity of the scapula; calcification of laryngeal and sternal cartilages and hyoid bone are also helpful. After the completion of bony union, exact age cannot be determined.

Q. What was the stature of the individual?

- Stature can be determined from long bones, such as femur, tibia, humerus or radius and using the formulae of *Pearson, Dupertuis and Hadden*; *Trotter* and *Gleser* for Americans; *Breitinger* for Germans or multiplication factors devised by Indian researchers.
- The principle of these formulae is to measure the length of long bone and multiply it with a given factor and then adding a fixed factor.
- The length of the humerus multiplied by five is a quick method of estimation of height.

> **NOTA BENE**
>
> Karl Pearson's formula for stature from dried long bones (in cms)
>
> | S.No. | Male | Female |
> |---|---|---|
> | 1. | $81.306 + 1.880 \times F$ | $72.884 + 1.945 \times F$ |
> | 2. | $78.664 + 2.376 \times T$ | $74.774 + 2.352 \times T$ |
> | 3. | $70.641 + 2.894 \times H$ | $71.475 + 2.754 \times H$ |
> | 4. | $89.925 + 2.271 \times R$ | $81.224 + 3.343 \times R$ |
>
> (F: Length of femur; T: Length of tibia; H: Length of humerus; R: Length of radius)

Q. What was the identity of the individual?

- It can be determined from fingerprints, tattoo marks, scars, moles, hair, teeth, flat feet, supernumerary ribs, congenital defects, deformities, implants **(Fig. 7.11)**, articles of clothing and superimposition technique (if skull is available).
- An X-ray of any bone, if taken during life, may be compared with an X-ray of the same bone, and it may help in identification **(Figs. 7.12A and B)**. Malunited fractures, healed fractures or deformities of bone, if present, are helpful.
- Determination of blood group antigens from teeth pulp might also help in establishing identity, if the blood group is known.

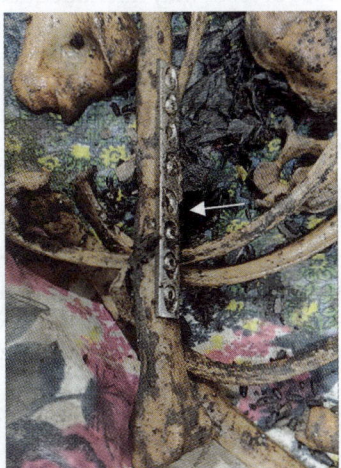

Fig. 7.11: Antemortem implant helped in identification of skeleton recovered from dump yard (arrow)
(*Courtesy:* Dr Charan Kamal, Civil Hospital, Ludhiana)

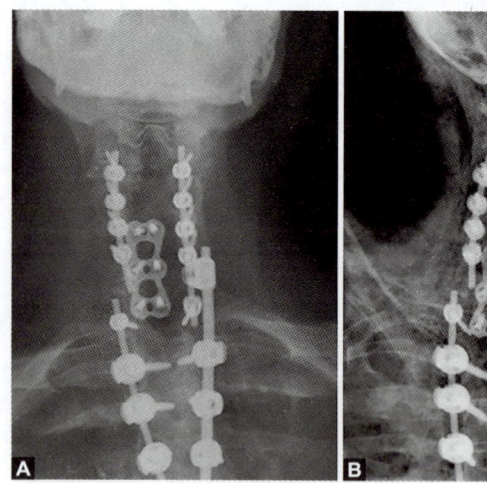

Figs. 7.12A and B: Positive identification using the X-rays of cervical spine: (A) Antemortem; (B) Postmortem
(*Courtesy:* Dr Carolyn V Isaac, Western Michigan University Homer Stryker MD School of Medicine, Michigan, US)

- Other methods include X-ray comparison of trabecular patterns and neutron activation analysis to distinguish the relative mineral contents.

Q. Whether DNA can be extracted from the skeletal remains?

- A variety of environmental and intrinsic factors (like bone type and density) act to create differential preservation in different skeletons and in different bones within the same skeleton.
- Low humidity, less oxygen, low temperature, neutral pH and the absence of microorganisms favor the preservation of DNA.
- The dense cortical portions of lower limb bones and the harder tissues of teeth may have adequately preserved DNA for analysis.
- With the advent of improved extraction buffers that provide complete demineralization of the osseous materials, extraction of total genomic DNA from nearly any skeletal remains is possible.

Q. What was the manner of separation of parts?

It can be found out by examining the margins of the parts and the ends of the long bones, and to look for whether they had been cleanly cut, sawn, hacked, lacerated, disarticulated at the joints or gnawed through by animals.

Q. What was the mode and place of disposal?

- The place of occurrence and disposal of the parts can be found out from trace materials attached with the parts from the place of disposal.

- A body buried in deep grave skeletonizes comparatively later. A body disposed off in open air dries up early. Bones of the bodies disposed in forest may be partly eaten by animals.

Q. Whether the injuries are antemortem or postmortem in nature?

Evidence of vital reaction is looked for at margins of the injured parts.

Q. What was the cause of death?

- The cause of death can be made out if there is evidence of fatal injury to some vital organ or large blood vessel, or marks of burning or deep cuts or fractures of bones, especially the skull, cervical vertebrae, hyoid bone or ribs. Foreign body, such as a bullet, when present is helpful.
- Bones or their charred remains may be subjected to chemical analysis for the detection of metallic poisons, such as arsenic, as these are not destroyed by heat.

Q. What type of weapon was involved?

In case of presence of antemortem injury, like fracture, or depending on the nature of injury of the bones, the weapon used to inflict the same and the type of weapon used to dismember the part, e.g., whether a hard blunt weapon, a light or heavy sharp cutting weapon, a pointed weapon or a firearm can be determined.

Q. What was the time of death?

The probable time since death (TSD) may be determined from the condition of parts and decomposition changes **(Table 7.8)**. The appearance of bones, unless they are very recent, is much more dependent upon the environment in which they have lain, than the passage of time. Bones left in a dry environment, such as sand, will last far longer than bones in a damp, acidic situation.

TABLE 7.8: Time since death from condition of body

Condition of body	Time since death
Soft tissues (fascia and ligaments) are still attached with bone	2 weeks to 2 months
No soft tissue attached, bone is not completely dry	1–3 months
Bone completely dry, putrid smell	Within 3 months
Bone dry with no putrid smell, retained its normal color	3 months to 1 year
Bone lighter, softer parts begin to crumble	>30–40 years

> **Recent Advances in Skeletal Age Estimation**
> - Total nitrogen content is >4–5 g% in bones less than 50 years old. Between 50–100 years, it is about 3.5 g%, and 2.5 g% when the bones are 350 years old.
> - The number of amino acids (initially about 15, glycine and analine are predominant) diminishes with age and hydroxyproline and proline tend to disappear after 50 years. A bone >100 years old will contain 7 amino acids.
> - Blood pigment tests using bone dust remain positive for up to 100 years.
> - Eluted bone dust solution tested for immunological activity against a human anti-Coombs serum test positive for 5–10 years.
> - **UV fluorescence:** The sawn shaft of a long bone, such as a femur is examined under an UV lamp; fresh bone will fluoresce across the whole surface from periosteum to marrow cavity. As time lengthens, the fluorescent zone narrows, breaks up and finally vanishes between 150–300 years.
> - **Bomb pulse dating** involves the analysis, comparison and interpretation of ^{14}C concentration within human tissues to atmospheric levels, and can provide an estimate of the year of death, which may assist in the identification process. Hair and nails have been found to have levels of ^{14}C consistent with either the year of death, or the year prior to death.
> - **Stable isotope analysis** is a technique to determine unidentified human remains for forensic profiling. Isotopic investigations on human remains have integrated the use of stable multi-isotope profiles (e.g., C, N, O, H, S, Sr, and Pb) as well as isotopic landscapes ("isoscapes") from multiple body tissues (e.g., teeth, bone, hair, and nails) to predict possible region-of-birth, long-term adult residence, recent travel history and dietary choices of unidentified human remains (e.g., isotopes oxygen and strontium isotopes reflect the source of drinking water and local geology, respectively).
> - **Transition analysis (TA)** is a multifactorial statistical method for estimating age at death in skeletons, which combines several correlated developmental traits (pubic symphysis, iliac auricular area, and cranial sutures) into one age estimate including a 95% prediction interval. TA calculates the probability of transitioning from one stage of skeletal aging to another since different parts of the skeleton age at different rates, hence the name transition analysis. TA does not require observations of all skeletal traits, and can therefore be used on partial skeletons, a common reality in both archaeological and forensic settings.

FM 2.17
Describe and discuss exhumation.

EXHUMATION

Definition: It is the lawful digging out of an already buried body from the grave for postmortem examination.
- Usually, it, involves a body (of any age group) that was not originally autopsied but which, for some reason, must be exhumed in order for an autopsy to be performed.
- It is infrequently done in India, because the bodies are disposed off by burning to ashes by most of the communities, except few.

Reasons

i. **Criminal cases**
   - Establishing the cause and manner of death in suspected homicide disguised as suicide.
   - Death as a result of criminal abortion and criminal negligence.
   - Retrieving some vital object which may throw light on the case, e.g., bullet from the dead body, if the person was killed by a firearm.
   - When new information or allegations suggest that the death was due to criminal action, either from injury or poison.

ii. **Civil cases:** Identification of the deceased for accidental death claim, insurance, workmen's compensation claim, liability for professional negligence, survivorship and inheritance claims, disputed identity, separation overseas, and burial of the wrong body inadvertently or by fraud.

iii. **Academic:** In ancient or historical circumstances, to investigate either the individual or a series of individuals for their identification and to study cause(s) of death or disease patterns and nutritional states.

Authorization: The body is exhumed only, when there is a written order from the First Class Magistrate/District Magistrate/Sub-Divisional Magistrate/Executive Magistrate [under **Sec. 176(3) CrPC**]; police cannot order exhumation.

Procedure (Fig. 7.13)

i. It should be done and completed in broad daylight, for which it should be started during the morning hours of the day.
ii. The body is exhumed under the supervision of a medical officer and Magistrate, in the presence of a police officer.
iii. Before opening the grave, it should be positively identified from location of burial plot, headstone and gravemarker, so that wrong body is not disinterred.
iv. Soil from above, below and two sides of the body or the coffin should be preserved in separate glass jars, with identification tags.
v. Disinfectants/pesticides should not be sprinkled on the body as it might interfere later with the determination of poison in the body.
vi. The doctor should note the position and appearance of the body inside the grave or the coffin. A drawing of the grave and body or skeleton should be made, noting all the details, whether the face is up, or to the side, arms are extended, or the lower limbs are flexed.
vii. The grave or the coffin with the body should be photographed.
viii. If decomposition is not advanced, a plank or a plastic sheet should then be lowered to the level of the earth on which the body rests.
ix. After this, the body is lifted and sent for postmortem examination, along with a requisition and a preliminary investigation report which contains the brief history of

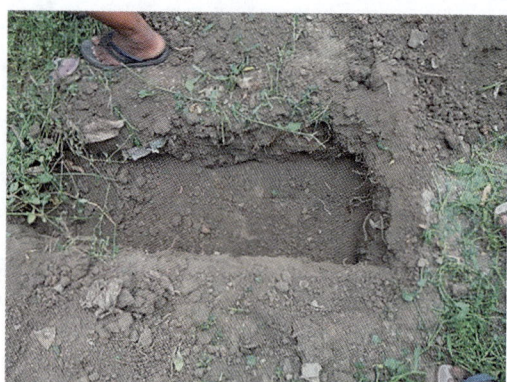 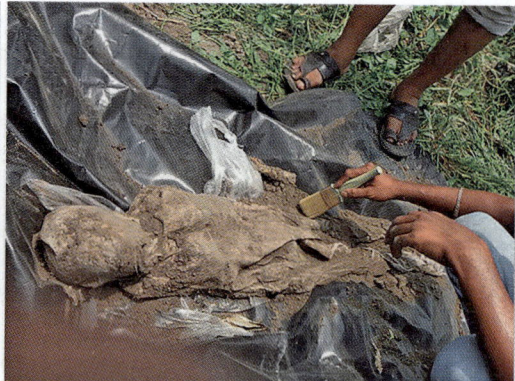

Fig. 7.13: Exhumation and examination being carried out

the case. In the mortuary, postmortem examination on the body is performed as in all other cases.

x. In highly putrefied bodies, an attempt should be made to establish the identity. Viscera should be preserved for chemical analysis. If the body is reduced to skeleton, the bones should be examined.

Time Limit

In India, there is *no time limit* for ordering of the exhumation, but many Western countries have well-defined time limit up to which exhumation can be done. For example, in France, the time limit is 10 years and in Germany, the time limit is 30 years. Thus in France, after 10 years of death, if some facts are found which may reveal foul play, even then the body cannot be exhumed.

NOTA BENE

- In Europe, exhumation services are carried out not only for forensic purposes but also for changing of graves, repartition to a different country and changing the type of disposal from burial to cremation.
- In Jewish and Islamic law, exhumation is forbidden except in certain circumstances.
- In Hong Kong, burial in government cemeteries are disinterred after 6 years under exhumation order. The remains are either collected privately or by the government for cremation and are reburied in an urn or niche.

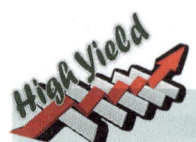

- Medico-legal autopsy is conducted when there is an official order from police or Magistrate.
- There is no provision in Indian law for a second autopsy.
- Autopsy is conducted by two doctors wherein a female has died within 7 years of her marriage.
- Body should not be embalmed before autopsy, since histopathological and toxicological examination will be impossible.
- After postmortem examination, dead body is handed over to police constable/IO.
- Last structure to be autopsied in asphyxial death: Neck.
- Method of autopsy in which organs are removed *en masse:* Letulle method.
- Method of autopsy in which organs removed one by one: Virchow's method.
- Black currant jelly and chicken fat thrombi are postmortem clots.
- Lines of Zahn are not seen in postmortem clots.
- Agonal thrombi: Firm, stringy pale-yellow thrombus on the right side of the heart in a person dying slowly due to circulatory failure.
- Sheehan's/subendocardial hemorrhages: Continuous, flame-shaped, confluent hemorrhages in left ventricle.
- **Berry aneurysms** are present at the junction of the posterior cerebral arteries, the posterior communicating vessels, and the middle cerebral arteries and the anterior communicating arteries.
- **Best method to remove spinal cord:** Posterior approach.
- Spinal cord is preserved in suspected poisoning with strychnine.
- **Test is used to demonstrate venous air embolus:** Pyrogallol test.

CHAPTER 7: Medico-legal Autopsy

- **Most useful sample for toxicological examination:** Blood.
- **Ideal site for collection of blood during autopsy:** Femoral vein.
- Vitreous humor is preserved at 4°C for confirmation of alcohol ingestion.
- Spleen is useful for finding toxins, such as CO and HCN that binds to hemoglobin.
- Viscera and specimens should be refrigerated at 4°C.
- **Most commonly used preservative for toxicological studies:** Saturated solution of common salt.
- In cases of alkali/acid poisoning (*except carbolic acid*), only rectified spirit is used.
- Rectified spirit is *not* used as preservative in case of poisoning with phenol, alcohol, kerosene, phosphorous.
- Blood is preserved using sodium/potassium fluoride and potassium oxalate. If required only for grouping, no preservative is used.
- Sodium fluoride is added to prevent glycolysis and inhibit growth of microorganisms.
- Fluoride used in the collection of blood samples inhibits the enzyme enolase.
- **Preservative used for tissues for virology study:** 50% glycerin.
- With respect to dating of a bone, a bone more than 100 years old contain: 7 amino acids.
- Body is exhumed under authorization from the Magistrate; police cannot order exhumation.
- Ideal time to start exhumation: Early morning.
- In India, there is *no time limit* for ordering of the exhumation.
- The best DNA profiling success rates can be obtained from femur and tooth.

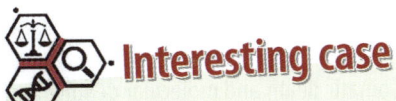

Interesting case

Mutilated Bodies ('Jigsaw Murders' Case, 1935)

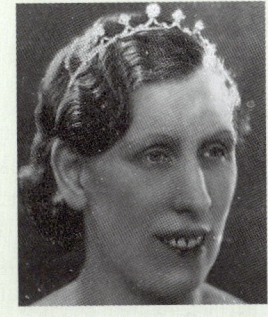

In 1935, Dr Buck Ruxton, an Indian-born physician residing in Lancashire, UK murdered his wife Isabella and her maid Mary, and then mutilated their bodies and scattered the parts, in an effort to make them unidentifiable and escape the law.

Isabella Ruxton was last seen on 14th September, 1935. Ruxton claimed that she had gone with her maid to Edinburgh, but her clothing was still in the house and the car that she used was parked outside. Prior to her disappearance, he had openly accused his wife of infidelity and threatened her with violence.

A passerby discovered some remains on 29th September, 1935 under a bridge in Scotland wrapped in a special edition of the *Sunday Graphic* newspaper that was only sold in the Lancashire area. The police were quick to investigate this lead. When first interviewed by the police, he had a deep cut on his hand, was agitated, and made inconsistent statements about where his wife and nursemaid had gone. Ruxton became the prime suspect. Their task was also made easier by the fact that, although he had worked hard to render the bodies unidentifiable (the fingers tips of the victims were cut off to prevent identification), but the skill with which the fingers were mutilated led police to hypothesize that the murderer had anatomical training and knew how to use a scalpel. Because the body parts of the two victims were jumbled and had to be reassembled, newspapers called the case the '*Jigsaw Murders*'.

The bodies were identified by a team of forensic experts consisting of pathologists, anatomists and entomologist using the evolving techniques of fingerprinting, anthropology and entomology. From the skull sutures, they determined the age of one of the bodies as between 35 and 45 and the second between 18 and 25. In reference to the cause of death, they opined that the older woman was strangulated and the second victim was hit by an unknown instrument and died due to blunt force trauma.

They reconstructed the mutilated parts and identified the bodies pioneering the use of photographic superimpositions. The skulls of the two victims were compared with multiple existing portraits to confirm the identifications.

To approximate the time of death of the victims, the entomologist identified the age of the maggots found upon the remains. He determined that the pupae had originated from the blowfly *Calliphora vicina* and the maggots were 12–14 days old. This indicated how long the bodies had been in the ravine—the window of time matched up with that of Isabella and her maid's disappearance. With the timeline narrowed down, police were able to gain access to Ruxton's home where traces of blood and human tissue were found in the bathroom.

The Ruxton case marked the first time entomological evidence successfully aiding an investigation. He was found guilty and hanged to death.

CHAPTER 8: Thanatology

LEARNING OBJECTIVES

Must know
1. Thanatology, death
2. Brain death and its certification
3. Clinical and molecular death
4. Cause, manner and mechanism of death
5. Writing cause of death (WHO)
6. Agonal period
7. Sudden death, causes
8. Coronary atherosclerosis

Desirable to know
1. Modes of death: Coma, syncope, asphyxia
2. Persistent vegetative state
3. Anoxia, types

 FM 2.1, 2.5
- Define, describe and discuss death and its types including somatic/clinical, cellular/molecular and brain-death, cortical death and brainstem death.
- Discuss moment of death.

Definitions

- **Thanatology** (Greek *thanatos*: death): Scientific study of death in all its aspects including its cause and phenomena. It also includes bodily changes that accompany death (postmortem changes) and their medico-legal significance.
- **Death:** The word 'death' denotes the death of a human being, unless contrary appears from the context **(Sec. 46 IPC)**.

DEATH

Death occurs in two stages **(Diff. 8.1)**:
i. Somatic, systemic or clinical.
ii. Molecular or cellular.

Somatic Death

The question of death is important in resuscitation and organ transplantation. Skin and bone remains metabolically active for many hours and these cells can be successfully cultured days after somatic death.

DIFFERENTIATION 8.1: Somatic death and molecular death

S.No.	Feature	Somatic death	Molecular death
1.	Definition	Permanent cessation of brainstem function	Progressive disintegration of body tissues with death of individual tissues and cells
2.	Onset	Precedes molecular death	Succeeds somatic death (1–2 h after stoppage of vital functions)
3.	Occurrence	Event	Process
4.	Tissues and cells of body	Alive and functioning	Dead and non-functioning with no metabolic activity
5.	Response to external stimuli	Muscle responds to thermal, electrical or chemical stimulus	Does not respond
6.	Confirmation	Flat ECG and EEG, and absent breath sounds	Rigor mortis, algor mortis, postmortem staining, putrefaction, etc.
7.	Resemblance	Suspended animation, coma, hypothermia	Does not resemble any condition
8.	Organ harvest	Possible	Not possible

Currently, somatic death is considered irreversible and permanent cessation of functions of the brainstem.

CHAPTER 8: Thanatology

> **NOTA BENE**
>
> According to *Bichat*, life could be compared to a tripod with its three legs representing the three vital systems—the nervous, circulatory and respiratory system—*tripod of life*. It is thought that all systems would fail if any one of the vital systems fails, and that is why these systems are known as '**atria mortis**' (*death's portal of entry or gateways of death*).

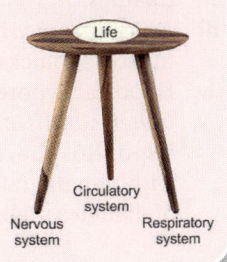

Molecular Death

- Molecular death occurs piecemeal. Initial changes occur due to metabolic dysfunction and later from structural disintegration.
- Nervous tissues die rapidly, the vital centers of the brain in about 3–7 minutes (min), but muscles survive up to 1–2 hours (h).

> **NOTA BENE**
>
> **Supravital reactions**
> - **Mechanical excitability of the skeletal muscle**
>   i. *Tendon reaction* (**Zsako's phenomenon**): Contraction of the whole muscle (e.g., quadriceps) due to propagated excitation following a mechanical stimulation, seen within 2–3 h after death.
>   ii. Localized idiomuscular contraction at the point of stimulation may be seen several hours after cessation of Zsako's phenomenon.
> - **Electrical excitability of the skeletal muscles** of the face may be observed for few hours after death.
> - **Pharmacological excitability** of the iris muscle resulting in change of pupil diameter following the administration of miotic or mydriatic solutions can be seen during the first hours of the postmortem period.

Whole-Brain Death–Cortical Death–Brainstem Death

- The **whole-brain death** concept states that 'an individual who has sustained irreversible cessation of all functions of the entire brain including the brainstem is dead'. This forms the standard for the determination of death by neurological criteria in the US and most European countries, and is based on the loss of *all brain function including but not limited to the brainstem*.
- **'Higher brain' or 'neocortical' death** is based on 'irreversible loss of personhood'. It is argued that an individual who has *irreversible loss of higher brain function in the cerebral cortex* rather than loss of whole-brain function should be considered dead, because consciousness, self-awareness, the potential for thought, applying reason and interactions with others are essential for being a person. In this view, persons in a persistent vegetative state (PVS) and anencephalic neonates would be considered dead. This concept has not been accepted by jurisdictions anywhere in the world.
- **Brainstem death** requires confirmation of the 'irreversible loss of the capacity for consciousness combined with the irreversible loss of the capacity to breathe', and relies on the fact that key components of consciousness and respiratory control—the reticular activating system and nuclei for cardiorespiratory regulation reside in the brainstem. The diagnosis of brainstem death *does not require confirmation that all brain functions have ceased*.

BRAIN/BRAINSTEM DEATH

The **moment of death** is the exact time when the person dies. The concept of the moment of death has changed through the years. The traditional cardiopulmonary standard (cessation of heartbeat and breathing) was the measure used during most of the 20th century to determine the presence of life.

As ventilator technology advanced, circulation and respiration could be maintained by means of a mechanical respirator, despite loss of all brain functions, and thus have brought the concept of **brain death**, i.e., irreversible loss of cerebral functioning.

- Brain death is the complete and irreversible cessation of functioning of the brain. Brain includes all the central nervous system (CNS) structures, except the spinal cord.
- Brain death is now accepted as brainstem death. The respiratory center which controls respiration lies within the brainstem. If this area is dead, the person is unable to breath spontaneously or regain consciousness.
- As the integrity of the reticular formation within the brainstem is essential for the proper functioning of the cortex, brainstem death can practically be considered to be sufficient for brain death. The crucial point in determining brain death is the demonstration of absence of all brainstem functions. Many countries, including India, now legally consider brainstem death as 'death'.

> **NOTA BENE**
>
> - **Harvard criteria of brain death (1968):** Laid stress on determining the activity of only brain to determine death.
> - **Minnesota criteria of brainstem death (1971):** Mohandas and Chou suggested that the most important part is brainstem and one must consider only brainstem death.
> - It may be argued by the defense when life-support machines are disconnected in brainstem death that the assailant did not 'kill' the victim, since 'death' was caused by the action of the doctors switching off the machine. In such a situation, it should be understood that death was diagnosed by the doctors before discontinuing artificial ventilation and the criminal act that initiated the chain of events was not remote enough to avoid culpability for the death.

Mechanism of Brain Death

Brain injury has a number of causes, such as traumatic or cerebrovascular injury and generalized hypoxia, all of which produce brain edema.

Edema is accompanied by an increase in intracranial pressure leading to gradual decrease in cerebral circulation to the level of almost cessation, causing aseptic necrosis of the brain. Within 3–5 days, there occurs widespread brain destruction or *pannecrosis* throughout the cerebrum and the brainstem, the brain becomes a liquefied mass, a condition known as '*respirator brain*'. Increase in the intracranial pressure compresses the entire brain including the brainstem resulting in whole brain infarction.

Diagnosing Brain Death (Box 8.1)

The two essential requirements for the diagnosis of brain death are:
1. *Establishment of cessation of all brain functions*, i.e., cerebral and mainly brainstem functions using primarily the clinical criteria and partly by confirmatory paraclinical/laboratory tests which include electro-encephalogram (flat isoelectric EEG) and somatosensory evoked potentials (SSEP) and tests to measure cerebral blood flow.
2. *Demonstration that cessation of these functions are irreversible and permanent*: Irreversibility is established by:
   - Determination of the cause of loss of brain function
   - Exclusion of reversible conditions
   - Demonstration that the cessation of brain functions persists for an appropriate period of observation.

Exclusion of Reversible Conditions

The most important reversible conditions/confounding factors that must be excluded are:
i. Hypothermia.
ii. Severe electrolyte, acid-base or endocrine abnormalities.
iii. *Drug intoxication*: Presence of sedation, neuromuscular blockade, or drugs causing CNS depression.
iv. Hypoxia, hypotension or shock.
v. *Other conditions*: Brainstem encephalitis, severe hypophosphatemia, encephalopathies associated with hepatic failure, uremia, or hyperosmolar coma of diabetes mellitus.

Brain Death Certification

- Two medical practitioners must perform the brainstem death tests.
- Patient's attending physician should participate in determination of death.
- Doctors involved should be experts in the technique of brain death assessment.
- Such tests *should not be performed* by transplant surgeons or any doctor in the transplant team.
- Each doctor should perform the tests twice.

Observation Period

- Neurological examination to determine brain death must not be done within 24 h after brain injury.
- All the tests are repeated after minimum interval of 6 h to ensure absence of 'observer/diagnostic error' and persistence of clinical state (not inconsistent with diagnosis of brain death).
- Second test essentially confirms brainstem death and the patient is declared brain dead.

Box 8.1 Diagnostic clinical brain death criteria (death by neurologic criteria)

A. **Prerequisites.** Brain death is the absence of clinical brain function when the proximate cause is known and demonstrably irreversible
   i. Clinical or neuroimaging evidence of an acute CNS catastrophe that is compatible with the clinical diagnosis of brain death
   ii. Exclusion of complicating medical conditions that may confound clinical assessment
   iii. No drug intoxication or poisoning
   iv. Core temperature >32.2°C (AAN guidelines require >36°C)
B. **The three cardinal findings in brain death** are coma, absence of brainstem reflexes and apnea
   1. **Coma** or unresponsiveness: No cerebral motor response to pain in all extremities. No grimacing to deep pressure on nail bed, supraorbital ridge, or temporomandibular joint (CN afferent V and efferent VII)
   2. **Absence of brainstem reflexes***
      a. *Pupils*
         i. Absent pupillary response to bright light (absent light reflex—CN II and III)
         ii. Size: Mid position (4 mm) to dilated (9 mm)
      b. *Ocular movement* (CN III, VI and VII))
         i. No oculocephalic reflex (Doll's eye phenomenon). No eye movements observed on brisk turning of head on either side
         ii. Absent oculovestibular reflex (Caloric test): No deviation of eyes to irrigation in each ear with 50 mL of cold water
      c. *Facial sensation and facial motor response*
         i. No corneal reflex to touch with a cotton swab (CN V and VII)
         ii. No jaw reflex (CN IX)
      d. *Pharyngeal and tracheal reflexes* (CN IX and X)
         i. No gag reflex: No response after stimulation of the posterior pharynx with tongue blade
         ii. No cough response to tracheobronchial suctioning
   3. **Apnea test:** It is based on the fact that loss of brainstem function definitively results in loss of centrally controlled breathing, with resultant apnea. The test requires removal of ventilatory support and monitoring of $PaCO_2$ levels. A positive test is total absence of respiratory movements and arterial $PaCO_2$ is ≥ 60 mmHg (when intense physiologic stimulation to breathe is present)

---

* Spinal reflexes including deep tendon, plantar flexion, abdominal reflexes, toe/finger flexion and withdrawal reflexes may remain during the first 24 h after brain death.

Beating-heart donor or living cadavers: After brainstem death has been established, the retention of the patient on the ventilator facilitates a fully oxygenated cadaver transplant, the so-called *beating-heart donor or living cadavers*.
- The success of a homograft depends mainly upon the type of tissue involved and the rapidity of its removal after circulation has stopped in the donor.
- The best results are obtained if the organs are salvaged while circulation is present or immediately after cessation of the circulation.
- Cornea can be removed from the dead body within 6 h (opacity occurs within 2 h of death, but the changes are reversible), skin in 24 h, bone in 48 h and blood vessels within 72 h for transplantation. Kidneys within 45 min, heart within 1 h, lungs and liver within 15 min.

> **NOTA BENE**
>
> **Types of transplants**
> - **Autograft:** Tissue transplanted from one part of the body to another in the same individual. It is also called *autotransplant* or *homologous transplantation*.
> - **Allograft:** Organ or tissue transplanted from one individual to another of the same species with a different genotype. It is also called *allogeneic graft* or *homograft*.
> - **Isograft:** Organs or tissues are transplanted from a donor to a genetically identical recipient (such as an identical twin).
> - **Xenograft:** Organs or tissue transplanted from one species to another, e.g., grafting of animal tissue into humans.
> - **Split transplants:** Deceased-donor organ (specifically the liver) may be divided between two recipients, especially an adult and a child.

CAUSE, MECHANISM AND MANNER OF DEATH

Two of the most important functions of the forensic doctor are the determination of the cause and manner of death.
- **Cause of death** is any injury or disease producing physiological derangement, briefly or over a prolonged period, which results in the death of the individual, e.g., a gunshot wound to the abdomen, a stab wound to the chest, adenocarcinoma of the lung or coronary atherosclerosis.
- **Mechanism of death** is the physiological derangement produced by the cause of death that results in death, e.g., hemorrhage, septicemia, metabolic acidosis or alkalosis, ventricular fibrillation or respiratory paralysis. A particular mechanism of death can be produced by multiple causes of death and vice versa. Thus, if an individual dies of hemorrhage, it can be produced by a gunshot wound or a stab wound or a malignant tumor of the lung eroding into a blood vessel. A cause of death, e.g., a gunshot wound of the abdomen can result in many possible mechanisms of death, like hemorrhage or peritonitis.
- **Manner of death** explains how the cause of death came about. Manner of death can generally be categorized as natural (death due to disease), homicide, suicide, accident or undetermined **(Flowchart 8.1 and Table 8.1)**.
  - A cause of death may have multiple manners of death. An individual can die of massive hemorrhage (mechanism of death) due to stab wound of heart (cause of death), with the manner being homicide (someone stabbed him), suicide (stabbed himself), accident (fell over the weapon) or undetermined (not sure what happened).
  - For some deaths, the manner may be undetermined because the circumstances are unclear, e.g., whether drowning was accidental or suicidal.
  - Deaths from alcohol and drug abuse are difficult to classify and are sometimes described as 'unclassified'.
  - Postoperative death may fall into the category of 'obscure death' and one of the common diagnosis is cardiac arrest.
- **Agonal period** is the time between a lethal occurrence and death.

> **NOTA BENE**
>
> - **Dyadic death** (*murder-suicide, homicide-suicide*) refers to an incident where a homicide is committed followed by the perpetrator's suicide almost immediately or soon after the homicide. Homicide-suicides are relatively uncommon and vary from region to region.
> - **Complex suicide:** Use of more than one method together and sequentially to complete suicide. For e.g. ingestion of hypnotics followed by hanging, drowning or use of firearms.

FM 2.2, 3.7
- Describe and discuss natural and unnatural deaths.
- Describe wound as a cause of death: Primary and secondary.

Natural deaths: Death is due to aging process, disease or illness, and not directly influenced by external forces.
- If the doctor is unsure of cause and manner of death, he will not certify the death and will inform the police.

Flowchart 8.1: Manner of death

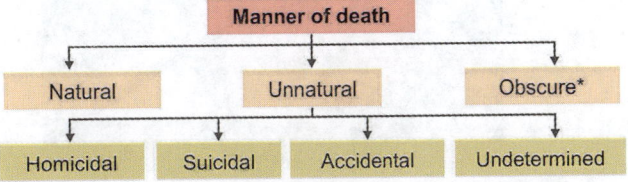

TABLE 8.1: Description of manners of death

Manner	Definition
Natural	Death resulting from disease
Homicide	Death resulting from the deliberate action of another
Suicide	Death intentionally self-inflicted
Accident	Death as a result of an environmental influence

---
*Not discovered or known about; uncertain.

- The police can then ask for postmortem which can help in determining the cause of death.
- If it reveals that the death is from natural causes, then no further inquiry is needed.

Unnatural deaths: All deaths that cannot be described as death by natural causes are categorized as unnatural deaths.
- This includes road traffic accidents, falls, drowning, poisoning, hanging, gunshot injuries, stabbing, etc.
- The police will ask for a postmortem and depending on the circumstances of the death, further investigation will take place.

Primary cause of death: The disease or event that started the chain of events that led to death.

Secondary cause of death is either a consequence or complication of the *primary cause*, or another disease which might have contributed to the death of the person.

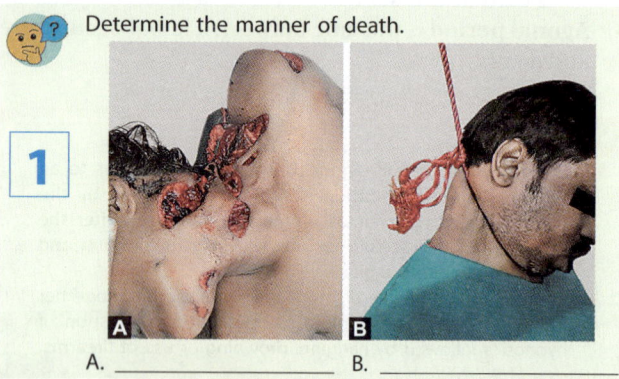

Determine the manner of death.

A. _____ B. _____

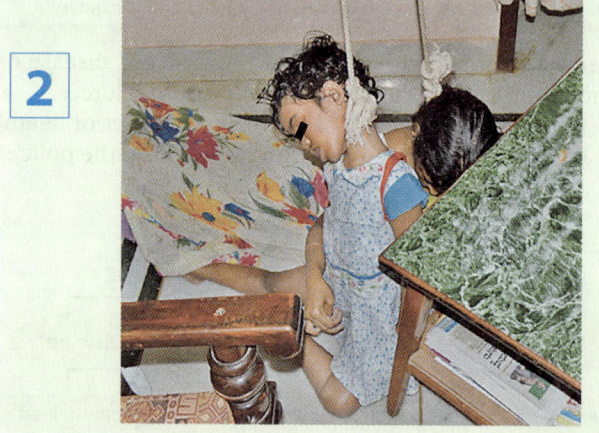

Mother and daughter were found hanging together from the same point. Such deaths are called:

CAUSE OF DEATH

The International format of certifying the cause of death is defined by the World Health Organization (WHO). The system divides the cause of death into two parts:
i. **Part I** describes the condition(s) that led directly to death (immediate cause). It is divided further into subsections, and generally four—(a), (b), (c) and (d). These are for disease processes that have led directly to death and that are causally related to one another, (a) being due to or consequent of (b) *(immediate cause)*, which in turn is due to or consequent of (c), and (c) due to or consequent of (d) *(antecedent causes)*.
ii. **Part II** is for other conditions, not related to those listed in Part I, that have also contributed to death (contributory cause), but should not be used as a basket for all the minor pathologies found at autopsy.

- It is important to realize that it is the disease lowest in the Part I list that is the most important, as it is the primary condition, the start of the events leading to death **(Table 8.2)**.
- It is not necessary to complete parts Ib, Ic or II, if there are no predisposing conditions.
- If a patient died suddenly due to intracerebral hemorrhage due to hypertension, the cause of death will be:

  Ia: Intracerebral hemorrhage.
  II: Hypertension.

- And, if the same patient survived for few days or weeks and developed pneumonia, the death certificate should record both processes:

  Ia: Bronchopneumonia.
  Ib: Intracerebral hemorrhage.
  II: Hypertension.

- Statistically, both certificates would record the primary cause as intracerebral hemorrhage.

FM 1.10, 1.11
- Select appropriate cause of death in a particular scenario by referring ICD-11 code.
- Write a correct cause of death certificate as per ICD-11 document.

International Classification of Diseases (ICD)

- The International Classification of Diseases (ICD) provides a common language that allows health professionals to share standardized information across the world.

TABLE 8.2: Cause, mechanism and manner of death

Cause of death	Mechanism of death	Manner of death
♦ Hemoperitoneum, as a consequence of – Laceration of the aorta, as a consequence of – Blunt thoracic trauma	Hemorrhagic shock	Accident
♦ Bronchopneumonia, as a consequence of – Stab wound of thorax	Septicemia	Homicide
♦ Cardiac tamponade, as a consequence of – Gunshot of thorax	Cardiac dysrhythmia	Homicide
♦ Pulmonary hemorrhage, as a consequence of – Advanced pulmonary tuberculosis	Hemorrhagic shock	Natural

- The ICD-11 is the 11th edition of a global categorization system for physical and mental illnesses published by the WHO. It replaces the ICD-10 for recording health information and causes of death. The ICD-11 officially came into effect on 1st January 2022.
- The ICD-11 catalogues known human diseases, medical conditions, and mental health disorders and is used for insurance coding purposes, for statistical tracking of illnesses, and as a global health categorization tool that can be used across countries and in different languages.
- The reported conditions are then translated into medical codes through use of the classification structure and the selection and modification rules contained in the applicable revision of the ICD.
- These coding rules improve the usefulness of mortality statistics by giving preference to certain categories, by consolidating conditions, and by systematically selecting a single cause of death from a reported sequence of conditions.
- A key feature of the revised system is that it provides a simple coding structure that makes it easier to record various conditions with specificity. The new ICD-11 was designed to be electronic and user-friendly for use by a global audience. It runs on a central platform and can connect to any software. In addition, it can be a machine-readable format, expanding its potential uses in the digital age.
- The ICD and the Diagnostic and Statistical Manual of Mental Disorders (DSM) share many similarities. Both are authoritative guidebooks for medical professionals to use for the diagnosis and treatment of diseases and disorders. They share a great overlap of material on mental disorders, with the DSM solely focused on mental health concerns, while the ICD covers all parts of the body and mind.
- The primary derivative is called the ICD-11 MMS, and is commonly referred to as simply 'the ICD-11' **(Table 8.3)**. MMS stands for Mortality and Morbidity Statistics.

TABLE 8.3: Chapters in ICD-11 for Mortality and Morbidity Statistics

#	Code	Description
1.	1A00–1H0Z	Certain infectious or parasitic diseases
2.	2A00–2F9Z	Neoplasms
3.	3A00–3C0Z	Diseases of the blood or blood-forming organs
4.	4A00–4B4Z	Diseases of the immune system
5.	5A00–5D46	Endocrine, nutritional or metabolic diseases
6.	6A00–6E8Z	Mental, behavioral or neurodevelopmental disorders
7.	7A00–7B2Z	Sleep-wake disorders
8.	8A00–8E7Z	Diseases of the nervous system
9.	9A00–9E1Z	Diseases of the visual system
10.	AA00–AC0Z	Diseases of the ear or mastoid process
11.	BA00–BE2Z	Diseases of the circulatory system
12.	CA00–CB7Z	Diseases of the respiratory system
13.	DA00–DE2Z	Diseases of the digestive system
14.	EA00–EM0Z	Diseases of the skin
15.	FA00–FC0Z	Diseases of the musculoskeletal system or connective tissue
16.	GA00–GC8Z	Diseases of the genitourinary system
17.	HA00–HA8Z	Conditions related to sexual health
18.	JA00–JB6Z	Pregnancy, childbirth or the puerperium
19.	KA00–KD5Z	Certain conditions originating in the perinatal period
20.	LA00–LD9Z	Developmental anomalies
21.	MA00–MH2Y	Symptoms, signs or clinical findings, not elsewhere classified
22.	NA00–NF2Z	Injury, poisoning or certain other consequences of external causes
23.	PA00–PL2Z	External causes of morbidity or mortality
24.	QA00–QF4Z	Factors influencing health status or contact with health services
25.	RA00–RA26	Codes for special purposes
26.	SA00–SJ3Z	Supplementary Chapter Traditional Medicine Conditions - Module I
27.	VA00–VC50	Supplementary section for functioning assessment
28.	XA0060–XY9U	Extension Codes

For e.g. if you click on 22, it will show the following

Chapter 22: Injury, poisoning or certain other consequences of external causes
- Injuries to the head
- Injuries to the neck
- Injuries to the thorax
- Injuries to the abdomen, lower back, lumbar spine or pelvis
- Injuries to the shoulder or upper arm
- Injuries to the elbow or forearm
- Injuries to the wrist or hand
- Injuries to the hip or thigh
- Injuries to the knee or lower leg
- Injuries to the ankle or foot
- Injuries involving multiple body regions
- Injuries to unspecified part of trunk, limb or body region
- Effects of foreign body entering through natural orifice
- Burns
- Frostbite
- Harmful effects of substances
- Injury or harm arising from surgical or medical care, not elsewhere classified
- Other or unspecified effects of external causes

This Block includes the following:
- Injuries of face [any part]
- Injuries of gum
- Injuries of jaw
- Injuries of oral cavity
- Injuries of palate
- Injuries of periocular area
- Injuries of scalp
- Injuries of temporomandibular joint area
- Injuries of tongue
- Injuries of tooth

- Internal chemical burn or corrosion
- External chemical burn or corrosion
- Burns from hot objects
- Burns from friction
- Burns from hot air and hot gases
- Burns from lightning

SECTION 1: Jurisprudence and Forensic Medicine

FM 2.5

Discuss modes of death—coma, asphyxia and syncope.

MODES OF DEATH (PROXIMATE CAUSES OF DEATH)

Definition: Mode of death refers to an abnormal physiological state that pertained at the time of death, e.g., coma, congestive cardiac failure, cardiorespiratory failure, cardiac arrest or pulmonary edema.

According to *Xavier Bichat*, a French physician, there are three modes of death depending upon the system most obviously affected, irrespective of what the remote cause of death may be **(Table 8.4)**:

1. **Coma:** It is a state of profound unconsciousness from which a person cannot be roused, with minimal or no detectable responsiveness to stimuli. This is death from failure of the function of the brain.
2. **Syncope:** This is death from failure of the function of the heart resulting in hypoxia and hypoperfusion of the brain.
3. **Asphyxia:** This is death from failure of the function of the lungs.
   Other features of asphyxia: Pronounced lividity, cardiac dilatation, or pathological changes which are dependent upon the type of death, like local injuries to the neck in hanging, strangulation and throttling, and color of blood in carbon monoxide poisoning.*

> **NOTA BENE**
>
> **Quintet of asphyxia** (*mnemonic FRCPC*): Fluid blood, Right heart engorgement, Cyanosis, Petechiae, Congestion

Doctors should not write the mode of death on the death certificate as these terms are cumbersome, immaterial, not useful and offer no information as to the underlying pathological condition. If used, it should be further qualified by the more fundamental etiological process, e.g., it is not possible to certify that a person died of coma, syncope or asphyxia without mentioning the cause which has produced them, e.g., coma due to head injury, syncope due to tobacco poisoning, or asphyxia due to hanging.

> **NOTA BENE**
>
> **Persistent vegetative state (PVS):** The individual has lost cognitive neurological function and awareness of the environment, but does have noncognitive function and a preserved sleep-wake cycle.
> - Spontaneous movements may occur and the eyes may open in response to external stimuli, but the patient does not speak or obey commands.
> - Patients in a vegetative state may appear somewhat normal.
> - It is usually seen in patients with diffuse, bilateral cerebral hemisphere disturbance with an intact brainstem, though it can occur with damage to the most rostral part of the brainstem.

TABLE 8.4: Modes of death

Mode	System	Causes	PM findings
Coma	Brain	Injury/disease of the brain; systemic disorders (diabetic ketoacidosis, heat stroke, eclampsia); alcohol, opium, cyanide or phenol poisoning	Inflammation of the meninges, compression from hemorrhage, tumor or vascular lesion
Syncope	Heart	Heart disease, hemorrhage, vagal inhibition, poisoning (digitalis, tobacco, aconite and oleander)	Non-specific findings; organs are pale and capillaries are congested
Asphyxia	Lungs	Pneumonia, paralysis of the respiratory center (opium), occlusion of air passages, traumatic asphyxia, etc.	**Triad of asphyxia:** Cyanosis; petechial hemorrhages (Tardieu spots) and visceral congestion

Identify the triad of asphyxia.

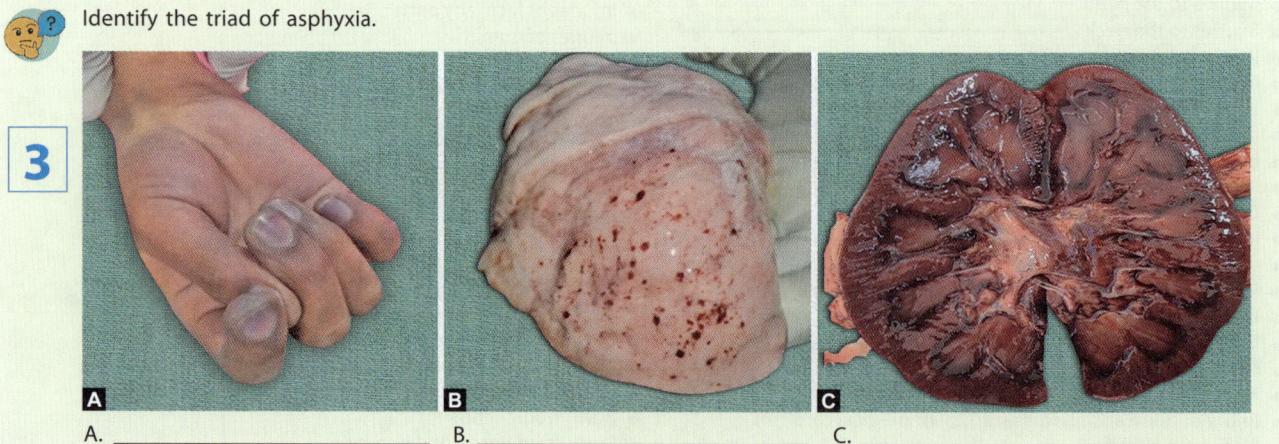

A. _____ B. _____ C. _____

---

* Fluidity of blood and dilation of right ventricle are not considered as pathognomonic of asphyxia.

ANOXIA

According to *Gordon*, cessation of vital functions is brought about by tissue anoxia.

- Anoxia means complete lack of oxygen, which ultimately leads to cardiac failure and death.
- The term 'hypoxia' is used commonly, which is shortage of oxygen in blood.

Anoxia is classified into four types (Flowchart 8.2):
  i. Anoxic anoxia
  ii. Anemic anoxia
  iii. Histotoxic anoxia
  iv. Stagnant/ischemic anoxia

Describe and discuss issues related to sudden natural deaths.

SUDDEN DEATH

Definition: Death occurring instantaneously or within 1 h of the onset of morbid symptoms (as per WHO, 24 h is the limitation period).

- It is the sudden and unexpected death of a person, who prior to death was not suffering from any dangerous disease, poisoning or injury.
- In such cases, it is usually not possible to ascertain the cause of death from an external examination of the body. Therefore, an autopsy is necessary to obviate the possibility of death due to foul play.
- A doctor who issues a death certificate in such a case runs the risk of being accused as an accessory to the crime, should the death be found to be due to foul play eventually.

Causes

1. **Cardiovascular** (44–50% of cases): Cardiovascular disease, particularly coronary artery atherosclerosis is the most common cause of sudden death.
   - Coronary artery disease
   - Valvular heart disease
   - Congenital heart disease
   - Hypertensive heart disease
   - Infection, e.g., myocarditis, pericarditis
   - Cardiac tamponade
   - Cardiomyopathies
   - Aortic aneurysm.
2. **Respiratory system** (15–23% of cases)
   - Pulmonary embolism
   - Lobar/bronchopneumonia
   - Massive hemoptysis
   - Obstruction by foreign body
   - Air embolism
   - Edema of glottis/lungs
   - Pneumothorax
   - Neoplasm.
3. **Central nervous system** (10–18% of cases)
   - Intracerebral hemorrhage
   - Cerebral thrombosis
   - Subarachnoid hemorrhage
   - Embolism
   - Meningitis
   - Tumor
   - Idiopathic epilepsy
   - Abscess.
4. **Gastrointestinal system** (6–8% of cases)
   - Hemorrhage from peptic ulcer, esophageal varices or malignancy
   - Strangulated hernia
   - Rupture of abdominal aneurysm
   - Ruptured diseased viscus
   - Acute hemorrhagic pancreatitis
   - Appendicitis
   - Fulminant hepatic failure
   - Ruptured liver abscess.
5. **Genitourinary system** (3–5%)
   - Chronic nephritis
   - Tuberculosis of kidney
   - Nephrolithiasis
   - Tumors of kidney/bladder.
6. **Reproductive system**
   - Toxemia of pregnancy
   - Rupture of ectopic pregnancy
   - Uterine hemorrhage due to fibroids
   - Carcinoma of vulva.

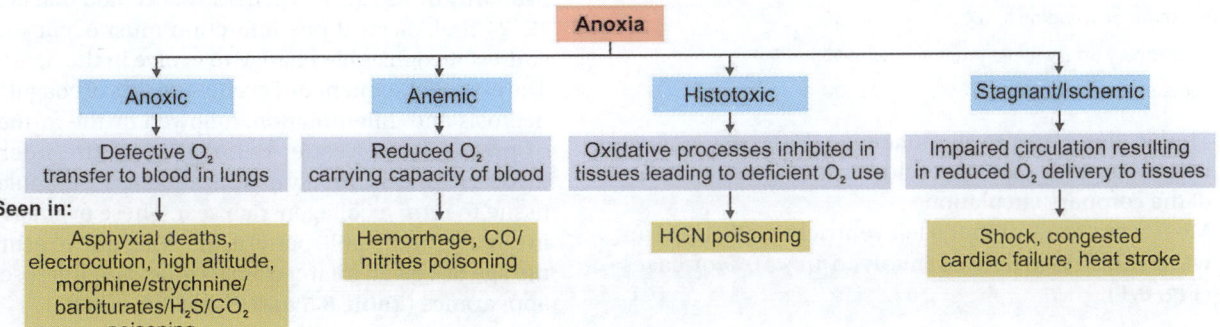

Flowchart 8.2: Classification of anoxia

7. **Endocrine**
    - Adrenal insufficiency or hemorrhage
    - Myxedemic coma or crisis
    - Diabetic coma
    - Parathyroid crisis.
8. **Iatrogenic**
    - Abuse of drugs
    - Mismatched blood transfusion
    - Sudden withdrawal of steroids
    - Anesthesia.
9. **Miscellaneous**
    - Anaphylaxis
    - Cerebral malaria
    - Alcoholism
    - Shock from dread, fright or emotion
    - Sickle cell crisis
    - Bacteremic shock.

Special Causes in Children

- Cot deaths or SIDS
- Mongols and others with congenital or mental abnormalities
- Concealed puncture wounds.

Indeterminate: Very rarely, the cause cannot be determined.

CORONARY ATHEROSCLEROSIS

The most common cause of death from cardiovascular disease is coronary atherosclerosis.

Almost all adults show atherosclerotic plaques scattered throughout the coronary arterial system. However, significant stenotic lesions that may produce chronic myocardial ischemia show more than 75% (three-fourth) reduction in the cross-sectional area of a coronary artery or its branch. Zones of occlusion are usually less than 5 mm in length, and the area of the severest involvement is about 3–4 cm from the coronary ostia, more often at or near the bifurcation of the arteries, suggesting the role of hemodynamic forces in atherogenesis.

Acute occlusion of coronary artery may result from thrombosis or hemorrhage within the wall of the artery. The frequency of occlusion of the coronary arteries is:

Coronary artery	Percentage (%)
Left anterior descending (LAD)	40–50
Right coronary artery (RCA)	30–40
Left circumflex artery (LCx)	15–20

- The location of myocardial infarction (MI) is determined by the site of the vascular occlusion and by the anatomy of the coronary circulation.
- Most infarcts occur in the left ventricle in the anterior wall. Right ventricle is involved in <10% of cases **(Fig. 8.1)**.

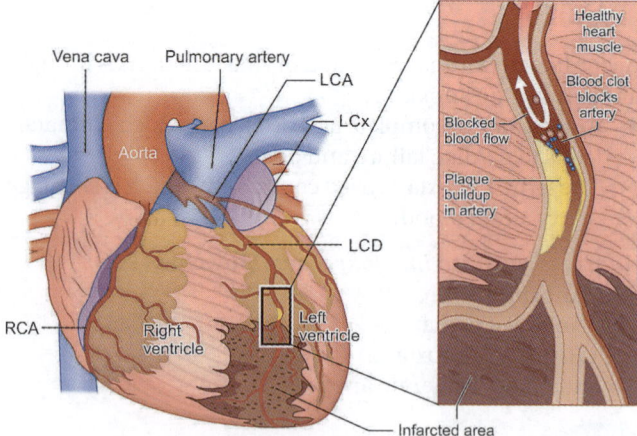

Fig. 8.1: Myocardial infarction

- Occlusion of the left anterior descending coronary artery causes an infarct in the anterior and apical areas of the left ventricle and the adjacent interventricular septum (anteroapical MI) **(Fig. 8.1)**.
- Occlusion of the right coronary artery is responsible for most infarcts involving the posterior and basal portions of the left ventricle.
- Posterior infarcts may be due to blockage of either the right vessel or the circumflex branch of the left artery.
- Myocardial infarcts which involve the entire thickness of the ventricular wall are referred to as *transmural infarcts*, while those restricted to the inner one-third of the myocardium are called *subendocardial infarcts*.
- Fresh thrombi are dark-brown and are attached to the vessel walls. Old thrombi appear as homogeneous yellowish or gray, firm plugs blocking the vessels.
- Significant obstruction of the coronary artery lumen (with 75% narrowing of the lumen) without MI or thrombosis may lead to sudden death.
- Hypoxic myocardium is electrically unstable, and liable to arrhythmia and ventricular fibrillation, especially at moments of sudden stress, such as exercise or during an adrenaline response, such as anger or emotion.

Postmortem Examination

- No naked eye change is seen for the first 12–18 h. The appearance of a myocardial infarct is determined primarily by its age. It is generally accepted that at least 12–24 h of survival postinfarction must occur for the earliest recognizable change to evolve in the heart.
- The essential sequence of events consists of coagulation necrosis and inflammation, followed by the formation of granulation tissue, resorption of the necrotic myocardium, and finally organization of the granulation tissue to form a collagen-rich scar. These events occur in a fairly predictable pattern, allowing one to estimate the age of a given infarct from its gross and microscopic appearance **(Table 8.5 and Figs. 8.2A and B)**.

TABLE 8.5: Sequential pathologic changes in myocardial infarction (MI)

S.No.	Duration	Gross changes	Microscopic changes
1.	0–6 h	No change; triphenyl tetrazolium chloride (TTC) test negative	No change; stretching and waviness of fibers
2.	6–12 h	No change or slight pallor	Coagulative necrosis and neutrophilic infiltration begins, minimal hemorrhage
3.	12–24 h	Slight pallor or mottling	Continuing coagulation necrosis, 'contraction band' necrosis at the periphery of the infarct,¥ neutrophilic infiltrate
4.	24–72 h	Pallor, hyperemic or alternate bands of red and pale areas—'tigroid appearance'	Complete coagulation necrosis of myofibers; neutrophilic infiltrate well developed with early fragmentation of neutrophil nuclei
5.	4–7 days	Central pallor with hyperemic border, soft	Macrophages appear, disintegration and phagocytosis of necrotic fibers, granulation tissue visible at edge of infarct
6.	10 days	Maximally yellow, soft, shrunken, purple periphery	Well-developed phagocytosis, prominent granulation tissue in peripheral areas of infarct, pigmented macrophages, eosinophils, lymphocytes and plasma cells present
7.	4–6 weeks	Thin, gray-white, hard, shrunken fibrous scar	Increased fibrocollagenic tissue, decreased vascularity, fewer pigmented macrophages, lymphocytes and plasma cells

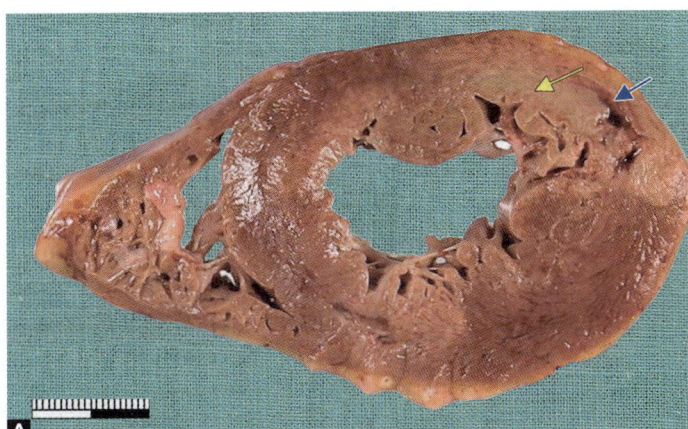 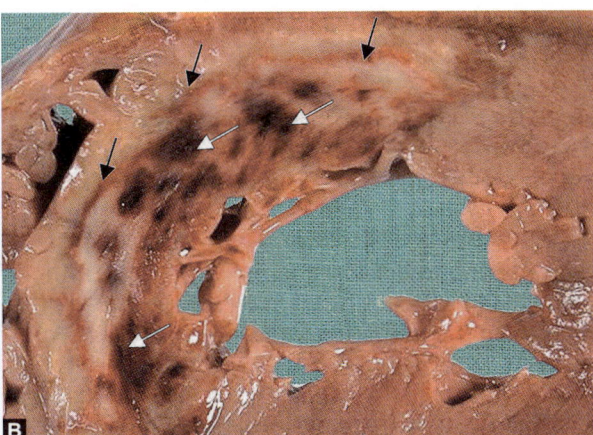

Figs. 8.2A and B: Myocardial infarction: (A) Pale infarcted area (yellow arrow) with hyperemic border (blue arrow); (B) Tigroid appearance between yellow infarcted areas (black arrows) with 'leopard rosettes' (white arrows)

- Immersion of tissue slices in a solution of triphenyl tetrazolium chloride (TTC) gives red color to the healthy area (where lactate dehydrogenase is preserved), but infarcted area appears pale,* and occur within 6–12 h after the onset of severe ischemia. This technique of demonstration of enzyme inactivity is useful up to 36 h of postmortem interval.
- Fresh thrombotic lesion is seen in less than 25% of the cases. Coronary artery spasm can cause death in patients suffering from angina without narrowing of the coronary arteries and without significant atherosclerosis or congenital anomalies.
- The lesions of the conducting system of the heart may sometimes cause arrhythmias and death.
- Any person with a heart in excess of 420 g is at risk of sudden death, even though the coronary arteries are normal.

> **NOTA BENE**
>
> - **Enzyme histochemistry** is the most reliable method of detecting early MI. Dehydrogenases—succinic, lactic, malic, hydroxybutyric and cytochrome oxidase are among those used. With *malate dehydrogenase*, normal myocardium stains dark blue-black and infarcted area is devoid of color.
> - **Periodic Acid-Schiff (PAS) stain:** In early infarcts (at least 28 h), damaged myofibers stain a pale purple-blue with PAS, compared with the pink color of healthy fibers.
> - **Hematoxylin-eosin (H&E) autofluorescence:** Routine formalin-fixed H&E sections are examined under UV light. Early infarcted fibers show a shift of their secondary emission towards yellow, away from the usual olive-green of healthy fibers.
> - **Acridine-orange fluorescent stain:** Slides are examined under UV light; normal myocardium is golden-brown/yellowish-brown with damaged fibers showing a shift to green.

---

* Because dehydrogenases leak out through the damaged membranes of the dead cells; an infarct appears as an unstained pale zone.
¥ Contraction bands (*myofibrillar degeneration, coagulative myocytolysis or Zenker necrosis*) are characteristic necrosis pattern representing hypercontraction and lysis of small groups of myocardial cells. They are also found in coronary occlusion, resuscitation attempts, drowning, burning and hypothermia.

Which of the statements is true?

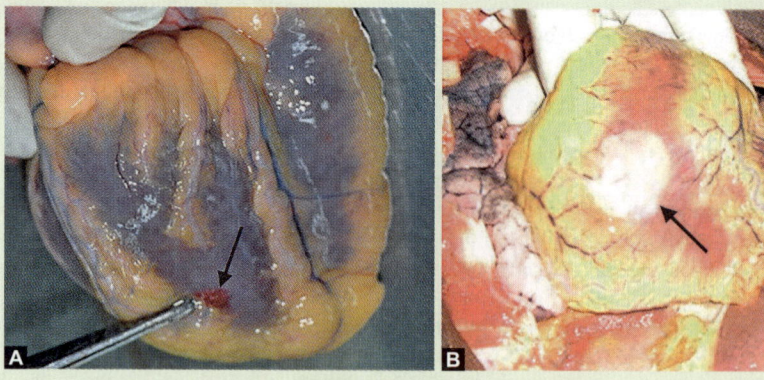

1. (A) is fibrosis of old myocardial infarction and (B) is contusion of heart
2. (A) is contusion of heart and (B) is fibrosis of old myocardial infarction
3. (A) is artefact and (B) is fibrosis of old myocardial infarction

Anaphylactic Deaths

Most anaphylactic deaths seen by forensic pathologist are caused by insect bites, drugs or foods.

Signs and Symptoms

- A typical anaphylactic reaction results in acute respiratory distress or circulatory collapse.
- Faintness, itching of the skin, urticaria, tightness in the chest, wheezing, respiratory difficulty and collapse.
- In anaphylactic deaths, the onset of symptoms is usually immediate or within the first 15–20 min. Beyond that time, one would need a well-documented medical history of gradually developing symptoms to implicate an anaphylactic reaction, e.g., the development of itching or wheals and flares. Death usually occurs within 1–2 h.
- Obstruction of the upper airway can be caused by pharyngeal or laryngeal edema; of the lower airway by bronchospasm with contraction of the smooth muscle of the lungs, vasodilatation and increased capillary permeability.
- Cardiac arrest may be caused by respiratory failure.

Vagal Inhibition (Vasovagal Shock/Reflex Cardiac Arrest/Nervous Apoplexy)

- Sudden death occurring within seconds or minutes as a result of minor trauma or harmless peripheral stimulation may be caused by vagal inhibition.
- Pressure on the baroreceptors situated in the carotid sinuses, carotid sheaths and the carotid body (located in the internal carotid artery and situated near the angle of mandible) causes an increase in blood pressure in these sinuses with resultant slowing of the heart rate, dilatation of blood vessels and fall in blood pressure.
- Some individuals show marked hypersensitivity to stimulation of the carotid sinuses, characterized by bradycardia and cardiac arrhythmias ranging from ventricular arrhythmias to cardiac arrest.

Mechanism

- It acts through a reflex arc in which the afferent (sensory) nerve impulses arise in the carotid complex of nerve endings, but not in the vagal nerve trunk itself. These impulses pass through glossopharyngeal nerves to the tenth nucleus in the brainstem, then return through the vagus (efferent) supply to the heart and other organs.
- This reflex arc acts through the parasympathetic autonomic nervous system, and is independent of the main motor and sensory nerve pathways.
- Afferent fibers are present over the skin, pharynx, glottis, pleura, peritoneum and cervix, which pass into the lateral tracts of spinal cord and finally to the brain.

Causes

- Pressure on the carotid sinuses, as in hanging or strangulation.
- Unexpected blow to the larynx, chest, abdomen or genital organs.
- Impaction of food in the larynx or sudden inhalation of fluid into the upper respiratory tract.
- Sudden immersion of body in cold water.
- The insertion of an instrument into the bronchus, uterus, bladder or rectum.
- Puncture of a pleural cavity producing a pneumothorax.
- Sudden evacuation of pathological fluids, e.g., ascitic tap.

Postmortem examination: There are no characteristic postmortem findings. The cause of death can be inferred only by exclusion of other pathological conditions and from the observation of reliable witnesses, history and clinical findings concerning the circumstances of death.

CHAPTER 8 : Thanatology

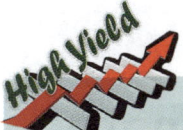

- **Thanatology:** Scientific study of death in all its aspects.
- **Sec. 46 IPC** defines death of a human being.
- **Tripod of life**—nervous, circulatory and respiratory system (as per *Bichat*).
- **Somatic death:** Complete and irreversible cessation of function of brainstem.
- **Molecular death:** Death of individual tissues and cells after somatic death.
- In somatic deaths, the muscle responds to thermal, electrical or chemical stimulus.
- **Brainstem death:** Complete and irreversible loss of *brainstem function*.
- In India, legally 'death' is considered *brainstem death*.
- **Cardinal findings in brain death:** Coma, absence of brainstem reflexes and apnea.
- Atria mortis is not a postmortem change.
- Xenograft is transplantation of tissue from a different species.
- **Moment of death:** Exact time when the individual dies.
- **Modes of death**: Coma, syncope and asphyxia.
- Gordon's clarification of death signifies modes of death.
- **Cyanide poisoning cause:** Histotoxic anoxia.
- **Carbon monoxide poisoning cause:** Anemic anoxia.
- **Agonal period:** Time between a lethal occurrence and death.
- **Sudden death:** Instantaneous death or within 1 h of the onset of morbid symptoms (24 h as per WHO).
- **Most common cause of sudden death:** Cardiovascular disease, particularly coronary artery atherosclerosis.
- **Most common site of occlusion of coronary artery:** Left anterior descending artery.
- **Most common site for infarcts:** Left ventricle in anterior wall.
- **Dye used to detect infarcted area:** Triphenyl tetrazolium chloride (TTC).
- In deaths due to myocardial infarction, color of healthy part of heart stained with TTC is red (lactate dehydrogenase is preserved).
- **Most reliable method to detect early MI:** Enzyme histochemistry.
- Myocardium infarct is easily identifiable when it is of more than 12 h of age.

Interesting case

Clinical Death (Case of Amitabh Bachchan, 1982)

In July 1982, while filming Coolie*, superstar Amitabh Bachchan suffered a near-fatal intestinal injury during the filming of a fight scene. Mr Bachchan was rushed to the hospital and he had to undergo multiple surgeries including an emergency splenectomy and remained critically ill in hospital for many months, at times close to death. In fact, he was reportedly clinically dead for eleven minutes before he was put on ventilator and was unresponsive of all treatment for a week. In a last ditch attempt to revive him, the doctors plunged an adrenaline injection into his heart which did the trick and he started recovering after that.

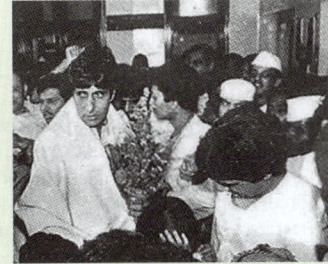

* The director altered the ending of Coolie after his accident. Mr Bachchan's character was originally intended to have been killed; but the character lived in the end. He said that 'It would have been inappropriate for the man who had just fended off death in real life to be killed on screen'.

CHAPTER 9

Signs of Death

LEARNING OBJECTIVES

Must know
1. Signs of death: Immediate, early and late changes
2. Suspended animation
3. Changes in eye after death
4. Postmortem staining, color of postmortem staining in different conditions
5. Algor mortis
6. Rigor mortis, factors affecting and conditions simulating rigor mortis, rule of 12
7. Cadaveric spasm
8. Cold and heat stiffening
9. Putrefaction, early and late putrefaction of organs
10. Time since death
11. PM staining and bruise (Diff.)
12. Rigor mortis and cadaveric spasm (Diff.)
13. Adipocere and mummification (Diff.)

Desirable to know
1. Congestion and postmortem staining (Diff.)
2. Nysten's law
3. Rigor mortis and heat stiffening (Diff.)
4. Rigor mortis and cold stiffening (Diff.)
5. Casper's dictum
6. Entomology
7. Adipocere and mummification, medico-legal importance
8. Embalming

The accurate determination of time of death is important due to its role in explaining possible criminal acts and determination of appropriate civil repercussions. The changes which occur after death that are helpful in estimation of the approximate time of death (and to differentiate death from suspended animation) can be classified into **(Table 9.1)**:
- Immediate changes
- Early changes
- Late changes.

TABLE 9.1: Changes after death

Immediate changes	Early changes	Late changes
Irreversible cessation of: ♦ Function of brain ♦ Circulation ♦ Respiration	♦ Loss of elasticity of the skin, and facial pallor ♦ Primary relaxation of the muscles ♦ Contact pallor and flattening ♦ Changes in the eye ♦ Livor mortis ♦ Algor mortis ♦ Rigor mortis	♦ Putrefaction ♦ Adipocere ♦ Mummification

FM 2.8
Describe and discuss postmortem changes including signs of death.

IMMEDIATE CHANGES (SOMATIC DEATH)

a. **Irreversible cessation of the function of brain including brainstem:** This is the earliest sign of death with stoppage of functions of the nervous system. There is insensibility, and loss of both sensory and motor functions. There is loss of reflexes, no response and no tonicity of the muscles. Pupils are widely dilated. This condition is sometimes seen in:
- Prolonged fainting attack
- Vagal inhibitory phenomenon
- Epilepsy, mesmeric trance, catalepsy, narcosis or electrocution.

b. **Irreversible cessation of respiration:** Complete stoppage of respiration for >4 minutes (min) usually causes death. The stoppage of respiration can be established by the following tests:
   i. *Inspection*: No visible respiratory movement.
   ii. *Palpation*: No respiratory movement can be felt.
   iii. *Auscultation*: Breath sounds cannot be heard from any part of the lungs.

iv. *Other tests:* Feather test, mirror test and Winslow's test are no longer utilized.

Respiration may stop briefly without death as in:
- Voluntary breath holding
- Drowning
- Cheyne-Stokes respiration
- Newborns.

c. **Irreversible cessation of circulation:** Stoppage of heart beat for >3–5 min is irrecoverable and results in death. The following tests may be performed to test circulation:
   i. Radial, brachial, femoral and carotid pulsations will be absent, if the circulation has stopped.
   ii. *Auscultation of heart:* Absence of the heart beat over the whole precordial area, and particularly, over the area of the apex.
   iii. *ECG:* In case of cessation of circulation, the ECG curve is absent and the tracing shows a flat line without any elevation or depression.
   iv. *Other tests:* Various tests, like diaphanous, magnus, Icard, pressure, cut and heat tests are now obsolete.

NOTA BENE

Tests to detect stoppage of respiration (obsolete)
- *Winslow's test:* No movement of reflection of light shone on mirror or surface of water in bowl kept on the chest.
- *Feather test:* No movement is seen, if a feather or fine cotton fibers are held before the nostrils.
- *Mirror test:* No haziness is seen on the reflecting surface of the mirror held in front of mouth and nostrils.

Tests to detect stoppage of circulation (obsolete)
- *Magnus test (ligature test):* Fingers fail to show bluish discoloration and edema to a ligature applied at their base.
- *Diaphanous test (transillumination test):* Failure to show redness in the web-space between the fingers on transillumination from behind.
- *Icard's test:* Fluorescein dye on being injected at a given site in a dead body fail to produce yellowish-green discoloration as seen in a living person.
- *Pressure test:* Fingernails appear pale and fail to show reddish color on removal of firm pressure over it.

Describe and discuss suspended animation.

SUSPENDED ANIMATION (APPARENT DEATH)

Definition: Suspended animation* is a condition in which vital signs of life (heart beat and respiration) are not detected by routine clinical methods, as the functions are interrupted for some time or are reduced to a minimum.

Mechanism: The metabolic rate is greatly reduced so that the requirement of the individual cell for oxygen is satisfied through the dissolved oxygen in body fluids.

Types

Two types:
   i. *Voluntary:* Seen in practitioners of yoga or in trance.
   ii. *Involuntary:* The causes and conditions leading to apparent death are summarized in **Box 9.1** and are called the '**AEIOU rule**'. Other conditions where apparent death may be seen are post-anesthesia, shock, insanity and newborns.

The patient can be resuscitated by cardiac massage or electric stimulator and artificial respiration. The death certificate should not be issued without an ECG or EEG record.

Medico-legal importance: It is necessary for doctors to diligently diagnose the systemic death as animated people has been wrongly declared dead on multiple occasions.

> **Recent Advances**
> Suspended animation can be lifesaving modality for the treatment of severe trauma victims. It has been observed that rapid induction of hypothermia (cryosleep) within 5 min of cardiac arrest is associated with better survival and improved neurological outcome. Recently, doctors have put humans into a state of suspended animation so as that surgeons can operate and treat traumatic injuries that would otherwise cause death. This **emergency preservation and resuscitation (EPR)** technique is being carried out on patients with an acute trauma (gunshot/stab wound) and have had a cardiac arrest.

EARLY CHANGES (MOLECULAR DEATH)

a. **Changes in the skin and facial pallor:** Skin becomes pale and ash-white due to stoppage of circulation and drainage of blood from the capillaries and the small vessels. The skin loses its elasticity, and the face looks younger due to loss of creases. The lips appear brownish, dry and hard due to drying.

b. **Primary relaxation or flaccidity of the muscles:** Muscles lose their tonicity and become flaccid, but the muscular tissues are still alive, their chemical reaction is alkaline and responds to electrical stimuli. The electric and mechanical stimulations of muscles are both useful to determine postmortem interval up to 13 hours (h).

c. **Contact flattening and pallor:** The areas which remain in contact with the ground become flat and the blood

> **Box 9.1** Causes and conditions of apparent death
> a. **A**lcohol, anemia, anoxemia
> b. **E**lectrocution, lightning strike
> c. **I**njury (head injury—cerebral concussion)
> d. **O**pium, barbiturates, anesthetics, neuropharmacology drugs
> e. **U**remia (and other metabolic coma), hypothermia, heat stroke, cholera

---

Cryptobiosis is the condition of inactive metabolic activity (reproduction, development and repair) during adverse environmental conditions. It is found in nature in some large mammals and amphibians like bears and frogs. In humans, this is known as suspended animation.

from vessels of these areas is pressed out, this continues even after the formation of postmortem staining over the surrounding areas.

d. **Changes in the eye**
- *Loss of corneal and pupillary reflexes:* It may be seen in all cases of deep insensibility and therefore is not a reliable sign of death. However, the pupils react for some time to miotic and mydriatic agents.
- *Pupils:* The pupils are dilated after death, because of the relaxation of muscles of the iris. Later, they are constricted with the onset of rigor mortis of the constrictor muscles and evaporation of fluid. As such, their state after death is not an indication of their antemortem appearance.
- *Opacity of the cornea*: There is opacity and haziness of the cornea due to drying and deposition of dust and debris over it. This may be delayed, if the lids are closed after death. If the lids are closed, the cornea remains clear for about 2 h. This haziness is transient and passes off, if a drop of water is poured on the cornea. But the cornea becomes permanently hazy after about 10–12 h of death due to decomposition.
- *Tache noire* (French, black line): If the eyelids remain open for 3–4 h after death, there is formation of two yellow triangles (base on the limbus, apex at the lateral or medial canthus and sides are formed by the margins of the upper and lower eyelids) on the sclera at each side of the iris, which become brown and then black.
  Cause: Drying/desiccation and deposition of cellular debris, mucus and dust on the exposed conjunctiva and the sclera underneath.
- *Loss of intraocular pressure (IOP):* IOP falls rapidly after death. It becomes zero in 4–8 h from 10 to 22 mmHg during life. The eyeballs look sunken in the orbit.
- *Changes in the retina:* The blood in retinal vessels appears fragmented or segmented (**cattle trucking or shunting**) within seconds to minutes after death, and persists for about an hour (**Kevorkian sign**) (**Fig. 9.1**). This occurs all over the body due to loss of blood pressure, but it can be seen only in retina by an *ophthalmoscope*.

  The retina is pale for the initial 2 h and the area around the optic disk look yellowish. At about 6 h, the disk outline is hazy, and becomes blurred in 7–10 h. By 12 h, the area for the disk can be known only by some convergent segmented vessels.
- ♦ *Vitreous potassium and hypoxanthine:* Steady rise in the values are seen after death. The rise is due to the autolysis of the vascular choroids and retinal cells of the eye.

Changes in the eye other than those in the *retina and vitreous humor* are less important for the purpose of estimation of time of death.

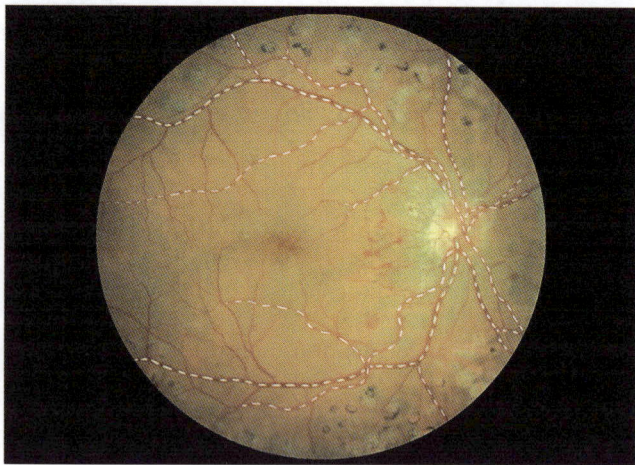

Fig. 9.1: Kevorkian sign

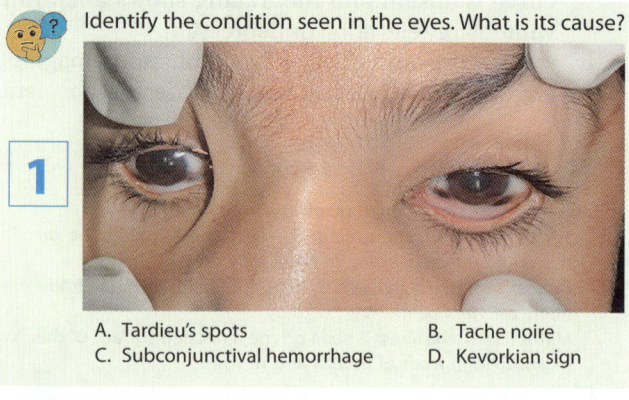

Identify the condition seen in the eyes. What is its cause?

1

A. Tardieu's spots B. Tache noire
C. Subconjunctival hemorrhage D. Kevorkian sign

FM 2.8

Describe and discuss postmortem changes—postmortem lividity.

POSTMORTEM STAINING (LIVOR MORTIS)

[*Synonyms:* Hypostasis, postmortem or cadaveric lividity, lucidity, cogitation, vibices, suggilation, darkening of death]

Definition: *Postmortem staining (PM staining) is bluish or purplish-red discoloration resulting from gravitational settling of blood in the toneless capillaries and venules of the dependant parts of the dead body.*

Site: It is present at the undersurface of skin in the superficial layers of the dermis.

Cause: After the stoppage of circulation, there is stagnation of blood in the vessels, and it tends to sink by force of gravity in the capillaries and venules of the dependent parts of the body.

- ♦ The upper portions of the body drained of blood are pale.
- ♦ The intensity of the color depends upon the amount of reduced hemoglobin in the blood.
- ♦ It is not possible to distinguish PM staining from cyanosis seen in the living. Therefore, one should not use cyanosis to describe postmortem appearances.

Development of PM Staining

In early stages (30 min to 1 h), it consists of discolored patches of 1-2 cm in diameter on the dependent parts of the body, having the same color as blood, which can be mistaken for bruises **(Fig. 9.2)**. Gradually, in 3-4 h, the small patches increase in size and coalesce with each other to form uniformly stained large areas. It is usually well-developed within 4 h, complete in 5-6 h.

- It begins immediately after death, but it may not be visible for about half to 1 h in normal individuals.
- When lividity is developing, applying '*thumb pressure*' against the skin for a few seconds will cause blanching. When the pressure is released, lividity will reappear.
- It is present in all bodies, but is more clearly seen in fair skinned people than in dark skinned ones. It may not be appreciated in infants and elderly.

Fixation of PM Staining

- After complete formation of the postmortem staining, if the body is undisturbed, the staining gets 'fixed' in 8-12 h and persists until putrefaction sets in **(Fig. 9.2)**. At this stage, lividity does not disappear, if finger is firmly pressed against the skin.
- If the position of the body is altered after fixation, the staining will not be changed and will remain as such, though the color may fade slightly in intensity.
- Fixation occurs earlier in summer, and is delayed in asphyxial deaths and in intracranial lesions.
- It is thought to be due to intravascular coagulation of the settled blood and blood leaking through the permeable vessels (as a result of decomposition). But practically, very little clotting of the blood is seen in the small veins and capillaries during postmortem examination.

Distribution of PM Staining

- It depends on the position of the body.
- In a body *lying supine*, it appears in the neck, and then spreads over the entire back with the exception of the areas directly pressed on the ground or the bed, i.e., occipital area, shoulder blades, buttocks, posterior aspects of thighs, calves and heels, which do not show any staining and appear rather pale. This phenomenon is known as *contact pallor/contact flattening/contact blanching* **(Fig. 9.3A)**. The vessels in these areas remain pressurized and the blood is compressed out. Similarly, any pressure that prevents the capillary filling, such as the collar band, waist bands, belts or wrinkles in the clothes remain free from color, and are seen as *stripes or bands*. Such pale areas may be mistaken for marks due to beating or strangulation, if they are seen on the neck.
- If the body is *lying prone*, as in drunken persons, intense lividity is seen in front and Tardieu's spots are common **(Fig. 9.3B)**. The eyes may suffuse and numerous hemorrhages may appear in the conjunctivae. This may give rise to suspicion of suffocation or strangulation.
- If the body has been *lying on one side*, the blood will settle on that side.
- If the body has been *suspended vertically,* as in hanging, postmortem staining will be most marked in the legs, and external genitalia, lower parts of forearms and hands *(glove and stocking)*, and upper margin of

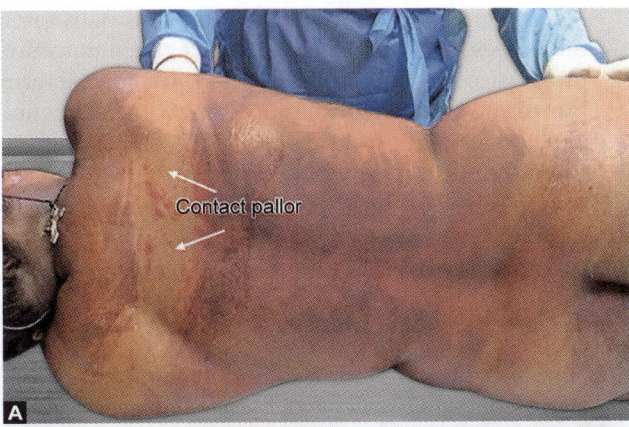

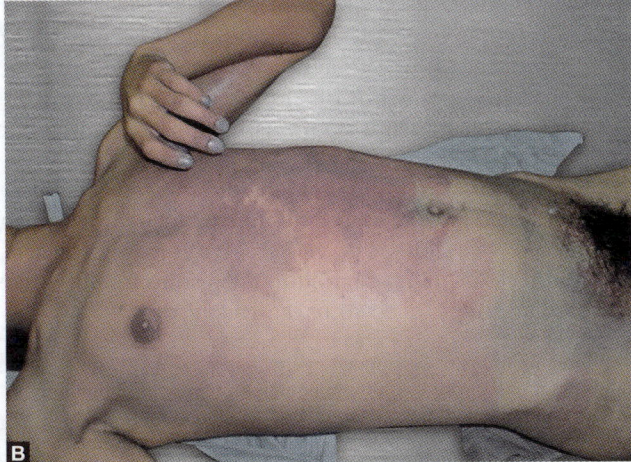

Figs. 9.3A and B: PM staining in dependent parts: (A) Back; (B) Front

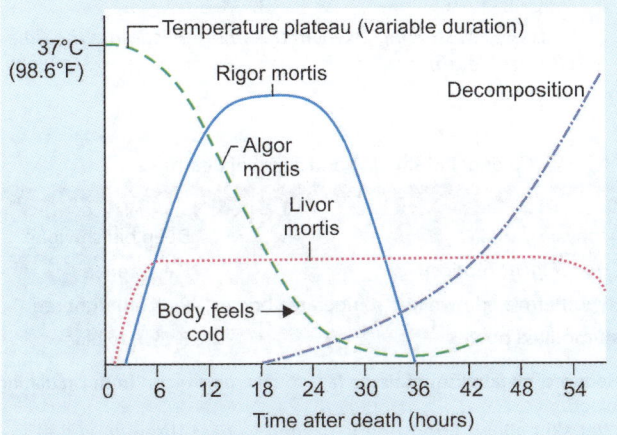

Fig. 9.2: Estimation of time since death

the ligature mark on the neck. In case of prolonged suspension, petechial hemorrhages are seen in the skin.
- When the body remains *submerged in water,* as in drowning, the head being the heaviest assumes a lower level in comparison with the rest of the body, and the staining is usually found on the face, the upper part of the chest, hands, lower arms, feet and the calves, as they are the dependent parts. If the body is in flowing water and constantly changing its position, staining may not develop.
- In case of electrocution in water (usually a bathtub), the PM staining is sharply limited to a horizontal line corresponding to the water level.

NOTA BENE

Vibices (PM ecchymoses/death spots): Tiny spots, sometimes confluent, round-to-oval bluish-black hemorrhages, limited to areas of lividity, due to postmortem mechanical rupture of subcutaneous capillaries.

Fate of PM Staining

- It merges with putrefactive changes.
- Initially, there is hemolysis of blood and diffusion of blood pigment into the surrounding tissues, where it undergoes secondary changes. Later, as decomposition progresses, the staining becomes dark in color and turns brown and green, before disappearing with destruction of blood.
- In mummification, staining becomes brown to black with drying of the body.

Features Related to PM Staining

- PM staining also occurs at the dependent parts of all the internal organs. Hypostasis in the heart can simulate myocardial infarction; in the lungs it may suggest pneumonia; dependent coils of intestine appear strangulated.
- If there has been excessive loss of blood during or before death, or in severely anemic individuals, PM staining may not be appreciable. It may not be appreciable in death from wasting diseases and lobar pneumonia.
- Congestion, resembling PM staining may be seen few hours before death in case of a person dying slowly with circulatory failure, e.g., cholera, typhus, tuberculosis, uremia, morphine or barbiturate poisoning, congestive cardiac failure, deep coma, and asphyxia.

Recent methods to determine time since death from PM staining is known as *calorimetry (color of staining measured by a colorimeter)*, which shows an increasing pallor of the hypostasis during the first 24 h. The rate of change of lightness decreases as PM interval increases. Linear regression analysis is performed to determine the relationship between PM interval and color of the skin.

Color of PM staining: The normal color of the PM staining is either bluish or purplish red. But in some specific causes of death, the color may be different, as given in **Table 9.2** (color changes seen in different poisoning is given in Chapter 35).

Medico-legal Importance of PM Staining

i. It is a sign of death.
ii. The time since death can be roughly estimated from the formation, extension and fixation of the PM staining.
iii. It indicates the posture of the body at the time of death.
iv. It may indicate the moving of the body to another position sometime after death.
v. Cause of death may be judged from the distribution and color of PM staining.
vi. In the early phase of its formation, it may be confused with bruise when patchy and small **(Diff. 9.1)**.
vii. Sometimes, it may be confused with congestion of the internal organs **(Diff. 9.2)**.
viii. Hemorrhagic spots on skin due to blood dyscrasias may be mistaken for PM staining.
ix. Some extraneous color or stain may be mistaken for PM staining; however, these can be easily wiped or rubbed off or washed out.

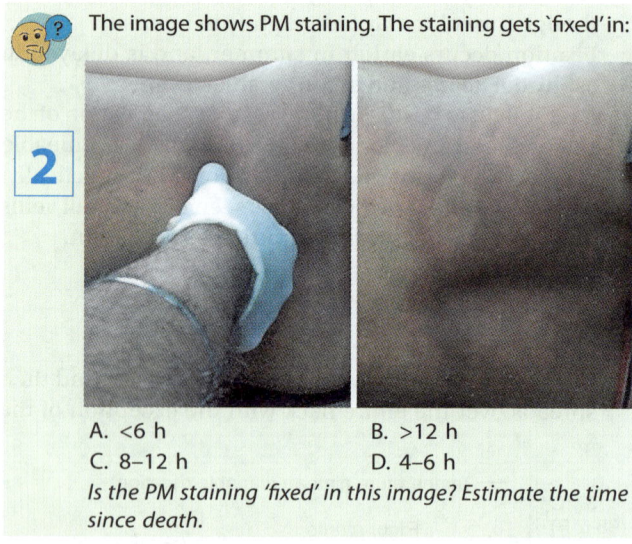

The image shows PM staining. The staining gets 'fixed' in:

A. <6 h B. >12 h
C. 8–12 h D. 4–6 h

Is the PM staining 'fixed' in this image? Estimate the time since death.

TABLE 9.2: Color of PM staining and cause of death

Cause	Color
Asphyxia	Deep bluish-violet
C. perfringens septicemia	Pale bronze
Hypothermia,[a] drowning,[b] refrigerated bodies	Pink or bright red
Mummified bodies	Brown to black

[a] Reduced metabolism of tissue fails to take up oxygen from circulating blood.
[b] Wet skin allows atmospheric oxygen to pass through, and at low temperatures hemoglobin has a greater affinity for oxygen.

CHAPTER 9 : Signs of Death

DIFFERENTIATION 9.1: Postmortem staining and bruise

S.No.	Feature	Postmortem staining	Bruise
1.	Situation	On the dependent parts	Anywhere
2.	Tissue level	Undersurface of the skin	Subcutaneous tissue level
3.	Surface	Not elevated	May be slightly elevated
4.	Margin	Sharp and clearly defined	Diffuse
5.	Color	Bluish or purplish red	Reddish when fresh, change in color occurs with time
6.	Cause	Capillo-venous distension with blood	Extravasation of blood from capillaries
7.	Nature of change	Postmortem	Antemortem
8.	Effect of pressure	Pressed spot appears pale	No change
9.	Cut section	Oozing of blood from the vessels, which can be cleaned by washing	Hemorrhage in the tissue, which cannot be washed
10.	Microscopically	Engorgement of capillaries infiltration	Extravasation of blood, cellular infiltration
11.	Enzymatic study	No change	Change in the level of certain enzymes
12.	Medico-legal importance	Time since death and position of the body may be known	Type of injury and weapon used may be known

DIFFERENTIATION 9.2: Congestion and postmortem staining

S.No.	Feature	Congestion	Postmortem staining
1.	Situation	Uniform, all over the organ	Irregular and in dependent parts
2.	Exudate	May be seen	No inflammatory exudate
3.	Mucous membranes	Normal	Dull and lusterless
4.	Swelling or edema	May be seen	None
5.	Hollow viscus	Uniform staining	Stomach and intestine when stretched show alternate areas of discoloration and pallor
6.	Cause	Due to some pathology in the organ	Passive capillo-venous distension
7.	Nature of change	Antemortem	Postmortem

PM staining can be seen on the hands, forearms and lower limbs. This is characteristic of deaths due to:

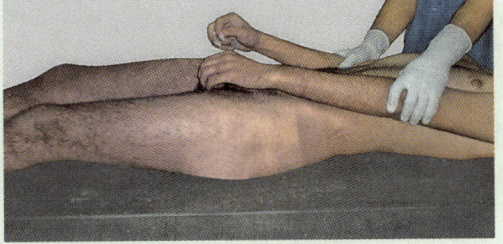

3

A. Strangulation B. Drowning
C. Traumatic asphyxia D. Hanging
It is also called _____ PM staining

FM 2.8
Describe and discuss postmortem changes—cooling of body.

■ ALGOR MORTIS (COOLING OF THE DEAD BODY)

Definition: *Algor mortis* (Latin *algor*: coolness, *mortis*: death) or *chill of death* is the cooling of the body that normally takes place after death, where the body temperature equilibrates with its environmental temperature.

♦ Sometime after death, the body temperature of the cadaver falls and after some hours, it tends to be equal to the temperature of its immediate environment (based on Newton's Law of Cooling). The surface (outer) temperature falls more rapidly for some time than the inner core temperature.
♦ The fall of temperature of the cadaver occurs due to cessation of energy production and inactivity of the heat regulating center after somatic death.
♦ Loss of the body heat occurs by conduction, radiation and evaporation when the body is in the atmospheric environment, and by conduction and convection when the body is in water.
♦ The curve of cooling pattern is **sigmoid, biexponential or inverted 'S' shaped (Fig. 9.2).**
  ■ Initial plateau (*isothermic phase*) indicates that there is no loss of heat or fall of the inner core (rectal) temperature for the first 1–2 h. This is due to the thickness of the skin and the subcutaneous tissue which are good insulators of heat.
  ■ Some hours after death, the fall of temperature at the inner core of the body achieves a regular, linear and constant pattern (*intermediate phase*).
  ■ Then, it gradually becomes slow as the temperature of the environment is reached. The last part of the

curve (*terminal phase*) is slightly above the base line which is indicative of bacterial activity.
- For the purpose of estimation of time passed after death, the measurement of the inner core temperature is important and is more reliable than the outer surface temperature.

Pearls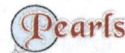

Sites to record the inner core temperature
- Rectum (8–10 cm above anus)
- External auditory meatus
- Subhepatic (inferior surface of liver)
- Nostrils up to cribriform plate
- Intracerebral (through the orbit)

- **Methods for measurement of core temperature:** Chemical (not clinical) thermometer 10–12 inches long with graduation ranging from 0–50°C is required. Nowadays, digital 'probe' thermometer is being used which has a temperature measuring range of –40°C to 110°C (with 0.5°C accuracy) **(Fig. 9.4).**
    - **Procedure:** For measurement of the temperature, the bulb/tip of the thermometer is introduced inside the rectum (*except in sodomy*), at least 10 cm above the anus.
    - Temperature can also be recorded by making an incision in the peritoneal cavity and inserting the thermometer against the inferior surface of the liver.
    - The time and temperature of the environment is also recorded.
    - Reading should be made at intervals, in order to obtain the rate of fall of temperature.
- The use of this method is useful in cool and temperate climates, because in tropical countries (like in India) there may be a minimal fall in body temperature postmortem, and in deserts the body temperature may even rise after death.

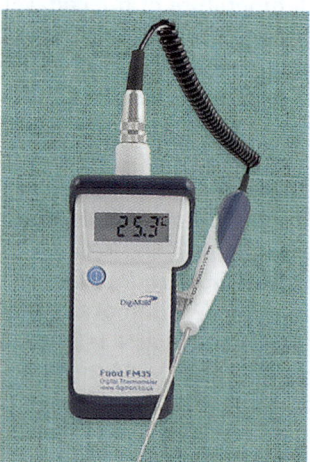

Fig. 9.4: Digital rectal thermometer

---
* Compensatory number for possible initial delay in cooling of the body.

- The average rate of fall of the body temperature is 0.4–0.7°C/h, and the body attains environmental temperature in 16–20 h after death.
- It is assumed that the body temperature at the time of death was normal, which varies between 35.7–37.7°C orally and 36.7–37.5°C in the rectum (in males).
- A rough estimate of time since death (TSD) in hours is obtained by the formula:

$$TSD = \frac{\text{Normal rectal temperature} - \text{Measured rectal temperature}}{\text{Rate of fall of temperature/hour}}$$

- For temperate countries, *Marshal and Hoare* formula is used. The rates of fall of temperature in an average built person is 1°F up to 3 h, 2°F up to 9 h and 1.5°F up to 12 h. The *rule of thumb is that the temperature falls at about 1.5°F/h.*
- Rectal temperature is higher in case of struggle or exercise prior to death.
- Low temperature is seen in congestive cardiac failure, hemorrhage, collapse and secondary shock.

> **Recent Advances**
> Various equations, algorithms and nomograms using rectal temperature have been developed. Examples of simple rule-of-thumb formulae (for temperate countries):
> - TSD = [Rectal temperature at time of death – measured rectal temperature (°F)] ÷ 1.5
> - TSD = [Rectal temperature at time of death – measured rectal temperature (°C)] + 3*
>
> Presently, **nomogram method** devised by *Henssge* is used. This method is based on experimental data, which can be carried out by a simple computer program or by a nomogram. Adjustments are built in for the body weight, ambient temperature and body temperature. It provides a 95% accuracy of estimating the TSD during the first 15 h (with an error of ±2.8 h).

Factors Affecting Algor Mortis

i. **Environmental temperature** *(major factor)*: Rate of fall of body temperature is directly proportional to the difference between the temperature of the dead body and the environmental temperature.
ii. **Air movement:** Air movement over the surface of the dead body causes a quick fall of temperature due to increased evaporation of body fluids. A body kept in a well-ventilated room will cool more rapidly than one in a closed room.
iii. **Humidity:** Cooling is more rapid in a humid rather than in a dry atmosphere, since moist air is better conductor of heat.
iv. **Media of disposal:** Cooling is earliest in water, and late in buried bodies. The ratio of the rates of fall of temperature in the three media, water: air: soil = 4:2:1.

The rate is thus maximum in water, moderate in air and minimum in a buried body.

v. **Built of cadaver:** Obese bodies cool slowly, and lean bodies rapidly, since fat is a bad conductor of heat.
vi. **Age and sex:** Rate of loss of heat is more in children and the elderly, compared to adults, because the surface area of the body is more in relation to the body volume. Females retain body heat for a comparatively longer period, because of their subcutaneous fatty tissue.
vii. **Clothing or coverings of the body:** A well-covered body retains heat for a longer period, compared to a naked or thinly clothed body, as clothes are bad conductors of heat.
viii. **Position and posture of the body:** If the body lies in supine and extended position, the loss of heat is rapid, because greater surface area of the body is exposed; whereas in curled fetal position, the loss will be slow.
ix. **Mode of death:** In case of sudden death in a healthy individual, the body tends to cool slowly, whereas in death due to long and wasting illness, the body cools rapidly.

Postmortem Caloricity

In this condition, instead of cooling, the temperature of the dead body remains high for the initial 2 h or so. This is due to:

a. *Postmortem glycogenolysis:* Compulsory phenomenon which occurs in all dead bodies, and which starts soon after death (produces up to 140 calories).
b. *Cause of death*
   - In deaths occurring due to infectious diseases, septicemia or bacteremia, heat is produced by the action of the infective organisms.
   - If death is preceded by a severe convulsion, as in tetanus and strychnine poisoning, it causes an increase in the body temperature.
   - In case of death due to heat stroke or pontine hemorrhage, the heat regulation is severely disturbed before death.
c. *High environmental temperature*: In tropical countries, when the environmental temperature is higher than the body temperature, the dead body may absorb some heat.

Medico-legal Importance of Algor Mortis

i. Algor mortis is a sign of death.
ii. It helps in the estimation of the time of death.
iii. Rapid cooling of a dead body delays the processes of rigor mortis and decomposition. If the heat is preserved for a longer period, then both the processes start early.

FM 2.8

Describe and discuss postmortem changes—rigor mortis, cadaveric spasm, cold stiffening and heat stiffening.

■ RIGOR MORTIS

Definition: *Rigor mortis* (Latin, stiffness of death) is that state of the muscles in the dead body when they become stiff or rigid with some degree of shortening.

The phase of primary relaxation of the muscles continues for about an hour which is followed by stiffening or rigidity. It indicates molecular death of the concerned muscles.

Mechanism: Muscle fibers contain bundles of myofibrils which consist of two types of protein filaments—actin and myosin. At rest, actin filaments interdigitate myosin filaments only to a small extent, and the muscle fibers also appear soft and supple. Maintenance of this condition of muscles is due to the presence of ATP (adenosine-triphosphate) above a certain level. On nervous stimulation, hydrolysis of ATP occurs to ADP (adenosine-diphosphate) and phosphate with the liberation of energy which causes contraction of the muscle fibers and extension of the actin filaments more inside the myosin filaments.

After death, there is continuous hydrolysis of the ATP, and as long as glycogen is available in the muscle, there is resynthesis of ATP. In this process, once the muscle glycogen is exhausted, no further resynthesis of ATP is possible and the muscle loses softness, elasticity and extensibility due to formation of viscid actomyosin complex giving rise to rigor mortis in the muscle **(Fig. 9.5)**.

After the pH of the muscle becomes 5.5, release of autolytic enzymes stored in lysosomes takes place. The major proteolytic enzymes are cathepsins and calpains. These enzymes act at the myofibrillar proteins and hydrolyze them. As a result, the actomyosin complex is broken down and muscles become soft again. This is known as *resolution of rigor* which occurs during the stage of secondary relaxation, due to decomposition.

Muscles Involved

- Rigor mortis occurs both in the voluntary and involuntary muscles.
- It occurs earlier in the involuntary or smooth muscles than in the voluntary or striated muscles.

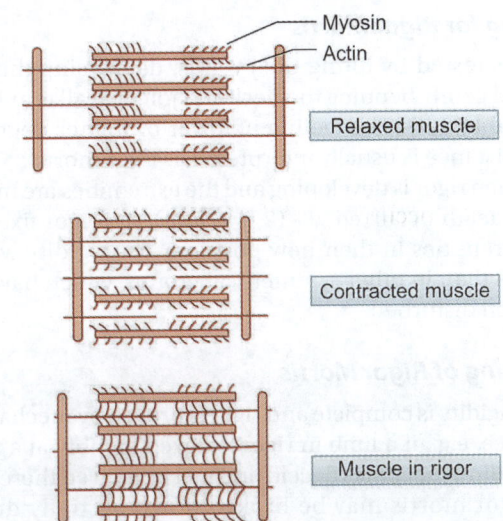

Fig. 9.5: Schematic representation of rigor mortis

Onset and Duration

- In tropical countries like India, roughly, it commences in 1–2 h after death, takes about 9–12 h to develop from head to foot, persists for another 12 h and takes 12 h to pass off **(Rule of 12) (Fig. 9.2)**.
- In Northern India, the usual duration of rigor mortis is 18–36 h in summer and 24–48 h in winter.

Order of Appearance

- Rigor mortis *first appears in the heart muscle (involuntary muscle)* within an hour after death.
- Among the voluntary muscles, rigor mortis usually develops sequentially and follows a descending pattern (proximo-distal progress), the so-called **Nysten's law**: it *first appears in the muscles of the eyelids* (orbicularis oculi) [3–5 h], then in jaw, facial muscles [4–5 h], neck, thorax [5–7 h] upper limb (from shoulder to the hand) [7–9 h], abdomen, lower limb (from the hip to the foot) [9–11 h], and lastly in the small muscles of fingers and toes [11–12 h].
- The rigidity disappears in the same order in which it has appeared. In the whole body, it stays for maximum duration in the muscles of the lower limbs.
- When rigor is fully established, the entire body is stiff; knees, hips, shoulders and elbows are slightly flexed, and fingers and toes often show a marked degree of flexion **(Fig. 9.6)**.
- It is independent of the integrity of the nervous system, though it is said to develop more slowly in paralyzed limbs.

> **NOTA BENE**
>
> **Nysten's law:** Rigor mortis affects first the muscles of jaw, followed by those of the face and neck, then muscles of the trunk and arms, and lastly the legs and feet.

Testing for Rigor Mortis

- It is tested by lifting the eyelids, depressing the jaw, and gently bending the neck and joints of all four limbs **(Table 9.3)**. The feeling of lower or higher degree of resistance is usually interpreted as rigor mortis.
- When rigor is developing and the extremities are moved (if death occurred <8–12 h before), the rigor fixes the extremities in their new position. The rigidity will be less than in other symmetrical groups, which have not been disturbed.

Breaking of Rigor Mortis

- If rigidity is complete and rigor is broken by mechanical force, e.g., if a limb in rigor is flexed forcibly at a joint, the limb becomes flaccid and will remain so thereafter.
- Rigor mortis may be broken down partially due to mishandling during the transit of the body from the scene of crime to autopsy table, which may misled the autopsy surgeon in estimating the time since death.

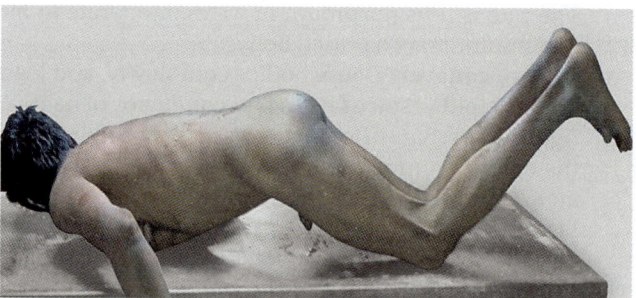

Fig. 9.6: Rigor mortis

TABLE 9.3: Interpretation of rigor mortis

Perception	Interpretation
Moves with little force	Present in moderate form
Moves with more force	Present in strong form
Free movement or not present in the part tested	Not developed yet or disappeared
• If only proximal parts show rigidity	Developing phase
• If only distal parts show rigidity	Developed, disappearing phase

Effects of Rigor Mortis

- There is goose skin appearance of the body due to rigor mortis of the erector pilae muscles.
- Rigor in the muscles of the seminal vesicles may cause postmortem ejaculation of seminal fluid.
- The iris is also affected so that antemortem constriction or dilatation is modified. Hence, the postmortem position of pupil is an unreliable indicator of toxic or neurological conditions during life.
- Contraction of the heart muscle due to rigor mortis should not be mistaken for myocardial hypertrophy.
- Rigor mortis in the uterine muscle cannot expel the fetus from the womb.

Factors Affecting Rigor Mortis

The major factors that influence the onset and duration of rigor mortis are the environmental temperature and the degree of muscular activity before death.

i. **Environmental temperature:** At high temperature, rigor mortis comes early and passes off early. In cold temperature, it comes late and stays longer.
ii. **Muscular activity:** Violent exercise prior to death may hasten the onset, as well as disappearance of rigidity.
iii. **Cause of death and condition of the body:** Refer to Table 9.4.
iv. **Built:** It comes early and passes off early in emaciated and thinly built subjects with weak musculature. In well-built subjects with strong musculature, it is well-marked, comes late and stays longer.
v. **Age:** It is claimed that rigor mortis does not occur in stillborn fetuses of <7 months old (muscles are not

TABLE 9.4: Cause of death and condition of the body affecting rigor mortis

Early onset of rigor	Late onset of rigor
Exhaustive or wasting diseases, like cholera, typhoid, tuberculosis, cancer	Asphyxia (CO, hanging)
Violent deaths, like cut-throat, electrocution, firearm and lightning injuries	Hemorrhage
Poisoning with strychnine, organophosphate, insulin or HCN	Cold, refrigerated bodies
Fatigue or exhaustion	Paralyzed muscles
Heat stroke	Pneumonia

developed enough to contribute appreciable degree of stiffness). However, complete rigor has been reported in infants dying of sudden infant death syndrome (SIDS). In healthy adults, rigor mortis develops slowly but is well-marked. It is weak, and comes early in children and elderly.

Medico-legal Importance of Rigor Mortis

- Rigor mortis is a sign of death and indicates molecular death of the muscle involved.
- During the early phase after death, it helps in estimating the time since death. During summer, if rigor mortis has not set in, death might have occurred within 2 h. If rigor mortis has involved the whole body then death might have occurred between 12–24 h back. In winter season, the above timings are roughly doubled.
- It indicates the position of the body at the time of death, e.g., if the body is lying on its back with its lower limbs raised in air, it indicates that the body reached full rigidity elsewhere while lying in a position where the legs were flexed.

Conditions which may imitate/simulate rigor mortis:
1. Cadaveric spasm
2. Heat stiffening
3. Cold stiffening
4. Gas stiffening or putrefaction

CADAVERIC SPASM (INSTANTANEOUS RIGOR)

Definition: *Cadaveric spasm* is a condition in which the muscles of the body that were in a state of contraction immediately before death, continue to be so after death without passing through the stage of primary relaxation.

It is a rare phenomenon of instantaneous rigor, which develops at the time of death with no period of postmortem flaccidity.

Predisposing conditions: It occurs especially in cases of sudden death, excitement, fear, severe pain, exhaustion, cerebral hemorrhage, electrocution, injury to the nervous system, firearm wound of the head or convulsant poisons, like strychnine.

Muscles Involved

The spasm is primarily a vital phenomenon; it originates by normal nervous stimulation of the muscles.

- It is usually limited to a single group of voluntary muscles, and frequently involves the hands.
- Occasionally, the whole body is affected, as seen in soldiers shot in battlefield when the body may retain the posture which it assumed at the moment of death.

No other condition simulates cadaveric spasm. A great force is required to overcome this stiffness.

Fate: It passes without interruption into normal rigor mortis and disappears when rigor disappears.

Mechanism

- It is unclear but may be neurogenic.
- It may be due to exhausted ATP in the affected muscles with persistence of contraction even after death and the resultant failure of the chemical processes required for active muscular relaxation to occur during molecular death.
- Adrenocortical exhaustion, which impairs resynthesis of ATP may be the possible cause.

Differentiating features between rigor mortis and cadaveric spasm are highlighted in **Diff. 9.3**.

Medico-legal Importance

Cadaveric spasm, being an antemortem phenomenon, reflects the last act of the subject performed before and at the time of his death. The *cause and the manner of death* may be judged.

- *In case of drowning*, the hand may firmly grip sand, mud, gravel or weed, which are present in the pond or lake from where the body was recovered **(Fig. 9.7)**.
- *In case of firearm/stab injury* over an approachable vital part of the body, the pistol/knife may be firmly grasped in the victim's hand, which is a strong presumptive evidence of suicide. Although, attempts may be made to simulate this condition in order to conceal murder, but rigor does not produce the same firm grip of a weapon.
- *In homicidal cases*, the deceased may grasp some part of clothing, button or hair of the assailant(s) with whom he had a struggle prior to his death.

HEAT STIFFENING

(*Synonyms:* Pugilistic attitude/fencing attitude/boxer's attitude/defense attitude)

- If the body is subjected to heat exposure at >65°C, rigidity is produced which is much more marked than that found in rigor mortis.
- There will be coagulation of the muscle protein in which the flexors are affected more, giving rise to a *pugilistic attitude* of the body **(Fig. 9.8)**.

SECTION 1: Jurisprudence and Forensic Medicine

DIFFERENTIATION 9.3: Rigor mortis and cadaveric spasm

S.No.	Feature	Rigor mortis	Cadaveric spasm
1.	Onset	Within 1–2 h after death	Instantaneous
2.	Production by other methods	Freezing and exposure to temperature >65°C can produce rigor	Cannot be produced by any method after death
3.	Mechanism of formation	Breakdown of ATP below critical level	Not known exactly
4.	Molecular death	Occurs	Does not occur
5.	Muscles involved	All the muscles of the body, both voluntary and involuntary	Usually restricted to selected group of voluntary muscles
6.	Seen in	All deaths	Rare phenomenon, in few cases only
7.	Primary flaccidity	Precedes rigor mortis	Not seen
8.	Muscle stiffening	Not marked	Marked
9.	Duration of stay	About 12–24 h	Few hours, until replaced by rigor mortis
10.	Predisposing factor	Nil	Sudden death, excitement, exhaustion, fear, fatigue
11.	Body temperature	Cold	Warm
12.	Muscle reaction	Acidic	Alkaline
13.	Reaction to electrical stimulus	Does not respond	Responds
14.	Medico-legal significance	Indicates time of death	Indicates the cause and manner of death

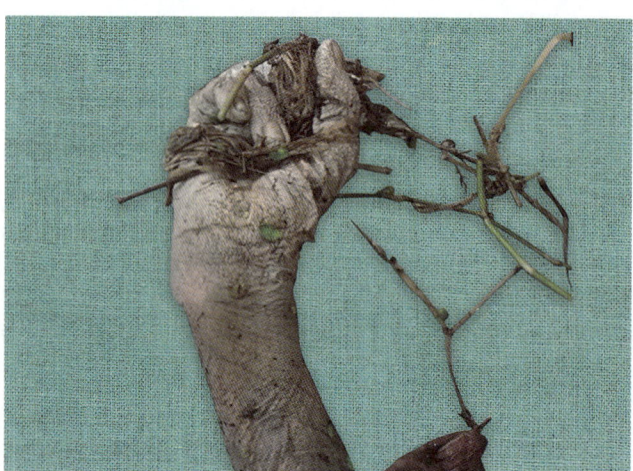

Fig. 9.7: Cadaveric spasm in drowning

- The muscles are contracted, desiccated or even carbonized on the surface. A zone of brownish-pink 'cooked meat' is seen under this, overlying normal red muscle.
- The stiffening remains until the muscles and ligaments soften from decomposition, and the normal rigor mortis does not occur.

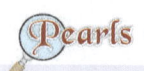

Normal rigor mortis is not seen in:
1. Heat stiffening
2. Embalmed body

Differentiating features between rigor mortis and heat stiffening are given in **Diff. 9.4**.

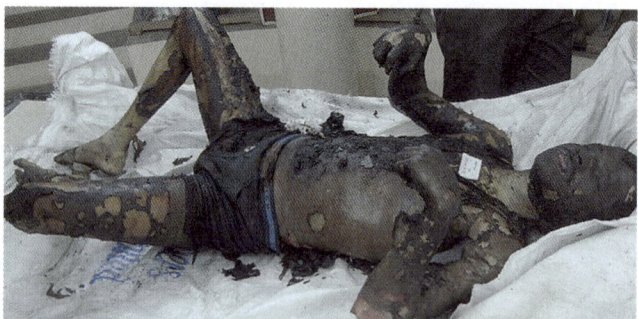

Fig. 9.8: Heat stiffening

 A 27-year-old male fell off from the bike. He was brought dead in the hospital. Lacerated wound present over the left side of face and the upper limbs raised in the front. What do you think caused this condition of the limbs?

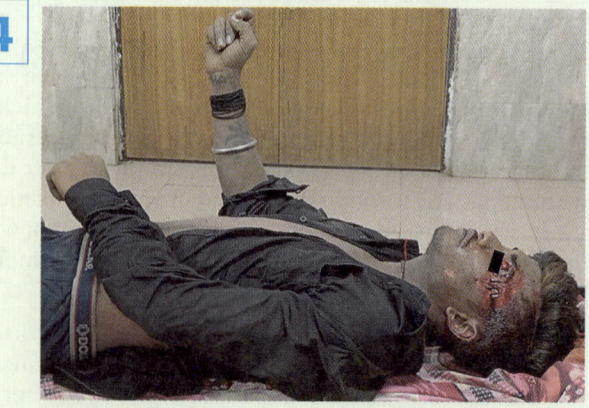

A. Cadaveric spasm B. Rigor mortis
C. Heat stiffening D. Gas stiffening

DIFFERENTIATION 9.4: Rigor mortis and heat stiffening (pugilistic attitude)

S.No.	Feature	Rigor mortis	Heat stiffening
1.	Mechanism	Due to breakdown of ATP of muscles	Due to heat coagulation of muscle protein
2.	Time of formation	2–12 h after death	Immediately when burnt
3.	Role of heat	High temperature enhances the process	Occur at a temperature >65°C
4.	Onset	In sequence	Rapid and diffuse
5.	Degree of stiffness	Moderate	High
6.	Mechanical pull at joints	Will revert to rigidity extension (if not fully developed)	Rupture of muscles may occur
7.	External features	Nothing specific	Signs of exposure to heat (burning, blackening, blisters)
8.	Disappearance	In sequence, at various duration	Uniform, with onset of putrefaction
9.	Medico-legal	Time since death	No significance (can be antemortem or postmortem)

COLD STIFFENING

This is seen when a body is exposed to freezing temperature for a reasonable period, the tissues becoming frozen and stiff, simulating rigor.

It occurs due to:
- Freezing of body fluids, particularly at the tissue level and in the synovial sacs of the joints
- Hardening of the subcutaneous fatty tissue.

*Differentiating features between rigor mortis and cold stiffening are given in **Diff. 9.5**.*

Gas stiffening occurs during putrefaction due to accumulation of gases in the tissues, which causes false rigidity resulting in stiff limbs **(Fig. 9.9)**. It is very obvious from the discoloration, swelling and foul smell.

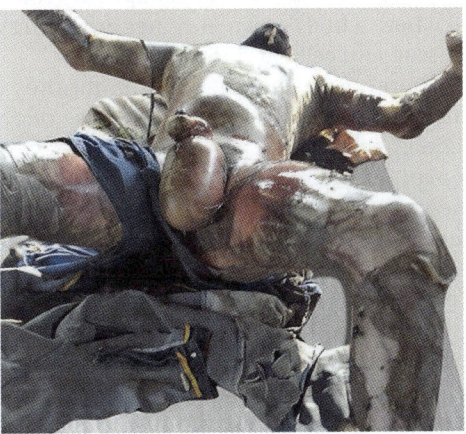

Fig. 9.9: Gas stiffening
(*Courtesy*: Dr Ashwani, AIMS, Mohali)

Secondary Relaxation of Muscles

- After some hours of stay, rigor mortis passes away and the body becomes relaxed or flaccid for the second time. This is secondary relaxation or secondary flaccidity of the muscles. It occurs with the onset of decomposition or putrefaction of the dead body **(Diff. 9.6)**.
- During this phase, other signs of putrefaction will be there. Apart from those signs, the reaction of the muscles

DIFFERENTIATION 9.5: Rigor mortis and cold stiffening

S.No.	Feature	Rigor mortis	Cold stiffening
1.	Cause	ATP loss	Temperature <0°C
2.	History	Non-specific	Exposure in ice caves, glaciers
3.	Body fluids	Liquid	Frozen
4.	Manipulation of joints	Will revert to rigidity extension (if not fully developed)	Crackling sound or crepitation is heard
5.	Disappearance	In sequence, at various duration	On thawing it goes, and rigor mortis appears

will again be alkaline due to breakdown of protein with liberation and accumulation of ammonia.

FM 2.9
Describe putrefaction and maceration.

PUTREFACTION/DECOMPOSITION

Definition: *Putrefaction* is a process by which complex organic body tissue breaks down into simpler inorganic compounds or elements due to the action of saprophytic microorganisms or due to autolysis.

- Putrefaction usually follows the disappearance of rigor mortis **(Fig. 9.2)**. During the hot season, it may commence before rigor mortis has completely disappeared from the lower extremities.
- After death, the body's protective functions are absent and its defense barrier is lost. Saprophytic microorganisms, which cannot invade the body during life, and physical and chemical agents which are present in the environment, all act on the dead body. Further, some body chemicals and enzymes which are helpful in different metabolic processes, in the absence of physiological control after death, start acting adversely.

DIFFERENTIATION 9.6: Primary and secondary relaxation of muscles

S.No.	Feature	Primary relaxation	Secondary relaxation
1.	Time of occurrence	Immediately after death	After rigor mortis passes off
2.	Molecular death	Has not occurred	Has occurred
3.	Response to stimuli	Responds	Does not respond
4.	Body temperature	Near normal	Cold
5.	External features	Nothing specific	Signs of decomposition present

Microorganisms involved: *Clostridium perfringens* (produces lecithinase), *Staphylococcus*, non-hemolytic *Streptococcus*, *diphtheroids*, and *Proteus* are the important ones.

Autolysis ('*auto*': self; '*lysis*': breakdown) refers to the situation where a body's own enzymes are acting on itself, causing tissue and cellular destruction.
- Immediately after death, cell membranes become permeable and breakdown, with release of cytoplasm containing enzymes.
- The proteolytic, glycolytic and lipolytic action of ferments causes autodigestion and disintegration of organs, and occurs without bacterial influence.
- The earliest autolytic changes occur in parenchymatous and glandular tissues, and in the brain.
- In adults, such digestion may start before death in cases of intracranial lesions and terminal pyrexias. Autodigestion of the gastric mucosa (*gastromalacia*) may occur from pepsinogen and HCl released, which may even cause perforation of stomach.
- In dead born, *maceration*—an aseptic autolysis of dead fetus *in utero* is seen. **Maceration** occurs when the dead child remains in the uterus surrounded with liquor amnii with exclusion of air. The macerated fetus is usually a brownish pink, rather than the greenish hue of putrefaction.

Gases produced: H_2S, phosphorated hydrogen, ammonia, CO_2, CO, mercaptans and methane.

External Changes due to Decomposition

> **Decomposition changes ('4 Ds')**
> 1. **Discoloration:** Greenish discoloration in the lower abdominal quadrants.
> 2. **Distension:** Various gases produced during decomposition permeate into skin, soft tissue and organs which manifests as crepitus and distension.
> 3. **Degradation:** Decomposition causes a loss of anatomic integrity of skin and other tissues, such as localized peeling of skin ('skin slippage'), loosening of skin of hands and feet ('degloving') and loosening of hair and nails.
> 4. **Dissolution:** Progressive decomposition leads to liquefaction and disappearance of tissues and organs, and eventual skeletonization.

Discoloration
- The **first external sign of decomposition** is usually a greenish discoloration *over the right iliac fossa* over the region of the cecum which lies superficially, and the contents of the bowel are more fluid and full of bacteria **(Fig. 9.10)**. *C. perfringens* are most abundant at the ileocecal zone of the intestinal tract.
- Internally, putrefaction is first seen as discoloration of aortic intima followed by undersurface of liver (as it is in contact with transverse colon).
- After death, when the tissue barrier is lost, microorganisms can invade through the intestinal wall and reach the blood vessels and produce H_2S gas. The gas combines with the hemoglobin of blood and forms *sulfhemoglobin (green pigment molecule),* which discolors the vessels and the surrounding tissue.
- *Onset*: In India, this change is seen by about 12 h after death in summer (or even earlier) and by 36–48 h in winter. The discoloration gradually spreads all over the abdomen, external genitalia, face, neck and thorax, and lastly on the limbs. In temperate conditions, these changes are seen in 24–48 h after death.

'Marbling' of Skin
- The blood vessels provide an important route through which the bacteria can spread with ease throughout the body.
- Their passage is marked by the decomposition of hemoglobin to sulfhemoglobin in the blood vessels,

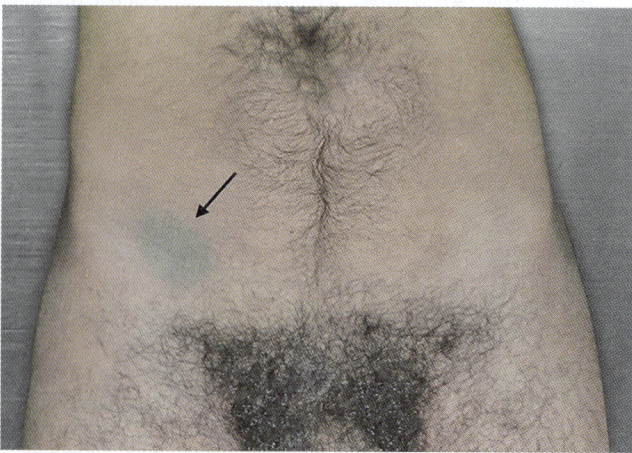

Fig. 9.10: First sign of external putrefaction (arrow)

which causes a greenish or reddish-brown staining of the inner walls of the superficial vessels.
- This is seen as linear branching patterns, which gives a 'marbled' ('*road map*') appearance of the skin (**Fig. 9.11**).
- *Areas where visible:* It appears first in the shoulder, roots of the limbs, thighs, sides of abdomen, chest and neck.
- *Onset:* In summers, 'marbling' is seen in 36–48 h after death.

Further decomposition changes seen in a dead body are given in **Table 9.5 (Figs. 9.12A to F)**. The changes describe the features seen in summer.

Internal Changes due to Decomposition

The organs composed of muscular tissue and those containing large amount of fibrous tissue resist putrefaction longer than the parenchymatous organs, with the exception of the stomach and intestine, which decompose rapidly because of their contents at the time of death.
- **Liver** softens and becomes flabby in 12–24 h, and blisters appear on its surface in 24–36 h. The liver assumes a '**honey comb**' ('**foamy**' or '**Swiss cheese**') appearance due to formation of air bubbles. It becomes greenish in color, and later changes to coal-black.
- **Brain** becomes soft, discolored pinkish-gray within 72 h, and liquefies in 5–10 days. Meningeal hemorrhage, hematoma and tumors may still be appreciated.
- **Heart** is moderately resistant, becomes soft and flabby with dilatation of cardiac chambers and thinning of the walls, making diagnosis of dilated cardiomyopathy impossible. Atheromatous stenosis in coronary arteries is possible. Heart may show white granularity consisting of calcium and soapy material on epicardial and endocardial surfaces known as '*miliary plaques*' (nodules are 1 mm or less in size).
- **Prostate and uterus** being the last organs to decompose, they help to identify the sex of the dead bodies in advanced state of decomposition.

As a general rule, the organs show putrefactive changes in the following order as given in **Table 9.6.**

> **NOTA BENE**
> - **Postmortem luminescence** is usually due to contamination by bacteria, like *Photobacterium fischeri*, the light comes from them and not from putrefying material. Luminescent fungi, *Armillaria mellea*, are other sources of light.
> - **Pink teeth:** In putrefied bodies, the teeth are sometimes seen to be pink in color, especially near the gum line as a result of hemolysis of extravasated blood in the dentinal tubules. It is independent of the cause of death and production of carboxyhemoglobin.

Factors Affecting Putrefaction

The factors can be divided into *external* and *internal* factors.

External Factors
i. **Environmental temperature** *(major factor)*: High temperature promotes early decomposition.
  - The optimum temperature for decomposition is 21–38°C. Beyond this range, decomposition occurs

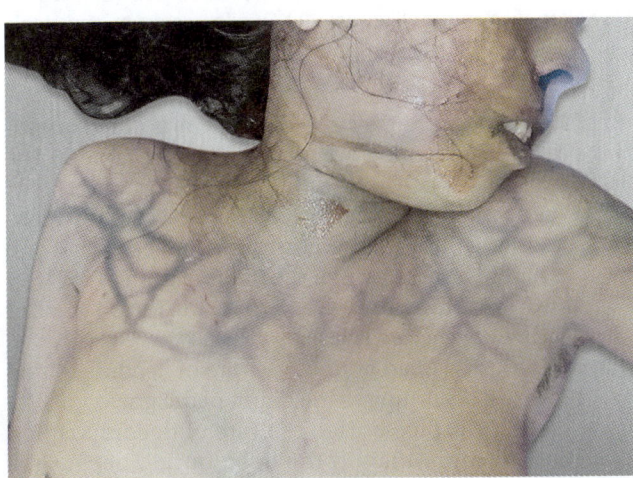

Fig. 9.11: 'Marbling' of the skin of shoulders and neck

TABLE 9.5: Putrefactive changes (in summer)

Duration	Changes
12–24 h	Gas accumulates inside the abdominal cavity making it tense. Blood-tinged froth comes out through the nostrils and mouth (*postmortem purge*). Eyes become soft and collapsed, cornea becomes white and flattened
24–48 h	Subcutaneous tissue becomes emphysematous. Breasts in females, scrotum and penis in males are swollen. Tongue is swollen and protruded. Blisters are formed on the lower surfaces of trunk and thigh, which contain fluid. Epidermis gets denuded
48–72 h	There is prolapse of uterus and anus. Postmortem delivery of fetus may take place. Postmortem staining gets displaced from the original stained areas. Eyes protrude. Face is swollen and discolored dark green to black with swelling of eyelids and lips, which take a '**fish-mouth-like**' appearance so that visual identification is difficult. Hair and nails become loose and may be taken out easily
3–5 days	Teeth (anterior and premolars) become loose. Skull sutures separate and the liquefied brain matter comes out, especially in children. Skin of hands and feet may come off in a '*glove and stocking*' manner, making identification by fingerprint difficult. Skin slippage also make tattoos more visible until the moist underlying dermis itself decomposes. Heavy maggot infestation will supervene with destruction of skin by innumerable holes and sinuses
5–10 days	Colliquative putrefaction (*liquefaction*) occurs during this period. Abdomen may burst open. Puffiness of the body passes over due to escape of gas through the damaged body parts. Soft, firm tissues change to thick, semisolid black mass. Finally, cartilages and ligaments are softened

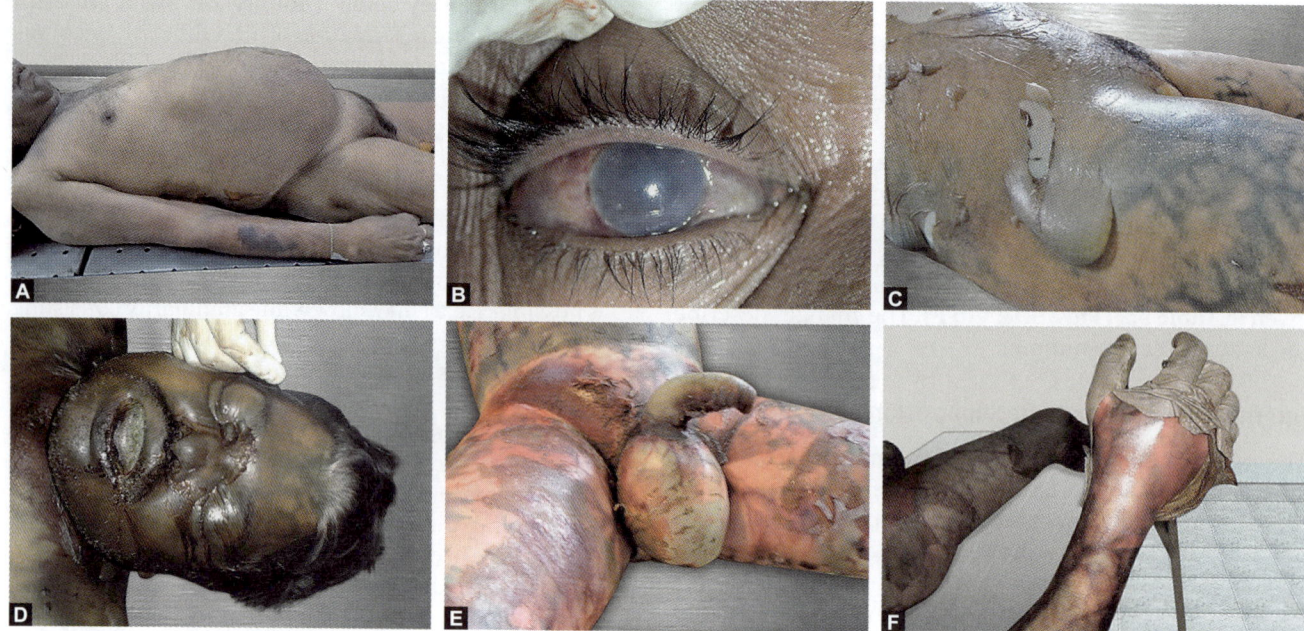

Figs. 9.12A to F: Putrefactive changes with increasing time: (A) Distended abdomen; (B) Opaque and flattened cornea; (C) Marbling of skin, formation of blisters and peeling off of skin; (D) Discolored, swollen, fish mouth-like face; (E) Swollen scrotum and penis; (F) Degloving of skin of hand

TABLE 9.6: Order of putrefaction

Early putrefaction	Late putrefaction
i. Larynx and trachea	i. Heart, lungs, kidneys
ii. Stomach, intestines	ii. Esophagus, diaphragm
iii. Spleen	iii. Blood vessels
iv. Liver	iv. Bladder
v. Brain	v. Prostate, uterus (non-gravid)
vi. Gravid uterus	vi. Skin, muscle, tendon

at a slow rate (delayed when the temperature is <10°C and >38°C).
- Decomposition nearly stops at <0°C and >48°C.
- The rate of decomposition is about twice as rapid in summer as in winter.
- Optimum temperature helps in:
  a. Chemical breakdown of the tissues
  b. Promoting the growth of microorganisms responsible for decomposition.

ii. **Moisture:** Presence of moisture promotes decomposition by promoting the growth of the organisms.
- If the body dries up quickly, putrefaction ceases and mummification occurs.
- Bodies recovered from water, if left in the air, decompose rapidly.

iii. **Air:** Free access of air hastens putrefaction, because the air conveys organisms to the body.
- Stagnant air promotes decomposition, whereas movement of air retards the process by evaporating the body fluids and cooling the dead body.

iv. **Clothing:** Clothing may reduce the rate of decomposition by preventing invasion of the body by airborne organisms.
- In winter, clothing hastens putrefaction by maintaining body temperature for a longer period and helping the growth of the microorganisms.

v. **Manner of burial:** If the body is buried soon after death, putrefaction is less.
- In buried dead bodies, the rate of decomposition varies according to the depth of the grave.
  - In surface burial, the rate of decomposition is more than in the deep burial, because of abundance of bacteria in surface soil in comparison to deep soil.
- Putrefaction is delayed if body is buried in dry, sandy soil or the body is placed in a coffin, because there is exclusion of water, air and action of insects and animals.

Internal Factors

i. **Age:** In stillborn fetuses or infants who are unfed or have not breathed, the process of decomposition is slow, since it occurs from outside as their bodies are sterile. Bodies of children putrefy rapidly, and of old people slowly.

ii. **Sex:** Sex does not have much to influence, but occurs faster in females, because of its abundant subcutaneous fatty tissue that contains moisture and retains body heat for a longer period.

iii. **Condition of the body:** Emaciated body decomposes later than a well nourished bulky, fatty body due to more fluid content in the latter, which promotes growth of microorganisms.
iv. **Cause of death:** When death is due to infection or septicemia, decomposition is rapid. Putrefaction is delayed in death due to wasting disease, anemia, poisoning by carbolic acid, zinc chloride, strychnine or heavy metal due to the preservative action of these substances on the tissues or their destructive/inhibitive effects on microorganisms.
v. **External injury on the body:** Dead body having external injuries (either antemortem or postmortem) will decompose earlier, because the injured areas will allow invasion of the body by bacteria.

Medico-legal Importance of Putrefaction

i. From decomposition changes, time since death can be assessed.
ii. In advanced decomposition, the identity of the deceased may be impossible.
iii. In advanced putrefaction, no opinion can be given as to the cause of death, except in case of poisoning, fractures and firearm injuries.

After few weeks to months, the softer tissues and viscera progressively disintegrate, leaving the more solid organs, such as uterus and prostate, together with the ligamentous and tendinous tissues attached to the skeleton.
- Often some areas of skin persist, especially where protected by clothing or under the body against the supporting surface.
- Eventually, the body will be reduced to a skeleton, but for some time, ligaments, cartilage and periosteal-tags will survive.

Skeletonization of the Body

Skeletonization of the dead body takes varying time depending on several factors (season of the year and location).
- In buried dead bodies, total skeletonization may take 1 year.
- When disposed off carelessly on land or water, skeletonization may occur within a few days to few months (may extend to 12–18 months).
- Destruction of bones ordinarily takes several years.

NOTA BENE

Decomposition changes can be divided into five stages—*fresh* (starts as early as 24 hours and as late as 7 days after death in colder winter months), *early decomposition* (begins with the onset of skin slippage and hair loss, maggots infestation, marbling, purging and strong disagreeable odor), *advanced decomposition* (begins with the appearance of loose, sagging skin and the collapse of the abdominal cavity, extensive maggot infestation, pupa, loss of internal organs, may progress directly to mummification or adipocere formation), *skeletonization* (exposure of more than half of the skeletal structure, with demonstrable soft tissue attached), and *extreme decomposition* (seen only in remains that have been exposed to the environment and lead to erosion of the skeleton).

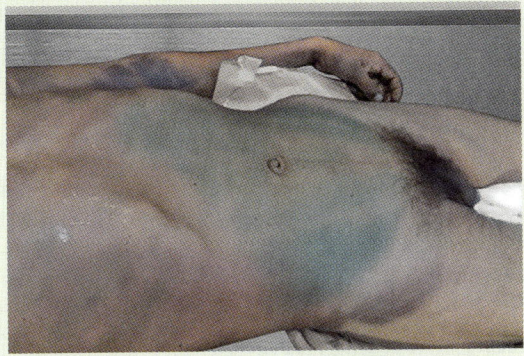

Cause of greenish discoloration of abdomen and blood vessels is due to the formation of:

A. Sulfhemoglobin B. Methemoglobin
C. Myoglobin D. Carboxyhemoglobin

DECOMPOSITION OF SUBMERGED BODY

- **Casper's dictum** is related to rate of putrefaction.
- One week of putrefaction in air is equivalent to two weeks in water, which is equivalent to eight weeks buried in soil, given the same environmental temperature.
- The rate of decomposition in air, water and deep burial is 1 : 2 (2 times slower) : 8 (8 times slower), it means decomposition changes seen in 8 weeks of burial in a body will be equivalent to 1 week of exposure in the air.
- Therefore, the deeper is the burial, better is the preservation.
- However, this dictum is not useful practically.

The process of decomposition in water is slow due to:
i. Exclusion of air
ii. Protection by clothes
iii. Early cooling of the body.

- After the body is removed from the water, the rate is rapid due to imbibition of water and optimum temperature for the growth of microorganisms.
- In submerged dead bodies, decomposition starts early in the head and face, because being heavy they assume the lowest level in the water and their blood content is maximum.
- As submerged cadavers float with the head lower than the trunk, gaseous distension and postmortem discoloration are first seen on the face and then spread to the neck, upper extremities, chest, abdomen and the lower extremities.

Factors Influencing Decomposition in Water

i. **Water, temperature and salinity:** Putrefaction is more in warm, fresh water than in cold, salt water.
ii. **Water current:** In stagnant water, decomposition is more rapid than in flowing water, since flowing water washes out the microorganisms from the surface of the body.
iii. **Quality of water:** Decomposition is slow in fresh water, and rapid in polluted water.
iv. **Aquatic animals:** Presence of aquatic animals including fish may cause mutilation of the dead body which accelerates the process of decomposition due to invasion by microorganisms.

FLOATATION OF A DEAD BODY ON WATER

In India, floatation of a dead body on water occurs usually by 24 h after death in summer. In winter, it takes about 2–3 days to float. In cold or temperate countries, time required for floatation is about 2–3 days in summer and 1–2 weeks in winter.

Factors Influencing Floatation

i. **Decomposition:** Early decomposition causes early floatation of the dead body, because accumulation of gas in the tissue increases the buoyancy of the body.
ii. **Salinity of water:** Floatation occurs early in salty water due to higher specific gravity.
iii. **Stagnant water:** Promotes early floatation by way of causing early decomposition.
iv. **Clothing:** It causes early floatation, as it is lighter than water due to air bubbles in between the spaces of the fabrics.
v. **Age:** Bodies of mature newly born float earlier than stillborn or immature ones.
vi. **Sex:** Female bodies are lighter, because of more fat content, so female bodies float early.
vii. **Season:** Floatation is early in summer than in winter, warm temperature being favorable for decomposition.

ENTOMOLOGY

Forensic entomology: It is the branch of science which deals with study of insects and other arthropods found in dead bodies that can shed light on time since death, the length of body's exposure, and whether the body was moved.

- It is important in entomological evidence for the identification of the insect species collected in association with the dead body or its surroundings.
- The forensic entomologist can use a number of different techniques including species succession, larval weight, larval length, and a more technical method—*accumulated degree hour technique* which can be very precise, if the necessary data is available.
- Invasion of the dead body by maggots is an important cause of early decomposition and destruction of the dead body. Maggots are larvae of flies. The most important insects that are typically involved in the process include the flesh flies (Sarcophagidae) and blowflies (Calliphoridae). The green bottle fly seen in the summer is a blowfly.
- Usually, three types of flies deposit or lay eggs, e.g., common house fly (*Musca domestica*), green bottle fly (*Lucilia sericata*) and blue bottle fly (*Calliphora vomitoria*). They lay eggs near the moist areas of the body, like the nose, mouth, near the canthi of the eyes or axillary folds. Laying of eggs may be as early as 8–9 h after death.
- *In case of common house fly*, hatching of the eggs occurs after about 8–12 h (first instar). The first change in the larva or the maggot occurs in 1–2 days (second instar), the second in another 1–2 days (3rd instar). They are pale-whitish, 3–9 mm long, thinner at the mouth end, and have no legs. The larva continues in this stage for 2–3 days. Then, it molds into a pupa (reddish or brown in color) and takes about a week to change to an adult fly **(Fig. 9.13)**.
- Thus, the maturation of these insects (egg-larva-pupa-adult insect) serves as a biological clock which takes 1–2 weeks following death (but depends on the species and on ambient temperature).

Hence, to determine time of death, one has to identify the variety of the maggot and the stage in which it is present in the body.

Under certain specific environmental conditions, modified decomposition of the body occurs, wherein instead of total destruction, the dead body is preserved for a pretty long period. The two varieties of modified decomposition are known as adipocere and mummification.

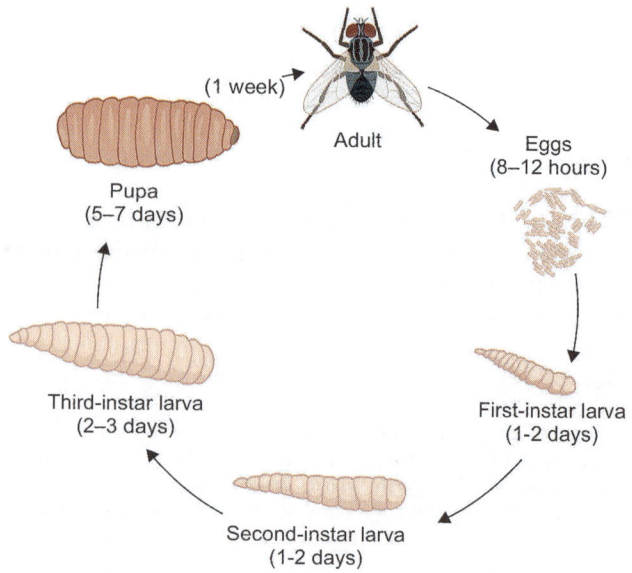

Fig. 9.13: Life cycle of house fly

> **FM 2.9**
> Describe adipocere.

ADIPOCERE (SAPONIFICATION)

Definition: Adipocere (Latin *adipo:* fat, *cire:* wax; 'grave wax') is formation of an offensive, sweet rancid smelling, soft, whitish or grayish white, crumbly, waxy and greasy material (similar to soap) occurring in fatty tissues of a dead body **(Fig. 9.14)**. It is a modification of decomposition.

Time required for formation: In warm and moist environment, it may occur by the end of 1 week (earliest recorded—3 days). In temperate countries, it starts in 3 weeks and completes in about 3 months.

Mechanism of Formation

- Adipocere consists mainly of fatty acids formed due to postmortem hydrolysis and hydrogenation of body fats.
- The process needs water which is provided by the body fluid of soft tissues.
- The chemical reaction essentially involves conversion of unsaturated liquid fats (oleic acid) to saturated solid higher fatty acids, like palmitic, stearic and hydroxystearic acid, mostly palmitic acid.

Distribution

It forms at any site where fatty tissue is present.
- The face, buttocks, breasts and abdomen are the usual sites. In case of a female body, this change will be seen almost all over the body due to presence of a good amount of subcutaneous fat.
- Internally, small muscles are dehydrated and become very thin, and have a uniform grayish color. The depths of large muscles have a pink/red color with complete conversion of the fat to adipocere.

- The intestines and lungs are usually parchment-like in consistency and thinness.
- The liver is prominent and retains its shape.

Fate of the body: Usual decomposition is prevented when the body remains submerged in water or buried in moist graves or damp soil, as the process of adipocere formation utilizes most of the fluid, and hence the body is not invaded by microorganisms. However, dry concealment may also led to adipocere formation; the internal body water providing for the hydrolysis.

Factors Influencing Adipocere Formation

A warm, moist and anaerobic environment favors adipocere formation.

i. **Environmental temperature:** Heat accelerates, and cold retards adipocere formation in a body.
ii. **Moisture:** Moisture is essential for chemical reactions to occur. It occurs rapidly in bodies submerged in water than in damp soil.
iii. **Bacterial infection:** Early activity by anerobes, such as *Clostridium perfringens* assist in the reaction. The bacteria produce lecithinase which facilitates hydrolysis and hydrogenation.
iv. **Built:** In obese people and mature newborn, it is formed quickly.
v. **Age:** Fetuses <7 months do not show adipocere formation.
vi. **Air current:** It retards adipocere formation by evaporation of the body fluid, and by reducing the body temperature.
vii. **Running water:** Adipocere formation is retarded as the electrolytes are washed away from the surface of the body, which is necessary for the change.

Medico-legal Importance

i. **Time since death:** It gives a rough estimate about the time since death.
ii. **Identification:** When the process involves the face, the features are well-preserved, which helps in identification.
iii. **Recognition of injuries:** The cause of death may be determined, since injuries can be recognized.
iv. **Place of disposable of body:** Some idea about the place of disposal of the body can be made, since its formation requires a warm place with high humidity or presence of moisture or water.

> **FM 2.9**
> Describe mummification.

MUMMIFICATION

Definition: It is the rapid dehydration/desiccation and shriveling of the dead body from evaporation of water,

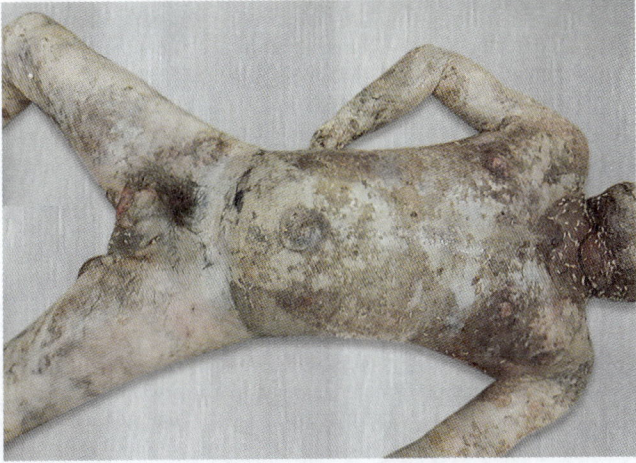

Fig. 9.14: Adipocere formation

with preservation of natural appearances and features of the body.
- It is a modification of putrefaction (*dry decomposition*).
- The entire body loses weight, becomes thin, stiff, brittle and odorless.
- The process of normal decomposition of the dead body is prevented, as the growth of the microorganisms is retarded.

Salient Features

- It begins in the exposed parts of the body, like face (lips, tip of nose), hands and feet, and then extends to the entire body including the internal organs **(Fig. 9.15)**.
- The *skin* may be translucent due to absorption of the liquefied subcutaneous fat. It is usually shrunken and contracted, dry, brittle, leathery and rusty-brown in color. The skin is stretched tightly across anatomical prominences, such as the cheek bones, chin, costal margins and hips, adheres closely to the bones, and often covered with fungal growths.
- The *internal organs* become shrunken, hard, dark-brown and black, and become a single mass, and may not be identifiable.
- Collagen, elastic tissues, cardiac and skeletal muscle, cartilage and bone are usually demonstrable histologically in the mummified material.
- Occasionally, a body may show evidence of mummification in certain parts and adipocere changes in others. Thus, there may be adipocere in cheeks, abdomen and buttocks with mummification of the arms and legs.

Time required for mummification: It varies between 3–12 months or longer.

Factors Favoring Mummification

i. **Hot environment:** As in the deserts.
ii. **Dry atmosphere:** Mummification cannot occur in humid conditions.
iii. **Free air movement:** It helps in rapid evaporation of body fluids.
iv. **Contact of the body with absorbing media:** A dead body lying in shallow grave, in dry sandy soils mummifies early due to absorption of body fluid rapidly.
v. **Poisoning:** Chronic arsenic or antimony poisoning favors the process of mummification.

Medico-legal importance: They are same as adipocere.

Major differences between adipocere and mummification are given in **Diff. 9.7**.

Summary of postmortem changes is given in Synopsis (beginning of the Unit).

Discuss estimation of time since death.

ESTIMATION OF TIME SINCE DEATH (TSD)/POSTMORTEM INTERVAL (PMI)

- **Postmortem interval (PMI):** It is the time that has elapsed since a person has died, i.e., it is the time interval between death and the examination of the body.
- **Thanatochemistry:** Techniques used to determine the time since death by chemical means.
- **Thanatomicrobiome:** Study of the microbes colonizing the internal organs and orifices after death.
- Determination of the time of death is important in both criminal and civil cases.
    - In civil cases, the time of death might determine who inherits property or whether an insurance policy was in force.

> **Postmortem interval is important in criminal cases:**
> - To know when crime was committed
> - It gives the police a starting point for their inquiries, and allows them to deal with the information available more efficiently
> - It might enable to exclude some suspects
> - To confirm or disprove an alibi
> - To check the suspect's statements.

DIFFERENTIATION 9.7: Adipocere and mummification

S.No.	Feature	Adipocere	Mummification
1.	Characteristic feature	Chemical change of fatty tissues into fatty acids	Dehydration or desiccation
2.	Basic difference	Moist putrefaction	Dry putrefaction
3.	Smell	Rancid smell	Odorless
4.	Moisture	Gains moisture and undergo hydrolysis	Looses moisture
5.	Ideal conditions	Warm temperature, moisture, less air, bacteria, and fat splitting enzymes	High temperature, dry condition, and free circulation of air
6.	External appearance	Pale, semi fluid material, waxy, greasy to touch	Discolored, leathery and stretched skin, colonization of molds
7.	Time since death	3 weeks to 3 months	3–12 months

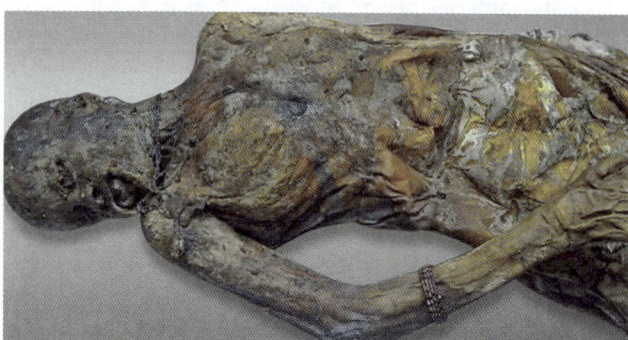

Fig. 9.15: Mummified dead body

- For all practical purposes, in many cases only gross estimation of TSD may be possible. In most cases in our country, time of death is usually estimated from the physical changes noticeable in the dead body. This necessitates *use of a range* for the estimated time of death, giving due consideration to the biological variable factors.
- The range of time provided is at best an educated guess, based on knowledge and experience, and is subject to error.

Physical Changes Useful for Estimation of TSD

Evidence for estimating the time of death may come from three sources **(Box 9.2)**:

1. *Corporal (physical) evidence*: present in the body.
2. *Environmental and associated evidence*: present in the vicinity of the body.
3. *Anamnestic evidence*: based on the deceased's ordinary habits, movements and day-to-day activities.

   i. **Changes in the eye**
   - **Eyeball** becomes flaccid due to fall in IOP within 4-8 h after death.
   - **Sclera:** If the eyelids remain open, there is deposition of dust particles which is triangular and dark brown-black in color (*tache noire*) and can be seen within 3-6 h after death.
   - **Cornea** becomes hazy and opaque within 6-8 h after death.
   - **Retina:** Segmentation of blood in retinal vessels (*Kevorkian sign*/cattle trucking) occurs immediately after death which can be seen with an ophthalmoscope.
   - **Vitreous humor:** There is an increase in potassium and hypoxanthine after death.

   ii. **PM staining:** The extent of appearance and its fixation give some idea about TSD. Mottled patches over the dependent parts occur within 1–3 h. These patches coalesce in 4–6 h. The lividity is fully developed and fixed in about 8–12 h.

   iii. **Algor mortis:** It is an useful single indicator of the PMI during the first 24 h after death in temperate countries. The body attains environmental temperature in about 16–20 h after death in temperate countries.

> **Box 9.2** Changes useful for determining the TSD **(Fig. 9.2)**
> i. Changes in the eye
> ii. PM staining
> iii. Algor mortis
> iv. Rigor mortis
> v. Putrefaction
> vi. Insect activity
> vii. Stomach and intestinal contents
> viii. Contents of urinary bladder
> ix. Bone marrow changes
> x. Biochemical changes
> xi. Circumstantial evidence

   iv. **Rigor mortis:** Appearance, distribution or its passing away are the most important physical changes, which are taken into account for estimation of TSD.
   - In tropical countries, it commences in 1–2 h after death, takes about 9–12 h to develop from head to foot, persists for another 12 h, and gradually passes off in the same order as it appeared.
   - In temperate countries, rigor mortis begins in 3–4 h, becomes fully established after 8–12 h, remains unchanged for up to 36 h, and then disappears in 2–3 days.

> **NOTA BENE**
> In temperate countries, rough guide to estimate TSD is as follows:
> ♦ If the body feels warm and is flaccid, death is within <3 h
> ♦ If the body feels warm and is stiff, death is 3–8 h back
> ♦ If the body feels cold and is stiff, death is 8–36 h back
> ♦ If the body feels cold and is flaccid, death has occurred >36 h back.

   v. **Putrefaction:** Among the delayed changes after death (and after rigor mortis), this change is the single best one for the purpose of estimation of TSD.
   - In India, greenish discoloration of the abdomen over the cecum and the flanks appears in about 12–24 h after death in summer.
   - It spreads over the whole of the abdomen and the rest of the body within the next 24 h.
   - Marbling commences after 24 h. Putrefactive odor is noticed at about the same time. By 36–48 h, marbling is prominent.
   - In 12–18 h after death, gases collect in the intestines and distend the abdomen. From 18–36 or 48 h, gas formation is abundant.
   - In about 36 h, in summer, the female genitalia appear pendulous. In about 48–72 h, the rectum and the uterus protrude.

   Adipocere and mummification: The time required for adipocere formation in our country is 5–15 days. The time required for the complete mummification of a body varies greatly from 3–12 months or longer.

   vi. **Insect activity:** By about 18–36 h, flies lay their eggs. The eggs hatch into maggots or larvae in about 12–24 h. In the course of 4–5 days, maggots develop into pupae, and in another 4–7 days pupae into adult flies. Lice usually die within 3–6 days after the death of the individual.

   vii. **Stomach contents:** From the state of digestion of food and the quantity of food substance in the stomach, it can be estimated for what period the person survived after taking his last meal. If the quality, quantity and the time of the last meal taken can be known, the approximate TSD can be made out indirectly.
   - Diet rich in carbohydrates leaves the stomach earliest, a protein meal leaves the stomach more rapidly than a fatty meal. Milk leaves rapidly, whereas meat and pulses are retained longer.

- A light meal usually leaves the stomach within 1–2 h, a medium-sized meal in 3–4 h, and a heavy meal within 5–8 h.
- If the stomach is full and contains undigested food, it can be said that death occurred within 2–4 h of eating of the last meal, and if the food is digested (indistinguishable) then >4 h.

viii. **Intestinal contents:** The head of the digested meal reaches the hepatic flexure in about 6–8 h, splenic flexure in 9–12 h, and pelvic colon in 12–18 h. In the pelvic colon, it may stay as feces for up to 12 h.

From the content of the pelvic colon and the rectum, it can be said if the person attended the nature's call within last few hours or not. If it contains feces, death may have occurred in the night and if empty, sometime after evacuation in the morning (depending upon the person's habit).

ix. **Contents of urinary bladder:** The amount of urine in the bladder may give some indication of TSD in some cases. If a body is found in the morning with the bladder full, then inference may be drawn that he might have died before the usual time of leaving his bed, since the first activity in the morning after leaving the bed is evacuating the bladder.

x. **Changes in the bone marrow:** Within 1 h of death, nuclei of the neutrophils in marrow start swelling, and by 4–5 h the nuclei become round. By 10–12 h, the outline of the neutrophils is lost.

xi. **Histological changes in kidney:** Within 12 h, architecture is maintained, there is mild cloudy swelling and disruption of tubular epithelium. Severe cloudy swelling, swollen/collapsed glomeruli, and disturbed architecture are seen by 24 h. By 36 h, these changes are marked and diffuse throughout the kidney parenchyma, and by 72 h, severe autolytic changes are seen.

xii. **Biochemical and enzymatic changes:** These changes are dependent on the cooling of the body. These are helpful and more suitable for cold or temperate countries.
- *Cerebrospinal fluid:* Cisternal fluid is examined. Lactic acid, non-protein nitrogen (NPN) and amino acid content increase in the first 15 h after death, but the rate is not uniform. Potassium, ammonia, creatine and uric acid increase, and glucose values decrease after death.
- *Blood:* Potassium and magnesium levels rise, whereas sodium and chloride fall after death. Lactic acid, creatine, NPN and amino acid nitrogen content increases after death. By about 12 h after death, the level of amino acid nitrogen is about 10 mg%, NPN is about 40 mg%, and that of creatine is about 10 mg%.

The enzymes acid phosphatase, amylase, serum glutamate-oxalate transaminase (SGOT) and lactate dehydrogenase (LDH) increase after death.

- *Vitreous humor:* Potassium, magnesium, ammonia, urea, creatinine, uric acid, hypoxanthine and lactic acid increase after death. Steady rise in vitreous potassium values occur up to 100 h after death, and linear rise of hypoxanthine up to 120 h. A combination of the two generate the greatest accuracy with respect to estimation of TSD.
  - Levels of calcium, sodium, ascorbic acid, glucose, enzymes and pyruvic acid in the vitreous fall after death.

NOTA BENE

Formulae used for vitreous potassium
- **Madea's formula:** TSD = 5.26 × [K$^+$]–30.9
- **Sturner's formula:** TSD = 7.14 × [K$^+$]–39.1

Where [K$^+$] is the potassium concentration (mmol/L)

- *Synovial fluid:* There is linear rise of potassium which doubles within 2 days.

xiii. **Facial hair growth:** Rate of growth of hair after shaving is 0.4 mm/day. Hair does not grow after death. If the time of his last shave is known, then survival time can be calculated, and the TSD can be estimated indirectly.

xiv. **Circumstantial evidences:** Pocket articles like letters, diary, cinema-show ticket, etc., may indicate in some way the date and time up to which the person survived.
- Degree of coagulation of milk, staleness of food on a table, and when the neighbor saw the person, etc. may be valuable.
- The dress should be noted as regards to whether the person is fully dressed or in the night dress.
- In some cases, the wrist watch may stop, and thus may indicate the date and exact time of death.
- Some idea about the earliest period of death can be made from the newspaper present by the side of the dead body.
- If a body is lying on the grass, it becomes pale due to non-exposure to sun for about 5 days.

When a dead body is still warm, not rigid, without any permanent haziness of cornea, the death of the person possibly has occurred within the last 1 h in summer and within last 2 h in winter.

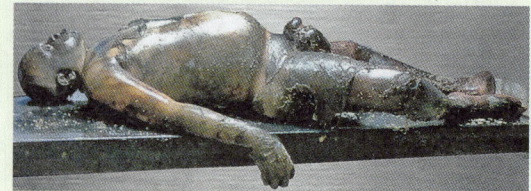

A discolored dead body was found in hot and humid climate, with absence of rigor mortis, non-descriptive PM staining, tongue protruding, peeling off skin (limbs), swollen penis and scrotum and maggot infestation. What could be the probable TSD?

A. 12–24 h
B. >1 week
C. 48–72 h
D. 3–5 days

Recent Advances for Estimating TSD (*Methods are still experimental*)
a. **Supra-vital reactions:** Supra-vital reactions can be used for estimation of TSD. Madea categorized the PMI into four stages:
   i. Latency period, where despite stoppage of circulation, the tissue still performs aerobic respiration till the depletion of its stores.
   ii. Survival period, where there is loss of tissue function, but they can be re-activated using external stimuli, e.g., electrical stimulation of nerves.
   iii. Resuscitation period, where the ability of the tissue to recover is completely lost.
   iv. Supra-vital period is the survival period of tissue after complete, irreversible ischemia.

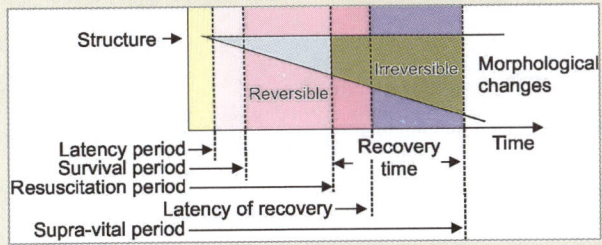

The survival period encompasses the latency period. The resuscitation period encompasses both the latency and survival periods, and the supra-vitality period includes all the other three. For e.g., the resuscitation period of skeletal muscle is about 2–3 h, but supra-vital period may extend to 20 h. Similarly, cardiac muscles have a resuscitation period of 3.5 to 4 min, while the supra-vital period may extend up to 2 h. A method for estimating the PMI was developed using the electric excitability of orbicularis oculi using surface electrodes.

b. **Thanatomicrobiome:** Majority of the microbes within the human body are the obligate anaerobes, *Clostridium spp*. Time-dependent changes in the thanatomicrobiome within internal organs can estimate the TSD as a human body decays. Current studies of thanatomicrobiome are based on 16S RNA sequencing for bacteria (microbial marker). Comprehensive knowledge of the number and abundance of each organ's signature microorganisms could be useful for estimating TSD.

c. After death, internal nucleases within the cells cause DNA to degrade into smaller fragments over time. If these fragments can be isolated and visualized, and if the fragmentation is proved to be measurable and quantifiable, it can be a good indicator of the PMI. Hence, it has been suggested that the *degree of DNA degradation* reflects the TSD.
   i. **Flow-cytometry:** In flow-cytometry, one correlates the degree of DNA degradation in tissue from the deceased with tissue from other individuals whose time of death is known, i.e., controls. Present analysis involves use of splenic tissue.
   ii. **Single cell gel electrophoresis (comet assay)** method is used to detect the relationship between the amount of degraded DNA and PMI in different tissues. It has been found that there is a linear relationship between the degradation rate of nuclear DNA and PMI in brain and liver cells.
   iii. **Fluorescence tissue spectroscopy** using time-dependent variations on the fluorescence spectrum and its correlation with the time elapsed after regular metabolic activity cessation has been investigated. The skin alterations occurring after death result in fluorescence changes (*skin autofluorescence*) that may be detected by spectroscopic measurement and correlated to the PMI.

d. **Cell death proteins (mRNA expression of proteins):** During decomposition, the cells are progressively destroyed and there is release and damage of cellular components and metabolites. Analysis is done of mRNA expression of Fas Ligand (FasL) and phosphatase and tensin homologue deleted on chromosome 10 (PTEN) by quantitative-PCR. A time-dependent increase in the mRNA levels of PTEN and FasL proteins (implicated in signaling pathways) and PMI up to 6 h after death has been found.

e. **Degradation of cardiac Troponin I (cTnI):** Cardiac Troponin I is a basic regulatory protein found as part of a ternary complex responsible for calcium dependent muscle contraction. Analyzing the degradation-banding pattern of cTnI in postmortem tissue is useful in the determination of PMI (0–5 days). The analysis involves extraction of the protein, separation by denaturing gel electrophoresis (SDS-PAGE) and visualization by Western blot using cTnI specific monoclonal antibodies.

f. **High-mobility group box-1 protein:** High mobility group box-1 (HMGB1), a nonhistone DNA-binding protein is released by eukaryotic cells upon necrosis, so its detection in serum by enzyme-linked immunosorbent assay (ELISA) may be related to PMI. The preliminary results indicate a time-dependent increase in the levels of HMGB-1 protein after death.

g. **Redistribution of blood components:** Postmortem chemical changes in compositions of the plasma are time-dependent, and various components including hemoglobin, proteins, lipids and nucleic acids may contribute to the discrimination of the samples at different time points. The technique of attenuated total reflection-Fourier transform infrared (ATR-FTIR) spectroscopy was used to monitor biochemical changes in plasma with increasing PMI and was useful to predict within 48 h PMI. Spectroscopic methods has also been used in pericardial fluid to assess variables associated with amide I, amide II, COO-, C-H bending, and C-O or C-OH vibrations arising from proteins, polypeptides, amino acids and carbohydrates respectively which can useful to estimate PMI.

h. **Chondrocytes' viability:** The structure and anatomical location together with its mechanical, physical and chemical properties enable chondrocytes to survive for several weeks after the individual's death. Therefore, cartilage could be used for PMI determination. A gradual decrease in chondrocytes' viability can be used for PMI determination.

i. **RNA degradation of dental pulp:** RNA degradation from the pulps of healthy wisdom teeth and premolars was determined as RNA integrity number (RIN) with Agilent Bioanalyzer and subsequently by amplification of different length products by PCR after reverse transcription. The RNA integrity analysis was able to determine the PMI in the first 21 days.

j. **Skin-specific mRNA marker:** The expression levels of skin-specific mRNA marker 'late cornified envelope 1C' (LCE1C mRNA) were serially detected and quantified using real-time PCR. The expression levels of LCE1C decreased with increasing the time interval in time-dependent manner, whereas changing the surrounding temperatures did not show any statistical significance which can be useful for estimation of PMI.

k. **Cellular changes in gingival tissue:** Light microscopic (homogenization and eosinophilia in the granular and spinous cell layer, cytoplasmic vacuolation, karyolysis, pyknosis etc.) and ultrastructure changes (lysis of desmosomes, increased intercellular space small spherical-shaped lysosomes, swollen mitochondria etc.) helps in estimation of early PMI.

l. **Non-invasive thermometry:** Early PMI reconstruction using skin thermometry in conjunction with a comprehensive thermodynamic finite-difference model has been developed. PMIs reconstructed using this approach deviated no more than ±38 minutes from their corresponding true PMIs (which ranged from 5 to 50 hours), significantly improving on the ±3 to ±7 hours uncertainty of the gold standard.

m. **Dental enamel in drowned decomposed bodies:** Diatoms attached to the surface of dental enamel increased with prolongation of immersion time. Further, as the immersion time increased, the quantity of O, Si, Mg, K, Al, and S detected on the

> surface of dental enamel increased, while the quantity of the main dental components (Ca and P) gradually decreased. A regression formula has been developed to estimate the immersion time and hence TSD.

PRESERVATION OF DEAD BODIES

Preservation of dead bodies may occur naturally, if disposed off in favorable environmental condition. Dead bodies may also be preserved artificially.

The methods are:
  i. *Use of dry ice (carbon dioxide ice):* It is a common and traditional technique for preservation at home. Dry ice is applied on different parts of the body, which freeze on contact. The ice must be changed every 24 h.
  ii. *Freezing* the body below 0°C, and at –20°C in refrigeration equipment (refrigerate lockers, beds or technical ramps) can preserve the body for years.*
  iii. The body is treated with *chemical agents,* like lead sulfide, arsenic and potassium carbonate which prevent bacterial action and autolysis.
  iv. Embalming.

Embalming or Thanatopraxia

- It is the art and science of preserving the dead body with antiseptics and preservatives to delay putrefaction.
- The three goals of embalming are sanitization, presentation and preservation (or restoration).
- This treatment results in coagulation of proteins, fixation of tissues, bleaching and hardening of organs and conversion of blood into a brownish mass. It produces a chemical stiffening similar to rigor mortis, and normal rigor does not develop.
- *Reason*: This may be required for public display at a funeral, religious reasons, for using as anatomical specimens, and legal requirements for international repatriation of human remains.
- *Anatomical embalming* is performed into a closed circulatory system. The fluid is usually injected with an embalming machine into an artery under high pressure. Then it is allowed to swell and saturate the tissues. These cadavers have a typically uniform gray coloration due to high formaldehyde concentration mixed with the blood known as 'formaldehyde gray' or 'embalmer's gray'.
- *Procedure*: The content of the intestine is syringed out or taken out by suction. Then, a six-point injection is made through the two iliac or femoral arteries, subclavian or axillary vessels, and common carotids, with the viscera treated separately with cavity fluid.

  The evacuation of the intestine clears out the prevailing microorganisms, and the formalin fixes the tissue protein and renders it unsuitable for bacterial invasion. Autolysis is also prevented due to chemical fixation of the tissue.
- Typical embalming fluid contains a mixture of formaldehyde, methanol, phenol, glycerin, oil of wintergreen (methyl salicylate), eosin and water. Other chemicals, like glutaraldehyde, sodium borate/citrate may be used.
- *Autopsy cases embalming* differ from standard embalming since postmortem irrevocably disrupts the circulatory system, due to removal of the organs and viscera.

Components of embalming fluid are given in **Table 9.7**.

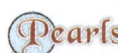

Disadvantages of embalming
- Difficult to interpret any injury or disease.
- Determination of cyanide, alcohol, alkaloids, organic poisons and drugs become difficult.
- Blood grouping may not be possible.
- Thrombi and emboli are dislocated/dislodged.

NOTA BENE

Natron was an important preservative for the Egyptians in their embalming process. Natron referred to a variety of chemical compounds—sodium chloride, sodium carbonate, sodium bicarbonate and sodium sulfate. Aside from mummification, natron was used to make soaps, blue color for ceramics, glass-making and metals, and application on wounds and cuts in 640 CE.

FM 2.6
Discuss presumption of survivorship and death.

PRESUMPTION OF SURVIVORSHIP

Two persons of one family may die in a common circumstance. In such cases, for the purpose of succession of properties of one or both of the deceased persons, it may be necessary to know who died earlier and who died later, i.e.,

TABLE 9.7: Embalming fluid components

Preservatives	Germicide	Buffers	Wetting agents
Formaldehyde Methanol Phenol	Phenol Zephiran chloride Glutaraldehyde	Sodium borate Sodium bicarbonate Sodium carbonate Magnesium carbonate	Glycerin Sorbitol Sodium lauryl sulfate
Anticoagulants	**Dyes**	**Vehicles**	**Other agents**
Sodium oxalate Sodium citrate	Eosin Ponceau	Water (commonly used) Glycerin Sorbitol Alcohol	Methyl salicylate Magnesium chloride Disinfectants

---
*The body of Ashutosh Maharaj, Head of DJJS sect who was declared 'clinically dead' on 28th January, 2014 continues to be preserved in a freezer at –20°C.

who survived whom. By postmortem examination, it may not be possible to say who died earlier and who later, if the deaths have occurred within a gap of a few minutes only. In such a case, it has to be presumed who might have survived whom, so that the problem of succession of property can be solved on that basis.

The case is decided by the facts and evidence available. In this regard, age (adults withstand better than young and elderly), sex (males withstand more than females), constitution (strong and robust withstand better than weak, debilitated and diseased), nature and severity of injuries (extent of hemorrhage, involvement of vital organs), and the mode of death (swimmer survives a nonswimmer) should be taken into consideration.

PRESUMPTION OF DEATH

This is a legal issue which does not have any medical implication or involvement. It is in connection with inheritance or succession of property of a person, missing for a long period, or for claiming insurance money when the individual is alleged to be dead and body is not found.

Sec. 107 IEA states that a person is presumed being alive, if there is nothing to suggest the probability of death within 30 years. **Sec. 108 IEA** states that, if it is proved that the said person has not been heard of for 7 years by them, who are expected to hear about him if he would be alive, then death is presumed.

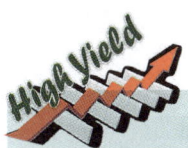

- **Obsolete tests to detect stoppage of respiration:** Winslow's, feather and mirror test.
- **Obsolete tests to detect stoppage of circulation:** Magnus, diaphanous, Icard's and pressure test.
- **Suspended animation:** Vital signs of life are reduced to a minimum; apparent death from which the person can be aroused. Seen in electrocution, head injury, shock, opium and barbiturates poisoning, insanity, heat stroke, newborns.
- **Tache noire:** Brownish to blackish triangles on the sclera at each side of the iris seen after death.
- **Kevorkian sign:** Segmented blood *(cattle trucking)* in retinal vessels.
- From vitreous humor, estimation of time since death is done using K^+ level.
- Algor mortis is cooling of the dead body.
- Curve of cooling pattern of dead body is *sigmoid or inverted 'S' shaped*.
- Rate of cooling of dead body is 1.5 F/h.
- Ideal place to record body temperature in dead body is rectum.
- **Postmortem caloricity:** Instead of cooling, temperature of dead body remains high for initial 2 h. Seen in: heat stroke, pontine hemorrhage, septicemia, tetanus, strychnine poisoning etc.
- **Synonyms of PM staining:** Hypostasis, lucidity, cogitation, vibices, suggillation, cadaveric lividity.
- **Color of PM staining:** Bluish or purplish-red.
- PM staining starts immediately after death, usually mistaken for contusion. Seen in dependent parts; even in internal organs and contact pallor seen in pressure points.
- Extravasation is not a feature of PM staining.
- PM staining gets 'fixed' in 8–12 h and disappears with putrefaction.
- **Recent methods to determine TSD from PM staining:** Calorimetry.
- **Rigor mortis:** Stiffening of muscles of dead body due to depletion of ATP.
- **Nysten's law:** Sequence of rigor mortis: Muscles of jaw → Face and neck → Trunk and arms → Legs and feet.
- Rigor mortis occurs earlier in involuntary muscles than in voluntary muscles.
- **Rigor mortis first seen in:** Heart muscle (involuntary) in 1 h.
- Among voluntary muscles, rigor mortis first appears in muscles of eyelids.
- After embalming, normal rigor mortis does not develop.
- Rigor mortis come early in high temperature, cholera, electrocution, strychnine poisoning.
- Rigor mortis not seen in: Stillborn fetuses <7 months old.
- Cadaveric spasm appears instantaneously after death (selected group of voluntary muscles) with no primary relaxation phase.
- Cadaveric spasm does not involve the involuntary muscles.
- Cadaveric spasm cannot be mimicked. Indicates the cause and manner of death.
- Cadaveric spasm may be seen in drowning.
- Heat stiffening occurs when body is exposed to >65°C.
- **Maceration:** Aseptic autolysis, seen in dead born fetus.

- **Earliest autolytic changes occur in:** Parenchymatous and glandular tissues and in brain.
- **First organ to undergo autolysis:** Pancreas.
- **Microorganisms involved in putrefaction:** *Clostridium perfringens* (most common).
- **Major bacterial enzyme responsible for putrefaction:** Lecithinase
- **'4 Ds' of decomposition:** Discoloration, distension, degradation and dissolution.
- **First external sign of decomposition:** Greenish discoloration over the right iliac fossa.
- **First internal sign of decomposition:** Discoloration of aortic intima.
- Marbling of skin is seen in 36-48 h.
- Liver assumes a *honey comb/Swiss cheese* appearance due to putrefaction.
- **Last organs to putrefy:** Prostate (males) and non-parous uterus (females)—help to identify sex of dead bodies.
- **Order of putrefaction:** Larynx→ Liver→ Brain→ Heart→ Bladder→ Prostate/Nulliparous uterus→ Skin→ Bone.
- Decomposition changes is most commonly dependent on the climate, season, body weight, and clothing.
- **Delayed putrefaction:** Seen in deaths due to poisoning with heavy metals, strychnine and phenol.
- **Casper's dictum:** Rate of putrefaction in soil: water: air = 1: 2: 8.
- **Floatation time of a dead body after drowning:** 24 h in summer (2–3 days in winter).
- Adipocere and mummification are modified forms of putrefaction.
- Adipocere is hydrolysis and hydrogenation of fats; mummification is drying and dehydration of tissues.
- Adipocere has rancid/ammoniacal odor; mummification is odorless.
- Formation of adipocere depends on the pH, temperature, moisture, and lack of oxygen in the environment.
- Arsenic, antimony and natron favor mummification.
- Early postmortem interval is most frequently estimated using the classical triad—livor mortis, algor mortis, and rigor mortis.
- **Most useful indicator to determine TSD during first 24 h:** Algor mortis.
- **Best method estimating TSD** in the early PM period: Temperature based nomogram method.
- **Best criterion for estimation of TSD among delayed changes:** Putrefaction.

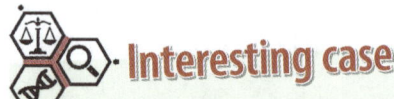 Interesting case

Time Since Death (Case of Joan Bent, 1986)

The frozen body of 47-year-old Joan Bent, a businesswoman in New York was found dead in the trunk of her snow-covered car in a parking lot. Her car keys were in the ignition and purse was on the front seat. She was not sexually assaulted. Frozen condition preserved the state she was in at the time of her death. The husband reported her missing 11 days back, claiming they had meal together before she went to work. When she did not return home that evening, he called the police.

During autopsy, the pathologist opined the cause of death was asphyxia—ligature strangulation. Manner of death was homicide. The pathologist also found intact potato fragments in her stomach. Digestion had not yet occurred. Since potatoes are quick to digest, the condition of her stomach contents indicated that she died less than an hour after her last meal. Circumstantially, this means her husband was still with her when she died. Joan's stomach contents provided critical evidence to establish the murder timelines. Based on this evidence, the husband was convicted of murder and sentenced to 25 years of imprisonment.

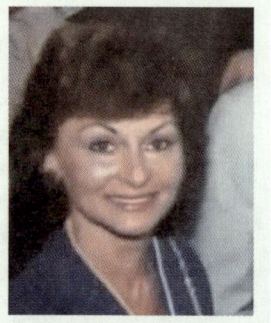

CHAPTER 10

Asphyxial Deaths

LEARNING OBJECTIVES

Must know
1. Asphyxia, etiology, Tardieu spots
2. Judicial hanging, lynching
3. Classification of strangulation; mugging, garroting, bansdola
4. Throttling, PM changes
5. Smothering
6. Choking, gagging, café coronary, Burking
7. Traumatic asphyxia, PM findings
8. Gettler's and Diatom test
9. Sexual asphyxia
10. Hanging, classification, PM changes
11. Ligature strangulation, PM changes
12. Drowning, classification, PM changes
13. Hanging and strangulation (Diff.)
14. Antemortem and postmortem hanging (Diff.)

Desirable to know
1. Hyoid bone fractures
2. Antemortem drowning and postmortem submersion (Diff.)
3. Autoerotic asphyxia and suicide (Diff.)

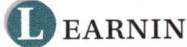

Define, classify and describe asphyxia and medico-legal interpretation of postmortem findings in asphyxial deaths.

Definition: Asphyxia (Greek, 'pulselessness' or 'absence of pulse') is a condition caused by interference with the exchange of oxygen and carbon dioxide in the body.

Asphyxia literally means 'defective aeration of blood' due to any cause.

Pathophysiology of Asphyxia

Pathophysiology of asphyxia is depicted in **Flowchart 10.1**.

Flowchart 10.1: Pathophysiology of asphyxia (vicious cycle)

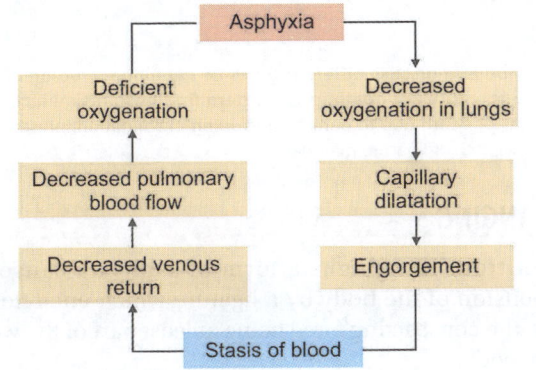

ETIOLOGY OF ASPHYXIA (TABLE 10.1)

It can be:

i. **Mechanical/violent:** Mechanical interference to the passage of air into the respiratory tract by (Fig. 10.1):
   - Closure of the external respiratory orifices by closing the nose and the mouth (e.g., smothering).
   - Closure of the air passages by external pressure on the neck (e.g., hanging, strangulation and throttling), or impaction of foreign bodies (e.g., gagging and choking).
   - Occlusion of the respiratory tract and lungs by fluid (e.g., drowning).
   - Pressure on the chest in a stampede or collapse of a building (e.g., traumatic asphyxia).

ii. **Pathological:** Entry of oxygen to the lungs is prevented by disease of the upper respiratory tract or lungs, e.g., laryngeal edema, spasm, tumors or abscess.

iii. **Toxic or chemical:** Cessation of the respiratory movements due to paralysis of the respiratory center in poisoning with morphine, barbiturates or strychnine. Inhibition of oxidative processes in the tissue preventing the use of oxygen in the blood, e.g., cyanide poisoning.

iv. **Environmental:** Breathing in vitiated atmosphere, as in high altitude, climbing or flying, or inhalation of carbon monoxide (CO), sewer gas or pure helium.

SECTION 1: Jurisprudence and Forensic Medicine

TABLE 10.1: Asphyxial conditions

Classification	Level of obstruction	Cause
Strangulation/hanging	Neck (including larynx, trachea and major blood vessels)	Occlusion of the internal airways by external pressure
Smothering	Mouth and nose	Blockage of the external orifices
Gagging	Nasopharynx	Blockage of the internal airways
Choking	Larynx	Blockage of the internal airways
Overlaying	Mouth, nose, chest	Occlusion of mouth and nose, and blockage of the internal airways by external pressure
Traumatic asphyxia	Chest	Restriction of chest movement due to external mechanical fixation
Wedging	Neck and chest	Occlusion of the internal airways by external pressure
Drowning	Upper and lower respiratory tract	Occlusion of the internal airways by fluid
Toxic asphyxia	Lung	Failure of oxygen transportation/utilization; CO or cyanide poisoning

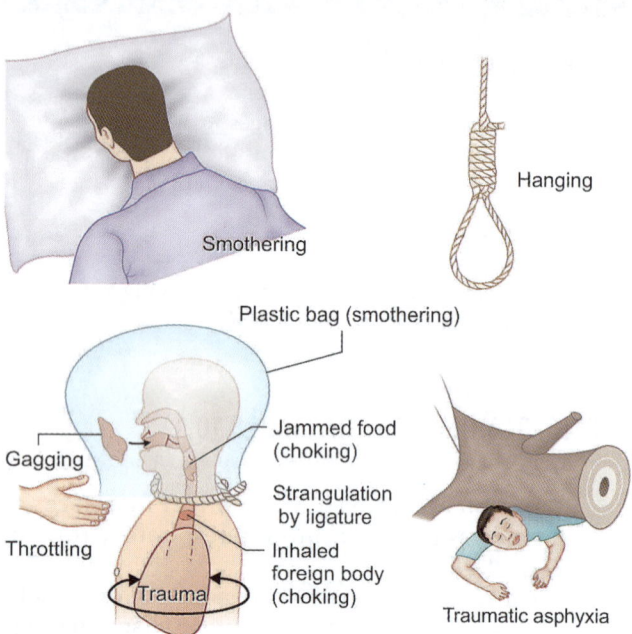

Fig. 10.1: Mechanism of asphyxial deaths of common occurrence in the medico-legal field

v. **Traumatic:** Blunt trauma to the thorax may result in pneumothorax, hemothorax or pulmonary embolism that will interfere with oxygenation and ventilation by compressing otherwise healthy parenchyma.

vi. **Positional/postural:** Positional asphyxia is due to abnormal body position that prevents adequate gas exchange.
- In alcoholics or addicts, where the person is unconscious and the upper portion of the body is lower than rest, or neck is forcibly flexed on the chest, or the body is in a jack-knife position which prevents normal respiratory movements. Deaths in such cases are diagnosed based on circumstantial evidence in combination with excluding other significant underlying causes of death.
- Positional/restraint asphyxia may occur in *hogtying* (individual is placed in a prone position, their hands are cuffed together behind their back, and their ankles are bound and tied to their wrists).

vii. **Iatrogenic:** It is seen during anesthesia.

CLINICAL EFFECTS OF ASPHYXIA

Clinical effects of asphyxia are shown in **Flowchart 10.2**.

Tardieu's or Bayard's ecchymoses/spots: They are usually round, dark-red, well-defined, pin-head sized spots, found in those parts where capillaries are least supported, e.g., conjunctiva, face, epiglottis, subpleural surface of lungs, heart, meninges and thymus.
- They tend to be better made out in fair skinned persons, readily visible in fresh bodies, and disappear with putrefaction.
- They are not pathognomic of asphyxia, and their absence does not exclude asphyxia (rarely seen in drowning).
- It can be seen in other forms of death—electrocution, poisoning, coronary thrombosis, in persons on anticoagulants, with bleeding disorders such as scurvy, leukemia and thrombocytopenia, but distribution is more generalized.

> **NOTA BENE**
>
> **Cyanosis** (Greek, dark blue): It is due to diminished O_2 tension in blood and increase in reduced hemoglobin (≥ 5 g/dL). Blood appears purple or dark in color; usually seen in the lips, tip of nose, and ears lobules, and internally in the lungs, meninges, liver, spleen and kidneys.

FM 2.21
Describe and discuss different types of hanging including clinical findings, causes of death, postmortem findings and medico-legal aspects of death due to hanging including examination, preservation and dispatch of ligature material.

HANGING

Definition: Hanging is a form of asphyxia caused by suspension of the body by a ligature which encircles the neck, the constricting force being at least part of the weight of the body.

CHAPTER 10: Asphyxial Deaths

Flowchart 10.2: Clinical effects of asphyxia

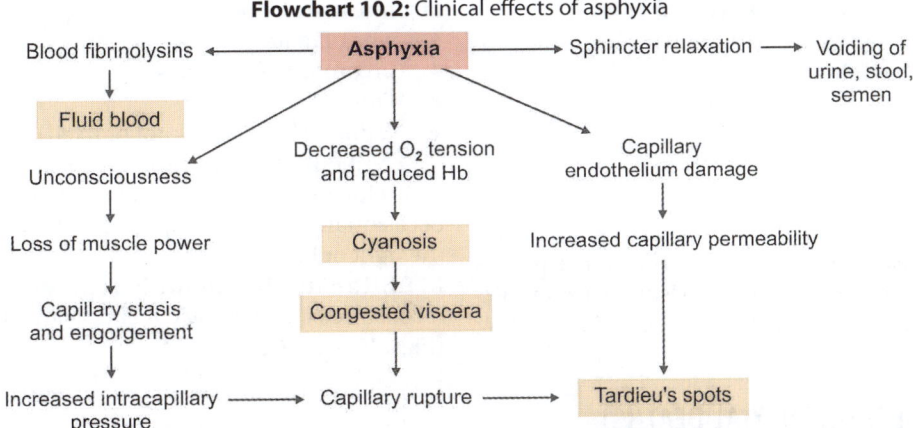

- **Near-hanging:** Patients who survive a hanging injury long enough to reach the hospital.

Classification

Based on Position of the Knot (Figs. 10.2A and B)
- **Typical hanging:** When knot is at nape of neck on the back.
- **Atypical hanging:** Knot of ligature is anywhere other than on occiput.

Based on Degree of Suspension (Figs. 10.3A and B)
- **Complete hanging:** Body is fully suspended and no part touches the ground. Constricting force is weight of the body.
- **Incomplete/partial hanging:** Lower part of the body (toes/feet) is touching the ground, in sitting, kneeling or prone position. Constricting force is weight of the head.

Based on Intent
- Suicidal
- Accidental
- Homicidal
- Autoerotic

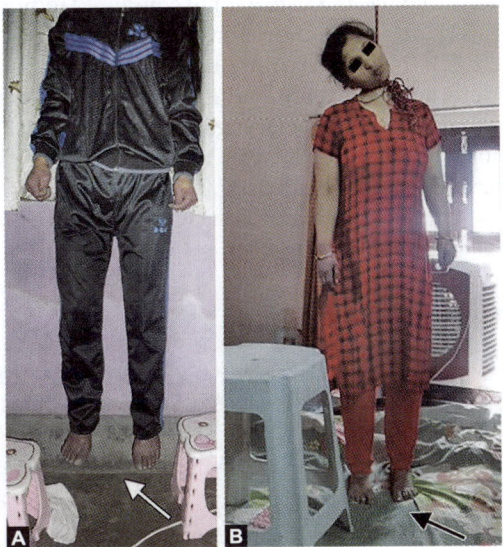

Figs. 10.3A and B: Classification of hanging (degree of suspension): (A) Complete; (B) Incomplete (partial)
[*Courtesy*: (B) Dr Shalender Sharan, Bikaner, Rajasthan]

Cause of Death

i. *Asphyxia:* Constricting force of ligature causes compressive narrowing of laryngeal and tracheal lumina, leading to asphyxia.
ii. *Venous congestion:* Jugular veins are blocked by the ligature, which results in stoppage of cerebral circulation; occurs if ligature is made up of broad and soft material.
iii. *Combined asphyxia and venous congestion.*
iv. *Cerebral ischemia:* It occurs when ligature is made of thin cord.
v. *Reflex vagal inhibition* leading to sudden cardiac arrest.
vi. *Fracture/dislocation of cervical vertebrae:* It is seen in judicial hanging.

Asphyxia is considered as the cause of death in *complete hanging,* and occlusion of neck vessels leading to venous congestion and cerebral ischemia in *incomplete hanging.*

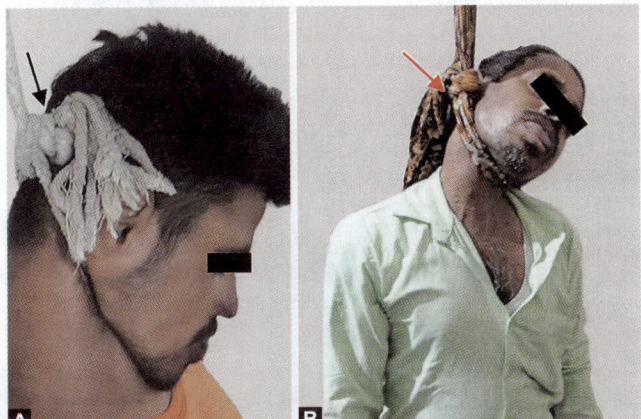

Figs. 10.2A and B: Classification of hanging (position of knot): (A) Typical; (B) Atypical

Delayed deaths are rare which may be due to:
- Aspiration pneumonia
- Edema of lungs, larynx
- Infections
- Infarction of brain
- Hypoxic encephalopathy
- Abscess of brain.

Fatal period: Death is *immediate*, if cervical vertebrae are fractured or if the heart is inhibited, *rapid* if cause is asphyxia and *least rapid* if coma is responsible. Usual period is 3–5 min, which may extend to 5–8 min of suspension leading to death.

AUTOPSY OF NECK (ASPHYXIAL DEATHS)

- When available, multislice spiral computed tomography (MSCT) or magnetic resonance imaging (MRI) of the neck may be carried out before any dissection to determine the state of the soft tissues of the neck, cervical spine and the laryngeal cartilages.
- If not available, then X-ray of the isolated larynx before dissection should be done.
- Photograph of the victim along with ligature (if present) is recommended.

External Examination

General features
- Clothing and personal effects.
- Distribution of lividity, rigor mortis and algor mortis.
- Bleeding from any sites, discharge of semen, urine or fecal matter.
- Ocular or facial petechiae, congestion, cyanosis.
- Tongue protrusion between clenched teeth, and dribbling of saliva.
- Evidence of any other trauma.

Ligature
Is ligature present in situ or removed?

Knot: If in situ, note knot position, number of loops.

Ligature description
- Type of material
- Circumference of noose
- Width
- Nature of knot (slip-knot or fixed).

Frequently, the knot is in the form of a simple slip-knot to produce a running noose, or fixed by granny or reef-knot; occasionally a simple loop is used. Usually, it is present on the right or left side.

If, in situ, it should be cut away from knot and reconstructed by joining cut ends with tape or another cord **(Figs. 10.4A to C).**

Description of ligature mark or furrow
- Course (angled or straight)
- Width
- Associated skin changes or trauma
- Relation to thyroid cartilage
- Pattern
- Neck circumference at level of furrow (to determine degree of neck constriction)
- Transfer of ligature material.

Internal Examination

i. Anterior neck structures are examined at the end of autopsy—following removal of tissues and organs, and collection of toxicology samples—to allow drainage of blood and reduce the possibility of artifactual hemorrhage.
ii. Modified Y-shaped incision is preferable to expose the neck structures.
iii. Anterior neck structures (tongue, larynx, trachea with thyroid gland, attached strap muscles including sternocleidomastoid muscles and submandibular glands) are inspected before removing them.
iv. Tongue is inspected and cut through (tip to base) to observe hemorrhage.
v. It is noted whether hemorrhages are present in the submandibular glands and strap muscles.
vi. The thyroid gland is removed and sectioned.

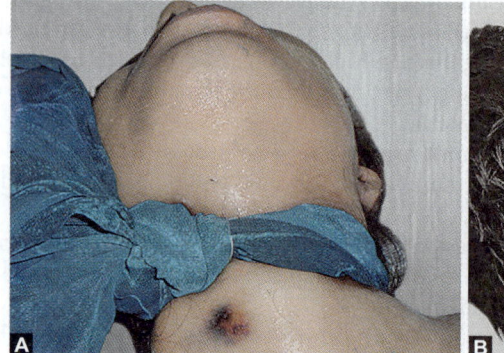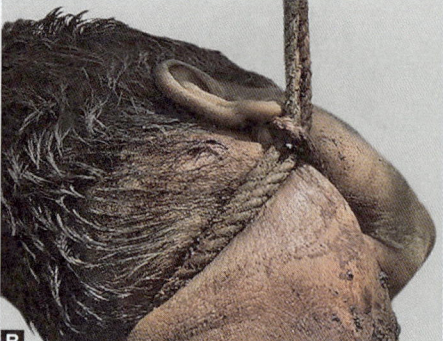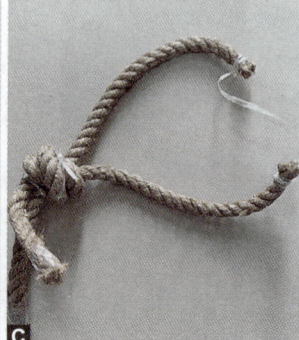

Figs. 10.4A to C: (A) Fixed noose; (B) Running noose; (C) Method of cutting the noose and preserving the cut ends and the knot.
[*Courtesy*: (B) Dr Chandresh Ishwarbhai Tailor]

vii. Any hemorrhage or fracture is noted in the muscle around the cricoid, laminae of the thyroid cartilage and superior horns.
viii. Hyoid bone is palpated, and hemorrhages adjacent to the hyoid or thyrohyoid ligament are also noted. Dissect away the hyoid (note that the lesser cornua are variably long and may be inadvertently cut).
ix. Longitudinal sections through the larynx may be done to note intracartilaginous hemorrhages—in suspected hanging cases.
x. The esophagus and larynx-trachea are dissected posteriorly to observe any submucosal hemorrhage or petechiae, mucosal injuries and aspiration.

Match the following:

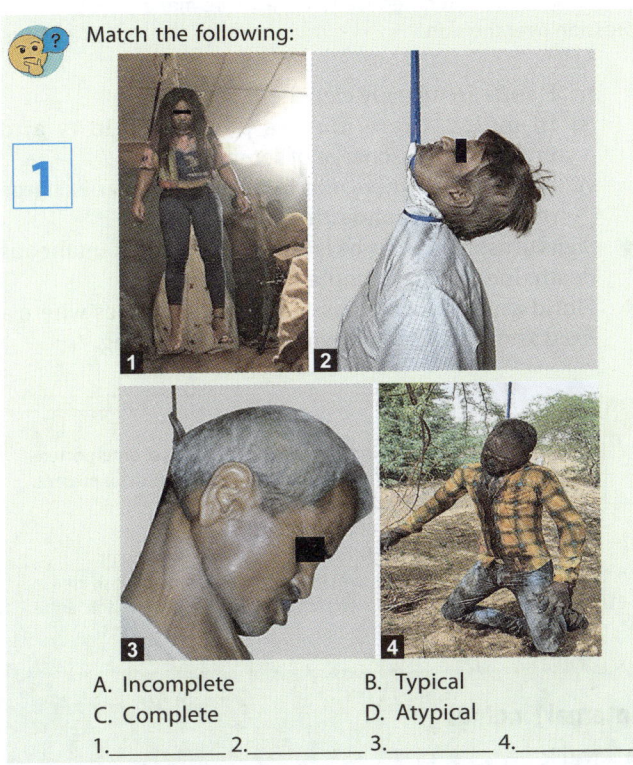

A. Incomplete
B. Typical
C. Complete
D. Atypical
1._____ 2._____ 3._____ 4._____

POSTMORTEM FINDINGS IN HANGING

External Findings

1. **Face**
   i. **Swollen, cyanosed face** due to impaired venous return and accumulation of blood.
   ii. **Prominent eyeballs** due to increased pressure resulting from passive accumulation of blood.
   iii. **Dilated pupils:** If the knot presses on cervical sympathetic, eye of the same side may remain open and pupil is dilated (**la facie sympathique**).* It indicates antemortem hanging.
   iv. **Subconjunctival hemorrhages.**
   v. **Protrusion of tongue** due to pressure on floor of the mouth by ligature. It is usually swollen and blue. Injuries include bite marks with or without underlying small hemorrhages (*'marginal'* hemorrhages).
   vi. **Bleeding from nose/ears** due to impaired venous return and increase in pressure resulting in passive flow of blood.
   vii. Lips and mucous membrane of mouth are blue.
   viii. **Dribbling of saliva:** *Surest sign of antemortem hanging* (**Fig. 10.5**). Excessive salivation occurs when the person is alive, due to pressure and friction caused by ligature material on the submandibular glands. Dribbling of saliva occurs from the angle of mouth which is at a lower level, i.e., from angle opposite to the side of knot. When the knot is on the nape of the neck, it occurs across the middle of lower lip.

2. **Neck**
   i. **Ligature mark ('furrow')**
      • *Site*: Usually above the hyoid bone.
      • *Size/shape:* Depends on the type of material used.
      • *Direction:* It runs obliquely, backwards, non-continuous, upwards and towards the point of suspension. Mark is non-continuous because of a gap at the nape of neck, and hair intervening between ligature material and the skin underneath. When the knot is in contact with the skin, it is usually inverted 'V' shaped, due to extension of ligature material downward on both sides from the knot above (**Fig. 10.6A**).
      • *Skin at the site:* Usually depressed/grooved, pale in color, but later becomes yellowish brown, dry, hard and parchment like with small abrasions at its edges, corresponding to the thickness and edges of the rope (**Fig. 10.6B**). These abrasions, known as *rope burns,* are due to frictional force.

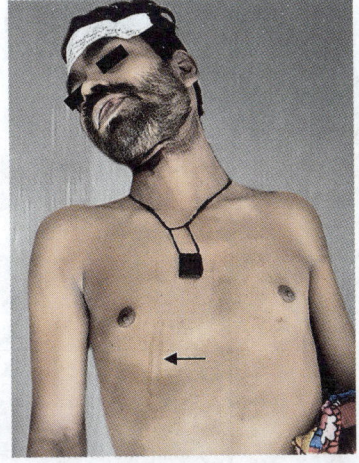

Fig. 10.5: Dribbling of saliva (arrow)—surest sign of antemortem hanging

* First described by Etienne Martin in 1899, it referred to unilateral miosis, with or without ptosis, at opposite side from the knot due to compression and/or stimulation by stretching of the cervical sympathetic trunk.

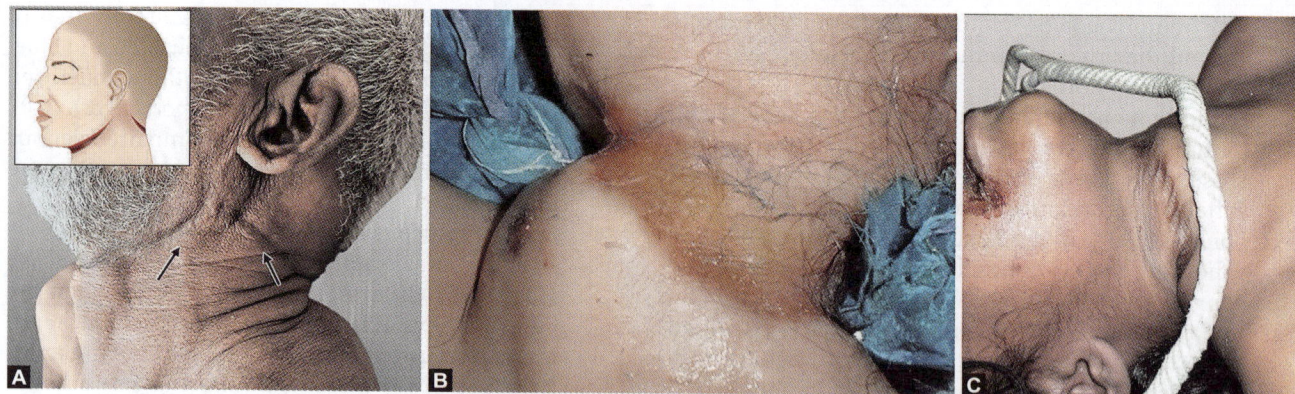

Figs. 10.6A to C: Ligature mark in hanging: (A) Inverted 'V' shaped; (B) Parchmentization of ligature mark; (C) Pattern of ligature impression over the skin

- The pattern of ligature may be reproduced in the furrow (**Fig. 10.6C**).
- Postmortem blisters may be seen on skin squeezed adjacent to the furrow.
- An abraded area below the furrow may indicate upward slippage of the ligature, usually seen when suspension is complete.
- Neck veins above the furrow may be distended.

ii. **Dimension of neck:** Due to prolonged suspension, the neck becomes slender and increases in length.

iii. **Bending of neck:** Neck gets flexed to the side opposite to the knot.

3. **Other parts of body**
   i. *Tardieu's spots:* May be present on forehead, over the eyelids, under the conjunctiva and near the temple.
   ii. Cyanosis of fingernails.
   iii. Purple colored postmortem staining in the lower limbs and lower regions of upper limbs (hands/forearms)—*glove and stocking PM staining* (**Fig. 10.7**).

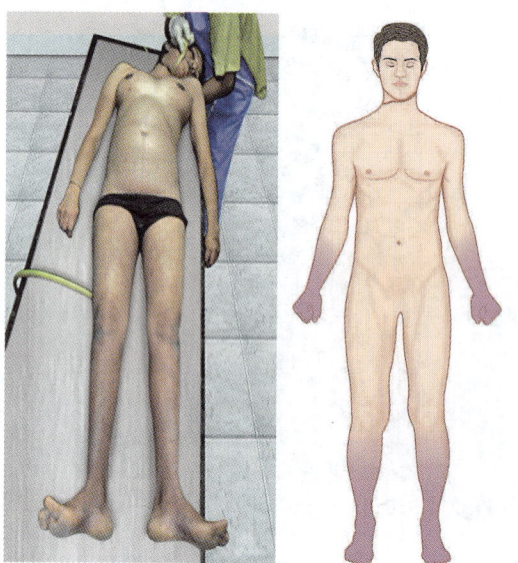

Fig. 10.7: Glove and stocking PM staining in hanging

   iv. Hands are usually clenched.
   v. In males, there may be penile turgidity and involuntary discharge of semen.
   vi. In both sexes, there may be an involuntary discharge of fecal matter and urine.

- Signs of asphyxia may be lacking in case of instantaneous death due to vagal stimulation.
- Florid asphyxial changes can be seen in cases where a fixed knot was used or in incomplete hanging.

NOTA BENE

Based on the ligature mark in the neck, the diagnosis of antemortem hanging can be made if the following triad of characteristics is present:
 i. Streaks or bands of reddened or pink tissue
 ii. Imprint of the pattern of the ligature in the furrow
 iii. Sloping or upward angle towards the suspension point.
Microscopically, engorgement in the reddened and pinkish area in contrast to the adjacent non-engorged and non-hemorrhagic areas may be demonstrated.

Internal Findings

- **Neck**
   i. Subcutaneous tissue underneath the ligature mark is dry, white, firm and glistening (**Fig. 10.8**). Platysma and sternomastoid may show hemorrhages and are sometimes ruptured.
   ii. Hyoid bone may be fractured in persons, more commonly above the age of 40 years. The fracture is usually due to ligature forcing the hyoid bone backwards, which results in increased divergence of greater horns (*anteroposterior compression fracture*), but it can be a traction fracture.
   iii. Transverse carotid intimal tears may be seen in obese victims, long drops and posteriorly placed knots (**Amussat's sign**).
   iv. Vertebral artery injuries—rupture, intimal tear and subintimal hemorrhage (most frequent) may be present.

CHAPTER 10 : Asphyxial Deaths

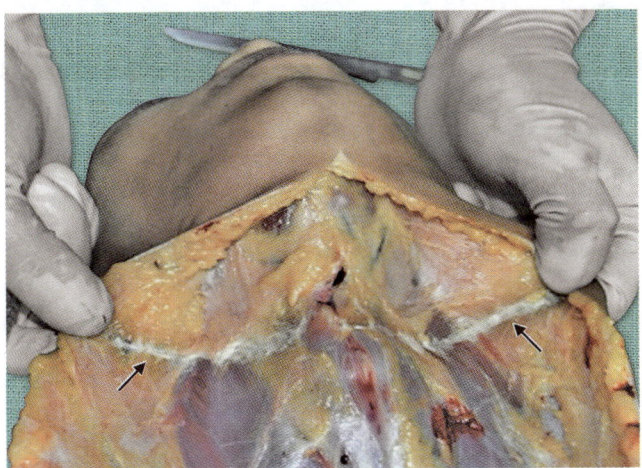

Fig. 10.8: Subcutaneous tissue underneath the ligature mark in hanging—dry, white, firm and glistening (arrows)

v. Larynx and trachea are congested.
vi. Fracture of superior horn of the larynx may be present.

- **Lungs:** They are congested, distended and emphysematous with plenty of Tardieu's spots subpleurally, particularly at the interfaces of the lobes.
- **Brain:** Congested and shows multiple petechiae.
- **Viscera:** All the abdominal organs are congested.
- **Blood:** Fluid and purplish in color.

NOTA BENE

- There may be hemorrhages on ventral surface of the intervertebral disks beneath the anterior longitudinal ligament in the lumbar spine (**Simon's sign**—a vital sign of hanging). It may also be seen in other traumatic elongation or overextension of spinal column (e.g., traffic accidents), drowning and putrefaction ('false positive').
- Pneumomediastinum and cervical soft tissue emphysema has been observed in postmortem MSCT, as well as visible in gross neck dissection in a hanged person. It is seen as frothy air, soap bubble-like formations in superficial and/or deep connective tissue between the neck muscles up to the ligature mark, and interpreted as a vital sign (if putrefaction is ruled out).

- Complete toxicological investigation of hanging deaths should be done, even when the 'obvious' cause of death is asphyxia due to hanging.
- Some of these cases may involve psychoactive substances (most often alcohol and cannabis).

MEDICO-LEGAL QUESTIONS

Q. Whether the hanging was suicidal, homicidal or accidental?

- **Suicide:** Hanging is a common method of asphyxial suicide in many countries. Person can be between 10 and 80 years of age, more common in males. Point of suspension remains approachable to the suicider. Partial hanging is almost always suicidal in nature. A history of a previous attempt may be present, and generally committed in a secluded place (victim's home is the most frequent site). Suicidal note may be left behind. There should be a motive for committing suicide. Fibers of ligature material may be present in the clenched hand.
- **Homicide:** Very rare. Not ordinarily possible in an adult victim, unless intoxicated or made unconscious or the victim is either a child or a debilitated person. Homicide should be suspected where:
  i. There are signs of violence/disorder of furniture
  ii. Clothing of deceased is torn or disarranged
  iii. There are injuries, either offensive or defensive.
- **Postmortem hanging/postmortem suspension:** Person may be murdered and the body suspended to simulate suicide. Look for signs of dragging to the place of suspension. Beam or branch of tree shows evidence of the rope having moved from below upwards, as the body has been pulled up. *In true suicidal hanging, the rope moves from above downwards* (**Diff. 10.1**).
- **Accidental hanging:** Hanging deaths in children <6 years are usually accidental. It has been reported among children while 'playing hanging' (e.g., pretending to be a cowboy) or playing 'Lasso' or getting suspended from playground equipment, and sometimes even in adults (e.g., autoerotic hanging).

 A 26-year-old man was found hanging from a tree. What characteristic feature do you observe? Which side was the knot?

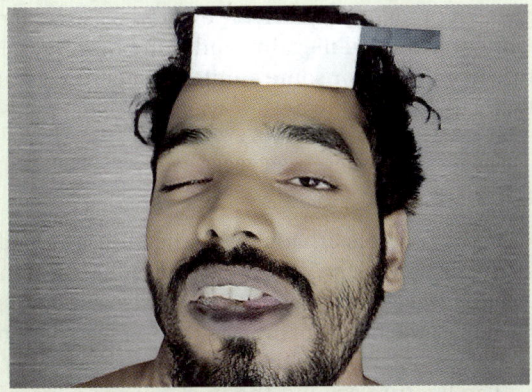

NOTA BENE

Factors which influence the appearance of ligature mark

- *Ligature material:* If it is tough and narrow, then the mark is deep and prominent. If it is soft and broad, then mark is less prominent or deep.
- *Period of suspension:* Longer the suspension, deeper is the groove, and it is more prominent and parchmentized.
- *Degree of suspension:* Mark becomes more prominent and deep in case of total suspension.
- *Weight of the body:* Heavier the body, more marked is the ligature impression.
- *Position of knot:* Main force applied to the neck by ligature is opposite to the point of suspension.
- *Slipping of ligature during suspension:* Produces double impression of ligature.

DIFFERENTIATION 10.1: Antemortem and postmortem hanging

S.No.	Feature	Antemortem hanging	Postmortem hanging
1.	Salivary dribbling mark	Present	Absent
2.	Fecal/urinary stains	May be present	Absent
3.	Ligature mark		
	♦ Direction	Oblique	Circular
	♦ Continuity	Non-continuous	Continuous
	♦ Level in the neck	Above thyroid	At or below thyroid
	♦ Parchmentization	Present	Absent
	♦ Vital reaction	Present	Absent
4.	Knot	Single, simple, on one side of neck	Multiple, granny or reef type on occiput/chin
5.	PM staining		
	♦ Above ligature mark	Present	Absent
	♦ In lower limbs	Present	Absent
	♦ Glove-stocking like	Present	Absent
6.	Evidence of injury		
	♦ Self-inflicted	Present	Absent
	♦ Struggle	Absent	Present
	♦ Tear of carotid artery intima	Present	Absent
	♦ Imprint abrasion	Present	May/may not be present
7.	Elongation of neck	Present	Absent
8.	Cyanosis	Deeply positive	Absent or faintly present
9.	Emphysematous bullae on lungs	Absent	Present
10.	Point of suspension	Compatible with self-suspension	Not so
11.	Histochemistry of ligature mark	Increased serotonin and histamine	Not so

Lynching

Lynching is a form of *homicidal hanging*. A suspect, an accused or an enemy is overpowered by several persons, acting jointly and illegally, and hung him by means of a rope from a tree or some similar object. It was prevalent in North America, where it was practiced by whites on blacks.

Judicial Hanging

♦ In case of judicial hanging, the ligature is looped around the neck with the knot under the chin (submental), but subaural (below auricle) knot is also used. The drop is at least the height of the person (5–7 feet, depending on the weight) and the hanging is complete.
♦ The ligature around the neck causes a forceful jerky impact on the neck at the end of the fall, so as to cause fracture of cervical column (fracture dislocation of C2 from C3, rarely C3 and C4 vertebrae—*hangman fracture*) **(Fig. 10.9)** with stretching or tearing of cervical spinal cord, but not decapitation.*
♦ In judicial hangings, odontoid process is usually not fractured.
♦ However, such fractures are the exception, and the cause of death can be attributed to a range of head and neck injuries, particularly compression or rupture of the vertebral and carotid arteries leading to cerebral ischemia.

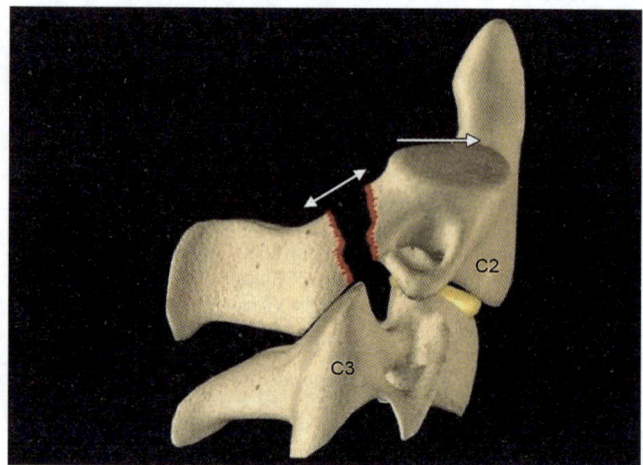

Fig. 10.9: Hangman's fracture

> **FM 2.21**
> Describe and discuss different types of strangulation including clinical findings, causes of death, postmortem findings and medico-legal aspects of death due to strangulation.

STRANGULATION

Definition: It is a form of violent asphyxial death caused by constriction of air passage at the neck by means of a ligature or by any means other than suspension of the body.

---
*There is fracture of the pedicles/lamina of C2 vertebra and a traumatic spondylolisthesis of the C2 over C3 (anterior subluxation/dislocation); can be seen in motor-vehicle accidents, diving injuries or contact sports.

Classification

- **Ligature strangulation:** When ligature material is used to compress the neck.
- **Manual strangulation or throttling:** When human fingers, palms or hands are used to compress the neck.
- **Mugging:** Strangulation caused by holding the neck of the victim in the bend of elbow or knee of the assailant. It is an attack, usually from behind, and may leave no external or internal injury mark. It is also known as *chokehold*. This hold is not permitted in wrestling, because of its danger.
- **Bansdola:** A bamboo or stick is placed across the back of the neck and another across the front. Both the ends are tied with a rope due to which the victim is squeezed to death. A bruise is seen in the center, across the trachea corresponding to the width of the object used.
- **Garroting:** Strangulation is caused by compression of the neck by a ligature which is quickly tightened by twisting it with a lever (rod, stick or ruler) known as *Spanish windlass*. This results in sudden loss of consciousness and collapse. Garroting as a mode of execution was practiced in Spain, Portugal and Turkey. An iron collar was tightened by a screw for strangulation.

A 37-year-old patient presented with severe neck pain and without any focal deficits. He was involved in a motor vehicle collision. A radiograph was taken. Identify the type of fracture (arrow)?

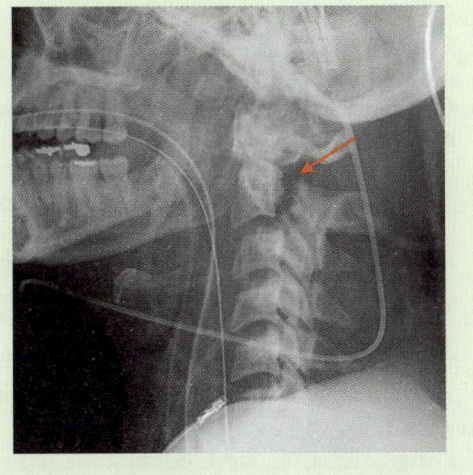

LIGATURE STRANGULATION

Cause of Death

- *Asphyxia* due to elevation of the larynx and tongue closing the airway at pharyngeal level.
- *Cerebral anoxia* due to venous congestion.
- *Vagal inhibition.*
- Rarely, *fracture dislocation* of cervical vertebrae.

POSTMORTEM EXAMINATION

External Findings (Figs. 10.10A and B)

1. **Face**
   i. Face is congested, swollen and cyanosed. Tardieu's spots are present on the forehead, temples, eyelids and conjunctiva; more abundant than in hanging.
   ii. **Eyes** are prominent, wide open, conjunctiva congested, pupils dilated, and subconjunctival hemorrhages are present (**Fig. 10.11**).
   iii. Lips, fingernails and ear lobules are cyanosed; marked postmortem staining on the skin above the ligature.
   iv. **Tongue** is swollen, dark colored, may protrude out of mouth, and bitten by teeth.
   v. Bloodstained frothy fluid and mucus may escape from mouth and nostrils.
2. **Neck**
   Ligature mark ('furrow')
   - Ligature mark is a well-defined groove, which is slightly depressed and of same width as that of ligature material. Groove may be narrow at parts due to folding of ligature.
   - The furrow is usually *horizontally placed* across the middle or lower part of neck, at or below the level of thyroid cartilage. The mark is transverse, circular and continuous.

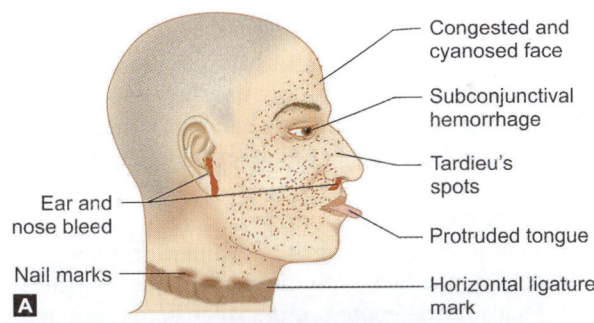

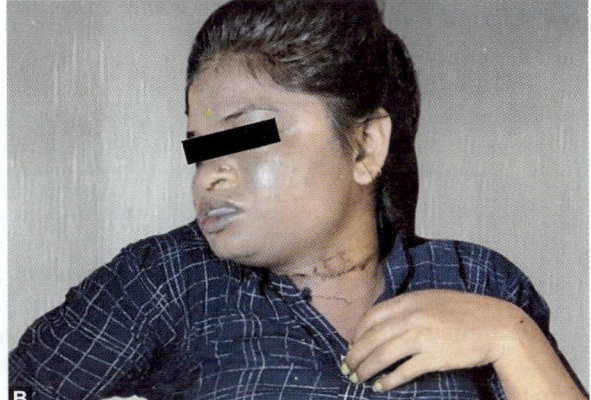

Figs. 10.10A and B: Postmortem findings in ligature strangulation

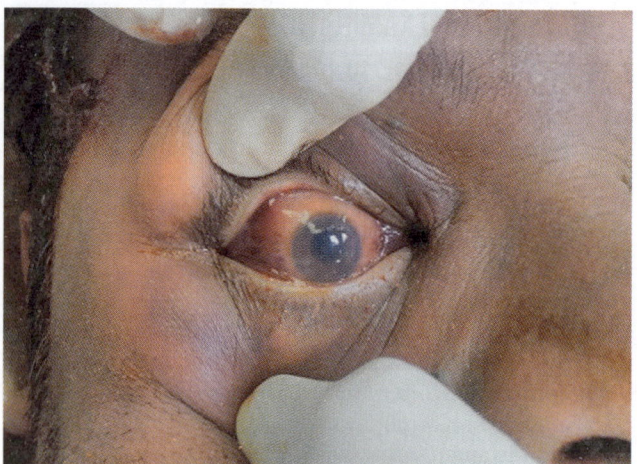

Fig. 10.11: Congested conjunctiva in strangulation

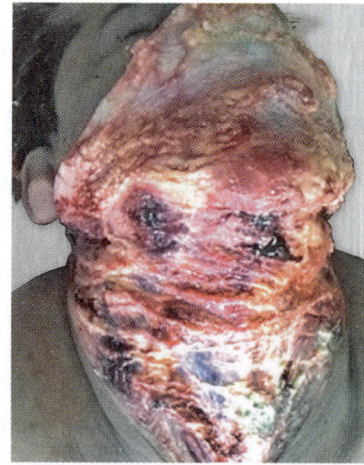

Fig. 10.12: Subcutaneous tissue underneath the ligature mark in strangulation—soft, reddish, bruising

- Mark, though completely encircling the neck horizontally, is more prominent on the front and sides, than on the back of the neck (as the underneath skin is thick).
- The base of the furrow is usually red, accompanied with congested or ecchymosed margins. Base may show imprint pattern of the ligature material used.
- It may be very indistinct or altogether absent, if the ligature was soft and broad, and was removed soon after death, and may need to be examined under UV light.
- Sometimes, a narrow cord or electric wire may be used, the so called '*cheese cutter method*', the ligature mark may appear deeply embedded, and on removal, a deep groove may be seen in the skin.
- Mark may be oblique as in hanging, if the victim has been dragged by a cord, after being strangled in a recumbent posture.

3. **Other parts of body**
   i. Postmortem staining is deep and prominent.
   ii. There may be involuntary discharge of urine and fecal matter—more common than in case of hanging. Seminal ejaculation is less common than in case of hanging.
   iii. Hands are usually clenched and genitals turgid.
   iv. In case of struggle, there may be evidence of abrasions, fingernail scratch marks, and contusions over the face, arms and other parts of the body.
   v. Scratches may be found on the skin of the neck near the ligature. They are usually horizontal, may be irregular or crescentic abrasions, consequent of the victim's attempts to pull the ligature away from the neck. Fingernails of the deceased should be examined for fragments of skin and blood.

Internal Findings

Neck
   i. Bruising of the subcutaneous tissue and muscles of neck, especially underneath the ligature and knot (Fig. 10.12). There may be bruising or laceration of the sheath of carotid arteries.
   ii. Injury of hyoid bone is not commonly noticed, because the level of constriction is well below, and traction on the thyrohyoid ligament is negligible.
   iii. Fracture of thyroid cartilage, one or both the superior horns may be seen.
   iv. Subcapsular and interstitial thyroid hemorrhages are common.
   v. Fracture of cricoid cartilage is less common.
   vi. Rings of trachea may sustain fracture when considerable force is applied.
   vii. Bruising of the root of the tongue and floor of the mouth may occur.
   viii. Lymphoid follicles at the base of the tongue and the palatine tonsils are congested.
   ix. Mucous membrane of the pharynx, pyriform sinuses, epiglottis and larynx usually show areas of hemorrhagic infiltration.
   x. Larynx, trachea and bronchi are congested, and contain frothy, often bloodstained mucus.
   xi. Fracture/dislocation of cervical vertebrae is not common, may occur in infants if associated with twisting of the neck.

Other Findings
   i. **Lungs** are congested, edematous with numerous subpleural petechial hemorrhages.
   ii. **Brain** is congested with petechiae in white matter.
   iii. All other organs are congested.

MEDICO-LEGAL QUESTIONS

Q. Whether death was caused by strangulation?

- General asphyxial features of death are present. The findings in the head and neck are strongly presumptive of strangulation, which is confirmed by ligature mark on the neck.

CHAPTER 10 : Asphyxial Deaths

- In absence of ligature mark in neck or deeper injury, it will be difficult to form an opinion, except from circumstantial evidence.
- The mere presence of cord or ligature around the neck of a dead body does not confirm the diagnosis, for it may be put around the neck for a malicious purpose.
- Strangulation by ligature has to be differentiated from hanging (Diff. 10.2).

DIFFERENTIATION 10.2: Hanging and strangulation

S.No.	Feature	Hanging	Strangulation
1.	Age	Young or elderly adults	No age limit
2.	Face	Usually pale, petechiae less common	Congested, livid with petechiae
3.	Signs of asphyxia	Less marked	Well marked
4.	Tongue swelling and protrusion	Less marked	More marked
5.	Bleeding from nose, ears, mouth	Less common	More common
6.	Neck	Stretched, elongated	Not so
7.	Ligature mark ('furrow') ♦ Direction ♦ Continuity ♦ Level in the neck ♦ Base	 Oblique Noncontinuous Above thyroid Pale, hard, parchment-like	 Transverse (Horizontal) Continuous Below thyroid Soft and reddish
8.	Knot	Single, simple, slip knot, on one side of neck	Multiple, granny or reef type, tied with force
9.	Abrasions and ecchymoses about the edges of mark	Not common	Common
10.	Involuntary discharge of feces and urine	Less common	More common
11.	Involuntary discharge of seminal fluid	More common	Less common
12.	Bruising of neck muscles	Less common	More common
13.	Subcutaneous tissue under the mark	White, hard, glistening	Ecchymosed
14.	Hyoid bone fracture	May occur	Uncommon
15.	Thyroid fracture	Unlikely	More common
16.	Larynx and trachea fracture	Unlikely	May be found
17.	Emphysematous bullae on lungs	Sometimes present	Very common
18.	Carotid arteries	Damage may be seen in intima	Rare
19.	Design	History of previous unsuccessful attempts of suicide may be available	No such history is available
20.	Suicide note	Usually present	Not present
21.	Place of occurrence	Usually in own bed room with doors and windows bolted from inside	Any place, not necessary inside room, not bolted from inside
22.	Signs of struggle	Absent	Always present, unless taken unaware

Which of the statement is true?

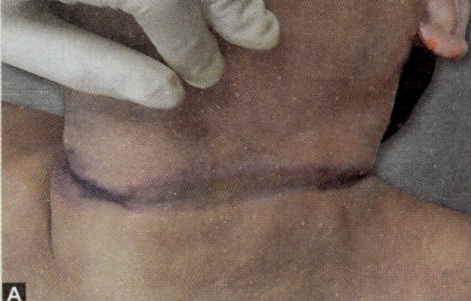
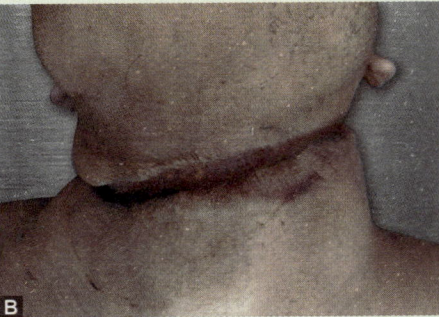

A   B

1. (A) is ligature mark of hanging and (B) is ligature mark of strangulation
2. (A) is ligature mark of strangulation and (B) is ligature mark of hanging
3. Both (A) and (B) are ligature marks of strangulation
4. Both (A) and (B) are ligature marks of hanging

Q. Whether the strangulation was suicidal, homicidal or accidental?

Suicidal Strangulation
- Suicide by strangulation is rare. The victims employ various methods of tightening the ligature, but the person can apply a single or double knot before consciousness is lost.
- In suicidal strangulation, signs of venous congestion are very well-developed above the ligature and are especially prominent at the root of tongue.
- The ligature should be found *in situ*; body should not show any signs of violence or marks of struggle. Laryngeal fractures are rare, and injuries are mild and often confined to the single ligature mark around the neck. Bleeding in the neck muscles is rare.
- Detailed examination of the scene and of the deceased person, along with circumstances leading to the death should be investigated.

Homicidal Strangulation
Strangulation should be assumed to be homicidal, until the contrary is proved. Many of the victims are women, and frequently, strangulation in them is associated with sexual assault.

Homicide is suspected when:
- There are two or more firm knots, each on separate turns of the ligature.
- Abrasions and fingernail marks are seen.
- The clothing of the victim is torn or disarranged, indicating that a struggle has taken place.
- The ligature when removed is loose.
- Macroscopic bleeding in laryngeal muscles.

Sometimes, homicidal strangulation is feigned by an individual to bring a false charge against his enemy. Hysterical women sometimes feign it, without any obvious motive.

Accidental Strangulation
- Accidental strangling may occur in uterus, when the movement of fetus causes the umbilical cord to encircle the neck.
- Children may get entangled in ropes during play or strangled in their cots.
- Persons under the influence of alcohol, epileptics and mentally retarded may be strangled either by a tight scarf or collar or necktie.

> **NOTA BENE**
> - **Incaprettamento** is a homicidal ligature strangulation used by the Italian mafia. While the victim is in the prone position, he is bound by one end of a rope, creating a slipknot around the throat, while the other end is used to tie the limbs behind the back. The death is caused by self-strangulation, since it is impossible to maintain the legs in this forced position.
> - Accidental ligature strangulation may occur in the **'long-scarf syndrome'** in which a clothing around the victim's neck (scarf or '*chunni/dupatta*') becomes entangled, usually in a stationary or moving mechanical device (e.g., rickshaw or scooter wheel), and the clothing becomes increasingly constricted owing to the continued action of the machine.

Pseudo or False Strangulation Groove
- Sometimes, marks are seen on the neck of dead infants or children. Infants have short neck, and these marks are produced from folds in the skin due to bending of the head.
- They are also seen in decomposed bodies with tight collars, buttoned shirt at the neck or a necklace around the neck.

 A 25-year-old was found dead at his home. He was brought for autopsy. Give your comments regarding the ligature and manner of injury.

5

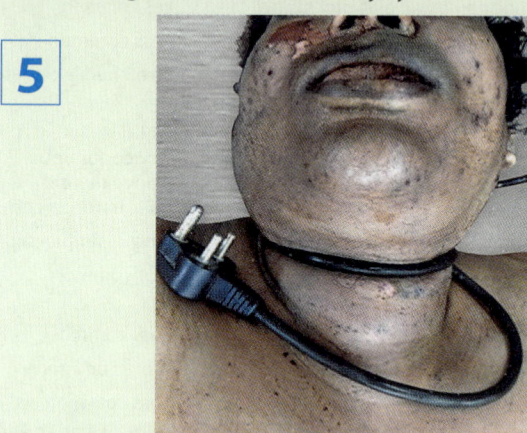

THROTTLING (MANUAL STRANGULATION)

Definition: Asphyxia produced by compression of the neck by human hands.

Cause of death
i. *Asphyxia* from obstruction of respiration.
ii. *Cerebral anoxia* from interference with cerebral circulation.
iii. *Vagal inhibition* from pressure on carotid nerve plexus consisting of fibers of vagus, sympathetic and glossopharyngeal nerves.
   - About half of the deaths are due to vagal inhibition.
   - The face will be pale as a result of rapid vasovagal cardiac arrest before congestive signs can develop.

Pressure must be applied for 2 minutes (min) or more to cause death.

POSTMORTEM EXAMINATION
- The external signs are abrasions and bruises on the front and sides of the neck, and are commonly at each side of the laryngeal prominence and just below the jaw-line.
- When pressure is prolonged, the classical signs of asphyxia may be seen—cyanosis, edema and congestion of the face, Tardieu's spot in the eyes and face, and sometimes bleeding from nose and ears.

The tips of the fingers produce bruises. They may be oval or round and 1.5–2 cm in size (may be more in case of continued bleeding). Presence and extent of fingertip bruising and nail scratch abrasions will depend upon:
  i. Relative position of victim and assailant.
  ii. Manner of grasping of neck, whether from front, back or sides.
  iii. Amount of pressure exerted.
  iv. Whether single or both hands have been used.
  v. Sex, age, condition of vessels and nutrition of individual.
  vi. Condition of nails of assailant.

Important to note that:
- Bruises made by tips of thumbs are more prominent than with other fingers.
- Multiple abrasions on the neck may also result from use of victim's hands in an effort to dislodge the assailant's grip. These curvilinear marks commonly lie close to areas of bruising and are often horizontally orientated. If these are from the assailant, they are usually vertical **(Fig. 10.13)**.

External Findings

  i. **If the assailant uses single hand from front:** Thumb will be applied on one side and other fingers on opposite side of neck. A grip from right hand produces a bruising due to bulb of pressing thumb over the cornue of hyoid/thyroid on anterolateral surface of right side of victim's neck and several fingertips bruising marks and overlying nail scratch abrasions over left side; being directed obliquely downwards and outwards, usually one below the other **(Fig. 10.13)**. Concavities of nail markings and their direction will indicate the relative position of victim and assailant.

  ii. **If the assailant uses both hands:** When both hands are used, evidence of pressure of thumb mark of one hand and finger marks of other hand are usually found on either side of throat. In case of grip from behind, the pressure is applied all around the neck, but some areas of bruising will be more prominent than others, because of pressing fingertips.

- Because of struggle and resistance, marks of bruising and abrasions may be found over the face, nostrils, lips, chin, cheeks, forehead, lower jaw and upper part of sternal area of the victim. These can also be caused in an effort to stop the victim from shouting or crying for help.
- It is, therefore, important to examine the nails of the victim and fingernail scrapings of the alleged assailant when possible, so that these can be compared with tissue type of the victim.

Internal Findings (Fig. 10.14)

  i. Extravasation of blood in subcutaneous tissues underneath the external marks of bruising and abrasions is the *most significant internal sign* **(Fig. 10.15)**.
  ii. Tear/laceration of platysma or sternomastoid muscles may be seen.
  iii. Tongue may be bruised/lacerated, may protrude out and bitten by teeth.
  iv. Hemorrhages, varying from pinpoint ecchymosis to extensive extravasation may be found in mucous membrane of larynx, epiglottis, pharynx and peritonsillar region.
  v. *Inward compression fracture of hyoid bone* is the most **diagnostic finding of throttling (Fig. 10.16)**.*
  vi. Fracture of superior horns of thyroid cartilage is common, though both horns do not get fractured simultaneously.*

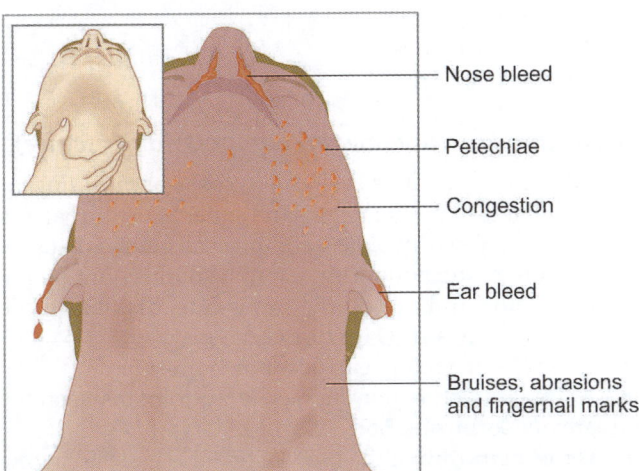

Fig. 10.13: Compression of neck with single hand along with findings

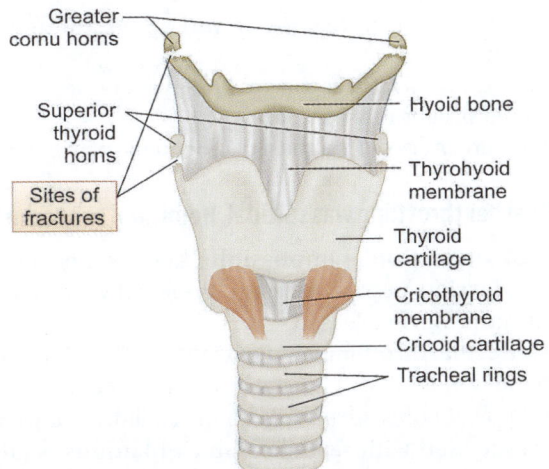

Fig. 10.14: Larynx: Sites of fracture from lateral compression (throttling)

---

*Antemortem nature of the fracture should be demonstrated by hemorrhage at the fracture site—both naked eye and confirmed histologically.

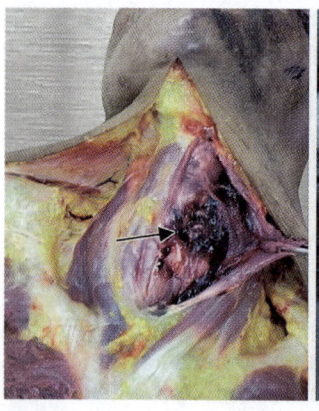
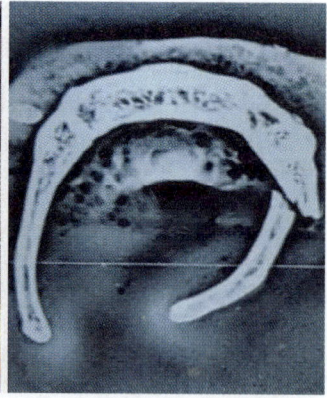

Fig. 10.15: Extravasation of blood (arrow) in subcutaneous tissue

Fig. 10.16: Inward compression fracture (X-ray) of hyoid bone
(*Courtesy*: Dr Prateek Karagwal, ESIC MCH, Alwar)

vii. Ribs may be fractured if murderer kneels on the chest of the victim.
viii. There may be laceration of carotid sheath and intima of carotid artery.
ix. Cricoid is usually not fractured.

> **NOTA BENE**
> Fractures of the superior horn of thyroid cartilage are not limited to fatal neck compression. Direct blunt trauma (e.g., motor vehicle impact or fall from height), resuscitation and poor autopsy technique can lead to this injury.

MEDICO-LEGAL QUESTIONS

Q. Whether death was due to throttling?

Diagnostic signs are:
 i. Bruising and abrasions on face and neck with or without rupture of neck muscles.
 ii. Engorgement of tissues at and above the level of compression.
 iii. Fracture of thyroid cartilages and hyoid bone.
 iv. General signs of asphyxia.
 v. Fracture of cricoid is almost pathognomic of throttling.

Q. Whether throttling was suicidal, homicidal or accidental?

- **Self-throttling** is impossible, because as soon as unconsciousness supervenes, the hand will relax and the grip will be released.
- **Homicidal throttling:** *Common mode of homicide* as the hand is immediately available, and method of choice in infants. Victims are usually infants, children or women (associated with sexual assault). In adults, signs of struggle are usually present, but if throat is seized firmly and compressed, victim cannot struggle. Adults can be throttled when under the influence of drugs/drinks or stunned or taken unaware. If contusions and fingernail abrasions are present on neck, the presumption must be of homicide.
- **Accidental throttling:** Sudden application of one or both hands on a person's throat as demonstration of affection, in joke or as a part of physiological experiment may cause death due to vagal inhibition.

Q. How much force an assailant could have used?

- If there is damage to neck structures, it indicates use of considerable force and is indicative of intent to injure, if not to kill.
- It there is fracture of hyoid bone/larynx, it indicates use of appreciable force and is homicidal in nature.
- Minor damage or absence of damage to the neck structures can kill, e.g., karate blow.
- If only slight changes are seen in neck structures, a guarded opinion should be given about the probable degree of force used.

> **NOTA BENE**
> The amount of force required to compress neck structures is estimated as—jugular vein: 2 kg-f (20 N assuming $g = 10$ m/s^2), carotid artery: 5 kg-f (50 N), trachea: 9 kg-f and vertebral artery: 30 kg-f. This implies that venous flow is decreased before arterial and airway obstruction occurs. For fractures of thyroid cartilage lamina: 14.3 kg-f and cricoid cartilage: 18.8 kg-f force is required.

HYOID BONE FRACTURES

Fracture of the hyoid bone occurs in 50–70% of cases in subjects above 40 years of age.

Classification

Fracture of hyoid bone can be classified as:
1. Adduction fracture
2. Abduction fracture
3. Avulsion fracture

Adduction Fracture (Inward Compression Fracture)

- Adduction fractures are seen in cases of *throttling*, as the fingers of the grasping hand squeeze the throat, the greater cornu of hyoid are compressed inwards causing fracture of the bone with tear of its periosteum on the outer side and not on the inner side, displacing the fragment inwards **(Fig. 10.17)**.
- This type of fracture can occur on both sides.
- A similar fracture may be seen at the joint between the greater cornu and body of hyoid.
- **Demonstration:** If the body of hyoid is grasped in one hand, and the distal fragment between the finger and thumb of the other hand, the distal fragment can be easily bent in inward direction, but outward movement is limited to normal position only.

Abduction Fracture (Anteroposterior Compression Fracture)

- It is seen in *hanging*; due to anteroposterior compression, hyoid bone is driven directly backward, divergence of greater cornu is increased causing fracture with outward displacement of the posterior fragment. As a result, periosteum on inner side of fracture is torn and the fragment can be easily moved outwards, but inner movement is limited to normal position only **(Fig. 10.17)**.
- This type of fracture can also occur in the greater cornu at its junction with the body, and it may be bilateral.
- They are also seen in ligature strangulation, run over motor vehicle accident and blows on front of neck by any means, e.g., rods, foot or stick.

Avulsion or Traction or Tug Fracture

It occurs due to hyperextension of the neck or muscular overactivity (e.g. in tetanus), as a result of traction on thyrohyoid ligament either by downward or lateral compression or when direct pressure is exerted between hyoid and thyroid by pressing fingers. The hyoid is drawn upwards and held rigid.

It may be noted that:
- Cartilaginous separations between the greater cornu and body, joints between lesser cornu and body, or the presence of incomplete bony union of hyoid parts should not be mistaken for fractures.
- A hyoid fracture should not be diagnosed as antemortem in origin, if there is no recent hemorrhage at alleged traumatized site.

NOTA BENE
- Chronic alcoholics are predisposed to hyoid fracture.
- Fractures of the hyoid can also be seen in natural deaths, presumably from intense muscle contractions during the agonal stages or following violent coughing.

FM 2.22
Describe and discuss pathophysiology, clinical features, postmortem findings and medico-legal aspects of traumatic asphyxia, obstruction of nose and mouth, suffocation.

SUFFOCATION

Definition: It is a form of asphyxia caused by mechanical obstruction to the passage of air into the respiratory tract *by means other than constriction of neck or drowning*.

Classification
i. Smothering
ii. Choking
iii. Gagging
iv. Overlying
v. Traumatic asphyxia
vi. Burking

Smothering

Definition: It is a form of asphyxia caused by mechanical occlusion of external air passages, i.e., the nose and mouth by hand, cloth, plastic bag or other material.

Postmortem Findings (Figs. 10.18A and B)
i. Abrasions and bruises around the mouth and nostrils. These may not be seen, if soft materials, like cloth or pillow has been used.

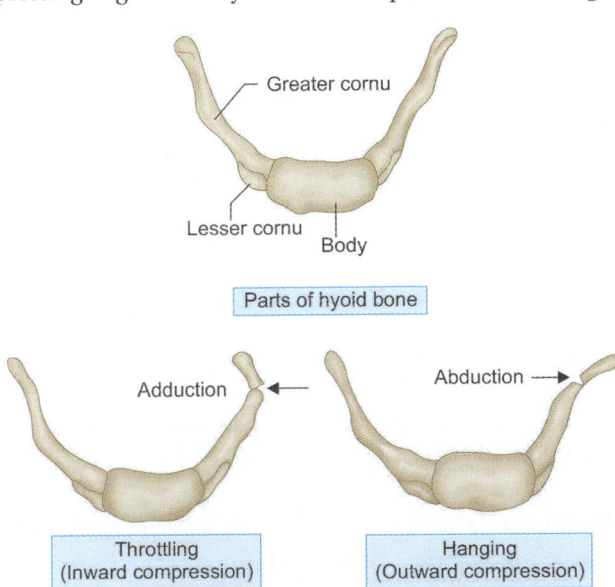

Fig. 10.17: Hyoid bone fracture (arrow)

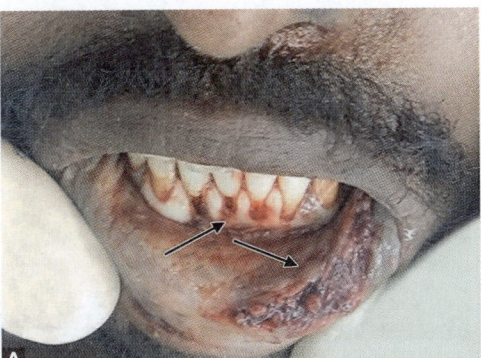
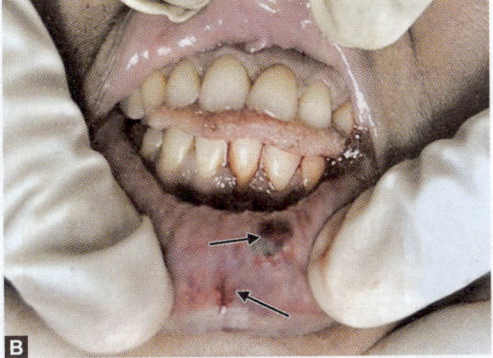

Figs. 10.18A and B: Bruising and lacerations inside the lips and gums in smothering (arrows)

ii. Injuries on the inside of the lips from pressure of teeth are seen.
iii. Bruising of gums or sometimes tears of delicate tissues are seen.

These findings may be missed, unless looked for.

Medico-legal Aspects

- Accidental smothering is common in alcoholics or epileptics, who may fall or roll over in a heap of mud or such other material.
- After birth, an infant may die from smothering, if he is born with membranes covering the nose and mouth (*cul-de-sac*) **(Fig. 10.19)**.
- Children may get smothered while playing with plastic bags over the face or head.

Choking

Definition: It is a form of asphyxia caused by an obstruction within the air-passages by a foreign object, like coin, fruit seed, toffees, candies, fishbone or any other material.

In an epileptic attack, tongue may fall back on to posterior pharyngeal wall causing choking.

The phases of acute fatal airway obstruction are:
i. Penetration of the object into the airway.
ii. Obstruction of the airway.
iii. Failure to expel once the obstruction has occurred.

Mechanism: Initially, there is stridor, respiratory distress, coughing and the inability of the victim to speak. This is followed by a rapid, deep inhalation, which causes the foreign object to pass further down the airway. Laryngospasm occurs, followed by vagal stimulation, leading to arrhythmia, apnea and death.

Cause of Death

i. Asphyxia.
ii. Vagal inhibition.
iii. Laryngeal spasm.
iv. Delayed death from pneumonia, lung abscess or bronchiectasis.

Postmortem Findings

i. Signs of asphyxial death. Subconjunctival hemorrhages without cutaneous petechiae may be seen.
ii. Presence of food items or foreign body in respiratory tract **(Figs. 10.20A and B)**. The food items are usually round and firm, yet pliable to allow molding in the airway.
iii. In an epileptic, tongue may show bite marks or bruising.

Medico-legal Aspects

Most choking deaths are accidental; suicide and homicide are rare.

- Accidental choking deaths are common in children <1 year of age. Ninety percent of choking deaths happen before the age of 5 years.
- Homicidal choking usually involves the aged, individuals debilitated by disease, alcohol or drugs, and infants. When objects are forced into the mouth, signs of a struggle, if the individual was conscious, may be noted. Perioral, teeth, tongue and other intraoral injuries can result.
- Suicidal choking is uncommon, and may occur in psychiatric patients and prisoners.

Café Coronary

This is a condition of *accidental choking* wherein a bolus of food produces complete obstruction of the larynx.

- It is called so, because it mimics a heart attack, and is usually seen in an intoxicated restaurant patron.
- Cause of death is due to reflex cardiac arrest from 'vagal inhibition' as a consequence of stimulation of laryngeal nerve endings. In such cases, asphyxial changes will not be found.
- The term, 'cafe coronary', was coined by *Dr Roger Haugen* in 1963.

Causes

Predisposing factors: Decreased protective airway reflex resulting from aging, poor dentition, tendency to swallow food whole, alcohol consumption, and ingestion of large

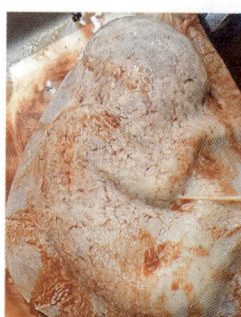
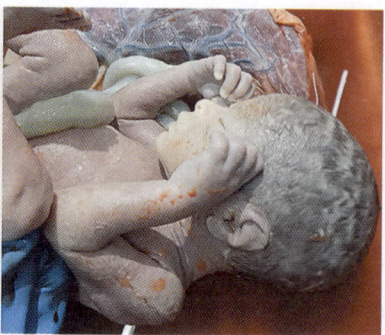

Fig. 10.19: Cul-de-sac delivery: Infant died from smothering
(*Courtesy*: Dr Ambreen Ejaz, Medical College, Kolkata)

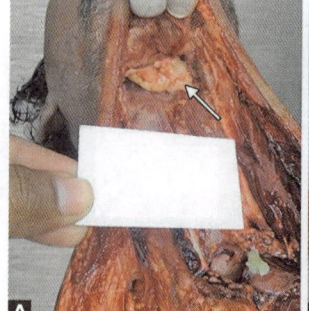
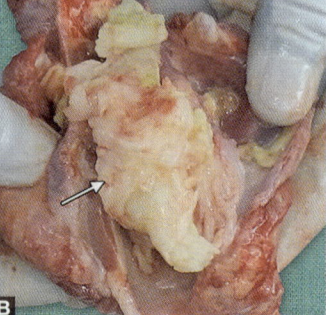

Figs. 10.20A and B: Food bolus in a case of choking: (A) Floor of the mouth (arrow); (B) In trachea (arrow)

doses of tranquilizers and other CNS depressants impairing the gag reflex.

Clinical findings: Victim who was apparently healthy, collapses suddenly turning blue while eating at a dining table.

Treatment (for choking)
i. If there is difficulty in breathing and cyanosis, give first aid by application of pressure on the abdomen (Heimlich maneuver) till the patient recovers or loses consciousness.
ii. A blow on the back or on the sternum may cause coughing and expel the foreign body.
iii. The victim is placed in a supine position and the mouth is opened to perform a finger sweep.
iv. If this is not successful, the foreign body should be removed from hypopharynx with the middle and index fingers or with forceps.
v. If the object cannot be removed, the person may need a tracheotomy/cricothyrotomy.

Postmortem Findings

Bolus of unchewed food or such material is found impacted in larynx or trachea. A litmus paper test of the bolus can be made to determine the acidity to ascertain its origin (mouth or vomitus). Blood for alcohol should be preserved.

> **NOTA BENE**
>
> **'Creche coronary':** Choking occurring in children aged 1–3 years as they are more vulnerable because of their increased mobility, putting inappropriate small objects in their mouth or unable to appreciate the size of a piece of food, small airways, inadequate dentition for chewing and weaker cough reflex.

Gagging

Definition: Gagging is a form of asphyxia which results from pushing a gag (rolled up cloth or paper balls) into the mouth, sufficiently deep to block the pharynx **(Fig. 10.21)**.
- It combines the features of smothering and choking.
- Initially, the airway may be patent through nose, but collections of saliva, excessive mucus with edema of pharynx and nasal mucosa causes complete obstruction.

Postmortem Findings

i. Same as choking.
ii. Injuries to nose and mouth with seepage of blood into the back of throat.

Medico-Legal Aspects

- Almost always homicidal, and the victim is usually an infant or an elderly person.
- Gagging is usually resorted to prevent the victim from shouting for help; death is usually unintended.
- Gags have been used to suppress screams by victims using a painful method of suicide (e.g., self-immolation).

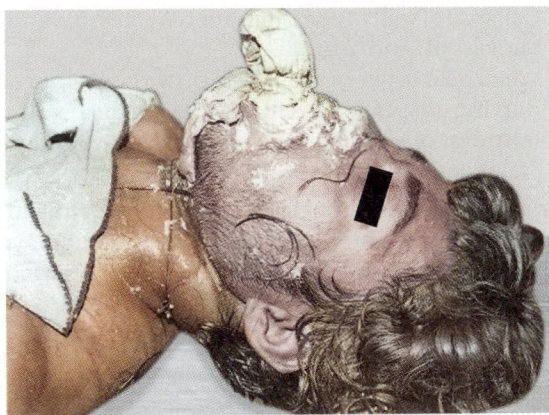

Fig. 10.21: Gagging

Overlaying

Definition: Overlaying or compression suffocation results from compression of the chest, nose and mouth, so as to prevent breathing.
- It is a form of accidental smothering of an infant by a nursing mother, sharing a bed with her child who may roll over during sleep and occlude the air passages.
- Ethanol intoxication or a medical condition can be a factor depressing an arousal response in the older bed-sharer.

Postmortem Findings

Face, nose and chest of the child may appear compressed and pale. Pressure marks from bedding or clothing may be seen on the victim, but these can happen postmortem. Usual findings of asphyxia will be seen along with intrathoracic petechiae.

Medico-legal Aspects

- Purely accidental in nature.
- It may also be a case of infanticide.
- These cases are likely to be victims of sudden infant death syndrome (SIDS).

Traumatic or Crush Asphyxia (Perthes Syndrome)

Definition: Asphyxia resulting from respiratory arrest due to mechanical fixation of chest, so that the normal movements of chest wall are prevented.
- Ollivier first described this condition in 1837 while doing autopsies on people trampled by crowds in Paris.

Causes

i. Due to house collapse, accidentally or in wars/earthquake.
ii. Stampede by crowd, running in panic, due to outbreak of fire in a movie hall/mall/public gathering.
iii. Run over by a vehicle or overturned vehicle (especially tractors).

iv. Collapse of wall inside a mine or trenches (cave-in), in bunkers of sand or grain.
v. When held between the buffers of two bogies of a train.
vi. Burying the person in sandy soil up to the neck.
vii. Restraint of suspects by *hogtying* practiced in some States in the US by police.

Mechanism: The essential feature is fixation of the thorax by severe compression or external pressure that prevents respiratory movements. An individual can die in seconds if there is considerable weight, but usually at least 2–5 min elapse before death ensues.

Postmortem Examination

External findings (Fig. 10.22)
Characteristic features seen are:
i. **Masque ecchymotique** refers to the classical appearance of:
   a. Cerebral vascular engorgement leading to congestion of face and neck with variable involvement of the upper thorax, back and arms.
   b. Craniocervical cyanosis.
   c. Subconjunctival hemorrhages.
ii. **Demarcation line:** Level of compression is indicated by a well-defined demarcating line between the discolored upper portion of body and the lower normal part.
iii. Areas of pallor seen at the level of collar of shirts, folds or creases in the garments.
iv. Facial edema.
v. External blunt trauma injuries can be seen on the head, neck and chest along with mud or other foreign material.

Internal findings
- **Eyes:** *Purtscher's retinopathy* (retinal hemorrhages).
- **Face:** Nose, ear or pharyngeal petechiae/ecchymoses that may result in external bleeding—mimic a basal skull fracture.
- **Bones:** Rib and clavicle fractures are common; extremity and pelvic fractures may be seen.
- **Upper respiratory tract:** Edema, epiglottic and laryngeal petechiae.
- **Lungs:** Congested, heavy, subpleural petechiae; contusions/lacerations and hemo-/pneumothorax may be present.
- **Heart:** Right heart and veins above aorta may be distended, injuries are rare.
- **Abdomen:** Hepatic and splenic lacerations may be found.
- **CNS:** Edema and petechiae can be seen.

Medico-legal Aspects

Mostly accidental, but fallen appliances or furniture particularly over children has been described as a means of homicide.

> **NOTA BENE**
> - In survivors, discoloration disappears within a few weeks and does not undergo the color changes seen with the healing of bruises. The color is not altered by the administration of oxygen. Petechiae disappear within days, but subconjunctival ecchymoses can persist for weeks, eventually fading to yellow and disappearing.
> - **Mechanism of masque ecchymotique:** Retrograde displacement of blood from superior vena cava into the subclavian veins and veins of the head and neck results from sudden compression of the chest or abdomen. Valves in the subclavian veins prevent the spread of hydrostatic force to the veins of upper limbs. But, the displacement of the blood into the valveless veins of the head and neck causes rupture of distal capillaries. Therefore, face and neck of the victim are deeply cyanosed; eyes bloodshot and numerous petechiae over scalp, face, neck and shoulders are seen.

Burking

- It is a combination of homicidal smothering and traumatic asphyxia **(Fig. 10.23)**.
- *William Burke* and *William Hare* killed 16 persons during 1827-28 in Scotland and sold their bodies to Dr Robert Knox for use as specimens in his anatomy classes in Edinburgh Medical School, in what became known as the case of the *Body Snatchers* (West Port murders).
- **Method:** A victim was invited to their house and given alcohol. When drunk, he was thrown on the ground. Burke would kneel or sit on the chest and close the nose and mouth with his hands, and Hare used to pull him around the room by the feet till he is dead.

> **NOTA BENE**
> - **Plastic bag asphyxia** results from decreased oxygen concentration in the available inspired air, and physical obstruction of the mouth and nose. The plastic bag becomes electrically charged and adheres to the face, aided by condensation **(Fig. 10.24)**. It is a common method of suicide among the elderly and debilitated individuals. It can also be seen in autoerotic asphyxia, drug misadventure—volatile inhalants (e.g., chloroform or propane), inhalation of volatile hydrocarbons (e.g., trichloroethane) or accidental deaths in children. Death can be rapid, leaving no signs of asphyxia.

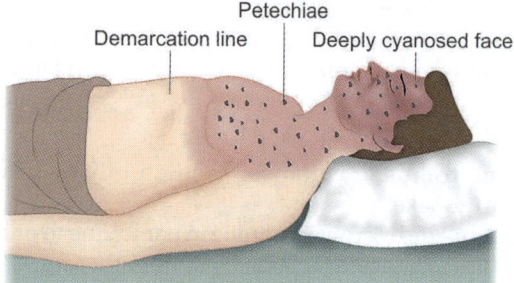

Fig. 10.22: Traumatic asphyxia

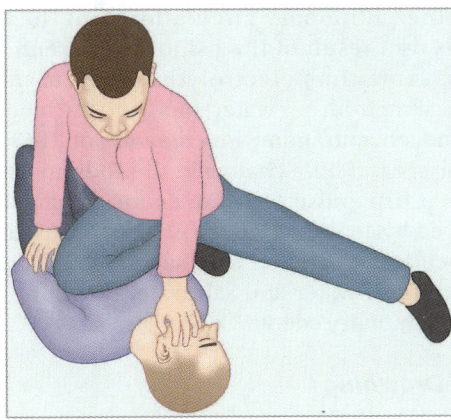

Fig. 10.23: Burking

- **Wedging** is a form of mechanical asphyxia in which the face, neck or thorax is compressed between two firm structures. It is common in 3–6 months old children when they start to move to the corners of beds and cribs, but they do not have the muscle development to free themselves out of a wedged position. They become wedged between the mattress and either the wall, bed frame, a piece of furniture, mesh or another mattress.
- **Confined space entrapment:** It occurs when there is inadequate oxygen in the enclosed space due to consumption or displacement by other gases. The mechanism of death is usually attributed to asphyxia from oxygen deprivation. Injuries identified at autopsy and damage to the inside of the structure indicate struggle to exit the cabinet. There are no specific autopsy findings or significant natural disease processes, and toxicology studies are negative.
- **Buried alive:** A person may be buried alive accidentally on the mistaken assumption that he is dead or intentionally as a form of torture, murder or execution. It is a form of suffocation wherein the victim typically dies of asphyxiation. Autopsy shows congestion of head and neck, petechial hemorrhages on the face, conjunctiva, neck and upper chest; congestion and hemorrhages in the cervical lymph nodes; emphysematous lungs; fine sand particles in nose, mouth and trachea till terminal bronchioles. The stomach will also reveal swallowed material of the same type inhaled. Histological examinations may be carried out to support the diagnosis.

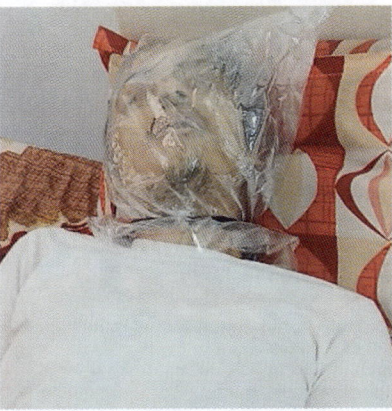

Fig. 10.24: Plastic bag asphyxia
(*Courtesy*: Dr Ashook Moondra, GMC, Kota)

 A 39-year-old man came to the ER after sustaining severe blunt chest trauma at a construction site. He had rapid shallow breathing, subconjunctival hemorrhages, injuries to chest and abdomen, and developed characteristic color change over chest, head and neck. What could be the diagnosis?

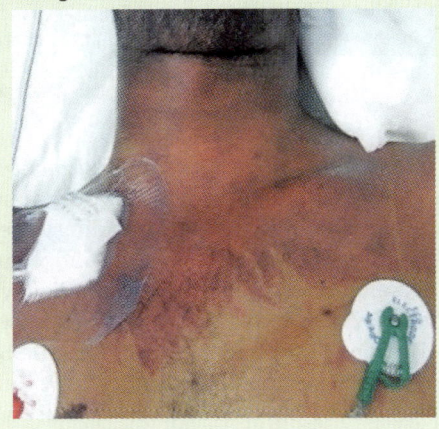

(*Courtesy*: Dr Hussein Lateef, Consultant Thoracic and Vascular Surgeon, Dubai, UAE)

FM 2.23

Describe and discuss types, pathophysiology, clinical features, postmortem findings and medico-legal aspects of drowning, diatom test and Gettler test.

DROWNING

Definition: Drowning is the process of experiencing respiratory impairment from submersion/immersion in liquid.
- Implicit in this definition is that a liquid-air interface is present at the entrance to the victim's airway, which prevents the individual from breathing oxygen.
- Outcome may include delayed morbidity, delayed or rapid death, or life without morbidity.
- Terms such as wet or dry drowning, active or passive drowning, near-drowning and secondary drowning would be discarded (World Congress on Drowning, Amsterdam, 2002).

NOTA BENE

Drowning was previously defined as immediate death secondary to asphyxia while immersed in a liquid, usually water, or within 24 h of submersion. The definition excluded aspiration of vomit, blood, saliva, bile or meconium.

Classification (Flowchart 10.3)

Typical or Wet Drowning

Fluid or water is inhaled into the lungs and the victim has severe chest pain (seen in 80–90% of cases). It is also known as *primary drowning*.

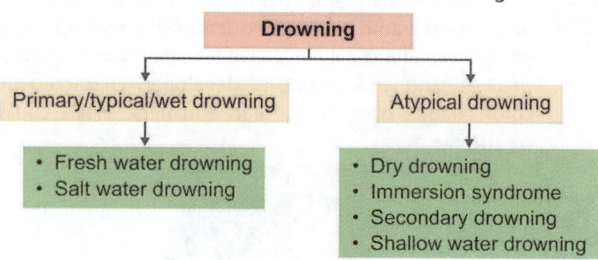

Flowchart 10.3: Classification of drowning

- *In fresh water and brackish water drowning* (0.5–0.6% NaCl), the aspirated water is rapidly absorbed from the alveoli into the circulation leading to hemodilution and hemolysis. Circulatory overload, hyponatremia, hyperkalemia, together with myocardial hypoxia result in fall of systolic blood pressure followed by ventricular fibrillation **(Flowchart 10.4 and Fig. 10.25)**.
- *In sea (salt) water drowning* (3–4% salinity), the aspiration of water results in withdrawal of water from the pulmonary circulation into the alveolar spaces as a result of the osmotic differential, while at the same time electrolytes (sodium, chloride, magnesium from sea water) pass into the blood. There is hemoconcentration with crenation of RBCs, but not hemolysis and little change in the sodium/potassium balance. The pulse pressure decreases slowly and is followed by atrioventricular (AV) dissociation, but not ventricular fibrillation **(Flowchart 10.4 and Fig. 10.26)**. In both fresh water and salt water drowning, there is terminal pulmonary edema.

Atypical Drowning

Conditions in which there is very little or no inhalation of water or fluid in the air passages.

1. **Dry drowning**
   - In dry drowning, water does not enter the lungs due to laryngeal spasm induced by small amounts of water entering the larynx.

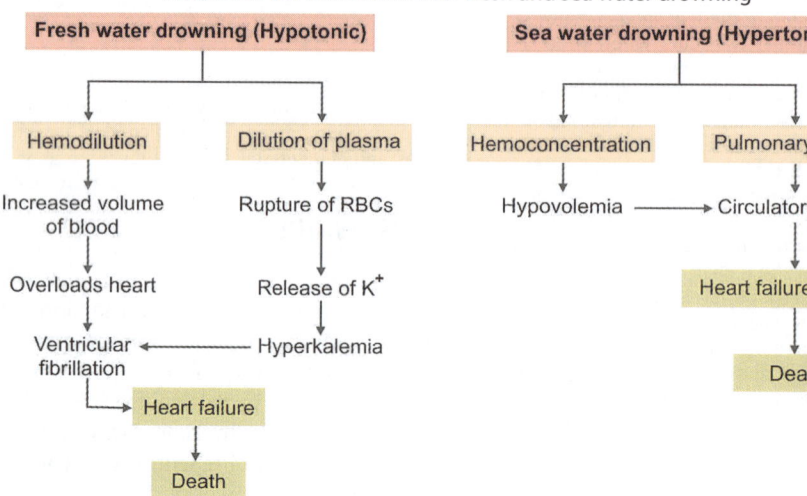

Flowchart 10.4: Mechanism of fresh and sea water drowning

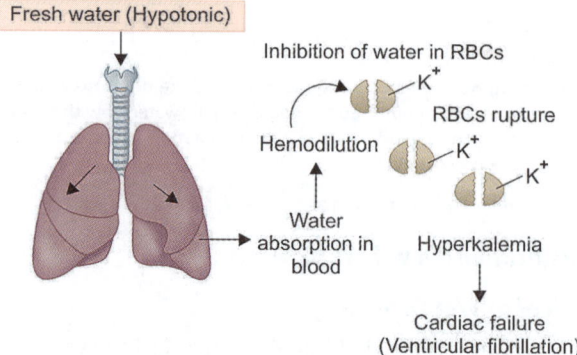

Fig. 10.25: Mechanism of death in fresh water drowning (RBCs: Red blood cells)

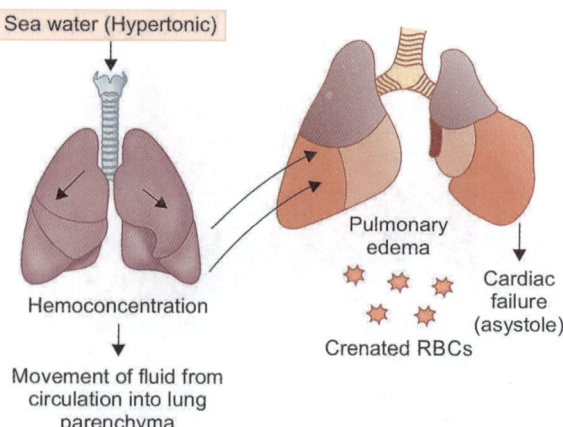

Fig. 10.26: Mechanism of death in sea water drowning (RBCs: Red blood cells)

- Seen in 1–2% of cases.
- Death may be extremely rapid and time elapsed is insufficient for typical drowning to occur. Two mechanisms have been postulated:
  i. Laryngeal spasm and airway closure causing lethal hypoxemia.
  ii. Reflex cardiac arrest due to vasovagal stimulation.
- In these cases, autopsy findings and tests for drowning are negative, and the lung fields are dry.

2. **Immersion syndrome** (*hydrocution, submersion inhibition or cold water drowning*): It refers to syncope resulting from cardiac dysrhythymias on sudden contact with water that is at least 5°C lower than body temperature.
   - The syndrome occurs as a result of:
     i. Cold water stimulating the nerve endings of the surface of the body.
     ii. Water striking the epigastrium.
     iii. Cold water entering eardrums, nasal passages, pharynx and larynx.
     iv. Falling or diving into water with feet first or *duck diving* by the inexperienced.
   - *Mechanism:* Vagal stimulation leading to asystolic cardiac arrest ('diving reflex'), or ventricular fibrillation secondary to QT prolongation after a massive release of catecholamine on contact with cold water. The resultant loss of consciousness leads to secondary drowning.
   - The findings of typical drowning are absent, and diagnosis of hydrocution is difficult because aspiration of water into the lungs does not occur.
   - The syndrome particularly affects the middle-aged or elderly men who have ingested some amounts of ethanol. Underlying cardiac disease could increase the risk of sudden collapse.

3. **Near drowning** (*post-immersion syndrome or secondary drowning*)
   - Near drowning refers to survival beyond 24 h after a submersion episode.
   - Death is caused by complications or sequelae (e.g., ARDS, pneumonia, sepsis, hypoxic-ischemic encephalopathy, cerebral edema and DIC).
   - *Secondary drowning* sometimes refers to a victim who initially responds well to resuscitation but then suffers respiratory decompensation.

4. **Shallow water drowning** (*submersion of the unconscious*): Alcoholics, drugged, epileptics, infants, children and unconscious persons may die due to drowning in shallow water in a pit or drain.

Epidemiology

- Drowning victims are predominantly male (>65%). It occurs in the summer months, more frequently seen in rivers, lakes, ponds and creeks.
- The age groups affected are the children (<4 years) and young adults (15–24 years). Drugs and alcohol abuse among the teenagers are other associated factors.

Cause of Death

i. *Asphyxia:* Most common cause of death.
ii. In fresh water drowning, death results from *ventricular fibrillation*. While in salt water, it is due to *cardiac arrest* from fulminant pulmonary edema and associated changes.
iii. *Vagal inhibition* due to impact with water.
iv. *Laryngeal spasm.*
v. *Concussion/head injury.*
vi. *Apoplexy:* Subarachnoid hemorrhage from rupture of berry aneurysm or cerebral hemorrhage due to rupture of cerebral vessels from sudden on-rush of blood to the brain due to excitement or sudden fall from height into cold water.
vii. *Secondary causes*
   - Septic aspiration pneumonia
   - Sudden bursting of aneurysm.

Symptoms: Apart from recalling of memory of past events, there may be mental confusion along with auditory and visual hallucinations, tinnitus and vertigo. In wet drowning, there is chest pain.

Treatment: First and immediate step consists of application of artificial respiration with closed chest cardiac compressions, even in absence of pulse and respiration and irrespective of injuries sustained during drowning. Defibrillator should be used when there is ventricular fibrillation.

Fatal period
- Fresh water drowning: 4–5 min.
- Sea water drowning: 8–12 min.

POSTMORTEM EXAMINATION

- The diagnosis of drowning is one of exclusion.
- Most of the signs are not specific of death due to drowning and are rather signs of submersion of body under water for some period. Any dead body, whatever the cause of death, will develop signs of immersion if left for a sufficient time in water.
- Moreover, some of the signs are not appreciable in case of putrefaction.

When freshly removed from water, the body and clothes will be wet. There will be sand and mud particles on the body, hair and clothes. This finding is not specific of antemortem drowning or death due to drowning.

External Findings

i. **Face** is pale, becomes bloated and discolored with putrefaction. Cyanosis may be present.

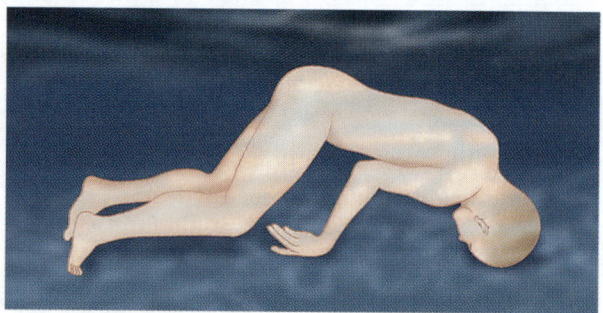

Fig. 10.27: Position of a submerged dead body

ii. **Eyes** are found half open or closed, conjunctiva suffused and pupils are dilated. Subconjunctival hemorrhages may be present in lower eyelids.
iii. **Tongue** may be swollen and protruded.
iv. **Postmortem staining**: Light pink in color, present over face, neck, front of upper part of chest, upper and lower limbs, as the body usually floats with face down, buttocks up, legs and arms hanging down in front of the body **(Fig. 10.27)**. With onset of putrefaction, skin of head and neck become dark with '*tête de négre*' appearance.*
v. **Froth**: Presence of *fine, copious white 'shaving lather-like' froth* at the mouth and nostrils is the **most characteristic antemortem external finding (Fig. 10.28)**. Production of this tenacious, fine, lathery foam is a vital phenomenon.
   - The mass of foam, consisting of fine bubbles, does not collapse when touched with the point of a knife.
   - It may be absent when wiped off, but reappears again by itself or by applying simple pressure on chest.

   Mechanism of production of froth: The inhalation of water irritates the mucous membrane of air passages due to which the tracheal and bronchial glands secrete large quantities of tenacious mucus, and the alveolar lining cell irritation produces edema fluid. Vigorous agitation of the seromucoid secretion, surfactant, aspirated water and retained air converts the mixture of endogenous and drowning medium into froth.

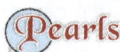

Other conditions in which froth can be seen:
- Strangulation
- Electric shock
- Putrefaction
- Acute pulmonary edema
- Epileptic fit
- Opium/OPC poisoning

In all these cases, froth is not fine, not of such large quantity or tenacious in nature as in drowning.

vi. **Cutis anserina** (*goose skin/goose flesh/goose bumps/horripilation*) is a state of puckered and granular appearance of skin of the extremities immersed in cold water due to contraction of erector pilorum muscles **(Fig. 10.29A)**. It can occur on submersion of the body in cold water immediately after death while the muscles are still warm and irritable, and also produced by rigor mortis of erector muscles.
vii. **Washerwomen's hand** is the wrinkled, sodden, bleached appearance of palms, palmer aspect of fingers and soles of feet including plantar surface of toes due to submersion of the body **(Fig. 10.29B)**. Maceration of skin occurs due to imbibition of water into its outer layers. It is first seen in the fingertips by 3–4 h and whole hand by 24 h.
viii. Scrotum and penis get retracted in contact with cold water during winter months.
ix. Grass, gravel, mud, sand, weeds or aquatic vegetations held firmly in clenched hands due to *cadaveric spasm* is a *vital proof of antemortem drowning* **(Fig. 10.29C)**. The material clenched in the hands indicates the place of submersion.
x. **Rigor mortis** appears early, especially when a violent struggle for life has taken place before death.
xi. **Antemortem injuries** might be sustained during fall into water, along the tank or by striking against a hard object while diving in shallow water. Examination of the skin for blunt injuries should be delayed until the body is dry. Abrasions are easily seen after drying, which becomes brownish in color.

Internal Findings

1. **Lungs**
   i. *Lungs are voluminous, distended and show ballooning*, i.e., bulge out of chest on removal of sternum **(Diff. 10.3)**. Tenacious, lathery froth in trachea and bronchi is present **(Fig. 10.30A)**. In case of laryngeal spasm, there will be no ballooning.
   ii. Distended lungs will show indentations of ribs on the pleural surface, because of pressure on increased volume of lungs.

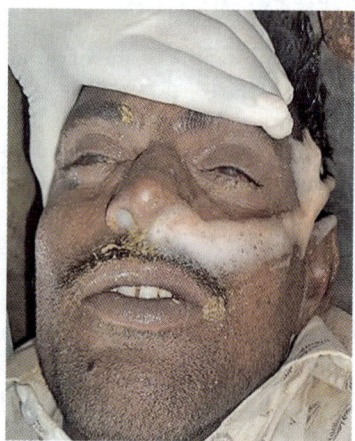

Fig. 10.28: White 'shaving lather-like' froth—surest sign of antemortem drowning

---

* Tête de négre is the French name for a dessert, a pastry covered with black chocolate, which means 'very dark brown' color.

CHAPTER 10 : Asphyxial Deaths

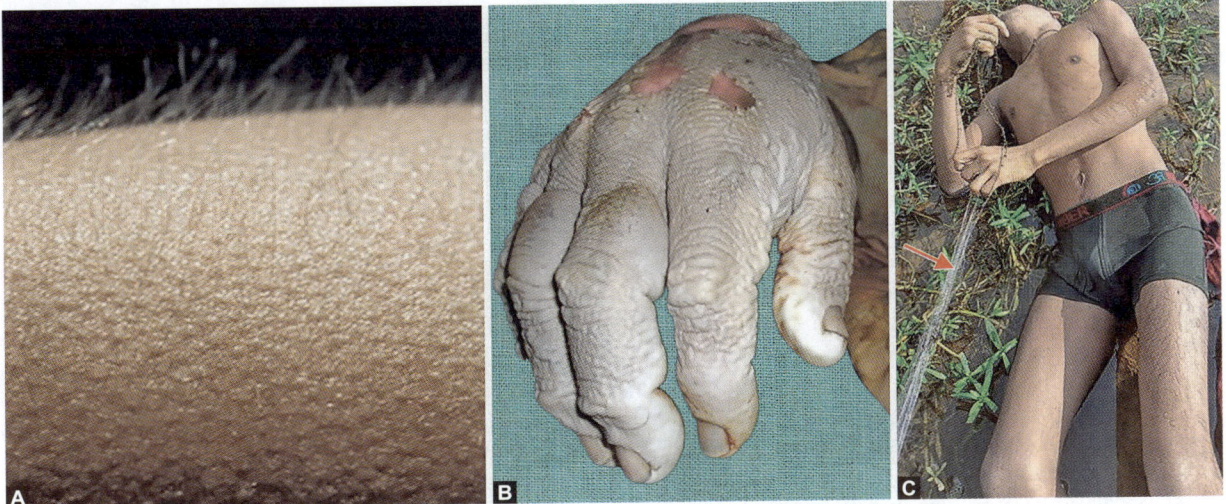

Figs. 10.29A to C: Features of drowning: (A) Cutis anserina; (B) Washerwoman hand; (C) Cadaveric spasm involving both hands. The fisherman grasped the fishnet in his left hand (arrow) and small vegetations in right hand

DIFFERENTIATION 10.3: Lungs in fresh water and sea water drowning

S.No.	Feature	Fresh water drowning	Sea water drowning
1.	Size and weight	Ballooned, but light	Ballooned and heavy
2.	Color	Pinkish	Purplish or bluish
3.	Consistency	Emphysematous	Soft, jelly-like
4.	Shape after removal from body	Retained, do not collapse	Not retained, tend to flatten out
5.	On cut section	Crepitus is heard, little froth and no fluid	No crepitus, copious fluid and froth

iii. Lungs feel heavy, boggy and doughy; will easily indent on pressure by fingers, because of water logging and edematous condition **(Fig. 10.30B)**.
iv. Lungs may be congested, but are often pale gray in appearance, because of forcing out of blood from lungs and compression of vessels in the interalveolar septa by the trapped air and water in lung alveoli.
v. Tardieu's spots over the subpleural tissues are few or none due to compression of blood vessels in interalveolar septa.
vi. There may be mottled areas of red and gray distended alveoli, alternating with few bigger areas of extravasation known as **Paltauf's hemorrhage**, from tracking of effused blood along the interlobular septa; mostly seen in the lower lobes on anterior surface and margins of lungs.
vii. Cut section of lungs will exude copious amount of frothy bloodstained liquid due to presence of water within alveoli and bronchioles **(Fig. 10.30B)**.
viii. Pleural cavities may contain bloodstained fluid, either by permeation through pleura or postmortem disintegration of lungs and pleurae.

♦ The overall picture of lungs and respiratory passage in *wet drowning* has been described as **emphysema**

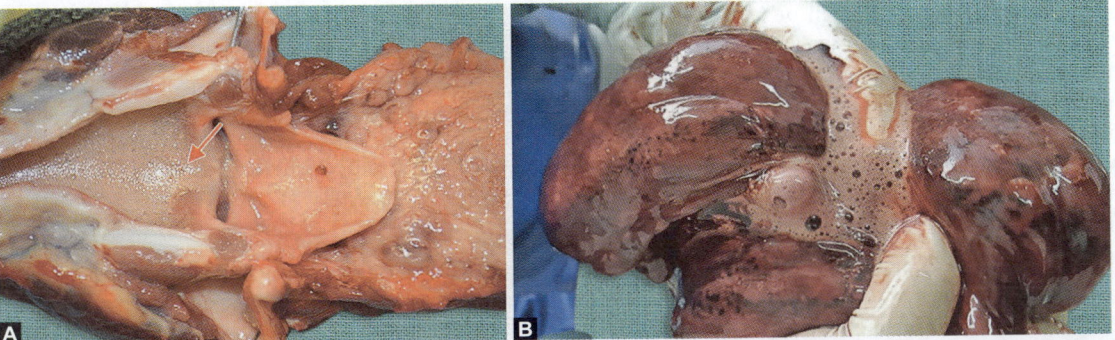

Figs. 10.30A and B: (A) Tenacious froth in trachea (arrow); (B) Heavy, congested, boggy distended lungs with copious lathery froth coming out of bronchi

aquosum *(emphyseme hydroaerique)* as it resembles the pulmonary hyperinflation seen in obstructive lung disease. There is dilation of alveoli, thinning of alveolar septae and compression of alveolar capillaries.
- When the person is unconscious at the time of drowning, **edema aquosum** develops. It is a state of mere flooding of lungs with the airless water and no formation of froth. Emphysema aquosum develops only when the conscious victim of drowning struggles for survival.
- When a dead body is thrown into water, even though *hydrostatic lungs* (due to hydrostatic pressure water passes into the lungs) are produced, yet there will be no classical signs of drowning lungs. A drowning lung together with frothy fluid is diagnostic.

2. **Larynx, trachea and bronchioles**
   - Presence of sand, mud, slit, dirt, aquatic vegetations, classical water flora, algae, and diatoms in the trachea and lower bronchial tree are characteristic *positive findings of antemortem drowning* **(Fig. 10.31A)**.
   - Fine white froth, at times blood tinged in the lumen of trachea and bronchi, interspersed with foreign material as above, is highly suggestive of death from antemortem drowning.
   - Mucosa of larynx, trachea and bronchioles may be red and congested.
   - Vomit reflex due to medullary hypoxia may result in regurgitation of gastric contents into larynx, trachea and bronchioles.

3. **Heart and blood vessels:** Like in other forms of asphyxia, left side of heart will be usually empty; the right heart will be full with the venous system engorged with dark blood, unusually fluid in consistency because of admixture with water.
   - In freshwater drowning, hemolytic discoloration of the endocardium of the left atrium and ventricle and hemolytic staining of the aortic root may be seen due to the phenomenon of *hemolytic imbibition*.

   Gettler test: Normally, the chloride content of the right and left side of heart is nearly same, about 600 mg/100 mL. If difference is 25 mg% or more, it is suggestive of antemortem drowning.
   - In case of *fresh water drowning*, the chloride content of the blood of left heart will be lower than that in right because of dilution by water.
   - In case of *salt water drowning*, chloride content of left heart will be greater than right heart because of hemoconcentration and mixing with salt water.
   - No change in chloride content of heart is seen in persons dying of laryngeal spasm or vagal inhibition, putrefaction, patent foramen ovale or the saline content of drowning medium approximates that of blood.

   Plasma magnesium: A high level of plasma magnesium in left heart blood is observed than in right heart blood and is due to absorption of magnesium from the drowning medium, particularly salt water.

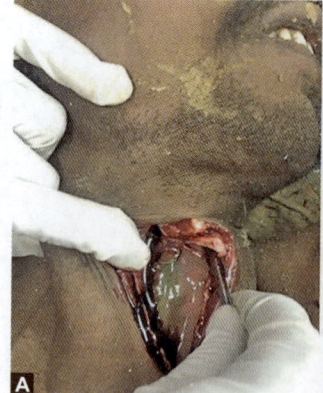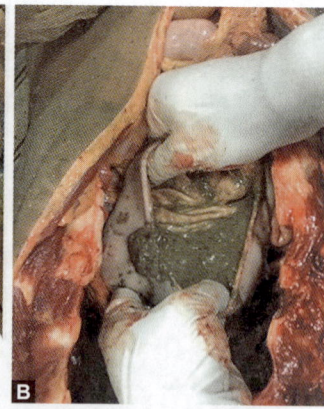

Figs. 10.31A and B: Presence of disagreeable liquid (e.g., muddy water) in (A) trachea and (B) stomach are indicators of antemortem drowning

Some researchers consider higher levels of *serum strontium* in left ventricle than in right as the best parameter for diagnosis of sea water drowning.

4. **Stomach and small intestines**
   - Stomach contains water in 70% of cases, but it is possible that the victim might have drunk the same water before death. When a disagreeable liquid is found, which could not be swallowed voluntarily and corresponds to drowning medium, like muddy water, it is a valuable indication of antemortem drowning **(Fig. 10.31B)**.
   - Water is not found in the stomach, if the person died from shock, syncope, putrefaction or was already dead (postmortem submersion).
   - Micro-ruptures of gastric mucosa due to over-stretching as a result of ingested fluid **(Sehrt's sign)** may be seen.
   - If the entire gastric content is collected in a beaker and allowed to stand for 1 h, it will form three layers—foam in uppermost, liquid in middle and sediment in lowermost **(Wydler's sign)**.
   - Small intestine may contain water in about 20% cases. This is regarded as *positive evidence of death by drowning* as it depends on peristaltic movement, which is a vital phenomenon.

> **NOTA BENE**
> Water may enter the mouth and pass down into the stomach passively if the water is turbulent, rather that the victim actively swallowing it. It may also be due to the postmortem relaxation of the gastroesophageal sphincter, which allows water to enter the stomach.

5. **Brain:** Congested gray matter, softening and loss of gray-white junction.
6. **Liver, spleen and kidneys** are congested. Spleen is small due to sympathetic stimulation with vasoconstriction and contraction of splenic capsule and trabeculae.

CHAPTER 10 : Asphyxial Deaths

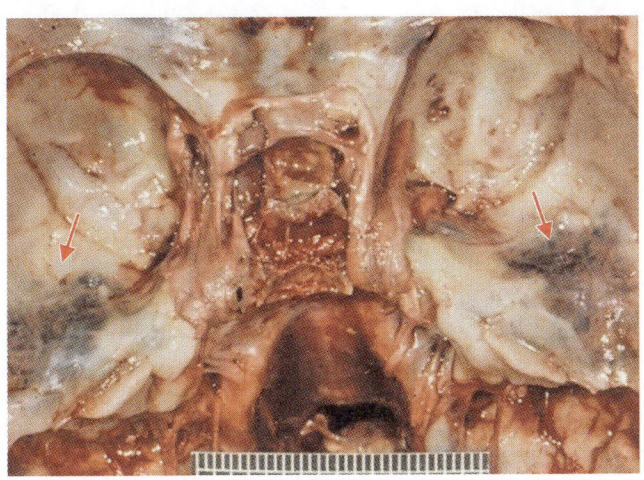

Fig. 10.32: Ueno's sign (petrous hemorrhages) (arrows)

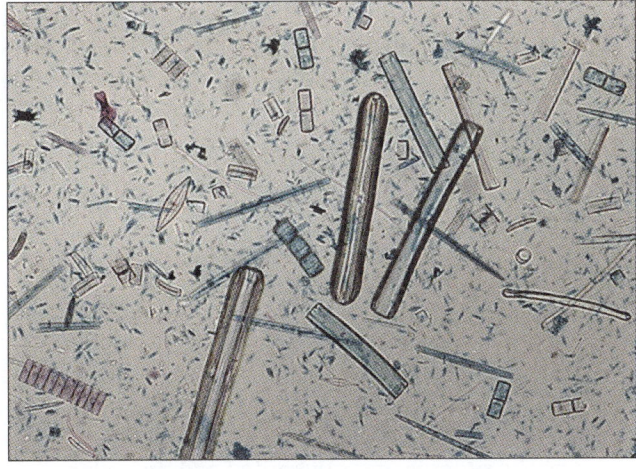

Fig. 10.33: Different types of diatoms

NOTA BENE

Drowning index = $\dfrac{\text{Weight of both lungs and pleural effusion}}{\text{Weight of spleen}}$

In drowning, the value is ≥14.1 and in non-drowning its much less.

7. **Middle ear:** Presence of water and hemorrhage in middle ear (petrous temporal bone) **(Fig. 10.32)** is claimed to be one of the positive proof of antemortem drowning **(Ueno's sign).**
   - Temporal bone hemorrhages are also seen in death due to hanging, head injury or carbon monoxide poisoning.

8. **Ethmoid and sphenoid sinuses:** Water may enter the respiratory sinuses **(Sveshnikov's sign)**; the jugum sphenoidale may be removed to expose the contents of the sphenoid sinus.

9. **Diatom test:** Diatoms belong to the class *Bacillariophyceae,* and are microscopic unicellular algae which secrete silicon skeletons called *frustules* **(Fig. 10.33).** They are chemically inert and almost indestructible, being resistant to strong acids. During drowning, diatoms (size up to 60 μ) enter the circulation via the lungs through the ruptured alveolar walls, lymph channels and pulmonary veins into left heart and then into general circulation, when the person is alive **(Fig. 10.34).**

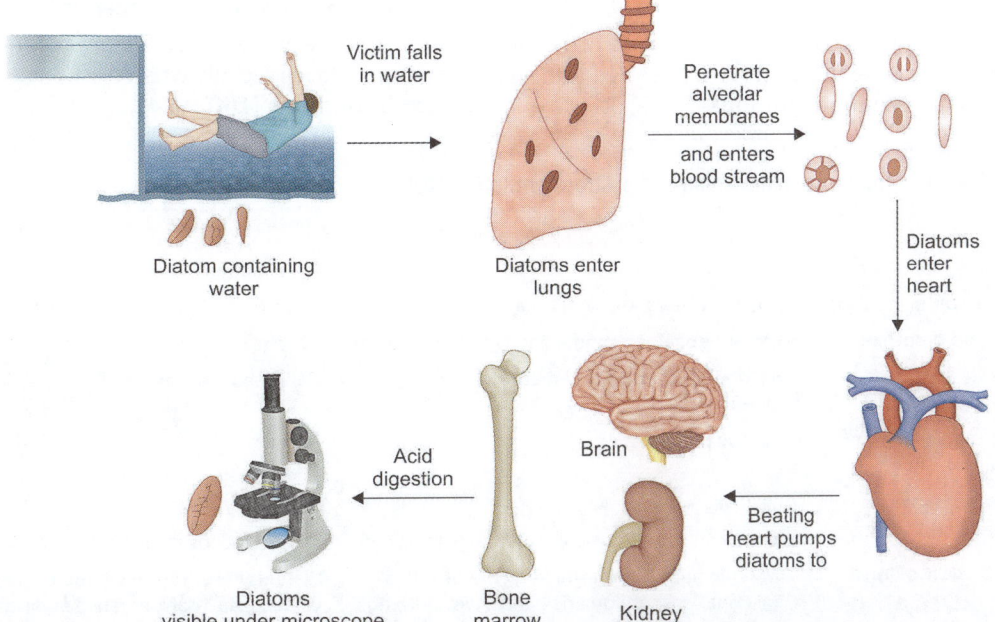

Fig. 10.34: Principle of diatom test

- Presence of diatoms in the lung substance, blood, brain, liver, kidneys, bone marrow of femur (*best site for analysis*) or humerus or in the skeletal muscle has been claimed to be *suggestive proof of antemortem drowning*.
- Since diatoms resist putrefaction, diatom test may have some value in examination of decomposed bodies.
- The test is negative in dead bodies thrown in water and in dry drowning.

Procedure: A sample of tissue is carefully retrieved to avoid surface contamination. Approximately 50 g of tissue is taken and placed in 50 mL of concentrated nitric acid in a boiling flask. The flask is heated for 48 h, cooled and the liquid is centrifuged for 20–30 min. The supernatant is discarded and the sediment is recentrifuged. The final residue is aspirated, placed on a clean glass slide and air dried. It is then examined for silica skeletons of diatoms, which are birefringent, using phase-contrast microscopy or dark ground illumination. A water sample is collected at the time of body retrieval in a clean container and similarity of different species of diatom is compared.

Interpretation

The presence of diatoms supports the diagnosis of drowning, while the absence of diatoms does not exclude it as a cause. The diatom test is valid only if it can be shown that:

- Deceased did not drink this water immediately before submersion or exposed to long-term repeated contact with the same source of diatom containing water.
- Species recovered from specimen are present in the sample from site of drowning.
- The various species are present in same order of dominance for the admissible size range and in approximately same proportions.

The test is limited by the difficulty of excluding the possibility of environmental contamination. Diatoms are ubiquitous in the environment and may enter the circulation via the GIT (as contaminants of foods, such as salads, watercress and shellfish) or via the respiratory tract (diatoms are normally present in small numbers in the air, in some paints, building plasters and dusts).

- Still, the diatom test is considered as the '*gold standard*' for diagnosis of 'typical drowning', particularly in decomposed bodies.
- The ideal diagnostic test as definite proof for drowning still needs to be established.
- At present, the combination of the autopsy findings and the diatom test is a good compromise in arriving at a conclusion.

> **Recent Advances**
> - **CT findings in antemortem fresh water drowning:** Frothy fluid in the trachea and main bronchi, many pulmonary nodular ground glass opacities or thickening in non-dependent regions of the lungs, differential level of hemidiaphragm, evidence of bronchospasm, hemodilution, presence of fluid and sediment in the paranasal sinuses, fluid in the ear, and swelling, fluid or sediment in the stomach.
> - **Molecular diagnosis of drowning:** Polymerase chain reaction (PCR) method for identifying diatoms by means of primers for chlorophyll-related genes has been developed. Other methods for identification of diatoms in tissue include amplification of planktonic or diatom DNA and RNA in human tissues, diatom cultivation in appropriate media and spectrofluorophotometry to quantify chlorophyll (a) of plankton in the lung, which is still in an experimental phase.

MEDICO-LEGAL QUESTIONS

Q. Whether death was due to drowning?

Drowning is one of the most difficult cause of death to prove at postmortem, especially when the body is not examined in a fresh condition **(Diff. 10.4)**.

DIFFERENTIATION 10.4: Antemortem drowning and postmortem submersion

S.No.	Feature	Antemortem drowning	Postmortem submersion
1.	Froth over mouth and nostrils	Fine, lathery froth, appears spontaneously	Absent, even if present, it is coarse, not spontaneous
2.	Cadaveric spasm in hands	Aquatic vegetations, mud may be present	Not observed
3.	Trachea and bronchioles	Presence of algae, mud along with frothy mucus	Absent
4.	Lungs	Ballooned up, bulky, edematous, bear indentations of ribs	Collapsed, decomposed
5.	Mud and algae in stomach and small intestine	May be present	Absent
6.	Diatom and Gettler tests	Positive	Negative
7.	Injuries	If present, need to be consistent with drowning	Injuries inconsistent with drowning
8.	Other suggestive signs	Water in middle ear, retracted genitals, cutis anserina, washerwoman's hands, wet clothing, mud and sand	Water is never present in middle ear; others are not valuable and corroborative findings

In doubtful cases, where definite opinion cannot be given, viscera and body fluids should be preserved for chemical analysis. Sometimes, the cause of death may have to be given as '*consistent with drowning*'.

Q. Whether drowning was accidental, suicidal or homicidal?

- **Accidental drowning** is most common, and seen in children, bathers, fisher men, dockworkers, intoxicated and epileptic subjects. Women may fall accidentally in a well, while drawing water. Accidental drowning may occur in precipitate labor, when the baby may fall into a bathtub or lavatory pan and die.
  - Information regarding inability to swim, trauma, seizure disorder, heart disease, exhaustion, and alcohol or drug abuse should be sought.
- **Suicide** by drowning is fairly common in India, especially among females.
  - Women usually make sure to tie up their clothes in such manner that their private parts are not exposed after death. Sometimes, a woman takes her child with her.
  - A determined suicider may tie his hands and legs together or attach weights to his body before immersion. Likewise, he may take poison, cut his throat and jump into a well.
  - If an adult is found drowned in shallow water, the presumption is usually suicide, unless proved otherwise.
  - Information/findings that may assist in the determination of suicide: Witnesses, clothes and personal effects found stacked by the water, a suicide note and suicidal ideation, a history of drug abuse, cancer or terminal illness, or unemployment, recent bizarre behavior or depression and associated self-inflicted wounds.
- **Homicidal drowning** is not very common, though it is one of the methods of choice in infanticide, especially of newborns.
  - While injuries may be found in a case of homicide, it is very easy to drown a person without leaving any suspicious mark behind, especially if the person is non-swimmer, intoxicated or already inside water taking a bath.
  - Victims of homicidal violence may be placed in the water after death in order to dispose off the body.

Hyperventilation Deaths

For long underwater swimming, the swimmer may hyperventilate before going down. While swimming, the oxygen gets utilized and the CO_2 produced, being low in tension is not sufficient to stimulate the respiratory center, and the swimmer may then suddenly become unconscious and get drowned.

In skin diving, a mask and fins are used, and it is an extension of swimming with similar hazards.

FM 2.22 Describe and discuss sexual asphyxia.

AUTOEROTIC ASPHYXIA (SEXUAL ASPHYXIA)

Definition: Autoerotic asphyxia is a paraphilia in which sexual arousal and orgasm depend on self-induced asphyxia up to, but not including loss of consciousness.

- Partial asphyxia caused by pressure on carotid vessels or obstruction of air passages causes cerebral ischemia, and may lead to hallucinations of an erotic nature in some men.
- The degree of asphyxia produced by mechanical means is controlled, i.e., the victim is in a position that allows self-release, but in some cases, death occurs accidentally.
- These cases are associated with some form of abnormal sexual behavior, usually masochism, cisvestism and transvestism.
- Victims are usually young males, scene is usually the victim's own house, bedroom, bathroom, basement, and the door is locked from inside (**Fig. 10.35**).

Methods

i. **Hanging:** Most frequent method. The presence of padding under the noose, nakedness of the victim, feminine attire and exposed genitalia are the hallmarks of these deaths. Frequently, the person ties his arms, legs and sometimes waist and genitalia (*bondage*) with a rope, string or chain.
ii. Sexual gratification may be obtained by **electrical stimulation**. For this, electrodes are applied to the genitals or on abdomen; usually a low voltage supply from a battery is used.
iii. *Other methods* include covering the head in plastic or some impervious bag, which may be secured around

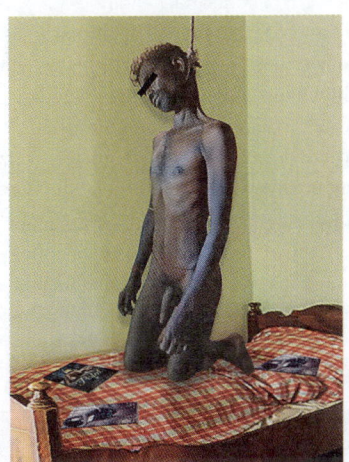

Fig. 10.35: Sexual asphyxia

the neck by an elastic band to achieve partial anoxia. It is sometimes combined with the inhalation of volatile solvents ('*glue sniffing*'). Carbon tetrachloride, paint thinners, petrol or amylacetate are either directly inhaled from container or re-breathed after placing in a plastic bag.

The scene should be examined for:
- Evidence of abnormal sexual behavior and nakedness of the deceased with presence of pornographic material. There may be mirror(s) positioned in such a way to allow viewing of the act.
- Evidence that the act has been practiced previously, such as worn grooves in rafter or door, where ropes or pulleys have been placed, from verbal communication with others regarding the nature of activities or from diaries, etc.
- Evidence of attempts to conceal the act by some method, or padding to prevent a ligature from leaving marks around neck.

There is no evidence to suggest it a suicidal act, and the situation is ruled as an accident **(Diff. 10.5)**.

DIFFERENTIATION 10.5: Death due to autoerotic asphyxia and suicide

S.No.	Feature	Autoerotic asphyxia	Suicide
1.	Salient feature	Asphyxia is due to a binding that was designed to cause hypoxia while he was engaged in some form of solitary sexual activity	Absence of any form of sexual activity
2.	Rescue mechanism	Often present in case they lose consciousness	Rarely seen
3.	History	No antemortem evidence of suicidal ideation or depression	There may be history of suicidal ideation or depression
4.	Association	Often accompanied with other paraphilias (e.g., bondage and transvestism)	Not so
5.	Sex	More among men relative to women	More in men relative to women

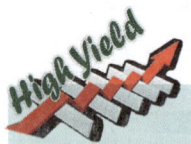

- **Tardieu's/Bayard's spots** are usually seen in conjunctiva, face, epiglottis, and subpleural surface of lungs in deaths due to asphyxia.
- Jack knife position causes death due to positional/postural asphyxia.
- In hanging, constricting force is at least part of the weight of body.
- **Most common method to commit suicide:** Hanging in males (firearm in the US) and pesticides and drowning in females.
- In typical hanging, knot is placed at the occiput.
- **Features seen in antemortem hanging**
    - Dribbling of saliva from the angle of mouth *(surest sign of antemortem hanging)*
    - *La facies sympathique* (eye remains open and pupil dilated, if the knot presses on cervical sympathetic on that side).
    - *Amussat's sign* (transverse carotid intimal tears).
    - *Simon's sign* (hemorrhages seen on intervertebral disks in the lumbar spine).
- **PM staining in hanging:** Lower limbs, forearms and hands—*glove and stocking type*.
- **Lynching:** Form of homicidal hanging.
- In judicial hanging, hangman's knot is placed beneath the chin *(submental)*.
- **Hangman fracture:** Fracture of pedicles/lamina of C2 and a traumatic spondylolisthesis of C2 over C3.
- Carotid intimal tear is seen in judicial hanging.
- Ligature mark in hanging is non-continuous, oblique and above thyroid cartilage.
- Ligature mark in strangulation complete, horizontal and below thyroid cartilage.
- Ligature mark (in hanging or strangulation) is an example of pressure abrasion.
- **Throttling:** Asphyxia produced by compression of neck by hands.

- **Diagnostic findings of throttling:** Fingernail marks, inward compression fracture of hyoid bone, and extensive bruising of neck tissues.
- *Adduction fracture* of hyoid bone is seen in throttling; *abduction fracture* in hanging.
- **Mugging:** Holding neck of victim in the bend of elbow *(chokehold)*.
- **Bansdola:** Form of homicidal strangulation with bamboo sticks placed across the front and back of neck and tightened with a rope.
- **Garroting:** Homicidal asphyxia caused by a ligature which is tightened around the neck by twisting it with a lever known as *Spanish windlass*.
- Smothering is a form of suffocation.
- **Choking:** Accidental asphyxia caused by an obstruction within the air-passages by a foreign object, like coin, candies, etc.
- **Café-coronary:** Accidental death wherein a bolus of food produces complete obstruction of the larynx. Occurs in intoxicated person.
- **Cause of death in café-coronary:** Vagal inhibition; if signs of asphyxia present then asphyxial death.
- Café-coronary should not be confused with *Caffey syndrome, i.e.,* battered baby syndrome or Caffey disease.
- **Traumatic asphyxia:** Asphyxia resulting from respiratory arrest due to mechanical fixation of chest preventing normal respiratory movements.
- In traumatic asphyxia, level of compression is indicated by a *demarcating line* between discolored upper portion and lower normal part.
- **Gagging** combines features of smothering and choking.
- **Burking:** Combination of homicidal smothering and traumatic asphyxia.
- **Overlaying:** Compression of the chest, nose and mouth, so as to prevent breathing.
- Convincing proof of burial alive is sand in trachea and bronchi.
- **Typical drowning:** Obstruction of air passages and lungs by inhalation of fluid.
- **Atypical drowning:** There is very little or no inhalation of fluid in the air passages.
- **Dry drowning:** Death due to laryngeal spasm (due to small amounts of water entering larynx; water does not enter the lungs).
- **Immersion syndrome:** Death from vagal inhibition on sudden contact with cold water.
- **Near drowning (post-immersion syndrome):** Death due to complications of submersion.
- Hemodilution is seen in freshwater drowning; hemoconcentration in salt water drowning.
- Death is earlier in fresh water drowning as compared to salt water drowning.
- **PM staining in drowning:** Face, chest, hands, lower arms, feet and calves.
- PM staining is usually *absent* in case of drowning in running water (rivers).
- **Positive proof of antemortem drowning (typical)**
  - Fine, copious white 'shaving-lather' like froth at the mouth and nostrils *(surest sign)*
  - Grass, gravel, weeds or aquatic vegetations held firmly due to *cadaveric spasm*
  - Sand, mud and aquatic vegetations in trachea and lower bronchioles
  - Presence of diatoms in blood, brain, liver, kidneys, bone marrow
- **Cutis anserina or goose skin:** Nonspecific sign in drowning.
- **Paltauf's hemorrhages:** Subpleural hemorrhages in lower lobes of lungs, seen in antemortem drowning.
- **Emphysema aquosum:** Seen in wet drowning (voluminous and distended lungs with dilation of alveoli and thinning of alveolar septae).
- **Gettler test** is done to differentiate fresh and salt water drowning based on chloride content of right and left side of heart.
- **Signs seen in antemortem drowning**
  - *Sehrt's sign* (micro-ruptures of gastric mucosa due to overstretching from ingested fluid).
  - *Wydler's sign* [gastric content forms 3 layers—foam (uppermost), liquid (middle) and sediment (lowermost)].
  - *Ueno's sign* (presence of water and hemorrhage in middle ear).
  - *Sveshnikov's sign* (water in ethmoid and sphenoid sinuses).
- **Gold standard for diagnosis of 'typical' drowning:** Diatom test.
- **Best specimen for diatom's test:** Bone marrow of femur.
- Diatoms test is negative in dry drowning and in dead bodies thrown in water.
- **Autoerotic asphyxia:** Paraphilia in which sexual arousal and orgasm depend on self-induced asphyxia.

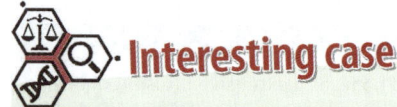 **Interesting case**

Hanging or Strangulation (Case of Jeffrey Epstein, 2019)

In July 2019, Jeffrey Epstein, a high-flying US financier was arrested and charged with sex trafficking by federal prosecutors. He was found dead in his Manhattan prison cell in August while awaiting trial. After his autopsy, the Chief Medical Examiner stated that the cause of death was hanging and the manner of death as suicide (initially did not classify the death as a suicide and listed the manner of death as 'pending'). Since then, conspiracy theories have flourished. Epstein was connected to a long list of rich and powerful people. Some suspect he was killed because of what he knew or what he threatened to tell. There are several inconsistencies in the evidence and the autopsy report as pointed out by the forensic pathologist hired by Epstein's family (who observed the autopsy too). The autopsy report mentioned:

a. Petechial hemorrhages of bilateral palpebral conjunctivae, face, head and oral mucosa
b. Confluent hemorrhages of right bulbar conjunctiva
c. Fractures of bilateral thyroid cartilage cornuae and left hyoid cornua with accompanying soft tissue hemorrhages
d. Abrasions of left forearm
e. Cutaneous contusions of wrists
f. Subcutaneous hemorrhage of left deltoid muscle

In October 2019, the pathologist issued a report stating that Epstein's neck injuries were much more consistent with 'homicidal strangulation' based on certain aspects of the autopsy, including the location of the ligature around his neck, injuries found on his body and the way PM staining settled.

Petechiae found on his face, mouth and eyes are often an indication of strangulation. The lower legs lacked PM staining suggesting that he did not die in an upright position. The ligature furrow was in the center of his neck, not under his mandibles as in a typical hanging—more common when a victim is strangled by a wire or cord. The 'furrow' was much thinner than the strip of bed-sheet which was supposedly used for suicide, and although there was blood on his neck, it was absent on the bed-sheet ligature. Epstein also had injuries on his wrists and left forearm, and deep muscle hemorrhage of his left deltoid which may suggest that he was 'handcuffed and struggled'.

Most importantly, the two fractures on the left and right sides of his thyroid cartilage as well as one fracture on the left side hyoid bone—very much unusual in suicidal hanging. Sometimes there is a fracture of the hyoid bone or a fracture of the thyroid cartilage in such cases.

The Medical Examiner's office disputed the pathologist's theory, saying that fractures of the hyoid bone and cartilage can be seen in suicides and homicides and they stand 'firmly' behind their finding of suicide by hanging.

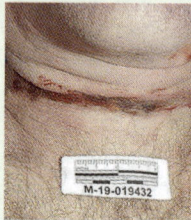
Ligature furrow

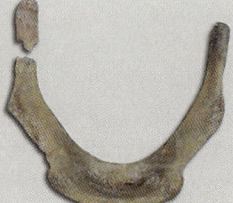
Hyoid bone fracture

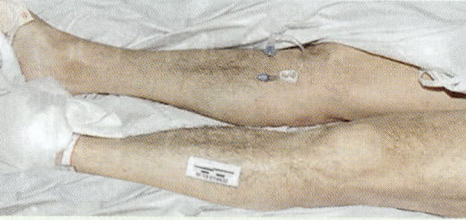
No PM staining on the legs

CHAPTER 11

Injuries

LEARNING OBJECTIVES

Must know
1. Injury (Sec. 44 IPC), classification of injuries
2. Abrasion, types, age, medico-legal importance
3. Bruise, types, color changes, ectopic bruise, patterned bruise, medico-legal importance
4. Which is more important medico-legally—abrasions or bruise?
5. Laceration, types, characteristics, medico-legal importance
6. Incised wound, characteristics, hesitation cuts, tailing, beveling, medico-legal importance
7. Langer's lines
8. Chop wounds
9. Stab wound, classification, characteristics, medico-legal importance
10. Defense wounds, fabricated wounds
11. Suicidal and homicidal cut throat wounds (Diff.)
12. PM staining and bruise (Diff.)
13. Suicidal and homicidal stab wounds (Diff.)

Desirable to know
1. Antemortem and postmortem abrasion and bruise (Diff.)
2. Age of incised wound and lacerated wound
3. Bevelling
4. Examination of a weapon

Define injury.

Define, describe and classify different types of mechanical injuries.

Definitions

- **Injury:** Any harm, whatever illegally, caused to any person in *body, mind, reputation or property* (**Sec. 44 IPC**).
- **Wound:** *Clinically*, it means any injury where there is breach of natural continuity of skin or mucous membrane. *In medico-legal practice,* the terms 'wound' and 'injury' are synonymous, but strictly wound will include any lesion, external or internal, caused by violence, with or without breach of continuity of skin.
  Different tissues have varying properties of elasticity (tendency of stressed material to regain its unstressed condition), plasticity (tendency to remain in stressed condition), and viscosity (resistance to change in shape when stressed).
  Different tissues, therefore, have different elastic limits (tolerance) and are vulnerable to different stresses. Injury occurs when energy applied exceeds the elastic limits of the tissues.

CLASSIFICATION OF WOUNDS/INJURIES

Injuries can be classified in many ways:

Based on Causative Factors

1. **Mechanical or physical injuries** (*produced by physical violence*, **Fig. 11.1**)
    i. Abrasion
    ii. Bruise or contusion
    iii. Lacerated wound
    iv. Incised wound
    v. Stab wound
    vi. Firearm wound
    vii. Fracture/dislocation of bone, tooth or joint.
- *Blunt force trauma* is caused when an object, usually without a sharp or cutting edge, impacts the body or the body impacts the object. Abrasion (can be caused by pointed objects too), contusion, laceration and fracture/dislocation of bone of tooth result from such an impact.

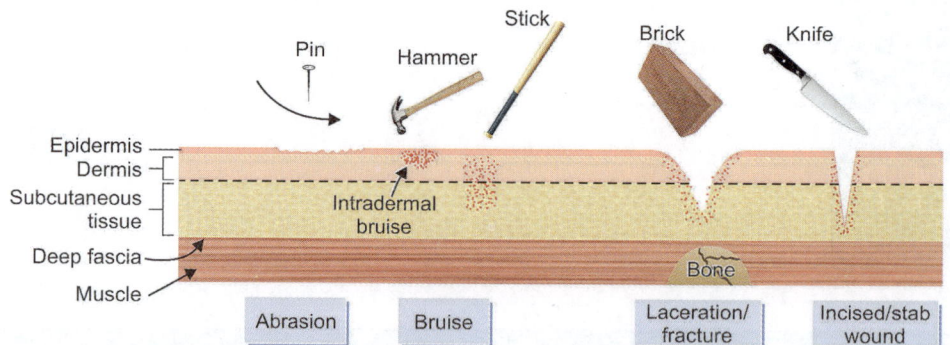

Fig. 11.1: Mechanical injuries caused by blunt and sharp objects

- *Sharp force trauma* occurs when an object with a sharp or sharpened edge impacts the body. Incised and stab wounds result from such trauma.
- For any given amount of force, the greater the area over which it is delivered, the less severe the wound (as applicable to blunt and sharp trauma).

2. **Thermal injuries**
   Due to application of heat
   a. General effects (may not cause any visible injury), e.g., heat cramps and heat stroke.
   b. Effects of local application, e.g., burns and scalds.
   Due to application of cold
   a. General effects, e.g., hypothermia.
   b. Local effects, e.g., frost bite and trench foot.

3. **Chemical injuries**
   a. *Irritation:* Due to application of weak acids, alkalis, plant or animal extracts.
   b. *Corrosion:* Due to application of strong acids or alkalis.

4. **Miscellaneous injuries**
   a. Electrical injury.
   b. *Radiation injury:* Due to X-ray, UV radiation, radioactive substances.
   c. Lightning injury.
   d. Blast injury.

   Injuries in category 1 are called *kinetic injuries* (caused by application of physical force), whereas the injuries in categories 2, 3 and 4 are called *non-kinetic* or *non-motion injuries*.

Based on Nature of Injury (Legally)

i. Simple
ii. Grievous.

Based on Manner of Injuries (Medico-legally)

i. Suicidal
ii. Homicidal
iii. Accidental
iv. Defense wounds
v. Fabricated or self-inflicted wounds.

Based on Time of Infliction

i. Antemortem—recent or old
ii. Postmortem.

FM 3.3, 3.6
- Define, describe and classify abrasion and its medico-legal aspects.
- Describe healing of injury with its medico-legal importance.

ABRASION

Definition: Abrasion is the removal of superficial epithelial layer of the skin, usually the epidermis and papillary dermis, by friction against rough surface.

Classification (Fig. 11.2)

i. **Scratch/linear abrasion**: It is caused by a sharp or pointed object passing across the skin, such as

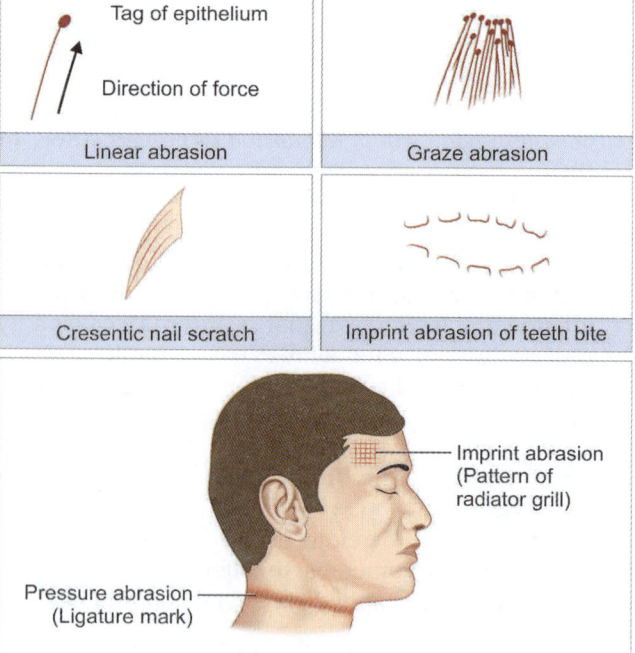

Fig. 11.2: Types of abrasions

fingernails, thorn or pin. Surface layers of skin are collected in front of the object, which leaves a clean area at the start, and tags at the end **(Fig. 11.3)**. Fingernail abrasions are seen in throttling, sexual assaults and child abuse.

ii. **Graze abrasion**
   - Grazes (*gravel rash*) are caused by horizontal or tangential friction between the skin and the hard rough surface. They show uneven, longitudinal parallel lines, which indicate the direction in which the force was applied (epidermis being heaped up at the opposite end) **(Fig. 11.3)**.
   - Most common type of abrasion, and commonly seen in road traffic accidents. Particles of glass, gravel or dirt may be embedded in such wounds.
   - **Brush burn:** Graze abrasion involving wider area such as the back, caused by violent rubbing against a surface, as in dragging along over the ground. Such injuries, when dry, become firm, even though no true 'scab' is present.
   - **Friction burn:** An extensive, superficial, reddened excoriated area with little or no linear mark, occurs when the skin is covered by clothing (element of thermal damage is present).

iii. **Pressure abrasion (crushing/friction abrasion):** It is caused by direct impact or linear pressure of a rough object over the skin. There is prolonged compression with minimal force resulting in crushing the superficial layers of the cuticle and bruising underneath, e.g., nooses or ligatures in hanging and strangulation.

iv. **Imprint abrasion (impact/patterned abrasion):** It is caused when a large force is applied perpendicular to the skin for a short duration, the cuticle gets crushed at the point of impact and bears the imprint of the object causing it.
   - The abrasion in slightly depressed below the surface.
   - It tends to be focal, and is commonly seen over bony prominences, where a thin layer of skin covers the bone.
   - Imprint abrasion becomes more defined when injured cuticle dries up and becomes brownish and parchmentized, in contrast with the surrounding uninjured skin surface.
   - Pattern abrasion is a variation of pressure abrasion.
   - When a person is knocked down by car, pattern of the radiator grill, headlamp rim or tyre-tread mark may be seen on the skin. Imprint of bicycle chain, serrated knife are other examples.
   - Teeth bite marks are included in this category, though they may produce contusion or laceration, depending upon the force applied.
   - UV light may be used to visualize the pattern injuries not apparent with visible light.

> **NOTA BENE**
> **Human bite** can occur during sexual behavior/assault, child abuse, self-defense, self-inflicted or a child biting another child. Bite may tear or crush, resulting in two U-shaped marks, corresponding to the upper and lower anterior six teeth (canine to canine) and separated by an open space of about 2.5–4 cm. Most victims of a criminal act are women, and breast is the most common location. Male victims are more frequently bitten on the arms.

Dating/Age of Abrasion

It produces minimum bleeding, heals rapidly (takes about 1 week) and leaves no permanent scarring on healing **(Table 11.1)**.

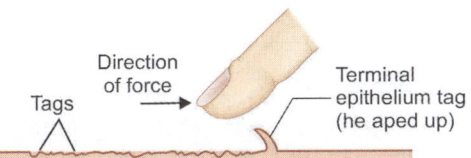

Fig. 11.3: Direction of force in an abrasion

Identify the type of abrasion:

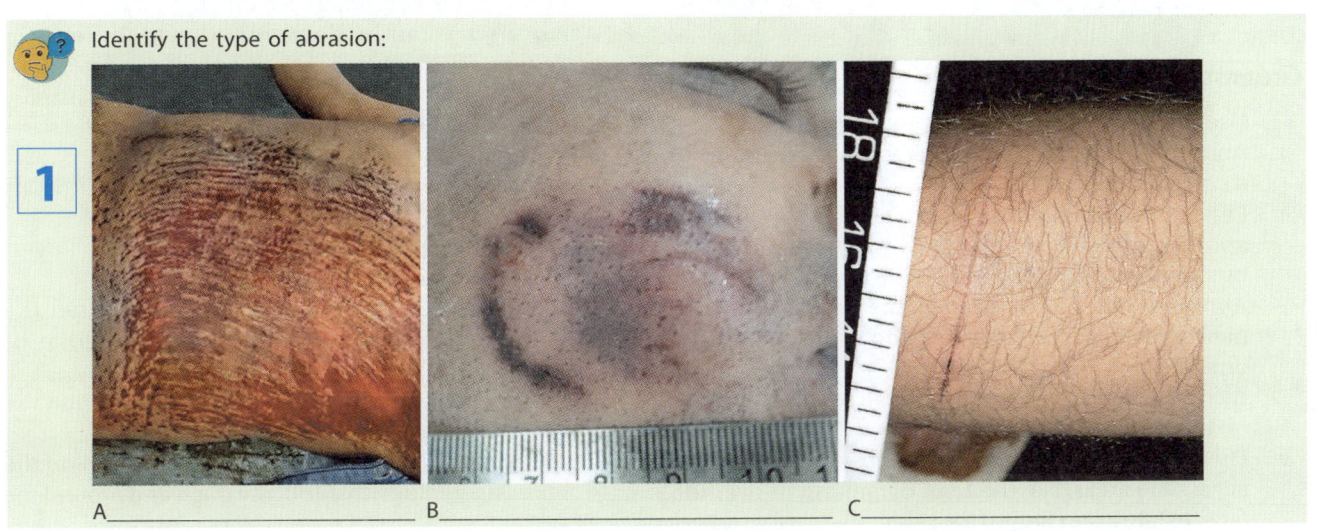

A_____ B_____ C_____

TABLE 11.1: Age of abrasion

Duration	Features
Fresh	Bright red, oozing of serum and some blood
2–24 h	Exudation dries to form a reddish scab, comprising blood, lymph and epithelial cells. Polymorphonuclear cells infiltrate (*scab formation*)
2–3 days	Reddish-brown scab, less tender
4–5 days	Scab is dark brown in color
5–7 days	Scab is brownish black and starts falling off from the margins. Epithelium grows and covers defect under the scab (*epithelial regeneration*)
7–12 days	Scab dries, shrinks and falls off, leaving depigmented area underneath. It gradually gets pigmented in due course of time (*subepidermal granulation*)
>12 days	Epithelium becomes thinner and atrophic. New collagen fibers are prominent. Basement membrane is present and vascularity of the dermis decreases (*regression*)

Differential Diagnosis

i. Postmortem insect bites of the skin caused by ants or cockroaches produce dry, pale brown lesions with irregular margins and are arranged in a linear pattern. Most commonly found at mucocutaneous junctions—around the eyelids, nose, mouth, ears, axilla, groins and genitalia. Vital reaction is absent.
   - It may also resemble tattooing (firearm injury).
ii. Excoriation of skin by excreta and diaper rash may be misinterpreted as abrasions.
iii. Dry skin of scrotum and vulva gives a reddish brown or yellow coloration when exposed to the open air.
iv. *Decubitus/pressure ulcers* (bed sores): These are due to pressure necrosis of the skin in a bedridden, caused by prolonged compression of soft tissue between bony prominence and external surface.
v. *Postmortem abrasions* (Diff. 11.1, and Figs. 11.4A and B): In doubtful cases, a histopathological examination may be needed.

Circumstances of Abrasions

i. Usually, it is seen in accidents and assaults.
ii. Abrasions on the face or body of the assailant indicate a struggle.
iii. Person collapsing due to a heart attack may fall forward and receive abrasions on the forehead, nose and cheek, but there will be no injuries on the upper limbs.
iv. Abrasions may be produced on the palmar surface of hands in a conscious person, who while falling puts out his hands to save himself.
v. Alcoholics tend to fall backwards and strike the occiput on the ground.
vi. Hysterical women may produce abrasions over accessible areas, like the front of forearm or over the face, to fabricate charge of assault.

DIFFERENTIATION 11.1: Antemortem and postmortem abrasion (Figs. 11.4A and B)

S.No.	Feature	Antemortem abrasion	Postmortem abrasion
1.	Site	Anywhere on the body	Usually, over bony prominences
2.	Color	Bright red	Yellowish, translucent and parchment-like
3.	Exudation	More, scab slightly raised	Less, no scab
4.	Vital reaction	Present	Absent
5.	Healing process	May be evident	Not seen

Note: Abrasions produced slightly before or after death cannot be differentiated even by microscopic examination.

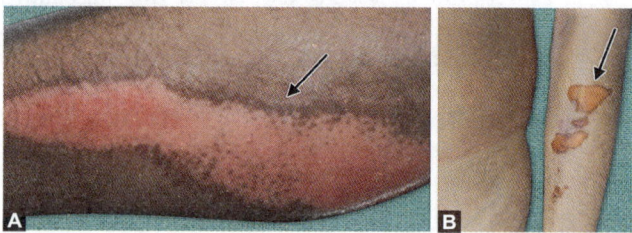

Figs. 11.4A and B: Abrasion: (A) Antemortem; (B) Postmortem

Medico-legal Importance

- Abrasions give an idea about the *site of impact and direction of force*.
- *Nature of injury*: Abrasions are superficial injuries and are mostly simple in nature. However, they may be the only external signs of serious internal injury. Abrasions over the cornea may cause corneal opacity, which may restrict vision permanently, amounting to grievous hurt (**Sec. 320 IPC**).
- Patterned abrasions are helpful in connecting the wound with the *causative weapon*.
- *Age of injury* can be determined, which helps to corroborate with alleged time of assault.
- In open wounds, dirt, dust, grease or sand is usually present which helps to connect the injuries to the *scene of crime*.
- *Character and manner of injury* may be known from its distribution:
   i. In *throttling*, crescentic abrasions made by fingernails are found on the neck.
   ii. Abrasions on the victim may show whether the fingernails of assailant were long, irregular or broken.
   iii. In *smothering*, abrasions may be seen around the mouth and nose.
   iv. In *sexual assaults*, abrasions may be found on the breasts, genitals, inside of the thigh and around the arms.

CHAPTER 11 : Injuries

> **NOTA BENE**
>
> **Patterned injuries** can be subdivided according to the type of force involved:
> i. **Blunt force injuries:** These are the most commonly seen group. Abrasions may preserve patterns well, especially if the force is applied perpendicular to the skin surface. Bruises may also reproduce patterns well, particularly if they are intradermal. Lacerations less frequently show a well-defined reproduction of the shape of the causative agent.
> ii. **Sharp force injuries:** Stab wounds may show characteristics of a specific type of blade. Distinctive patterns may be seen with the hilt, or a stab wound with screwdrivers or scissors.
> iii. **Gunshot wounds:** Contact entry wounds (may have sight marks) and shotgun wounds (e.g., wad marks) may produce distinct patterned injuries.
> iv. **Other miscellaneous wounds and marks,** e.g., fern-like pattern with lightning strikes, tool marks on internal structures (such as cartilage).
>
> *Medico-legal importance:* Connect a particular weapon or object to an injury, which may allow a perpetrator to be linked to the crime and/or enable better understanding of the events surrounding a death.

FM 3.3, 3.6, 3.7

- Define, describe and classify bruise and its medico-legal aspects.
- Describe healing of injury with its medico-legal importance.
- Describe factors influencing infliction of injuries and healing.

BRUISE/CONTUSION

Definition: Bruise is the extravasation of blood in the subcutaneous/subepithelial tissues due to rupture of blood vessels, usually capillaries, as a result of blunt force injury or pressure.

- Usually, there is no loss of continuity of the overlying skin.
- 'Bruise' implies that the lesion is observed through the overlying intact skin as bluish purple discoloration and swelling of the involved area, while a 'contusion' is a bruise within an organ or tissues, such as muscles, liver or mesentery.

Causes

i. By application of blunt force, such as blow with fists, sticks, iron-bar, cane, whip or chain.
ii. From compression, like pressing fingers.
iii. Medical intervention sometimes produces bruise—sternal and cardiac bruising, bruising around needle puncture marks and pinching skin to test conscious level (*butterfly bruise*).

Classification

Bruise is classified into three types depending on its situation:
i. **Intradermal bruise:** Bruise lies in the immediate subepidermal layer. It is made by impact with a patterned object, and hemorrhage is sharply defined.
ii. **Subcutaneous bruise:** It is situated in subcutaneous tissue, often in the fatty layer, and the edges are blurred. Most common type of bruise caused by a blunt object, and appears soon after injury as dark red swelling.
iii. **Deep bruise:** Bleeding deeper to the subcutaneous tissues. It may take hours to 1–2 days to appear at the surface (**delayed bruising**). Therefore, one more examination should be carried out 24–48 h after first examination. *Infrared photography* may demonstrate such bruises, if suspected initially.

Factors Influencing the Bruise

i. **Type of tissue/site involved**
- Soft, lax and vascular tissues, such as face, scrotum and eyelids develop large bruises with little force.
- In tissues which are strongly supported, contain firm fibrous tissue and are covered by thick dermis, e.g., abdomen, back, scalp, palms and soles, even a moderate violence may produce only a small bruise.
- Bruising of scalp is better felt than seen.

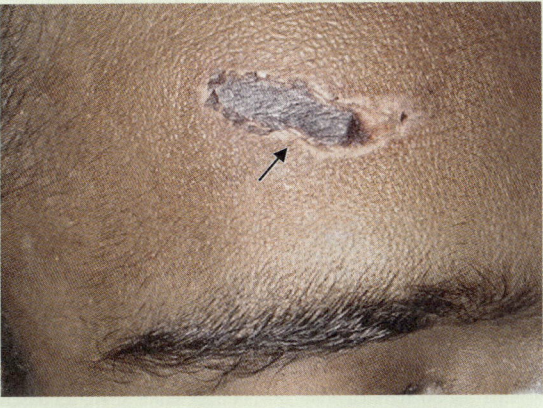

2 What could be the age of this abrasion?

A. 24 h B. 3–4 days
C. 4–5 days D. 5–7 days

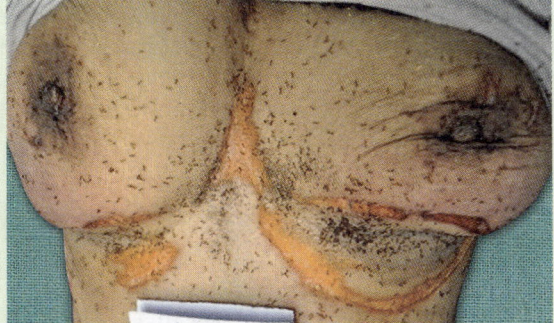

3 The surface injuries represents:

A. Early signs of death B. Healed abrasion
C. Postmortem ant bites D. Postmortem abrasions

- Bruising is more marked on tissues overlying bone.
- In boxers and athletes, bruising is much less, because of good muscle tone.
- Chronic alcoholics with cirrhosis and individuals taking aspirin bruise easily.

ii. **Age:** Children and elderly bruise more easily because of softer tissue and delicate skin in the former, and loss of subcutaneous supportive tissue and cardiovascular changes in the latter.

iii. **Sex:** Women tend to bruise more easily than men because tissues are more delicate and subcutaneous fat is more. Obese people bruise more easily than lean because tissues are more delicate.

iv. **Color of skin:** Bruising is more clearly seen and recognized in fair skinned persons than those with dark skin, in whom they may be better felt than seen.

v. **Natural diseases:** Prominent bruising following minor trauma is seen in persons suffering from atherosclerosis, purpura hemorrhagica, leukemia, hemophilia, scurvy, bleeding diathesis, vitamin K and prothrombin deficiency, and in phosphorus poisoning.

vi. **Gravity shifting of blood (ectopic/migratory bruise):** It is responsible for the appearance of bruises at a site other than the site of injury, e.g., black eyes **(Fig. 11.5)**. Blood will track along the fascial planes (or between muscle layers) along the path of least resistance and may appear where the tissue layers become superficial. Thus, site of bruise does not always indicate the site of injury.

> **NOTA BENE**
> - **Grey Turner's sign:** Ecchymosis seen over flank or side of abdomen, occurring due to extensive retroperitoneal hemorrhage. This sign takes 24–48 h to develop.
> - **Cullen's sign:** Bluish-black discoloration of the periumbilical skin due to extensive retroperitoneal or intra-abdominal hemorrhage. This may be caused by ruptured ectopic pregnancy or acute pancreatitis.

Patterned Bruise

Patterned intradermal bruise is due to impact with a hard, patterned object with ridges and grooves. Bruise may indicate the nature of the weapon, especially when death occurs soon after infliction of injury.

Mechanism: When the weapon sinks into the skin, there is little or no damage to the blood vessels over ridges where it compresses the skin. However, traction causes marginal dermal vessels to rupture in the skin forced into grooves. The resulting accumulation of a small amount of blood, near the epidermis may demonstrate the obvious pattern of the causal surface (tyre, rod, shoe tread, car bumper, clothing, or gun muzzle) **(Fig. 11.6A)**.

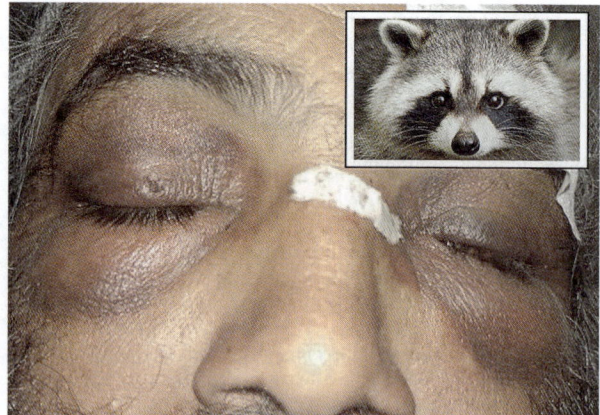

Fig. 11.5: Ectopic or migratory bruise (black eyes or raccoon eyes)

- A blow from a solid body, such as hammer or a closed fist produces a rounded bruise. *Doughnut bruise* is due to a spherical object (such as cricket ball).
- Blows with a rod, stick or a whip produce two parallel, linear hemorrhages (**railway line or tram-line type**). The intervening skin appears unchanged **(Fig. 11.6B)**.
- A woven, spiral or plaited ligature may produce a patterned bruise. A solid stick bruise is limited to the convexity of the body surface. A flexible strap or flex will wrap around the convexity producing a longer and often curved tram-line bruise.
- Suction or biting on the sides of the neck or the breasts during love making/sexual intercourse produces elliptical patterned bruises.*

Deep Tissue and Organ Contusion

- Internal organs can also get contused; contusion of the brain may cause confusion, coma and death.
- Contusion in vital centers, e.g., which controls respiration and blood pressure can be fatal even when very small.
- Small contusions of heart can cause serious disturbances of normal rhythm or stoppage of cardiac action and death.

Dating/Age of Bruise

Consistent, reliable microscopic dating is not possible and color changes in resolution of a contusion is not always a reliable indicator of its age. However, methods used to date a bruise are:
i. Histology (only in postmortem situation)
ii. Color changes (visual examination)
iii. Calorimetry
iv. Spectrophotometry.

- Bruises heal by destruction and removal of extravasated blood.
- The extravasation of blood is followed by an inflammatory reaction that causes vasodilation and

---

*Love bite (*hickey*) is not actually a true bite since there are no teeth marks. Bruise is caused by firm application of the lips against the skin, forming an air-tight seal, and oral suction cause a shower of petechial bruises from rupture of numerous small vessels.

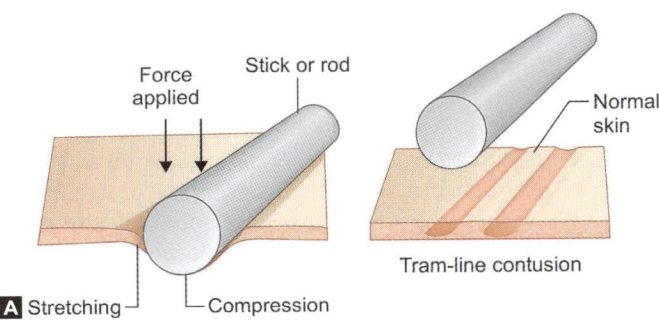
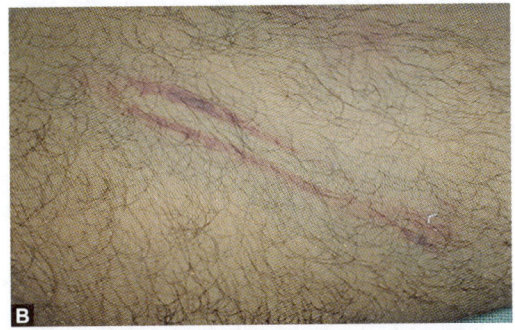

Figs. 11.6A and B: (A) Formation of 'tram-line contusion'; (B) Tram-line bruise

attracts macrophages, which breaks down hemoglobin to biliverdin. Biliverdin is then broken down by the enzyme *biliverdin reductase* to yellow color bilirubin. As hemoglobin is broken down, some of its iron is released and combines with ferritin, which gives rise to hemosiderin.

- Color change starts at the periphery and extends inwards to the center.
- The time required for bruising to clear is extremely variable (takes about 2 weeks) and is only a general guideline in interpreting the age of the bruise **(Table 11.2)**. It should only be stated whether the bruise is recent or old.
- **Subconjunctival hemorrhage** does not show similar color changes owing to hemoglobin being kept oxygenated by air. It is red at first, then becomes yellow and finally disappears **(Fig. 11.7)**. Similar changes are seen in **meningeal hemorrhages** owing to O_2 supplied from CSF.

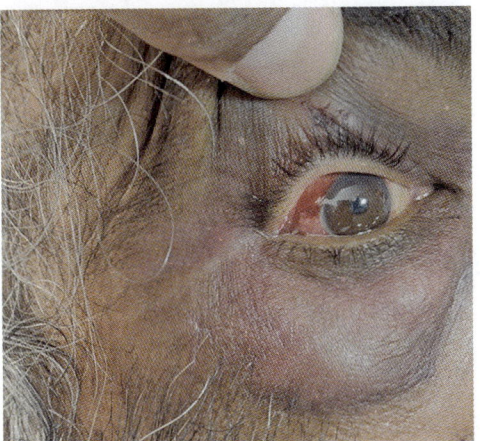

Fig. 11.7: Subconjunctival hemorrhage is reddish in color whereas the periorbital hemorrhage is bluish red. The patient sustained injury 36 h back

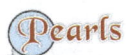

Color change is not seen in:
- Subconjunctival hemorrhages
- Meningeal hemorrhages
- Discoloration in traumatic asphyxia

- Healthier the individual, the more rapid will be the healing. A bruise takes a much longer duration to heal in the old than in the young. In old age, it may remain for 4–5 weeks. Bruises of soft loose tissues, like those surrounding the eye resolve faster.
- Environmental lighting may slightly alter the color of the bruise. Drugs, such as steroids may change the rate of bruise dispersion, and interventions, such as ice packs or heat treatment may add to variability.
- Bruises of the same age may show different color progression, so that variation in color does not necessarily mean that there have been multiple episodes of injury.
- Not all bruises pass through a yellow phase before they resolve.
- Dating a bruise may be helpful in determining the veracity of the informant and together with other data may justify further investigation into a particular case.

NOTA BENE

- Hemosiderin is a granular brown iron-storage complex composed of ferric oxide, commonly found in macrophages and derived from breakdown of hemoglobin.
- Biliverdin is a green pigment formed as a byproduct of heme breakdown.
- Bilirubin was discovered by Virchow in 1849, who called the yellow pigment '**hematoidin**'.

TABLE 11.2: Age of bruise

Duration	Color
Fresh	Red (oxygenated blood)
Few hours to 3 days	Blue (deoxyhemoglobin)
4–5 days	Bluish black to brown (hemosiderin)
5–6 days	Green (biliverdin)
7–12 days	Yellow (bilirubin)
2 weeks	Normal

Complications

i. Multiple contusions can cause death from shock and internal hemorrhage.

ii. Gangrene and death of tissue can result.
iii. Bacterial infections, especially by *Clostridia* can occur.
iv. Pulmonary fat embolism may occur.

Estimate the age of the bruise from its color:

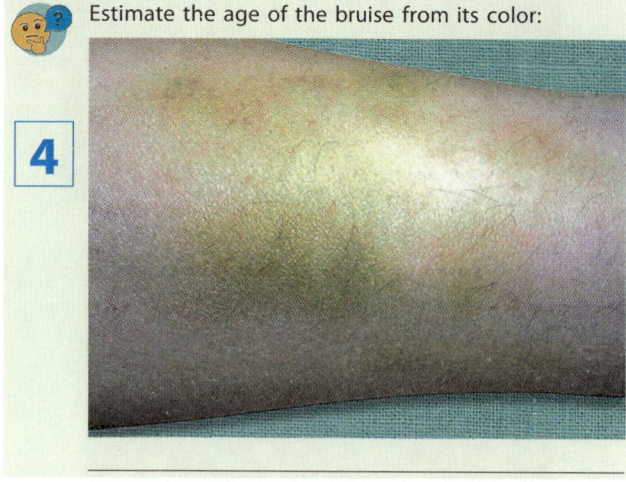

Medico-legal Importance

♦ It is advisable that a medical officer should re-examine the patient after 24 h, as by this time deep bruises are clearly visible.

♦ *Age of injury* can be determined by the color changes.
♦ *Degree of violence* may be determined from their size. Since, the appearance of bruise depends upon many factors, great caution must be used before giving any opinion regarding its appearance.
♦ Patterned bruises may connect the victim and the *object/weapon*, e.g., whip, chain, tyre, cane or ligature.
♦ *Nature of injury*: Bruises are generally simple injury. However, the impact responsible may result in injury to the vital organs underneath the bruised area. In such a situation, the bruise is grievous in nature.
♦ Contusions can be produced postmortem, if a severe blow is given to the body within few hours after death. To confirm at postmortem examination, deep incisions are made at suspected sites, which show ecchymosis **(Diff. 11.2)**.
♦ Sometimes, the autopsy surgeon needs to differentiate bruise from PM staining **(Diff. 11.3)**. Since in early phases of development of PM staining, it may look like a bruise, which may led to misinterpretation (assault/trauma).
♦ Bruises may be fabricated by applying juices of marking nut or calotropis to incriminate others, or in defense of a crime.
♦ Surgical removal of cornea can result in hemorrhage into the eyelids, identical with antemortem trauma.

DIFFERENTIATION 11.2: Antemortem and postmortem bruise

S.No.	Feature	Antemortem bruise	Postmortem bruise
1.	Swelling	Present	Absent
2.	Damage to epithelium	Present	Absent
3.	Extravasation of blood	Present	Absent
4.	Coagulation	Present	Absent
5.	Infiltration of the tissues with blood	Present	Absent
6.	Color changes	Seen	Uniform color
7.	Margins	Merge with surrounding area	Sharply demarcated
8.	Appearance	More marked in victims who survive for sometime	Less marked

DIFFERENTIATION 11.3: Postmortem staining and bruise

S.No.	Feature	PM staining	Bruise
1.	Cause	Distension of vessels with blood in dermis	Rupture of vessels which may be superficial or deep
2.	Cuticle	Not abraded	May be abraded
3.	Site	Occurs over extensive area of the most dependent parts	Occurs at the site of and surrounding the injury, may appear anywhere on the body
4.	Appearance	No elevation of involved area	Often swollen, because of extravasated blood and edema
5.	Margins	Clearly defined	Merge with the surrounding area
6.	Color	Uniform bluish-purple color	Different colors, depending on the age of bruise
7.	On incision	Blood is seen in blood vessels, can be easily washed away, subcutaneous tissues are pale	Extravasation of blood into the surrounding tissues, cannot be washed by water, subcutaneous tissues are deep reddish-black
8.	Effect of pressure	Absent in areas of the body which are under even slight pressure	Lighter over the area of pressure or support
9.	Superimposed abrasion	Not present	May be present
10.	Microscopically	Blood cells are found within the blood vessels and there is no evidence of inflammation	Blood cells are found outside the blood vessels, evidence of inflammation present

- *Character and manner of injury* may be known from its distribution:
    i. Bruising of the arm may be a sign of restraining a person. When arms are grasped, there may be 3–4 bruises on one side (corresponding to fingers) and one larger bruise on the opposite side (thumb).
    ii. Small bruises along with nail marks on the inner aspect of thighs of a woman may indicate sexual assault.
    iii. Typical small bruises (*six-penny bruises*) are produced by forcible poking or pressure of fingertips.
    iv. Bruising of the shoulder blades indicates firm pressure on the body against the ground or other resisting surface.
    v. In manual strangulation, position, number of bruises and nail marks give an indication of the position of the assailant.
    vi. Bruises found in 'soft' sites in a child such as cheeks or trunk, and multiple bruises in various stages of healing suggest abuse.

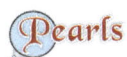

Bruises are of lesser value than abrasions because:
- Their size may not correspond to the size of the weapon.*
- They do not indicate the direction in which the force was applied.
- They may become visible after few hours or even 1–2 days after injury.
- They may appear at a distance away from the actual site of injury. It may not indicate the point of trauma.

NOTA BENE

Bone contusion refers to trabecular microfractures due to impaction of bone. It may occur due to blunt force from outside the body or more commonly from two bones striking each other after ligament injuries. Conventional X-rays may not detect bone contusion, and MRI is needed in acute stages.

 Name the type of injury. Can you identify the causative agent?

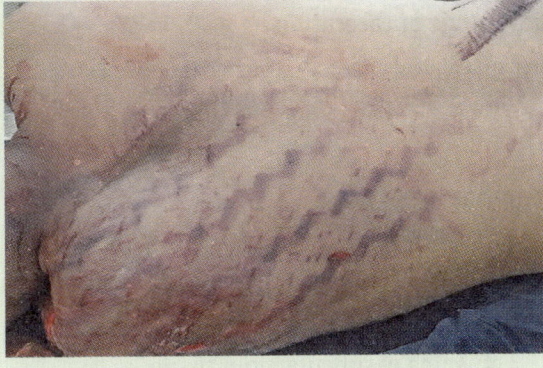

FM 3.3, 3.6
- Define, describe and classify laceration and its medico-legal aspects.
- Describe healing of injury with its medico-legal importance.

LACERATED WOUND

Definition: Laceration is the tearing or splitting of skin, mucous membranes, muscles or internal organs caused by either a shearing or a crushing force, and produced by application of a *blunt force* to a broad area of the body.

If the blunt force produces extensive bruising and laceration of deeper tissue, it is called *crush injury*.

Classification

i. **Split lacerations:** Occur when soft tissues are sandwiched between a hard unyielding deeper structure and the agent applying the force. Scalp lacerations occur due to the tissues being crushed between the skull and some hard object (**Fig. 11.8A**).
   - **Incised-looking lacerated wounds:** When the skin is closely applied to the bone and the subcutaneous tissue is scanty, blunt force may produce a wound which by linear splitting of the tissues resembles an incised wound.
   - *Sites:* Scalp, forehead, eyebrows, zygoma, iliac crest, lower jaw, perineum and shin.

ii. **Stretch lacerations:** Result from a heavy forceful frictional impact of blunt forces exercising localized '*pressure with pull*'.
   - Overstretching of the skin and subcutaneous tissues may cause lacerations with flapping of the skin, which may indicate the direction of application of force.
   - They are seen in run over by motor vehicle, kicking and in compound fractures.

iii. **Avulsion or grinding compression:** Produced by shearing force delivered at an oblique or tangential angle to detach (tear off) a portion of traumatized skin surface or viscus (tissue/organ) from their attachment.
   - Commonly seen in road traffic accidents where the rotating force of a wheel tears off the skin over a large area. This is called *flaying*, and most frequently occurs on the legs (**Fig. 11.8B**).
   - Amputation injuries are a type of avulsion injury in which an entire extremity or portion thereof is severed from the body.
   - The most severe is a decapitation injury, in which the head separates from the body.

iv. **Tears:** Tearing of skin and subcutaneous tissue can occur from localized impact by or against some hard, irregular object, like car door handle, radiator mascot or from blows with broken glass bottles (sometimes).

---

*The size of a bruise is not necessarily related to the size of the object. Thus, one cannot state that a bruise, 9 × 3 cm, was caused by an object of similar dimensions.

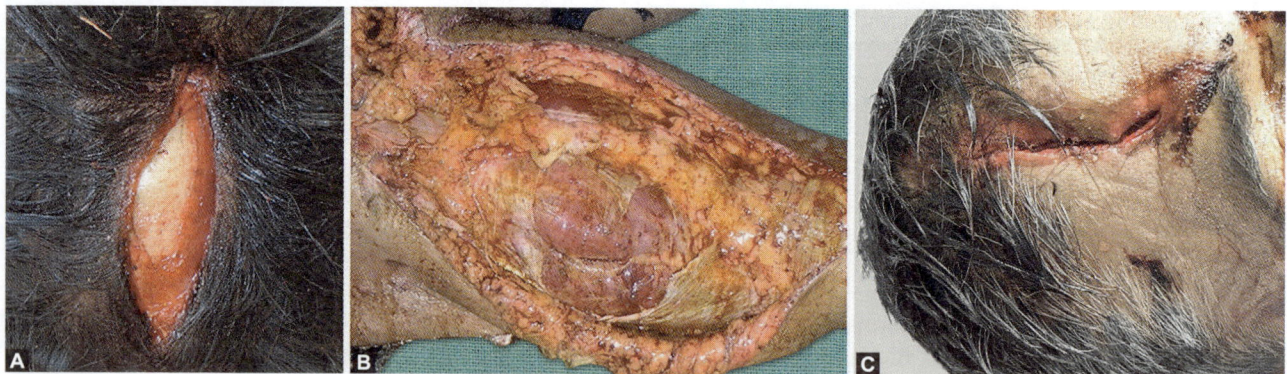

Figs. 11.8A to C: Laceration: (A) Split laceration; (B) Avulsed laceration; (C) Cut laceration

v. **Cut lacerations:** Sometimes, a heavy moderately sharp edged weapon causes a deep and wide cut over the body tissues **(Fig. 11.8C)**.

Characteristics (Fig. 11.9)

- **Margins:** Ragged, irregular and uneven; may show tearing of the extremities at angles diverging from the main laceration (*shallow tails*) **(Fig. 11.10)***; pieces of tissue are attached in between called *tissue tags*.
- **Site:** Occurs most commonly over bony prominences, such as the head where the skin is fixed and easily stretched and torn.
- **Bruising and abrasion:** Seen around the margin.
- **Edges:** May give an indication of direction in which the blow or force was applied.
- **Depth of wound:** Shows bridges of irregularly torn fibrous tissue, blood vessels and nerves across the interior of the wound. ¥
- **Soiling of wound:** Mud, wood splinters, sand, glass fragments or paint material of the vehicle involved, hair or fibers may get embedded in the wound, and are of great medico-legal importance.
- **Hair bulbs:** Crushed.
- **Hemorrhage:** Less, because the arteries are crushed and torn across irregularly; they retract and blood clots readily, *except* in the scalp where the temporal arteries bleed freely, as they are firmly bound and unable to contract.
- **Shape:** May correspond with the weapon or object which produced them.
- **Gaping:** Seen due to pull of elastic and muscular tissues.
- **Beveling:** Laceration caused by a blow directed tangentially or at an angle will produce undermining of the tissue on one side (indicates the direction of blow) and abrasion and beveling on the other (direction from which the blow was coming).
- **On healing:** Produces permanent scar.

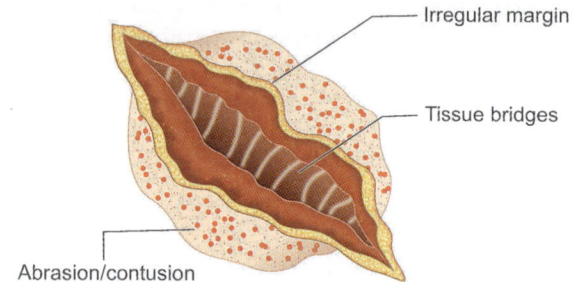

Fig. 11.9: Characteristics of lacerated wound

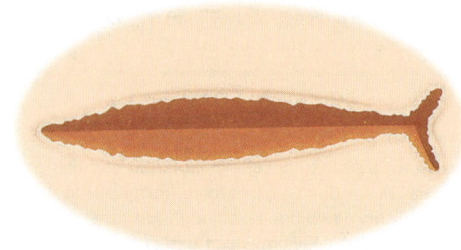

Fig. 11.10: 'Swallow tail' appearance of split laceration

Antemortem lacerations show bruising of margins, vital reaction, eversion and gaping of margins.

Dating/Age of Laceration

The gross findings are summarized in **Table 11.3** when healing occurs by first intention without any secondary infection.

Complications

i. Lacerations may cause severe and fatal bleeding leading to shock and death.
ii. Infection.
iii. Pulmonary/systemic fat embolism may occur due to crushing of subcutaneous tissue.

---

* Usually seen over parietal eminence as the bone at that point has two diverging planes.
¥ Tissue bridging results from the application of blunt force that overcomes the elasticity of the skin; as a result, the skin splits while underlying structures such as vessels, nerves, and connective tissue visibly span the wound.

TABLE 11.3: Healing of a lacerated wound

Duration	Gross findings
Fresh	Bleeding or fresh clot is attached; margins are red, swollen and tender
12–24 h	Margins swollen, red and covered by dried blood clots and lymph
3–5 days	Margins strongly adherent with each other and covered by dried crust
6–7 days	Crust/scab falls off or can easily be taken off, soft reddish tender scar
Few weeks	Scar is whitish, firm and painless

iv. If located where skin stretches or is wrinkled, e.g., over joints, repeated and continued oozing of tissue fluids and blood may cause irritation, pain and dysfunction.

Medico-legal Importance

- The type of laceration may indicate the *cause of injury and shape of blunt weapon*, e.g.,
  i. Blunt round end (hammer) may cause a stellate laceration.
  ii. Blunt object with an edge, such as hammer head, may cause crescentic laceration (patterned laceration).
  iii Long, thin objects, like pipes or sticks produce linear or elongated lacerations, while objects with a flat surface produce irregular, ragged or Y-shaped lacerations.
- *Nature of injury*
  - A laceration may be a simple injury.
  - Underlying fracture or injury to the vessels, nerves, muscles and organs should be ruled out before giving the opinion.
  - Extensive scar formation during healing of a laceration over the joint leading to restriction of joint movement is a grievous injury.
  - Similarly, scar due to laceration on the face resulting in disfiguration is also a grievous injury.
- Whether the laceration is *accidental/homicidal/suicidal*?
  a. **Accidental laceration**: Commonly seen anywhere on exposed parts of body.
  b. **Homicidal laceration**: Noticed on nonaccessible parts of the body, especially in assault cases. It is usually seen on the head.
  c. **Suicidal lacerations** are rarely seen, as they are painful to produce, and if present, they are seen on exposed parts of body and on same side.
- Sometimes, **human bites** can be a combination of deep lacerations and crushing and are associated with a high incidence of infection. It may be associated with avulsion of pieces of the nose or ear.*

- Foreign matter in the wound may give clues about the *object causing* it, e.g., paint material of vehicle may be transferred to the lacerated wound.
- Skin flap which overhangs the cut margin (avulsion cases) can indicate the *direction of force* applied.

> **Wounds caused by sharp edged and pointed weapons are of four types:**
> 1. Incised wound   2. Chop wound
> 3. Stab wound   4. Therapeutic/diagnostic wound

 Identify the type of wound. What could be the weapon causing this injury?

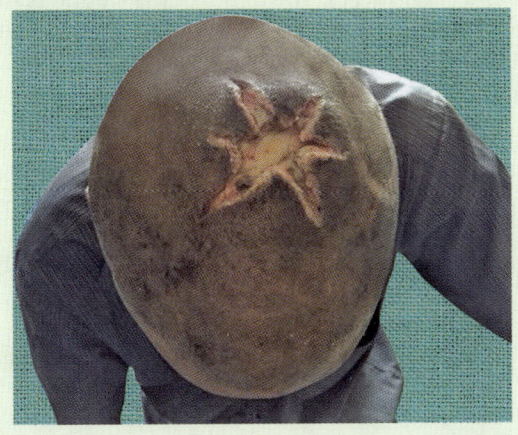

FM 3.3, 3.6

- Define, describe and classify incised wound and its medico-legal aspects.
- Describe healing of injury with its medico-legal importance.

INCISED WOUND (CUT/SLASH/SLICE)

Definition: Incision is a clean cut wound through the tissues (usually the skin and subcutaneous tissues including blood vessels), which is *more long than deep*, and caused by a sharp-edged instrument.

It is produced by pressure and friction against the tissue by an object having a sharp cutting edge or point, such as knife, box cutter, glass (thin glass causes incised wounds and thick glass will cause incised or lacerated wounds), razor or scalpel.

Description of a Sharp Wound

On the skin surface, the edges of a stab, incised or chop wound are referred to as the wound's '*margins*', whereas the ends or tips of the wound are referred to as '*angles*'. The '*length*' of a wound is measured from one angle to the other. The '*width*' of the wound is the widest measurement between the two margins. An imaginary line drawn between

---
* An accidental type of injury results from an attacker striking the victim's incisor teeth with his knuckles (metacarpophalangeal joint is usually involved).

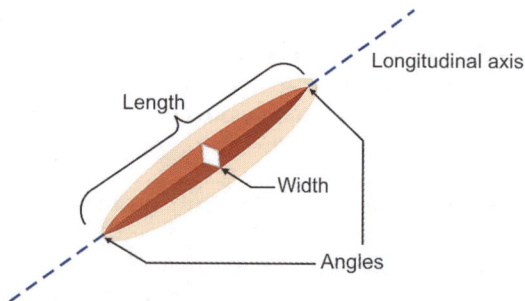

Fig. 11.11: Characteristics of a sharp wound

the two angles defines the '*long/longitudinal axis*' of the wound **(Fig. 11.11)**. The depth of the wound is measured from the skin surface to the deepest point of penetration.

Characteristics

- **Margins:** Edges are clean cut, well-defined and usually everted. They may be inverted, if a thin layer of muscle fibers is adherent to the skin as in the scrotum (due to the attached dartos muscle to the skin). The edges are free from contusions and abrasions. Wrinkled wounds are produced where the skin is wrinkled (i.e., folded), and more than one incised wound is seen.
- **Width/breadth:** Width is greater than the edge of the weapon causing it due to retraction of the divided tissues.
- **Length:** Length is greater than its width and depth and has no relation to the cutting edge of the weapon, for it may be drawn to any distance.
- **Shape:** Usually spindle-shaped due to greater retraction of the edges in the center **(Fig. 11.12)**. Gaping is more, if the underlying elastic fibers in the skin (*Langer's lines*) have been cut transversely or obliquely, and is less when cut longitudinally.
- **Depth and direction:** Usually deeper at the commencement, except in case of suicidal cut throat injuries, with hesitation cuts at the beginning. This is known as *head of the wound*. Towards termination, the cut becomes progressively shallow, known as *tailing of the wound* **(Fig. 11.12)**. Consequently, depth and tailing will suggest the direction in which the force was applied.
- **Hemorrhage:** As vessels are cut clean, hemorrhage is more.
- **Beveled cuts:** If the blade of the weapon enters obliquely, tissues will be visible at one margin and other margin will be undermined; if the blade is nearly horizontal, a flap wound is caused.

Dating/Age of Incised Wound

Refer to **Table 11.4** for dating of incised wound.

Medico-legal Importance

- Indicates the *nature of weapon* (sharp-edged). Although, the appearance of stab wounds may indicate the shape of

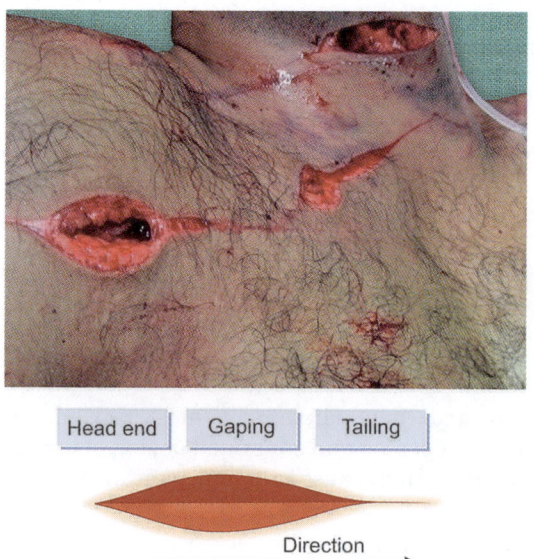

Fig. 11.12: Incised wound

TABLE 11.4: Dating of an incised wound

Duration	Gross findings
Fresh	Red with clotted blood
12 h	Margins red, swollen and adherent with blood and lymph
24 h	Continuous layer of endothelial cells cover the surface with a scab of dried clot
2–3 days	Reddish-brown color, edges are weakly adherent
4–6 days	Edges are firmly adherent
7 days	Scar formation

the weapon used, this is not possible with incised wounds. However, rarely, the appearance of incised wounds may provide some indication as to the weapon type.
- Give an idea about the *direction of force*.
- *Age of injury* can be determined.
- *Nature of injury*: Incised wounds are rarely life-threatening because they seldom penetrate deeply enough to damage a blood vessel of significant size. However, incised wounds over the wrist or neck, where major arteries lie in the superficial tissues, can prove fatal.
- Position and character of wound may indicate manner of production, i.e., *suicide, accident, or homicide* **(Diff. 11.4, and Figs. 11.13A and B)**.
  a. **Suicide:** Multiple incised wounds of varying depths on the neck or wrists suggest a suicide. Some features of suicidal wounds are:
     - Fatal wounds are present over limited accessible areas of the body, such as front of neck, groin, chest or back of legs. Suiciders usually do not injure the face.
     - **Hesitation cuts/marks or tentative cuts or trial wound:** These cuts are multiple, small and superficial often involving only the skin, and are seen at the beginning of the incised wound,

DIFFERENTIATION 11.4: Suicidal and homicidal cut-throat wounds

S.No.	Feature	Suicidal cut-throat	Homicidal cut-throat
1.	Situation	Left side of the neck and passing across the front of the throat	Usually on the sides
2.	Level	High, above the thyroid cartilage	Low, on or below the thyroid cartilage
3.	Direction	Obliquely, above downwards and from left to right in right-handed persons	Transverse or from below upwards
4.	Number of wounds	Multiple, may be 20–30, superficial, parallel and merge with main wound	Multiple, cross each other at a deep level
5.	Edges	Usually ragged due to overlapping of multiple superficial incisions	Sharp and clean cut, beveling may be seen
6.	Hesitation cuts	Present	Absent
7.	Tailing	Present	Absent
8.	Severity	Less severe, one wound is severe, but sometimes, there may be 2–3	More severe, all tissues including vertebrae may be cut
9.	Wounds in other parts of body	May be present across wrists, groin and thighs	No wounds on wrists, but severe injuries on head may be present
10.	Defense wounds	Absent, unintentional cuts may be found	Present, unless taken unaware
11.	Hands	Weapon may be firmly grasped due to cadaveric spasm	Fragments of clothing or hair of the assailant may be grasped
12.	Weapon at site	Usually present	Usually absent
13.	Vessels	As head is thrown back, carotid artery escapes injury	Jugular vein and carotid artery are likely to be cut
14.	Clothes	Not cut or damaged	May be cut, corresponding to injuries in the body
15.	Blood stains	If standing in front of mirror, then splashing on the mirror; stains running downwards on the clothes, front of body and feet	Found in both palms in an effort to cover the wound; if lying down, stains collect behind the neck and shoulder
16.	Circumstantial evidence	Quiet place, such as bedroom or bathroom; suicidal note	Disturbance at scene, footprints outside

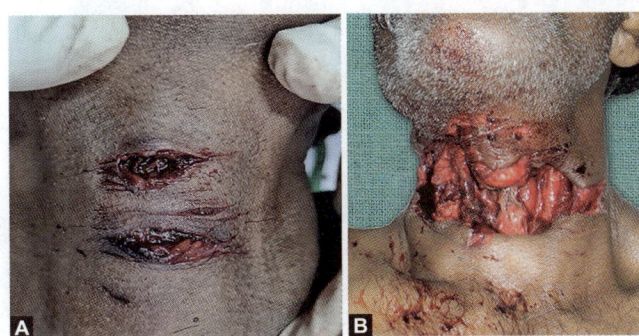

Figs. 11.13A and B: Cut throat wound: (A) Suicidal; (B) Homicidal

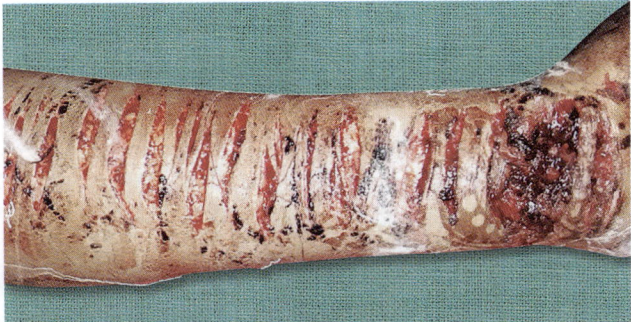

Fig. 11.14: Hesitation cuts on wrist and forearm

presumably hesitating while gaining courage to make a final decisive cut **(Fig. 11.14).***

- A person who commits suicide exposes his body by opening his clothes and then inflicts the wounds.
- When a safety razor blade is used, unintentional cuts are found on the fingers where the blade has been gripped.
- Most people have a vague knowledge of the anatomy and do not know where to cut a major blood vessel, and may cut their forearms vertically, rather than horizontally.

b. **Homicidal wounds:** They are deep and deliberate in character and are seen on the head and front of neck, and sometimes on the trunk. Incised wounds on nose, ears and genitals are usually homicidal, and may result from sexual jealousy, caused by a jilted lover, husband or wife.

c. **Accidental wounds:** Commonly seen around the hands.

---

* Multiple, superficial, roughly parallel incised wounds on the neck, adjacent to a deep, lethal incised wound, can be seen in victims of homicidal sharp force injury, particularly if torture was employed.

d. **Defense wounds:** Injuries are seen on the forearm and palm, when the victim may try to ward off an attack by raising hands and arms in defense or by grabbing the weapon.
e. **Self-mutilation:** Sometimes, injuries may be caused by an individual with a mental disorder as a form of self-mutilation or by one who deliberately harms oneself for motives of gain. They are found anywhere on the body; superficial, multiple and avoiding vital areas such as lips, nose and ears.

 A 35-year-old male was found unconscious in a pool of blood on the floor of his room. Body was lying supine and clothes were completely soaked in blood. A deep cut throat wound was present. Give your opinion regarding the same.

7

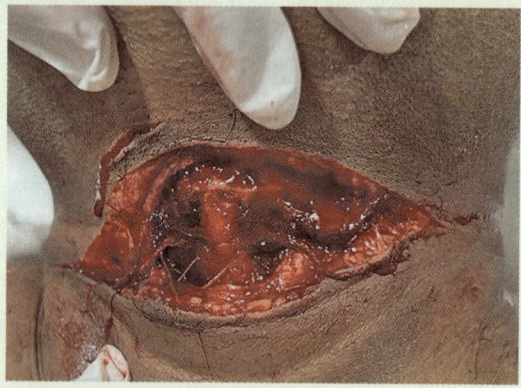

 Identify the type of wound. Give reasons.

8

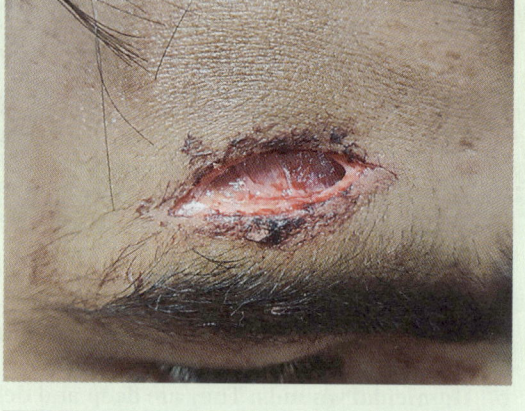

- A chop wound is considered a combination of blunt and sharp force injury.
- **Weapons used:** hatchet, axe, tomahawk, saber or meat cleavers.
- Presence of an incised wound on the skin with an underlying comminuted fracture or deep groove in the bone indicates wounds caused by such weapons **(Fig. 11.15)**.
- Dimensions of the wound correspond to cross-section of the penetrating blade.
- Margins are sharp, and may show abrasion, bruising and some laceration with severe injury to the underlying organs.
- Usually, the lower end (heel) of the axe strikes the surface first, which produces a deeper wound than the upper (toe) end. Deeper end indicates the position of the assailant **(Fig. 11.16)**.
- Undermining occurs in the direction towards which the chop is made **(Fig. 11.17)**. In the skull, the undermined edge of the fracture is the direction in which the force was exerted, and slanted edge is the side from which the force was directed.

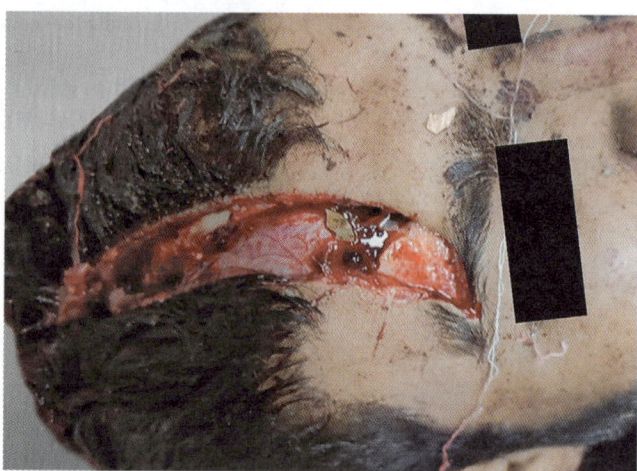

Fig. 11.15: Chop wound of head

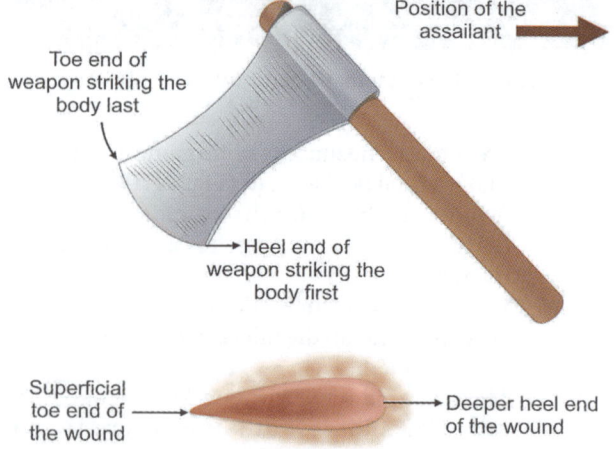

Fig. 11.16: Determining the relative position of the assailant from a chop wound

 FM 3.3
Define and describe chop wound and its medico-legal aspects.

CHOP WOUNDS

Definition: Chop wounds are deep gaping wounds caused by a blow with the moderately sharp cutting edge of a heavy weapon, applied with a significant degree of force.

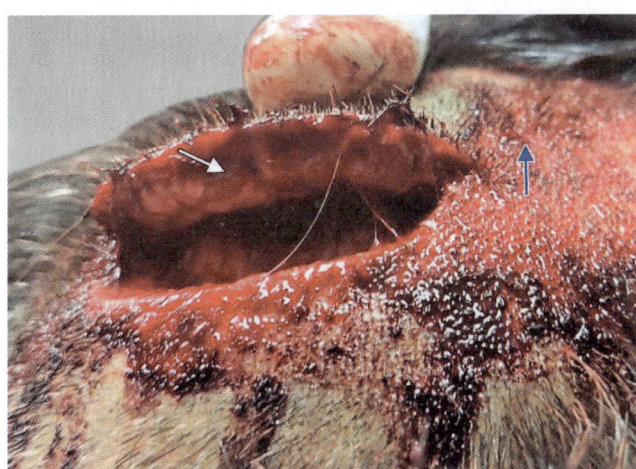

Fig. 11.17: Beveling due to oblique strike (blue arrow showing direction of force)

Medico-legal Importance

- Most of the injuries are homicidal, and usually inflicted on the exposed portions of the body, like head, face, neck, shoulders and extremities.
- Few are accidental due to machinery, like propeller injuries.
- Rarely, they could be suicidal.
- Wound examination could reveal clues regarding the causative weapon.

NOTA BENE

Bevel: A surface having a sloped or slanting edge. It is the angle or inclination of a line or surface that meets another at any angle but 90°.

Presence of a beveled margin indicates:
 i. Sharp cutting heavy or moderately heavy weapon was used.
 ii. Injury has been inflicted by striking the blade of the weapon. The chances of beveled margin by drawing or sawing the weapon are almost negligible.
 iii. Wound is homicidal in nature.
 iv. Direction of application of the weapon, and the relative position of assailant and the victim.

FM 3.3

Define, describe and classify stab wound and its medico-legal aspects.

STAB WOUND/PUNCTURED WOUND

Definition: Stab wounds are produced from penetration with long narrow instruments having pointed (sometimes blunt) ends into the depths of the body, which are *deeper than its length and width*.

- **Weapons used:** The most frequently used object is a knife (single-edged kitchen or pocket knives with a blade length of 10–13 cm). Less often, injuries are caused by pieces of glass (broken-off bottle necks), scissors, dagger, screwdrivers, pens, ice picks or forks.
- A stab wound is an open injury in which foreign material and organisms are likely to be carried deep into the underlying tissues.
- **Concealed punctured wounds:** These are punctured wounds caused on concealed parts of body, such as nostrils, fontanelles, inner canthus of eyes, axilla, vagina, rectum and the nape of the neck. They are caused by slender instruments, such as ice picks or knives with thin blades. Fatal penetrating injuries can be caused without leaving any easily visible external marks or bleeding.

Classification

Clinically, stab wounds are of two types (Figs. 11.18A and B):
 i. **Penetrating wound:** Weapon enters into the body cavity producing only one wound, i.e., wound of entry.
 ii. **Perforating wound** (through and through punctured around): Weapon after entering into one side of the body will come out through the other side, producing two wounds:
  - *Wound of entry:* Through which the weapon enters the body. It is larger and with inverted edges.
  - *Wound of exit:* Through which the tip of weapon emerges out of the body. It is usually smaller with everted edges.

Characteristics (Figs. 11.19A and B)

In describing a stab wound, the wound length, width, and directionality, appearance of the wound's margins and angles should be described.

- **Margins:** Edges of the wound are clean cut, usually no abrasion or bruising of the margins, but in full penetration of the blade, a patterned abrasion or bruising may be produced by the hilt-guard striking the skin (Fig. 11.20). The margins are regular, sharp and well-defined. However, injuries caused by a pointed or conical instrument have lacerated edges.
- **Length:** Length is slightly less than the width of the weapon because of stretching of the skin.

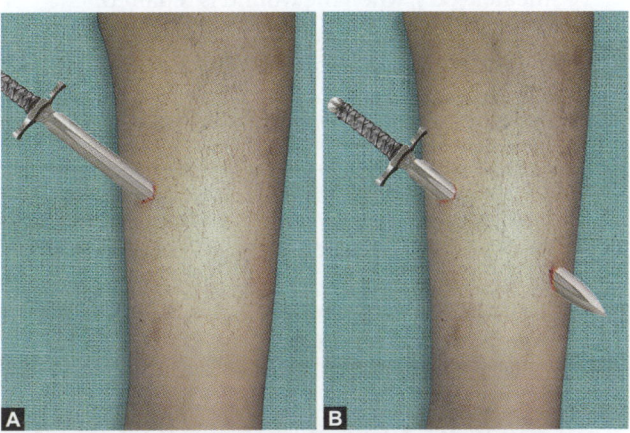

Figs. 11.18A and B: Classification of stab wounds: (A) Penetrating; (B) Perforating

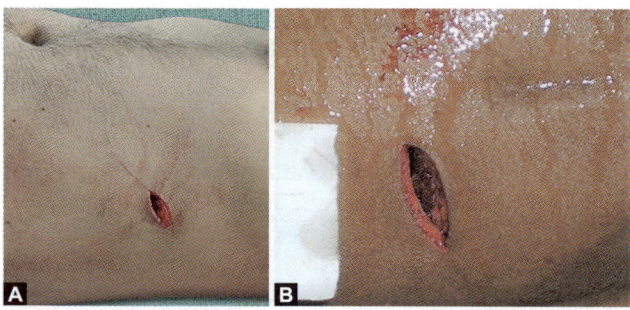

Figs. 11.19A and B: Stab wound: (A) With tailing; (B) With beveling

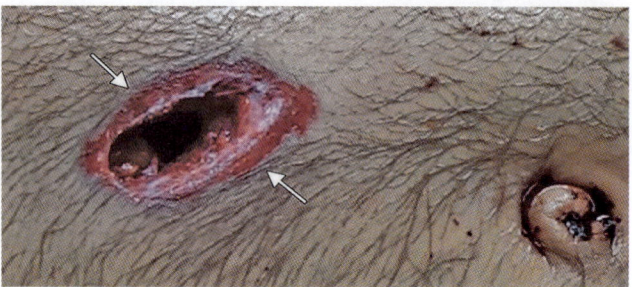

Fig. 11.20: Stab wound: Hilt-guard abrasion

- **Breadth:** It is more than thickness of the blade due to gaping. Approximation of the edges is needed to get the actual measurement.
- **Depth:** Depth is the greatest dimension of a stab wound. Depth corresponds to the length of the blade of the weapon entering the body, when the whole length of the weapon enters the body, but has not produced any wound of exit.
  - It is not safe to find out the depth of a stab wound by introducing a probe in the emergency room because it may disturb a loose clot and may lead to fatal hemorrhage.
  - The probe may easily pass between the fascial planes or within the muscle producing a false track.
  - Depth should be determined in the operation theater (OT), when the wound is repaired.

> **NOTA BENE**
>
> **Depth of stab wound depends on:**
> - *Condition of the knife:* Sharpness of the tip of the knife is the most important factor in skin penetration. Once the tip has perforated the skin, the cutting edge is of little importance.
> - *Resistance offered by the tissues and organs:* Apart from bone and calcified cartilage, the skin is most resistant to knife penetration. Once the skin has been penetrated, the blade slips easily through the underlying muscle, internal organs and uncalcified cartilage, without the need for further application of force.
> - *Clothing:* Multiple layers of tough cloth or leather jackets require greater force to penetrate.
> - *Force applied:* Speed of thrust of the knife.
> - *Location:* Stretched skin is easier to penetrate than lax skin, e.g., chest wall.
> - *Angle of strike:* A knife striking the skin at a right angle penetrates more deeply, than when it strikes from some acute angle.

- **Direction**
  - The directionality of a stab wound can be described as 'vertical', 'horizontal' or 'oblique', with a general or specific measurement of the angulation. One method is to describe the directionality based on a clock-face configuration. For example, the long axis of the stab wound is between the 10 and 4 O'clock positions.
  - Direction of the track of the wound should be determined in the OT. It should be described in three terms of description, e.g., when a weapon has been used from above, back and left side, the direction of the track of the wound will be downward, forward and from left to right.
  - When a knife penetrates at an angle, the wound will have a beveled margin on one side with undermining (undercut) on the other, so that subcutaneous tissue is visible, indicating the direction from which the knife entered **(Fig. 11.19B)**. In solid organs, like liver, the track made by the weapon is seen well.
- **Shape:** It is slit-shaped or gape depending on their location and their orientation, with regard to the cleavage lines of Langer.
  - A stab wound which runs parallel to the cleavage lines will remain slit-shaped and narrow, and the dimensions of the blade will be represented with considerable accuracy.
  - A stab wound which enters through the cleavage lines transversely will gape.
  - Some specific patterns seen with common weapons are described below **(Fig. 11.21)**:
    i. If a single-edged weapon is used, the surface wound will be triangular or wedge-shaped, and one angle of the wound will be sharp and the other rounded, blunt or squared off. Blunt end of the wound may have small splits in the skin, so-called '*fish-tailing*' **(Fig. 11.22)**. *Virtually all stab wounds are made with single-edged weapons.* Sometimes, this is not always the case, as the blunt edge of the knife may split the skin and resemble a double-edged knife wound.
    ii. If a double-edged weapon is used, the wound will be elliptical or slit-like, and both angles will be sharp or pointed.
    iii. A round object, like a spear may produce a circular wound.
    vi. A flat head screwdriver head will produce a slit-like stab wound with squared ends and abraded margins.
    v. A Phillips head screwdriver may produce a cross-shaped injury, each of the four edges tearing their way through the tissues (stellate or 'X' shaped).

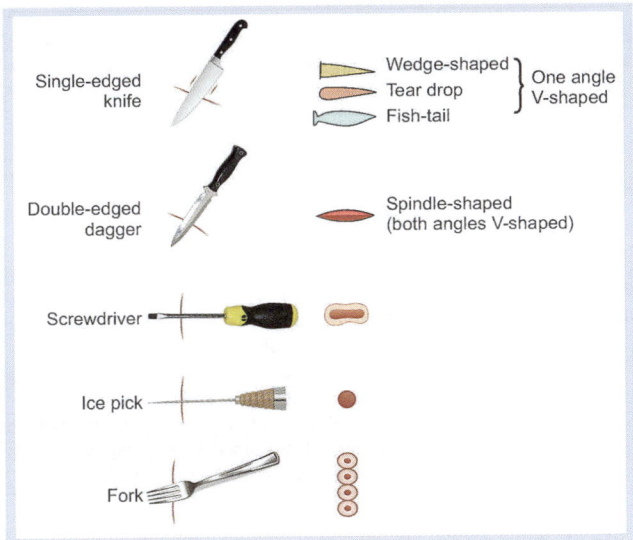

Fig. 11.21: Shape of stab wounds

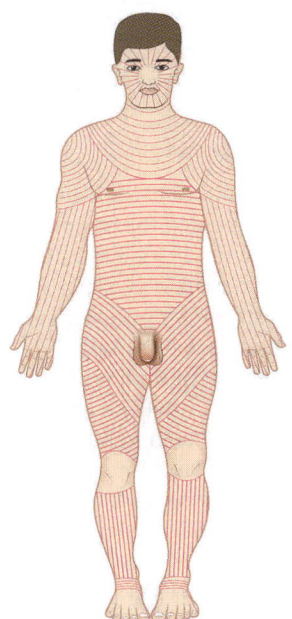

Fig. 11.23: Cleavage lines of Langer (similar lines are present at the back also)

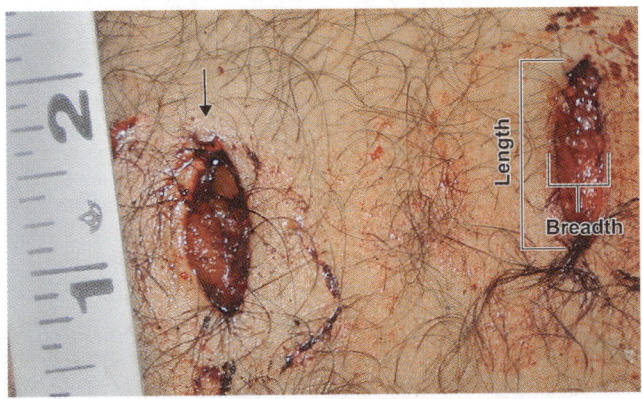

Fig. 11.22: Stab wound: Fish tailing (arrow)

vi. Stabs produced with a broken bottle appear as clusters of wounds of different sizes, shapes and depths with irregular margins.
vii. Skin wound made by closed scissors produces a flat 'Z' shaped wound. If the blades were open, the injuries may look similar to those produced by a knife.
viii. Ice picks produce small, round or slit-like wounds, which may look like 0.22-caliber bullets or shotgun pellets.
ix. A fork will produce clusters of 3–4 wounds depending on the number of prongs on the fork.

NOTA BENE

◆ The pattern of arrangement of the dense network of intimately intermingled dermal collagen and elastic fibers is called the *cleavage direction* or *lines of cleavage* of the skin and their linear representation on the skin are called *Langer's lines* (**Fig. 11.23**).

◆ *Nonlinear or irregularly shaped stab wounds* can result from irregularly shaped or jagged weapons, from intersecting wounds or from a twisting weapon/body interaction, since both the assailant and victim are in a highly charged state during an altercation. The latter can result in combined stab/incised wounds which can be 'V' shaped or irregular- shaped wounds—also referred to as 'twisting cuts'. It cannot be determined based on the configuration of these wounds whether the assailant twisted the knife while it was in the body or if the victim twisted while impaled, unless there is clear evidence that the wound occurred postmortem.
◆ **'Hilt mark' injuries:** An accurate measurement of the depth of the wound in case of stab wounds with hilt mark injuries can help estimate the length of the blade. However, because of the elasticity of skin, subcutaneous tissues and internal tissues, the depth can still be greater than the blade length. It is entirely possible for a knife with a 4-inch-long blade to produce a wound that is 5 or 6 inches deep. Obviously, it is also possible for a 6-inch-long blade to penetrate less than 6 inches.

Complications/Cause of Death

i. Hemorrhage leading to hypovolemic shock due to injuries of major vessels (most frequent cause).
ii. Cardiac tamponade (less common). Death is due to hemopericardium if heart is involved, but cardiac tamponade can occur (accumulation >150 mL of blood is fatal).
iii. Aspiration of blood into lungs and air embolism—when the stab is located on the neck (injury to jugular vein).
iv. Infections due to foreign matter embedded in the wound.

v. Asphyxia from airway obstruction from hematoma formation in the neck.
vi. Pneumothorax and hemothorax.

Medico-legal Importance

- Shape of the wound may indicate the *type of weapon*, which may have caused the injury.
- Depth of the wound will indicate the *force of penetration*.
- Direction and dimensions of the wound indicate the relative *positions of the assailant and the victim*.
- *Age of injury* can be determined.
- If a broken fragment of weapon is found, it will *identify the weapon* or will connect an accused person with the crime. Sometimes, glass fragments may be found within the depths of wound, and X-ray examination is valuable, since glass in common use is radiopaque.
- Position, number and direction of wounds may indicate manner of production, i.e., *suicide, accident or homicide*.
    - The major differences in suicidal and homicidal stab wound are given in **Diff. 11.5**.
    - **Accident:** Rare. It is caused by falling against any projecting sharp objects, like glass or nails or gored by horns of an animal (bull). It is usually a single large deep wound on front or back going straight inside.
- In case of multiple stabbing, to assess which surface wounds are responsible for which internal injuries.

> **NOTA BENE**
>
> - **Physical activity following fatal stab wound:** Whether a victim after receiving fatal stab can perform any physical activity, like running away from the assailant or shouting for help depends on the organs injured, extent of the injury, the amount and rapidity of blood lost. When bleeding is profused, physical activity is limited, and with slow bleeding, the victim may be able to run a few meters from the assailant or climb stairs before they collapse.
>   - After stab injuries to the heart, the ability to act is maintained at least for a short period of time. A stab wound through the left ventricle may almost completely seal itself by contraction of the cardiac muscle around the defect. Death will only occur if continued leakage of blood into the pericardial sac interferes with the pumping action of the heart (cardiac tamponade). A stab wound through the thin-walled right ventricle, atrium or coronary artery is unlikely to re-seal itself and will bleed out into the pericardium with fatal results.
>   - Wounds involving the great vessels of the thorax (aorta, vena cava, pulmonary arteries and veins) bleed profusely with no chance of closure. In lesion of the abdominal aorta, the ability to act may be maintained over prolonged periods of time, whereas in injuries of the thoracic aorta, incapacitation generally occurs within seconds. Most victims with heart and great vessel injuries are dead within 1 h.
>   - Injuries of the lungs or abdominal organs do not lead to immediate incapacitation.
> - **Degree of force involved in the stabbing incident:** Forensic experts are sometimes asked to estimate or quantify the degree of force used so as to determine an alleged assailant's intent to cause harm. It is considered to be a difficult area due to the large number of variables present, such as sharpness of the weapon, the area of the body and alignment with cleavage lines of the skin, the angle of attack and the relative movement of the person stabbing relative to the victim being stabbed. It is generally not possible for the expert to determine this with any reliable degree of certainty. However, a rough estimate of 'mild pressure', 'moderate force' or 'extreme force' is often used, and the forensic pathologist may utilize the presence of hilt-guard bruising or the penetration of bone as a guide to their description of force.
> - The amount of blood loss necessary to cause death is variable from seconds to hours, and depends on the rate of bleeding, amount of blood loss, nature of the injury and body's physiological response.

DIFFERENTIATION 11.5: Suicidal and homicidal stab wounds

S.No.	Feature	Suicidal stab wounds	Homicidal stab wounds
1.	Location	Accessible areas of body, mostly chest (precordial region) and abdomen	May be injured anywhere, most often chest, neck and back
2.	Direction	Descending, backwards and to the right (right-handed persons)	May be any direction, often at an angle from left-to-right and from above downwards
3.	Number of wounds	Single	Multiple
4.	Grouping	Regularly placed	Irregularly placed
5.	Multiple deep wounds	Unlikely	Common
6.	Tentative wounds	Common	Not seen
7.	Defense wounds	Not seen	Frequent
8.	Other fresh marks of self-injury (trial cuts)	Sometimes seen	Not seen
9.	Older marks of self-injury	Sometimes seen	Not seen
10.	Body disfigurement	Unlikely	May be seen
11.	Exposure/undressing of stab region	Common; clothes are spared	Unusual; wounds are through clothing
12.	Signs of disturbance of scene	Unlikely, body not moved	Common, body may be moved
13.	Weapon close to body	Found in almost all cases	Not found in most cases

- Arteries carry blood at higher pressure than veins of similar size and, therefore, bleed more rapidly when cut. A partially transected vessel is less likely to seal off than one which is cleanly cut.
- Arterial hemorrhages from major vessels may lead to death relatively fast. A loss of >1 liter of blood from a major vessel may be fatal.
- Sudden blood loss causes interference with activity when it exceeds 20–25% of the total blood supply. A person can lose over a third of his blood volume before progressing to irreversible hemorrhagic shock.
- A person who is elderly or frail has little reserve to withstand blood loss may succumb quickly.

♦ **Harakiri (seppuku):** It is an unusual type of suicidal disembowelment connected with Japanese Samurai warriors. The victim with a short sword inflicts a single large abdominal stab wound into the left side, drawing the blade across to the right side and then turning it upwards producing an L-shaped cut. The sudden evisceration of the internal organs causes immediate decrease of intra-abdominal pressure and cardiac return resulting in collapse and death.
  - The *jigai* ritual is a traditional method of female suicide, carried out by cutting the jugular vein using a knife called a *tantō*. It is the feminine counterpart of *seppuku*.

NOTA BENE

Examination of the weapon

When examining a weapon, such as a knife, it should be noted whether the blade is 'single-edged' (having a single sharp edge, with the opposite edge being 'blunt' or squared-off), 'double-edged' (having 2 sharp edges), or a combination of single and double edges, and whether or not the blade is serrated (having teeth). Serrated knives produce wounds that are indistinguishable from wounds caused by other single-edged knives. The same knife can produce differing wounds at different levels of penetration **(Fig. 11.24)**.

It is important to note that the terminology used to describe the dimensions of the knife (length, width and the thickness of the blade) and the wound do not correspond with one another **(Fig. 11.11)**. When comparing a stab wound to the weapon, the thickness of the blade produces the 'width' of the wound, the width of the blade produces the 'length' of the wound, and the length of the blade produces the 'depth' of the wound. It should also be noted that wound width *does not necessarily equal* blade thickness, wound length does *not necessarily equal* blade width, and wound depth *does not necessarily equal* blade length; because of the elasticity and flexibility of human tissues, as well as the fact that the weapon can move within the wound path. The wound width, length and depth may actually be *smaller* or *larger* than the corresponding dimensions of the weapon.

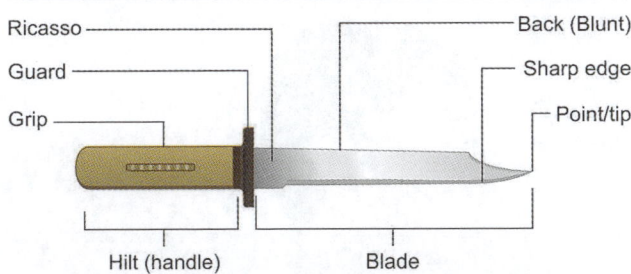

Fig. 11.24: Parts of a single-edged knife (one edge sharp and the other blunt)

Observe the injury and describe the findings. Name the type of injury.

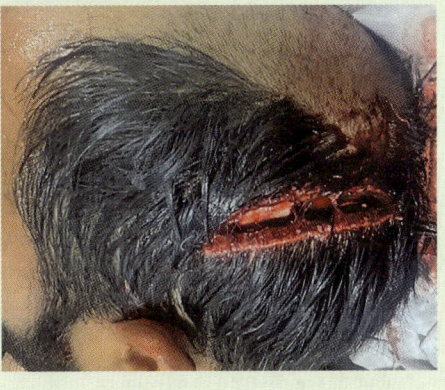

FM 3.3
Define, describe and classify defense wounds, self-inflicted/fabricated wounds and their medico-legal aspects.

■ DEFENSE WOUNDS

Definition: Defense wounds are wounds of the extremities, which result from the immediate and instinctive reaction of the victim to ward off an attack.

Classification

They are usually classified into two types:
  i. **Active defense injuries:** They are seen when the victim tries to seize the weapon, and the injuries are sustained on grasping the weapon **(Fig. 11.25A)**. Injuries are usually located on the palms, the flexor sides of the fingers and the interdigital spaces, more common in the web between the base of the thumb and index finger.
  ii. **Passive defense injuries:** These are seen when the victim raises the hands or arms for protection **(Fig. 11.25B)**. They are located on the extensor or ulnar surfaces of forearms, wrists, knuckles and the back of the hands.

Usually, the victim's right forearm and hand are involved since it is nearest to the perpetrator and preponderance of right-handed individuals in a population.

Injuries

♦ If the weapon is blunt, bruises and abrasions are produced.
♦ If the weapon is sharp, the injuries will depend upon the type of attack, whether stabbing or cutting.
  - In stabbing with single-edged weapon, if the weapon is grasped, a single cut is produced on the palm of the hand or on the bends of fingers.
  - If weapon is double-edged, cuts are produced on the palm and fingers.
  - Cuts are usually irregular and ragged because skin tension is loosened by gripping of the knife.

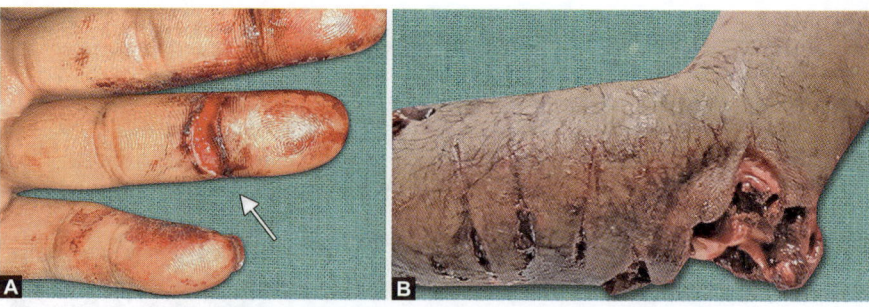

Figs. 11.25A and B: Defense wounds: (A) Active; (B) Passive
[*Courtesy:* (A) Dr Rajiv Joshi, Dr Karan and Dr Samuel, GGSMC, Faridkot]

Pearls

Defense wounds are absent if the victim is:
- Unconscious
- Taken by surprise
- Attacked from behind
- Under the influence of alcohol/drugs

NOTA BENE

Therapeutic/diagnostic wounds
These are produced by medical personnel during the treatment of the patient, e.g., surgical wounds on the chest and abdomen for insertion of tubes for drainage, laparotomy incisions, cutdowns on antecubital fossa or wrists, tracheotomy and thoracotomy incisions. Sometime, they may be mistaken for primary traumatic injury, e.g., chest tube drainage wound may be mistaken a homicidal stab wound.
To avoid misinterpretation, therapeutic tubing should never be removed prior to sending the body for postmortem examination.

FABRICATED/FICTITIOUS/FORGED WOUNDS

Definition: Fabricated wounds are produced by a person on his own body or by another with his consent.

Classification

It can be:
i. **Self-inflicted wounds** are those inflicted by a person on his own body. Self-inflicted injury without conscious suicidal intent is a form of self-mutilation.
ii. **Self-suffered wounds** are those inflicted by another person on the alleged victim.

Motive

The reasons for fabricating injuries are:
i. To simulate a criminal offense for false charge
   - By women, to bring a charge of rape.
   - Charge an enemy with assault or attempted murder.
   - Convert simple injury into grievous one.
   - By prisoners, to bring a charge of beating against officers.
ii. To avert suspicion
   - Destroy evidence of certain injury which might connect a person with crime.
   - Assailant may pretend self-defense.
   - Policemen/watchmen may feign robbery or alleged attack.
iii. By soldiers and prisoners to escape difficult task.
iv. Suicidal gestures, attempted suicide.
v. For the purpose of insurance frauds.

Diagnosis

The diagnosis can be done by careful history taking and examination of injuries **(Box 11.1)**.
- **Types of wound:** Mostly incised wounds, sometimes contusions, stab wounds and burns. Chop wound of little finger of left hand may be seen too. Lacerated wounds are rarely fabricated. Burns are superficial and usually seen on left upper arm.
- **Most commonly used object** is a knife. Razor, glass piece, scissors and ice pick are some of the other objects used.
- **Body parts where found:** Top of the head, forehead, neck, outer side of left arm, front and outer side of thighs, and front of abdomen and chest **(Fig. 11.26)**.

Box 11.1 Typical features of fabricated injuries **(Fig. 11.26)**
- History of assault incompatible with injuries.
- Multiple shallow, non-penetrating cuts or fingernail abrasions.
- Uniform in shape, linear or slightly curved course of lesions.
- Grouped and/or parallel and/or criss-cross arrangement.
- Location is easily reachable—usually on the left side (non-dominant side).
- Avoidance of pain sensitive regions of the body.
- Absence of defense injuries.
- No damage to clothes or inconsistent damage.

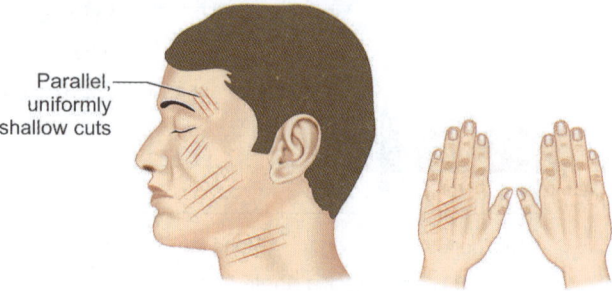

Fig. 11.26: Characteristics of self-inflicted injuries (seen mostly in left side and avoid eyes, nose, mouth and ears)

CHAPTER 11 : Injuries

 A 23-year-old man presented with history abduction, looting and assault by group of five unknown persons with sticks and knives. He was later dumped on the roadside. There were multiple superficial injuries over his back and right upper arm. Describe the injuries and give your opinion regarding the manner of injury. The police found that he was under duress as he was not able to repay a loan.

10

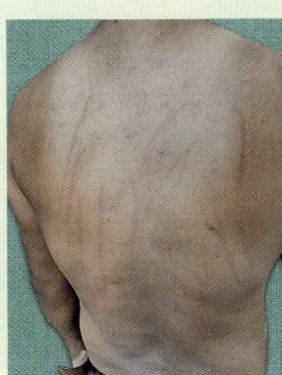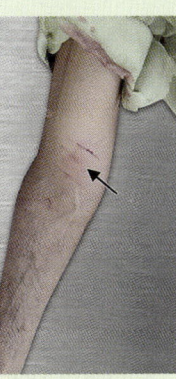

(*Courtesy:* Dr Rajiv Joshi, Dr Karan and Dr Samuel GGSMC, Faridkot)

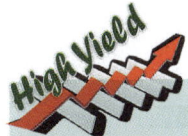

- **Injury:** Any harm, whatever illegally, caused to any person in body, mind, reputation or property (Sec. 44 IPC).
- **Commonest type of abrasion:** Graze abrasion (seen in road traffic accidents).
- **Brush burn:** Graze abrasion over back, caused by sliding over ground.
- Tyre and bite marks are examples of patterned abrasion.
- Epithelial tags are seen at the tail end of abrasion.
- Nail scratch causes crescent shaped abrasion.
- UV light can be used to visualize the pattern injuries not apparent with visible light.
- Reddish-brown abrasion is seen in 2-3 days.
- Abrasion heals in 1 week with *no permanent scarring on healing*.
- Medico-legally, abrasions are more useful than bruises.
- **Railway line/tram-line bruise:** Blows with a rod/stick produce two parallel, linear hemorrhages with intervening normal skin.
- **Ectopic/migratory bruise:** Bruises at a site other than site of injury due to gravity shifting of blood, most commonly seen in the eyes as *black eyes (raccoon eyes)*.
- Bruise showing bluish discoloration is <3 days old.
- Brown color of contusion is due to formation of hemosiderin.
- Multiple bruises of varying colors are seen in child abuse.
- **Crush injury:** Blunt force producing extensive bruising and laceration.
- **Incised-looking wounds:** *Split lacerated wounds* seen on the scalp, forehead, zygoma, iliac crest etc (subcutaneous tissue is scanty).
- Flaying is seen in avulsed lacerated wounds.
- **Chop wound:** Deep gaping wound caused by *moderately sharp cutting edge of a heavy weapon*, applied with significant degree of force.
- Chop wounds are combination of blunt and sharp force injury.
- Beveling cut has one margin undermined; usually homicidal in nature.
- **Incised wound:** Clean cut wound through the tissue which *longer than its depth*.
- **Stab wound:** Clean cut wound through the tissue which is *deeper than its length and width*.
- Length is the maximum dimension in incised wound.
- Depth is the maximum dimension in stab wound.
- Gaping of a wound is dependent on cleavage lines of Langer.
- Hemorrhage is more in incised wound compared to laceration.
- **Commonest type of injury fabricated:** Incised wounds.

- **Hesitation/tentative cuts:** Multiple, small, superficial incised wounds; seen at the beginning of *suicidal wound*.
- Incised wounds on nose, ears and genitals are usually homicidal.
- **Types of stab wound:** 2 types—penetrating (only entry) and perforating (both entry and exit).
- **Shape of stab wound using single-edged weapon:** Triangular or wedge-shaped.
- **Shape of stab wound using double-edged weapon:** Elliptical with both angles sharp.
- Presence of hilt mark in stab wound indicates full penetration of blade.
- **Harakiri:** Type of suicidal abdominal stab wound (seen among Japanese Samurai warriors).
- Right atrium stab wounds are immediately fatal.
- Defense injuries are absent when unconscious, unaware, under influence of alcohol or attack from behind.

Characteristic injury	Seen in
Swallow tail	Laceration
Tailing	Incised wound
Fish-tail	Stab wound

Type of injury	Caused by (weapon)
Abrasion	Blunt/pointed
Contusion	Blunt
Laceration	Blunt
Incised wound	Sharp
Stab wound	Sharp pointed

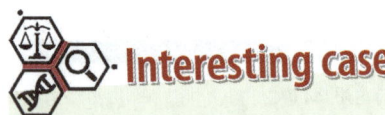

Interesting case

Perforating Wound (Case of Phineas Gage, 1848)

Phineas Gage, a railroad worker in Vermont sustained a freak accident in the mid 19th century when an iron tamping rod *perforated* through his entire skull which damaged his frontal lobe **(Figs. A and B)**. He unbelievably survived the accident but was changed as a result and many described him as a different man entirely. He is often referred to as one of the most famous patients in neuroscience.

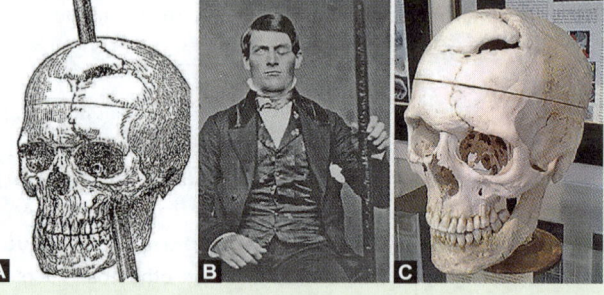

After sustaining the initial injury, Gage was able to speak and walk to a nearby cart so that he could be taken to a doctor in the town. He was conscious and able to recount the names of his co-workers. After developing an infection, Gage then spent a week in a semi-comatose state. After two weeks, his intellectual functioning began to improve, but had difficulty estimating size and amount of money. Within a month, he ventured out of the house and into the street. When the doctor saw Gage again the following year, he had lost vision in his eye and was left with scars from the accident, but he was in good physical health and appeared recovered.

Prior to the accident, Gage was a hardworking, pleasant man. Post-accident, he was a changed man, as the injury had transformed him into a surly, aggressive drunkard who was unable to hold down a job. The injury led to a loss of social inhibition, leading Gage to behave in ways that were seen as inappropriate.

He died in 1860 due to an epileptic seizure that was related to his brain injury. Seven years later Gage's body was exhumed, and his skull and the tamping rod are on display at the Harvard Medical School's Warren Anatomical Museum in Cambridge, Massachusetts **(Fig. C)**.

Gage's case had a tremendous influence on early neurology. The specific changes observed in his behavior pointed to emerging theories about the localization of brain function. Today, scientists better understand the role of frontal cortex in important higher-order functions such as reasoning, language and social cognition. In those years, while neurology was in its infancy, Gage's extraordinary story served as one of the first sources of evidence that the frontal lobe was involved in personality.

In a 1994 study, researchers utilized neuroimaging techniques to reconstruct Gage's skull and determine the exact placement of the injury. Their findings indicate that he suffered injuries to both the left and right prefrontal cortices, which would result in problems with emotional processing and rational decision-making. Another study conducted in 2004 involved using three-dimensional, computer-aided reconstruction to analyze the extent of Gage's injury. They found that the effects were limited to the left frontal lobe. In 2012, new research estimated that the iron rod destroyed approximately 11% of the white matter in Gage's frontal lobe and 4% of his cerebral cortex.

CHAPTER 12

Firearm Injuries

LEARNING OBJECTIVES

Must know
1. Ballistics, bore/caliber, cartridge, classification of firearms
2. **Bullet:** Dum-dum, hollow point, incendiary, green, armor piercing, ricochet, tandem, duplex, frangible, souvenir
3. Tattooing, blackening; abrasion and grease collar
4. Choke and cylinder bore, paradox guns, wad
5. Advantages of rifling, choking and wads
6. Types of gunpowder
7. Components of a cartridge
8. Characteristic of shotgun and rifle injuries at varying ranges
9. 'Billiard ball' ricochet effect
10. Kennedy phenomenon
11. Multiple exit wounds from single bullet
12. Entry and exit wound of a bullet (Diff.)
13. Bullet and shotgun cartridge (Diagram)
14. Preservation of evidence in case of firearm injury
15. Tests to determine gunshot residues

Desirable to know
1. Parts of a firearm
2. Shored exit wound
3. Yawing and tumbling of a bullet
4. Double tap
5. PM examination in firearm injuries
6. Class characteristics and secondary markings
7. Puppe's rule
8. Suicidal, homicidal and accidental firearm injury (Diff.)
9. Medico-legal aspects related to firearm injury

Definitions

- **Ballistics:** It is the science of projectile units (bullets, missiles and bombs), encompassing the physical phenomena involved and the movement of the projectile.
- **Forensic ballistics:** Science which deals with the investigation and identification of firearms, ammunition and the problems arising from their use.

> **NOTA BENE**
> Ballistics is subdivided into:
> - *External ballistics:* Study of the passage of the projectile through space or the air.
> - *Internal ballistics:* Study of the projectile in the firearm.
> - *Terminal ballistics:* Study of the interaction of a projectile with its target.
> - *Wound ballistics:* It is concerned with the motion and effects of the projectile in tissue.

- **Firearm:** Any instrument or device that discharges a missile by the expansive force of gases produced by burning of an explosive substance.

It consists of **(Fig. 12.1)**:
  i. **Barrel:** A hollow metal cylinder in which the propellant charge is placed. It is long in rifles and shotguns, and short in pistols and revolvers. The lumen is known as *bore*. The rear end where the cartridge is inserted is known as the *breech end*, and the front end where the bullet/shots comes out is the *muzzle end*.
  ii. **Action:** It consists of a bolt, a striker or hammer and a trigger.
  iii. **Extractor** is a part of a gun's action which serves to remove brass cases of fired ammunition after it has been fired from the chamber of the gun.
  iv. **Butt/grip:** Rear portion of stock in a shoulder arm or bottom of a handgun containing a magazine.
  v. **Magazine:** The receptacle for the cartridges in a repeating type of weapon from which the cartridges are fed automatically into the chamber by the action of mechanism.

- **Range of fire:** The shortest distance between the point of discharge and the point of explosion of a projectile (bullet/pellets), i.e., the distance from which a gunshot was fired to the target.

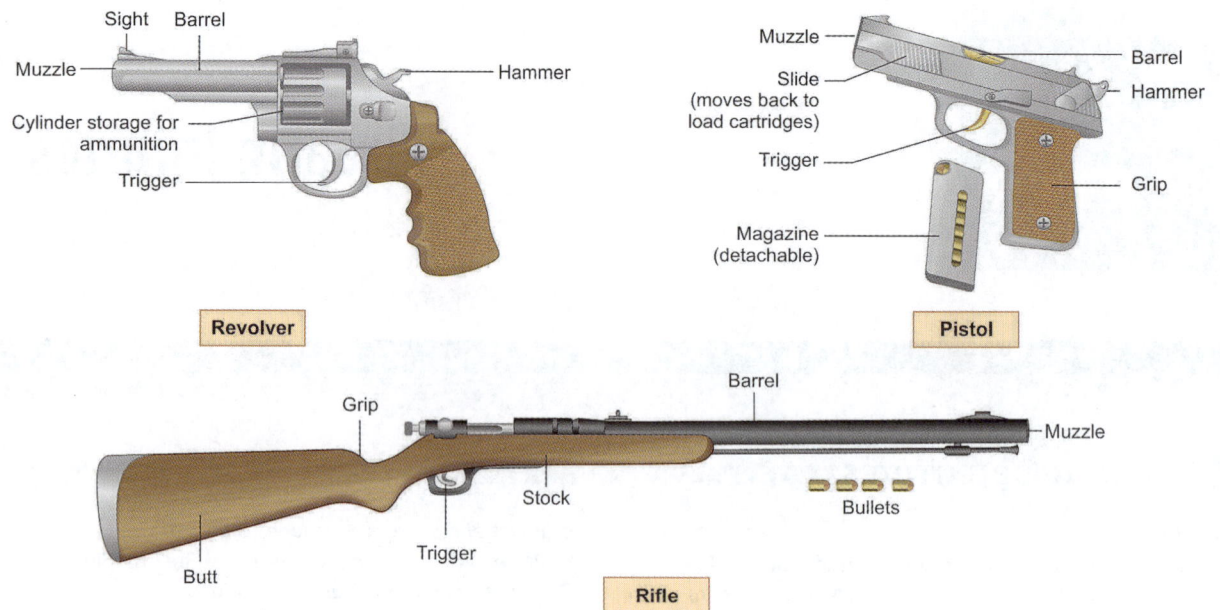

Fig. 12.1: Parts of rifled weapon

Velocity
- *Muzzle velocity*: The velocity of the projectile as it emerges from the muzzle end. Depending on it, firearms can be of low, medium and high velocity.
- *Striking velocity*: Velocity of the projectile at the point of impact. The velocity diminishes as the missile travels ahead to strike the target.

Trajectory: Path traced by the projectile during flight.

> FM 3.9
> - Describe different types of firearms including structure and components.
> - Describe various terminology in relation of firearm—caliber, range, choking.

CLASSIFICATION OF FIREARMS

Firearms are broadly classified into two categories depending on the type of barrel:
  i. **Rifled weapons**
      - Rifles: 0.22, single shot, lever action, bolt-action, pump action, auto-loading
      - Revolvers: Swing-out, break-top, solid-frame
      - Single shot and auto-loading pistols
      - Submachine and machine guns
  ii. **Smooth bore weapons (shotguns)**
      - Single-shot and double barrel
      - Bolt action, pump-action, and lever action
      - Auto-loading
- Broadly, single-shot pistols, derringers (variant of single-shot pistols), revolvers and auto-loading pistols are considered as *handguns*.
- Country made firearms (*katta* or improvised firearms) are mostly 12 bore smooth bore weapons.

RIFLED FIREARMS

The bore is scored internally with number of shallow spiral grooves varying from 2 to 22, most common are 4, 5 or 6, which run parallel to each other, but twisted spirally from breech to muzzle end. These grooves are called '*rifling*' and the projecting ridges between the grooves are called '*lands*' **(Figs. 12.2 and 12.3).***

- Rifles, pistols, revolvers, submachine guns and machine guns—all have rifled barrels.
- The direction of rifling can be either right (clockwise) or left (counter-clockwise)—majority of handguns have a right-hand twist.

When the bullet passes through the bore, its surface comes in contact with the projecting spirals, which gives the

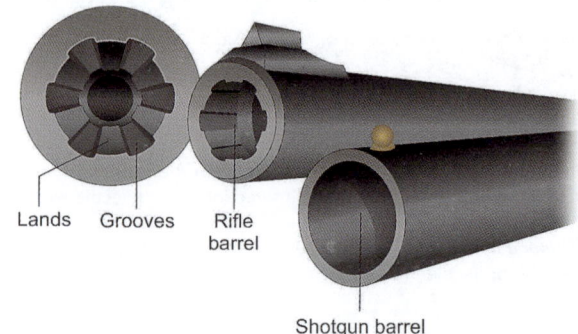

Fig. 12.2: Rifle and shotgun barrel

---

* **Helixometer** (developed by Goddard and Fisher), a magnifier probe is used to examine the interior of firearm barrels and accurately measure the pitch (twist rate) of rifling.

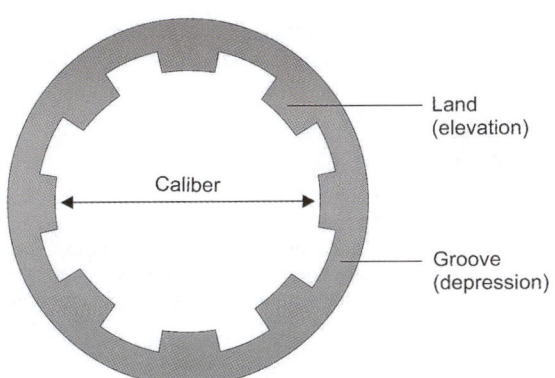

Fig. 12.3: Caliber of rifled firearm (distance between two opposite lands)

bullet a rotational spinning or spiraling motion along its longitudinal axis. Rifling gives the bullet a signature marking that is unique to the weapon that fired it.

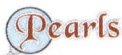

Advantages of rifling
- Imparts gyroscopic stability
- Increases accuracy and range
- Prevents wobbling or tumbling end-over-end
- Gives greater power of penetration

NOTA BENE

- **Fully-automatic:** Small firearm, which after first cartridge is manually loaded and fired, will eject the fired case, load the next cartridge from the magazine, fire and eject that fired case and repeats the process indefinitely, as long as trigger is held pressed or until cartridge supply from magazine is exhausted.
- **Semi-automatic:** A weapon which fires, eject and reloads on trigger being pressed, but does not fire again until the trigger has been released and pressed again. Auto-loading pistols are semi-automatic wherein the empty cartridge is ejected after firing.
- **Revolver** has a revolving cylinder that contains several chambers, each of which holds one cartridge.
- **Rifle** is a firearm with a rifled barrel which is designated to be fired from the shoulder.
- **Handgun** is a firearm capable of being carried and used by one hand, such as a pistol or revolver.
- **Zip guns:** Crude home made single shot rifled firearm.
- **Stud guns:** Tools used to fire metal studs into wood, concrete or steel.

SMOOTH BORE FIREARMS/SHOTGUNS

In smooth bore firearms, the bore or the inner surface of the barrel is uniformly smooth **(Fig. 12.2)**. It is intended to be fired from the shoulder, and is designated to fire multiple pellets from the barrel.
- Barrel lengths of shotgun range from 18–36 inches; 26 and 28 inch being most common.
- Shotgun barrel is divided into three sections: Chamber, forcing cone and bore.

- **Musket** is a muzzle-loaded, smooth bore long gun. It is usually fired from the shoulder.

Choking

Choking: An interior constriction of a shotgun bore at the muzzle for the purpose of controlling the pattern of the fired shot.

Cylinder bore (unchoked): Entire barrel from breech to muzzle is of same diameter.

Choke bore: A shotgun slightly constricted at the muzzle, usually distal 7–10 cm of the barrel is narrow.
- Usual degrees of choke in descending order are full, modified, improved cylinder and cylinder **(Fig. 12.4)**.
- *Advantages of choking:* Lessens the rate of spread of shot (keep the pellets from spreading too quickly), increases the explosive force and velocity, and thus increases the range.
- Dispersion of pellets in fully choked is about half that of cylinder bore.
- *For cylinder bore,* an old 'rule of thumb' for the range of discharge is by measuring the diameter of the wound from the outermost individual pellet wound, in cm and dividing it by three, giving the result in meters.

Balling or welding of shot: In shotguns, there may be conversion of shots (pellets) into compact mass* which may cause a circular or oval large entry wound of 5–10 mm and several small circular punctures, suggesting use of two weapons—one rifle and the other a shotgun.

Paradox guns: Some shotguns which have small portion of their bore near the muzzle end rifled **(Fig. 12.5)**.

Shotgun pellets fall into two categories depending on the size: Birdshot and buckshot (larger shot). There are three types of lead shot depending on the composition:
  i. Drop/soft shot: Made with pure lead.
  ii. Chilled/hard shot: Lead is hardened by the addition of antimony.

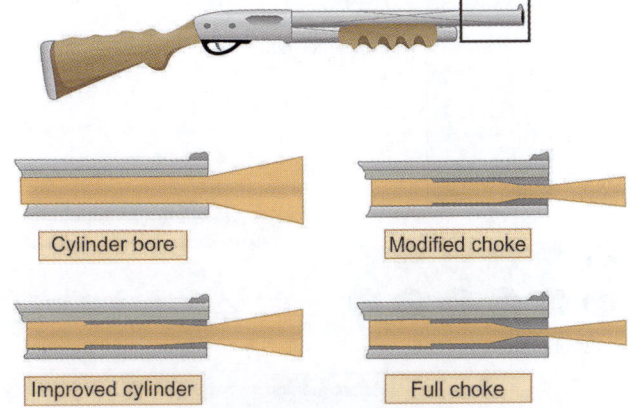

Fig. 12.4: Choking of shotgun

---

*Occurs due to faulty or old ammunition, too much of powder, incorrect wads or high sealing pressure of the wads.

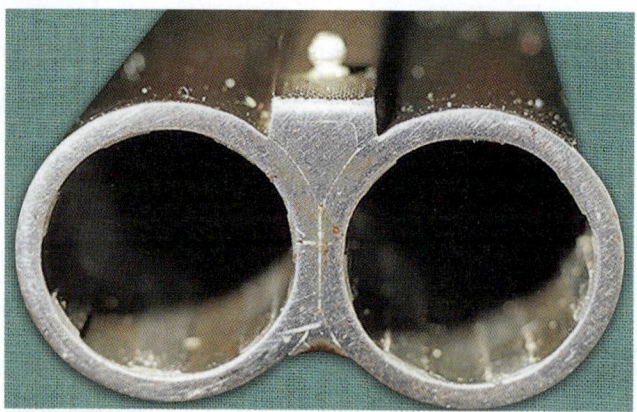

Fig. 12.5: Paradox guns. Note the rifling near the muzzle end in double barrel shotgun

iii. **Plated shot:** It is coated with a thin coat of copper or nickel to minimize distortion on firing—maintains good aerodynamic shape and increase the range.

CALIBER (GAUGE/BORE)

Rifle

It is the diameter of the interior of the barrel of a *rifled firearm* measured between diagonally opposite lands, expressed in inches or millimeters, e.g., .22", .32", .38" **(Fig. 12.3)**. It represents the diameter of the barrel before the rifling grooves are cut.

Shotgun

For shotguns, bore is the number of spherical lead balls of size fitting the barrel of a shotgun which can be made from one pound of lead (454 g), e.g., 12, 16, 20 bore **(Fig. 12.6)**.* Barrel of 12 bore gun will pass a ball that weighs 1/12 lb [12 gauge is the most popular shotgun round (largest shot)].

> **NOTA BENE**
>
> The *European system* of cartridge designation which uses metric system is more thorough and logical than the Indian system. It specifically identifies a cartridge by giving the bullet diameter and the case length in millimeters, as well as the type of cartridge case, e.g., 7.62 × 54 mm R, indicates the diameter, length and rimmed bullet respectively.

FM 3.9

Describe different types of cartridges and bullets.

BULLET

Bullet is the projectile of a rifled firearm that leaves the muzzle when it discharges.

- Traditional bullet is made of soft metal and has a rounded nose. The metal used is lead with varying amounts of antimony and/or tin added to provide hardness. This is known as *round nose soft bullet* **(Fig. 12.7)**.
- Wadcutter is a cylindrically shaped projectile that has a flat nose, and designed for cutting perfect holes in paper targets.
- Semiwadcutter is a compromise between a round nose and a wadcutter. It has a truncated cone or a slightly curved ogive and can be used in autoloaders.
- Caliber of a bullet is the cross-sectional diameter.
- In revolver and pistol, the bullet is short, and the point is usually round **(Fig. 12.8)**.
- In a rifle, the bullet is elongated with a pointed end **(Fig. 12.8)**.

Modern bullets fall in two categories: Lead- and metal-jacketed.

Jacketed bullets: A tough metal envelope [made of brass (copper 90% and zinc 10%) or copper and nickel with steel] covering the outside of the bullet—thickness ranges from 0.0165–0.030 inches.

It is of two types:

i. *Full metal jacket (FMJ):* Covers all, but the base **(Fig. 12.9A)**.

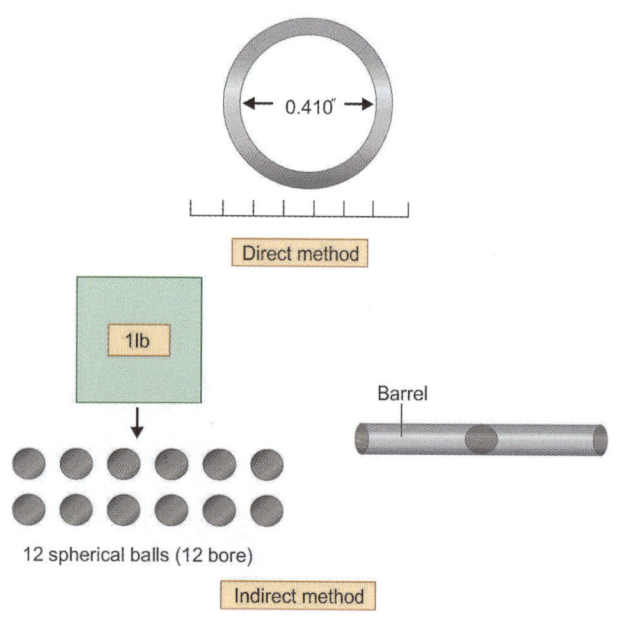

Fig. 12.6: Caliber of a shotgun

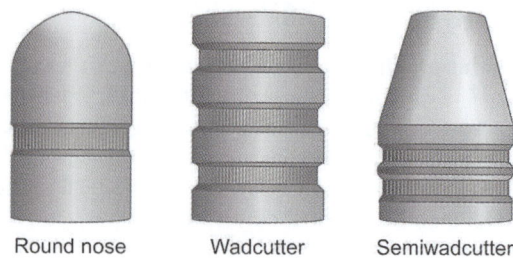

Fig. 12.7: Lead bullets

---

* The only exception to this nomenclature is the .410 bore which has a bore .410 inch in diameter (smallest gauge of shotgun shell).

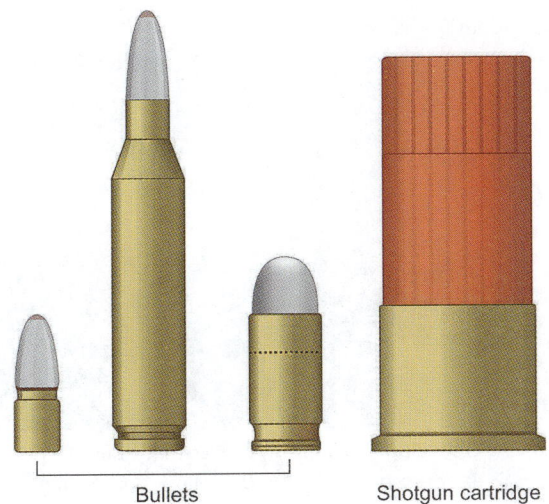

Fig. 12.8: Cartridges of rifled and shotgun weapons

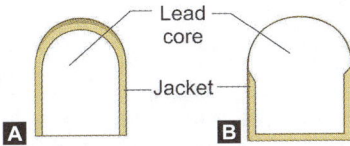

Figs. 12.9A and B: (A) Full metal jacket; (B) Semi-jacketed bullet

ii. *Partial metal-jacketed bullet (semi-jacketed):* Covers the base and cylinder portion of the bullet, leaving the nose partly or fully exposed; designed to expand or mushroom **(Fig. 12.9B)**.

Advantages of jacket: It prevents:
♦ Deformation of the bullet in the barrel from dirt overpressures or damage outside the gun, and reduces misfires.
♦ Fragmentation or melting.
♦ Damage to the gun barrel from 'leading'—lead fouling of the barrel.

Types of Bullet (Fig. 12.10)

i. **Dum-dum bullet (expanding bullet):** Jacketed bullet (.303 centerfire rifle) which does not cover the entire bullet, an area near the nose is left uncovered to expose the core.
ii. **Hollow-point bullet:** Modern version of dum-dum bullet. There is a pit present in front of the nose. When the bullet strikes a target, the pressure in the pit forces the ring of lead around it to expand into a mushroom-shape. This causes more soft tissue damage, and has higher incapacitation index on the target.
iii. **Soft-point bullet:** Jacketed bullet that is left open at the tip, exposing some of the lead inside. They are designed to expand upon impact, but slowly, as compared to the hollow-point bullets.
iv. **Tandem bullet (Piggyback bullet):** Bullets ejected one after the other, when the first bullet having been

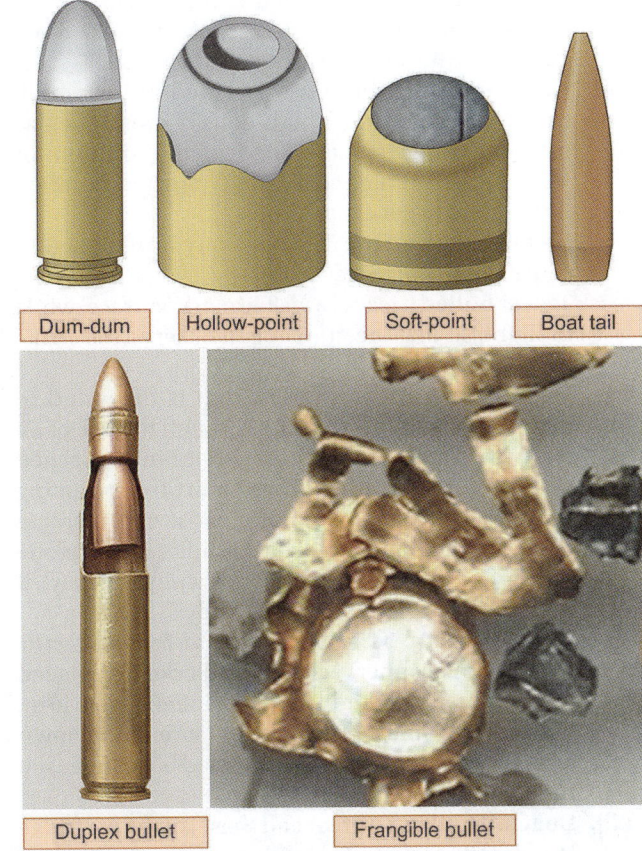

Fig. 12.10: Different types of bullets

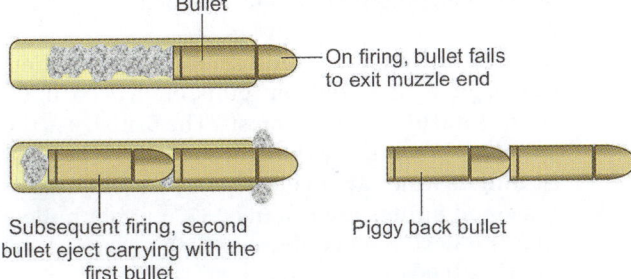

Fig. 12.11: Piggy back bullet

struck in the barrel, fails to leave the barrel and is ejected by a subsequently fired bullet **(Fig. 12.11)**. *Cause:* Faulty ammunition or loaded firearm unused for years.

v. **Duplex bullet:** Contains two projectiles by design, used in military rifles and enter a target at different points.
vi. **Frangible bullet:** Designed to fragment upon impact, often to the point of disintegration, made mostly of copper, powdered tungsten, lead or iron. They do not ricochet.
vii. **Souvenir bullet:** Bullet present in the body for long time with no fresh bleeding around it and surrounded by a dense fibrous tissue capsule. It was not removed

as it was not causing any harm or it was located in an area from where its retrieval could cause more damage to the body, e.g., bullet in the spine.

viii. **Armor piercing bullet:** A jacketed bullet which has inner core of hard, high-density metal such as tungsten, tungsten carbide, depleted uranium or steel, and a truncated cone. This type of ammunition is designed to penetrate armor.
ix. **Incendiary bullets:** Type of army bullet used to cause fire in the target.
x. **Tracer bullet:** It leaves a visible mark or 'trace' while in flight, so that the gunner can observe the strike of the shot.
xi. **Exploding bullet:** A bullet that is designed to detonate or forcibly break up through the use of an explosive or deflagrant contained within or attached to such bullet. These bullets, apart from causing extensive damage in the victim, pose considerable danger to the doctor because the bullet may explode during any procedure (ultrasonography/autopsy), if it had failed to detonate in the body.
xii. **Nontoxic shot:** This is a new *lead-free projectile* wherein the copper-jacketed lead core is replaced with copper-jacketed tungsten, steel, strontium, antimony, bismuth, tin or nylon core. It is known as the **'green bullet'** since toxic lead is not released into the environment.
xiii. **Boat tail bullet:** The rear end (base) of the cartridge is tapered instead of squaring off to stabilize the projectile in flight. The boat shape reduces drag on a bullet, helping it to retain velocity, and resist deflection from crosswinds.
xiv. **Rubber bullets** are usually non-lethal rubber-coated projectiles fired from guns, often used in riot control and to disperse protests. The British use the term *baton round*. They have been replaced by **plastic bullets** which are made of polyvinyl chloride.
xv. **Poisoned bullets** are usually 0.177 caliber bullets (the smallest in general use) which carry curare, ricin or aflatoxin.

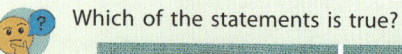

Which of the statements is true?

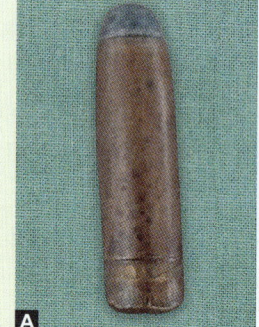
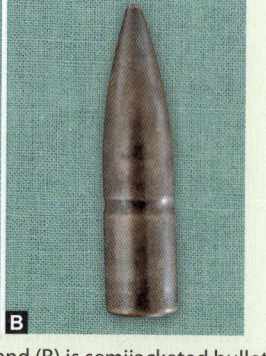

1. (A) is full metal jacketed and (B) is semijacketed bullet
2. (A) is semijacketed and (B) is full metal jacketed bullet
3. Both (A) and (B) are full metal jacketed bullets

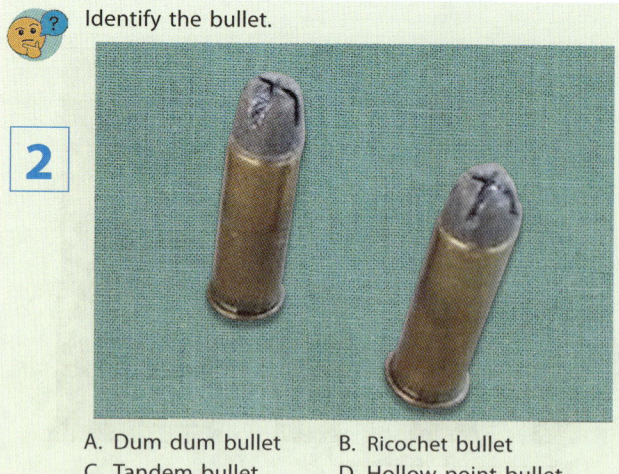

Identify the bullet.

A. Dum dum bullet B. Ricochet bullet
C. Tandem bullet   D. Hollow point bullet

NOTA BENE

♦ Originally, dum-dum bullet referred to a new type of ammunition produced at the Dum-Dum arsenal in British India (near Kolkata) in the early 1890s.
♦ In frangible bullets, class characteristics can be demonstrated but individual markings are lost which is necessary for bullet-to-gun comparison. X-ray picture produced will be similar to the '*lead snowstorm*' seen with hunting bullets.

CARTRIDGE

Cartridge is one unit of ammunition.

Cartridge consists of:
i. Cartridge case with percussion cap containing primer
ii. Propellant charge (gunpowder)
iii. Projectile (bullets/pellets)
iv. Wads (in smooth bore weapons only)

Use of cartridge case
♦ Keeps various components together
♦ Prevents backward escape of gases
♦ Provides waterproofing for gunpowder

Cartridge of shotgun and rifle consists of the following as shown in **Figures 12.12 and 12.13.**

Percussion cap: It is made of either zinc or copper or a compound of both, so as to be malleable and deformable under the blow of the firing pin.

Cartridge cases in rifled firearms are usually made of brass. Sometimes, they are made of steel, nickel or aluminum. Cartridge cases are classified into:

♦ Five types based on configuration of their bases: Rimmed, rimless, semi-rimmed, rebated and belted. Rimmed cartridge has a base with projecting rim and used in revolvers. Rimless cartridge is used in pistols.

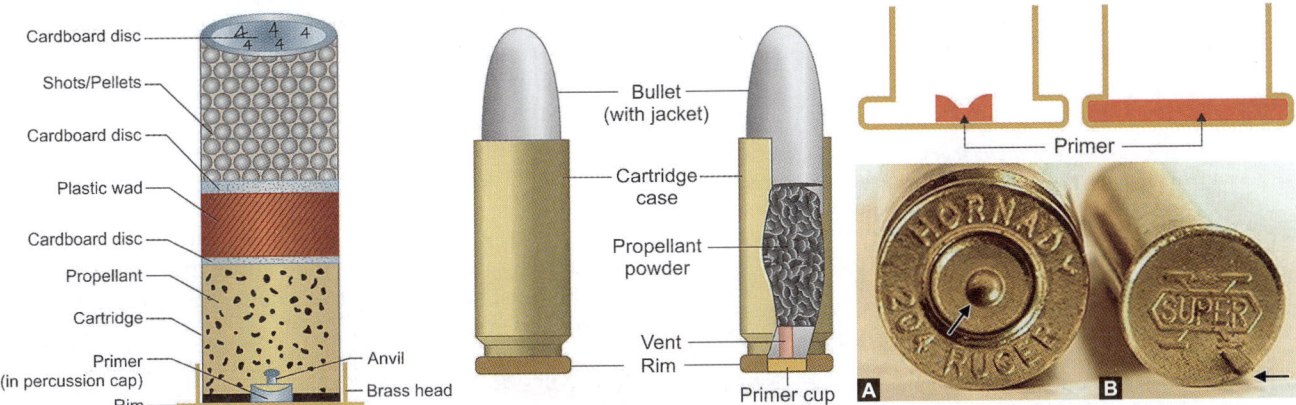

Fig. 12.12: Parts of a shotgun cartridge

Fig. 12.13: Parts of a rifled cartridge

Figs. 12.14A and B: (A) Centerfire; (B) Rimfire cartridge

- Two types depending on location of primer: Centerfire or rimfire **(Figs. 12.14A and B)**:
    - *Centerfire*: The primer is located in the center of the base of the cartridge case.
    - *Rimfire*: Cartridges with priming mixture inserted in the hollow rim. Firing pin gives a hit mark on the circumference.

Blank cartridge: Cartridge with primer, gunpowder and wadding, but without any bullet. It is used in:
- Starter pistol in sports
- Stage/movie performance
- Army maneuvers.

Wad: Wad is made of some soft material, like disc of felt, cardboard, plastic, cork or straw. It is placed between powder and shot or over the shot. The cardboard disc behind the shot charge prevents the pellets from getting lodged in the felt wad **(Fig. 12.12)**.

Pearls

Advantages of wad
- Allows optimum pressure to develop
- Seals the bore effectively
- Helps in lubrication
- Prevents the escape of gas from the breech end
- Separates propellant from the projectiles

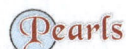 A person came to the emergency with history of gunshot injury. Following was recovered during the operation. Can you identify it? What type of firearm was used?

3

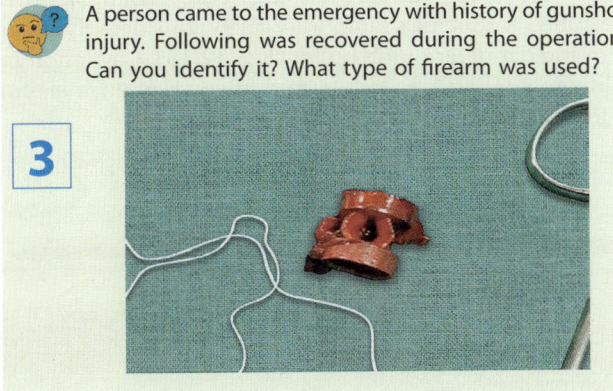

FM 3.9 Describe ammunition propellant charge and mechanism of firearms.

GUNPOWDERS (PROPELLANT CHARGE)

Gunpowder consists of any of several low-explosive mixtures used as propelling charges in guns and as blasting agents in mining.

i. **Black powder:** It produces flame, smoke and heat, and consists of granular ingredients, like sulfur, charcoal and saltpeter (potassium nitrate).

  The optimum proportions for gunpowder and its function is given in **Table 12.1**.

ii. **Smokeless powder:** It is more effective than black powder as it burns more efficiently and produces much less smoke, resulting in less blackening and tattooing around the entry wound.

Types
a. **Single base powder** consists of nitrocellulose (gun cotton). It is the *most common type of* commercial powder, because of its simplicity, adequate power and low flame temperature.
b. **Double base powder** consists of nitrocellulose and nitroglycerin. It is more powerful than single base because of nitroglycerin, but has a flame temperature that may melt the steel of the barrel.
c. **Triple base powder** consists of nitrocellulose, nitroglycerin and nitroguanidine. The quantity of nitroglycerin is small, but sufficient to give power; the nitroguanidine lowers the flame temperature while adding an active explosive constituent.

TABLE 12.1: Composition of gunpowder with its function

Chemical	Percentage (%)	Function(s)
Potassium nitrate	75	Oxygen supplier or oxidizer
Sulfur	10	Makes the mixture more denser and readily ignitable
Charcoal	15	Fuel

iii. **Semi-smokeless powder:** It consists of mixture of 80% black and 20% smokeless type.

> **NOTA BENE**
>
> - When black powder burns properly, it produces 44% of its original weight in gases and 56% in solid residues (potassium carbonate and potassium sulfate). These residues appear as a dense, white smoke. A grain of black powder gives rise to 200–250 mL of gas composed of CO_2, CO, N_2, hydrogen, H_2S and traces of methane and O_2, whereas a grain of smokeless powder forms 800–900 mL of gas with nearly 100% conversion of powder to gases [about 15.1 grains = 1 gram and 7,000 grains = 1 pound (approx)].
> - **Grading of black powder:** The term grading refers to grain size. There are two separate categories of gunpowder grades, 'C' and 'F'. 'C' grade is for cannon and large capacity explosive devices. Powder meant for small arms uses the letter 'F' to denote the grain size. It correlates to the size of the screen mesh which it falls through for sorting. Ranges are course FG (used in large bore rifles), FFG (used in medium and small bore arms, such as muskets), FFFG (used in small bore rifles and pistols) and FFFFG (used in short pistols) which is very fine. Small particles, higher FG numbers burn much faster.

Primer: The primer is a small charge of impact-sensitive chemical that may be located at the center of the case head (centerfire ammunition) or at its rim (rimfire ammunition) **(Fig. 12.14)**. It ignites the powder or propellant charge by impact of gun's firing pin.

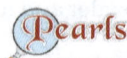

Composition of primer
  i. Lead styphnate
 ii. Barium nitrate
iii. Antimony sulfide
 iv. Lead peroxide
  v. Potassium chlorate
 vi. Tetrazine

MECHANISM OF DISCHARGE OF PROJECTILE

A firearm is fired when the trigger is pulled. The trigger releases a pin or hammer whose tip strikes the percussion cap at the base of the cartridge. The primer contained in it explodes by the heat created by the firing pin. This sends a flash through a tiny hole into the main body of powder filled case, and powder charge or propellant is set on fire instantaneously producing a large amount of gas and heat under pressure. The cartridge case swells outwards, due to which the hold on the bullet (missile, pellets) is released; the bullet is forced into the barrel and passes out.

- When the bullet emerges from the barrel, it is accompanied by:
  i. Unburnt propellant particles
 ii. Partially burnt propellant particles
iii. Soot from combustion of propellant
 iv. Nitrates and nitrites from combustion of propellants
  v. Particles of primer residue (oxides of lead, antimony and barium)
 vi. Vaporized metal and metallic particles stripped from the bullet and cartridge case.
- Varying the length of the barrel also affects how much powder exits the muzzle. Shortening the barrel causes more unburned powder to emerge and vice-versa.
- The confined gas left behind gives recoil thrust to the gun.
- Noise of gun firing is caused by the muzzle blast or sudden release of gases disturbing the air.
- The blast has the shape of a cone, the apex of which is located at the muzzle.

> **NOTA BENE**
>
> - **Muzzle blast** is the release of gases under high temperature and pressure from the muzzle of a firearm when it is discharged.
> - **Muzzle flash** is the visible light of the muzzle blast.

WOUND BALLISTICS AND MECHANISM OF INJURY

As a missile traverses the body, it causes injury by transferring some or all of its energy. This is manifested as laceration and crushing of tissues in its path, and sometimes away from its path. The amount of energy transferred is given by the formula:

$$KE = \tfrac{1}{2} M (V_1^2 - V_2^2)$$

where KE = Kinetic energy
M = Mass of the bullet
V_1 and V_2 = Velocities at entry and exit

It shows that velocity rather than its weight plays a greater role in determining the amount of kinetic energy possessed by a bullet. Doubling the weight doubles the kinetic energy, but doubling the velocity quadruples the kinetic energy.

In general, bullets fired from handguns are propelled at a low velocity, have low energy (50–100 J) and result in *low energy transfer wounds* which are characterized by injuries confined to the wound track. Missiles with high available energy (2000–3000 J) include high-velocity assault rifle bullets, and have the potential to cause *high energy transfer wounds*. As a bullet moves through the body, it crushes and shreds the tissue in its path, while at the same time flinging outward (radially) the surrounding tissue from the path of the bullet, producing a temporary cavity considerably larger than the diameter of the bullet **(Fig. 12.15)**. Cavitation in solid organs, like liver, kidney and spleen is often fatal, but in the bones, it creates *secondary missiles*.

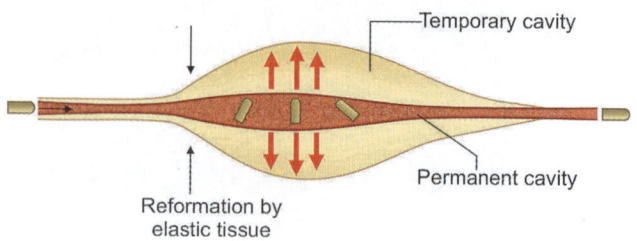

Fig. 12.15: Shock waves from a gunshot result in cavitation.

FM 3.10

Describe and discuss wound ballistics, different types of firearm injuries and their interpretation.

FIREARM WOUNDS

Gunshot wounds are either penetrating or perforating.
- *Penetrating wounds*: The bullet enters the body and does not exit **(Fig. 12.16A)**.
- *Perforating wounds*: The bullet passes completely through the body **(Fig. 12.16B)**.

For example, a bullet striking the head may pass through the skull and brain before coming to rest under the scalp, producing a penetrating wound of the head, but perforating wound of the skull and brain.

> **Characteristics of firearm wounds depend upon:**
> - Nature of the firearm, whether shotgun or rifle
> - Shape and composition of the missiles
> - Range (distance) of firing
> - Part of the body struck (head or trunk)
> - Direction of firing

- **Tattooing:** It consists of unburnt or partially burnt powder particles that are embedded in and under the skin through the force of their impact (when the weapon is near enough for the powder grains to strike) **(Fig. 12.17A)**.
    - Tattooing is an antemortem phenomenon and indicates that the individual was alive.
    - It cannot be wiped away with a wet cotton.
    - It consists of numerous reddish-brown punctate abrasions surrounding the wound of entrance.
    - The greater the range, the larger and less dense the powder tattooing.
    - Marks usually heal completely if the individual survives (involves the superficial layer of the epidermis).

- **Stippling:** It is the visible mark powder grains leave, when it does not get embedded on the skin (when the range increases). It may also be produced by other material, e.g., shotgun filler or fragments of intermediary targets. The term 'stippling' is sometimes used synonymously with 'powder tattooing'.

- **Blackening (soot or smoke soiling/smudging):** Deposition of powder soot (carbon) produced by combustion of gunpowder **(Fig. 12.17B)**.
    - As the range increases, the size of the zone of blackening will increase, whereas the density will decrease.
    - It can be easily removed with a wet cotton.

- **Fouling:** Tiny lesions around the entry wound caused by fragments of metal expelled by the discharge.
    - These fragments may come either from the surface of the bullet or from the interior of the barrel.
    - It cannot be wiped off from the skin.

- **Abrasion collar/ring:** As the bullet strikes the skin, it first indents and then stretches the skin surface so that perforation takes place through a tense area which produces a rim of flattened reddish-brown zone of abraded epidermis, surrounding the entrance wound **(Fig. 12.17C)**.* The abrasion ring can vary in width, depending on the caliber of the weapon, the angle and site at which the bullet entered.
    - A bullet striking perpendicularly will produce a concentric ring, and if the bullet penetrates at an oblique angle, the zone will be eccentric with the wider zone on the side from which the bullet came **(Figs. 12.18A and B)**.
    - Entrance wounds in the skin overlying the clavicle have a wider abrasion ring than those in the other parts of the body.
    - The entry wound on the palms and soles usually lack abrasion collar due to the thickness and keratinization of the epidermis in these areas, and may be stellate instead of round.

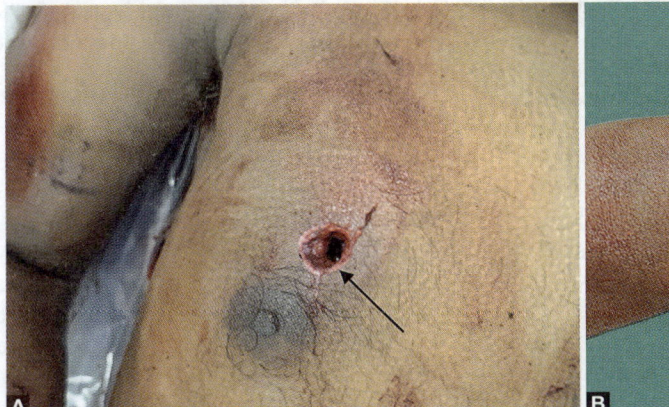
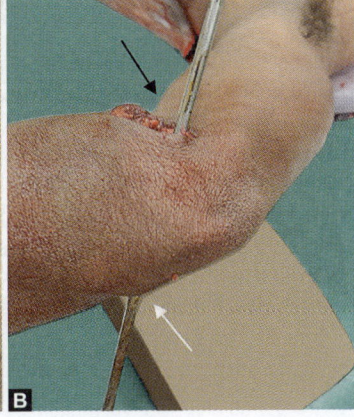

Figs. 12.16A and B: (A) Penetrating; (B) Perforating wounds
(*Courtesy*: Dr Praveen Kumar Tiwari, IMS, BHU, Varanasi)

---

* According to German researchers, abrasion collar is not caused by friction or overstretching, but by superficial tissue particles being thrown back against the direction of the fire, since the collar is seen even when shots are fired at non-biological, layered objects.

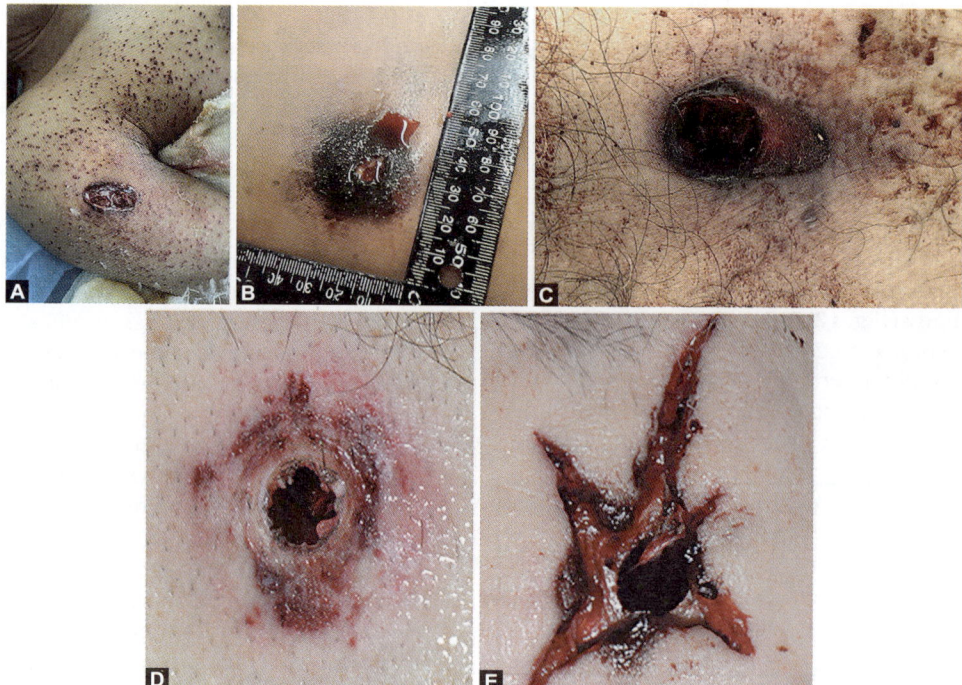

Figs. 12.17A to E: Characteristics of gunshot injuries: (A) Tattooing; (B) Blackening and grease collar; (C) Abrasion collar; (D) Muzzle imprint; (E) Wound due to blow back phenomenon

- Some contusion is present in abraded collar and as such, it is also called '**contusion collar**'.
- **Grease/dirt collar (bullet wipe):** A black/gray colored ring is seen lining the defect, sharply outlined, caused from removal of substances from bullet as it passes through the skin **(Fig. 12.17B)**. It consists of bullet lubrication, paraffin, lead from surface of bullet, barrel debris and gun oil from interior of the barrel.
    - The ring of dirt is more pronounced in shots from freshly oiled weapons than in shots from lubricant-free barrels.
    - By contrast, soot is dark in the center and fades towards the periphery.
    - Abrasion collar surrounds the dirt collar.
    - This gray rim is more prominent in clothing, where it is called '*bullet wipe*'.
    - Abrasion and dirt collars are proof of an entry wound.
- **Muzzle imprint**[+] (described by *Werkgartner* in 1922) is regarded as a patterned abrasion/intradermal contusion caused by the expansive power of the gases lifting the skin forcibly up against the muzzle **(Fig. 12.17D)**.
    - This is a sign of a contact shot.
    - Its shape depends on the firearm, the ammunition and the anatomical conditions, but does not require a bullet.
    - Characteristic imprint marks can provide clues to the type of the firearm and its position at the time of discharge.

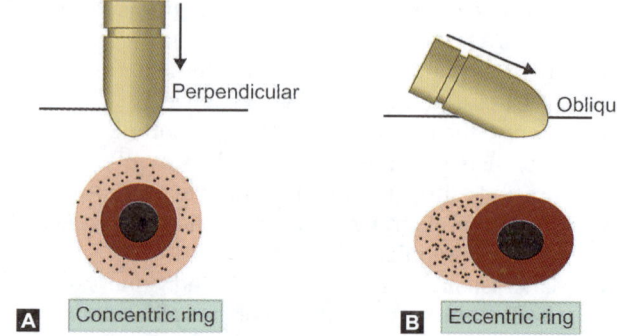

Figs. 12.18A and B: Abraded collar when bullet struck: (A) Perpendicularly; (B) At an angle. The wider side determines the direction of fire

- **Back spatter:** In a contact shot, the muzzle blast and negative pressure in the barrel may suck blood, hair, fragments of tissues and cloth fibers back into the barrel.
- **Blowback phenomenon:** Cruciate, stellate or ragged laceration is seen, especially if there is a thick bone immediately under the skin, such as the skull **(Fig. 12.17E)**. This occurs as a result of expansion of gases beneath the skin and their exit through the entry wound (in contact wounds).
- **Point blank:** When the range is very close to, or in contact with the surface of the skin.

[+] Some consider the muzzle impression is due to the recoil of the gun. Recoil takes the muzzle away from the skin, not towards it.

Deduce the direction of fire from the given image. What other feature can you observe?

 4

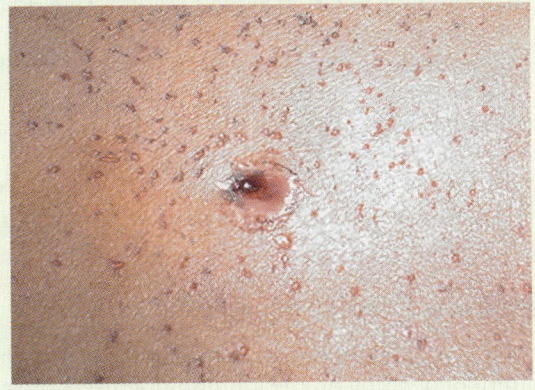

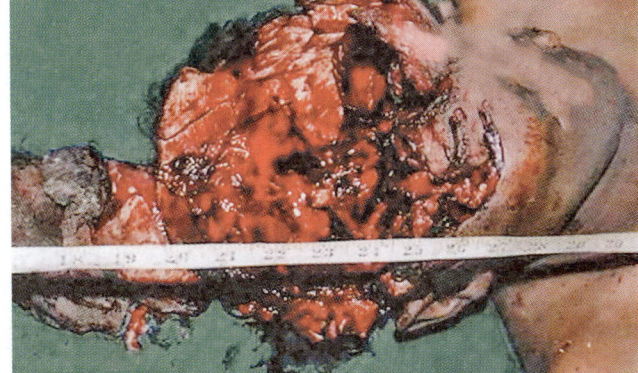

Fig. 12.19: Contact shotgun injury of head

CHARACTERISTICS OF SHOTGUN WOUNDS

♦ The following constituents of shotgun cartridge that emerge during discharge may contribute to the wound: flame and hot gases (about 760°C), soot, unburnt and burnt propellant particles, lead pellets, wads, carbon monoxide, detonator constituents and fragments of the cartridge case.

♦ When a shotgun is fired, the projectile travels as a compact mass. As the range increases, the individual pellets spread out, collectively travel in a cone-like manner and their velocity decreases with distance. A rough estimate of the rate of spread is about 1 inch/yard from the muzzle of a full choke gun.

Contact or Near Contact Shot

Contact wound: Muzzle of the weapon is held against the body at the time of discharge. Contact wound can be hard (muzzle held tightly against the skin), loose, angled or incomplete.

♦ Contact wounds differ in appearances, depending upon the site, whether it is the head or the non-resisting parts, e.g., chest or abdomen.

♦ Contact shotgun wounds of the *head* are the most mutilating firearms wounds. Extensive destruction of bone and soft tissue structures occurs with bursting rupture of the head and evisceration of the brain, since the gases have restricted space for expansion **(Fig. 12.19)**. Soot is seen around the entrance in most contact wounds of head.

♦ Contact wound of the *trunk* appear circular in shape, and have diameter usually equal to that of the bore of the weapon as shot enters as a mass.

♦ If the muzzle is pressed firmly, soiling or burning is absent, but the edges of the wound is seared and blackened by the hot gases, and a muzzle impression may be found.

♦ If the muzzle is not pressed firmly or is loosened by recoil; flame, gas and soot may escape sideways and soil the adjoining skin **(Fig. 12.20)**.

♦ If clothing interposes between the muzzle and skin, soot will be found on the clothing, as well as the skin. Clothing may be singed, and there may be burning around the skin wound.

♦ The gases cause laceration of deeper tissues and even fragmentation of bone.

♦ Wad is often found in the wound, and this may prove to be an important clue to the type of cartridge used.

♦ Wound track and adjacent tissues appear cherry-red due to carboxyhemoglobin and carboxymyoglobin from absorption of carbon monoxide (CO) formed from combustion of the gunpowder (can spread up to 15 cm or more from the entrance).

♦ Usually, shotgun projectiles do not exit out of the body.

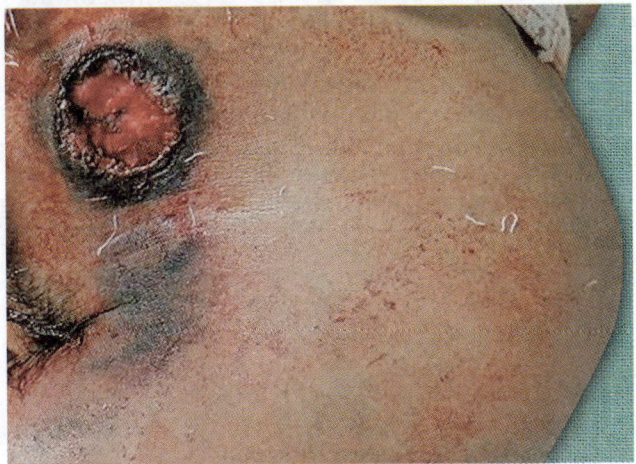

Fig. 12.20: Contact shotgun injury with the muzzle not firmly pressed

Close Range (Between Contact and 3 ft)

- Close range shotgun wounds of the head are almost as mutilating as contact wounds, because the pellets are still traveling in a single mass. Large gaping tears of the scalp are present.
- When clothing is present, it traps most of the soot and powder grains and may reduce the flame effect.
- Depending on the angle of firing, the wound is circular or elliptical. There are no separate pellet holes.
- Singeing of hair, scorching, blackening and tattooing (less with smokeless powder) of skin is seen. Blackening and tattooing can be demonstrated by *infrared photography*.
- No burning is seen beyond 1 ft (30 cm).
- Soot soiling is less and disappears at over 1–3 ft.
- Wound track and adjacent tissues appear cherry-red due to absorption of CO.
- Wads or plastic cups from cartridge may be found in the wound.

NOTA BENE

- Powder tattooing from a shotgun is less dense than the tattooing a handgun produces at the same range, due to more complete combustion of powder caused by the greater barrel length.
- If the wad also contains the pellets, then the shot cup peel open between 1–2 feet in the form of petals and the circular entrance wound is surrounded with a **Maltese cross abrasion (Fig. 12.21)**. Twelve, 16 and 20 bore shells have four petals; .410 bore has three petals. By 3 feet, air resistance folds back the petals and a single hole of entrance will be produced. The plastic wad may or may not accompany the shot column into the body.

Mid/Near Range (Up to 7 ft)

As the muzzle of the shotgun moves further from the body, tattooing disappear and the diameter of the circular wound of entry increases in size until a point is reached where individual pellets begin to separate from the main mass.

- No burning and soot soiling is there, but tattooing can be seen up to 3–4 ft (90–125 cm).
- Between 3 ft, the shots enter the body in one mass, producing a round hole. The edge of the wound is abraded and crenated/scalloped (**rat hole or cookie cutter appearance**) **(Fig. 12.21)**.

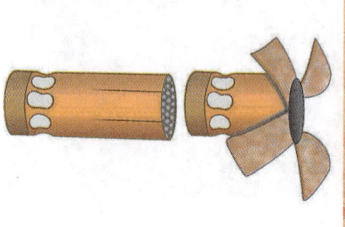
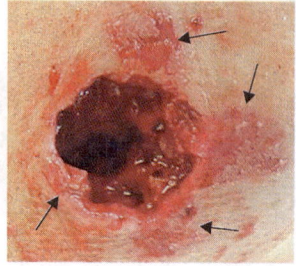

Fig. 12.21: Close range shotgun wound (cross-like abrasion formed by wad with rat hole appearance of entry wound)

- At a distance of 4 ft, the shot mass spreads and individual pellet holes may be seen which are round with surrounding abrasion at their margins **(Fig. 12.22A)**.
- At a distance of 6–7 ft, the central aperture is surrounded by separate openings in an area of 8–10 cm in diameter.
- As distance increases, the main entrance wound progressively becomes smaller and individual pellet wounds increases in number.
- Beyond 4–5 ft, the wads often strike the body below the main wound leaving a circular or oval imprint on the skin.

Long Range (Beyond 7 ft)

Beyond 7 ft, great variation occurs in the size of the pellet pattern depending on the ammunition used, the choke of the gun and the range.

- Charge of shot progressively spreads, so that small openings due to separate pellets appear around the main wound. With further increase in range, there is a more even distribution of pellet injuries with disappearance of the central aperture **(Fig. 12.22B)**.
- At far longer ranges, the shots, depending upon its size and velocity, may not lodge in the body.
- Wadding injury may be seen up to 15–20 ft. Wad may cause an independent impact abrasion.

All these figures presuppose the lack of clothing, since it will absorb soot and powder, making close range wounds appear to be distant by examination of the body alone.

The characteristic features seen in shotgun injury at varying ranges is summarized in **Table 12.2** *and* **Fig. 12.23**.

 A 45-year-old male was brought to mortuary with alleged history of gunshot injury. Determine the range of fire. Comment on the type of weapon.

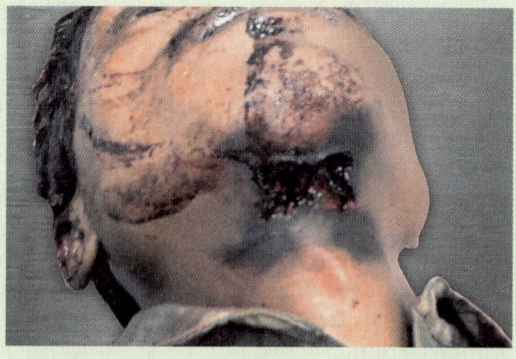

CHARACTERISTICS OF RIFLED FIREARMS WOUNDS

- Handguns are most commonly used form of firearm both in homicides and suicides.
- The presence and extent of tearing of the skin depends on the caliber of the weapon, the amount of gas produced by the combustion of the propellant, the firmness

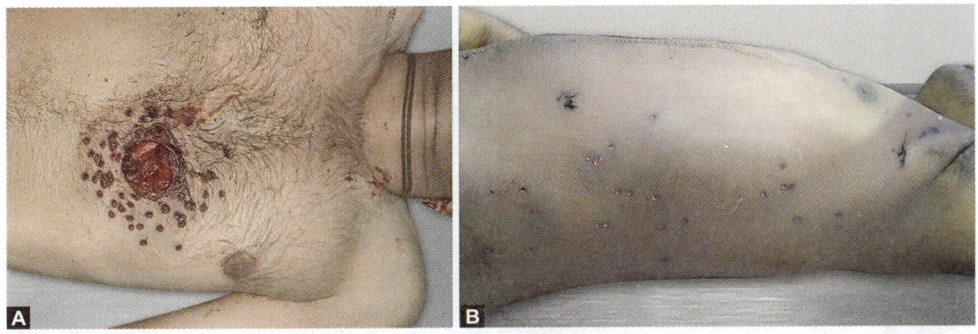

Figs. 12.22A and B: Shotgun injury: (A) Mid range (rat hole appearance with satellite pellet pattern); (B) Long range

TABLE 12.2: Features of shotgun injuries at different range

Features	Contact shot	Close range (contact to 3 ft)	Mid range (Up to 7 ft)	Long range (>7 ft)
Wound	Circular, equal to bore of weapon (mutilation and evisceration of brain, if in head)	Circular/elliptical with no separate pellet holes (mutilating in head)	Round, edges crenated (rat hole appearance) with satellite pattern pellet holes around it	Uniform distribution of pellet with no central aperture
Muzzle impression	+	–	–	–
Burning	–	+	–	–
Blackening/soot	– (+ in contact wound of head)	+	–	–
Singeing	–	+	–	–
Tattooing	–	+	+/–	–

'+': Present; '–': Absent

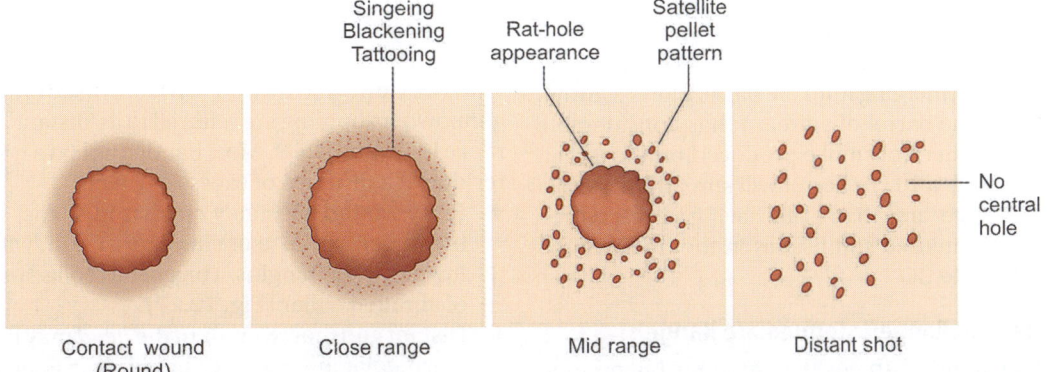

Fig. 12.23: Shotgun wounds at varying distances

with which the gun is held against the body and the elasticity of the skin.

Contact Shot

Whole of the discharge containing flame, gases, powder smoke and metallic particles will be blown under pressure into the track taken by the bullet through the body, often leaving little evidence that one is dealing with a contact wound.

- In case of contact shot over *forehead or mastoid* region (head) where the bone is thick, entry wound will be large and irregular, stellate or cruciform shaped having everted margins because of expansion of gas between the skull and scalp **(Fig. 12.24A)**. Back spatter may be seen.
- In contact wounds of the *trunk*, stellate/cruciform entry wound usually do not occur because the gas is able to expend into the abdominal or chest cavity or soft tissue.
- Contact wound over *abdomen* will show cavitations, because of blast effect.
- There is little or no evidence of burning, singeing, blackening and tattooing.
- Muzzle impression may be present around the wound **(Fig. 12.24B)**.
- Muscles around the track taken by bullet will be cherry-red due to presence of CO.
- Burning, blackening and powder grains deposits will be found in the depths of the wound (examination of the wounds with dissecting microscope is of value).
- Hair nearby may get burnt or clubbed by fire/heat.

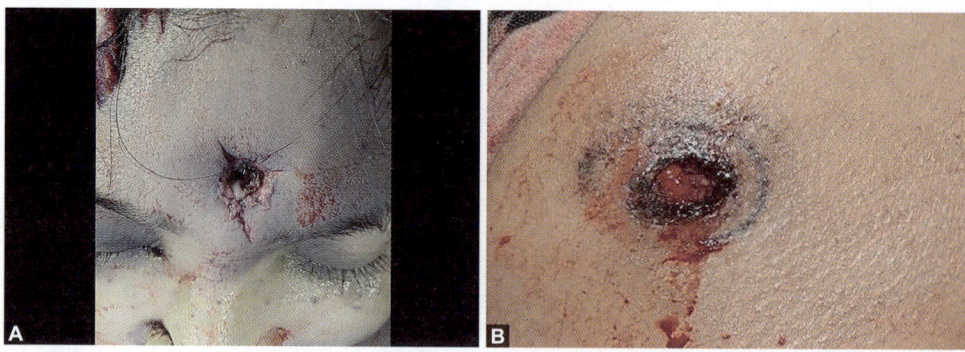

Figs. 12.24A and B: Contact wounds: (A) Stellate wound; (B) Muzzle imprint

Close Shot (Flame Range)

Body lies within the range of flame, smoke and powder blast, i.e., within 2–3 inches (5–8 cm).
- Entry wound is small and circular in shape having inverted and contused lacerated margins.
- Skin adjacent to the entry wound shows evidence of grease/dirt collar on the inner zone, and abraded-contused collar on the outer zone **(Fig. 12.25)**.
- Evidence of burning, singeing, blackening and tattooing of the skin in and around the entry wound **(Fig. 12.25)**.
- Clothings over the part will be burnt from flame of discharge.
- Hair, in and around, show singeing and will look clubbed, shriveled and swollen at intervals (rarely seen, because the gas emerging from the barrel blows it away).
- The length of the barrel of a firearm has considerable effect on the pattern of smoke produced on the target, e.g., a pistol with a 10 cm barrel will spread the smoke over a much larger area than a rifle having a 2 feet barrel.
- The blood and injured soft tissues in the track will be cherry-red due to CO.

Near Shot (Medium Range/Intermediate Range)

Gunshot entry wounds with powder tattooing, but no soot, are commonly referred to as 'near-shot' or 'intermediate range' wounds, i.e., when the range is within 24 inches (60 cm) **(Figs. 12.26A and B)**.
- Entry wound will be circular in shape, approximately the same size as the bullet, with lacerated, inverted edges surrounded by a narrow zone of grease and abrasion collar, with no evidence of any burning and singeing.

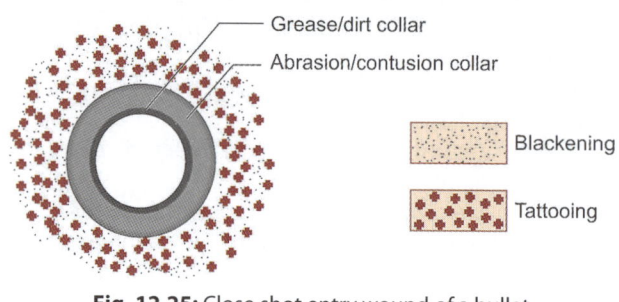

Fig. 12.25: Close shot entry wound of a bullet

- Entry wound looks like a distant shot when the range is beyond 6 inches (15 cm). Beyond 15 cm, the burning effects of gases and singeing of hair is absent.
- Zone of blackening will be present when the range is within 6–8 inches (15–20 cm), and zone of tattooing will be present around it. In case of handguns, soot is absent beyond 30 cm.
- Tattooing becomes discrete as the range increases, no trace of powder marks will be found when the range is beyond 24 inches, i.e., normally beyond arm's length. For handguns, powder tattooing extends to a maximum distance of 18–24 inches (45–60 cm).

Distant Shot

Gunshot entry wounds with no associated soot or gunpowder stippling are referred to as 'distant' wounds, i.e., range is beyond 2 feet. Most handguns leave no gunpowder residue at a distance of excess of 2 feet.
- Entry wound is usually circular in shape, smaller than the bullet, because of elasticity of skin, with lacerated, inverted skin margins, a bigger dirt collar and usual zone of abraded collar **(Fig. 12.27)**.
- Distant gunshot wounds of the *head* may have a stellate or irregular appearance simulating a contact wound.
- There will be no evidence of any burning, singeing, blackening and tattooing.
- Wound of exit will be slightly bigger than the wound of entry.
- Sometimes, the term *'indeterminate'* is used since closer range shots where the soot and gunpowder is totally blocked by an interposed target may produce identical appearing wounds.

The characteristic features seen in rifle firearm injury at varying ranges is summarized in **Table 12.3**.

NOTA BENE

Irregular, cruciform or stellate entry wounds can occur in individuals shot at intermediate or distant range when the bullet perforates the skin underlying a bony prominence. Head is the most common site—forehead, top and back of the head, supraorbital ridges and cheek bone. Uncommon site is the elbow.

CHAPTER 12 : Firearm Injuries

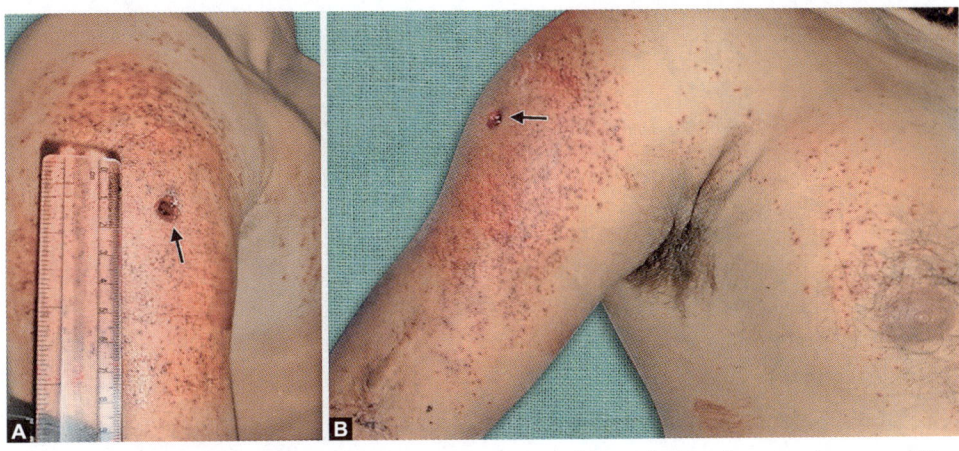

Figs. 12.26A and B: Near shot rifled firearm entry wound (arrow). Note the tattooing around it

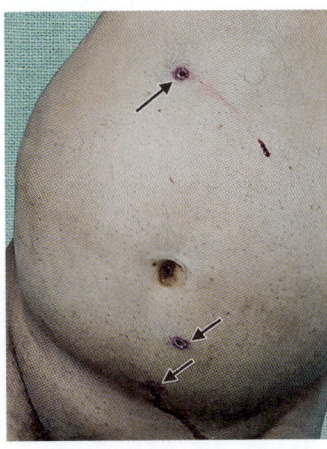

Fig. 12.27: Distant shot rifled firearm entry wounds (arrows)

TABLE 12.3: Features of rifled firearm injuries at different range

Features	Contact shot	Close range (2–3 inches)	Mid Range (<2 ft)	Distant shot (>2 ft)
Wound	Large, irregular, stellate shaped (in head)	Small and circular	Circular, same size as bullet	Circular, smaller than bullet
Margins	Everted	Inverted	Inverted	Inverted
Muzzle impression	+	–	–	–
Grease collar/abrasion collar	–	+	+	+
Burning	–/+	+	–	–
Blackening/soot	–	+	+/–	–
Singeing	–	+	–	–
Tattooing	–	+	+	–

'+': Present; '–': Absent

 A 27-year-old female presented in the emergency with alleged history of gunshot injury. Estimate the range of fire. Give reasons.

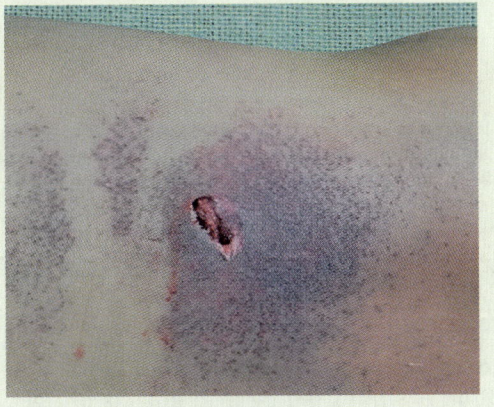

FIREARM WOUNDS ON SKULL

- **The entry wound** shows a punched in hole (clean cut) on the outer table and beveled appearance on the inner table (as it remains unsupported, chipping of the bone occurs) **(Fig. 12.28)**. Fissured fracture may radiate from the hole. The piece may be driven inside causing injury to the brain. Dura shows irregular tear. In contact wounds, shattering of skull wound may occur.
- **The exit wound** shows clean cut hole on inner table and beveling on the outer table **(Fig. 12.28)**. The wound is larger than the entry wound due to the deformity and tumbling of the bullet on entering the skull. The beveling helps to assess the angle of fire.

Tangential entrance wounds (*gutter wound*) into bone may produce 'keyhole' defects with entrance and exit side-by-side; the skin is torn or lacerated by the bullet **(Fig. 12.29).**

Puppe's Rule

This rule states that when two fracture lines intersect each other, the second fracture line never crosses the first one **(Fig. 12.30)**. It determines the sequence of shots when several bullets have struck the cranium, and is also applicable to the multiple blunt force impact on the skull.

EXIT WOUNDS

Shotguns

- The appearance of shotgun exit wound depends upon the part involved and the nature of tissues encountered during its passage in the body.

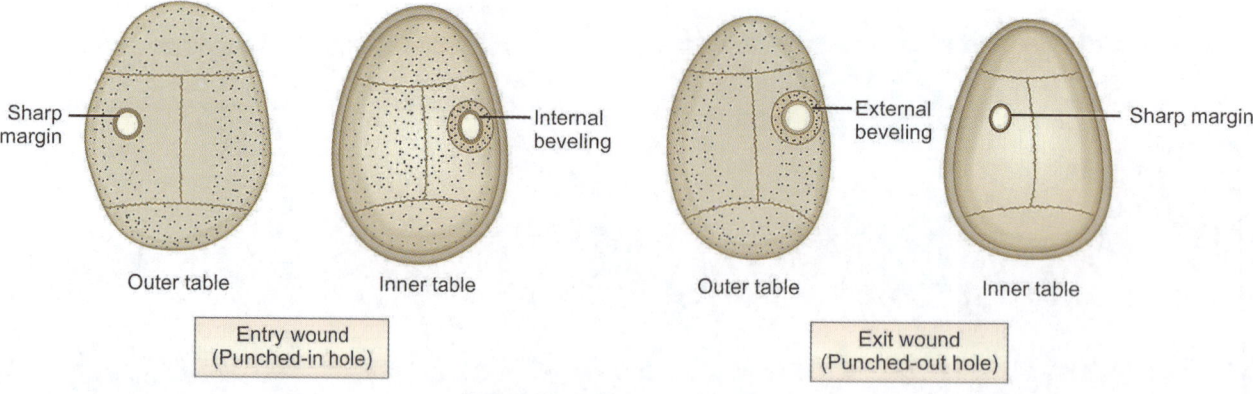

Fig. 12.28: Bullet wounds in skull

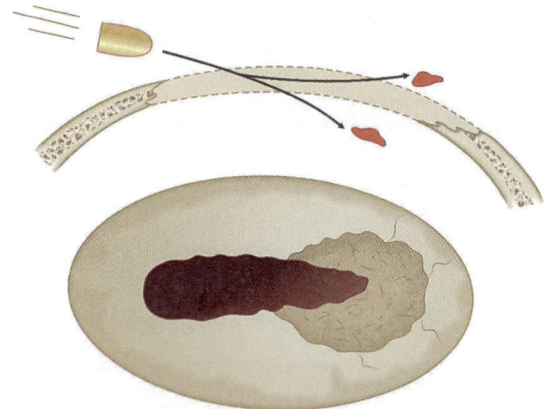

Fig. 12.29: 'Key-hole' defect on the outer bone table when a bullet strikes it tangentially

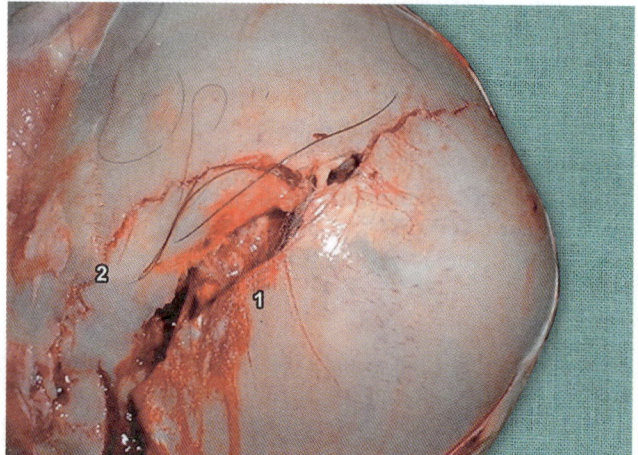

Fig. 12.30: Puppe's rule: (1) First (initial) fracture; (2) Subsequent (later) fracture

- Exit wounds with shotguns are uncommon, especially when they involve the chest or abdomen.
- When present, it is in the form of serrated, irregular laceration with everted margins through which some tissues or bone fragments may be seen protruding.
- Sometimes, the pellets may accumulate immediately beneath the skin opposite the entry wound, after they have traveled through the body and trapped by the skin.

Rifled Firearms

Exit wounds, whether they are from contact, intermediate or distant firing, all have the same general characteristics.
- It may be stellate, circular, elliptical, cruciate, star shaped or slit-like as bullet gets deformed when struck by a bone (common in head and shoulders)—may be confused with contact wounds.
- In contact wounds and very close range, exit wound is smaller than entry wound due to elastic nature of the skin. However, as range increases, the size of exit wound also increases.
- Exit wounds do not show burning, blackening, tattooing, abrasion or contusion collar. The edges are everted, torn or puckered with pieces of contused, hemorrhagic subcutaneous fat or muscle protruding out of the defect.

> **NOTA BENE**
> **Variations in shape and size of exit wounds occur when:**
> - Bullet tumbles in the body and fails to exit nose-end first
> - Bullet exits as multiple pieces after breaking up
> - Bullet is deformed
> - Unsupported skin tends to tear and break into pieces
> - Fragments of bone are blown out along with the bullet (*secondary missiles*).

Shored or supported exit wound: If the skin at the exit wound is supported by firm objects or tight garments, e.g., belt, waist band, bra or tie, or body leaning against a hard object, such as wall or floor, the exit wound appears as a circular defect surrounded by a margin of abrasion resembling an entry wound. The pattern of the material overlying the shored exit may be imprinted on the edges of the wound.

Diff. 12.1 tabulates the differences between entry and exit wound of a rifled firearm (**Figs. 12.31A and B**).

DIFFERENTIATION 12.1: Entry and exit wound

S.No.	Feature	Entry wound	Exit wound
1.	Definition	Wound that results from a projectile entering a body	Wound that results from a projectile exiting a body
2.	Size	Smaller than the diameter of the bullet (except contact shot)	Bigger than the bullet
3.	Edges	Inverted	Everted, puckered
4.	Skull	Clean cut on outer table and beveled in the inner table	Beveled in the outer table and clean cut on inner table
5.	Bruising, abrasion and grease collar	Present	Absent
6.	Burning, blackening, tattooing	May be seen	Absent
7.	Bleeding	Less	More
8.	Condition of hair	Singeing or breakage of hair	Hair may overlie the wound
9.	Fat	No protrusion	May protrude
10.	Wound track	May be cherry-red due to carboxyhemoglobin and/or carboxymyoglobin	No color change
11.	Fibers of clothes	Turned in	Turned out
12.	Histopathology	Coagulative necrosis of keratinocytes associated with subepidermal crack and tattooing	Presence of adipose, muscular and bone tissue
13.	Radiological/micro-chemical examination	Lead ring may be seen	Absent
14.	Spectrograph	More metal is found	Less metal

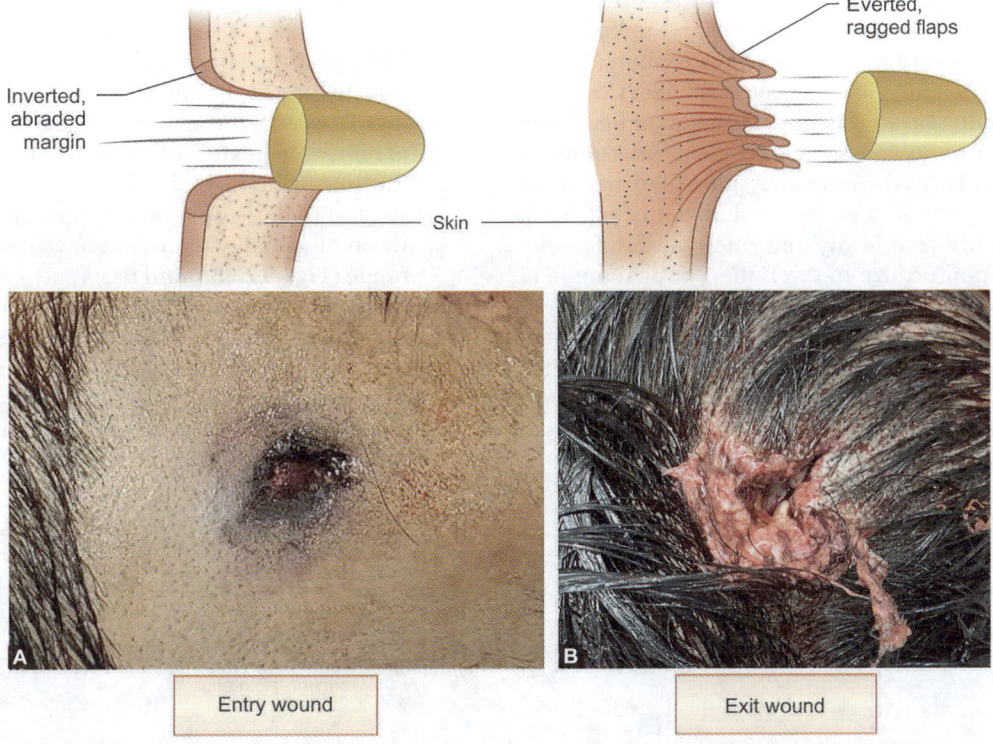

Figs. 12.31A and B: Firearm entry and exit wounds. (A) Entry wound over temple (note inverted margins, abrasion collar, blackening and muzzle impression); (B) Exit wound over parietal eminence (everted margins, no abrasion collar, grease collar, blackening)
(*Courtesy*: Dr Praveen Kumar Tiwari)

Which of the statements is true?

7

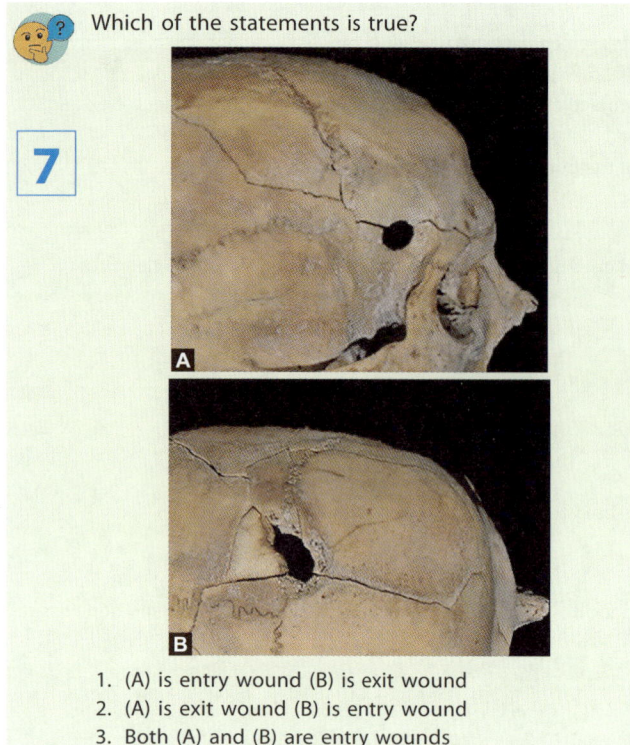

1. (A) is entry wound (B) is exit wound
2. (A) is exit wound (B) is entry wound
3. Both (A) and (B) are entry wounds

PECULIAR EFFECTS OF FIREARMS

Atypical gunshot entrance wounds are created when the bullet is destabilized prior to entering the body and consequently does not enter the body nose first but sideways or at an angle. The most common cause is bullet ricochet.

- **Ricochet bullet:** It is a rebound, deviation or deflection of a bullet from its course by striking an intermediate surface **(Fig. 12.32A)**. Sometimes, the bullet may strike the surface, but fail to penetrate and glance off. Such projectiles are commonly deformed, and deformity depends upon texture of the bullet, critical angle of impact* and intermediary object.
    - Round nose bullets are more likely to ricochet than flat nosed; FMJ than lead, and low velocity than high velocity.
    - A bullet having ricocheted off another object would be subjected to all the secondary movements of a missile: 'yawing', 'wobbling' and 'tumbling'. This will cause an atypical entry wound.

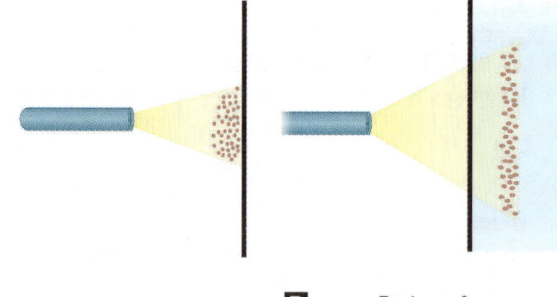

Figs. 12.33A and B: 'Billiard ball' ricochet effect: (A) If shot is fired at close range, the leading pellets are slowed as they enter the body and are stuck by trailing pellets; (B) The colliding pellets ricochet to spread the shot pattern giving the impression of longer-range fire

- **Tumbling bullet:** Bullet rotates end-to-end during its path **(Fig. 12.32B)**.
- **Tail wobble or tail wag:** It occurs for few microseconds after the bullet leaves the muzzle and may cause great damage.
- **Yaw:** Deviation between the long axis of the bullet and axis of the path of the bullet **(Fig. 12.32C)**. The projectile can yaw in two ways—precession and nutation.
- **'Billiard ball' ricochet effect**: This is seen in relation to ricochet of shotgun pellets from an intermediate target surface, such as door, windows, clothes or within the body itself.
    - When a mass of shotgun pellets enters tissue, the first pellets which penetrate are slowed and struck from behind by the following pellets which can cause them to scatter through the tissue much like a cluster of billiard balls struck by the cue ball.
    - Radiographically, the dispersal of pellets may suggest that the weapon was fired from a distance, when in actuality the weapon was fired from close range **(Figs. 12.33A and B)**.
- **Kennedy phenomenon:** The evaluation of whether the wound was an entrance or an exit becomes difficult due to surgical alteration or suturing of the gunshot wound. It is in reference to the late US President John F Kennedy who was shot, and surgical alteration of the gunshot wound on the neck made it difficult to evaluate as to whether it is an entrance or exit wound *(refer to the Case study given at the end of the chapter)*.

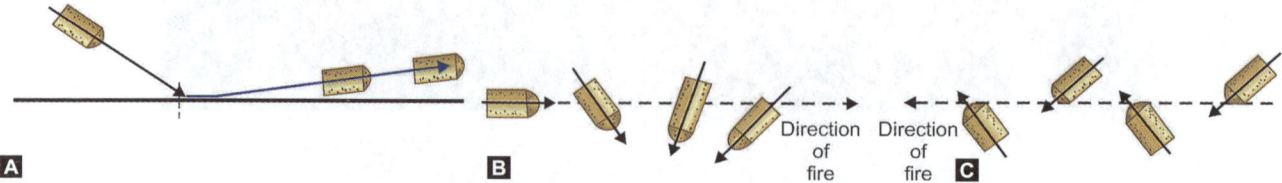

Figs. 12.32A to C: (A) Ricochet bullet; (B) Tumbling; (C) Yaw

---

* It is the angle of incidence below which a bullet striking the surface will ricochet rather than penetrate which is determined by the nature of the surface, the construction and velocity of the bullet.

- **Double tap:** Tactical shooting technique commonly employed by Special Forces by which the trigger is pulled in a quick succession allowing two shots to be fired in the same target zone.
  - The shots will cluster within 1–2 inch of each other (similar to tandem shot) and have an 8-shaped defect in which two coalescing, round defects are formed.
  - Although they have same area of entrance wound, but do not exit from the same location.
  - They are the hallmark of extrajudicial executions because it is considered to be an 'insurance shot' to the intended target.

NOTA BENE

- **Graze/slap wound:** Bullet strikes the skin at so acute angle that it produces an elongated area of abrasion without actually perforating or tearing the skin.
- **Superficial perforating wound:** Shallow through-and-through wounds in which the entry and exit are close together.
- **Krönlein shot** is a very rare injury of the skull caused by a high-velocity bullet. In this close-range shot, there is bursting of the skull and laceration of the dura mater with complete evisceration of the brain. The autopsy cannot determine with certainty the appearance of the primary gunshot wound, and the entrance and exit wounds.
- **Rayalaseema phenomenon:** It is an artifact. Sometimes, to fake a firearm injury, a bullet is planted in an individual killed initially by stab injury or deliberate mutilation of firearm injury may be done like cutting or stabbing through it to mislead the investigating agency. These cases were reported from the district of Rayalaseema in Andhra Pradesh.

FM 3.10
Describe and discuss preservation and dispatch of trace evidences in cases of firearm.

POSTMORTEM EXAMINATION

Scene of crime: Before any object is removed, the following photographs must be taken with identifying labels and rulers:
- Bullet holes in the walls, floor, ceiling or in the furniture.
- Body of the victim before and after undressing.
- After removing the clothes, entrance and exit bullet holes along with bullets, pellets or wads found in the body. X-ray examination should be done before autopsy to avoid prolonged search for the bullet in the body.

NOTA BENE

Usefulness of X-rays
- To see whether the bullet/any part of if it is still inside the body
- To locate the bullet
- To retrieve small fragments deposited in the body by a exited bullet
- To identify the type of ammunition/weapon used prior to autopsy
- To document the path of the bullet

Clothing

All the clothing is removed, the condition and the extent of blood staining is noted. Location, number, size of the bullet hole, the extent of soot and powder distribution, and the density of tattooing around the bullet hole is noted. Sometimes, a single bullet may produce several holes due to the presence of folds in the garment, and simulate more than one shot. Note whether the fibers of the clothing are turned inwards or outwards. Clothing may be forced into the tissues in shotgun wounds.

- The holes in the clothing should be connected to those in the body to determine the direction of fire.
- *If exit wound is present* in the body but no corresponding tear in the clothes, then either the clothing did not cover the area of the exit or the bullet may be in the clothing or has fallen away.
- The powder grains adherent to clothing should be carefully removed with forceps and preserved in a glass vial as they may be lost from the clothes due to rough handling.
- The clothes should be air dried, and then sealed in clean brown paper.
- *Infrared photography* can be used to find out soot deposit on dark colored or black fabrics. X-ray can be used to search for larger metallic fragments.

Bullet wounds: Multiple wounds should be numbered. On the body diagrams, wounds are drawn as they appear on the body including burning, blackening, tattooing and abrasion collar.

Description of Bullet Wounds (Entry or Exit)

i. The exact location of each wound in relation to its distance from:
   - The top of the head or the sole of the foot, as it gives the direction of the track and also the height above the ground at which the bullet entered and left the body, if the person was in standing position when struck.
   - Midline of the body.
   - A fixed anatomical landmark.
ii. The shape (stellate, round, slit-like or irregular) and size, abrasion collar and powder markings surrounding the borders of the wound. The difference in the width of the abrasion collar at different points is noted, as they indicate the angle at which the bullet struck the skin.
iii. The presence or absence of blackening and tattooing should be noted. If the entry wound is soiled with blood, it should be sponged carefully, so that any tattooing of the skin is not disturbed.
iv. Muzzle imprint (if present).
v. Metal deposition, if any.

Alteration by medical care personnel: If surgical alterations are made on entry or exit wound of the victim, the surgeon should make adequate documentation of their location and nature in the hospital records. This prevents confusion, if subsequently the patient dies and an autopsy is performed.

Track taken by the bullet through the body: It is advisable to record the wound in the skin and the wound track through the body in one section. Probes should not be introduced through the track. The path taken by the bullet through the body should be carefully traced by dissection with the organs *in situ*.

The bullet track should be described in relation to the planes of the body:
- From front to back or from back to front
- From left to right or from right to left
- From above downwards or from below upwards
- Angular estimates, i.e., vertical, horizontal and sagittal planes of the body.

Frequently, the track of the bullet is unpredictable due to its deflection by bone, and the bullet may be found in an unexpected situation.

Next to bone, the skin offers the greatest resistance to the penetration of a bullet. A bullet passing through the body may come to rest just underneath the skin on the opposite side.

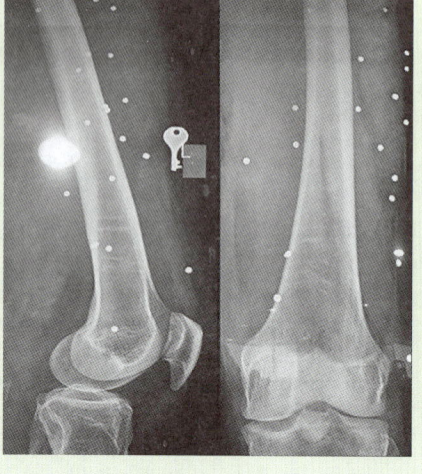

Identify the type of firearm from the X-ray. Comment on the range of fire.

8

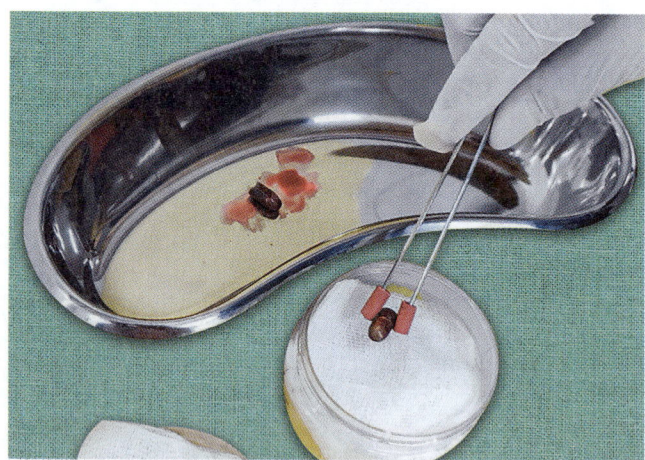

Fig. 12.34: Handling and preservation of bullet

identification of the bullet difficult. It should be removed with fingers or with a forceps protected with rubber tubing **(Fig. 12.34)**. The recovered bullet should be dried and not washed, since washing removes the powder residue.

Description of the bullet should include its:
- Weight
- Caliber (diameter of the base)
- Whether intact, deformed, fragmented or jacketed

iii. **Pellets:** In a shotgun injury, the forensic pathologist need not recover every pellet. A few pellets and all wadding should be recovered for the ballistic expert to determine the shot size, gauge and type of ammunition. The size of pellets is difficult to measure after the shot is fired, as they become deformed.

Preservation

a. **Fired cartridge cases:** Identification mark should be scratched on the inside of the open end. It should be wrapped in cotton and packed in cardboard boxes.
b. **Fired bullets:** Identification marks should be scratched on the base, or just above the riflings on the ogive, but not on the end of the nose, for the nose may pick up trace evidence. It is wrapped in cotton and packed in cardboard box.
c. **Pellets, slugs and wads:** They may be packed in a cardboard box with cotton, after drying.
d. **Clothes:** The bullet holes should be encircled and signed. The area of the powder tattooing should be preserved by fastening a cellophane paper over it and packed in a box.

PRESERVATION AND MARKING OF EXHIBITS

i. After the wound has been examined, the skin around the entrance and exit wounds should be cut out including at least 2.5 cm of the skin around and 5 mm beneath the wound. They should be sealed separately in rectified spirit.
ii. **Bullet:** All bullets and recognizable parts of bullets in the victim must be recovered from the body and preserved with correct labeling of each bullet to the corresponding wound and placed in a separate envelope. Marks due to artefacts such as, scratches should not be produced on the bullet while removing it from the body. Such markings may make subsequent

Collection of evidence
i. Clothes with trace evidence.
ii. Victim's hair, clothing, fibers and blood.
iii. Gunpowder and other evidence on the hands.
iv. Unspent ammunition and empty cartridges.
v. Gun used in the crime.

MEDICO-LEGAL QUESTIONS

Q. Is the injury caused by firearm?

- It is recognized by the appearance of clothing, entry and exit wounds, track of bullet and presence of bullet or pellets and residual matter in the clothing or around the entry wound and in tissues.
- Stud guns injuries may mimic firearm injuries, and have been responsible for both accidental and even homicidal deaths. Similarly, injuries with air gun (not a firearm in the strict sense of the word) may also mimic firearm injury (abraded collar is seen in pellet injuries) and can be fatal (rarely).
- It may be difficult to both find and determine the nature of gunshot wounds in a decomposed body. Extensive care should be taken to avoid misinterpretation of wounds and artifacts.

Q. From what distance was the shot fired?

The distance can be determined by **(Table 12.4)**:
- Presence or absence of marks of soot, burning, singeing and tattooing on the body of the victim.
- Effect of wads.
- Diameter of dispersion of pellets over the body.
- Muzzle impression.

When the range is greater, the distance can be determined only approximately.

Test firing with the suspect weapon using the same ammunition is useful for estimating the range.

Q. From which direction was the shot fired?

The direction of the firing depends upon the posture of the body at the time of impact.

It can be determined by:
- The position of entrance and exit wounds and the track, bearing in mind the possibility of deflection of bullet and the different relationships of the parts of the body in movement.
- Pattern of dispersion of pellets in case of shotguns, and from abrasion/contusion and grease collars in cases of rifled firearms.
- Pellets disperse over a wider area as they travel more. Hence, the victim is shot from the side opposite to the side of wider dispersion.
- From the direction of the track of the wound inside the body; useful only in cases of bullet injury, but the track may change on striking against a bone. In a shotgun, individual pellets take divergent routes, which will not help in finding the direction.

Q. What kind of weapon fired the shot?

The kind of weapon can be determined by the size, shape and composition of the bullet, and examination of the cartridge, shots and wads left in the body or found at the scene of the crime and from the appearance of the wounds.

In case of **shotguns,** appearance of wound is characteristic.
- The wad consists of either plug of paper/cloth, plastic or circular discs of felt/cardboard from which the bore of the gun can be determined.
- Stains on the clothes or skin may show whether black or smokeless powder was used.
- Evidence of recent fire can be made by examination of weapon under *mercury vapor*.

The **rifled firearm** leaves its signature on the cartridge case and on the bullet. With all rifled firearms, the bullet is slightly larger than the barrel, and as it passes through the barrel, its sides are marked by the rifling ('lands') of the barrel (*primary marking/class characteristics*) **(Fig. 12.35)**

> **NOTA BENE**
> - **Class characteristics** are determined by manufacturing specifications, design and dimensions. They are most useful in identifying the make and model of the gun involved. Class characteristics in fired bullet identification would be:
>   i. Number, diameter and width of lands and grooves
>   ii. Depth of grooves
>   iii. Direction and degree of rifling twist
> - **Secondary markings or individual/accidental characteristics** are produced on the surface of the bullet by imperfection on the inner surface of the barrel. These irregularities are produced by sticking of particles of the bullet to the bore when shots are fired and is known as *metallic fouling*. They also result accidentally during the manufacturing process, usually microscopic in nature and have random distribution. They are useful in identifying the specific gun which was fired.

- Each firearm sold has a manufacturer's serial number stamped into it, which may be used to identify the weapon.

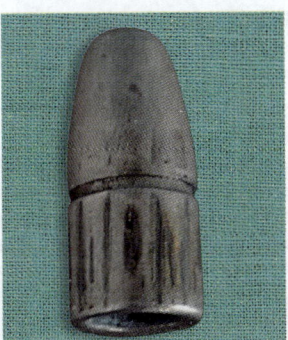

Fig. 12.35: Primary markings on fired bullet

TABLE 12.4: Estimation of range from effects produced by firearms

Effects produced	Shotguns	Handguns	Rifles
Flame	1 ft	2–3"* (5–8 cm)	6–8"
Smoke (soot)	1–3 ft	12" (30 cm)	12"
Tattooing	3–4 ft	18–24" (45–60 cm)	24–30"
Cardboard	6–7 ft	—	—
Wads	15–20 ft	—	—

* (") Indicates inches

- Examination of a fired cartridge having primary and secondary markings may make it possible to identify the weapon in terms of type, make and model.
- Class characteristics may be identical on bullets fired by two different weapons; the individual characteristics will be different.
- Individual characteristics are more pronounced where the grooves score the lead bullet, but for jacketed bullets, the land marking are more pronounced.
- In addition to markings on the bullets, the appearance of the firing pin imprint from centerfire weapons may indicate the make of weapon used (most important identifying mark).
- Gas chromatography has been used to identify gun oils in targets and is very sensitive.
- Bullets recovered from decomposed bodies may show partial or complete loss of individual characteristics, depending upon the tissue from which the bullet was recovered and the construction of the bullet.
- The individual characteristics may also be destroyed by rust, corrosion, accumulation of dirt and grease from multiple firings or firing of thousands of rounds of jacketed ammunition.
- The bullet found in the body, known as *crime bullet*, is compared under a *comparison microscope* with one fired from a suspected weapon known as *test bullet*. The suspected weapon is fired using the same brand and type of ammunition into a roll of wool/bag of rags/sand bag/oiled saw-dust/blocks of ice or water tanks. Cleanly shaven, fresh pork skin is ideal for comparison with patterns on human skin.

Q. Is it possible to identify the victim/assailant from a recovered bullet?

- A bullet found at a scene may be linked to the specific individual through which it had passed by examining the tissue deposited on its surface (usually not visible) which can be removed by swabbing and performing DNA fingerprinting by STR analysis. This can be compared to the DNA of the individual (living/dead) through which the bullet is thought to have passed.
- **Fingerprints:** It is usually rare for an identifiable fingerprint to be left on a firearm, especially a handgun. But latent fingerprints may be obtained from fired cartridge cases which should be collected from the crime scene.

NOTA BENE

- **Secondary target wounds and trace evidence:** If a bullet passes through a body or intermediary target or ricochet off a hard surface, fragment of tissue, target or foreign material may adhere to or be imbedded in the bullet which can be identified by histological/cytological examination (for large tissue) and SEM-EDX (for non-organic material and small tissue). Glass and clothing are common secondary targets.

- **"Back spatter" phenomenon** can offer the amount of DNA and RNA recovered from the surface of the firearm following firing at a victim. DNA was recoverable up to 5 cm from the target with a revolver and up to 15 cm with pistols. RNA was recoverable up to 30 cm. Both mRNA and miRNA can be recovered, but the latter is smaller and more stable for greater likelihood of recovery.

Q. If multiple wounds of entrance and exit are present, could a single bullet have produced them?

Single entrance and multiple exits: If a bullet splits up within the body and divides itself into 3–4 pieces, there will be only one entry and several exit wounds **(Fig. 12.36)**.

Q. If multiple wounds are present, were they produced from the same or different weapons?

This is determined by examination of the wound, bullet(s), cartridge, shots and wad(s).

Q. When was the firearm discharged?

- Smokeless powder leaves a dark gray deposit in the barrel of a recently discharged firearm. It forms a neutral solution with distilled water and contains nitrites and nitrates, but *no sulfates*. The mixture of gases of explosion has a peculiar smell, which can be noticed for several hours after the discharge of a gun.
- If black powder was used, H_2S may persist in the barrel for few hours, if breech is closed. Gunpowder washings from barrels are alkaline; contain nitrite, sulfate and thiosulfate.

Q. How long did the victim survive after the injury?

- It depends on the cause of death, i.e., whether from shock and hemorrhage, injury to a vital organ or septic complications.

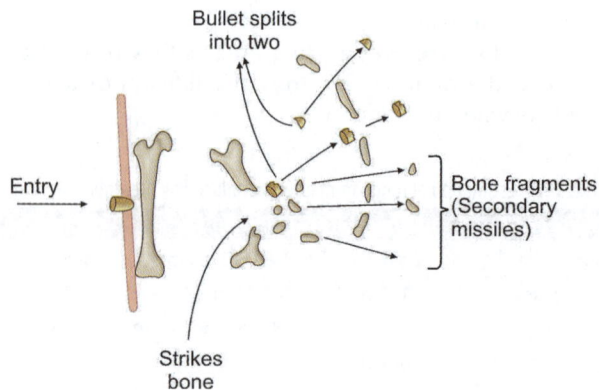

Fig. 12.36: Single entry and multiple exit wounds

- An individual can function without a heart for a short time. The limiting factor for consciousness is the O_2 supply to the brain. When the O_2 in the brain is consumed, unconsciousness occurs.

Q. How much activity could the victim perform following the injury?

This varies considerably depending on the site of injury and the organ involved (Refer to Chapter 11 also).
- The victim may not be aware of the injury initially. Pain is suppressed by the adrenaline response of 'fight or flight', and vigorous activity may be maintained for a period of up to a few minutes when the will exists. Such activity will cease when physical factors such as blood loss lead to immobility, loss of consciousness or death.
- Young adult will survive longer and capable of greater activity than an elderly, infirm individual.
- Extensive destruction of the frontal lobes of the brain may permit some activity before death occurs.
- If the injury involves the motor area of brain, brainstem, basal ganglia, medulla or cervical cord, or there is laceration of the heart or aorta, the victim becomes incapacitated immediately.
- In order of fatality, wounds of the auricles are most rapidly fatal, followed by wounds of the right ventricle and then the left ventricle.
- The amount and rapidity of blood loss will also help to form an opinion about the extent of physical activity possible.
- In injury to other parts of the body, the victim may be able to walk about.

Q. Is it a case of suicide, accident or homicide?

- The differentiating features are tabulated in **Diff. 12.2**.
- Most contact shotgun wounds of the head are suicidal in origin. The individual tends to use his dominant hand to press the trigger, steadying the muzzle against the head with the non-dominant hand. So, powder soot may be visible on the non-dominant hand.
- *Path of the bullet:* Suicide victims are typically in a stable and comfortable situation, allowing them to point the gun in a predetermined way. In contrast, the dynamic situation of homicide creates multiple different paths.
- Gunshots to right temple show a front-to-back or upward path in suicides. Therefore, a downward shot or a back to front should raise suspicion despite typical shot location.
- Gunshots to the left chest tend to show a right-to-left path and in the mouth, an upward trajectory in suicides.

NOTA BENE

For suicides, the sites of preference are (in decreasing order of occurrence) **(Fig. 12.37)**:
- Temple (60% of cases)
- Center of forehead
- Roof of mouth
- Midline behind the chin
- Left side or front of chest (precordium)

Hands of suicide victims may have orange-brown stain from contact with gun barrels following death, presumably from perspiration coupled with a prolonged postmortem interval of contact.

Suicidal/accidental deaths in adolescents/young adults may sometimes occur from playing **Russian roulette.** It is a lethal game of chance in which a player places a single round in a revolver, spins the cylinder, places the muzzle against his head, and pulls the trigger. Since only one chamber is loaded, the player has only one in 'n' chance of hitting the loaded chamber, where n is the total number of chambers in the cylinder.

Q. Can there be multiple wounds of entry and exit from a single shot?

Yes, it may be seen in re-entry wounds where the bullet passes through one part of the body and then re-enters

DIFFERENTIATION 12.2: Suicidal, homicidal and accidental firearm injury

S.No.	Feature	Suicide	Homicide	Accident
1.	Site of entry wound	Head or heart	Any area	Any area
2.	Shot distance	Contact or very close range	Any range, usually distant	Close or very close
3.	Direction	Upward or backward	Usually upward/back-front	Any direction
4.	Number of wounds	Usually one	Any number	One
5.	Powder residue on hand pressing trigger	Present	Absent	Present
6.	Cadaveric spasm	May be seen with the weapon firmly grasped	Not so	Not so
7.	Weapon at scene	Found	Not found	Found
8.	Scene	Usually his house, suicide note, previous psychiatric illness	Any place, evidence of struggle, body may be moved	In his house or while hunting/handling
9.	Exposure/undressing site	Not shot through clothing	Shot through clothing	Shot through clothing
10.	Sex	Usually males	Any sex	Usually males
11.	Motive	Insanity, illness, financial loss	Gang feuds, robbery, revenge	Nil

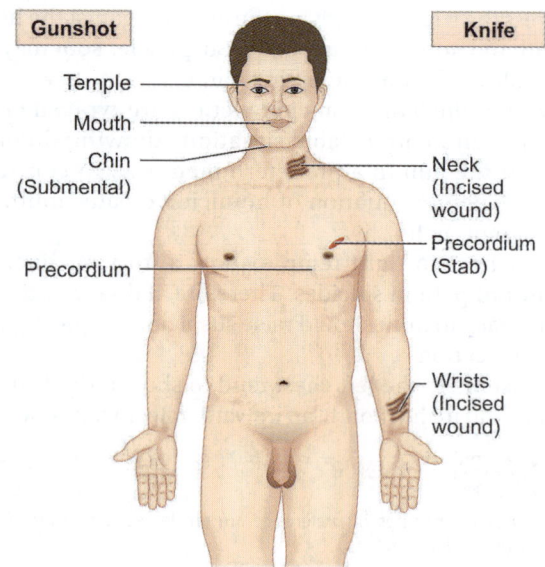

Fig. 12.37: Sites of election in suicide with firearm and knife

another part **(Figs. 12.38A and B)**. For example, a bullet may pass through and through:
- An arm and the chest, so that four wounds would result (most common).
- The chest or abdomen and thigh and lower leg, producing six wounds. This occurs when the person is running or sitting in an unusual position (thigh and leg flexed).

Q. Is it possible that entry wound is present but the bullet is not found in the body?

It may occur when the bullet entering the:
- Stomach, may be vomited out.
- Windpipe, may be coughed up.
- Mouth, may be spat out.
- Body and coming in contact with the bone, and exiting by the same wound from where it entered.

 FM 3.10

Describe and discuss the various tests related to confirmation of use of firearms.

DETECTION OF GUNSHOT RESIDUES

Gunshot residues (GSR) may be deposited by two mechanisms:
 i. Impact deposition from particles propelled by the force of the blast.
 ii. Fallout deposition of drifting particles that settle on a surface.

Shooters have GSR from impact and bystanders from fallout.

- The deposition of GSR particles following initial firearm discharge is *primary transfer*. *Secondary transfer* of these particles to other surfaces occur from contact with the surface or person on whom the particles have deposited such as shaking of hand or contact with clothing.
- GSR deposition may vary by gun used to fire the bullets viz. greater particle deposition with revolvers than with automatic rifles; greater with non-jacketed than jacketed.
- Sample must be obtained from the skin surface of the victim at the scene. Delay in obtaining residues, movement or washing of the body prior to autopsy will diminish or eliminate GSR. A rapid loss of GSR occurs from 1 to 3 hours post firearm discharge.
- The two methods of collection of GSR include collection onto a carbon-coated adhesive stub or with an alcohol swab **(Fig. 12.39)**. In causality and during autopsy, residues should be collected by tape lift method involving adhesive tapes that can easily trap the samples or swabbing using some adsorbent surface. Various methods for collecting GSR from hair include the comb method, swab, and tape lifting for particles settled on hair.
- The analysis techniques applied for detecting GSR includes conventional (color test, instrumentation) and advanced (electro-chemical sensor based) methods.

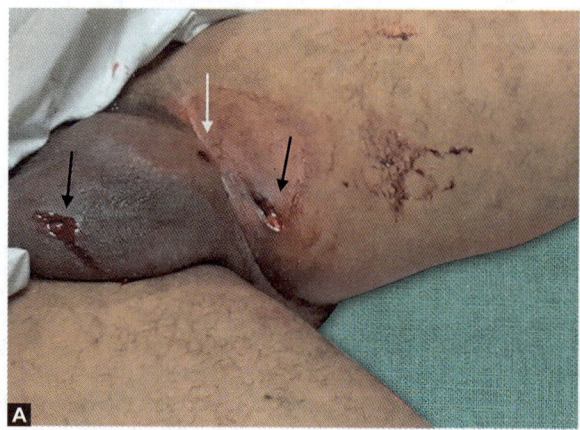
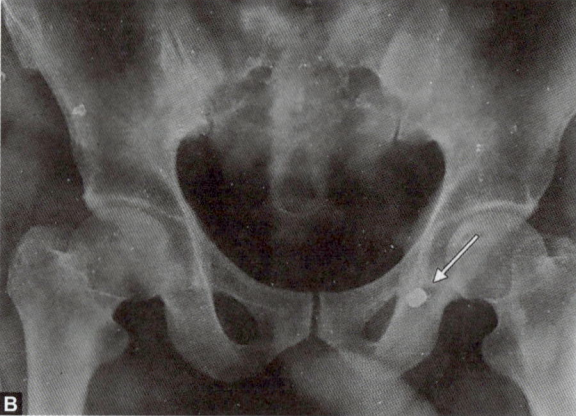

Figs. 12.38A and B: (A) The bullet entered through the scrotum on the right and exited from left (white arrow) to re-enter the medial side of thigh (two entry wounds and single exit wound); (B) Corresponding X-ray showing the bullet (arrow)

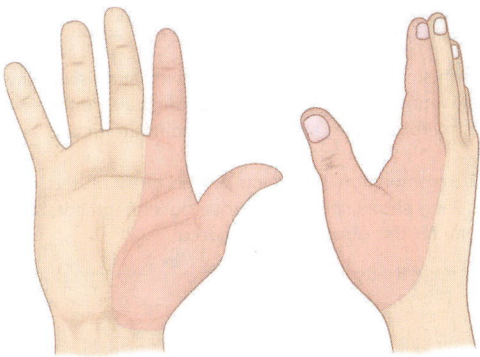

Fig. 12.39: Areas to be swabbed for GSR in case of suicidal victim or a suspected assailant

- Color spot tests include dermal nitrate test, Walker or Griess test, modified Griess test, Marshal and Tiwari test, Harrison and Gilroy test, sodium rhodizonate test.
- Instrumentation for organic residues—GC-MS, HPLC, TLC, Raman spectroscopy and for inorganic—AAS, NAA, inductively coupled plasma mass spectrometry, SEM/EDX.
- Electro-chemical methods include cyclic voltammetry, nitrite test based on amperometry, and abrasive stripping voltammetry.

Some of these tests are:

i. **Dermal nitrate or paraffin test:** It is an obsolete and non-specific test. It detects GSR (nitrates) from the suspect's hand by removing it in a paraffin cast or cotton swab and treating with diphenylamine dissolved in strong H_2SO_4. A positive test is indicated by blue flecks in the paraffin.

ii. **Harrison and Gilroy test:** It is a qualitative calorimetric chemical test, and not specific for firearm discharges residues, but detects the presence of antimony (Sb), barium (Ba) and lead (Pb).

> **NOTA BENE**
> A cotton swab moistened with HCl is used to swab the hand and then treated with triphenylmethylarsonium iodide for detection of antimony, and sodium rhodizonate for the detection of barium and lead.

iii. **Neutron activation analysis:** This chemical method is useful in identifying minute traces of elements present in the hair, nails, soil, glass pieces, paints, GSR and drugs. It is based on the detection and measurement of characteristic radioisotopes formed by irradiation in a nuclear reactor. Sb and Ba residues (from the primer) are detected from the suspect's hand. The test is most sensitive, non-destructive, and effective method with a detection sensitivity of about 1 ng only.

iv. **Atomic absorption spectroscopy (AAS) and Flameless atomic absorption spectrophotometry (FAAS):** This analytical method utilizes high temperatures to vaporize the metallic elements of the primer residues, to detect and quantify them. AAS is very sensitive for detection of Pb in GSR samples but less sensitive in detecting Ba and Sb. FAAS help to analyze these metals. Measuring the antimony, barium and lead from the primer and copper vaporized from either the cartridge case or the bullet jacketing helps in determining:
- Holes in clothing and tissues as bullet holes.
- Range of fire.
- Common origin of bullet fragments or shotgun pellets found at different places.
- Whether or not a person has fired a gun.

v. **Scanning electron microscope-energy dispersive X-ray spectrometry (SEM-EDX):** It is the *most sophisticated tool* which can detect minute traces of GSR found on the body of suspect. The instrument is non-destructive and allows the highest specificity in detection of gunshot residue (Pb, Sb, Ba, etc.). However, it is a qualitative, not a quantitative analysis.

> **NOTA BENE**
> **Other tests for GSR**
> - **Griess test or Walker's test** performed for detecting nitrites present in GSR. It uses chemicals (alpha-naphthol) to produce a dark red color spot.
> - **Modified Griess test** is for detecting nitrites present in GSR. A pink color indicates the presence of nitrites.
> - **Sodium rhodizonate test** is helpful in determining lead in any form whether it is in vapor form, particulate lead, in primer residues, in lead bullet, or shot pellet.
> - **Marshall and Tewari tests** are used for detecting propellant particles for estimation of a range of firing cases.

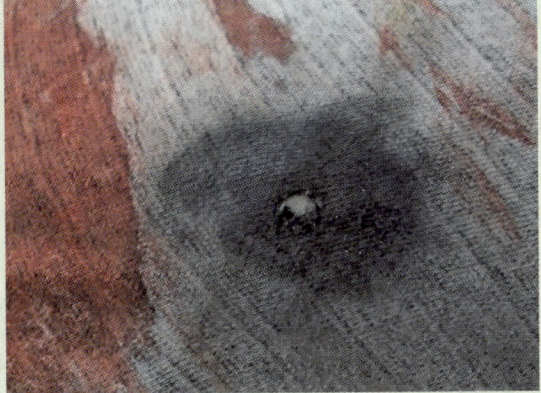

Test to detect gunshot residue on clothes:
A. Dermal nitrate   B. Modified Greiss test
C. Harrison and Gilroy test   D. Marsh test

NOTA BENE

- **Bullet emboli/Wandering bullet:** Vascular embolization is usually associated with small caliber, low velocity bullet, and usually involves the arterial system. It should be suspected whenever there is a penetrating bullet wound with failure to discover the bullet in the expected region or to visualize the bullet on routine X-ray. The most common sites of entry for a bullet are the aorta, right atrium and ventricle, pulmonary artery and the inferior vena cava.
- **Lead snowstorm:** This is seen in radiograph of an individual shot with centerfire ammunition. Fragments of lead break off the lead core as the bullet moves through the body and gets lodged into surrounding tissue. X-ray shows small radiopaque bullet fragments scattered along the wound track—'*lead snowstorm*'. A rifle bullet need not have to hit bone for this phenomenon to occur.

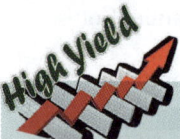

- **Parts of firearm:** Barrel, action (hammer, bolt and trigger), extractor, grip, magazine.
- **Types of firearms:** 2 types—Rifled and smooth bore weapons (shotguns).
- **Rifled firearms:** Shallow spiral grooves in the bore running parallel to each other from breech to muzzle end.
- Bullets are used in rifled firearms; lead pellets are used in shotgun.
- **Bullet:** The projectile of a rifled firearm.
- **Associated with shotguns only:** Wads.
- Choking is seen in shotgun.
- **Cylinder bore:** Shotgun whose entire barrel is of same diameter.
- **Choke bore:** Shotgun slightly constricted at muzzle, usually distal 7–10 cm.
- **Paradox guns:** Shotguns where small portion of the bore near muzzle end rifled.
- **Caliber:** Diameter of bore measured between diagonally opposite lands (in rifles), or the number of spherical balls exactly fitting the barrel which can be made from one pound of lead (in shotguns).
- **Caliber of a bullet:** Cross-sectional diameter.
- Traditional bullet is made of soft metal and has a rounded nose *(round nose soft bullet)*.
- Metal used in bullets is *lead with antimony and/or tin* added to provide hardness.
- Modern bullets are divided into two categories: Lead and metal-jacketed.

Type of bullet	Features
Dum-dum	Jacketed bullet wherein nose is cut to expose the core.
Hollow-point	Semi-jacket bullet that has a hole drilled into its nose.
Soft-point	Jacketed bullet wherein tip is left uncovered to expose some core.
Tandem	Bullets ejected one after the other.
Duplex	Contains two projectiles by design.
Frangible	Designed to fragment upon impact; do not ricochet.
Souvenir	Bullet present in body for long time.
Ricochet	Deflection of a bullet from its course by striking an object.
Incendiary	Type of army bullet used to cause fire in the target.

- **Primer:** Small charge of impact-sensitive chemical. It ignites the powder or propellant charge by impact of gun's firing pin.
- Most common compounds used as primer: Lead styphnate, barium nitrate and antimony sulfide.
- **Gun powders**
    - Black powder (potassium nitrate, sulfur, charcoal)
    - Smokeless powder (nitrocellulose, nitroglycerin and nitroguanidine)
    - Semi-smokeless powder (mixture of black and smokeless powder)
- Burning of black powder produces 44% gases and 56% solid residues.
- FG, FFG, FFFG is used to indicate black powder grain size.
- Contact shotgun wounds of the head may cause bursting of the head and evisceration of the brain.
- Wound track appear cherry-red due to carboxyhemoglobin from absorption of CO formed from combustion of the gunpowder.
- 'Rat hole' appearance of entry wound is seen in near/mid-range of shotguns (up to 7 feet).
- **Tattooing/stippling:** Consists of unburnt gun powder particles that are embedded in skin.

- Tattooing around the entry wound is seen in close shots.
- **Blackening/soot soiling:** Deposition of powder soot produced by combustion of gunpowder.
- **Abrasion collar:** Narrow rim of abrasion surrounding the bullet entry wound (rifled firearm) caused by friction and indentation.
- Direction of fire is determined from the shape of abrasion collar.
- **Grease or dirt collar/bullet wipe:** Black/gray colored ring lining the entry wound caused from removal of substances from bullet as it passes through skin.
- **Signs of contact shot head:** Muzzle imprint and stellate shape entry wound.
- **Muzzle/recoil imprint** is a patterned abrasion/contusion.
- Abrasion collar may be seen in the exit wound *(shored exit wound)*.
- Puppe's rule gives the sequence of fractures—which fracture followed which.
- **Yaw:** Deviation between long axis of bullet and axis of path of bullet.
- **Tumbling bullet:** Bullet rotates end-to-end during its path.
- **Kennedy phenomenon:** Evaluation of whether the wound was an entry or an exit becomes difficult due to surgical alteration.
- **Graze/slap wound:** Abrasion seen when a bullet strikes at acute angle without penetrating the skin.
- **Resistance offered to penetration of a bullet:** Bone → skin.
- Beveling of inner table of skull is seen in entry wound and beveling of outer table is seen exit wound of rifled firearm.
- Primary markings/class characteristics on bullet are caused by lands of rifled firearm.
- Secondary markings are specific to an individual firearm, produced by imperfection on inner surface of barrel.
- Class characteristics may be identical on bullets fired by two different weapons; individual characteristics will be different.
- Helixometer is an instrument to examine the interior of barrel.
- Blackening, tattooing and soot deposit on dark colored fabrics can be demonstrated by *infrared photography*.
- **Tests to detect of gunshot residues:** Dermal nitrate/paraffin test & Harrison and Gilroy test.
- **Test to identify gun oils:** Gas chromatography.

Interesting case

Single Bullet—Multiple Entry and Exit (Case of John F Kennedy, 1963)

US President John F Kennedy was assassinated by former US Marine Lee Harvey Oswald while he was riding in an open limousine with Governor Connally in Dallas, Texas in 1963. Governor Connally was seriously wounded in the attack.

President Kennedy sustained two bullet wounds fired from above and behind him. The first shot entered his upper back, penetrated his neck and exited his throat nearly midline just beneath his larynx and damaging the trachea and nicked the left side of his suit tie knot **(Fig. A)**. According to the Warren Commission's single bullet theory **(magic bullet)**, the same bullet penetrated Governor Connally's back just below his right armpit (who was sitting at the front). The bullet created an oval-shaped entry wound, impacted his right fifth rib, and exited his chest just below his right nipple and then entered his arm just above his right wrist and fractured his right radius bone. The bullet exited just below the wrist at the inner side of his right palm and finally lodged in his left inner thigh.

The second shot that hit Kennedy ('the fatal missile') entered the rear of his head and passed in fragments through his skull; this created a large, 'roughly ovular' hole (more than five inches in its largest dimension) on the rear right side of the head **(Fig. B)**.

The first bullet made a small hole at the base of the back of the neck, which was not found until autopsy. The autopsy doctors were initially puzzled by the fact that there was a clear entrance wound on Kennedy's upper back, but no visible exit wound. This wound's original dimensions were distorted by surgeons by the tracheostomy done at hospital **(Fig. C)**. The autopsy report ended any confusion about the number of bullet wounds the President suffered.

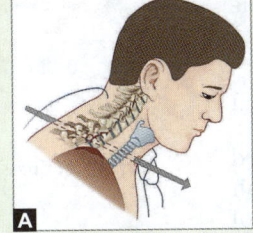

A

First bullet

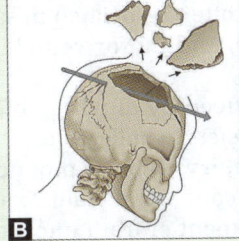

B

Second bullet

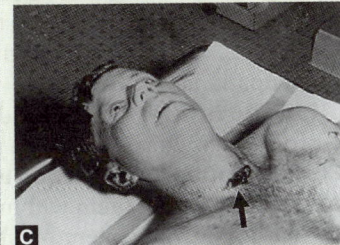

C

Exit wound of first bullet and tracheostomy wound (arrow)

CHAPTER 13

Regional Injuries

LEARNING OBJECTIVES

Must know
1. Classification of craniocerebral injury
2. Black eyes
3. Types of skull fracture
4. Closed and open head injury
5. Coup and contrecoup injury (Diff.)
6. Concussion
7. Berry aneurysm
8. Whiplash injury
9. Railway spine
10. Flail chest
11. Cardiac concussion
12. Greenstick fracture
13. Healing of fracture
14. Intracranial hematomas, causes, features
15. Drunkenness and concussion (Diff.)
16. Hematoma and depressed skull fracture (Diff.)

Desirable to know
1. Biomechanics of head injury
2. Chronic traumatic encephalopathy
3. Diffuse axonal injury
4. Contusion of brain
5. Age of subdural hematomas
6. Traumatic and non-traumatic intracerebral hemorrhage (Diff.)
7. Cerebral edema
8. Complications of chest and abdominal injury
9. Open, closed and comminuted fracture

Definitions

- **Traumatic brain injury (TBI):** Traumatically-induced structural injury and/or physiological disruption of brain function as a result of an external force.
- **Closed head injury (non-penetrating):** Damage to the brain without any fracture of the skull and/or penetration of dura; most often results from blunt trauma.
- **Open head injury (penetrating):** Disruption of cranial vault with opening through skin and cranial bones to expose damaged brain; most often associated missile wounds, stab/chop wounds, and motor vehicle or occupational accidents.
- **Missile injury:** Injury produced by moving object striking cranium; most often refers to bullet injury.
- **Acceleration/deceleration injury:** Damage produced by movement of brain within confines of cranial vault (tearing during violent movement or from impact of striking interior of skull or dural folds).

CRANIOCEREBRAL INJURIES

- There are three main components of the head: scalp, skull and brain (Fig. 13.1).

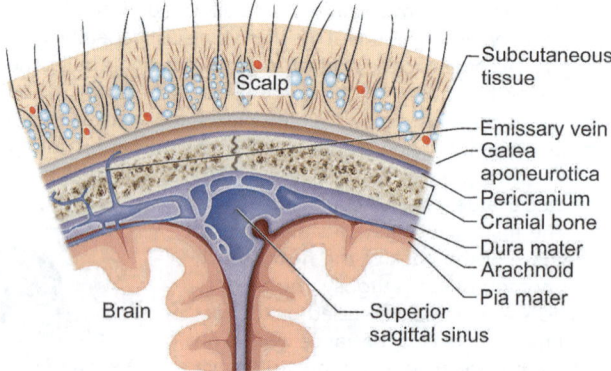

Fig. 13.1: Cross section of the scalp, skull and meninges

- The term 'craniocerebral injuries' is used to describe the presence of skull ('cranio') and brain ('cerebral') injury.
- Craniocerebral injuries to the head can be grouped into two types: 'focal' or 'diffuse' in the sense that they are localized or widespread (Table 13.1).

TABLE 13.1: Classification of craniocerebral injury

Focal	Diffuse
Scalp lacerations	Axonal injury
Skull fractures	Ischemic injury
Contusions/lacerations	Vascular injury
Intracranial hemorrhage	Brain swelling
Lesions secondary to raised intracranial pressure	

BIOMECHANICS OF HEAD INJURY

Head injury can be broadly classified into two types based on mechanical loading **(Flowchart 13.1)**:
  i. Static/contact
  ii. Dynamic/inertial

- **Static/contact injuries:** Contact injuries occur both at the site and remote from the point of impact on the head. It results in skull fractures and contusions. The length and direction of a skull fracture depends on the amount of contact energy absorbed by the skull and its thickness at the impact site.
- **Dynamic/inertial injuries:** Dynamic loading is usually the result of an impact, such as the head being struck a blow by a moving object or the moving head itself striking a relatively stationary surface. Inertial injuries are commonly called 'acceleration' or 'deceleration' injuries which biomechanically can be considered as the same phenomenon. The brain is damaged by one or both mechanisms: through strains produced within the brain tissue itself, and through differential movements between the brain and the skull.

Strain within the brain tissue is the deformation that it undergoes when a mechanical force is applied. *Tensile strain* refers to elongation of neural tissues and is the most important mechanism in head injury. *Compression* wherein constituent units are being forced together and *shear or sliding strains* which move adjacent strata of tissue laterally also occur. The brain is virtually incompressible, and has a low tolerance to tensile and shear strains.

FM 3.11
Describe and discuss regional injuries to the head—scalp wounds and fracture skull.

SOFT TISSUE INJURY

- **Injuries:** Scalp wounds are caused by falls, blows, sharp cutting instruments or discharge of a firearm. It can be:
  i. **Abrasion:** It caused by a lateral rubbing action by a blow, a fall on a rough surface or by being dragged in a vehicular accident. They are simple injuries, bleed slightly and heal rapidly.
  ii. **Contusions:** Presence of scalp contusion is indicative of contact injury. In superficial fascia, they appear as localized swelling due to the dense fibro fatty tissues, but contusions deep into the galea aponeurotica are diffuse on account of loose aponeurotic tissues, and difficult to make out on examination.
     - The easiest way to detect scalp injuries is by palpation, but shaving is necessary for proper documentation and photography.
     - During postmortem examination, autopsy surgeons are able to visualize this subgaleal hemorrhage after reflection of the scalp **(Fig. 13.2)**.
     - Scalp hematoma may be associated with an underlying linear skull fracture.
  iii. **Lacerations:** They resemble incised wounds (incised looking lacerations). Careful examination in the depths of the wound will reveal the bridging fibers with surrounding band of abrasion.
  iv. **Incised wounds:** They have clean cut margins; hair bulbs are cleanly cut.
- An effusion of blood over the top of the head or forehead may gravitate down to the loose tissues causing **black eyes (periorbital hematoma)**.

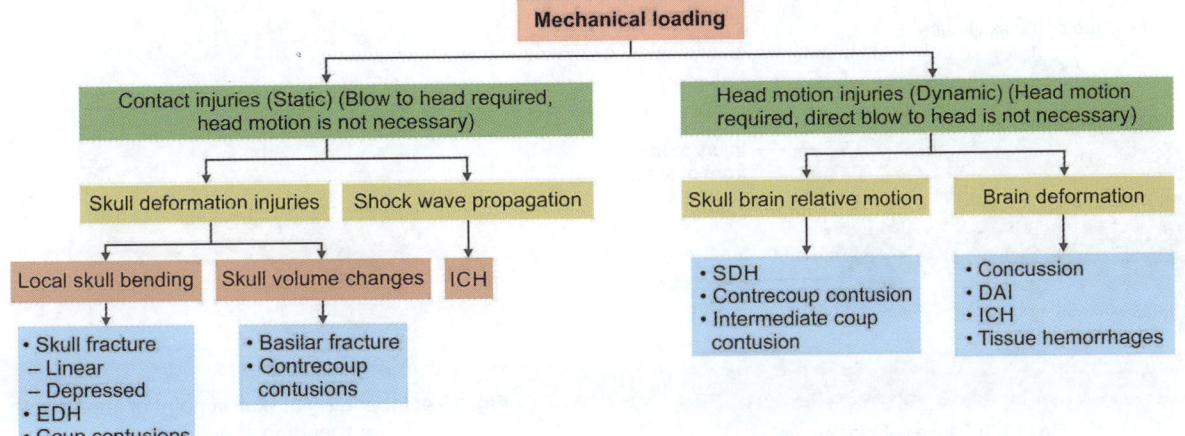

Flowchart 13.1: Pathological changes depending on mechanism of injury

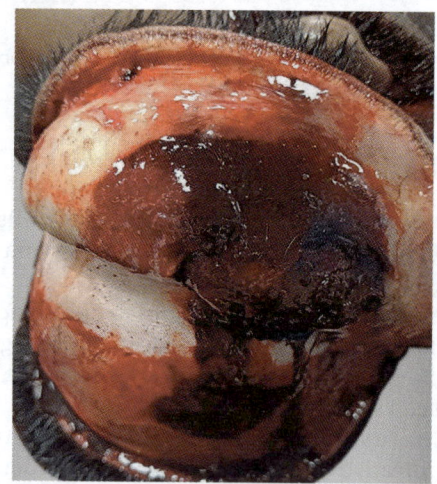

Fig. 13.2: Subgaleal hemorrhage (reflected scalp)

Pearls

Causes of black eyes (*spectacle hematoma, 'panda sign' or raccoon eyes*) **(Fig. 13.3)**
  i. Most commonly due to *local violence* causing subcutaneous extravasation of blood into the lids, occurs soon after injury to upper and lower eyelids.
  ii. Bleeding into the layer of loose connective tissue after a *blow on the skull*; the blood gravitates under the frontalis muscle and appears first in the upper eyelid and then the lower eyelid over the course of a couple of days.
  iii. *Fracture of the orbital plate of the frontal bone* results in hemorrhage into the orbit, the blood tracks under the conjunctiva, appearing as a triangular, flame-shaped hemorrhage, the apex of which is at the margin of the cornea and the posterior limit cannot be seen, which distinguishes it from the subconjunctival hemorrhage.

♦ Wounds of the scalp bleed freely (blood vessels in the fibrous layer, superficial to galea aponeurotica, being held open once cut), but heal rapidly. If an injury extending through the galea gets infected, it may spread through the emissary veins to involve the sagittal, lateral and cavernous sinuses causing septic complications, like meningitis and brain abscess.

SKULL FRACTURES

Motor vehicle accidents and falls are the most common causes of skull fractures.

Mechanism: The skull is not a completely rigid structure, and it is able to bend and distort when force is applied to it. A blow to the skull causes '*inbending*' of the bone at the site of impact, and asymmetric and variably localized '*outbending*' at a distance from the impact **(Fig. 13.4)**. If the forces applied exceed the elastic properties the skull, fracture will occur.

♦ In general, if force is applied over a small area (e.g., a blow from a weapon), a fracture occurs at the site of inbending, whereas an impact over a larger skull area leads to fractures at the site of outbending.
♦ Fractures also represent the point of maximum stress upon the skull, which may not be at the immediate site of impact.
♦ Skulls of infants and children are thinner than those of adults and may be able to distort more before fracturing.
♦ The fracture of skull can occur either by direct or indirect violence.
  i. **Direct violence:** The forces act directly on the bone to produce a fracture, e.g., head crushed under the wheels in road traffic accidents or an object like stick/rod/bullet striking the head.
  ii. **Indirect violence:** The forces act indirectly on the skull through some other structure, which receives primary impact, e.g., fall on buttocks from height which transmits the force to occipital bone through vertebral column or a blow to the chin resulting in fracture of base of the skull.

During autopsy, prior to cutting the skull cap off, the skull should be visually inspected and palpated for the presence of fractures.

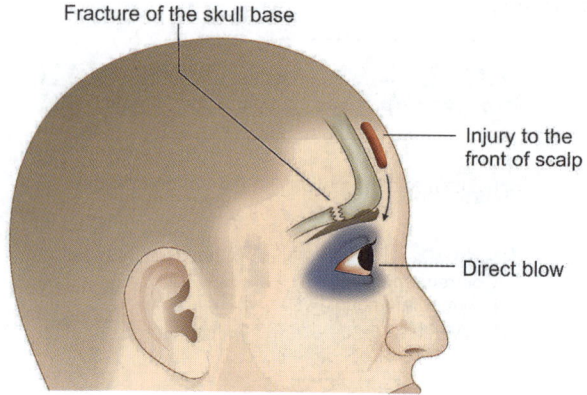

Fig. 13.3: Causes of black eyes

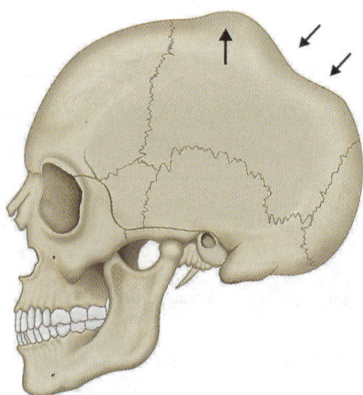

Fig. 13.4: Inbending of skull at point of impact with outbending at periphery

Types

There are several types of skull fractures based on location and/or mechanism of injury:

1. **Linear/fissure fractures:** These are linear cracks passing over the vertex or across the skull base without any displacement of the fragments, and either involves the whole thickness of the bone or the inner or outer table alone **(Figs. 13.5 and 13.6)**.
   - These fractures are usually caused by:
     i. Forcible impact against a broad resisting surface, like hard ground surface, as in road traffic accidents.
     ii. When knocked to the ground by the blow of a fist.
     iii. Blows with a hard blunt object having a relatively broad striking surface.
   - The fracture line tends to follow an irregular course, and is no more than a hair's breadth.
   - They are difficult to detect, may not be seen on X-ray, and can only be detected at autopsy.
   - The line of fracture runs parallel with the axis of compression.
   - Depression of bone fragments is not seen.
   - An injury of the head sustained by a fall is mostly situated at the level of the margin of the hat, while an injury due to blow is commonly situated above this level.

2. **Depressed fracture:** When a portion of fractured bone is driven inwards to a distance equivalent to the thickness of the skull table, it is known as depressed fracture **(Figs. 13.5 and 13.7A to C)**. It is also called *'fracture-a-la-signature'* (**signature fracture**), as the shape often points towards the shape of the offending weapon.
   - They are caused by blows with a heavy weapon having small striking surface, such as hammer, axe, brick or chopper.
   - The part of the skull which is first struck shows maximum depression; usually seen in the left frontal region.
   - This type of fracture often suggests the probable manner of application of violence, and also the relative position of the victim and the assailant at that moment.
   - Depressed fracture is considered to be *compound* if an associated scalp laceration extending through the pericranium is present, and *penetrating* if a dural laceration exits.
   - The soft fluctuant centers of scalp hematomas can masquerade as depressed skull fractures **(Diff. 13.1)**.
   - The risk of post-traumatic epilepsy following depressed skull fracture and cortical laceration is about 15%.

DIFFERENTIATION 13.1: Hematoma and depressed skull fracture

S.No.	Feature	Hematoma	Depressed skull fracture
1.	Relation with skull surface	Raised above the surface	At or below the level of skull surface
2.	On pressure	Will pit	Will not pit
3.	Pulsation	May have pulsation, if any artery is involved	No arterial pulsation felt
4.	Shape	Circular in shape and movable over skull surface	Margins sharper, irregular, less evenly circular

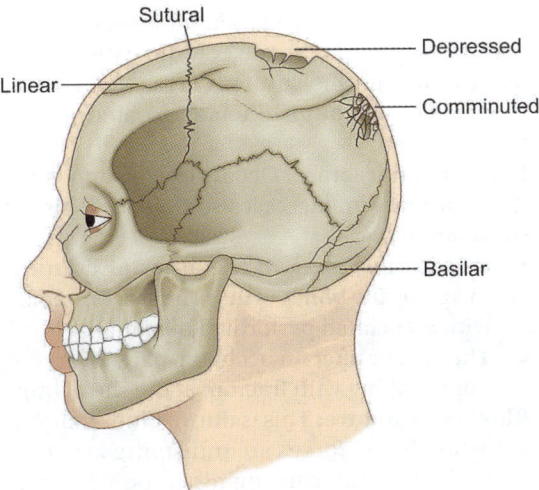

Fig. 13.5: Types of skull fractures

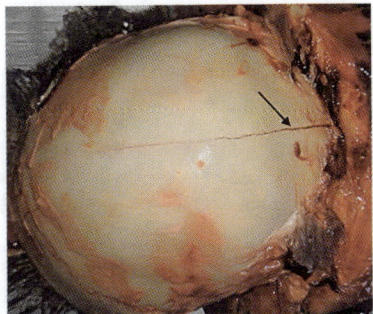

Fig. 13.6: Linear fracture (arrow)

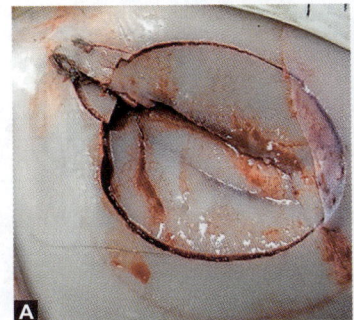
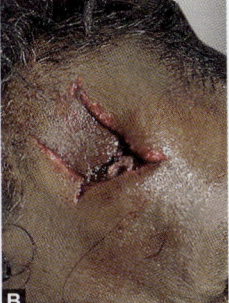
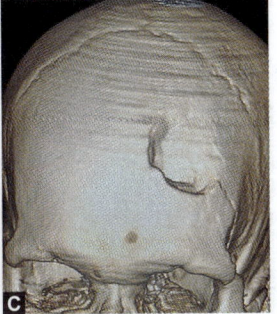

Figs. 13.7A to C: (A) Depressed fracture; (B and C) Patient hit by a brick on the forehead with corresponding CT showing depressed fracture

Some variants:
   a. **Elevated fracture:** One end of fractured fragment is elevated above the surface of skull, while the other end may dip down into cranial cavity resulting in injury to the brain.
      - It is caused by a blow from sharp, heavy object (e.g., an axe) which elevates the skull fracture by lateral pull of the weapon while retrieving it.
      - These fractures are rare, and are usually associated with injury to the dura also.
   b. **Pond or indented fracture:** This is a smooth concave depression without a fracture line, resulting from in-buckling of skull, occurring usually in the elastic skull of infants and children (prior to 4 years of age) **(Fig. 13.8)**.
      - Inner table is not fractured, meninges and brain are not damaged.
      - It may also be caused by forcible compression with an obstetric forceps or impact against some protruding objects, e.g., sacral promontory during delivery.
      - It is also known as **ping-pong fracture**, as it looks similar to a dent in ping-pong ball.
3. **Comminuted fracture (spider-web/mosaic fracture):** Two or more intersecting lines of fracture divide the bone into three or more fragments resembling a *spider web or mosaic pattern* **(Figs. 13.5 and 13.9)**.
   - Skull bone gets broken into multiple pieces by fracture lines, which are haphazardly or concentrically arranged, or stellate if they radiate from the site of impact.
   - It is caused by vehicular accidents, fall from height on a hard surface or by blows with weapons having large striking surface, such as heavy iron bar, or from a bullet.
   - Comminuted fractures may be a complication of fissure fracture, and the fragments of bone if displaced inward, form a depressed skull fracture.
4. **Gutter fracture:** It is formed when part of the thickness of the bone is removed so as to form a gutter, e.g., oblique bullet wounds. It is usually accompanied by comminuted depressed fracture of the inner table of skull, and the fragments causing injury to the meninges and brain.
5. **Ring fracture:** This is a type of fissure fracture that encircles the base of skull around the foramen magnum **(Fig. 13.10)**, running from the sella turcica, partly through petrous ridges and then going posteriorly and medially, joining in the posterior fossa. In the front, the fracture may pass through the middle ear and roof of the nose. As a result, the skull gets separated from the spine. These fractures do not occur commonly.
   Seen in:
   - Fall from a height on feet or buttocks, when the force of the fall is transmitted upwards through the spinal column.
   - Vault of skull being driven against vertebral column by fall of heavy load or by a heavy blow over the vertex.
   - Violent twisting of the head on the spine, shearing the vault from base.
   - Heavy blow directed underneath the occiput or chin.
6. **Diastasis or sutural fracture:** Usually occurs in young children following a forcible blow on the head with a heavy hard blunt object where the fracture line passes through the sutures **(Figs. 13.5 and 13.11)**. It occurs alone, but is often associated with fissure fracture.
7. **Contrecoup fracture:** Occurs exactly opposite to the site of primary impact or 'coup violence'. This is due to shear strain.
   - It is usually seen in the anterior cranial fossa involving the bones of the orbital or ethmoid plates with associated periorbital hematoma.
   - They occur after an occipital, parietal or temporal impact along with fracture at the site of impact.
8. **Blow-out fracture:** This is due to blunt trauma to the eye wherein the forces are transmitted via the globe to the bony orbit, causing disruption of the orbital walls.

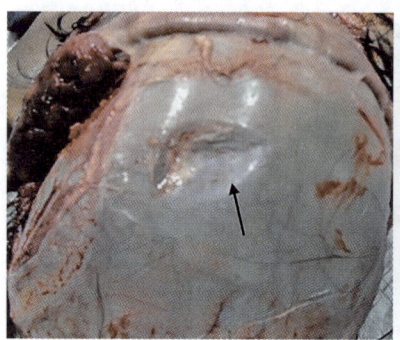

Fig. 13.8: Pond fracture (arrow)

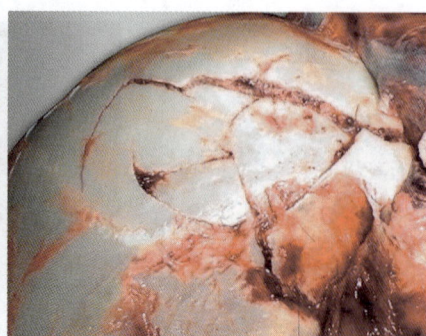

Fig. 13.9: Comminuted fracture

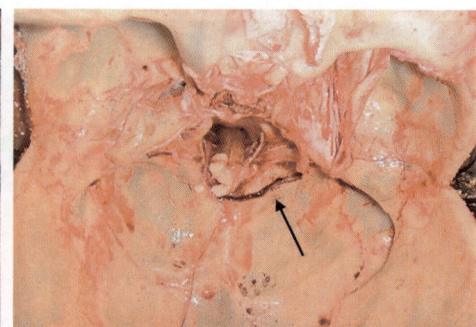

Fig. 13.10: Ring fracture (arrow)

> **NOTA BENE**
>
> **Teardrop sign**: The blow-out fracture most commonly involves the thin medial wall and/or orbital floor that results in orbital contents such as periorbital fat and inferior rectus muscle herniate downwards into the maxillary sinus resulting in pain, restricted eye movements and diplopia. Radiographically, a soft tissue 'teardrop' or polypoid mass in the roof of the maxillary antrum may be seen.

9. **Basilar fracture:** The base of the skull is weak, and hence any diffuse impact to the vertex of the skull will produce basilar fracture **(Fig. 13.5)**. These fractures may be missed on X-ray examination.
    - *Fracture of anterior cranial fossa:* Usually due to direct impact, although fissure fractures in orbital or cribriform plate may be due to contrecoup injury. The patient presents with epistaxis, CSF rhinorrhea (at times from mouth), anosmia, nasal tip paresthesiae, black eye, or occasionally caroticocavernous fistula.
    - *Fracture of middle cranial fossa:* It is seen due to direct impact behind the ear or crush injuries of the head. It manifests by CSF otorrhea if petrous part of temporal bone is fractured (or rhinorrhea via Eustachian tube), hemotympanum, ossicular disruption, Battle sign, or VII and VIII nerve palsy **(Fig. 13.12)**.
    - *Fracture of posterior cranial fossa:* It is commonly due to direct impact of the back of the head on the ground, and clinically diagnosed by escape of blood and CSF through the mouth **(Fig. 13.13)**.
10. **Hinge/transverse fracture:** Fracture of the base of skull occurs that completely splits it, creating a hinge (*'nodding face' sign*); frequently occurs with side impacts. It is sometimes referred to as *'motorcyclists fracture'*. Most common form is the one which extends from the petrous bony ridge through sella turcica to lateral end of the contralateral petrous ridge **(Fig. 13.14)**.

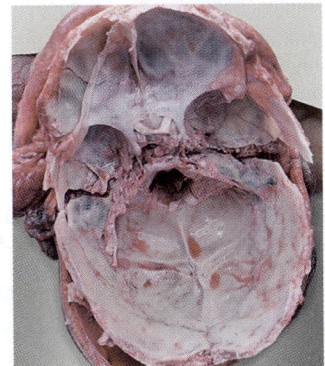

Fig. 13.14: Hinge fracture

> **NOTA BENE**
>
> - **Compound skull fracture**: Laceration of scalp associated with skull fracture.
> - **Growing skull fracture:** Expanding linear fracture (usually in young children) associated with dural tear which allow leptomeninges to herniate into fracture site and expand with cerebrospinal fluid pressure (leptomeningeal cyst).
> - **Halo or ring sign:** Blood from head injured patients may mix with CSF and mask the recognition of a leak. CSF will separate from blood when the mixture is placed on filter paper resulting in a central area of blood with an outer ring or halo.
> - **Glucose estimation:** CSF has a greater concentration of glucose than mucus or lacrimal secretions. The quantitative determination of a glucose level in nasal fluid not contaminated by blood can be diagnostic of CSF rhinorrhea, if the nasal fluid contains >30 mg/dL.
> - **Immunoelectrophoretic identification:** β-2-transferrin assay is the most widely used test and is considered the standard criterion for diagnosis of CSF rhinorrhea.
> - **Battle's sign** (*retro-auricular or mastoid ecchymosis*): Bruising behind the ear appearing 36 h after head injury as a result of extravasation of blood along the path of the posterior auricular artery; may be confused with retro-auricular scalp bruise. It is associated with fracture of middle cranial fossa (petrous part of temporal bone, at junction of middle and posterior cranial fossa).
> - With basilar fracture, intracranial passage of a nasogastric tube or nasopharyngeal airway can happen. These fractures may be visible on plain radiographs or on bone window axial CT scans, but confirmed radiologically by pneumocranium or air-fluid levels in the sinuses.

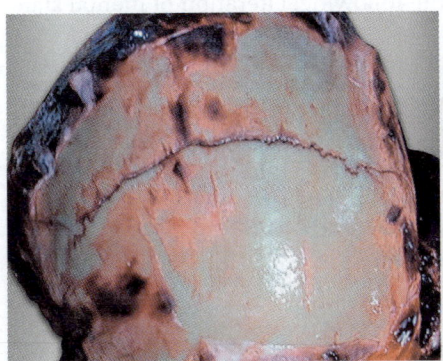

Fig. 13.11: Sutural fracture

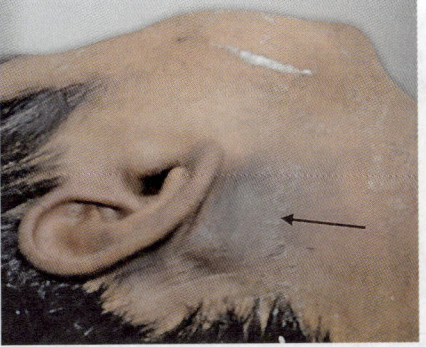

Fig. 13.12: Features of fracture of middle cranial fossa: Battle sign (arrow)

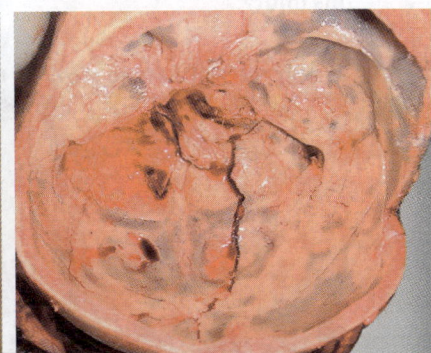

Fig. 13.13: Posterior cranial fossa fracture

- **Skull X-rays** have a limited role in head injuries, since they do not identify intracranial injury. However, it may be helpful when CT scan is not available. Plain X-rays can detect a skull fracture, and its presence is helpful in predicting the presence of intracranial injury. However, a normal skull series does not rule out a brain injury.
- **Skull fractures** may occur in utero, during labor, with forceps delivery, vacuum extraction, excessive manipulation during Cesarean section or during a prolonged, difficult labor with compression and battering of the fetal skull against the maternal ischial spines, sacral promontory or symphysis pubis.

Complications of Skull Fractures

i. **Injury to the brain** which may be dangerous to life.
ii. **Hemorrhage:** If middle meningeal artery is ruptured, fatal hemorrhage may occur.
iii. **Infections:** It may be direct spread from compound fracture or spread from fracture of paranasal sinuses, like frontal or ethmoidal.
iv. **Traumatic epilepsy:** More common with open head injuries. Usually seen 1–2 years after the episode, and manifests as tonic or clonic fits.

BRAIN INJURY

- Traumatic brain injury (TBI) is usually caused by motor vehicle accidents, falls and assaults.
- TBI can be classified based on severity (mild, moderate or severe, **Table 13.2**) mechanism (missile or blunt) and pathology (primary or secondary, **Flowchart 13.2**).
- **Primary brain injury** is the injury caused at the time of impact (e.g., contusion, laceration).
- **Secondary brain injury** is brain damage arising from events developing subsequent to primary injury.
    - Some secondary injuries occur almost instantaneously (e.g., hemorrhage as a consequence of tearing of vessel), whereas others evolve over hours to days (e.g., delayed hemorrhage, inflammation, brain swelling, and axonal swelling secondary to paralysis of axonal transport or tearing of axons).
    - Excitatory neuropeptides, cytokines, free radicals, metabolic and oxygenation insufficiencies cause this injury.

TABLE 13.2: Severity of brain injury stratification

Criteria	Mild/concussion	Moderate	Severe
Structural imaging	Normal	Normal or abnormal	Normal or abnormal
Loss of consciousness	0–30 min	>30 min and <24 h	>24 h
Alteration of consciousness/mental state	A moment up to 24 h	>24 h	Severity based on other criteria
Post-traumatic amnesia	≤1 day	>1 and <7 days	>7 days
Glasgow Coma Scale (best available score in first 24 h)	12–15	9–12	3–8

Flowchart 13.2: Classification of brain injury

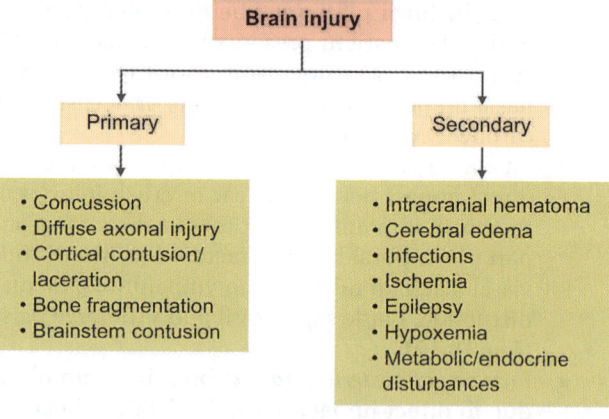

- Primary
  - Concussion
  - Diffuse axonal injury
  - Cortical contusion/laceration
  - Bone fragmentation
  - Brainstem contusion
- Secondary
  - Intracranial hematoma
  - Cerebral edema
  - Infections
  - Ischemia
  - Epilepsy
  - Hypoxemia
  - Metabolic/endocrine disturbances

- Little can be done about primary injury once it has occurred. However, medical management attempts to minimize the damage caused by secondary injury.
- Acute injury to the brain causes increase in glutamate, potassium and calcium levels with decrease in glucose metabolism and level of magnesium.

CEREBRAL CONCUSSION

Definition: Concussion is physiological disruption of brain functions as a result of a traumatic event. It is manifested by at least one of the following: alteration of mental state,

Identify the skull fracture shown in the images:

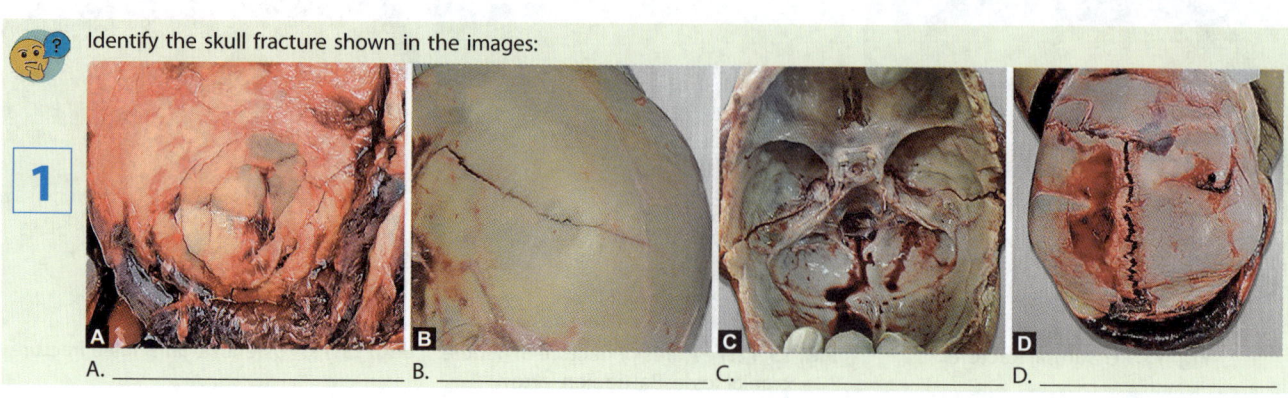

A. _____ B. _____ C. _____ D. _____

loss of memory or focal neurological deficit, that may or may not be transient.
- Concussion, also known as mild traumatic brain injury is a clinical diagnosis.
- It results from acceleration/deceleration of the head.
- Violent head movement causes shearing or stretching of nerve fibers and axonal damage.
- It may resemble drunkenness **(Diff. 13.2)**.
- Concussion is common among contact and collision sports participants. Football players and boxers are particularly exposed to repetitive concussions, leading to the condition known as *chronic traumatic encephalopathy*.

Signs and Symptoms

Unconsciousness, bradycardia, hypotension and sweating, and is always followed by retrograde or post-traumatic (antegrade) amnesia, temporary lethargy, irritability and cognitive dysfunction. Muscles are flaccid, pupils are dilated and unreacting, pulse is weak and slow, and respiration is shallow.

Findings: Gross and light microscopic changes in the brain are usually absent, but biochemical and ultrastructural changes—mitochondrial ATP depletion, local disruption of blood-brain barrier occur. CT and MRI scans are usually normal.

NOTA BENE

- **Post-traumatic automatism:** It is intimately associated with amnesia. After an accident, the patient may speak and act in a purposive manner, but does not remember anything later on.
- **Retrograde amnesia:** Loss of memory preceding the event.
- **Anterograde amnesia:** Loss of memory subsequent to the event that caused the amnesia.
- **Post-concussion syndrome:** Seen in patients who returned to work too early after head injury. It consists of headache, vertigo, lassitude, irritability and depression which may persist for months.
- **Second impact syndrome** is characterized by rapid death due to a second concussion prior to a return to baseline functioning after an initial one.

- **Chronic traumatic encephalopathy** *(previously called Punch drunk syndrome, dementia pugilistica or boxer's encephalopathy):**
A condition occurring late in American football players, rugby players and boxer's career or years after retirement, which is the cumulative result of recurrent cerebral concussions.
Signs and symptoms: There may be deterioration of speed and reflexes, and incoordination along with personality change associated with social instability and sometimes paranoia and delusions. Later, memory loss progresses to full dementia, often associated with Parkinsonian signs, ataxia or intention tremors, shuffling, broad-based gait and dysarthria.
Autopsy: Chronic SDH, attenuation of corpus callosum, DAI and cortical atrophy may be seen. There is deposition of hyperphosphorylated tau (p-tau) protein around small blood vessels of cortical sulci.

There are four forms of diffuse TBI: axonal injury, vascular injury, hypoxic ischemic encephalopathy and brain swelling. These categories overlap and they are often accompanied by various forms of focal TBI.

DIFFUSE AXONAL INJURY (DAI)

Definition: Diffuse axonal injury (DAI) is a condition representing a spectrum of severity in which the victim is unconscious from the time of injury, and then either remains in a coma or enters a persistent vegetative state.
- In severe cases, patients may expire depending on the severity of concurrent secondary injury.
- DAI is a clinical syndrome with supporting neuro-radiological changes.
- **Cause:** It results from relative movement (shearing) at the gray-white matter interface following sudden rotational acceleration/deceleration forces which cause disruption and tearing of axons, myelin sheaths and blood capillaries. With concussions, the axonal damage is considered as reversible; however, when sufficient vital axons are severely injured then death can occur.
- Ninety percent of cases are due to road traffic accidents and 10% due to falls and assaults.

DIFFERENTIATION 13.2: Drunkenness and concussion

S.No.	Feature	Drunkenness	Concussion
1.	Skin	Flushed, congested and warm	Pale, cold and sweating
2.	Pulse	Rapid and bounding	Slow and feeble
3.	Pupils	Dilated; contracted in coma	Contracted in pontine hemorrhage
4.	Light reflex	Sluggish	May be brisk
5.	Respiration	Sighs, puffs, eructates	Shallow, irregular, slow
6.	Memory	Confused, disoriented	Retrograde amnesia, unrelieved by time
7.	Behavior	Uncooperative, abusive, talkative, sulky	Quiet and retracted, curled up in bed, photophobia
8.	Urine/blood	Examination will be helpful	Retention of urine, urine may contain albumin
9.	History	History of having consumed alcohol, smell of alcohol	History of head injury with features of concussion

* Bennet Omalu was the first to highlight the link between concussions sustained by American football players and long term neurological effects. The movie '*Concussion*' shows his efforts to study and publicize CTE in the face of National Football League where the lead actor Will Smith played the part of Omalu.

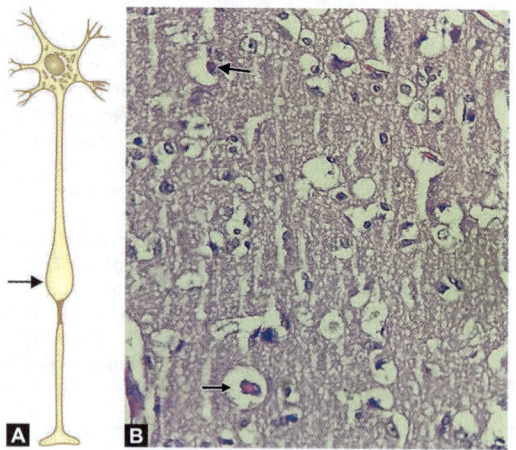

Figs. 13.15A and B: (A) Axonal swelling/ballooning (arrow); (B) Brain showing shrunken red neurons with neuronal swelling and clearing (arrow)

Autopsy Findings

i. Contact injuries to the scalp and skull may be absent.
ii. Thin subarachnoid hemorrhage may be seen.
iii. **Brain:** Cut sections may be normal to the naked eye or there may be minimal gross alterations—focal necrosis or petechial hemorrhages in the corpus callosum, focal lesions in the dorsolateral aspect of the rostral brainstem in the vicinity of the superior and middle cerebellar peduncles. Gliding contusions are common, and hemorrhages in the thalamus and basal ganglia are frequent.

> **NOTA BENE**
>
> **Diagnosis**
> - *CT scan*: Characteristic CT findings may be absent but in severe DAI, focal lesions are seen as petechial hemorrhages in the corpus callosum, cerebellar peduncle and evidence of diffuse injury to axons.
> - *MRI* with its high sensitivity for parenchymal injury, DAI is diagnosed in patients with non-hemorrhagic areas of T2 signal within the white matter or at the gray-white junction.
> - *Histologically*, it is diagnosed by demonstrating scattered microglial accumulates and debris-laden macrophages along with numerous axonal swellings ('**retraction balls/bulbs**') in the internal capsule, corpus callosum and superior cerebellar peduncle (**Figs. 13.15A and B**). They can be seen as eosinophilic-pink swellings on H&E stained sections and can be also detected by silver stains, but a survival of 15–18 h is required before they can be identified using this technique.
> - *Immunohistochemistry* is the most sensitive technique, and currently immunostaining for β-*amyloid precursor protein* (BAPP) has proven to be a sensitive and specific method of detecting axonal swellings.

CEREBRAL CONTUSION AND LACERATION

Definition: Areas of hemorrhagic disruption (tearing lesions) of the CNS that are superficially located in the brain are called *contusions* if the pia mater is intact, and *lacerations* if the pia is torn.

Location: Contusions occur usually in the frontal and temporal poles, inferior surfaces of the frontal (orbital gyri) and temporal lobes, and the cortex above and below the Sylvian fissure (**Fig. 13.16**).
- Typically, it involve the crests of gyri and often involve the gray matter only; may extend into underlying white matter and form a hematoma.
- In severe cases, extensive laceration with underlying parenchymal hemorrhage may be associated with subdural hemorrhage, forming a so-called *burst lobe*—often seen in the temporal lobes.

Pathogenesis

Contusions are the sites where the brain tissue comes in contact with the bony protuberances and dural coverings, sites of forcible separation of the brain from the dura, and sites of differential movement between the brain and dura and between adjacent areas of the brain.
- Contusion produces focal neurological deficits that persist for >24 h. Since, the damage is focal, patients may recover uneventfully, provided that they did not develop complications leading to other types of brain damage, and did not sustain DAI at the time of injury.
- Intoxication by alcohol is associated with unduly large contusions as they tend to fall more heavily because of their blunted protective locomotor reflexes. Moreover, associated liver disease and acute alcohol intoxication hinder hemostasis.

Types

There are several types of brain contusions based on location and/or mechanism of injury:
i. **Coup contusion:** Occurs at the site of impact due to inbending bone rebounding and injuring the brain.

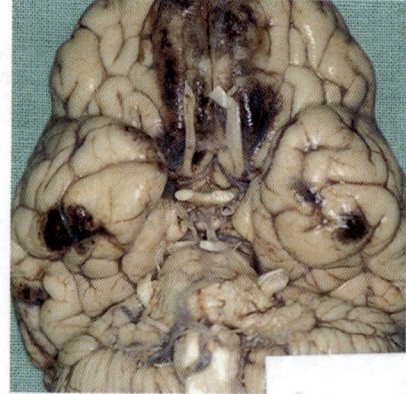

Fig. 13.16: Location of contrecoup contusions on undersurface of frontal and temporal lobes

They have a *wedge-shaped appearance* whose base is at the pial surface and the tip pointing towards the white matter **(Fig. 13.17A)**.

ii. **Contrecoup contusion:** It is associated with falls and occurs at a site diametrically opposite to the point of impact. It is due to the brain rebounding backward from the skull following impact. It is seen most commonly in the frontal (orbital gyri) and temporal lobes **(Figs. 13.16 and 13.17B)**.

iii. **Fracture contusion:** Related to fractures of the skull and bears no relation with the point of impact.

iv. **Intermediary coup contusion:** Present in deeper structures of the brain, like the white matter or basal ganglia. It is present along the line of impact between coup and contrecoup points.

v. **Gliding contusion:** Usually associated with DAI, and independent of site and direction of impact. It is a focal hemorrhage in the cortex and underlying white matter of the dorsal surface of cerebrum, particularly the frontal region. It is seen in falls and road traffic accidents.

vi. **Herniation contusion:** It is due to the impact of medial side of temporal lobe with the edge of the tentorium, or the cerebellar tonsils against the foramen magnum. It is independent of the site and direction of impact.

Clinical features: The GCS is often low, and focal neurologic symptoms, loss of consciousness and visual changes are present. Secondary injury may further complicate the clinical picture by producing infarcts due to local vasospasm. Prognosis is usually poor.

Diagnostic tool: CT scan shows a mixture of hypo- and hyperdense lesions within the brain parenchyma.

Autopsy Findings

i. In early stages, small contusions appear as linear hemorrhages perpendicular to the pial surface and associated focal swelling. Large contusion-lacerations appear as fragmented and irregularly shaped hemorrhagic areas. Frequently, there is associated subarachnoid hemorrhage.

ii. With time, it shrinks and takes a golden brown color secondary to hemosiderin deposition.

iii. Old contusions are frequent incidental autopsy finding, particularly in chronic alcoholics, which are seen as depressed yellow gliotic scars (***plaque jaune***).

> **FM 3.11** Describe and discuss injuries to the head—coup and contrecoup injuries.

COUP AND CONTRECOUP INJURY

- **Coup injury** is one which occurs immediately beneath the area of impact, and results directly by the impacting force.
    - Smaller the impact area, greater is the likelihood of a coup injury.
    - Effects are immediate, resulting in contusion and hemorrhage.
    - For example, if the head is fixed (person standing still) and there is violent impact over the frontal bone, fracture and underlying brain damage will be located beneath the site of impact **(Fig. 13.18A)**.
- **Contrecoup injury** (French *contre*: opposite, *coup*: blow) means that the lesion is present in the brain opposite to the site of impact.
    - It is caused when the moving head is suddenly decelerated by hitting a firm surface, e.g., striking of the head on the ground during a fall, usually seen in road traffic accidents.
    - For example, when a person falls with his occiput striking the ground, he may sustain injury at the occipital lobes (coup injury) and a more prominent injury to the frontal lobes (contrecoup injury) **(Fig. 13.18B)**.

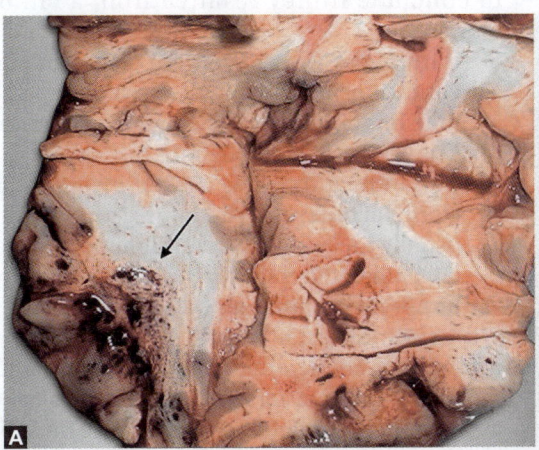
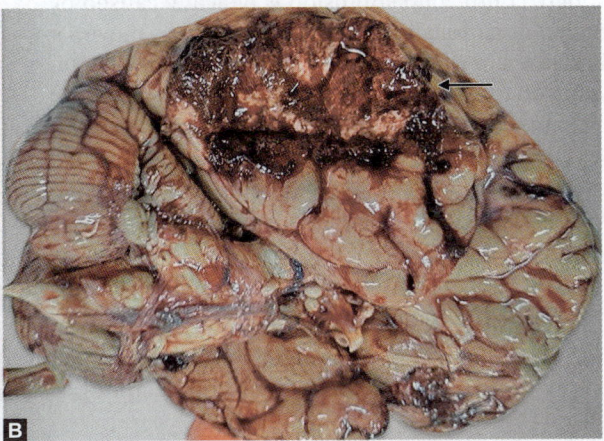

Figs. 13.17A and B: (A) Wedge-shaped coup contusion (arrow); (B) Contrecoup contused laceration of right temporal lobe of brain (arrow). The deceased had impact over left side of head with skull fracture

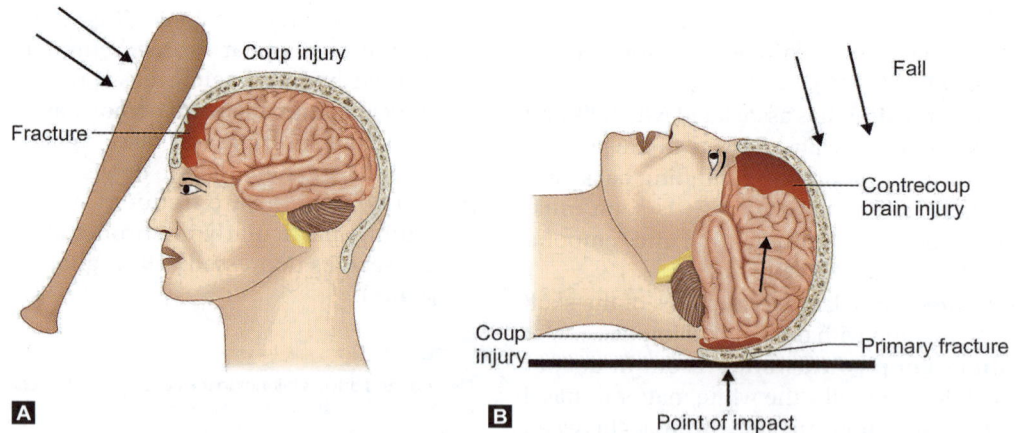

Figs. 13.18A and B: Mechanism of: (A) Coup; (B) Contrecoup injury of the brain

Mechanism

There are several hypotheses to explain this phenomenon and most are correct in some aspect.
- When head strikes the ground, a transient deformation of the skull occurs with increase in pressure which may impinge on the underlying brain causing compression—*coup injury*.
- Simultaneously, opposite area of the skull will bulge outward to accommodate the deformation—the so-called '*struck-hoop*' action. There is formation of vacuum or rarefaction (due to negative pressure gradient) as brain lags behind the moving skull. The vacuum exerts a suction/cavitation effect that causes tension and shear strain by pulling apart of the constituent of the brain—*contrecoup injury*.

The following points should be considered:
  i. Contrecoup injury is rare before the age of 3 years.
 ii. There may be only contrecoup injury without any coup injury.
iii. There may be no fracture of skull, even in the presence of severe coup and contrecoup lesions.
iv. Though, contrecoup contusion is typically caused by deceleration of a falling head (head is free to move), it can also occur when a fixed head is struck. If the victim is lying on the ground, a heavy blow on the upper side may cause typical contrecoup lesions either in the contralateral temporal or parietal cortex, or against the falx on the inner side of the ipsilateral lobe. In such cases, there is often coup injury as well.

Site

- The most common site for contrecoup injury is the frontal lobes (tips of the frontal poles/orbital surface) and may be symmetrical, if a fall on the occiput has occurred **(Fig. 13.16)**.
- In temporal or parietal impacts, the contrecoup lesions are usually on the contralateral surface of the brain.
- It is rare for a fall on the frontal region to produce occipital contrecoup. This is thought to be due to the anatomical configuration of the floor of the cranium.

Differentiating features between coup and contrecoup injury are highlighted in **Diff. 13.3.**

DIFFERENTIATION 13.3: Coup and contrecoup injury

S.No	Feature	Coup injury	Contrecoup injury
1.	Site	At site of impact	Opposite to site of impact
2.	Severity of injury	Mild	Severe
3.	Produced due to	Direct impact on brain	Vacuum and suction force
4.	External injury	Present	Absent
5.	Head in motion	No, head fixed	Yes, moving head strikes
6.	Most common site	Occipital lobe	Frontal and temporal lobes

Medico-legal Importance

i. On the basis of localization of injuries, it is possible to conclude if they resulted from a fall or from blows.
   - With *blows (assault)*, brain shows much larger contusions underlying the area of impact (coup) than on the site opposite to impact (contrecoup). Contrecoup lesions are rare.
   - But, in head injuries caused *by falls* (e.g., road traffic accidents), the contrecoup injuries are usually located in inaccessible portions and are larger than the coup contusions. Coup lesions may be absent or minimal.
ii. With severe frontal contrecoup from a fall on the occiput, the transmitted force may cause fracture of the floor of the anterior fossa resulting in 'black eyes'. In assaults where a fall has occurred, care must be taken not to attribute such periorbital bleeding to direct punches.

CHAPTER 13 : Regional Injuries

2 A 27-year-old came to the emergency with alleged history of road traffic accident. She was unconscious with multiple episodes of vomiting with no history of seizures. On examination, GCS: E1V1M5, pulse: 80/min, BP: 120/70 mm Hg, SpO$_2$ (blood oxygen level): 96%, pupils reacting to light, right ear bleed present and moving all limbs. What could be the reason of her ear bleed? What is the type of contusion shown in the CT? Make a diagnosis.

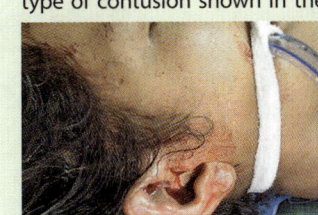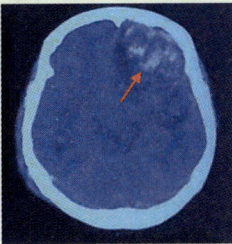

Describe and discuss injuries to the head—intracranial hemorrhages.

INTRACRANIAL HEMATOMA

Intracranial hemorrhages are classified by anatomical location.

Types of intracranial hematoma	
♦ Extradural	♦ Subarachnoid
♦ Subdural	♦ Intracerebral

- Intracranial hemorrhage is a common complication of head injury, and is the most common cause of death in patients who experienced a lucid interval, '*talk and die*', or '*talk and deteriorate after injury*'.
- Clinical complications associated with a hematoma are related to the size/volume of the lesion, the anatomical location and the rapidity with which it develops.
- Hypovolemic shock cannot happen from intracranial bleeding; there is not enough space inside the head for the amount of blood loss needed to produce shock.
- *Expanding hematomas* should be distinguished from *delayed hematomas*, which are as lesions that occurs 24–48 h after the time of injury and are not evident on initial imaging studies. It reflects increased blood flow or pressure through a vascular capillary network that was focally damaged, compounded by post-traumatic coagulopathy.
- In several cases of death due to blunt force head trauma, the only intracranial injuries that are evident at autopsy include subdural and subarachnoid hemorrhage.

NOTA BENE
- **Hemorrhage:** Copious discharge of blood from the blood vessels.
- **Hematoma:** Localized collection of blood in the tissues, usually clotted or partially clotted.
- **Apoplexy:** Sudden large effusion of blood in an organ or tissue. The term is synonym for cerebral hemorrhage.

EPIDURAL/EXTRADURAL HEMATOMA (EDH)

Definition: It is the bleeding occurring between the inner table of the skull and meninges (dura) (**Fig. 13.19A**).

Causes

Mostly traumatic in origin, and unilateral. EDH is seen in falls and road traffic accidents (up to 10% of severe head injury cases).

Salient Features

- EDH occurs usually on the side of the impact, and common in adults between 20–40 years as the dura is able to strip more readily off the underlying bone.
- It is infrequent in the elderly and young (<2 years) due to greater adherence of dura to the skull in both these age groups, and absence of a bony canal for the artery in the young.
- It shows typical limitation due to the dural attachments at the suture lines.
- Fracture (*linear* type) is present in most of the cases (90–95%).
- In children, EDH may be seen even without skull fracture.
- It forms a circumscribed ovoid or disk-shaped blood clot that progressively indents and flattens the adjacent brain.
- Size and extent of an EDH is determined by the source of bleeding (arterial or venous) and the strength of attachment between the outer layer of the dura and the cranium.
- Artifactual EDH can occur in fire victims, related to heat-induced postmortem skull fractures.

Site and Vessels Involved

i. It may be due to impact over:
   - Lateral convexity of head, resulting in linear fracture of squamous temporal bone with rupture of underlying middle meningeal artery (direct branch of internal maxillary artery)—*commonest cause*.
   - Forehead—tear the anterior ethmoidal artery.
   - Occiput—tear the transverse sigmoid sinus.
   - Vertex—cause hemorrhage from sagittal sinus.
ii. Fracture of skull with tear of diploic veins and middle meningeal veins.

Types

i. *Acute* onset is within few minutes to few hours or even a day (arterial bleeding).
ii. *Chronic:* Symptoms are slower in onset (48–72 h) after trauma. It is rare, and commonly associated with tears of venous structures.

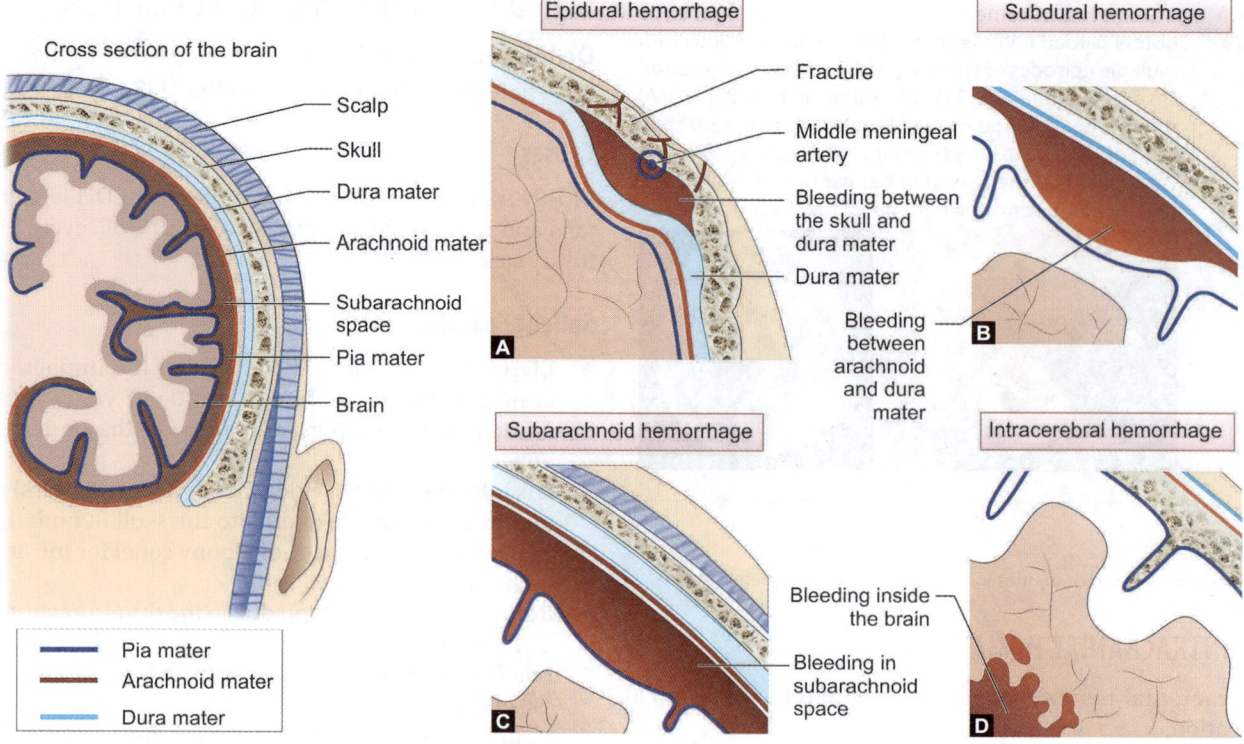

Figs. 13.19A to D: Intracranial hematomas

Clinical Features

i. Loss of consciousness due to concussion.
ii. Dilation of pupil (*Hutchinson's pupil*) on the side of hemorrhage with conjugate deviation of eyes to opposite side.
iii. Bilateral fixation of pupils.
iv. **Lucid or latent interval** is seen.* It is a state of consciousness between two episodes of unconsciousness. *Mechanism*: Since, the initial brain injury is only a concussion, subsequent middle meningeal bleed cause the ensuing decompensation from the expanding blood collection, causing increased intracranial pressure and a reduction in cerebral perfusion (a secondary injury).
v. Features of cerebral compression supervene and may lead to coma.
vi. Decerebrate rigidity and death due to respiratory failure.

Frequently, patient presents in coma and requires an urgent craniotomy. It is a *surgical emergency*, and early diagnosis and intervention usually saves the patient, since the brain itself is not significantly injured, and the bleeding originated from outside the brain parenchyma.

Diagnostic tool: CT head.
♦ It produces a biconvex lenticular-shaped hemorrhage, due to adherence of the dura to the inside of the cranium (**Fig. 13.20A**).
♦ Isolated EDHs of ≥2 cm or about 30 mL in volume may cause an alteration in the level of consciousness or a focal neurologic deficit.

Autopsy Findings

i. Temporal scalp contusion on the side of the hematoma.
ii. Hematoma in the epidural space on removal of the skull cap along with linear fracture of the temporal bone and a small thrombus on the surface of the middle meningeal artery may be seen (**Fig. 13.20B**).
iii. Diffuse brain swelling and cerebral contusions may be seen.
iv. Subfalcine herniation extending from the side of the hematoma to the opposite side, and transtentorial herniation which is usually more marked on the side of the hematoma (effects of intracranial 'space occupancy').
v. Swelling of the cerebral hemisphere under the hematoma causes effacement of sulci and flatness of the crests of the gyri, which gives a smooth appearance of the brain.

Medico-legal Aspects

♦ Prognosis is good with proper treatment. Hematoma on the contralateral side should be carefully excluded.
♦ Patient may be discharged from hospital during lucid interval and die at home; doctor may be charged with negligence.

---
* Patients with lucid interval are often not associated with other types of brain injury. If the patient is in coma from the time of injury, other types of brain injury are likely to be present.

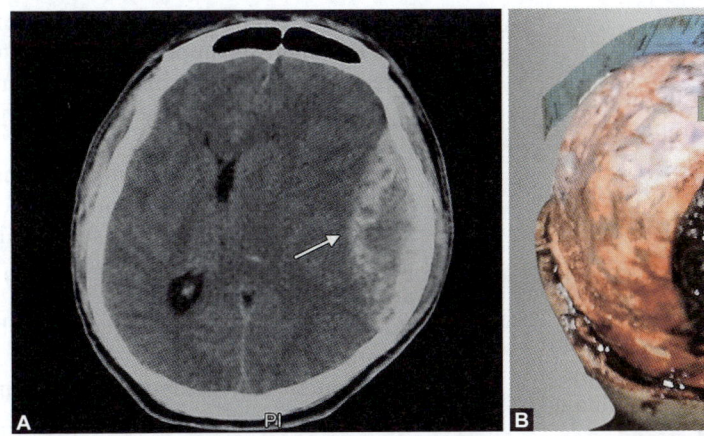
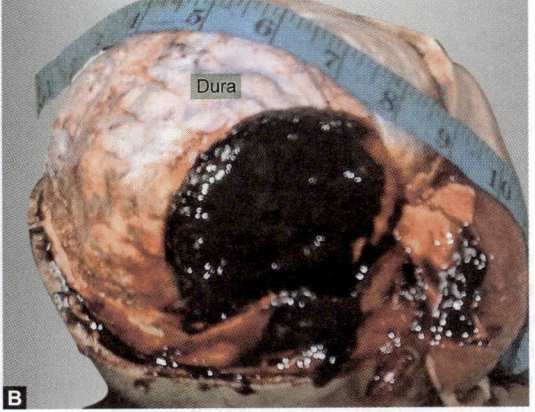

Figs. 13.20A and B: Epidural hematoma: (A) CT head (convex lens appearance); (B) Autopsy appearance

- Most complications occur within the first 24 h following the injury. Patient's attendants should be instructed on what signs to look for and when to return for further care.
- The condition may resemble drunkenness and patient may die in police custody.
- Presence of an EDH may or may not cause death—the possibility increasing with increasing volume of blood, duration of injury and the presence of herniation phenomenon.

NOTA BENE

Non-traumatic spontaneous EDH may be seen in sickle cell anemia, coagulopathies, infectious diseases of the skull like sinusitis, vascular malformations of the dura, metastasis to the dura or skull, and chronic kidney disease. In this category of patients, typically there is no evidence of head trauma, skull fracture or lucid interval.

SUBDURAL HEMATOMA (SDH)

Definition: It is the bleeding occurring between the undersurface of dura and outer surface of arachnoid mater **(Fig. 13.19B)**. It is essentially a venous or capillary bleeding, and not an arterial bleeding.

Cause

It is usually traumatic, following an assault or fall (70–75%), accidents account for another 20–25% of cases, but it can be due to secondary causes including alcoholism and anticoagulant therapy **(Table 13.3)**.

Salient Features

- One of the *most common head injuries ending fatally*. SDH is caused due to acceleration-deceleration injury in which there is significant primary damage to brain parenchyma.
- Hematoma often not associated with a fracture of the skull.
- Commonly seen in elderly and alcoholics.

TABLE 13.3: Causes of subdural hematoma

Causes	Comment
Trauma	Blunt force head injury (accident/assault)
Neurosurgical complication	Neurosurgical management of hydrocephalus
Perinatal	Following labor (rarely significant)
Vascular	Aneurysms, a rare childhood cause
Hematological disorders	Inherited and acquired coagulation disorders, and hematological malignancies
Metabolic disorders	Glutaric aciduria, Menkes disease, and galactosemia
Hypernatremia	Associated with intracerebral hemorrhages
Raised central venous pressure	Intradural bleeding may lead to subdural collections

- Location of a SDH does not necessarily correlate to the location of the blunt force impact site.
- In infants <1 year, the subdural space is narrower and less tolerant of space occupying lesions.

Vessels Involved

i. Rupture of bridging or communicating veins traversing the subdural space to drain into parasagittal sinus.
ii. Tears in the dural venous sinuses.
iii. Cerebral contusions/lacerations after a fall.
iv. Fresh tear of old adhesion between dura and brain.

Site

- It is commonly seen over the upper lateral surface of cerebral hemispheres and most commonly supratentorial (frontotemporal region).
- The blood presses on both the crests and depths of the gyri, hence the cerebral convolutions retain their normal contours.
- It causes displacement of the cerebral hemispheres with flattening of the convolutions of the opposite hemispheres.

Types

SDHs are classified in clinical terms as acute, subacute, chronic or acute on chronic depending on the length of history, the neuroimaging findings and the appearance of the blood when the hematoma is drained.

i. **Acute SDH:** Signs are evident within 3 days of injury. It occurs due to rupture of large bridging veins or the cortical artery or due to cerebral laceration.
   - It is mostly unilateral, may be bilateral with mortality—90%.
   - *Clinical features:* Drowsy or comatose (one-third patients have a *lucid interval*) from the moment of injury. Unilateral headache, hemiparesis, dilated pupil on the same side are frequent.
   - It is a rapidly evolving lesion and burr (drainage) holes or emergency craniotomy is mandatory.
   - Blood tends to accumulate in the base of skull, especially in the middle cranial fossa, is reddish in color and clotted.

ii. **Subacute SDH:** The signs are evident between 4–21 days.
   - It is due to rupture of smaller bridging veins.
   - It is associated with minor cerebral contusions or swelling.
   - *Clinical features:* Drowsiness, headache, confusion, forgetfulness or mild hemiparesis.
   - It may be mistaken in the young for schizophrenia and in the old for presenile and senile dementia.
   - Mortality is less.
   - Blood is partly clotted and partly fluid due to hemolysis or dilution with CSF.

iii. **Chronic SDH or *Pachymeningitis hemorrhagica interna chronica***
   - Signs and symptoms of alteration in mental state or progressive focal neurological deficits (usually headache, cognitive decline, gait abnormalities and hemiparesis) appear >3 weeks after trauma.
   - It is most common in infants (<6 months) and in the elderly (>60 years). A history of head trauma may be elicited.
   - Blood is liquefied, mixed with proteins and CSF.
   - *Risk factors:* Cerebral atrophy, alcohol abuse, seizures, coagulopathies, subdural structural abnormalities, intraventricular shunts, CSF fistulae and dehydration.
   - It is usually seen over the parietal lobe and near the midline.
   - It is frequently an incidental finding during autopsy in old persons.

Diagnostic tool: CT head. It appears as concavo-convex crescentic opacity **(Fig. 13.21A)**.

> **NOTA BENE**
> - Acute SDH appears hyperdense to brain tissue, subacute appears isodense and chronic appears hypodense on noncontrast CT.
> - Acute SDH >120 mL is invariably fatal, between 50–120 mL is likely to cause death (particularly if there is significant subfalcine herniation and uncal herniation), and <50 mL is unlikely to be fatal. Usually 50 mL of rapidly accumulating subdural blood is sufficient to be life-threatening.
> - 'Acute on chronic' SDHs are chronic SDHs into which there has been recent bleeding to the extent that new neurological symptoms are precipitated in a patient who previously had no symptoms or trivial symptoms.
> - When a child presents with unexplained vomiting, lethargy and/or head trauma, and subdural hematoma is found, the possibility of non-accidental injury (child abuse) must be explored.

Age of Subdural Hematoma

- **Grossly,** during the first 4 days, hematoma undergoes clotting, and gradually becomes dark red to brownish in

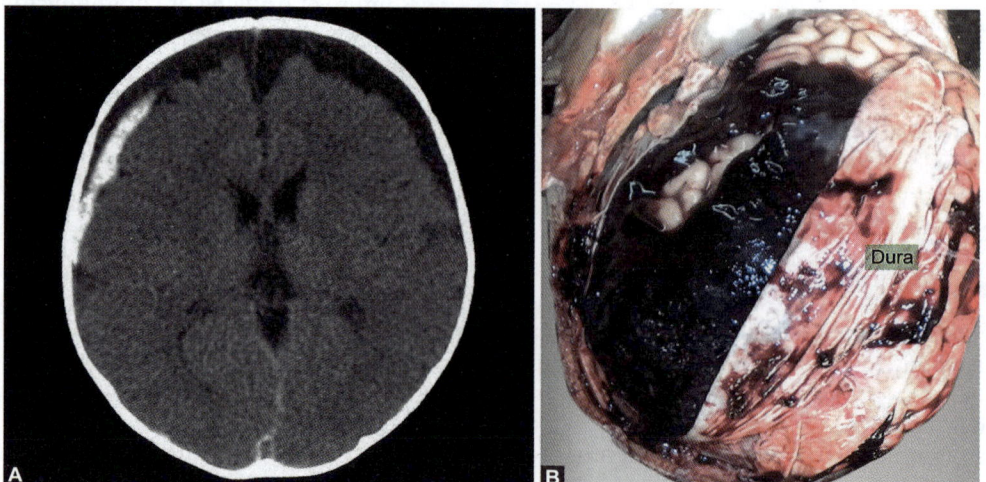

Figs. 13.21A and B: Subdural hematoma: (A) CT head (concave lens appearance); (B) Autopsy appearance

TABLE 13.4: Histological timing of subdural hematoma

Interval	Features
36 h	Intact RBCs, fibroblastic activity at the margins
4–5 days	Loss of RBC contour, neomembrane adjacent to dura is 2–5 layers of thickness
6–10 days	Laked RBCs, clot liquefies, 12–14 layers of fibroblasts, hemosiderin laden phagocytes seen, neomembrane visible grossly
11–14 days	Fibroblasts, capillaries and fibrin subdivide the clot, fibroblasts migrate around the edges of clot, siderophages present on arachnoid side
15–20 days	Capillary formation, original RBCs lysed, membrane $\frac{1}{3}$ to ½ dural thickness on the side of dura, but variably thin on arachnoid side
3–4 weeks	Liquefied clot, membrane same thickness as dura on dural side and ½ dural thickness on arachnoid side. Siderophages in membranes
1–3 months	Hyalinization of membranes, more of collagen and of same thickness as dura on arachnoid side
3–6 months	Hyalinized neomembrane resembling dura

color by 5–10 days. Discrete fragile membrane becomes obvious by 2nd week. Liquefaction of clot occurs by 3 weeks. After 1 month, a firm capsule containing a dark brown watery fluid is formed.
♦ **Histologically,** age of subdural hematoma can be estimated as given in **Table 13.4**.

Autopsy Findings

i. Externally, evidence of blunt force injury, more commonly to the face than to the head may be seen.
ii. Skull fractures may be present.
iii. Clotted or partly liquefied hematoma extending for a considerable distance in the subdural space, producing an accentuation of the gyral pattern on the affected side with flattening of the opposite side (in contrast to the smooth brain surface under an epidural hematoma) **(Fig. 13.21B)**.
iv. In acute SDH, there are no enclosing membranes. Chronic SDH may present 'classically' as typical *hematoma* surrounded by a clearly defined membrane that includes original dura, and an *inner* and *outer* 'neomembrane' which contains bloodstained fluid of variable color (usually yellow).
v. Transtentorial herniation (more marked on the same side of the hematoma), and tonsillar herniation and subfalcine herniation directed away from the side of the hematoma may be seen.

Medico-legal Aspects

♦ When an infant or a child has SDH, the diagnostic priority is to exclude physical abuse following shaking or shaking impact injury.

♦ The presence of any amount of SDH is usually interpreted by forensic experts as an indicator that the amount of force sustained by the individual was likely sufficient to cause lethal brain injuries. However, it is possible for individuals to survive a SDH.
♦ Histopathology of SDH, both acute and chronic is used as a basis for estimating the period between injury and death, which helps in correlating the events prior to death.

Subdural Hygroma

It is an accumulation of CSF in subdural space. When arachnoid is torn, CSF may pass from subarachnoid space into subdural space. A large collection of fluid may accumulate and cause cerebral compression.
♦ It is usually seen in infants and children.
♦ This chronic lesion has all the features of subdural hematoma, except trauma is not recorded and amount of blood is minimal.
♦ It may develop as a complication of meningitis, hydrocephalus and head trauma with/without skull fracture.

SUBARACHNOID HEMATOMA (SAH)

Definition: It is the hemorrhage in the subarachnoid space between the arachnoid and pia mater, mixed with CSF **(Fig. 13.19C)**.

Causes

It is mostly venous in origin.
a. **Non-traumatic/natural causes**
   i. Rupture of a developmental aneurysm of the vessels in the circle of Willis [Berry (saccular) aneurysm]. Excluding head trauma, it is the most common cause (70% of cases) of SAH especially in young adults **(Figs. 13.22A and B)**. Aneurysm size and site are important in predicting risk of rupture. Rupture is likely with aneurysms that are large (7–10 mm in diameter).
   ii. Arteriovenous malformations (10%).
   iii. Atherosclerotic changes in blood vessels associated with hypertension in elderly subjects.
   iv. Leaking intracerebral hemorrhage.
   v. Disease conditions, like purpuric states and leukemia.
b. **Traumatic causes**
   i. Cerebral contusions or lacerations.
   ii. Explosive blast.
   iii. Asphyxia by strangulation.
   iv. Traumatic asphyxia.
   v. Blows to the neck, accidents, falls, and cervical manipulations causing damage to the vertebral or basilar arteries.
   vi. Rupture of a traumatic ICH into the subarachnoid space or into the cerebral ventricles with flowing of the blood through the foramina of Magendie and Luschka into the subarachnoid space.

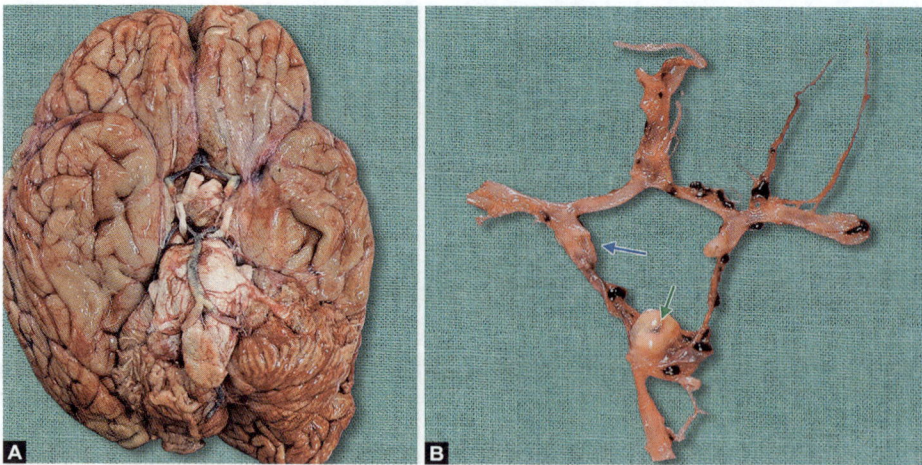

Figs. 13.22A and B: (A) Circle of Willis; (B) Multiple aneurysms in the circle of Willis. Root of the internal carotid artery (blue arrow) and bifurcation of the basilar artery (basilar apex) (green arrow)
(*Courtesy:* Dr Dinesh Fernando, Color Atlas in Forensic Pathology)

vii. Prolonged hyperextension of the head during bronchoscopy, bleeding originating from rents in basilar or vertebral arteries (may lead to a charge of negligence).

NOTA BENE

In acute alcoholism, traumatic SAH is common due to:
- Loss of muscular coordination resulting in excessive rotational forces within the head
- Increased bleeding from congested vessels
- Bounding pulse of the drunken person

Salient Features

- SAH is common in TBI. Even in minor head trauma, small amount of localized SAH over the cerebral convexities is almost invariably seen.
- Like SDH, the location does not correlate with the site of impact in blunt force trauma, but usually SAH is most prominent close to its source.
- SAH is extensive because CSF and unclotted subarachnoid blood flow freely in the subarachnoid space.

Site

- SAH has a predominantly basal distribution.
- It is usually found over the orbital surface of the frontal lobe, parietal lobe and anterior third of the temporal lobes.
- It can be unilateral or bilateral, localized or diffuse.

Types

i. Immediate.
ii. Delayed/reactionary hemorrhage—until the initial contraction and retraction of vessels has subsided (delayed post-traumatic SAH).

Clinical Features

i. Sudden onset of severe, unusual headache ('*thunderclap headache*').
ii. Nausea and vomiting.
iii. Neck stiffness, photophobia, drowsiness or agitation.
iv. Depressed consciousness.
v. There may be ocular findings (e.g., intraocular hemorrhages) or focal findings (e.g., unilateral loss of motor function, loss of visual field, aphasia).

Physical findings: Meningism and a positive Kernig's sign.

Diagnosis: Non-contrast CT head. It shows hyperdense blood collections along the falx, and in the basilar cisterns **(Figs. 13.23A and B)**. Lumbar puncture (LP) should be performed, if CT scan is not yielding sufficient information. LP will reveal CSF intimately mixed with blood coming under increased pressure.

Differential diagnosis: Bacterial meningitis.

Autopsy Findings

- Most cases show evidence of abrasions/bruises/lacerations to the head, side of face/jaw or neck.
- SAH is usually found over frontal, occipital and basal areas of the brain—most common site being the base.
- The hemorrhage cannot be washed away under water during autopsy since the arachnoid membrane remains firmly attached to the brain.
- Careful dissection of circle of Willis may show evidence of aneurysm. Results of prior angiography if available, greatly facilities the location of aneurysm.
- There may be multiple infarcts with perifocal edema scattered throughout the cortex and subcortical white matter of the whole brain.

CHAPTER 13 : Regional Injuries

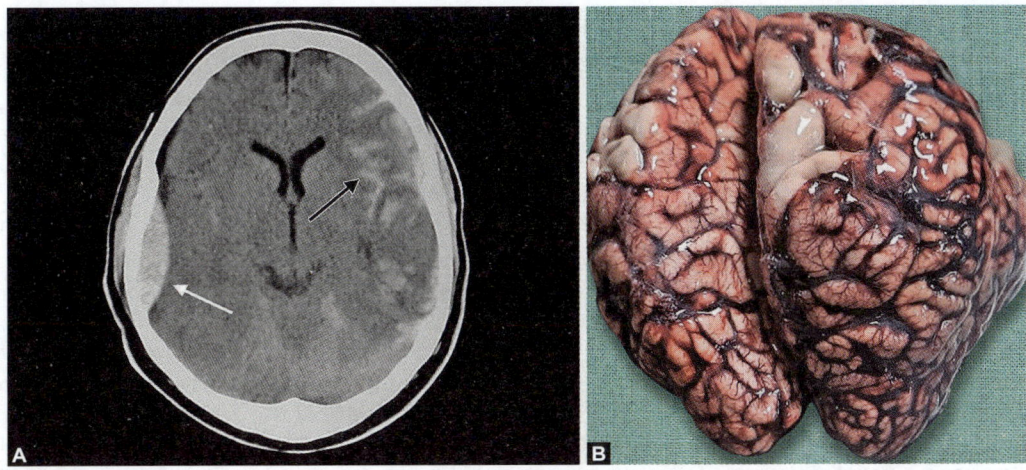

Figs. 13.23A and B: Subarachnoid hematoma: (A) CT head [including epidural hematoma (white arrow)]; (B) Autopsy appearance

Medico-legal Aspects

♦ Atherosclerotic vessels in older persons with high blood pressure rupture more easily than normal ones. The condition of blood vessels must therefore receive most careful consideration.
♦ It is possible to testify that trauma has caused or precipitated the rupture of developmental Berry aneurysm when head injury is followed at once by symptoms of unexplained acute neurologic deficit (headache, hemiparesis, stupor or confusion).
♦ SAH can be produced postmortem, secondary to decomposition, with lysis of blood cells, loss of vascular integrity and leakage of blood into subarachnoid space. It can also be produced during the process of removing the brain.

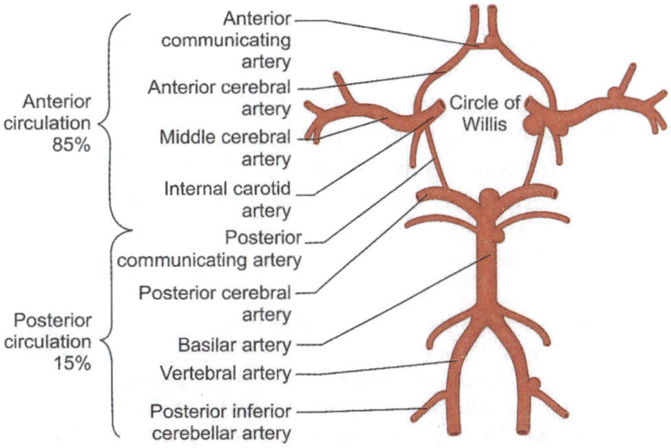

Fig. 13.24: Common sites of Berry aneurysms in circle of Willis

> **NOTA BENE**
>
> ♦ **Berry aneurysms** usually occur at a point where an artery is branching from a parent artery close to the circle of Willis, and develop where the vessel wall is abnormal due to congenital defect or a degenerative change producing a thin-walled out-pouching **(Fig. 13.24)**. The wall of an aneurysm lacks an internal elastic lamia and muscularis layer. Only the intimal layer and adventitia of the artery form the dome of the aneurysm.
> ♦ **Thunderclap headache**: Headache that reaches its maximum intensity in <1 min. SAH is the most common cause.
> *Other causes:* Sentinel headache, cerebral venous sinus thrombosis, unruptured cerebral aneurysm, cervical artery dissection, pituitary apoplexy and ischemic stroke.

*Important differentiating features of epidural, subdural and subarachnoid hemorrhages are given in **Diff. 13.4**.*

INTRACEREBRAL HEMATOMA (ICH)

Definition: Hemorrhage found within the cerebral parenchyma that is not in contact with the surface of the brain **(Fig. 13.19D)**.

Causes

♦ Hypertension, trauma and cerebral amyloid angiopathy cause the majority of these hemorrhages. Advanced age, and heavy alcohol and cocaine use increase the risk. Usually, it is due to disease of cerebral vessels; hypertension is often a contributory cause.
♦ Common causes are:
   i. Spontaneous hemorrhage in the region of basal ganglia due to rupture of lenticulostriate artery (Charcot's artery) which is a branch of middle cerebral artery.*

---

* Charcot-Bouchard aneurysms are minute aneurysms (microaneurysms) in the brain that arise from arterioles usually less than 300 μm in diameter. Hypertensive hemorrhage frequently involves deep gray matter but can occur anywhere in the brain.

DIFFERENTIATION 13.4: Epidural, subdural and subarachnoid hemorrhage

S.No.	Feature	EDH	SDH	SAH
1.	Location	Between skull and dura	Between dura and arachnoid	Between arachnoid and pia
2.	Cause	Always due to head injury	Mostly due to injury but not always	Both natural and traumatic
3.	Incidence	2% of head injuries	5% of all head injuries; 50% of fatal head injuries	Extremely common in head injuries
4.	Vessel involved	Middle meningeal artery	Bridging veins, cortical contusions	Leakage from vessels on brain surface
5.	Externally	Often swelling under the scalp	Often no external manifestation	No external manifestation
6.	Confusion with other condition	Can be confused with heat artifact	Seldom confused with other bleeding	Can be artifact from opening the skull
7.	Space occupying	Can be space occupying	Often space occupying	Space occupying, if it is arterial
8.	Effect on brain	Brain surface ironed out by dura (*ruler straight appearance*)	Brain compressed, but less ironed out (*undulating appearance*)	Brain surface not distorted
9.	Situation	Usually on one side, but can be bilateral	Unilateral or bilateral	Focal, diffuse or bilateral
10.	Clinical course	Classic lucid interval	Less well-defined	Depends on cause, location, vessel
11.	Autopsy	Save a portion for alcohol and drugs	If fresh, save a portion for alcohol and drugs	Blood seldom sufficient or helpful for analysis

ii. Capillary hemorrhage in anoxia, arterial thrombosis, blood dyscrasias, fat embolism and asphyxial states.
iii. Angioma or malignant tumor of the brain.
iv. Hypertensive cerebral vascular disease.
v. Laceration of the brain.
vi. Puerperal toxemia.

> **NOTA BENE**
>
> **Traumatic and nontraumatic ICH (Diff. 13.5)**
> The cause of ICH is at times remains uncertain, and a coincidental hypertensive hemorrhage or a hemorrhage associated with cerebral amyloid angiopathy may be difficult to exclude.
> - The exclusion of a hypertensive hemorrhage is presumptive, based on the lack of a history of hypertension and the absence of gross (e.g., cardiomegaly and renal tubular atrophy) and microscopic features (hypertensive vascular changes in the basal ganglia and dentate nucleus) of hypertension.
> - Hemorrhage owing to cerebral amyloid angiopathy is excluded when microscope sections stained with Congo red do not show amyloid in the cerebral vessels.

Salient Features

♦ Traumatic ICH is seen in 15% of all patients who sustain fatal head injuries.
♦ Most likely result from a direct rupture of intrinsic cerebral blood vessel in relation to contusions at the time of injury.
♦ May be single or multiple.

Sites

ICH are well demarcated homogenous collection of blood seen most frequently in the white matter of the frontotemporal lobes when superficially located and are most likely related to extensive contusional injury; more deeply seated hematomas are seen in impacts of greater force, such as road traffic accidents.

Clinical Features

i. Abrupt onset of focal neurologic deficit.
ii. Diminished level of consciousness.
iii. Signs of increased intracranial pressure, such as vomiting and headache.
iv. Seizures are uncommon.
v. Contralateral hemiparesis.

Large intracerebral hematomas should be evacuated, unless the patient's neurological state is improving. Small multiple hematomas need not be removed.

DIFFERENTIATION 13.5: Traumatic intracerebral hemorrhage and non-traumatic (spontaneous) cerebral hemorrhage (apoplexy)

S.No.	Feature	Traumatic cerebral hemorrhage	Non-traumatic cerebral hemorrhage
1.	Cause	Head injury	Hypertension, atherosclerosis or aneurysm
2.	Age	Young individuals	Adults (past middle age)
3.	Onset	Distinct interval after injury	Sudden
4.	Position of head	In motion	Any position
5.	Mechanism	Blunt force injury, coup and contrecoup	Rupture due to disease
6.	Site/location	White matter of frontal or temporo-occipital region	Ganglionic region
7.	Concussion	May be seen	Not present
8.	Coma	Variable; coma from beginning, or concussion → consciousness → coma	Deep unconsciousness and no such sequence

CHAPTER 13: Regional Injuries

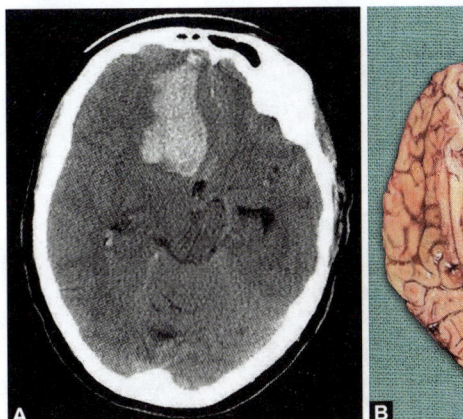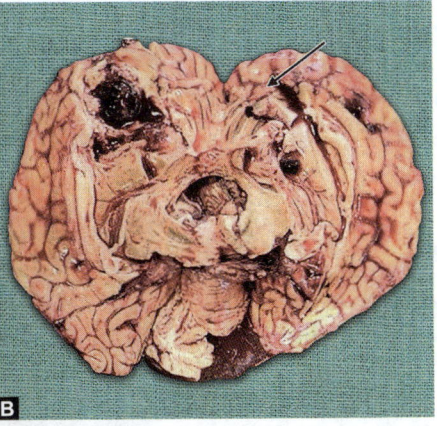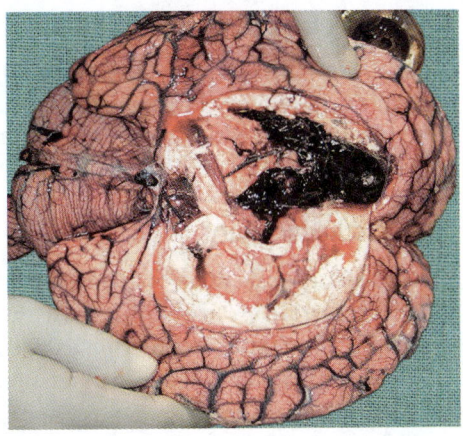

Figs. 13.25A and B: Intracerebral hematoma: (A) CT head; (B) Autopsy appearance (arrow)

Fig. 13.26: Intraventricular hemorrhage (IVH)

Diagnostic tool: CT head. ICH appear as hyperdense lesions (small foci, typically at gray/white matter interface or more centrally in the white matter) and are associated with mass effect and midline shift **(Fig. 13.25A)**.

Autopsy: There may be extensive edema and softening, and hemorrhage within the brain substance, right and left ventricles and in both putamen **(Fig. 13.25B)**.

NOTA BENE

Intraventricular hemorrhage (IVH)
The presence of copious blood in the fourth ventricle, seen through the foramina of Luschka and Magendie before the brain is sectioned, can be taken as indirect evidence of IVH which is confirmed when the brain is sectioned **(Fig. 13.26)**. Traumatic IVH can be primary or secondary.
- *Primary traumatic IVH* is rare, but occurs after motor vehicle accidents and assaults.
- *Nontraumatic primary IVH* originates from a ruptured Berry aneurysm or vascular malformation, or can be associated with hypertension, anticoagulant therapy or methamphetamine abuse.
- *Secondary IVH* is common after trauma which is usually self-evident when the brain is sectioned and a hematoma is found in continuity with the ventricles.

Pearls

- Most common type of intracranial hemorrhage: Intracerebral hemorrhage.
- Least common type of intracranial hemorrhage: Epidural hemorrhage.
- Most common non-traumatic intracranial hemorrhage: Intracerebral hemorrhage.
- Most common intracranial hemorrhage following head trauma: Subdural hemorrhage.
- Most common cause of subarachnoid hemorrhage: Head trauma.
- Second most common cause of subarachnoid hemorrhage: Rupture of Berry (saccular) aneurysm.
- Most common cause of intraparenchymal hemorrhage: Hypertension.
- Most common artery involved in intraparenchymal hemorrhage: Lenticulostriate artery.
- Most common sites of hypertensive hemorrhage: Basal ganglia [putamen (most common site, 55%), thalamus (15%) and adjacent white matter (10%)], deep cerebellum (10%), and pons (10%).
- Sites of hemorrhage following head trauma: Intraparenchymal (inferior frontal lobes, anterior temporal lobes), subarachnoid, subdural and epidural spaces.
- Commonest sites of rupture of Berry aneurysm: Anterior circulation (85%), with the most common locations at the origin of the anterior communicating artery, origin of the posterior communicating artery and the bifurcation of the middle cerebral artery **(Fig. 13.24)**. Vertebral artery is the least common site.

Match the following:

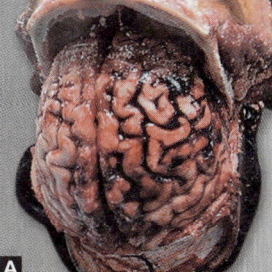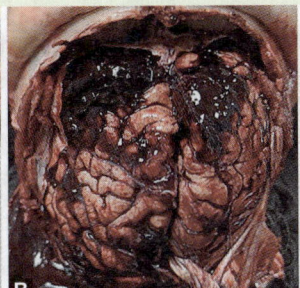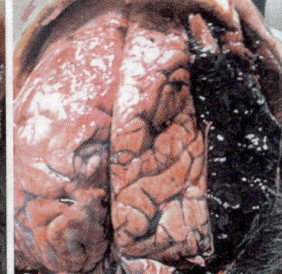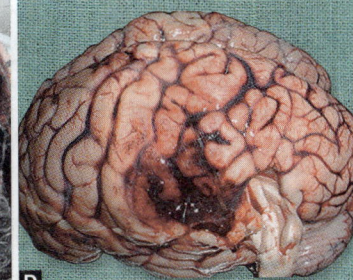

1. Contusion of brain   2. Epidural hematoma   3. Subdural hematoma   4. Subarachnoid hematoma

A. _____   B. _____   C. _____   D. _____

DIFFUSE INJURY TO THE BRAIN

Diffuse axonal injury (DAI) has already been discussed. Ischemic and hypoxic brain damage, and an increase in the volume of all or part of the brain are common pathology seen in autopsy of fatal TBI.

Diffuse Ischemic Injury

- Diffuse ischemia injury can develop as a consequence of increasing cerebral swelling secondary to cardiorespiratory arrest, or as a consequence of profound hypotension due to other injuries, particularly fracture of long bones.
- More common in patients with high intracranial pressure [(ICP), >60 mm Hg is fatal].
- Ischemic damage is another cause of traumatic coma in the absence of an intracranial mass lesion.
- *Histologically*, neuronal ischemic injury can be identified using H&E stain: neuronal nucleus is shrunken and the cytoplasm undergoes eosinophilic change, appearing red.

Diffuse Vascular Injury

- Diffuse vascular injury is caused by the same type of forces that cause DAI, but the force is more severe and produces extensive disruption of neuronal function, so that death occurs before axonal swellings can develop.
- *Autopsy findings*: Contact head injuries may not be apparent. Brain reveals thin SAH and widely scattered petechial hemorrhages. The hemorrhages are prominent in subependymal regions, lateral pons and midbrain, and midline of the hypothalamus and rostral brainstem.

> **NOTA BENE**
>
> **Differential diagnosis of multiple brain petechiae**
> The petechiae of diffuse vascular injury may be confused with vascular congestion which is common and often marked in the brain after fatal TBI.
> - Petechiae in vascular congestion can be identified by its preference for dependent areas of the brain, its localization to the walls of the third ventricle, and its tendency to be absent or inconspicuous in the brainstem.
> - Widespread petechiae are also seen in many non-traumatic conditions including DIC, thrombotic thrombocytopenic purpura, air and fat embolism, and cerebral malaria.

Brain Swelling

- Swelling may be severe enough to raise the ICP and cause death from brain shift, herniation and secondary damage to the brainstem.

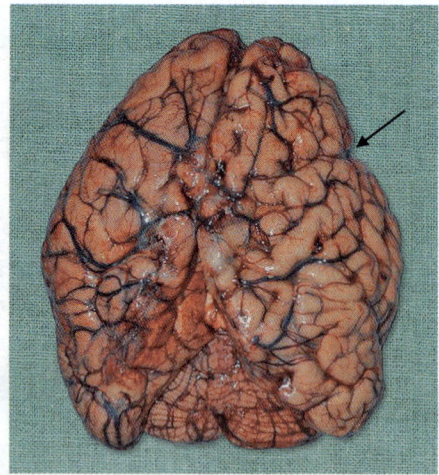

Fig. 13.27: Cerebral edema. Note: compression of the right cerebral hemisphere associated with midline shift to the left (arrow)
(*Courtsey:* Dr Dinesh Fernando, Color Atlas in Forensic Pathology)

- The unmyelinated infant brain with its higher water content more rapidly produces life-threatening cerebral edema.
- *Types*: It can be classified into three types:
  i. Swelling adjacent to contusions (focal).
  ii. Diffuse swelling in one cerebral hemisphere seen in association with ipsilateral acute SDH which becomes evident after surgical removal of the hematoma.
  iii. Diffuse swelling involving both cerebral hemispheres due to global ischemic injury which tends to occur in young patients.
- *Pathogenesis*: It is caused by vasodilation secondary to loss of cerebrovascular autoregulation causing increase in the cerebral blood volume (i.e., congestive) or an increase in water content of the brain tissue (*cerebral edema*).*
- *Features*: Flattening of the surface of the gyri and narrowing, effacement of the sulci causing a smooth, flat outline on the normal undulations of the surface of the cerebral hemisphere (**Fig. 13.27**). Brain swelling also causes narrowness of the cerebral ventricles, and when it is localized, it may cause herniation (**Fig. 13.28**).
- In rare cases, the only intracranial injury identified at autopsy is a markedly swollen brain. The swelling may be diffuse or it may be localized to a single side with an associated 'midline shift' which is referred to as '*malignant cerebral edema*'.

> **NOTA BENE**
>
> - **Cushing ulcer** is one of the complications seen in 50–75% of patients with TBI. It is a form of gastroduodenal stress ulceration similar to *Curling's ulcer* seen in severe burns. The ulcers are usually small and multiple.

---
* Cerebral edema is defined as a pathological increase in the amount of total brain water content leading to an increase in brain volume.

CHAPTER 13 : Regional Injuries

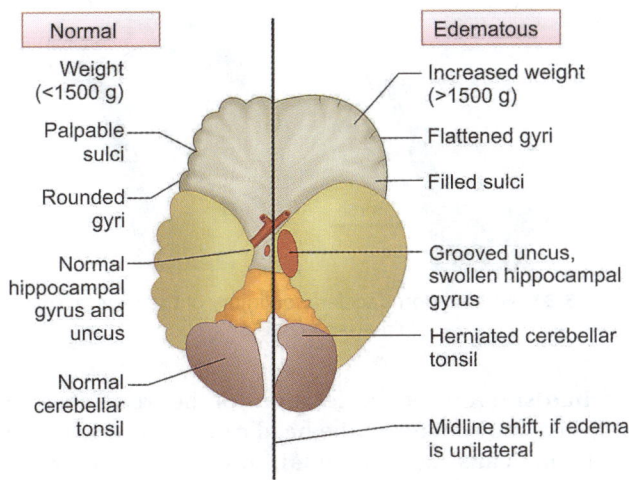

Fig. 13.28: Features of brain swelling

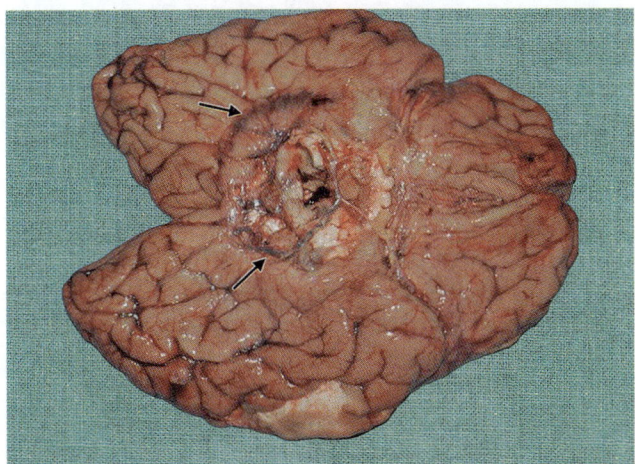

Fig. 13.29: Base of brain showing herniation of the uncus. Note: the hematoma caused by the free margin of the tentorium cerebelli on the hemisphere (arrows)
(*Courtsey:* Dr Dinesh Fernando, Color Atlas in Forensic Pathology)

- **Brain herniation** may extend under the falx cerebri damaging the cingulate gyrus (*subfalcine or supracallosal hernia*), under the tentorium cerebelli damaging the parahippocampal gyrus/medial temporal lobe (*tentorial or uncal hernia*), and through the foramen magnum damaging the tonsil of the cerebellum (*tonsillar hernia*) **(Fig. 13.29)**.
- An intracranial mass lesion is usually associated with a contralateral hemiplegia due to either cortical dysfunction or compression of the ipsilateral cerebral peduncle. However, a supratentorial mass lesion can cause shift of the midbrain to the opposite side. The contralateral cerebral peduncle can then impinge on the tentorium cerbelli, causing the unexpected finding of an ipsilateral hemiplegia. At autopsy, this can be seen as the **Kernohan-Woltman notch** indentating the midbrain **(Fig. 13.30)**. This can be seen in SDH, EDH and cerebral tumors with midline shift. The process explains how clinical signs may appear on the same side of damaged cerebral hemisphere and has been referred to as *false localizing sign*.
- **Duret hemorrhages** are delayed, secondary brainstem hemorrhages (seen in midbrain and pons) **(Fig. 13.30)**. They occur in cranio-cerebral trauma victims with rapidly evolving descending transtentorial herniation. *Diagnosis:* CT head.

NOTA BENE

Evaluation of head injury case
- Initial neurological assessment should evaluate the patient's level of consciousness and symmetry of neurologic function from head to toe. This should include a determination of the patient's GCS, cranial nerve examination that evaluates pupillary function, extraocular movements, facial symmetry, and vital cranial nerve reflexes, as well as motor examination.
- Noncontrast head CT scan.

Surgical management
- Patients with an EDH >30 mL in volume, or EDH in coma (GCS <9) with pupillary asymmetry, or an acute SDH with thickness >10 mm or a midline shift >5 mm on CT should be surgically evacuated.
- A 10 mm thickness and midline shift <5 mm should undergo evacuation, if GCS score decreases since admission.

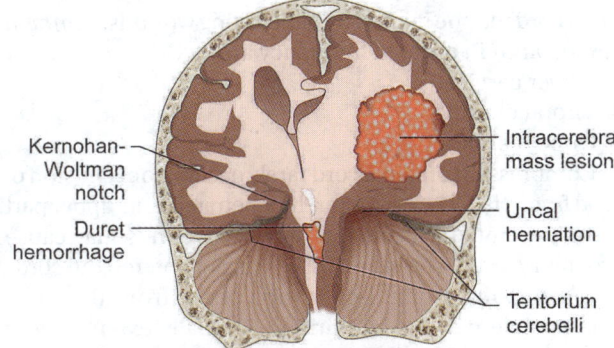

Fig. 13.30: Effect of brain herniation and midline shift

- Patients with parenchymal mass lesions (contusions and intracerebral hematomas) and signs of progressive neurological deterioration due to the lesion or signs of mass effect on CT scan should be treated operatively.
- Patients with GCS scores of 6–8 with frontal or temporal lesions <20 mL in volume with a midline shift of at least 5 mm and/or cisternal compression on CT scan, and patients with any lesion >50 cc in volume should be treated operatively.

FACIAL INJURIES

Facial injuries are also seen along with head injury. However, they are rarely fatal by themselves, unless the victim has asphyxiated from the blood entering into the air passages. The face has many prominences with complex contours such as chin, nose, cheekbones, eyebrows, ears and lips. They may be the first ones to receive the blows directed at the face producing characteristic injuries.
- Eyebrows are injured during falls and blows producing abrasions, lacerations and fractures of the frontal bone and orbital margin.

- Although the cartilaginous part of the nose escapes from being damaged, nasal bone is frequently fractured causing excessive and serious bleeding into the nasal passages, if the victim is unconscious.
- Direct impacts on the face can cause fractures of the mandible and maxilla. This also can cause dangerous bleeding into the air passages. Severe impacts like kicking and road traffic accidents may totally detach the maxilla from the face.
- Injuries to the mouth and lips are very common in physical assaults, including child abuse and wife battering. Punching or kicking on the mouth injures the lips when compressed between the inflicting object and teeth.

FM 3.11, 3.12
- Describe and discuss injuries to the spinal cord.
- Describe and discuss railway spine.

SPINAL CORD

Spinal cord may be injured by penetrating wounds; *common sites involved* in order of frequency are:
- Lower cervical
- Thoracolumbar
- Upper cervical

Compression of spinal cord rarely occurs from effusion of blood from a fall. The cord is rarely penetrated in its upper part by sharp-pointed instruments. Firearm wounds may cause cord injury, even when the missile has not entered the cord.

Contusion of spinal cord may occur from direct or indirect violence. The hemorrhages usually extend in the axis of the cord. Bleeding may occur either into the spinal meninges (*hematorrhachis*) or into the substance of the spinal cord (*hematomyelia*).

Whiplash Injury

- Whiplash injury is an acceleration-deceleration mechanism of energy transfer to the neck that may result in bony and soft injuries.
- Commonly seen in road traffic fatalities, which are due to the hyperextension of the neck. Hyperflexion injuries are less likely but can be caused if heavy weights are dropped onto the bent back of an individual—may be seen in roof collapse.
- This injury is sustained commonly by occupants of the front seat in a motor vehicle.

Causes

- Rear-end or side-impact motor vehicle collisions and sometimes in front impact collisions (**Fig. 13.31**).
- Blow on the chin.
- Blow against the spinous process of upper cervical vertebrae (rabbit punch).

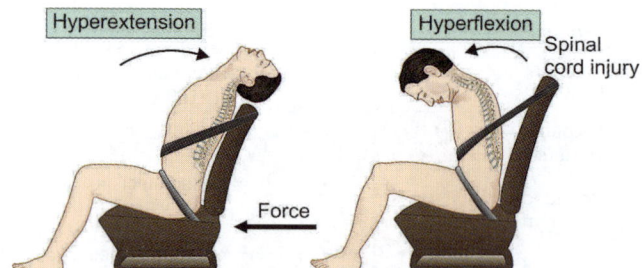

Fig. 13.31: Acceleration-deceleration injury of the cervical spine in rear-end collision

Mechanism: Abrupt accelerations of the trunk causing whip-like movements of the head can occur in rear end collisions causing a maximal, unchecked backward thrusting of the head, followed immediately by a forward rebound (**Fig. 13.31**), if there is no/poorly adjusted head rest. In case of side impact collision, the cervical spine will be forcibly bent in the frontal plane or in an intermediate plane (frontal and sagittal).

Signs and Symptoms

- Pain and/or stiffness of neck and lower back immediately or within 24 h after trauma (*cardinal manifestation*)
- Headache, dizziness, tinnitus, vertigo
- Irritability, nausea and fatigue
- Blurred vision
- Numbness and tingling
- Pain in the arms, legs, feet and hands
- Difficulty in swallowing
- Pain between the shoulder blades
- Concentration and memory problems
- Psychological problems

NOTA BENE

Imaging
- *Plain X-ray*: New degenerative changes may be seen.
- *CT scan*: Rotatory instability with increased rotation at C0–C1 and/or C1–C2.
- *MRI*: Disc herniations, ligamentous lesions at the craniovertebral junction, especially at the alar ligaments and transverse ligaments.

Autopsy Findings

- Facet joint (cervical zygapophysial joint), yellow ligament, uncovertebral and disc/endplate lesions may be seen.
- An area of hemorrhagic discoloration on the surface or in substance of the cord, or subthecal effusions of blood may be found.

Medico-legal aspects: A rising percentage of car accidents result in a refund claim based on whiplash. This is partly due to an increased awareness and documentation, though few false claims cases are also there.

Concussion of Spinal Cord (Railway Spine)

Causes
i. In railway and motor vehicle collisions (most common).
ii. Severe blow to the back.
iii. Compression from dislocation/fracture of vertebrae.
iv. Damage by effusion of blood.
v. Fall from height.
vi. Bullet injury.

Symptoms appear immediately or after some hours and include headache, giddiness, restlessness, sleeplessness, neurasthenia, weakness in limbs, amnesia, loss of sexual power and derangement of special senses.
- It produces paralysis, affecting the arms and hands or bladder, rectum or lower extremities.
- Paralysis is temporary, and recovery occurs in about 48 h.

Describe and discuss injuries to the neck.

NECK

The neck can be the site of many different types of injury. Its importance in forensic medicine is due to the presence of a large number of vital structures, and the fact that it is of a size that can be grasped and easily held.
- Fractures of the hyoid bone or thyroid cartilage may occur due to fall injuring the neck, or when the neck comes in forcible contact with the handlebar of a cycle or the dashboard of a motor car.
- A blow to the side of the head or face, with a resultant abrupt twisting or sideways flexion motion of the neck can result in a laceration of the vertebral artery.
- A blow on the front of the neck may cause unconsciousness or even death due to vagal inhibition or by fracture of the larynx, usually involving the thyroid and cricoid cartilages, and resultant suffocation from hemorrhage or edema of the larynx.
- The mucous membrane of the trachea or larynx may be torn producing surgical emphysema and cause death by asphyxia.
- Suicidal incised wounds are more common than homicidal, but punctured wounds are usually homicidal.
- In wounds of the trachea and of the larynx below the vocal cords, speech is not possible. Wounds of the larynx and trachea are not fatal, if the large blood vessels are not damaged.
- Wounds of the sympathetic and vagus nerves may be fatal, those of the recurrent laryngeal nerves cause aphonia.
- Fractured neck by blunt force can cause spinal cord contusion, laceration or transection. Disruption of the atlanto-occipital junction can result in similar injuries.

VERTEBRAL COLUMN

- The spine is commonly injured in major trauma such as road traffic accidents or falls from a height.
- Force applied to the spine may result in damage to the discs or to the vertebral bodies.
- Fractures of the vertebral column are caused by direct violence or by indirect violence, as by forcible bending of the body or by a fall on buttocks or feet.
- Hyperflexion is the most common mechanism of fracture of spine. Falling from a height, diving and being thrown from automobile are the common causes.
- The *common sites of fracture* are upper and lower cervical regions and the junction of thoracic and lumbar segments. Fracture-dislocation and fracture of the laminae can damage the spinal cord.

Fracture of vertebral bodies: Compression (wedging) of vertebral body is the most common fracture of the thoracic, thoracolumbar or lumbar spine. It may occur with a fall from a height. Injuries to the atlas and axis are more dangerous than lesions in the lower cervical vertebrae, because of involvement of the respiratory center.

Describe and discuss injuries to the chest.

CHEST

Injuries of the chest can be:
- **Non-penetrating or closed,** i.e. they do not open up any part of the thoracic cavity. Usually caused by blunt force.
- **Penetrating or open,** if an injury damages the parietal pleura, it will produce an open pneumothorax, communicating directly with the external air.

Children and young adults whose chest is elastic, may sustain severe injuries to the intrathoracic viscera without fractures of sternum or ribcage.

In some cases, absence of injuries may be due to clothing worn by the victim.

Ribs

Blunt injury may result in fractures of the ribs. The fracture of a few ribs is unlikely to have much effect, other than causing pain in a healthy adult. In children, rib fractures are more resilient and they are able to cope better.
- If compression is front to back, lateral rib fractures may occur, and if back to front, the ribs tend to fracture near the spine.
- If compression is from side to side, the ribs may fracture near the spine and sternum. The middle ribs from 4–8th are usually fractured. In fractures due to direct violence,

the fragments are often driven inwards and lacerate the underlying structures.
- In case of run over by a motor vehicle, the ribs are fractured symmetrically on both sides, in front near the costal cartilages and at the back near the angles.
- Multiple unilateral or bilateral rib fractures give rise to a *flail or 'stove-in' chest*, with consequent paradoxical respiration (the area of chest around the fractures may be seen to move inwards on inspiration) which interferes with respiratory exchange and also with return of the blood to the right atrium, resulting in severe dyspnea. *Flail chest occurs when at least three successive ribs are fractured at two points.*

Sternum: Fractures of the sternum are not common.

Complications of rib fracture: Flail chest, lacerations of intercostal blood vessels with hemothorax, laceration of lungs with pneumothorax or hemopneumothorax, impaling wounds of heart, pleurisy and pneumonia.

Rib fractures can also be *artifactual* due to cardiopulmonary resuscitation, which may result in sternal and parasternal fractures.
- They are usually identified by their symmetrical, parasternal pattern and relative lack of hemorrhage at fracture site which indicates postmortem origin.
- Sometimes, fractures are seen in the left side only and may involve the first six ribs and sternal fracture may occur at the level of third or fourth intercostal space.

LUNGS

- Compression of the chest or blunt weapon trauma produces contusions or lacerations.
- After severe head injury, where victim has been maintained for some time in a respirator, areas of collapse and hemorrhage with the formation of hyaline membrane is seen—*'respirator lung'*.
- A wound of the lung causes frothiness of blood, which issues from the mouth and nose or during coughing.
- Sudden compression of the chest may produce contrecoup contusions due to violent displacement of air in the lungs to the posterior surfaces near the angles of the ribs. The contusions may extend laterally or forwards into the substance of the lungs.
- Stab wounds of the lungs are usually not fatal, unless a major pulmonary blood vessel has been severed.
- *Spontaneous pneumothorax* may occur following rupture of an emphysematous bulla. *Tension pneumothorax* is seen when the leak in pleura has a valve-like action, air is sucked into the chest wall at each inspiration, but cannot escape on expiration. *Iatrogenic pneumothorax* may occur by external cardiac massage, percutaneously introduced subclavian catheters and continuous ventilatory support.

Complications of chest injuries
- Pneumothorax
- Chylothorax
- Hemothorax
- Interstitial emphysema
- Air embolism
- Cardiac tamponade
- Intraparenchymal hemorrhage
- Infection

Diaphragm: Traumatic rupture of diaphragm is seen with blunt trauma of the lower anterior chest and is more common on the left (right side is protected by liver).

HEART

- Contusions and lacerations of the heart may be caused by direct violence to the chest or by compression of the thorax, or when a driver is forcibly thrown against the steering wheel. Cardiac contusions are usually seen on the anterior surface of either ventricle or the interventricular septum. Recent cardiac contusions are dark-red hemorrhagic areas, which are usually subepicardial.
- The commonest pincer lesion is a contusion of the right atrium at the entrance of the inferior vena cava. This is seen in compression injuries. It may cause sudden death, several days after the injury.
- Contrecoup contusions of the heart are seen over the posterior wall of the left ventricle. They are seen in traffic accidents in which the driver is thrown forward against the steering wheel and the heart is compressed against the vertebrae. Contusions may cause sudden death from ventricular fibrillation, or they may cause progressive circulatory failure and death after few hours or days.
- Foreign bodies, e.g., bullet, may remain embedded in the myocardium for years without producing any symptoms.
- The *common sites of traumatic cardiac rupture* in order of diminishing frequency are: right auricle, right ventricle, left auricle, ventricular septum and valves.
- The only *natural cause of rupture of the heart* is softening or thinning by infarction, which invariably occurs in the left ventricle.
- Stab wounds of the heart are dangerous. If the left ventricle is pierced, the thickness of the muscle wall may restrict the bleeding, allowing time for surgical treatment. A stab of the right ventricle is more rapidly fatal, blood escaping through the wound to cause hemopericardium and **cardiac tamponade (Figs. 13.32A and B).** Even 150 mL (average 400–500 mL) of blood can cause death by increasing intrapericardial pressure and producing mechanical interference with ventricular contractility. The right ventricle is more likely to be wounded, as it exposes its widest area towards the front of the chest.

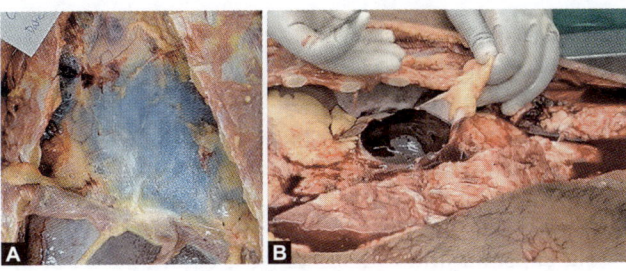

Figs. 13.32A and B: Cardiac tamponade

> **NOTA BENE**
>
> **Cardiac tamponade** presents with three signs (*Beck's triad*). They are—low arterial blood pressure, increased central venous pressure and distant heart sounds. Hypotension occurs because of decreased stroke volume, jugular-venous distension due to impaired venous return to the heart, and muffled heart sounds due to fluid inside the pericardium.

Cardiac concussion or commotio cordis: It refers to sudden cardiac death following a blunt trauma to the chest. It is often associated with sports and in young athletes.

Mechanism: The impact occurs at an electrically vulnerable phase of the cardiac cycle (during early ventricular repolarization; 15–30 msec before the peak of the T wave).

Aorta: Wounds of the aorta or the pulmonary artery are rapidly fatal.
- The rupture of the aorta commonly occurs at the junction of the arch and the descending parts, just beyond the origin of the left subclavian artery, and is due to violent compression of the chest.
- It is common in traffic accidents, and less common in fall from height and crushing chest injuries.
- Spontaneous rupture of the aorta may occur from local disease.

Describe and discuss injuries to the abdomen.

ABDOMEN

Abdominal organs are vulnerable to a variety of injuries from blunt trauma because lax and compressible abdominal walls can transmit the force to the abdominal viscera.

Injuries of the abdomen can be classified into:
- **Non-penetrating or closed**, i.e. peritoneum is intact. It is caused by blunt force; seen in falls, traffic accidents and assault by blunt weapons.
- **Penetrating or open**, i.e. when peritoneum is ruptured, it is open to infections.
  Profuse subcutaneous or deep-seated bleeding of the abdominal wall may track along the muscular and fascial plane to become more diffuse, and may cover a large area of abdominal wall, especially in the lower segment. Blood may track down the inguinal canal and appear in the scrotum or labia.

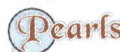

In order of frequency, *the structures most likely to be damaged in blunt abdominal trauma are:* spleen, liver, kidneys, intestines, abdominal wall, mesentery, pancreas and diaphragm.

Injuries of the stomach and intestines may be caused by:
  i. Compression or crushing forces which produce contusions or lacerations.
  ii. Traction or tearing forces.
  iii. Disruption or bursting forces.
- Hollow visceral injuries are less common in blunt trauma compared to penetrating injuries.
- Children have proportionally larger solid organs, less subcutaneous fat, and less protective abdominal musculature than adults. They suffer relatively more solid organ injury from both blunt and penetrating mechanisms.
- Small intestine is more commonly injured by forces of compression than the stomach and the large intestine.
- The proximal jejunum is the commonest site of rupture, followed by the ileum, duodenum, cecum, and large intestine. Transverse colon is usually involved in case of large intestinal rupture.
- The small bowel is most common intra-abdominal organ involved on penetrating trauma (e.g., stab or gunshot wounds) followed by colorectal injury and duodenal and gastric perforations.
- The intestinal wound may be situated at some distance from the external wound due to the compression and mobility of the intestines, and the depth of the wound is greater than the length of the penetrating object.

Pancreas: Wounds of the pancreas are very rare. The pancreas may be injured by compression forces, usually where it overlies the second lumbar vertebra.

Spleen

- Most common organ to be injured in blunt abdominal trauma.
- Penetrating wounds of the spleen are less common than those of liver, but bleeding is more profuse. The spleen may be injured by forces of compression or traction forces. Compression forces produce lacerations. Traction forces may tear the spleen from its pedicle.
- The spleen is ruptured usually in its concave surface (visceral), and is generally associated with injuries to other organs and rib fractures. Lacerations are usually transcapsular and may occur at the hilar or convex surfaces. They are often multiple and may simulate the

alphabetical figures, Y, H or L. Death from rupture of spleen is usually rapid due to profuse hemorrhage.
- A relatively mild trauma or even the contraction of the abdominal muscle may predispose the spleen to rupture, when it is diseased and enlarged, e.g., infectious mononucleosis, malaria, kala-azar or leukemia.

Liver

- It is the *second* most frequently damaged abdominal organ in blunt trauma. The liver is commonly ruptured by motor accidents, blow, kick or by a sudden contraction of the abdominal muscles.
- The liver is more susceptible than spleen to penetrating injury.

Blunt force to the abdomen may produce the following lacerations:
  i. *Transcapsular laceration:* Both capsule and parenchyma are torn, and the laceration is present over the convex surface of the liver. It may cause rapid death from hemorrhage and shock.
  ii. *Subcapsular laceration:* Capsule is intact and injury is beneath the capsule or intraparenchymal, and present over the convex surface of the liver. It may rupture few days after the injury and cause fatal delayed intraperitoneal hemorrhage.
  iii. *Non-communicating or central lacerations* are seen in the substance of the liver.
  iv. *Coronal lacerations* are seen over the superior surface due to distortion.
  v. *Lacerations* of the inferior surface are due to distortion.
  vi. *Contrecoup lacerations* involve the posterior surface of the right lobe, at the point where it rests against the vertebral column.

- The right lobe is five times more commonly affected than the left.
- Convex surface and inferior border are commonly involved.
- Mild degree of external violence may rupture the liver, if it is diseased, e.g., fatty change, abscess formation, malaria or bilharziasis.

> **Complications of abdominal injuries**
> - Laceration of the liver produces slow, but considerable bleeding over a period of time.
> - Laceration of the spleen produces rapid and profuse hemorrhage leading to hypotension.
> - Peritonitis is more common in rupture of the large intestine than with rupture of the small intestine due to the presence of pathogenic organisms in the colon.
> - *Chemical peritonitis* is caused by leakage of gastric contents or pancreatic juice into the peritoneal cavity.
> - Multiple contusions of the intestines may produce paralytic ileus.

KIDNEYS

Injuries to the kidneys are uncommon as they are situated in relatively well-protected part of the body. Contusions and lacerations usually result from blunt force applied directly to the posterior or lateral aspect of the kidneys, such as blows to the loins or in motor vehicle accidents and fall from a height.

- Lacerations of the kidneys may be transcapsular, subcapsular and transrenal (tear extending from the capsule to the renal pelvis). These may cause hemorrhage into the perinephric fat and form a large perirenal hematoma.
- Penetrating wounds are produced by bullets or pointed weapons, usually through the loin, and other viscera are also injured with retroperitoneal hemorrhage.
- *Complications* may be sepsis and the extravasation of urine into the surrounding tissues with the development of urinary fistula.

Bladder

The bladder may be lacerated from a fall, a kick or a blow on the abdomen.

Ruptures are of two types:
  i. **Extraperitoneal:** It occurs when the bladder is empty or contains little urine and lies within the pelvis. It is usually associated with pelvic fractures. The urine may extravasate upwards to the level of the kidneys or downwards along the spermatic cord into the scrotum which may produce cellulitis and death.
  ii. **Intraperitoneal:** It occurs when the bladder is full of urine. Any blunt trauma to the lower abdominal wall can compress the bladder against the sacrum, resulting in rupture due to increased pressure with the urine entering the abdominal cavity.

Stab wounds of the lower abdomen may penetrate the bladder and cause rapid death from hemorrhage. There may be extraperitoneal extravasation of urine.

The male urethra may be ruptured usually under the pubic arch by a kick in the perineum, fall on a projecting substance, fracture of pubic bone or a foreign body. Forcible catheterization or cystoscopy, especially in the presence of some obstruction can cause rupture of urethra from within.

Describe and discuss injuries to the genital organs.

Reproductive Organs

Female genital organs: Contusions and lacerations of the vulva and vagina may be due to kicks during assault or fall on a projecting substance. Wounds of vulva caused by a blunt weapon may resemble incised wounds. Lacerated wounds of the vulva may bleed profusely.

- The non-gravid uterus is usually not injured.
- The gravid uterus may be ruptured by a blow or kick on the abdominal wall, by instrumental criminal abortion, or in obstructed labor. Placenta may separate from uterus causing death of fetus.

Male genital organs
- The penis may be injured by a squeeze or crush, and the engorged erected penis may be completely avulsed from the pubes by forceful pull.
- Accidental injuries are rare, but the penis may be injured or amputated in revenge (bobbitization).*
- Penile strangulation may occur by application of a constricting apparatus around the penis.
- Compression or crushing of the testes may cause sudden death from cardiac inhibition.

FM 3.6, 3.11
- Describe healing of fracture with its medico-legal importance.
- Describe and discuss injuries to the limbs and skeleton.

BONES AND JOINTS

Fractures may occur from falls, blows or by muscular hyperactivity.
- In **simple or closed fracture,** there is no communication between the bone and the air. A fall on the outstretched hand will cause Colles fracture (fracture of the distal end of radius).
- In **compound or open fracture,** there is a communication between the bone and the air through a wound.
- **Comminuted fractures:** The bone breaks into fragments which may impact into each other or separate and become displaced.
- **Partial or green-stick fractures:** These occur because bones in children are very flexible and bend or partially break, instead of breaking cleanly when overloaded. There may be discontinuity in one cortex of the bone, but not in the other.
- In childhood, slipping of an epiphysis is common, e.g., in distal end of the radius, medial epicondyle of the humerus, capitulum and distal end of the tibia.
- Fracture at the neck of the fifth metacarpal bone occurs, usually by striking the closed hand (fist) against a firm surface **(boxer's/brawler's fracture).**

NOTA BENE
- Fractures of the mandible, maxilla, zygoma and zygomatic arch are produced by assaults and motor vehicle accidents.
- The frequency of fracture of different parts of mandible in decreasing order is: condyle (36%), body (21%), angle (20%), parasymphyseal (14%), alveolar (3%), ramus (3%), coronoid (2%) and symphysis (1%).

- Maxillary fractures can be divided into five categories:
  i. *Dentoalveolar*: Separation of fragment of maxilla containing number of teeth.
  ii. *LeFort I*: Transverse fracture of maxilla, above the apices of the teeth, through nasal septum and maxillary sinuses, the palatine bone and the sphenoid bone.
  iii. *LeFort II*: Fracture has same track posteriorly, anteriorly it curves upwards near the zygomatic-maxillary suture, through the inferior orbit rim onto the orbital floor, across the nasal bones and septum.
  iv. *LeFort III*: High transverse fracture of the maxilla that goes through the nasofrontal suture, through the medial orbital wall and fronto-zygomatic suture, across the arch and through the sphenoid.
  v. *Sagittal*: Fracture line runs through a sagittal plane through the maxilla.

Direct Fractures

Fracture of the extremities caused by **direct application of force (Fig. 13.33)**:
  i. *Penetrating fractures* are caused by large force acting on a small area; seen in gunshot wounds.
  ii. *Focal fractures* are *transverse* fractures results from a small force applied over a small area. It is usually seen in the forearms produced by weapons, like rods, when the person tries to ward off blows. Overlying soft tissue injury is relatively minor.
  iii. *Crush fractures* result from large force applied over a large area with extensive soft tissue injuries and often *comminuted fractures* of the bone. Mostly seen on the legs in motor vehicle-pedestrian accidents.

Indirect Fractures

Indirect fractures result from force acting at a distance from the site of fracture, e.g., a fracture of the head of the radius or of the lower end of the humerus caused by a fall on the extended palm.

Classification (Fig. 13.33)
  i. *Avulsion or distraction fracture:* In this, the bone is pulled apart by traction, e.g., transverse fracture of patella due to violent contraction of the quadriceps muscle.
  ii. *Spiral fracture:* The bone is twisted and a spiral fracture is produced. It occurs only when the bone is subjected to torsional force.
  iii. *Vertical compression fracture* produces an oblique fracture of the body of long bones with the hard shaft driven into the cancellous end.
  iv. *In angulation and compression fracture*, the fracture line is oblique.
  v. *Angulation, rotation and compression fracture* causes fracture with a triangular butterfly fragment.

---

* To remove/cut off someone's penis; usually out of rage (after Lorena Bobbit who cut off her husband's penis in 1994).

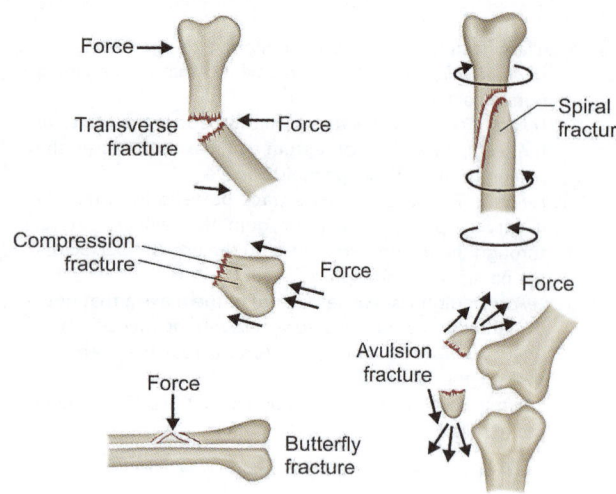

Fig. 13.33: Classification of fracture

TABLE 13.5: Estimation of age of skull fractures

Features	Age (weeks)
Edges stick together	1
Calcification of inner table and rounding of sharp edges	2
Bands of osseous tissue running across	3–4

TABLE 13.6: Estimation of age of tooth dislocation

Features	Age
Bleeding stops from its socket, edges sharp and feathered	1–2 days
Clot obliterated by fibrous tissue	14 days
Socket completely filled with new bone (as seen on X-ray)	1 year

Complications of fracture
- Shock
- Hemorrhage
- Infection
- Crush syndrome
- Fat embolism
- Venous thrombosis with pulmonary embolism

NOTA BENE
- Teeth most often affected by trauma in order of decreased frequency: Maxillary central incisors (60%), maxillary lateral incisors (22%), mandibular central incisors and mandibular lateral incisors.
- In permanent dentition, tooth fractures result from trauma whereas dislocation is common in primary dentition (due to elastic structures of the alveolar process).

Pelvic fractures

Classified by the direction of force:
i. Anterior-posterior compression: 'Open-book' pelvic fracture (diastasis and/or fracture of the pubic rami with posterior pelvic disruption of the sacroiliac joint) may be seen.
ii. Lateral compression.
iii. Shear.
iv. Complex fractures.

Healing of Fracture

- Fractures of cancellous bone unite faster than those of cortical bone.
- In children, a callus (osteogenic granulation tissue) is visible on X-ray within 2 weeks of fracture, and the bone is consolidated in 4–6 weeks, though it takes 2–3 months to solidly. In adults, callus formation is visible on X-ray by about 3 weeks, consolidation takes about 3 months, and for femur it may take 4–5 months.
- *Histologically*, signs of clot organization are seen in about 48 h, the formation of osteoid matrix in about 3 days and formation of soft callus by about 1 week.
- In comminuted fractures, where edges are not in apposition, bone formation does not occur. The gap is filled by fibrous tissue in 1–3 months depending on the size of the gap. The fracture line remains permanently visible on X-ray.
- Age of skull fracture can be estimated as given in **Table 13.5**.
- In case of fracture of the skull, healing occurs without formation of a visible callus, because the injured periosteal vessels impede the formation of an external callus.
- In case of tooth being knocked out, age is estimated as given in **Table 13.6**.

At autopsy, a fracture may be suspected when there is extensive swelling and discoloration of the skin, or when there is abnormal mobility or crepitus is found. The tissues surrounding a suspected fracture should be dissected to determine injuries to the soft parts.

Antemortem or Postmortem Fracture

- Fracture produced just before death or just after death will have similar characteristics, except in the former there may be comparatively greater effusion of blood which will infiltrate the surrounding tissues.
- Antemortem fracture few hours prior to death will show edema and active cellular infiltration into the adjacent tissues and between the fractured edges of the bones.
- Antemortem fracture of long bones may result in fat emboli traveling to distant parts of the body producing characteristic lesions (punctate hemorrhages in skin, eyelids, conjunctiva) which are seen grossly and microscopically.

These changes are *not seen* in postmortem fractures.

CHAPTER 13 : Regional Injuries

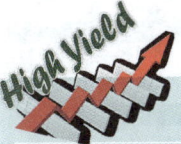

- **Closed head injury (non-penetrating):** Damage to the brain *without any fracture of skull and/or penetration of dura*; most often results from blunt trauma.
- **Open head injury (penetrating):** Disruption of cranial vault with exposure of damaged brain; most often associated missile wounds, RTAs or occupational accidents.
- **Focal lesions:** Scalp lacerations, skull fractures, contusions/lacerations and intracranial hemorrhage.
- **Diffuse lesions:** Axonal injury, ischemic injury, vascular injury, brain swelling.
- **Black eye** *(periorbital or spectacle hematoma/raccoon eyes):* Seen in fracture of anterior cranial fossa.
- **Battle's sign:** Mastoid ecchymosis associated with fracture of middle cranial fossa (basilar fracture).
- Fracture of middle cranial fossa causes injury to VII and VIII cranial nerves.
- Fall from a height on feet or buttocks may cause ring fracture.
- CSF rhinorrhea is due to fracture of cribriform plate.
- CSF otorrhea is due to fracture of petrous temporal bone.
- Concussion resembles drunkenness.
- Unconsciousness immediately following head injury is due to concussion.
- **Characteristic histological finding in DAI:** Axonal swellings *('retraction bulbs')* in the internal capsule, corpus callosum and superior cerebellar peduncle.
- **Most sensitive technique to diagnose DAI:** Immunohistochemistry [staining β-amyloid precursor protein (BAPP)]
- Coup contusions are wedge-shaped contusion.
- *Plaque jaune* are old contusions seen in chronic alcoholics.
- **Commonest cause of EDH:** Rupture of middle meningeal artery.
- **Commonest cause of SDH:** Rupture of cortical bridging veins.
- Artifactual EDH is seen in burns associated with heat-induced PM skull fractures.
- **Commonest cause of thunderclap headache:** SAH.
- **Commonest hemorrhage following head injury:** SDH.
- **Most common cause of intracerebral hemorrhage:** Hypertension.
- **Most common location of hypertensive intracranial hemorrhage is:** Basal ganglia.
- **Investigation of choice for evaluation of acute head injury:** Non-contrast CT scan.
- **Diagnosis of EDH:** CT scan (biconvex lenticular-shaped).
- **Diagnosis of SDH:** CT scan (crescentic opacity).
- **Diagnosis of SAH:** CT scan (hyperdense blood collections along the falx and basilar cisterns).
- **Cushing ulcer:** Form of gastroduodenal stress ulceration; seen in patients with TBI.
- **Duret hemorrhages:** Delayed, secondary brainstem hemorrhages, seen in patients with TBI.
- **Lucid/latent interval:** State of consciousness between two episodes of unconsciousness. Seen in EDH and SDH. Also seen in insanity.
- **Kernohan-Woltman sign (notch) is seen in** uncal herniation.
- **Whiplash injury:** Acceleration-deceleration injury due to the hyperextension of neck. Seen in RTAs.
- **Concussion of spinal cord (railway spine):** Seen in railway and motor vehicle collisions *(most common)*.
- **Flail chest** occurs when three successive ribs are fractured at two points separating a segment.
- **Contrecoupe injury** is seen in brain, heart, liver and lungs.
- **Minimum amount of blood causing cardiac tamponade:** 150 mL.
- Rupture of aorta occurs at junction of arch and descending parts, just beyond the origin of left subclavian artery; common in RTAs.
- **Most common site of spontaneous cardiac rupture:** Left ventricle (softening due to infarction).
- **Most common site of traumatic cardiac rupture:** Right auricle.

- Most common organ injured in blunt abdominal trauma: Spleen (not the liver).
- Most common organ injured in penetrating injury: Liver.
- Most common site of splenic rupture: Concave surface.
- Alphabetic lacerations are seen in spleen.
- **Boxer's/brawler's fracture:** Fracture at the neck of the fifth metacarpal bone occurs, usually by striking the fist against a firm surface.
- LeFort's fracture does not involve the mandible.
- **Most common site of mandible fracture:** Condyle.

Skull fracture	Characteristic feature
Fissure/linear fracture	Linear cracks without any depression of bone fragments. *Most common.*
Depressed fracture	Portion of fractured bone is driven inwards (**signature fracture**).
Pond/ping-pong fracture	In-buckling of skull without fracture and without any damage to the brain, seen in *infants and children.*
Comminuted/spider web fracture	Two or more intersecting lines of fracture divide the bone into three or more fragments.
Gutter fracture	Part of bone is removed so as to form a gutter.
Ring fracture	Fissure fracture that encircles foramen magnum.
Diastasis/sutural fracture	Fracture line passes through sutures; seen in *young children.*
Blow-out fracture	Fracture of orbital walls—medial wall and/or orbital floor (**teardrop sign**).
Hinge/motorcyclists fracture	Fracture of base of skull that completely splits it ('**nodding face' sign**).

Hemorrhage	Most common etiology	Source of bleeding
EDH	Trauma (associated skull fracture)	Arterial (Middle meningeal artery)
SDH	Trauma	Venous (Bridging veins)
SAH	Aneurysm rupture	Arterial (Berry aneurysm)
ICH	Hypertension	Arterial (Lenticulostriate artery)

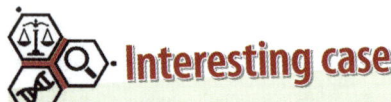

Subdural Hemorrhage (Case of Hrithik Roshan, 2013)

Superstar Hrithik Roshan suffered a traumatic brain injury on the sets of his movie *Bang Bang* while performing a stunt in Phuket. The actor started experiencing headaches soon after the accident. He was given painkillers as initial CT scan did not show a clot.

After a month, the actor was unable to move his legs and hands in a coordinated manner on treadmill or sign properly; complained of severe headache and developed weakness in the right arm and hand. CT scan and MRI done after 2 months revealed left sided subdural hematoma. He successfully underwent a surgery to remove the clot.

He must have had an impact on the left skull which did not result in skull fracture or frank bleeding, but might have produced a small tear in one of the veins. Blood started oozing out of it slowly and started pushing the brain inside, leading to weakness on his right arms and hand.

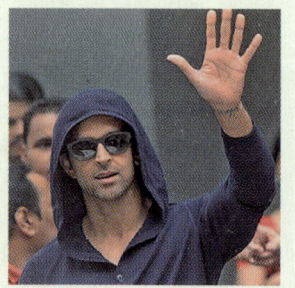

CHAPTER 14: Thermal Injuries

LEARNING OBJECTIVES

Must know
1. Hypothermia, clinical features and postmortem findings
2. Frost bite, trench foot (immersion syndrome)
3. Heat cramps, heat stroke, heat syncope
4. Burns, types, rule of nine, classification, cause of death, postmortem changes
5. Pugilistic attitude
6. Scalds, classification, features
7. Joule burn, crocodile skin, current pearls, wax drippings
8. Arborescent marks (Litchenberg's flowers)
9. Antemortem and postmortem burns (Diff.)
10. Pugilistic attitude and rigor mortis (Diff.)
11. Dry heat, moist heat and chemicals burns (Diff.)

Desirable to know
1. Paradoxical undressing
2. 'Hide and die' syndrome
3. Chilblains
4. Heat exhaustion
5. Heat hematoma
6. Heat ruptures
7. Epidural hematoma due to burns and blunt force (Diff.)
8. Judicial electrocution

FM 2.24
Describe the clinical features, postmortem finding and medico-legal aspects of injuries due to physical agents like cold—systemic and localized hypothermia, frostbite, trench foot, immersion foot.

Definition: Thermal injury is tissue injury due to application of heat or cold in any form to the external or the internal body surfaces.

Classification: Refer to **Flowchart 14.1**.

Flowchart 14.1: Classification of thermal injuries

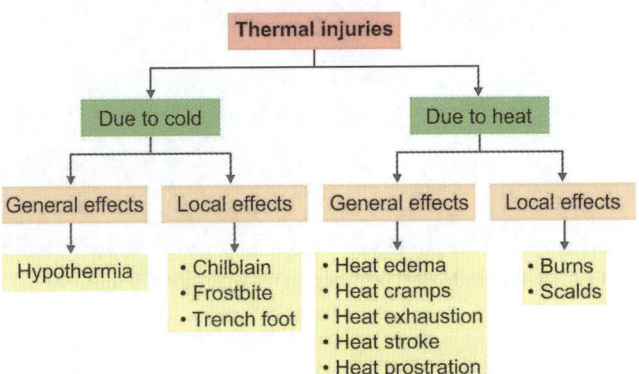

COLD INJURY

Hypothermia

- Exposure to cold produce hypothermia which is defined as core temperature below 35°C (95°F).
- It is classified into mild (35–32°C), moderate (32–30°C) and severe (<30°C).
- An esophageal or rectal probe that measures temperatures as low as 25°C is required; oral or axillary thermometers are inaccurate.
- Risk factors:
  - Low environmental temperature.
  - Extremes of age (infants, children and elderly ≥60 years).
  - Immersion in water, and wet clothing.
  - Pre-existing diseases, such as hypothyroidism, atherosclerosis, dementia, or inadequate nutrition.
  - Intoxicated persons (alcohol, tranquilizers or opiates) or persons engaged in activities like mountaineering and sailing.
- Effects of hypothermia:
  - Direct effects are prominent in fatty tissues and myelinated nerve fibers.
  - Indirect effects are mostly ischemic.

Clinical Features

- When the temperature falls below 32°C to 24°C, there is disorientation, dulling of consciousness, loss of reflex, and fall in respiration, heart rate and blood pressure.
- Red patches and pallor of the skin, edema of the face, and stiffness of neck muscles may be seen.

Death is common due to ventricular fibrillation or asystole.

Complications: Patient who survives for a short time may develop hemorrhagic pancreatitis, pneumonia, ulcers or focal hemorrhages in the GIT, acute tubular necrosis and myocardial fiber necrosis.

Postmortem Examination

There are no definitive autopsy findings of hypothermia. However, there are several features which are taken together, and in the presence of history (scene and circumstances) allow a reasonably confident diagnosis.

External Findings

- Patches of pink to brownish-pink discoloration may be seen on the external surface, most often present over the extensor surfaces of large joints (usually on knees, elbows or outside of the hip joint).
- Postmortem staining is pink/bright red due to antemortem binding of oxygen to hemoglobin and its postmortem diffusion through skin.
- The extremities may be cyanosed or white (*white deaths*).
- Edema of feet and blistering of skin may be seen.

Internal Findings

- *Blood*: Bright red in color.
- *Trachea*: Frothy and sanguineous fluid.
- *Lungs*: Congested, edematous and shows hemorrhages.
- *Heart*: Dilatation of right atrium and ventricle.
- *Stomach*: **Wischnewsky spots*** may be seen.
- *Kidneys*: Acute tubular necrosis with accumulation of lipid in epithelial cells of proximal renal tubules.
- *Liver and spleen*: Congested. Fatty changes in liver and contracted spleen.
- *Muscles*: Hemorrhages into core muscles like iliopsoas.
- *Pancreas*: Hemorrhages in parenchyma and mucosa of the pancreatic duct.
- *Intestines*: Ulceration of the colon and ileum, and hemorrhagic infarction of the colon.

Moreover, the autopsy is helpful to rule out other causes of death, collect evidence as necessary and contribute to the identification process.

Viscera should be sent for blood alcohol and toxicological analysis.

NOTA BENE

- **Paradoxical undressing:** In deaths due to hypothermia, the body is found either partially or fully undressed (**Fig. 14.1**). During hypothermia, the victim becomes disoriented, confused and combative, and may begin discarding the clothing he/she is wearing, which in turn increases the rate of temperature loss. This sometimes results in the assumption that the deaths are associated with sexual assault (homicide).
- **'Hide and die' syndrome:** In some hypothermic deaths, bodies are found in some strange places—under a bed or bench, on a shelf or behind a wardrobe, or alternatively may pull down household articles into a heap on top, which may give the impression of their attempt to 'hide' (protective '*burrow-like*' or '*cave-like*' situation). This may also lead to the assumption of a homicide or robbery. It is due to mental confusion from hypothermia and may be related to hibernation reflex.

Cold or freezing temperature can produce localized effects, e.g., chilblain, trench foot/immersion foot and frostbite, which are phases of the same process.

Chilblains (Erythema Pernio)

These are red, itching, skin lesions, usually in the extremities, caused by exposure to cold. They may be associated with edema and blistering, and are aggravated by warmth. On continued exposure, ulcerative or hemorrhagic lesions may develop.

Treatment: Elevation of the affected part and allowing it to warm gradually at room temperature. The areas should not be rubbed or massaged or subjected to heat application.

Immersion Syndrome (Trench/Immersion Foot)

- Immersion foot, trench foot and trench hand are types of immersion syndrome injuries.

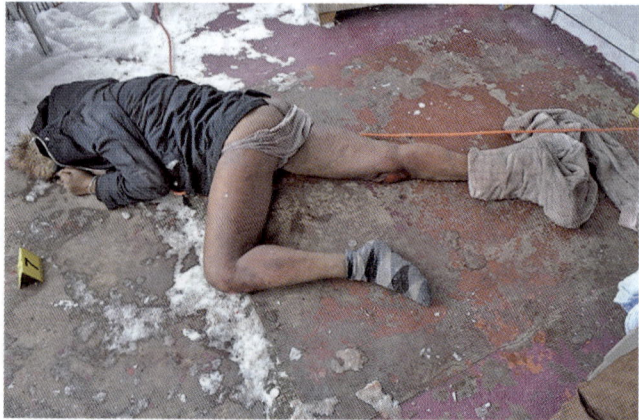

Fig. 14.1: Paradoxical undressing in hypothermia mimicking sexual assault

---

* Wischnewsky spots are blackish-brownish color gastric mucosal erosions/ulcerations seen in hypothermia (vary from 1 mm to 2 cm in size and from few to >100). Similar changes are seen in drug/alcohol abuse and in stress/shock.

- Immersion foot/hand results from prolonged exposure to severe cold (<10°C) and dampness; seen in soldiers during warfare, especially in trenches, and in persons exposed to prolonged immersion or exposure at sea.
- Extremities are affected in these conditions.

Clinically, it is divided into:
  i. **Pre-hyperemic stage:** The affected parts are cold and anesthetic.
  ii. **Hyperemic stage:** The parts are hot with intense burning and shooting pains.
  iii. **Post-hyperemic stage:** Area is pale or cyanotic with diminished pulsations.

Treatment: Air drying, protecting the extremities from trauma and secondary infection, and gradual rewarming by exposure to air at room temperature (not heat) without massaging or moistening the skin or immersing it in water.

> **NOTA BENE**
> - **Warm water immersion foot:** Exposure of the feet to warm, wet conditions for ≥48 h may cause maceration, blanching, and wrinkling of the soles and sides of the feet. Itching and burning with swelling may persists for a few days.
> - **Tropical immersion foot** is seen after continuous immersion of feet in water or mud (temperature >22°C) for 2–10 days. This was known as 'paddy foot' in Vietnam. Symptoms are erythema, edema, pain of dorsal feet, fever and adenopathy.

Frostbite

- Frostbite (*congelatio*) is injury due to freezing and formation of ice crystals and obstruction of blood supply within tissues.
- It occurs due to exposure to great extremes of cold (≤−2.5°C).
- This is typically evident as blue-black discoloration of fingers, toes or other susceptible body parts such as the nose, ears and face **(Fig. 14.2)**.
- In **mild** cases, only the skin and subcutaneous tissues are involved, and symptoms are numbness, prickling and itching.
- **Deep** frostbite involves deeper structures, and there may be paresthesia and stiffness. Thawing causes tenderness

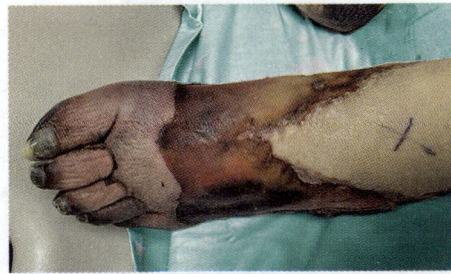

Fig. 14.2: Frostbite of the toes. The patient survived for few days before dying

and burning pain. The skin is white or yellow, looses its elasticity and becomes immobile. Edema, blisters, necrosis and gangrene may appear beyond the line of inflammatory demarcation.
- Frostbite is only produced during life and cannot be caused postmortem.

Treatment
  i. *Rewarming*: For superficial frostbite (frostnip): Firm steady pressure is applied with warm hand (without rubbing), by placing fingers in the armpits; and for the feet, by covering with dry socks.
  For deep frostbite: Frozen extremity is immersed for several minutes in a moving water bath, heated to 40–42°C, until the distal tip of the part being thawed, flushes.
  ii. *Protection of the part*: Pressure or friction is avoided and physical therapy contraindicated in the early stage.
  iii. *Anti-infective measures*: Tetanus prophylaxis and antibiotics for deep infection are given.

> **FM 2.24**
> Describe the clinical features, postmortem finding and medico-legal aspects of injuries due to physical agents like heat—heat cramps (miner's cramp), heat exhaustion, heat stroke (sun stroke/heat hyperpyrexia), heat prostration.

HEAT INJURY

> **NOTA BENE**
> **Heat edema:** Mildest form of heat illness which manifests as dependent soft tissue swelling (typically involves the lower extremities).
> - Commonly seen in sailors who roam on hot decks to kill time (*deck ankles*).
> - There is peripheral vasodilatation with pooling of interstitial fluid into the third space.
> - *Clinical features:* Swelling or puffiness of the tissues with shoes getting tight, stretched or shiny skin.
> - *Treatment:* Elevation of leg and proper acclimatization.

Heat Cramps (Miner's/Stoker's/Fireman's Cramps)

- They are due to fluid and electrolyte depletion.
- It usually occur in workers in high temperature when sweating has been profuse.
- Cramping results from dilutional hyponatremia, as sweat losses are replaced with water alone.
- There is a history of vigorous activity just preceding the onset of symptoms.

Clinical features
Onset is sudden.
- Severe and painful paroxysmal skeletal muscle contractions ('cramps') and severe muscle spasms

lasting 1–3 min, usually of the muscles most used (arms, legs and abdomen) occur. Involved muscle groups are tender, hard and lumpy.
- Face is flushed, pupils dilated, and patient complains of dizziness, tinnitus, headache and vomiting.
- Skin is moist and cool.
- Body temperature may be normal or slightly increased.

Treatment: Patient should be moved into a cool environment and given oral saline solution to replace both salt and water, and advised rest for 1–3 days.

Heat Exhaustion

- It results from prolonged strenuous activity with inadequate water or salt intake in a hot environment.
- Heat exhaustion is characterized by dehydration, sodium depletion or isotonic fluid loss with accompanying cardiovascular changes.
- Symptoms associated with heat syncope and heat cramps may be present. If untreated, it may progress to heat stroke (Fig. 14.3).

Clinical features
- Nausea, vomiting, malaise and myalgia may occur.
- The patient may be quite thirsty and weak with CNS symptoms, such as headache, dizziness, fatigue.
- In cases due chiefly to water depletion—anxiety, paresthesias, impaired judgment, hysteria and occasionally psychosis.

Diagnosis: Prolonged symptoms, rectal temperature >37.8°C (but ≤40°C), increased pulse and moist skin.

Treatment: Patient is treated in a cool environment, adequate hydration (1–2 liters over 2–4 h), oral salt replenishment and active cooling (fans, ice packs). Normal saline or isotonic glucose solution should be administered IV, if necessary.

HEAT STROKE/HEAT HYPERPYREXIA

- Heat stroke is a life-threatening medical emergency resulting from failure of the thermoregulatory mechanism.
- It is characterized by cerebral dysfunction with impaired consciousness, hyperthermia (rectal temperature >40°C) and anhydrosis (absence of sweating).
- The term *thermic fever or sun stroke* is used when there has been direct exposure to the sun.

Classification

Heat stroke presents in one of the two forms:
1. **Classic:** Seen in patients with compromised homeostatic mechanisms.
2. **Exertional:** Seen in healthy persons undergoing strenuous exertion in a thermally stressful environment.

Predisposing Factors

- *Environmental causes:* High temperature, increased humidity, lack of acclimatization and physical exertion.
- *Non-environmental causes:* Extremes of age (infants, and elderly ≥65 years), obesity, alcoholism, brain hemorrhage, malignant hyperthermia, chronically infirm, underlying medical conditions like thyrotoxicosis or sepsis, salicylate overdose, patients receiving medications like anticholinergics, antihistamines or phenothiazines, and reactions to certain drugs of abuse such as cocaine.

Clinical Features (Fig. 14.4)

Onset is sudden, with sudden collapse and loss of consciousness.
- *Prodromal symptoms* include dizziness, weakness, nausea, vomiting, confusion, faintness, staggering gait, purposeless movements, disorientation, drowsiness and irrational behavior.

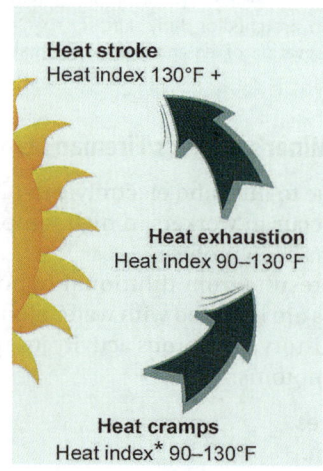

Fig. 14.3: Progression of heat illnesses.

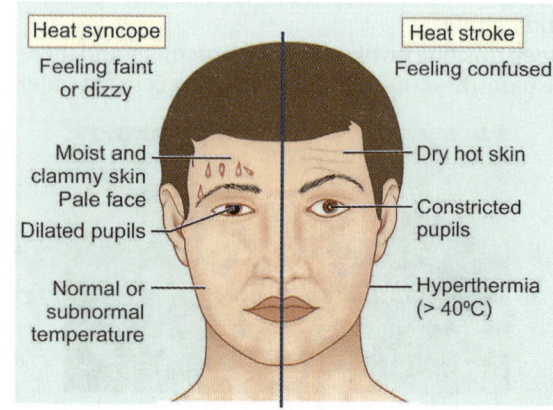

Fig. 14.4: Difference between heat syncope and heat stroke

---
* Heat index (apparent temperature) is what the temperature feels like to human body when relative humidity is combined with the air temperature.

- Skin is hot, and initially covered with perspiration, later it dries. Pulse is strong initially (160–180/min).
- Tachycardia and hyperventilation (with subsequent respiratory alkalosis) occur.
- Blood pressure may be elevated in early stages, but later hypotension develops.
- The core temperature is usually >40°C.
- Pupils are constricted.
- Delirium, blurred vision, convulsions, collapse and unconsciousness occur.

Morbidity or even death can result from cerebral, cardiovascular, hepatic or renal damage.

Treatment

Immediate measures should be taken to lower the core temperature (Fig. 14.5).
  i. The patient is unclothed to the minimum and sprayed with water (20°C) while air is passed across the patient's body. Immersion in an ice-water bath is very effective. Treatment should be continued until the rectal temperature drops to 39°C.
  ii. Chlorpromazine (25–50 mg IV) or diazepam (5–10 mg IV) is given every 4 hourly to control shivering.
  iii. Fluid administration to ensure high urinary output (>50 mL/h), mannitol administration (0.25 mg/kg) and alkalinization of urine (IV bicarbonate administration, 250 mL of 4%) are recommended.

Complications: Patients who survive >24 h may show lobar pneumonia, acute tubular necrosis of kidneys, hepatic necrosis, myocardial fiber necrosis, disseminated intravascular coagulation, pancreatitis, adrenal hemorrhage and myoglobinuria (due to rhabdomyolysis).

Postmortem Findings

Deaths related to hyperthermia have no specific autopsy findings. When the body temperature is not available, but the circumstances of the death suggest hyperthermia, then it can be listed as the cause of death.

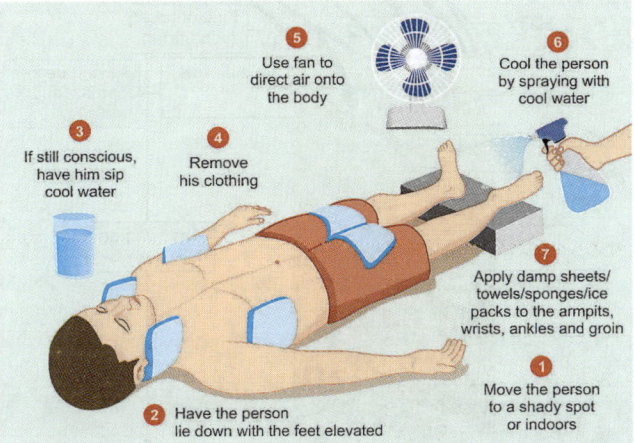

Fig. 14.5: Emergency treatment in case of a victim of heat stroke

External: Early occurrence and rapid development of postmortem changes (due to high body temperature).

Internal
  i. **Lungs:** Congested and edematous. Intrathoracic petechiae may be present, particularly in infants and children.
  ii. **Heart:** Right sided cardiac dilation. Subendocardial hemorrhages in the left ventricle may be seen.
  iii. **Brain:** Congested and edematous. Convolutions are flattened, and scattered petechiae are found in the walls of the third ventricle and floor of the fourth ventricle.

NOTA BENE

In *brain*, nonspecific degenerative changes in cortical neurons may be visible in light microscopy in individual who survives for some period. There may also be marked changes in the cerebellum, including necrosis of Purkinje cells (which appear dense, red and eosinophilic) and a marked decrease in the number of Purkinje cells.

Medico-legal aspects: Deaths are usually accidental. Postmortem is done to rule out any other cause of death or contributory cause of death.

Heat Prostration (Heat Syncope/Collapse)

- It results from salt depletion and dehydration due to excess of sweating and cutaneous vasodilation with consequent systemic and cerebral hypotension, but without any rise of temperature, despite exposure to excessive heat.
- The condition is usually seen in the tropics and deserts.
- **Precipitating factors** are overexertion, heavy muscular work and use of unsuitable clothing.

Clinical features (Fig. 14.4)
- Patient suddenly feels weak, giddy and sick.
- Nausea, dizziness, flushing of face, throbbing headache in temples, dimness of vision may occur.
- Face is pale, pulse is weak and feeble, respiration sighing, skin cool and moist, and temperature sub-normal.
- Systolic BP is usually <100 mm Hg.

Patient usually recovers and consciousness is never lost.

Treatment consists of rest and recumbency in a cool place and rehydration by mouth (or IV, if necessary).

NOTA BENE

Anhidrotic heat exhaustion (*tropical anhidrotic asthenia or thermogenic anhidrosis*): It is characterized by depression of sweating, exhaustion and vesicular skin lesions on the trunk (*miliaria profunda*). The illness can occur in newcomers or even in normal acclimatized persons on prolonged exposure to heat. It involves failure of the normal sweat mechanism due to occlusion of the sweat ducts. There is tachycardia, tachypnea, mild pyrexia, anhidrosis and polyuria. The patient is shifted to cool surroundings and recovery is generally rapid. This syndrome must be differentiated from heat stroke and heat exhaustion, and malingering should be ruled out.

Describe types of injuries, clinical features, pathophysiology, postmortem findings and medico-legal aspects in cases of burns.

BURNS

Definition: Burn is an injury caused by heat, or by a chemical or physical agent having an effect similar to heat.

Characteristics/Types of Burns

i. *Contact burns:* There is physical contact between the body and a hot object, like heated solid or molten metal. When applied momentarily, it produces a blister with erythema corresponding to the shape and size of the agent.

ii. *Flame burns:* There is actual contact of body with flame. It may produce vesication, singeing of the hair and blackening of the skin.

   Flash burns are a variant of flame burns which are due to initial ignition from flash fires (sudden ignition or explosion of gases or petrochemicals). It burns the exposed surfaces to the flash, and not the folds of skin and other protected areas.

iii. *Scalds:* They are caused by contact with hot liquids, most commonly water, and usually occur on exposed skin.

iv. *Radiant heat burns:* They are caused by heat waves, a type of electromagnetic wave. There is no contact between the body and flame or hot surface. Initially, the skin appears erythematous and blistered, and later it is light brown and leathery.

v. *Ionizing radiation burns* (X-rays, radium, UV rays): It can be localized or may involve the whole body depending on radiation exposure. The burn varies from redness of skin to dermatitis with shedding of hair and epidermis, and pigmentation of the surrounding skin. Fingernails may show degenerative changes and wart-like growth.

vi. *Chemical burns*: Classified into acids, alkalis and vesicants (blister forming). Characteristically, there are ulcerated patches, no blisters, hair is not singed and the red line of demarcation is absent. Sometimes, the burn shows distinct coloration, and is usually uniform in character.

vii. *Electric and lightning burns.*

viii. *Microwave burns:* The waves create heat through molecular agitation. The greater the water content of a particular tissue, the greater the heat produced, e.g., muscle tends to be heated more than fat. Burns caused by microwave ovens tend to be indirect, like the person ingests liquid without realizing how hot it is. Medico-legal implications are rare.

- Most burns are produced by dry heat, and result from contact with a flame or a heated solid object or exposure to radiant heat of an object.
- The majority of burns in children are scalds caused by accidents, and most electrical and chemical injuries occur in adults.
- Cold and radiation are very rare cases of burns.

Classification

Burns can be classified in many ways, but two classifications are given in **Table 14.1 (Fig. 14.6)**.

Other types of classification: Heba's (similar to Wilson's, but uses the symbol of degree); and *Evan's* which categorizes burns into superficial, partial and full thickness.

Clinically, burns are classified as first degree (superficial), second degree (partial and deep partial) and third degree (full thickness) burns **(Diff. 14.1 and Figs. 14.6 and 14.7A to C)**.

Effect of Burns

Effects will depend upon factors like:

i. **Degree of heat applied:** Effects are severe, if heat applied is very great.

TABLE 14.1: Classification of burns

Degree of damage	Dupuytren's	Wilson's
Erythema	1°	Epidermal
Vesication with blister formation	2°	Epidermal
Destruction of superficial skin	3°	Dermo-epidermal
Destruction of whole skin including dermis	4°	Dermo-epidermal
Destruction of deep fascia, muscles	5°	Deep
Complete charring involving vessels, nerves and bones	6°	Deep

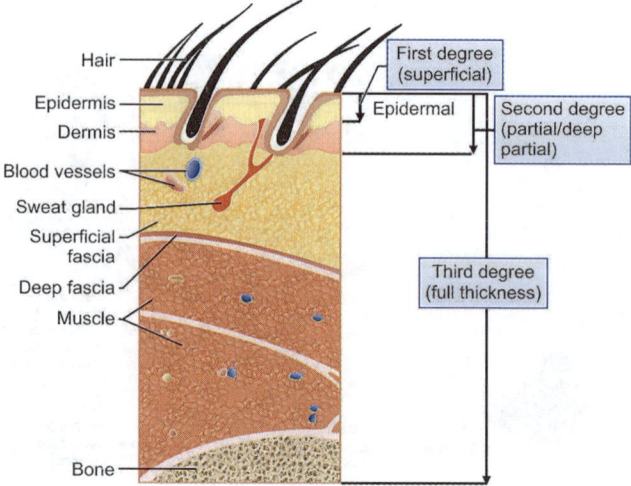

Fig. 14.6: Classification of burns

CHAPTER 14 : Thermal Injuries

DIFFERENTIATION 14.1: Classification of burns (degree of burns)

S.No.	Feature	First	Second	Third
1.	Depth	Epidermis	Epidermis and dermis	Deeper to dermis
2.	Color	Red/pink	Dark red	White/gray/black (charring)
3.	Pain to stimuli	Painful, tender	Very painful	Painless (destruction of nerve endings)
4.	Blanching	Yes	Yes, but slow	No
5.	Blisters	Not present	Present	May or may not be seen
6.	Appearance	Dry	Moist	Dry/leathery
7.	Healing time	3–6 days; skin peeling	3 weeks	Small areas take months; large areas need skin grafting
8.	Scar	No scar, slight discoloration	Yes	Yes
9.	Cause	Sunburn, scald, flash flame	Scalds, flash burns, chemicals	Flame, hot liquids, chemical, electric
10.	Medico-legally	Simple	Grievous	Grievous

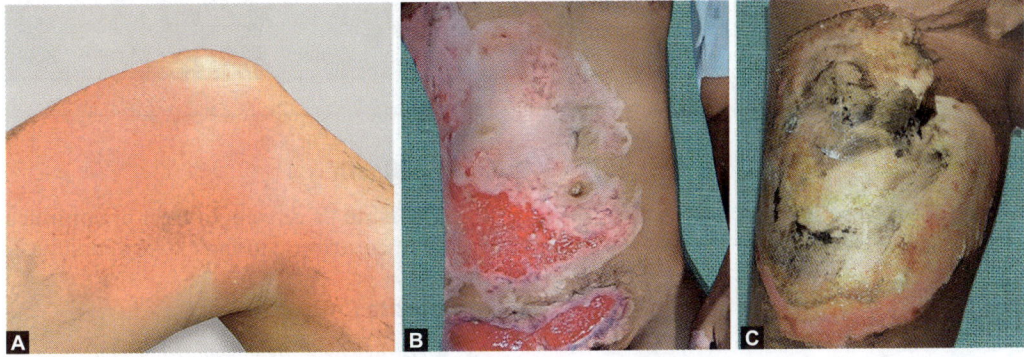

Figs. 14.7A to C: Degree of burn: (A) First degree (sunburn); (B) Second degree; (C) Third degree (firecracker burn)
[Courtesy: (B and C) Dr Ish Kumar Garg, SPS Hospital, Ludhiana]

ii. **Duration of exposure:** More prolonged the exposure, more severe will be the effect as burning of human skin is temperature and time dependent. Indication of burn depth comes from history.

iii. **Assessing the size** (*extent of body surface affected*): The total body surface area (TBSA) involved is usually worked out by the **Wallace Rule of Nines** wherein each upper limb is 9% of TBSA, 9% each for the front and back of lower limb, 9% for the front and back of chest, 9% for the front and back of abdomen, the head and neck 9% and 1% for the perineum **(Fig. 14.8)**. The above area distribution is to be used for adults.
- When burn surface involves 1/3rd of body surface area or more (usually 30–50%), the result is nearly always fatal.
- It is common error to underestimate the depth and to overestimate the extent.
- Estimation of the TBSA using the Wallace's Rule of Nines is not accurate in children because of the relatively larger head surface area. **Lund and Browder** described a method for compensating for the differences.
  - In children <1 year, head is 18% of TBSA and each leg is 14% of TBSA. Trunk and arms represent the same percentages as in adults.
  - For each year above 1 year old, add 0.5% to each leg and reduce 1.0% to the head until adult values are reached.
- **Rule of palms:** The surface area of a patient's palm (including fingers) is roughly 1% of TBSA. Palmar surface can be used to estimate small burns (<15% TBSA) or very large burns (>85%, when unburnt skin is counted).

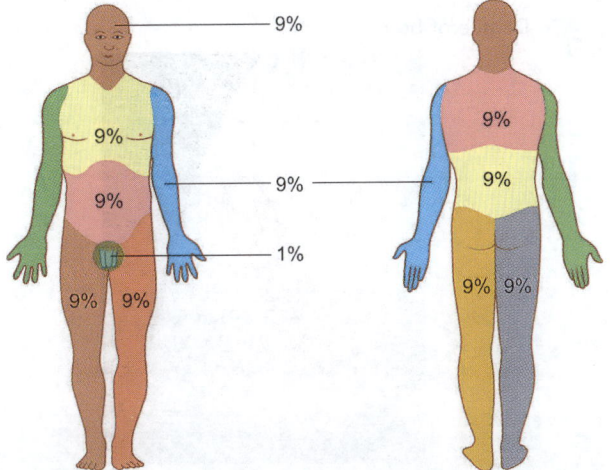

Fig. 14.8: Wallace rule of nines

iv. **Site:** Burns of head and neck, chest and abdomen, especially anterior abdominal wall including genitals and perineum, even when superficial are more dangerous than deep burns involving the extremities or back.
v. **Age:** Children ≤2 years and elderly (>60 years) are more susceptible (≥20% surface area involvement carries poor prognosis).
vi. **Sex:** Women are more susceptible.
vii. History of natural disease or concomitant trauma, electrical injury or inhalation injury also results in poor outcome.

NOTA BENE

- **Fluid resuscitation:** In children with burns over 10% and in adults over 15% TBSA, IV fluid is needed to prevent circulatory shock. Volume of fluid lost is directly proportional to the area of burn. If fluids are given orally, they should not be salt free. The key is to monitor urine output (50–60 mL/h).
- The ideal fluid for resuscitation in burn is the one that restores plasma volume without any adverse effects. Isotonic crystalloids, hypertonic solutions and colloids have been used for this purpose, e.g., Ringer lactate (RL), plasma, human albumin solution, dextran and Hartmann's solution.
- Most commonly used fluid for burn resuscitation in India and the UK is Hartmann's solution, and RL is mostly used in the US and Canada.
- Commonly used formulas:
  - **Parkland formula (Baxter formula):** It calculates the fluid (Ringer lactate) to be given in the first 24 h (4 mL/kg/TBSA% burn for adults and 3 mL/kg/TBSA% burn for children). Half of this is given in the first 8 h, and the second half in the next 16 h.
    TBSA (%) × Weight (kg) × 4 = Volume (mL) to be given
  - **Muir and Barclay formula:** Amount of fluid that needs to be infused during the first 36 h. Initially, freeze-dried plasma and 5% dextrose were used which was replaced by human albumin solution [TBSA (%) × Weight (kg)/2 = Volume (mL) per period].
  - **Brooke formula:** RL solution 1.5 mL/kg/% burn plus colloids 0.5 mL/kg/% burn plus 2,000 mL glucose in water for initial 24 h.

Degree of burn?

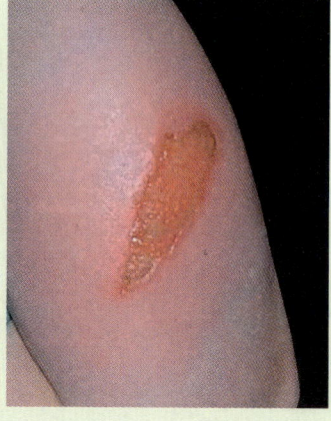

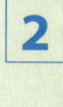

A 29-year-old female sustained burns to her face and chest, entire left arm, anterior portion of her right arm, and upper 1/3 of her abdomen while cooking food in the kitchen. Calculate the total body surface area burnt.

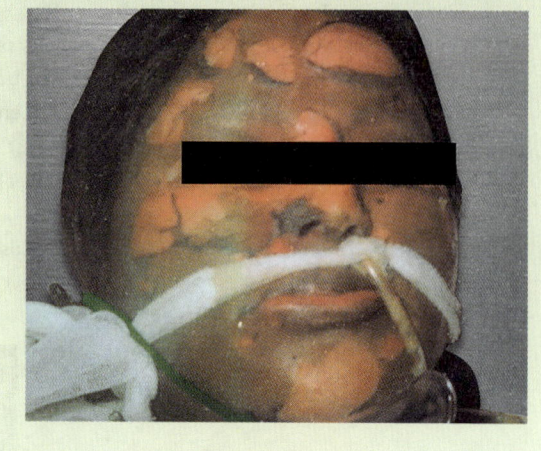

Cause of Death

Burn individuals develop a host of complications; one or more can contribute to the cause of death.

Immediate Causes

i. *Primary or neurogenic shock:* Due to pain or fright.
ii. *Asphyxia:* Suffocation may result from inhalation of CO, CO_2, or cyanide (produced by burning of materials containing nitrogen compounds such as polyurethane in vinyl, wool or nylon) or falling of the building on the body during attempt to escape.
 - CO poisoning is an important cause in most fire deaths (COHb ≥50% is confirmatory).
iii. Smoke- or heat-induced laryngospasm, respiratory arrest, and/or a vagal reflex-caused cardiac arrest are other proposed mechanisms of rapid death.

Delayed Causes

i. *Hypovolemic, burns or secondary shock:* More than half of the deaths occur due to secondary shock within 24–48 h due to loss of fluid and protein, causing decrease in cardiac output and multiorgan failure.
ii. *Acute edema of glottis* occurs from inhalation of irritant smoke or hot gases with or without pulmonary edema. Respiratory failure (inhalation injury, pneumonia or ARDS) is also a significant cause of death within 3 days.
iii. *Toxemia* due to absorption of toxic products from the burnt surface. Death occurs in about 3–4 days.
iv. *Sepsis:* **Most important cause** of death, occurring in 4–5 days or longer after burn. Septicemia can be caused by burn wound infections (e.g., *Pseudomonas aeruginosa* and other Gram-negative bacteria, *Staphylococcus aureus*), pneumonia, urinary tract

infection following catheterization, infected IV lines and infection of skin donor sites.

v. *Infective complications:* Bronchitis, bronchopneumonia, enteritis may cause delayed death.

Remote Causes

i. *Complications:* Anorexia, hematemesis, indigestion, respiratory complications or melena.
ii. *Suppurative discharges* from infected burn areas lasting for weeks or months can result in disease of the internal organs and death.
iii. Gangrene, tetanus, anemia, edema of dependant parts and jaundice.

Sequelae of burns: Scars, keloid, Marjolin's ulcer, Curling's ulcer, corneal capacity, obliteration of external auditory meatus, joint deformity or ankylosis can occur.

A 30-year-old female was brought dead to the emergency with alleged history of thermal burns. What could be the cause of death?

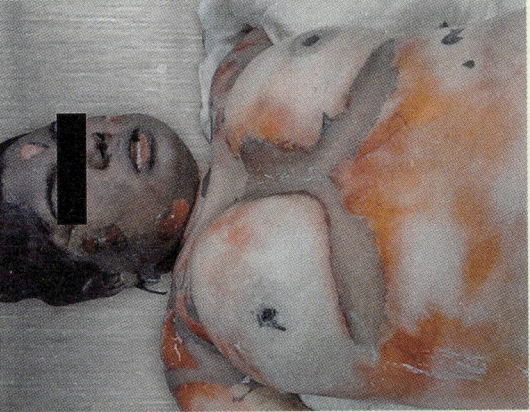

A. Asphyxia B. Neurogenic shock
C. Hypovolemic shock D. Both A and B

A 32-year-old female patient was admitted in burns ICU with 65% burns. She died 5 days after the admission. Most common cause of death in this case?

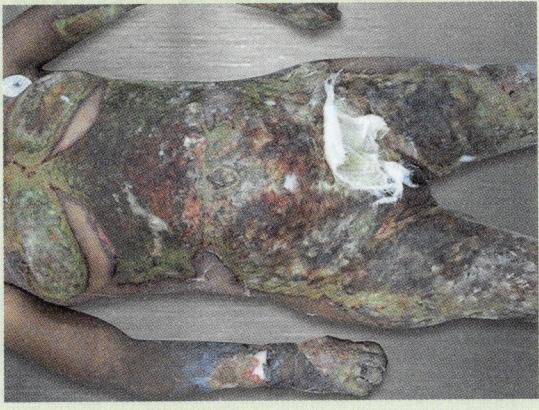

POSTMORTEM EXAMINATION

An autopsy not only helps determine the cause of death, but also reveals findings unsuspected clinically.

Before commencing with the autopsy, the following should be done:

♦ Photographic documentation.
♦ Clinical history is reviewed and information is obtained from other sources (e.g., police) depending on the circumstances of the death.
♦ X-ray to rule out any other trauma.
  ▪ Any radio-opaque material such as bullets or lead shots may be detected.
  ▪ Antemortem fracture may be found.
  ▪ Sometimes, gunshot or stab wounds are often identifiable, although they may be shrunken to a small size.

External Findings

i. **Clothing** should be carefully removed and examined for presence of accelerants like kerosene, petrol or any other inflammable substance.
   ▪ Evidence of medical procedures (if any) is recorded including fasciotomies/escharotomies.
   ▪ Tight fitting clothes may protect the underlying skin from burns, and these areas will be spared.
ii. **Site, distribution and extent** of burning are recorded. Distribution is important in the analysis of whether the burns are appropriate for the position in which the body was found.
iii. **Face:** Usually distorted and swollen. Tip of the tongue is usually burnt as it protrudes due to contraction of the tissues of the neck and face **(Fig. 14.9A)**. Froth, often pink stained, may appear at the mouth and nose due to irritation of the air passages by smoke, producing copious mucus in the airway as a result of acute pulmonary edema—a vital reaction.
   ▪ There may be absence of burns and/or soot deposits in the corners of the eyes (**'crow's feet'**) and incompletely singed eye-lashes, suggestive of squinting or closing of the eyes owing to smoke irritation **(Fig. 14.9B)**.
   ▪ In case of severe burns of neck and/or thorax, petechial hemorrhages may be found on the lids and conjunctivae, which may be regarded as vital sign.
   ▪ In charred bodies, corneas acquire a white translucency and the lenses became opaque.
iv. **Skin:** Antemortem burns will show redness (hyperemia)—a vital reaction.
   ▪ Kerosene oil burns gives characteristic odor and sooty blackening of the parts **(Fig. 14.9B)**.
   ▪ Where the burns are more severe, the skin may be stiffened, yellow–brown and leathery and becomes

parchment-like after death. Owing the effect of heat on blood, the veins stand out, giving a marbled appearance **(Fig. 14.9C)**.

v. **Postmortem staining** is cherry red in color from presence of carbon monoxide (CO), if the individual was alive and breathing during fire.

vi. **Blisters,** either ruptured/collapsed or filled with fluid may be seen.
- They are either in the main burn or as islands beyond the periphery and have a marginal red zone of variable width, usually 5–20 mm across **(Fig. 14.9D)**.
- Most antemortem blisters have a bright red base when burst and an erythematous areola.

> **NOTA BENE**
>
> **Blisters of a 2° burn may be seen in:**
> - CO poisoning
> - Antemortem/postmortem gasoline exposure
> - Deep coma
> - Peeling of skin in early putrefaction

vii. **Degloving/destocking** may be seen due to cuticular peeling **(Fig. 14.9E)**.

viii. **Hair:** It may be singed, or partially/completely burnt **(Fig. 14.9B)**. The changes occur at temperature >150°C.
- Gray hair becomes reddish or brown, but black hair stays black.
- Singed hair looks curly/clubbed at its tip and is highly fragile.
  - *Cause of singeing*: Keratin of the hair at the distal end melts and resolidify forming a terminal bob.
  - *Sites where it can be seen*: Scalp hair, eyebrows and eyelashes.

ix. **Pugilistic attitude (boxing, fencing or defense attitude):** It is due to heat stiffening. The legs are flexed at the hips and knees, the arms are flexed at the elbows and held out in front of the body and the fingers are hooked like claws **(Fig. 14.9F)**.
Cause: Due to coagulation of proteins of muscles and dehydration which causes contraction. Flexor muscles being bulkier than extensor, contract more and a position of generalized flexion is adopted.
It occurs *whether the person was alive or dead at the time of burning and has therefore no medico-legal significance.*

> **NOTA BENE**
>
> Extreme version of this phenomenon is reported in funeral pyres where the body may be seen to 'sit up' (**'sit up and beg attitude'**) due to the intense action of the heat on the muscles during open air cremation.

x. **Heat ruptures:** These are splits occurring in the skin due to prolonged exposure to heat, and the resultant breaches may simulate incised or lacerated wounds **(Diff. 14.2)**.

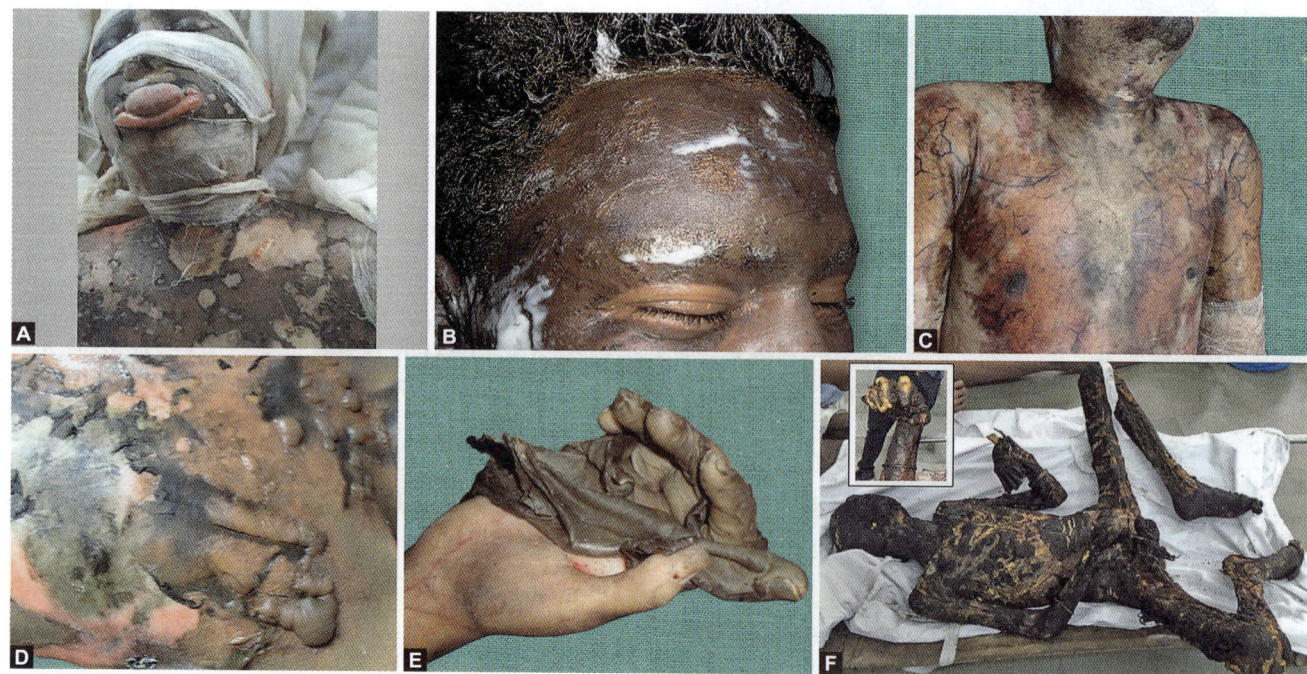

Figs. 14.9A to F: Postmortem findings in burns: (A) Protruding tongue; (B) Blackening of skin, singeing of hair and 'crow feet' appearance of eyes; (C) Marbling and leathery skin; (D) Blisters; (E) Degloving of skin; (F) Pugilistic attitude: Heat flexures of the limbs

DIFFERENTIATION 14.2: Heat rupture and lacerated wound

S.No.	Feature	Heat rupture	Lacerated wound
1.	Cause	Exposure to heat	Blunt force
2.	Site	Fatty tissue	Anywhere
3.	Vessels and nerves	Intact	Torn
4.	Bruising around the margins	Absent	Present

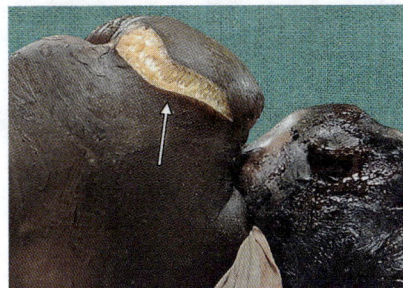

Fig. 14.10: Heat ruptures near shoulder joint. Note there is no clotted blood or vital reaction

- It is usually seen over the area of severe burning, over fleshy areas, like calves and thighs, and over extensor surfaces and joints **(Fig. 14.10)**, as well as on the scalp.

Pearls

Heat ruptures may be distinguished from the effects of violence by:
- Presence of nerves, blood vessels and connective tissue running across the split from side to side.
- There is no clotted blood in these fissures and no extravasation of blood in the surrounding tissues, since heat coagulates the blood in the vessels.
- Presence of irregular margins.
- Absence of bruising or other signs of vital reaction in the margins.

Internal Findings

i. **Skull**
   - **Heat hematoma** is not a vital sign but an artifact and has the appearance of *epidural hematoma* **(Diff. 14.3 and Fig. 14.11)**.
     - It is large, thick (about 1.5 cm) and contains 100–120 mL of blood.
     - *Cause:* The blood may come from the longitudinal venous sinuses or the diploic veins. The heat may force blood out of the marrow of the calvarium through veins and out over the surface of the dura.
   - Skull bones may be fractured and burst open along the sutures due to intense heat. The latter may be difficult to interpret from gunshot injury.

ii. **Brain:** Congested and appears swollen with widening and flattening of the gyri and obliteration of the sulci due to the contraction of the coagulating dura against the surface of the brain. Subdural hemorrhage may be present.

iii. **Neck:** Hemorrhage in the root of the tongue and neck muscles—considered vital reactions in burn victims.

iv. **Larynx, trachea and bronchioles:** Contain carbon and soot particles, and the mucosa is congested with frothy mucus secretions **(Fig. 14.12)**. This is **the surest sign of antemortem burns**, which is due to inhalation of gases.
   - However, soot usually disappears by the 2nd day of hospitalization.
   - Detachment of the mucosa of the tracheobronchial tree, pharynx, epiglottis or esophagus; and epiglottic swelling—indicators of vitality (air is a poor conductor of heat and thermal injury is usually limited to the upper airways).

v. **Pleura:** Congested and inflamed with serous effusion.

vi. **Lungs:** Congested and edematous, may be shrunken, cherry red in color due inhalation of CO **(Fig. 14.13)**.

DIFFERENTIATION 14.3: Epidural hematoma (EDH) due to burns and blunt force

S.No.	Feature	EDH due to burns	EDH due to blunt force
1.	Cause	Charring of the skull due to intense heat	Blunt force to the head
2.	Situation	Anywhere	Usually adjacent to Sylvian fissure
3.	Position	Usually bilateral	Usually unilateral
4.	Distribution	Diffuse	Localized
5.	Origination	Dural venous sinuses and emissary veins	Middle meningeal artery
6.	Characteristics	Evenly distributed or sickle-shaped; honeycomb appearance; soft, granular, foamy, friable clot; chocolate brown in color (pink, if CO is present)	Disc shaped; uniform, smooth, rubbery; reddish-purple color
7.	Skull fracture	Eggshell fracture—elliptical, mosaic or circular defect without radiating fracture lines, seen above the temple	Fracture line radiating from a skull defect present in temporal area
8.	Crossing of suture lines	It may cross suture lines and overlie the frontal, parietal and temporal area	Hematoma do not cross sutures as the dura is anchored at the suture lines
9.	Injury to brain	Absent	May be present

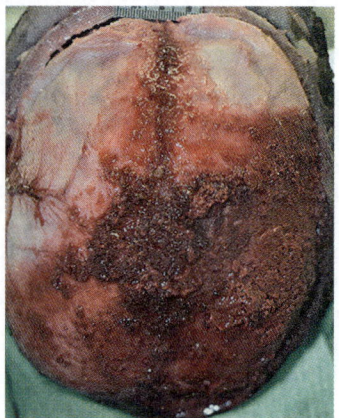

Fig. 14.11: Heat hematoma.

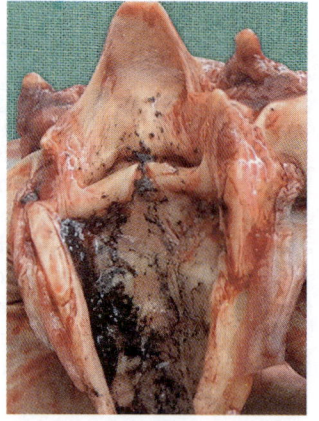

Fig. 14.12: Soot particles in larynx and trachea: Surest sign of antemortem burns

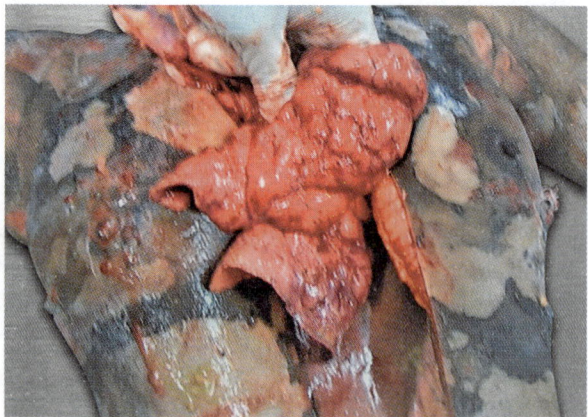

Fig. 14.13: Shrunken and cherry red color lungs

vii. **Heart:** Chamber full of blood, cherry red in color due inhalation of CO.
viii. **Vessels:** Intense red discoloration of the intima of the vessels may be seen due to hemolysis occurring at >52°C. If circulation was intact, fragmented erythrocytes can be demonstrated microscopically in other organs also—a vital sign.
ix. **Stomach and intestines:** Stomach may contain carbon particles impregnated in mucous membrane. It may be red in color. There is inflammation and ulceration of Peyer's solitary glands of intestines.
   - *Curling's ulcers* (acute gastroduodenal ulcer) may be seen in severely burnt patient's gastric antrum and first part of duodenum after 72 h* (3–10 days post-survival). It develops due to mucosal ischemia as a result of stress and shock, and not related to acidity.
x. **Spleen:** Enlarged and softened.
xi. **Liver:** Cloudy swelling and fatty liver or necrosis of the cells, if death is delayed. Jaundice may occur.
xii. **Kidneys:** Show signs of nephritis, thrombosis and infarction.
xiii. **Adrenals:** May be enlarged and congested.
xiv. **Fractures:** Fine, linear, superficial fractures of the cortical surface of bones are characteristics of heat-induced fractures. Thermal amputations occur as fire consumes the distal extremities and may be difficult to distinguish from traumatic amputations. The findings are rounded, burnished edges of the bone as against sharp well-demarcated edges of traumatic amputation.
- The prolonged exposure of the body to high temperatures (results in vaporization of body fluids) along with the direct effect of the heat cause shriveling of the internal organs which became firm, hardened and cooked by heat—the so-called '**puppet organs**'.
- Samples of heart and femoral blood are collected in tubes containing sodium fluoride. Blood can be obtained even from a badly burnt body. If no blood is available, sections of the spleen or skeletal muscle may be used.

*Sometimes it develops within 24 h of severe burn.

NOTA BENE

Histological findings: Vesicular detachment of tracheal and bronchial mucosa, pseudogoblet cells, massive secretion of mucus, nucleic elongation and palisade arrangement of the mucosal epithelium in trachea and bronchi, and hyperemia and edema of the tracheal and bronchial mucosa.

Heat artifacts
- Remnants of clothing around neck mimic ligature strangulation.
- Pugilistic attitude.
- Splitting of skin.
- Fractures not associated with soft tissue hemorrhage (right-angled fractures of long bones—'*street and avenue fractures*').
- Bilateral epidural hemorrhage.
- Shrunken, firm and light brown colored ('*cooked*') brain.
- Introduction of soot into the trachea during incision of the charred neck at autopsy.

A dead was brought to the civil hospital, which shows charring and flexion of the limbs. This condition is due to:

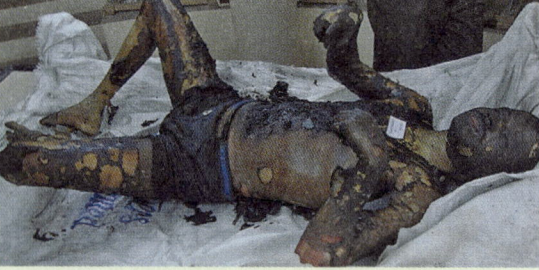

A. Muscle proteins coagulation
B. Formation of actomyosin complex
C. Muscle hyperactivity
D. Cadaveric spasm

MEDICO-LEGAL QUESTIONS

Q. In case of a living patient, whether the burn injury is simple or grievous in nature?

- A person with burn injury on the face will result in scarring/tattooing and permanent disfiguration—grievous injury. Grievous hurt can occur when burn injuries involving the skin lead to the person being admitted to the hospital and unable to follow his/her ordinary pursuits or be in severe bodily pain, for a period of at least 20 days.
- Injuries dangerous to life can also occur due to potentially life threatening burn injuries (risk of hypovolemic shock). Three risk factors for death after burns are: age >60 years, burn size >40% of body-surface area (TBSA) and inhalation injury. Patient's mortality is 0.3% with no risk factors, 3% with one risk factor, 33% with two risk factors, and nearly 90% with all three risk factors.
- Potentially life threatening burns can occur in persons either <10 years of age or >50 years of age who have partial thickness burns involving >30% of the TBSA and in those between 10–50 years of age with partial thickness burns involving >35% TBSA.

> **NOTA BENE**
>
> The **Baux Score** is the *sum of age and the TBSA burned*. There is a strong association between this score and case fatality for both men and women. A score of 110 is associated with death in 50% of cases. Baux Score of 140 or more is non-survivable. For patients with an inhalation injury, a score of 100 is associated with death in nearly 50% of cases, compared with 110 for those without. Thus, a revised Baux Score, i.e., Age + Percentage burn + 17 has been suggested for those with inhalation injuries. Therefore, doctors should desist from using only 40% of TBSA burnt to classify the burns as simple or grievous, since inhalational injuries and age of the person also play a significant role in assessing whether burns are endangering life.

Q. What is the identity of the deceased?

Identification is difficult when the body is completely burnt, however the following may be helpful:

- *Sex of the deceased:* It can be assessed by external and internal sexual characteristics. Prostrate and nulliparous uterus may not be burnt even at high temperatures.
- *Race:* Individuals from Afro-Caribbean origin have a dark gray deposit of melanin in the arachnoid of the medulla oblongata. Microscopic analysis of residual hair for melanin deposition and hair structure may be required.
- *Age:* It is usually established by teeth and ossification of bones.
- *Dental identification:* Dental charts should be prepared and X-rays of the jaws obtained, which can be compared with the dental X-rays and charts of the individual who is believed to be deceased.
- Clothing* (it is retained in body folds where the fire has not reached) and personal effects like watches, spectacles, dentures, hearing aid, SIM card[†], jewelry and keys, and nonspecific characters like scars, tattoos (may show up well, despite the loss of the epidermis) or absence of organs can help in identification. A clenched hand resulting from heat contracture preserves fingerprints.
- X-ray examination of a charred body (e.g., evidence of prior surgery, old fracture) can assist in identification by comparison of postmortem X-rays with antemortem X-rays of the individual the deceased is suspected of being. Surgical implants, and skeletal diseases and injuries may be helpful for identification.
- If conventional comparison methods are not possible, teeth or bone can be used for DNA analysis.

Q. When did the victim sustain the burn injury?

The question arises as to when the burns were caused and whether all the burns were caused simultaneously. Features which help in estimating the age of burns is given in **Table 14.2**.

Q. Whether the burns are antemortem or postmortem?

- It is sometimes impossible to differentiate between antemortem and postmortem burns when they are sustained near to the time of death.
- The exposed skin surface may be reddened in both in antemortem and postmortem burns, the classical signs of a 'red erythema' or 'vital reaction' may be unsafe to conclude its antemortem nature.
- Some of the important differences are given in **Diff. 14.4**.

Q. Whether the burns are the cause of death?

- Presence of carbonaceous or soot particles in the respiratory tract, esophagus and stomach.
- Cherry red discoloration of blood due to CO confirm burns as cause of death.

TABLE 14.2: Age of burns

Features	Age
Redness	Immediate
Vesication	1–2 h
Exudates begins to dry	12–24 h
Dry brown crust formation and pus formation	48–72 h
Superficial slough separates	4–6th day
Deep slough separates	15th day
Granulation tissue begins to cover	>15 days
Formation of cicatrix and deformity	Several weeks

---

* It helps to determine the race of the individual from underlying intact skin and also useful for accelerant analysis.
† Data from SIM cards can be retrieved even after exposure to 450°C.

DIFFERENTIATION 14.4: Antemortem and postmortem burns

S.No.	Feature	Antemortem burns	Postmortem burns
1.	Line of redness	Present	Absent
2.	Vesicles	Contain serous fluid, rich in albumin, chloride and some polymorphs	Contain air; if fluid is present, it is thin and clear, and contain little albumin and no chloride
3.	Base of vesicles	Red and inflamed with erythematous areola	Dull, dry, hard and pale yellow with no erythematous areola
4.	Soot in upper respiratory tract	May be present	Absent
5.	Mucus secretions in air passages	May be present	Absent
6.	Inflammation and repair	Present along with pus and slough	Absent
7.	Healing	Granulation tissue seen in old cases	Absent
8.	Carboxyhemoglobin	Present	Absent
9.	Enzyme reaction	Increase in enzymes in the periphery of burns	No such increase

NOTA BENE

- If the hemoglobin saturation is >10% CO, then the person was alive and inhaled the air during the fire. If death occurs due to the toxicity of CO, the blood carboxyhemoglobin (COHb) saturation is in the range of 50–80%. The COHb saturation level will not be artificially elevated in a dead person by being in or near a fire, i.e., CO will not diffuse through the skin or otherwise be absorbed by a dead body.
- Cyanide concentration >0.2 ng/mL may be seen in antemortem burns (although significant concentration is produced during decomposition).

Q. Whether the burns are suicidal/accidental/homicidal/self-inflicted?

- **Suicidal burns** are common among Indian women. They pour kerosene over their heads and clothes before setting fire to themselves. Burns may be absent from the feet and lower legs, if the body is in upright position. Some women stuff clothes inside the mouth to prevent their shouts from being heard by others. Classic religious examples were seen in certain Buddhist sects or the rite of '*sati*' performed in some parts of India (now prohibited).
- **Accidental burns** are common among children and elderly people. Accidental kerosene stove bursting is also reported. Accidents may result from smoking in bed, especially under the influence of alcohol or drugs, using faulty equipments and playing with fire.
- **Homicidal burns** are quite common in India. Custom of dowry leads to young brides being murdered by pouring kerosene on them and setting them on fire by the husband and in-laws, and later claimed to be accidental burns.
  - Sometimes, a homicide victim may be burned to conceal murder by other means in an attempt to cover up or destroy the evidence. Diagnosis require the presence of fatal injuries inflicted by another person and the absence of classical vital parameters.
  - In case of traumatic EDH produced before the fire began, it should contain no COHb. A heat hematoma formed contains COHb if the victim has absorbed this gas during the fire.
- **Self-inflicted burns** for false accusation: These burns are usually seen on accessible parts of body.

Q. Is it possible to extract DNA from burnt bones?

- Exposure to heat in the presence of moisture breaks the phosphodiester bonds leaving sheared DNA in bone cells. This will make an amplification of genetic markers difficult or even impossible.
- Moreover, heavily burnt bones are very prone to contamination with external DNA.
- This limits the possibility of generating a complete profile of the victim.
- Identification is reliably and reproducibly possible from well preserved and semi-burnt bones.

NOTA BENE

- **Preternatural combustion:** It is a rare phenomenon where a putrefying dead body catches fire spontaneously due to formation of inflammable gases, such as hydrogen, H_2S and methane formed in the bowel. A flame is necessary for ignition.
- **Spontaneous human combustion** refers to a situation when a human body is found with significant burns with minimal damage to the direct surroundings of the body. Typically, no observable source of ignition is found in the vicinity of the victim. A tear in the skin has to occur for the melted fat to impregnate the charred clothes, igniting a wick effect that produces localized heat for extended period.
- **Necklacing** is a method of homicidal burning which involves placing petrol filled vehicle tyre around the neck of the victim and setting it alight. It was followed in South African black townships during the apartheid period as a form of punishment for political opponents.
- **Arson** is the willful and malicious burning of the dwelling of another or burning of one's own property for an improper purpose, e.g., to collect insurance. The presence of several points of ignition and liquid fire accelerants, such as petrol or paraffin provides strong evidence of fire has been ignited deliberately.

CHAPTER 14 : Thermal Injuries

6 A 25-year-old female was found dead in room having 98% burns with tongue protruding out, body in pugilistic attitude, heat ruptures, peeling of skin, and heat hematoma and heat fractures of skull. COHb was 25% and soot particles were present in trachea. Two findings to establish that the burns were antemortem in nature:

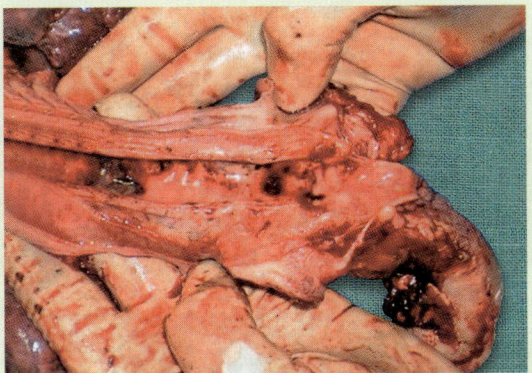

A. Heat hematoma and heat ruptures
B. Heat fracture of skull and COHb in blood
C. Protruding tongue and pugilistic attitude
D. COHb and soot particles in trachea

Describe types of injuries, clinical features, pathophysiology, postmortem findings and medico-legal aspects in cases of scalds.

■ SCALDS

Definition: A scald is a form of thermal injury which results from application of liquid >60°C or from steam, and involves only the superficial layers of skin. An actual skin temperature of 44°C (lowest) is considered to cause damage to the skin.

Types

It is of three types:
  i. **Immersion burns:** Accidental or deliberate immersion in hot liquid, usually water. This is characterized by a straight, horizontal burn pattern corresponding to the level of the liquid.
 ii. **Splash or spill burns:** Usually accidental.
iii. **Steam burns:** Exposure to superheated steam.
♦ Hot water accounts for most of the immersion or splash burns.
♦ Scalds show uniform injury pattern of all the affected skin, sharp demarcation with trickle marks, soddening and bleaching, but do not singe the hair or blacken/char the skin.
♦ With inhalation, there is laryngeal, tracheal and respiratory burns that may progress to adult respiratory distress syndrome.

Classification

Clinically, it is classified into three degrees:
  i. **Erythema or reddening** by vasoparalysis.
 ii. **Vesication or blister formation** due to increased permeability of the capillaries.
iii. **Necrosis** of the dermis when deeper layer of skin is involved **(Fig. 14.14)**.

As the temperature applied in moist heat is usually lower than dry heat (water boils at 100°C), it does not produce destruction of muscles, charring or amputations.

Medico-legal Aspects

♦ It is usually accidental due to splashing or pouring of fluid during cooking.
♦ Accidents are common in children and elderly.
♦ Boiling water may be thrown intentionally, usually domestic homicide intent with the husband being the victim.
♦ Deliberate scalding by hot water is common form of child abuse. Dipping injuries of the limbs appear as well-demarcated *'glove and stocking'* distribution of scalds reflecting the flow of hot liquid under the influence of gravity. Areas of scalding round the buttocks with clear, unaffected areas on the upper thighs occur when the child is forcibly made to sit in a hot liquid **(Fig. 14.15)**.

Important differentiating features of dry and moist heat and chemical burns are given in **Diff. 14.5 and Figs. 14.16A to C**.

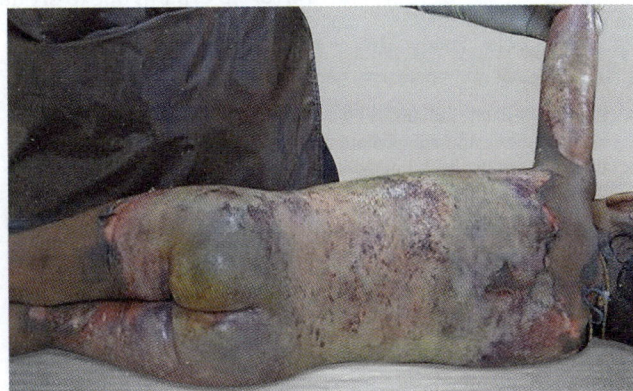

Fig. 14.14: Scalds due to boiling water

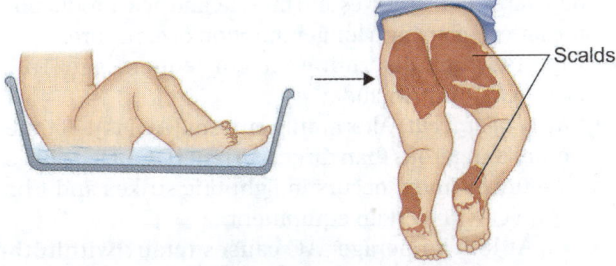

Fig. 14.15: Scalding (child abuse)

DIFFERENTIATION 14.5: Dry heat, moist heat and chemical burns (Figs. 14.16A to C)

S.No.	Feature	Dry heat burn	Moist heat burn	Chemical burn
1.	Cause	Flame, heated body or X-rays	Solid steam or liquid >60°C	Corrosives
2.	Site	At or above the site of contact	At and below the site of contact	At or below the site of contact
3.	Splashing	Absent	Present	Present
4.	Skin	Dry, wrinkled and may be charred	Sodden, bleached	Corroded and devitalized
5.	Vesicles	At the circumference of burnt area	Over the burnt area	Usually not present
6.	Red line	Present	Present	Absent
7.	Color	Black	Bleached	Distinctive coloration
8.	Charring	Present	Absent	Absent
9.	Singeing	Present	Absent	Absent
10.	Ulceration	Absent	Absent	Present
11.	Scar	Thick, contracted	Thin, less contracted	Thick, contracted
12.	Clothes	Burnt	Wet, not burnt	May be burnt, with characteristic stains

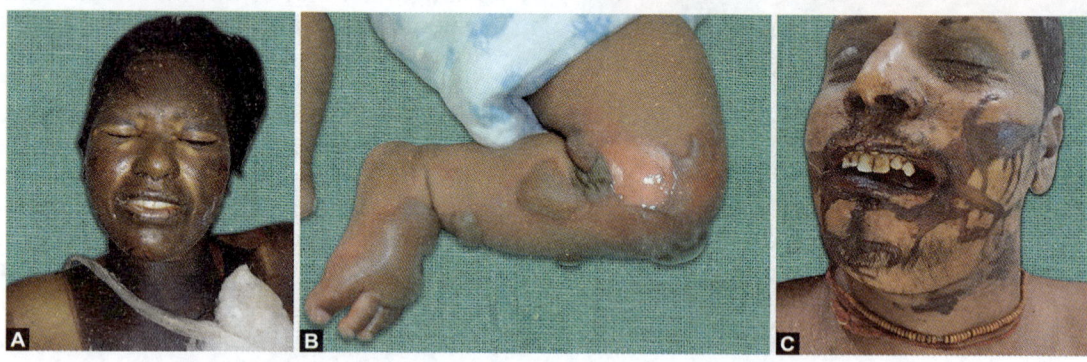

Figs. 14.16A to C: Burns due to dry heat, moist heat and corrosives (chemicals)

> **NOTA BENE**
>
> **Pleura sign:** If hot steam is inhaled, the parietal pleura is reddened, whereas the costodiaphragmatic angles are pale. In deaths caused by the effects of dry heat, this sign is absent. It is useful to differentiate deaths due to hot steam and dry air at autopsy.

FM 2.25

Describe types of injuries, clinical features, pathophysiology, postmortem findings and medico-legal aspects in cases of electrocution.

ELECTRICAL INJURIES (ELECTROCUTION)

- Electricity exerts two major effects on the body: cellular depolarization of nerves and muscle, and heat production, the latter reflecting a longer duration of exposure.
- Factors which determine the consequent pattern of electrical injury include:
  i. *Kind of current:* Alternating current (AC) is 4–5 times more dangerous than direct current (DC). DC injuries are uncommon, occurs in lightning strikes and from contact with certain equipment.
      - At low amperage, AC causes tetany within the flexor muscles of hand and forearm, and hence the patient is unable to release the device until the power is turned off. It also interferes with the normal cardiac pacing causing cardiac arrest.
      - In contrast, DC tends to cause a single muscle contraction, throwing the victim, and resulting in a shorter duration of exposure to the electrical source, but increasing the chance of blunt trauma.
  ii. *Amount of current:* The amount of current is expressed as Ohm's law: $I = V/R$, where 'I' is current (amperes [A]), 'V' is voltage (volts [V]) and 'R' is resistance (ohms). Flow of the current is great, if voltage is high or if resistance is low. Electrocution is rare at <100 V and most deaths occur at >200 V. Amperage is more important, as it indicates the actual intensity/amount of electricity which passes through the body.
  iii. *Path of current:* Death is more likely to occur, if the brainstem or heart is in the direct path of the current.
  iv. *Duration of current flow:* Severity is directly proportional to the duration of current flow. For an electric shock to occur, the body must be in contact with both the positive and negative pole or with the earth.
  v. *Resistance:* The principal bodily barrier to an electrical current is the skin, and once beyond the dermis, the current passes easily through the electrolytes-rich

fluids.* The greater the resistance, the more likely that burns will result. Dry skin offers high resistance (1000–1500 ohms), but resistance is decreased when the skin is moist or covered with sweat (200–300 ohms). Blood has low resistance, and as such within the body, electricity tends to be conducted along blood vessels **(Fig. 14.17)**. With high voltage, condition of the skin plays no significant role.

vi. *Site of contact:* Electrical injuries on the face and arms are more serious than those on the palms.

Predisposing factors: Unexpectedness of the shock, anxiety, fear and emotions, exhaustion, cardiovascular and other diseases.

Effects due to Passage of Electricity

Electrical injuries are divided into low tension and high tension injuries (threshold 1000 V) **(Fig. 14.17)**:

i. **Low-tension injuries:** Skin burns results from heating of the tissues by the passage of the electric current.
   - Most common sites of low-voltage contact injury (entry) are the hands (fingers), and that of grounding (exit) is the foot or opposite hand.
   - Tissue damage from this heating effect may be insufficient to produce a visible injury, if the surface contact area is broad and the conductivity of the skin is high because of high water content—seen in bathtub electrocutions. Torture by electricity may be done using broad wet electrodes in order to avoid leaving evidential marks.

ii. **High tension injuries:** Injuries can be caused by three sources—*flash, flame or the current itself.* In overhead lines, the person acts as a conduction rod to the earth, causing damage to the subcutaneous tissues and muscles along with entry and exit points. Burns may be severe with confluent areas of third-degree burns or charring of the body. There can be massive destruction of tissue with loss of extremities and rupture of organs.

Characteristics of Injuries

Local Effects

i. **Burns and blisters:** Characteristically, these are seen as puckering of the skin around the edges of the burns with surrounding areola of pallor. There is *no red line* surrounding the burns or reddening of the base at the point of entry and exit. The characteristic marks seen are called *Joule burns,* also known as *electrical burns/mark* which is **specific and diagnostic of electric burns,** and is found at the point of entry.

Joule burns: These marks are round, oval or irregular, chalky white, shallow, centrally collapsed blister, from few millimeters to 1–1.5 cm in diameter and have a raised border of about 1–2 mm around, part or the whole circumference **(Figs. 14.18A)**.
   - The crater floor is lined by pale flattened skin. There may be mild hyperemia of the adjacent intact skin, due to rapid dilatation of the pre-capillary vessels.
   - The blister is created by the steam produced in the heating of the tissues by the electric current, the so-called *endogenous burns*. When the current ceases, the blister cools and collapses to leave a crater with a raised rim. It may sometimes reproduce the shape of the conductor.
   - When contact is more prolonged, skin mark becomes brown and with further contact—charring occurs.
   - Joule burn is commonly found on exposed parts of the body, especially on the palmer aspects of hands.

> **NOTA BENE**
>
> *Microscopically*, the epidermis shows a **Swiss cheese appearance**. There is vacuolization of epidermis and dermis, subepidermal blistering, nuclear streaming, elongation of epidermal cells and eosinophila of dermal collagen. There is streaming of nuclei—thin, elongated and lie parallel to each other (*palisade-like appearance*).

Exit marks: Variable in appearance, but some features are those of the entry mark **(Fig. 14.18B)**. Often seen as splits in the skin at points where the skin has been raised into ridges by passage of the current.
   - In high-voltage current, the exit often appears as a 'blowout' type wound.

ii. **Flash or spark burns:** Where the contact is less firm, so that an air gap exists between skin and conductor, the current jumps the gap as a spark and causes the

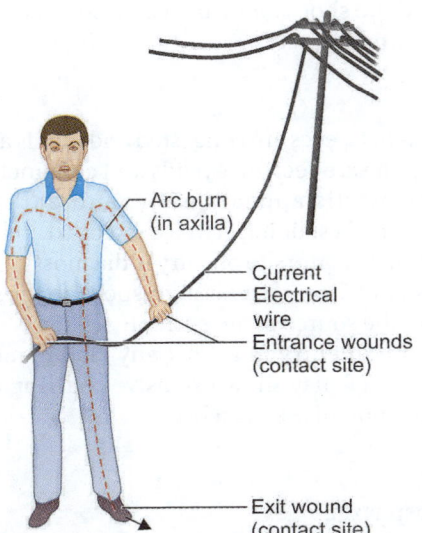

Fig. 14.17: Mechanism of electrical injury: Current passing through the body follow the path of least resistance to the ground

---
* Order of increasing resistance of tissues for electrical current: Blood vessels, nerves and muscle, skin, tendon, fat and bone.

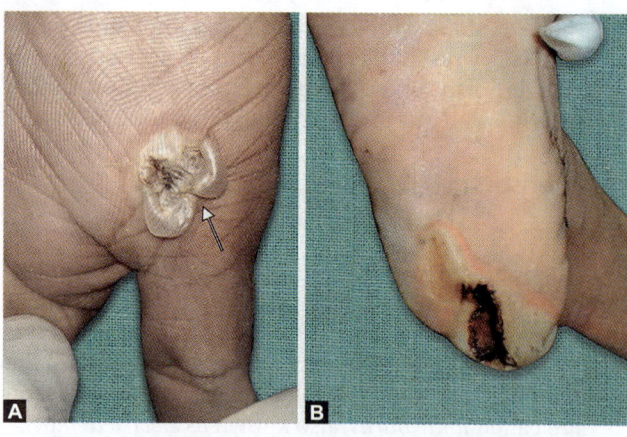

Figs. 14.18A and B: (A) Joule burn (entry mark). Note the hyperemia around the margin (arrow); (B) Exit mark

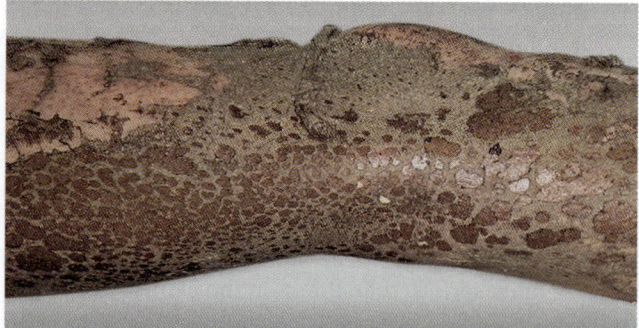

Fig. 14.19: Crocodile skin lesions due to high voltage electrocution

outer skin keratin to melt over a small area. On cooling, the keratin fuses into a hard brownish nodule, usually raised above the surrounding surface, the so-called *'flash/spark burn.'*
- In high-voltage burns, such as those sustained from high-tension grid transmission cables, sparking may occur over many centimeters. It causes numerous individual and confluent areas of third-degree burns or red/brown punched-out spark lesions which are called as '**crocodile skin**' lesions, and typically involve exposed areas of the body **(Fig. 14.19)**.
- Flash burns are also called *exogenous burns* as the flame is produced outside the body. The flash can ignite the patient's clothes causing flame burns along with singeing of hair.

iii. **Wounds:** These are lacerated or punctured with contusions of the margins.

- The heat generated at the site of entry may cause atomization of the metallic wire, which may give a metallic lustre.
- Small balls of molten metal derived from the metal of the contacting electrode, so-called **current pearls**, may be carried deep into tissues, which can be identified by *scanning electron microscopy.*
- Heat generated by the current may melt the calcium phosphate, which is seen in X-rays of limbs as typical round dense foci, known as **bone pearls or wax drippings**.

Systemic Effects

i. Immediate death from shock.
ii. **CNS:** Hemiplegia or paraplegia, aphasia, headache, vertigo and convulsions.
iii. **Eye:** Cataract, optic atrophy and choroido-retinitis may occur. In case of close range electrical flash, singeing of eyelash along with first degree burn of the skin of face may occur (*arch eye*).
iv. Pulseless, hypotensive, loss of response to external stimuli, cold and cyanotic and without respiration—*suspended animation*-like state may occur.

With recovery, there may be muscular pain, fatigue, headache and irritability.

Cause of Death

- Ventricular fibrillation (low voltage current)—most common cause.
- Less commonly, paralysis of the respiratory muscles (asphyxia), and rarely, a direct effect on the brainstem as a result of current passing through the head and neck.
- Inhibition of respiratory center, electrothermal injury or ventricular asystole (in high voltage).
- *Secondary causes:* Complications, like infection or septicemia (due to burns) or from mechanical injuries like fall from height.

Postmortem Findings

- Before autopsy, it is important to examine the scene and the tools, appliances or machinery involved in the incident.
- Examination of the entire body, particularly the hands and especially the fingers, along with examination of the feet and the shoes for evidence of electrical burns is of utmost importance.

External

i. Face is pale, eyes are congested and pupils are dilated. Petechiae are seen on eyelids and conjunctiva.
ii. Rigor mortis appears early, and dark blue-red postmortem staining is well developed.
iii. Joule burn at the site of entry is diagnostic. The shape and size of the mark may correspond to the shape and size of the source of the current.
iv. The site of entry may lack any visible marks or in some cases may show extensive charring with heat coagulation of the muscles.

Internal

Those of asphyxia.
i. *Lungs:* Congested and edematous.
ii. *Heart:* Focal necrosis with variable hemorrhage and acute contraction bands in the myocardium and conduction system may be seen.

iii. Brain, meninges and parenchymatous organs are congested.
iv. Petechial hemorrhages may be found along the line of passage of the current, under the endocardium, pericardium, pleura, brain and the spinal cord.

> **NOTA BENE**
> - **'Electrical petechiae':** The petechiae seen in electrocution are not caused by asphyxia but by a combination of venous congestion due to cardiac arrest and a sudden rise in blood pressure induced by muscle contractions. Consequently, it represents a nonspecific but typical finding in electrocution. Unlike electrical burns, petechiae also indicate the vital origin of the events.
> - **Acro-reaction test:** It is a micro-chemical test for metals at the site of entry of electric current. The test is applicable for detection of metals which are soluble in HCl or HNO_3.

Medico-legal Aspects

- Deaths are usually accidental. Suicides are rare and homicides are even rarer.
  - Common method of homicide is to drop a plugged-in electrical device into a bucket/bathtub while the individual is taking a bath. There is usually no electrical burn, and if the electrical device is removed, the cause of death will be missed.
- Iatrogenic accidents may lead to a charge of negligence. Traumatic injury may be sustained from electric shock itself during electroconvulsive therapy in treatment of mental disorder or through improperly earthed instruments in the operation theater.
- It is not possible to differentiate between antemortem and postmortem electrical burns.

> **7** A 45-year-old male was found unconscious by the side of an aluminum ladder at a construction site. He was declared brought dead in the hospital. The autopsy surgeon found these marks on his fingers. What are these marks? What could be the cause of his death?

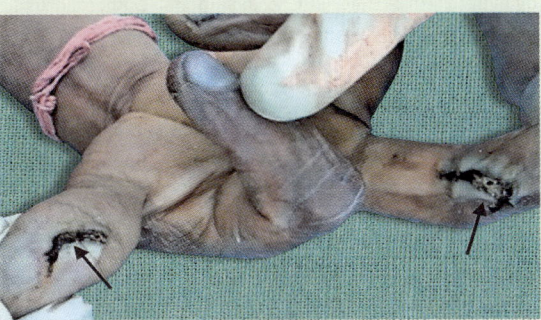

JUDICIAL ELECTROCUTION

- Death penalty is carried out using the electric chair in some States in the US.
- The condemned man is strapped to a wooden chair, and one electrode is put on the shaven scalp and the other on the right lower leg (head and body shaved to provide better contact with the moistened copper electrodes) by the executioner.
- The voltage varies in power from State to State, and is also determined by the convict's body weight. The first jolt is followed by several more in a lower voltage. In Georgia, executioners apply alternating current of 2,000 V for 4 seconds, 1,000 V for the next 11 seconds and then 208 V for 2 min.
- The findings during autopsy are: an annular burn on the head due to the scalp electrode and a burn on the right calf due to the anklet, both due to electrical current flow.

FM 2.25
> Describe types of injuries, clinical features, pathophysiology, postmortem findings and medico-legal aspects in cases of lightning.

LIGHTNING STROKE

Lightning bolt (DC >1000 million V) is produced when the charged undersurface (which is mostly negatively charged) of a thundercloud sends its electrical charge to the ground. It may injure or kill an individual by direct strike, a side flash or conduction through another object. Death is caused by high-voltage direct current due to cardiopulmonary arrest or electrothermal injuries.

Lichtenberg Flowers/Arborescent Markings

- Lichtenberg flowers can be seen in *lightning strike*, but are rare.
- These are superficial, several inches long, thin, irregular, tortuous, dendritic red marks on the skin **(Fig. 14.20)**. These marks have a resemblance to the branches of a tree.
- This fern-like pattern of erythema in the skin is usually found over the shoulders or flanks.
- It is not associated with burning.
- They indicate the path taken by the discharge and tend to follow skin creases and the long axis of the body. It appears within 1 h, and disappears in 24–48 h, if the person survive.

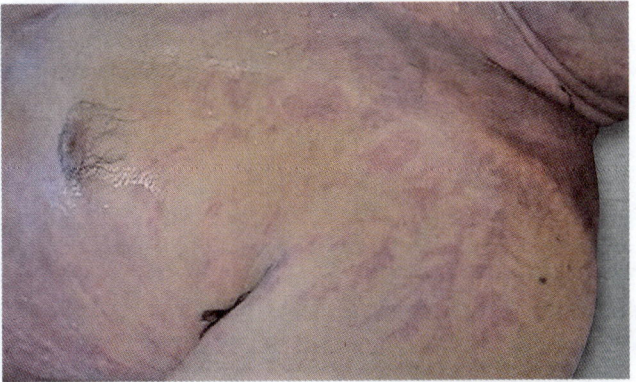

Fig. 14.20: Lichtenberg flowers/Filigree burns

Cause: The exact mechanism has not yet been determined. There are various theories:
- Static electricity discharges along superficial vasculature (or perhaps nerves).
- Hemoglobin staining the tissues in the pattern of a tree due to break down of RBCs within the capillaries of the skin.
- Electron showers eliciting an inflammatory response in the skin.
- Current following lines of perspiration and skin moisture.
- Minute deposits of copper in the skin.

Medico-legal aspects
- Its recognition may be lifesaving in the unaccompanied comatose patient, and is important because even delayed resuscitation of lightning victims can be very successful.
- Death is accidental.
- It can help differentiate a natural death from murder.
- Appearance is *pathognomonic* for injury by lightning, but may closely resemble those produced by criminal violence.

Other Features of Lightning
- Development of edema of skin at the point of entry wound in those who survive due to paralysis of capillary and lymphatic vessels.
- As the exit is often in the feet, shoe may be ripped apart or blown off the foot. Articles of clothing may be found some distance from the body with the body partly stripped which may suggest sexual assault, particularly when the body is found in the open.
- Linear burns and surface burns.
- Fusing and magnetization of metallic articles, such as rings, spectacle frames, pen-knives, keys and watches due to tremendous heat liberated by the electrical discharge. These are useful signs for eliminating suspicion of foul play.
- Injuries like contusions, lacerations, rupture of tympanic membrane and organs, and spinal cord damage.
- Additional findings—singed hair, and patterned skin burns marks underneath metal article of jewelry.

> **NOTA BENE**
>
> **Lichtenberg flowers:** It is known by different names like 'arborization', 'feathering', 'ferning', 'filigree burns' or 'keraunographic markings'. The phenomenon is also known as '*keraunographism*' from Greek *keraunos*, a thunder bolt.

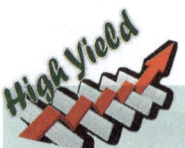

- **Hypothermia:** Core temperature <35°C.
- In hypothermia, depression of consciousness level starts when the core body temperature falls below 32°C.
- Paradoxical undressing, 'hide and die' syndrome, Wischnewsky spots in stomach are seen in hypothermic deaths.
- In hypothermia, cause of death is cardiac arrest.
- **Color of PM staining in hypothermic deaths:** Bright pink.
- Immersion foot, trench foot and trench hand are types of immersion syndrome injuries from prolonged exposure to severe cold (<10°C) and dampness.
- In frostbite, injury is due to formation of ice crystals with obstruction of blood supply.
- Heat cramps/miner's cramps are due to fluid and electrolyte depletion.
- **Heat stroke:** Failure of thermoregulatory mechanism characterized by hyperthermia (>40°C), CNS dysfunction and anhidrosis.
- Burn is due to dry heat whereas scald is due to moist heat (liquid >60°C or steam).
- First degree (epidermal) burns heal without scar and are simple in nature.
- Second and third degree burns heal by scar formation.
- Third degree (deep) burns are relatively painless (due to damage of nerve endings).
- Dupuytren's and Wilson's classification are used to assess the degree of burns.
- **Wallace Rule of Nines** is used to calculate the total body surface area (TBSA) burnt.
- Lund and Browder chart is used in children to calculate TBSA.
- **Rule of palms:** Surface area of a patient's palm is roughly 1% of TBSA.
- Minimum temperature to produce burns: 44°C.
- **Parkland formula (Baxter formula):** Calculates fluid to be given in first 24 h.
- **Immediate cause of death in burns:** Neurogenic shock or asphyxia.
- **Delayed cause of death in burns:** Hypovolemic shock (within 24-48 h) and sepsis (>4–5 days).
- **PM staining in burns:** Cherry red in color due to CO.
- Pugilistic attitude is due to heat stiffening; seen in extensive burns with flexion of hips, knees and arms.

CHAPTER 14 : Thermal Injuries

- Pugilistic attitude can be antemortem or postmortem—*no medico-legal significance*.
- **Heat ruptures:** Splits occurring in skin due to prolonged exposure to heat; simulate incised/lacerated wounds *(artifacts)*.
- **Heat hematoma in skull:** It is an artifact and has the appearance of EDH.
- **Surest sign of antemortem burns:** Carbon and soot particles in larynx, trachea and bronchioles.
- **Curling's ulcers** in gastric antrum and first part of duodenum develop after 72 h of burns.

Ulcer type	Seen in
Curling's ulcers	Burns
Cushing ulcer	Brain injury

- Intense heat causes shriveling of internal organs which became firm, hardened and cooked—'**puppet organs**'.
- **Necklacing:** Method of homicidal burning by placing petrol filled tyre around the neck of the victim and setting it alight.
- **Characteristic of scalds:** Sharp demarcation with trickle marks, soddening and bleaching, but do not singe hair or blacken/char the skin.
- AC is 4–5 times more dangerous than DC. Electrocution is rare at <100 V and most deaths occur at >200 V.
- Most resistant body tissue to electrical injury: Bone → Skin → Blood vessel.
- There is *no red line* surrounding the electrical burns or reddening of base at the point of entry and exit.
- **Characteristic feature of electrocution:** Joule burns at the point of entry.
- Joule burn is produced in heating of tissues by electric current—*endogenous burns*.
- Microscopically, the epidermis in Joule burn shows a *Swiss cheese appearance*.
- In high-voltage burns, '*crocodile skin lesions*' (confluent areas of 3° burns or red/brown punched-out spark lesions) are seen.
- Flash burns are also called *exogenous burns* as the flame is produced outside the body.
- **Current pearls:** Small balls of molten metal derived from the electrode carried deep into tissues (identified by *scanning electron microscopy*).
- **Bone pearls/wax drippings:** X-rays of limbs show round dense foci caused by melting of calcium phosphate due heat generated by electric current.
- **Most common cause of death in electrocution:** Ventricular fibrillation (in low voltage current).
- **Acro-reaction test:** Micro-chemical test for metals at site of entry of electric current.
- **Characteristic of lightning burns:** Lichtenberg flowers/arborescent markings/filigree burns.

Interesting case

Postmortem Burns ('Tandoor' Murder Case, 1995)

Naina Sahni was killed and burnt in the Tandoor of a restaurant by her husband Sushil Sharma who was a political leader and member of legislative assembly. Policemen patrolling the area saw thick smoke coming from the tandoor and found her charred body, with both legs severed below the knee and arms cut below the elbow.

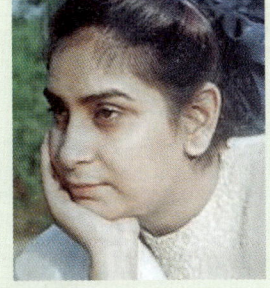

The first postmortem (PM) report gave the cause of death as 'excessive bleeding' and was probably unconscious when she was dismembered. The autopsy also found alcohol in her stomach. Dissatisfied with the first PM report (as the police recovered fired cartridge cases from the victim's flat), the second PM was ordered by Lieutenant Governor Delhi, which was conducted by a team of three doctors. The doctors got a PM X-ray done (which was not done in the first autopsy) and detected two bullets in head and neck region. As per the second PM report 'the cause of death was due to coma consequent upon firearm injury on the head which was found to be sufficient to cause death in the ordinary course of nature'. The ballistic expert also gave a report confirming that the fired cartridge cases came from the .32 Arminus revolver which was in possession of accused. The case also involved the use of DNA evidence to establish the identity of the victim.

The PM and ballistic reports led the lower court sentencing the accused to death. He appealed against the lower court verdict in the High Court which upheld the lower court judgment. He then appealed to the Supreme Court which upheld his conviction, but commuted his death sentence to life imprisonment. The 'tandoor murder case' is one of the landmark cases for the use of *second autopsy* to establish the guilt of the accused.

CHAPTER 15

Transportation Injuries

LEARNING OBJECTIVES

Must know
1. Pedestrian injuries (primary and secondary impact and secondary injuries)
2. Front impact injuries for vehicle occupants
3. Steering wheel impact injury
4. Role of seat belt, seat belt injuries

Desirable to know
1. Motorcycle injuries
2. Railway injuries
3. Postmortem examination of death due to road traffic injury

Definitions

- **Transportation injuries** are blunt force injuries that occur from travel on the ground, in the air and on water. The most frequent of these are motor vehicle collision and pedestrian injuries. Less common cases are associated with railway accidents and aircraft crashes.
- **Motor vehicle collision or road traffic accident** occurs when a vehicle collides with another vehicle, pedestrian, animal, road debris or other stationary barrier, such as a tree or utility pole.
- **Hit-and-run:** Failure to stop at scene of accident by the driver of a motor vehicle without giving assistance or informing the police.

Those injured by accidents can be divided into three broad groups: pedestrians, cyclists (pedal or motor) and the drivers and passengers of vehicles.

- Pedestrians (most common), cyclists, children and the elderly are among the most vulnerable of road users.

Describe and discuss injuries related to vehicular injuries—primary and secondary impact, secondary injuries.

PEDESTRIAN INJURIES

- Most pedestrian crashes involve the bumper and front of the vehicle.
- In a typical situation, an adult sustains bumper injuries on the legs. These injuries may be severe, with fractures and extensive soft tissue damage, or may be minimal or even absent on external examination of the body. Moreover, in winters, when heavy garments are worn, injuries caused by impact of car bumpers may be inconspicuous, since much force is absorbed by clothing.
- Severity of injury depends upon:
  a. speed of the vehicle
  b. shape of the bumper
  c. amount of clothing over the area struck
  d. age of the pedestrian

Three patterns of injuries are seen (**Fig. 15.1**):
  i. Primary impact injuries
  ii. Secondary impact injuries
  iii. Secondary injuries

Primary Impact Injuries

- Primary impact injuries indicate that part of the body which has been struck first by the vehicle, and often form recognizable patterns.
- Injuries include abrasions, contusion (sometimes patterned car's headlight) and lacerations on legs, thighs or buttocks due to overstretching, along with fractures of the tibia and fibula, and rarely, of the femur and pelvis (**Figs. 15.2A to C**).
- When an adult is hit by the front of a car, the front bumper or radiator usually strikes the victim at about knee level. The exact point of contact, whether on the front, side or back of the leg(s) will depend on the orientation of the victim. It also depends on the type of car, possible lowering of the car's front end (from braking) and pedestrian height.

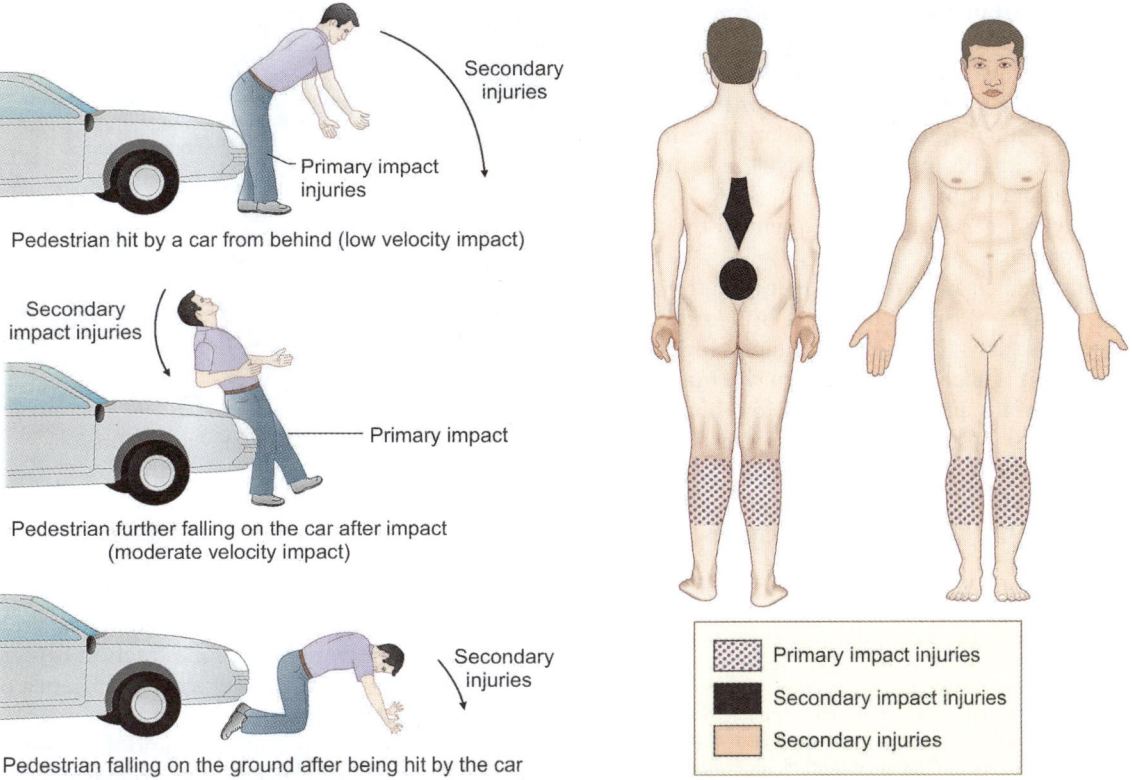

Fig. 15.1: Dynamics of pedestrian injuries and sites of primary impact, secondary impact and secondary injuries

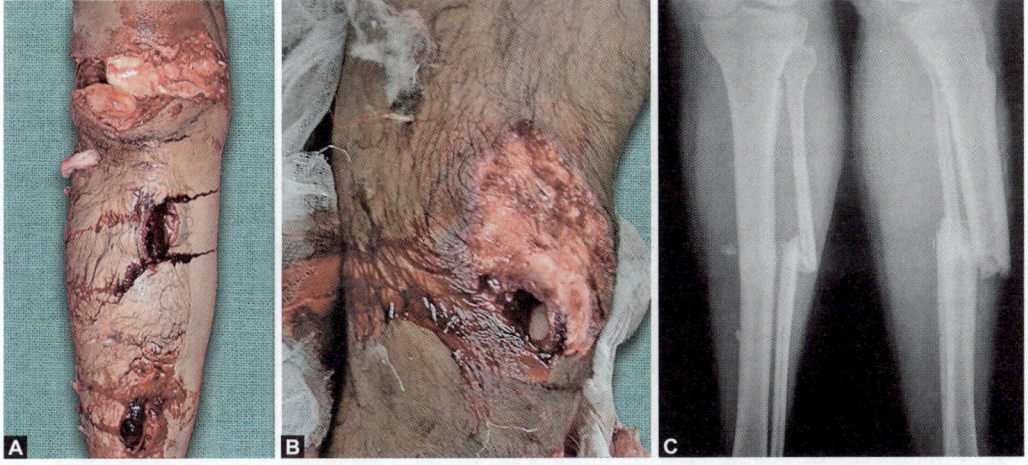

Figs. 15.2A to C: (A and B) Primary impact injury; (C) X-ray showing fracture of tibia and fibula

- They help to establish the position of the victim at the material moment when struck, and help towards identification of the offending vehicle.

Behavior of the body and disposition of injuries will be modified by factors like:
- Whether both the feet were firmly placed on the ground or one of them was raised at the time of impact.
- *Speed of the vehicle*: At low speeds (e.g., 20 kph), the victim is usually thrown off the bonnet either forwards or to one side. Between 20 and 60 kph, the victim may be tipped onto the bonnet, and the head may strike the windscreen or the metal frame that surrounds it. At higher speeds (60–100 kph), the victim may be projected into the air ('scooped-up'); sometimes pass completely over the vehicle and avoid hitting the windscreen and other points on the vehicle.
- *Nature of road surface*: Smooth, rough, full of gravel or mud and its skidding resistance.
- Point of impact in relation to the center of gravity.

When the pedestrian is knocked down from behind with both feet fixed to the ground: There will be fracture of the bones of the lower limbs, the buttocks and back of the pedestrian on being hit by head lamps or the radiator of the car. It may result in fracture dislocation of the lumbar or thoracic spine, and this injury may drive the femoral head through the acetabulum.

- Stretch-type lacerations are frequent in the inguinal (groin) regions.
- Where the vehicle is relatively larger than the victim—adults impacted by a truck or a bus and children impacted by cars—the point of contact is higher up the victim, and it is likely that the victim will make contact with more of the front of the vehicle. This pattern of contact may be result in primary injuries to the pelvis, abdomen, chest and head. Usually, the victim is projected along the line of travel of the vehicle, which may increase the risk of 'run-over' injuries.

> **NOTA BENE**
>
> **Waddell's triad** is a classic pattern of injury seen in pedestrian children who are struck by motor vehicles. It comprises of fractured femoral shaft, intra-thoracic or intra-abdominal injuries and contralateral head injury. Mechanism of injury is an initial impact causing injury to the pelvis and femur (bumper injury) instead of the knees and tibias; followed by the chest and abdomen (grill, fender or hood). Then the child is thrown on the ground and sustaining injury to the opposite side of the head.

On being struck from behind and feet not firmly on the ground: The victim's feet will fall backward and may be propelled upwards and backwards, so that the head may sustain *secondary impact injury* by striking against the windscreen. The victim can also be 'scooped-up' or fall to one side and may sustain head injuries by striking the ground on falling.

If the victim is struck from front, he may sustain injuries to the chest and abdomen with fracture of ribs or vertebrae. Victim can also sustain fracture of pelvis or fracture dislocation of sacroiliac joint from the impact of a mudguard, and fracture of tibia and fibula of one or both legs can be sustained from impact by a bumper.

- *Bumper impacts* usually cause soft tissue damage and comminuted wedge-shaped fracture of the tibia with forward displacement of the bony fragments **(Figs. 15.3A and B)**. Base of the triangular fractured fragment will suggest the site of impact and its apex will point to the direction of the moving vehicle.*
  Bumper injuries at different levels in two legs or when absent on one leg, will suggest that the victim was walking or running while struck.

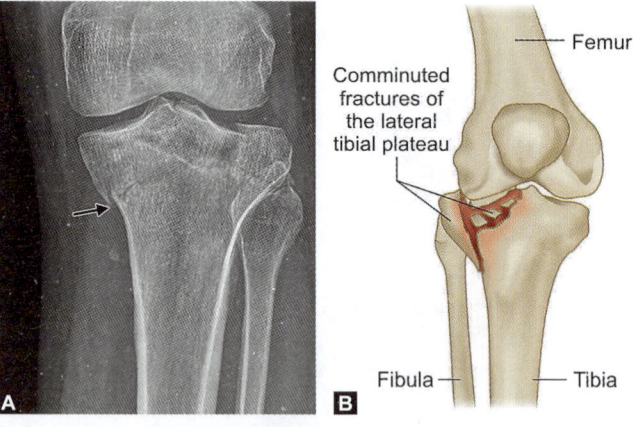

Figs. 15.3A and B: Bumper fracture

- Bumper fracture when present, the measurement of the distance from the heel to the fracture site will give an idea about the height of the bumper of the offending vehicle. When brakes are applied before the accident, the distance from heel to the fracture is less than the height of the bumper (presence or absence of braking may help to determine the driver's intent).¥
- The lack of 'bumper injuries' and the presence of tyre marks could indicate the pedestrian was already prone or supine on the road when 'run over'.

When the pedestrian walks onto the side of a moving vehicle: He will sustain glancing abrasions or crushing lacerations on the side or front of the face, chest and arms. Due to *primary impact injury* over the elbow, there may be fracture of ribs with/without laceration of the lungs. The victim on being struck on the side will be pushed forward or to the side, and will sustain *secondary injuries* on striking the ground.

Fracture of the skull occurs due to direct impact of the vehicle on the head or when the head strikes the ground following secondary injuries.

Secondary Impact Injuries

- These are often seen in case of 'scooped up' victim being thrown over the bonnet, i.e., further injuries caused by the vehicle following primary impact. He may sustain injuries by hitting his head against the windscreen, its rim or side-pillars.
- Extensive abrasions, bruises and lacerations may be seen.

Secondary Injuries/Tertiary Impact Injuries

These result from body parts striking the ground following the primary and secondary impact. They are more lethal than the primary injuries, especially to the head, chest and pelvis.

---
* Strictly, bumper fracture is a fracture of the lateral tibial plateau.
¥ Bumper fracture do not occur unless the vehicle was traveling at ≥25 kph.

- When the pedestrian is thrown to the ground, he sustains abrasions (skidding *brush burns* are common), bruises or lacerations over the bony prominences, such as elbows, knees, etc. which is most pronounced over unclothed areas.
- Brain damage is frequent without any associated skull fractures. This is due to the moving head of the victim being suddenly stopped on impact (*contrecoup injury*)—diffuse damage to axons may be caused by the rotational or shearing forces acting upon the brain.
- Fracture of the skull and ribs due to direct contact with a surface, and fracture of the spine due to hyperflexion or extension may be seen. Fractures of the spine, especially in the cervical and thoracic segments may lead to cord damage.
- Fractures of the limbs are common but apart from those of the legs (primary impact sites), they are rather unpredictable because of the random movements of the limbs.
- Sometimes, pedestrians are 'run over' if knocked down by the vehicle. This will tend to occur if the pedestrian's center of gravity is lower than the impact site, or scooped-up victim being run-over by other vehicles. Injuries are variable, depending on the area of the body involved, the weight of the vehicle and the surface area of the contact.

There may be:
  i. Tyre tread marks over the unclothed or not very thickly clothed areas on one surface of the body, with graze-like abrasions on the opposite side, i.e., pavement side **(Figs. 15.4A and B)**.
  ii. The head may be crushed causing gross distortion and externalization of the brain, or severe injuries may occur to the chest, pelvis or abdomen **(Fig. 15.4C)**.
  iii. Compression of the chest may result in multiple rib fractures, causing a 'flail chest' with rupture of internal organs along with fracture of the spine, sternum and ribs.
  iv. Avulsion injury occurs when the wheel moves over a fleshy part causing degloving of skin and subcutaneous tissue, by tearing it away from underlying tissues. It is also called '*flaying injury*', and is seen mostly in legs, arms and scalp **(Fig. 15.5)**.
  v. Burning and singeing of skin and hair resulting from discharge of hot exhaust.
- Usually, it is very difficult to classify the injuries as primary impact, secondary impact or secondary injuries.
- Typical injuries seen in car vs. adult pedestrian collision at moderate speed is given in **Table 15.1**.
- A rear impact pedestrian is often associated with fracture of the spine, often fracture/dislocation at base of the skull at the atlanto-occipital joint.
- In pedestrian accidents, the common cause of death is head injuries and fracture dislocations of cervical spine, mainly at the atlanto-occipital joint. Injuries to the chest and abdomen are minimal or absent.

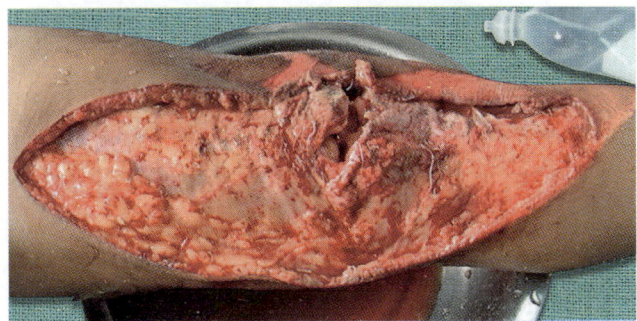

Fig. 15.5: Avulsion injury of thigh and leg

TABLE 15.1: Typical injuries in car vs. adult pedestrian collision

Phase	Site of impact	Injuries
Primary impact	Bumper	Lower extremity
Secondary impact	Vehicle hood, pillar, windscreen	Head and torso
Secondary	Ground and fixed object	Head and torso
Run-over	Crushing, car or another vehicle	Abdominal and thoracic

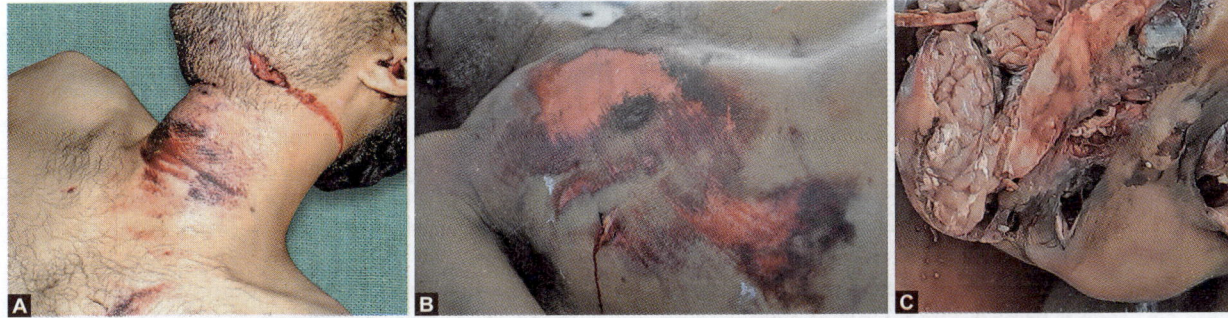

Figs. 15.4A to C: (A) Tyre treadmark over neck; (B) Graze abrasion on the chest; (C) Crush injury of head
[*Courtesy*: (B) Dr Chaitanya Mittal, BCRMMRC, IIT Kharagpur; (C) Dr Mukul Sharma AIIMS, Raebareli]

> **NOTA BENE**
>
> For injury documentation, incision should be made in areas of the body known to be frequently traumatized, even in absence of external evidence of injury. Incision and reflection of the skin of both calves and exploration of the calf muscles is vital to determine the presence of bumper impact. The incision should be vertical and extend from above the popliteal fossa to the entire length of each calf. Deep exploration of the hips may help to document a subcutaneous pocket filled with blood and crushed fat.

Identify from X-rays whether it is primary imact, secondary impact or secondary injury. Give reasons.

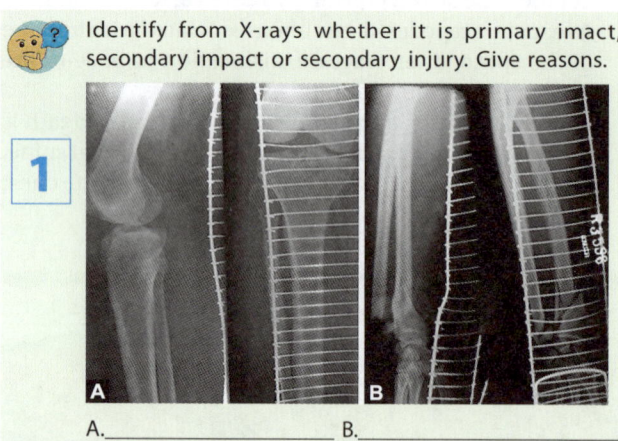

A. _____ B. _____

INJURIES SUSTAINED BY VEHICLE OCCUPANTS

- After pedestrians, the driver is the most frequent casualty in road traffic accidents as a high proportion of vehicles are occupied only by a driver. Next in frequency is the front seat passenger, followed by rear seat passengers.
- Ejection of both driver and passenger from a vehicle is associated with significantly severe injuries or fatality as the doors often burst open.
- Unbelted rear seat occupants are also at increased risk of serious injury in motor vehicle accidents; they may be ejected or thrown forward against the front seat.
- The driver and passenger injuries depend upon the type of impact crash.

Types of impact	
i. Front impact	iii. Side impact
ii. Rear impact	iv. Roll-over

Front Impact Crash

This happens when one car strikes another car head-on or strikes a stationary object, like an electric pole/tree (approx. 80% of impacts). While the vehicle rapidly decelerates and stops, the occupants continue to move forward striking against the interior of the vehicle, unless they are restrained. If the head impacts against the windshield, the victim does not sustain severe cuts from the fragments of glass which used to happen when it was made exclusively of glass. Windshields, nowadays, are made of a thin outer and inner layer of glass with thick plastic core.

The driver tends to receive a different pattern of injury as compared to either the front seat or rear seat passenger.
- The driver may receive a momentary warning of the impending collision and brace himself against the steering wheel.
- Fractures of the wrists and arms may thus occur, as well as fractures or dislocation of tibia, fibula and pelvis may occur from transmission of the force of impact from pressing on the brake and clutch pedals.
- If the driver is *unaware*, his knees will impact against the dashboard, his chest against the steering wheel, and his head against the windshield.
- An impact of the knees against the dashboard commonly causes fractures of the tibia, fibula, femur and pelvis.
- Severe impact against the windshield pillar may cause avulsion of the skin of the forehead, basilar skull fractures, closed head injury and fracture or dislocation of the atlanto-occipital junction (**Fig. 15.6A**).

Steering Wheel Impact Injury

- The circular rim of the steering wheel may cause fractures of the jaws and facial bones, as well as imprint abrasions, minor bruises and contusions of the chest or bilateral rib fractures (**Fig. 15.7**).
- Transverse fracture of sternum is usually seen at 3rd intercostal space.
- Damaged steering wheel spokes may penetrate the chest and lacerate the heart and lungs. Flail chest may occur.
- With severe thoracic compression, partial or complete transection of aorta may occur usually at the junction of the aortic arch with descending aorta—*classical injury*. The rupture is circular, clean cut and with multiple transverse intimal tears, adjacent to main wound (*ladder tears*).
- Lacerations of liver and spleen may be seen.
- Serious steering wheel injuries are less frequent, if the car is fitted with energy absorbing compressible steering wheel column.

Front Seat Passenger

- The most dangerous place in the car is the *front passenger seat*. He may not get the momentary warning of the impending collision. Without a seat belt, he is at risk of severe impaction of his head against the windshield with its consequences (**Fig. 15.6B**). The occupant may be ejected out of the vehicle through the windscreen, increasing the risks of secondary injuries or running over.
- There may be peculiar facial lacerations due to contact with the shattered windscreen known as '**sparrow foot marks**' (similar to dicing injuries mentioned below)

Rear Impact Crash

Low velocity rear impacts are relatively common. Usually, they cause whiplash injury. Neck fractures are rare. A high velocity rear impact crash can deform and rupture the gas tank with ignition of the fuel.

Side Impact Crash

The vehicle strikes on the side of another vehicle or skids sideways into a fixed object. This is a common pattern in an intersection, and is therefore a frequent occurrence in urban areas.

Injuries are often severe, because the side of a car has a thin metal wall door and no other components to absorb the force of impact. Since, the occupants of the vehicle move toward the side of impact, the persons sitting on that side run the greatest risk.

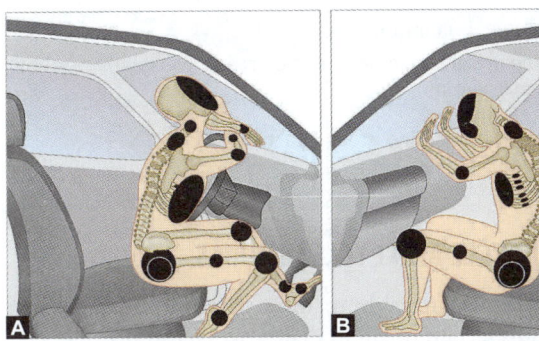

Figs. 15.6A and B: Major sites of injury (black shaded) in: (A) Unrestrained driver; (B) Front seat passenger of a car

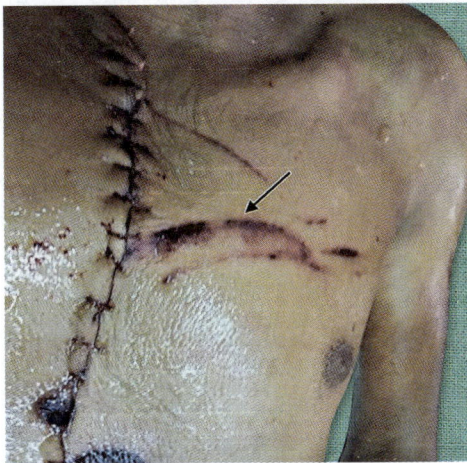

Fig 15.7: Steering wheel marks on chest

- **Dicing injuries** may occur which are superficial cuts of the skin caused by fragments of tempered glass (designed to shatter into small glass cubes on violent impact).
- They are produced when the side and the back windows of a car shatter.
- They are linear, right angled or V-shaped laceration seen typically on the face, forehead and arm on the right side of the driver and left or right side of passengers. Fragments of tempered glass embedded in the wound may be seen.
- They help to locate the position occupied by the victim in the automobile.

- Cervical spine fracture, fractured ribs, contusions, lacerations and explosive tearing of the lungs on the side of the impact are common.
- External injuries tend to be on the right side of the driver, the right arm and leg may be fractured.
- Internally, fractures of ribs on the right side are seen. In the abdomen, a lateral impact on the right side commonly causes lacerations of the right lobe of the liver and right kidney. An impact on the left frequently lacerates the spleen, left kidney and left lobe of the liver. The pelvis may be fractured from impact on either side.

(Fig. 15.8). Contact with the dashboard may cause injuries to the knee **(Fig. 15.6B)**.

Passengers of the rear seat often escape such injuries because of the absence of impact against the windshield and dashboard, and of the cushioning effect of the front seat. However, they may be injured against internal fittings, like door handles or ejected through burst-open doors.

Roll-over Crash

Although, the automobile may suffer severe damage in a roll-over crash, the occupants receive surprisingly moderate impact, if the vehicle is not brought to a sudden stop and the impact is spread over a period of time. It is usually less lethal than front or side impact collision. The crashing of different sides of the vehicle absorbs the forces of impact, if the passenger compartment remains intact, the belted occupants frequently survive the crash (anything that prevents ejection of occupants). Non-belted occupants are involved in two types of injury:

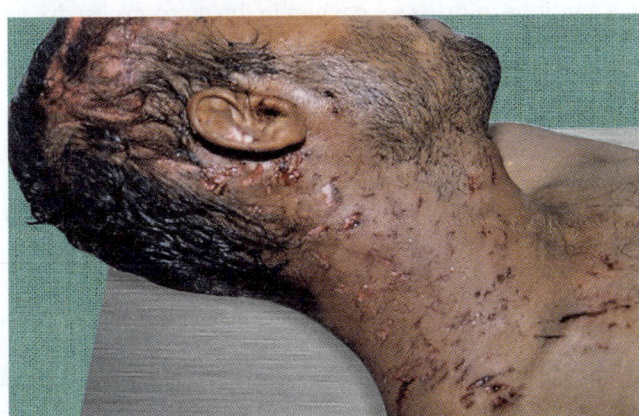

Fig. 15.8: Facial lacerations due to shattered tempered glass

1. Tumbling around inside and striking the interior of the vehicle
2. Ejection out from the vehicle.

There is no specific injury pattern.

ROLE OF SEAT BELTS AND AIR BAGS

Numerous safety features such as safety belts, airbags, collapsible steering columns, softened interior dashboards and antilock brakes have contributed to the saving of lives.

The air bag system has reduced the gravity and incidence of chest and facial trauma, especially in those individuals not using seat belts. These are intended to provide protection only in frontal crashes and to be used in conjunction with seat belts. Compared to three-point seat belts, air bags are significantly less effective.

Seat belts offer the greatest benefits in frontal and rollover crashes. Wearing seat belts reduces the risk of fatalities to front seat occupants by 45%, since:

- Injuries are of less severity, except whiplash injury.
- Probability of severe head injury is lower.
- Probability of being ejected from the vehicle is lower.
- There are fewer fatal/major injuries to head, neck, chest and abdomen.

Although, seat belts reduce mortality, they cause a specific pattern of internal injuries.

- **Seat belt syndrome** is a collective term that includes a seat belt mark, an intra-abdominal organ injury (e.g., bowel perforations) and/or thoracolumbar vertebral fractures (*Chance fractures*). It is a result of the pressure that the belt causes along its course, and is associated with lap-belt restraints.
- The presence of a seat belt mark (skin abrasions of the neck, chest and abdomen) indicates that the possibility of injury to the chest and abdomen to be four and eight times more respectively compared with those without seat belt mark.
- Injuries caused by seat belt are given in **Box 15.1**.

NOTA BENE

- There are three forms of automobile belt restraints: Lap belts, shoulder (diagonal) belts and three-point belts (lap plus shoulder). Lap belts were the first form of restraint used in automobiles. The most popular and efficient seat belt is the three-point belt which consists of both a diagonal and transverse strap set in inertia recoil housing.
- **Chance fractures (seat belt fractures)** are flexion-distraction type injuries of the spine that extend to involve all three spinal columns (anterior, middle and posterior). These are unstable injuries and have a high association with intra-abdominal injuries. This fracture is most commonly seen in the upper lumbar spine (thoracolumbar junction).

Box 15.1 Seat belt injuries

- Lacerated mesentery, omentum, bowel and liver
- Abdominal wall injuries
- Fractured spine
- Chest injuries including sternal fracture
- Blood vessel injuries
- Myocardial contusion

MOTORCYCLE AND CYCLE INJURIES

- An accident that might result in minor injuries with an automobile, can result in death with a motorcycle.
- The common causes of motorcycle accidents are alcohol, drugs, environmental factors (bumps or potholes), reckless driving and failure by drivers of cars to see the motorcycle. The most common cause of motorcycle fatality is running off the road.
- Most injuries are due to ejection from the vehicle into the roads, due to high speed and instability of the vehicle. In a high speed impact of a motorcycle, there may be primary injuries due to the initial impact, followed by secondary injuries from striking the ground. Head and leg injuries are common.
    - *Primary injuries* are mostly open fractures of the tibia and fibula.
    - *Secondary injuries* are mostly fractures of the skull, ribs and cervical spine, as well as contusions of the brain. There are graze abrasions due to sliding across the road.
- **Fracture of the skull:** Transverse fracture of the base of the skull—the *hinge fracture* is common, sometimes referred to as '*motorcyclists fracture*'. Temporoparietal fractures are also quite common. Ring fracture around the foramen magnum may be seen in some cases by an impact of the crown of the head.
- Passengers falling off the backs of the motorcycle will have lacerations of the back of the head, fractures of posterior cranial fossa, contrecoup contusions of frontal lobes of the brain, and abrasions of back and elbows. If they fall forwards, there will be abrasions of the face.
- A unique injury is seen wherein the motorcyclist drives under the rear of the truck, causing head injuries and even decapitation, which is known as **'under-running'** or **'tail-gating'**.*

Pedal cycle injuries are common in India, but severity is less due to slow speeds. Primary injuries may occur from impact by cars and trucks, but secondary injuries involving the head and chest are common from falling. A unique injury seen among bicyclists is stripping of the skin from the leg due to limb being forced between the wheel spokes.

---

* This injury has been reduced by the presence of bars at the sides and rear of trucks to prevent both bikes and cars passing under the vehicle.

> **NOTA BENE**
> - *Motorcyclists* experience a death rate 35 times greater than occupants of cars. Helmets reduce the risk of fatal head injury by 1/3rd and reduce the risk of facial injury by 2/3rd. Fractures of the lower extremities are common, occurring in approximately 40% of motorcyclists hospitalized for non-fatal injuries.
> - *Injuries to bicyclists*: Children aged 5–14 years have the highest rates of injury and head injury accounts for 75% of the deaths. Helmets have been shown to reduce the risk of brain injury for bicyclists by 88%.
> - *Injuries to pedestrians occur* disproportionately among school going children, the elderly and the intoxicated.

■ POSTMORTEM EXAMINATION

Photographs of the scene, clothing and injuries should be taken routinely. Since, some countries limit the damages to be recovered if the victim was not wearing a seat belt, any injuries consistent with seat belt injuries should be noted. The role of the automobile to commit homicide is also postulated.

History

The history should include the condition of the eyes (corneal opacities), blindness, if the victim was suffering from any disease, e.g., heart, epilepsy or diabetes, drugs that he was using (or abusing), and if he was depressed or under unusual stress.

Clothing

The clothing should be described with special attention to tyre imprint marks, tears, amount of bleeding and foreign bodies, especially glass particles, metal, grease marks or oil stains and paint which may indicate the part of the vehicle that struck the victim and provide valuable evidence with respect to the suspected vehicle (hit and run cases). Similarly, hair, blood and other tissues can be transferred from the pedestrian to the vehicle. For this reason, autopsy surgeon should preserve hair and blood samples for comparison.

Injuries

External injuries: It should include:
i. The type of the wound, i.e., whether it is a bruise, abrasion or laceration.
ii. The wound dimensions, viz. length, width and depth. It is helpful to take a photograph of the wound with an indication of dimension (e.g., a tape measure placed next to the wound).
iii. The position of the wound in relation to fixed anatomical landmarks, e.g., distance from the midline or below the clavicle.
iv. The height of the wound from the heel (i.e., ground level)—this is important in cases where pedestrians have been struck by motor vehicles, so that the height of an impact point can be compared with any suspect vehicle.

Internal injuries: The distribution of fatal injuries is mostly related to the head and chest. Due to extraordinary resilience of the skin, serious internal injuries may be present without any evidence of corresponding external injury. It is therefore necessary to incise suspected areas of impact.

Laboratory Specimens

A blood sample (of the driver or pedestrian) should be analyzed for the presence and amount of alcohol (taken from peripheral vein and not from heart or viscera, if death occurred within 12–24 h of accident) and drugs, since the question of contributory negligence may subsequently arise. If sufficient blood is not obtainable, vitreous fluid from the eye can be analyzed for alcohol. The urine should be screened for commonly abused drugs.

Medico-legal Issues

Whether the Victim was the Driver or a Passenger?

Sometimes, it is necessary to know who was driving the vehicle for insurance purpose. Following can assist the autopsy surgeon in determining if a particular occupant was the driver:
- **Steering wheel impact abrasions** may be seen on the chest.
- **Dicing injuries** on the right side of the body.
- **Patterned seat belt abrasion** is seen on the right side of shoulder going diagonally across the chest to the left. In front seat passenger, it is on the left going diagonally to the right **(Fig. 15.9)**.
- **Imprint marks** of the brake and clutch pedals on the soles of shoe if pressed at the time of impact (patterns on the accelerator and brake pedals are purposefully different from one another).

Whether it is a Case of Accident, Suicide or Homicide?

In different jurisdictions, autopsy surgeons may rule the manner of death in hit-and-run pedestrian fatalities as 'homicide', 'accident', 'suicide' or 'undetermined' depending on the existing protocol.

Suicide with a car is difficult to prove. However, following maybe helpful:
i. History of previous suicidal attempts/depression/domestic quarrels/financial crisis.
ii. Evidence of over speeding.

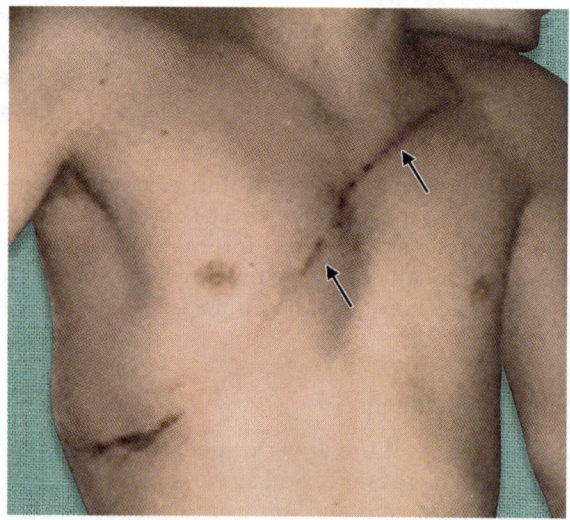

Fig. 15.9: Patterned seat belt abrasion over chest (arrows)

iii. Impact on a tree/bridge usually on the front of vehicle in its center.
iv. Single occupancy of the car.
v. Imprint of accelerator pedal pattern on the sole.
vi. Absence of evidence of applying brakes with absence of skid marks leading to the site of collision.
vii. Recovery of suicide note.

 Two persons met with a fatal accident in the early hours of the day. One of the occupants sustained multiple injuries and died on the spot. The other person was arrested by the police for negligent driving. But he claimed that he was sitting next to the driver. Dicing injuries sustained by him are shown below. Whether this person was the driver or a passenger?

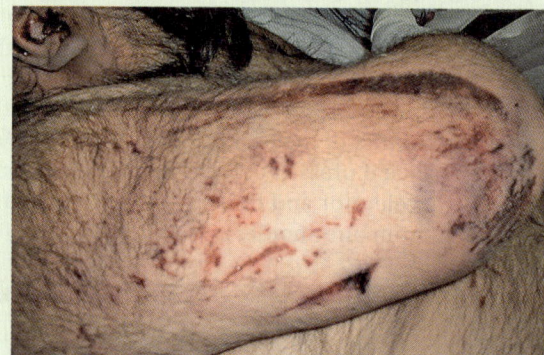

ALCOHOL, DRUGS AND TRAUMA

Alcohol and substance abuse are major associated factors in all forms of trauma. About 10% of the drivers with blood alcohol level higher than the legal limit account for nearly 1/3rd of non-fatal and half of fatal driver deaths. Injury to drunken pedestrians shows even greater association, as pedestrian accidents account for nearly 3/4th of adult traffic accidents. There is a strong association with alcohol, drug dependency and dangerous driving, violent and aggressive behavior.

- Drugs tested for should include alcohol, carbon monoxide, acid, basic and neutral drugs. Marijuana and opiates testing are indicated in select cases.
- Blood used for testing should be the one which has been drawn prior to starting of IV fluids and blood transfusion.
- In case of death, analysis of vitreous fluid is valuable as it reflects the alcohol and drug levels 1–2 h prior to death.

RAILWAY INJURIES

These are common in India and China because of a wide network and unprotected crossings. It is a common mode of suicide, but accidents are common in children. There is nothing specific about railway accidents, except the frequency of severe mutilation.

- The body may be severed into many pieces and soiled by axle grease and dirt from the wheels and track.
- When passengers fall off from the train, multiple injuries along with abrasions are seen due to contact with coarse gravel along the line ballast.
- Suiciders either jump in front of a moving train from a platform, bridge or other structure near to the track, or place their head across a rail causing transected neck, either partial or complete with black soiling at the crushed decapitation or amputation site **(Fig. 15.10)**.
- There may be 'flail chest' along with traumatic asphyxia when the victim is crushed between the buffers of two bogies.
- A careful search for unusual injuries (stabs, gunshots), and for vital reaction to the severe blunt force injuries should be made, as there many occasions when the victim of a homicide has been placed onto the rail track in an attempt to make it appear like an accident.

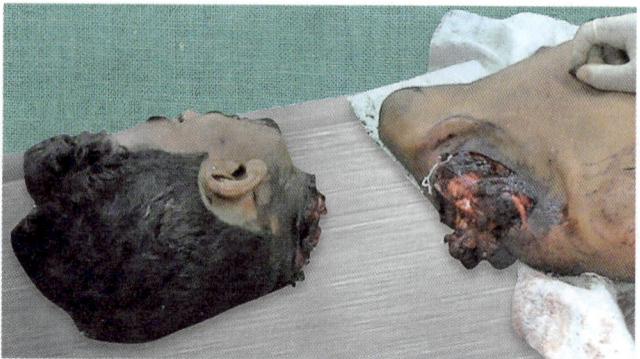

Fig. 15.10: Decapitation in railway track (suicide)

CHAPTER 15 : Transportation Injuries

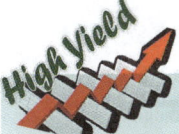

- Pedestrians (most common), cyclists, children and elderly are most vulnerable to road traffic injuries.
- **Primary impact injuries:** Part of body which has been struck first by vehicle; most commonly seen in the legs.
- **Secondary impact injuries:** Further injuries caused by the vehicle following primary impact.
- **Secondary injuries:** Result from body striking the ground following primary and secondary impact.
- Extensive abrasions found on the body of a pedestrian are example of secondary injury.
- **Common cause of death in pedestrian accidents:** Head injuries and fracture dislocations of cervical spine, mainly at the atlanto-occipital joint.
- **Waddell's triad:** Fracture femur, thoracic/abdominal injuries and contralateral head injury—seen in pedestrian children who are struck by motor vehicles.
- **Bumper fracture:** Fracture of tibial plateau; occurs when bumper of a car hits lateral side of knee.
- **Steering wheel impact injury:** Imprint abrasions, bruises and contusions of chest, fractures of jaws and facial bones, bilateral rib fractures. Transverse fracture of sternum is usually seen at 3rd intercostal space.
- Severe thoracic compression may cause transection of aorta at the junction of aortic arch with descending aorta *(classical injury)*.
- Ladder tears are seen in aorta around the transected artery.
- **'Sparrow foot marks'** facial lacerations are seen due to contact with the shattered windscreen.
- **Dicing injuries:** Superficial cuts of the skin caused by fragments of tempered glass (*right side of driver and left/right side of passengers*).
- **Most common injury caused by seat belt:** Lacerated mesentery and omentum.
- **Seat belt syndrome:** Seat belt mark plus an intra-abdominal organ injury (e.g., bowel perforations) and/or thoracolumbar vertebral fractures *(Chance fractures)*.
- **Motorcyclists fracture/hinge fracture**: Transverse fracture of base of skull seen in motorcyclists.
- **Under-running/'tail-gating'**: Injury seen in motorcyclist when he hits the rear of truck, causing head injuries.
- In case of driver of a vehicle, patterned seat belt abrasion is seen on the right side of shoulder going diagonally across the chest to the left.

Interesting case

Driver or Passenger (Case of Billy Martin, 1989)

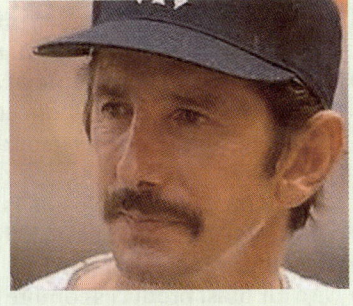

Alfred 'Billy' Martin was a legendary baseball player and was killed in a low speed pickup truck crash during an ice storm in New York on Christmas Day in 1989. He suffered a broken neck, a compressed spinal column and multiple internal injuries and was pronounced dead at the hospital. As per request of the family, no autopsy was done.

Reports of the crash indicated that Martin had been drinking earlier and his friend William Reedy, and hence he was driving him home. Neither Martin nor Reedy was wearing a seat belt. Reedy too suffered a broken hip and was charged with driving while intoxicated. Reedy at first stated that he was driving the vehicle with Martin as co-passenger. But after learning that Martin had died, changed his story, saying that he had lied to protect Martin against the consequences of a drunk driving conviction.

The Medical Examiner was allowed to examine Martin's body who also investigated the accident scene, including the pick-up truck in which he died. The forensic pathologist opined that Martin's impact injuries were all on the right side, and that hair and other DNA found on the right side of the shattered windshield belonged to Martin, who was not wearing a seat belt at the time of the accident (vehicles are left-hand driven in US). Reedy was also seen holding the car keys as the two left the bar, and the positions of the men when rescuers arrived pointed to Reedy being the driver. The final conclusion was that Reedy drove the pick-up and Martin was the passenger.

Reedy was convicted in a jury trial of driving with a blood alcohol level of .10% (above the New York State legal limit) was fined and his license suspended. A subsequent civil trial also found he was the driver.

CHAPTER 16

Explosion Injuries and Fall from Height

LEARNING OBJECTIVES

Must know
1. Characteristics of bomb blast injuries
2. Blast lung
3. Preservation and dispatch of evidences in blast injury
4. Marshall's triad

Desirable to know
1. Postmortem in blast injury deaths
2. Injuries sustained in fall from height and its medico-legal aspects

FM 3.10

Describe and discuss blast injuries and their interpretation, preservation and dispatch of trace evidences in cases of blast injuries.

EXPLOSION INJURIES

Definitions

- **Bomb** is a container filled with an explosive mixture and missiles which is fired either by detonator or a fuse.
  - **Incendiary bombs**, e.g., napalm bombs primarily cause burns. Usually phosphorus and magnesium are added. Temperature of 1000°C is produced.
  - **Molotov cocktail** is an incendiary bomb which is thrown by hand. In its crude form, a bottle is filled with gasoline, and a rag to serve as a wick. The wick is lit and thrown at the target.
- **Blast injury** is a complex type of physical trauma resulting from direct or indirect exposure to an explosion causing sudden increase or decrease in atmospheric pressure.

If the force of the explosion is transmitted through the air, the term 'air blast' is used; if through water, 'immersion blast', if through solids it is called 'solid blast'.

- An **air blast** produces compression of the body towards the side of the explosion. The injuries are less severe compared to immersion blast as force is dissipated in all directions and the molecules of the medium are less densely packed.
- In **immersion blast**, the body is compressed from all direction as the molecules of the medium are closely situated and the damage produced will be diffuse. If the liquid is in closed space, the shock wave from the air outside the liquid surface amplifies the shock waves in the medium and the injury will be severe.
- In case of **solid blasts**, the force is transmitted through part of the body in contact with the vibrating solid structure. Effects of primary and/or secondary impacts and secondary injuries may be seen on the body.

Mechanism of Action

The explosive pressure that accompanies the bursting of bombs or shells, ruptures their casing and imparts a high velocity to the resulting fragments. These fragments have the potential to cause more devastating injury to tissues than bullets.

In addition, all explosives are accompanied by a **complex wave**. The two main components of this wave are a **blast wave** (known as *dynamic overpressure*) with a positive and negative phase, and the **blast wind** (*mass movement of air*) **(Fig. 16.1)**. Injuries are mainly due to the initial shock wave, but are aggravated by the sub-atmospheric phase.

- The positive pressure phase of the blast wave lasts a few milliseconds, but close to an explosion it may rise to over 7000 kN/m². As the tympanic membrane ruptures at about 150 kN/m², the effects on the human body of such an explosion can be devastating. Like sound waves, the blast pressure waves flow around an obstruction and affect anyone sheltering behind a wall or a trench. Also, any person standing in front of a wall or any surface facing an explosion is subjected to the added effect of a reflected pressure.

CHAPTER 16: Explosion Injuries and Fall from Height

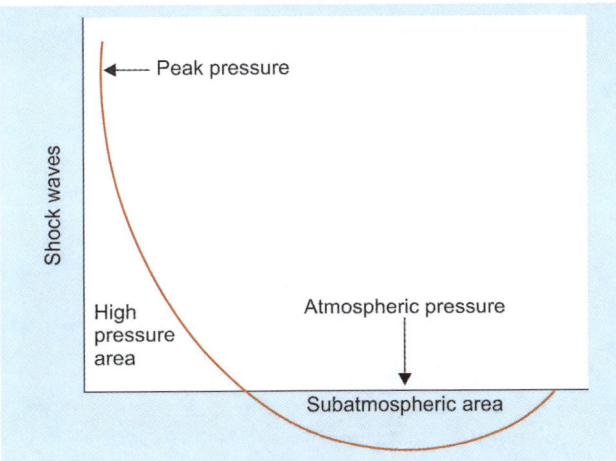

Fig. 16.1: Pressure changes occurring in bomb explosion

- The mass movement of air (*blast wind*) disrupts the environment, throwing debris and people. This phenomenon results in injuries ranging from traumatic amputation to disruption.
- When the body is impacted by a *blast pressure wave*, it couples into the body and sets up a series of stress waves which are capable of injury, particularly at air-fluid interfaces. Thus, injury to the ear, lungs, heart and the gastrointestinal tract (GIT) is notable.

Classification of explosives (based on material used)
i. **High-order explosives (HEs)** undergo detonation producing an instantaneous blast wave under extremely high pressure causing severe primary blast injury, e.g., TNT, dynamite, ammonium nitrate and C-4 'plastic' explosives.
ii. **Low-order explosives (LEs)** undergo deflagration rather than detonation, and thus lacking in blast wave—uncommonly to cause the pulmonary and central nervous system injuries unique to primary blast injury. They are composed of propellants such as black powder, pyrotechnics such as fireworks, and oil- or petroleum-based explosives such as Molotov cocktails.

CLASSIFICATION OF INJURIES

Blast injuries are divided into four categories: primary, secondary, tertiary and quaternary (**Table 16.1 and Fig. 16.2**).

i. **Primary:** Primary injuries are characterized by the absence of external injuries. They are usually internal injuries which are often unrecognized and their severity underestimated. The *ears are most often affected* by the overpressure, followed by the lungs and the hollow organs of the GIT. GIT injuries may present after a delay of hours or even days. Primary blast injuries are:
   - **Acoustic barotrauma** commonly consists of rupture of the tympanic membrane, dislocation of the ossicles or widespread disruption of the inner ear leading to permanent deafness.
   - **Lungs:** Considerable disruption at the alveolar-capillary membrane (air-fluid interface) leads to capillary leakage, resulting in extensive hemorrhage in both lobes of lung. There is pulmonary contusion, systemic air embolism and free radical-associated injuries such as thrombosis and DIC, or a combination of all these—**blast lung**. ARDS may be a result of direct lung injury or of shock from other body injuries.
     - Blast lung is the most common cause of death among people who initially survive an explosion.
     - Clinically characterized by the triad of dyspnea, bradycardia and hypotension, and the patient

TABLE 16.1: Classification of blast injury

Category	Characteristics	Body part affected	Type of injuries
Primary	Unique to HEs, results from the blast wave (over-pressurization wave)	Gas filled structures—lungs, GI tract, and middle ear	◆ Tympanic membrane rupture and middle ear damage ◆ Blast lung ◆ Abdominal perforation and hemorrhage ◆ Concussion ◆ Globe (eye) rupture
Secondary	Results from flying debris and shrapnel and bomb fragments	Any body part may be affected	◆ Penetrating or blunt injuries ◆ Eye penetration (can be occult)
Tertiary	Results from individuals being thrown by the blast wind against solid objects	Any body part may be affected	◆ Fracture and traumatic amputation ◆ Closed and open brain injury
Quaternary	Injuries not included in the first three categories. Includes exacerbation or complications of existing conditions	Any body part may be affected	◆ Burns (flash*, partial, and full thickness) ◆ Crush injuries ◆ Closed and open brain injury ◆ Asthma, COPD or other breathing problems from dust, smoke or toxic fumes ◆ Angina ◆ Hyperglycemia, hypertension

*When the bomb explodes, the temperature of the explosive gases can exceed 2000°C, and the heat radiated momentarily can cause flash burns.

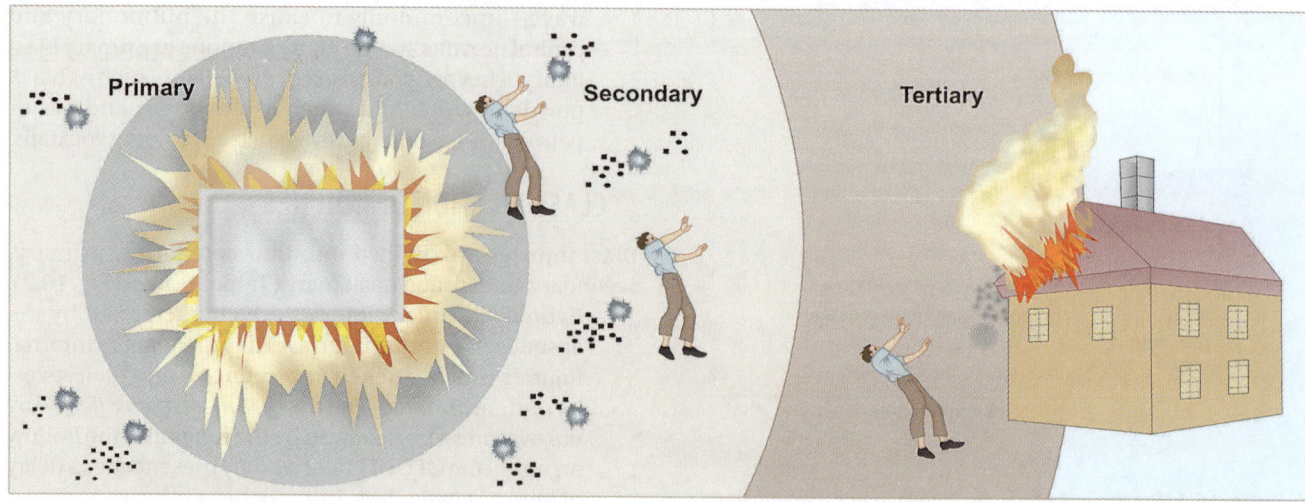

Fig. 16.2: Blast injuries

may present with dyspnea, cough, hemoptysis or chest pain.
- Chest radiographs in the initial stages may show localized contusion injury, but as the time passes, the effect becomes generalized with bilateral fluffy infiltrates spreading out from the hilum of both lungs—'*butterfly*' pattern.
- **GIT:** Injury to gas-filled viscera is more common in underwater explosions than in air blasts. Although the colon is most commonly affected, perforation of the stomach, small intestine and cecum are also seen.
- **Brain:** It can cause concussion or mild traumatic brain injury, without a direct blow to the head. There may be headache, fatigue, poor concentration, lethargy, depression, anxiety, insomnia or other constitutional symptoms.

ii. **Secondary injuries:** Most casualties are caused by secondary injuries. Some explosives, such as *nail bombs*, are purposely designed to increase the likelihood of secondary injuries.
   - Penetrating thoracic trauma, including lacerations of the heart and great vessels is a common cause of death.

iii. **Tertiary injuries:** Tertiary injuries may present as combination of blunt and penetrating trauma, including bone fractures and coup contrecoup injuries. Children are at particular risk because of their lesser weight.

iv. **Quaternary (miscellaneous) injuries:** Psychiatric injury (due to neurological damage sustained during the blast) is most common, and post-traumatic stress disorder (PTSD) may affect people who are otherwise completely uninjured.

Sequelae of traumatic injuries:
- Crush syndrome and acute renal failure may occur in patients rescued from collapsed structures.
- Increasing extremity pain after an explosion may indicate developing compartment syndrome.

Work up

The most common urgent clinical problem in survivors is usually the penetrating injury caused by blast-energized debris and fragments from the casing of the exploding device. Many of those exposed will have blunt, blast and thermal injuries, in addition to more obvious penetrating wounds (referred to as *combined injury*). The soft-tissue wounds are heavily contaminated with dirt, clothing and secondary missiles, such as wood, masonry and other materials from the environment (**flying missiles**).

Medico-legal Aspects

Forensic pathologist may encounter blast injuries in both routine case work and as part of mass casualty events. Therefore, recognition, proper interpretation and documentation of these types of injuries would assist with reconstruction of the incident.

a. **Whether a bomb explosion has caused the injuries?**
   - Full body photographs and complete X-rays of the whole body are indicated before the clothes are removed. Any radiopaque fragments and radiolucent material (paper fragments, wood and plastic) may be components of an explosive device.
   - 3D CT bony reconstruction and even soft tissue injuries from projectiles with foreign bodies in them may help reconstruct the explosion.
   - Residues are either burnt (black or gray) or unburnt (yellow, brown, gray) material. Swab the soiled skin and hands. Collect hair and fingernail scrapings.
   - Foreign body (shrapnel or empty shell) may be found during autopsy.
   - Toxicological analysis may also help.

- Extensive burns are usually not caused by localized bomb explosion.
b. **Number of dead persons:** A major initial problem, correct fragments are to be allocated to the right individuals.
c. **Identification of the dead:** The injuries can be extreme, and thus make identification and inter-pretation difficult for the autopsy surgeon. All body parts and clothing are recovered (clothing is submitted in airtight containers).
   - Dentition, dentures and artificial teeth also help in identification.
   - Fingerprinting may also help.
d. **Enlisting the injuries:** External and internal injuries are described in detail.
   External injuries
   Total body disintegration indicates high-order condensed explosive at close range.
   - There may be mangling of body near explosion with parts of extremities amputated; craniofacial injuries are seen in case of suicide. Lower limb amputation is typical of standing or seated individual. Hand injuries are seen, if explosive device was held **(Fig. 16.3)**.
   - There may be projectile injury.
   - Punctate lacerations, dust tattooing and black soiling from explosive materials may be seen. **Marshall's triad** of bruises, abrasions and punctate lacerations with tattooing of the body indicates bomb explosion **(Figs. 16.4A and B)**.
   - Injuries may be seen due to fallen rubble.
   - Burns (flash burns and singed hair seen on victims in immediate vicinity).
   Internal injuries have been described earlier.
e. **Cause of death:** Death may result from variety of causes, viz. complete disintegration of body, blast shock, burns, blunt force injuries and crush asphyxia.
f. **Circumstances of death** need to be looked for.

> **NOTA BENE**
> Recognizing the *'suicide bomber'* may be difficult. The nature of suicide bomber injuries is vital in locating and identifying these types of offenders. The hands are examined to determine whether he was holding the explosive **(Fig. 16.3)**.

Describe and discuss injuries related to fall from height.

FALL FROM HEIGHT

Introduction

- Deaths due to fall from height are common in urban settings. In occupational settings, it is the most common type of accident. Builders, electricians, miners and

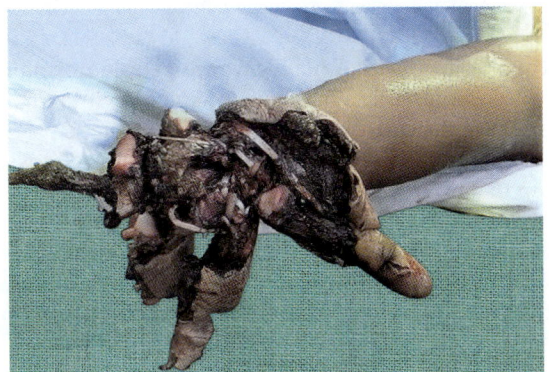
Fig. 16.3: Hand injury in case of hand held explosive

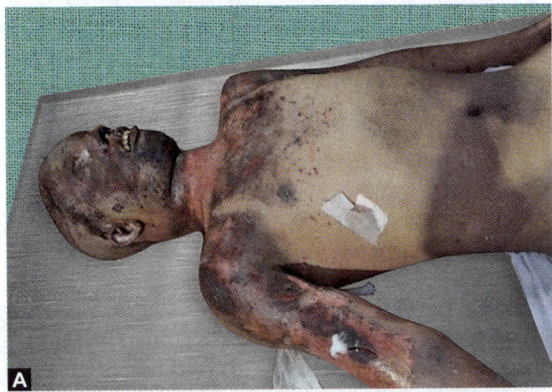

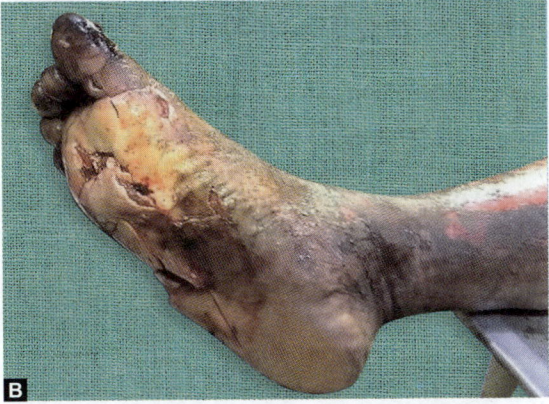
Figs. 16.4A and B: Marshall's triad of bruising, abrasion, laceration with soot soiling and tattooing

painters are particularly at risk. It is also a major cause of personal injury, especially for the children and the elderly.
- Factors contributing to falls from heights include faulty equipment, such as ladders and scaffold structures and human factors, such as intoxication and inattention.

The evaluation of injuries alone during autopsy is not sufficient to assess whether the manner of death is suicide, accident or homicide. Findings at the scene of death, and medical, psychiatric, social history and toxicology results of the victim should also be taken into account to determine the manner of death.

Investigation of the Scene

- Falls or jumps from places where people normally do not go are highly suspicious of suicide. Suicide notes are also indicative of a suicidal fall.
- Dangerous work-places like building sites—most falls are usually accidental.
- Signs of a fight at the death scene always suggest homicide. Distance of the body from the jumping site can be used as an additional tool to determine the manner of death. In intentional jumps, the distance to the jumping site is likely to be higher than in accidental falls.
- There are now established mathematical formulae for computing distance from superstructure to site of impact, and thus the question of fall vs. pushed can be determined. CT reconstruction of the pattern of fall and animation of the 3D bony window images may help in understanding the mechanism of fall and impact.

Psychiatric history: A history of psychiatric illness is most frequently found in suicidal falls from height which often includes depression, schizophrenia and/or substance abuse.

INJURY PATTERNS

It is dependent on the part of the body that hits the ground first, the height of fall, ground composition, and age, clothing, body weight and physical condition of the victim in the form of preexisting medical condition (e.g., osteoporosis or an enlarged spleen) **(Fig. 16.5)**.

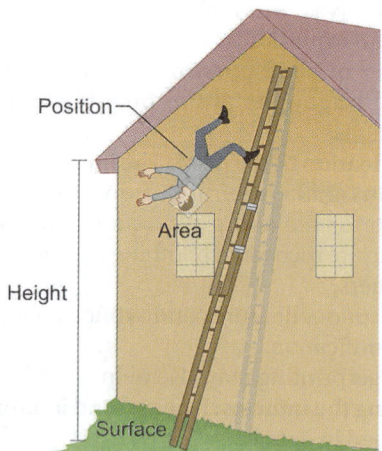

Fig. 16.5: Factors affecting injury patterns

External Examination

Examination of the clothing can provide some clues about the nature of a fall from a height. In feet-first impacts, longitudinal tears in the loin region of trousers may be seen due to inguinal stretching.

i. Postmortem staining is sparse due to loss of blood.
ii. In feet-first impacts, longitudinal tears of the inguinal regions may be seen. Plantar injuries with open fractures of the ankle joint or calcaneus are characteristic **(Figs. 16.6 and 16.7)**. Bruising in the perineal region is sometimes misinterpreted as a sign of sexual abuse prior to the fall.
iii. Palmar skin tears and open comminuted fractures of the wrists and knees are common in free falls wherein the victim may have attempted to cushion the impact.
iv. Blunt injuries such as abrasions and hematoma at the site of primary impact (plantar impacts) are a frequent finding.
v. Depending on the impact surface, the ground texture might be reflected as patterned injuries.
vi. Palmar injuries such as abrasions ('*rope burns*'), resulting from the attempt of the victim to hold on to objects preventing a fall, suggest a homicidal or an accidental fall, or fresh wrist incisions ('*hesitation marks*') are indicative of a suicidal intention.

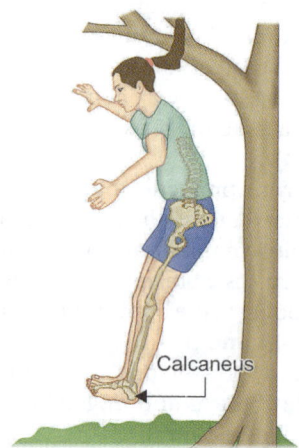

Fig. 16.6: Feet-first impact

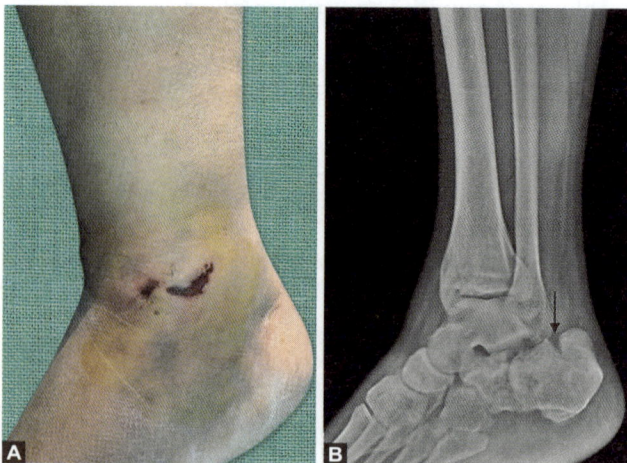

Figs. 16.7A and B: Fall from height: (A) Feet-first impact; (B) Fracture calcaneum (arrow)
(*Courtesy:* Dr Shekhar Singhal, Associate Professor, Department of Orthopedics, DMCH, Ludhiana)

Internal Examination

Severe injuries of the internal organs and/or the musculo-skeletal system can be found in all fatal falls from height.

Head injuries

All types of brain hemorrhages—subarachnoid, subdural, epidural and intracerebral, and brain contusion, as well as severe disruption and complete or partial loss of brain structures may be seen.

- In head-first impacts, there is usually open comminuted skull fractures with additional facial bone fractures and externalization of the brain over wide areas, and rarely severe internal organ injuries.
- If feet-first impact, forces transferred upward can result in significant pelvic trauma, as well as a 'ring fracture' of the skull, as forces drive the spinal column upward into the cranial cavity **(Fig. 16.8)**. Brainstem injuries such as laceration, contusion or transection are frequent.
- Traumatic subarachnoid hemorrhage can be seen, where there is no evidence of direct head trauma is present.

Neck Injuries

If neck injuries along with subconjunctival hemorrhages are present, then possibility of strangulation prior to the fall should be considered. However, blunt force neck injuries directly related to the fall are frequent. Mild to moderate hemorrhage in subcutaneous and muscular layers, thyroid hematoma along with fractures of hyoid bone may be seen in falls from >10 meters.

Chest Injuries

Thoracic cage injures like abrasions and bruises of the chest wall, and rib fractures are found in all fatal falls. Rib fractures are mostly bilateral; multiple fractures of the whole thoracic cage, including the sternum and thoracic spine are found when height of fall is >25 meters.

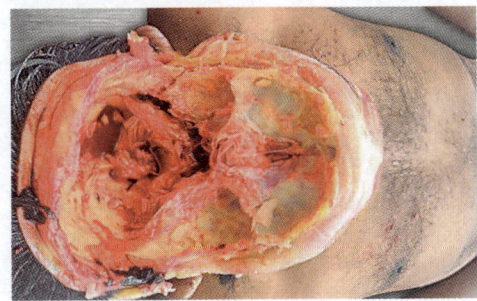

Fig. 16.8: Fall from height: Ring fracture

- **Heart:** Cardiac injuries are frequently seen in fatal falls from height.
  - Pericardial tears are most common, and occur in the right posterior part of the pericardium and tend to be of longitudinal orientation. Endocardial tears are more likely to be found in falls from greater heights.
  - Complete or incomplete transmural tears of the heart affect the right heart (atrial posterior wall) more often than the left heart. Tears of the interatrial septum are more common than interventricular septal tears.
  - In falls from great heights, the heart can be completely or subtotally torn off from the great vessels which usually results in immediate death.
- **Thoracic blood vessels:** Ruptures of the thoracic aorta are a common finding in free fall victims and are mostly located in the isthmus area (aortic arch). The frequency of aortic rupture increases with the increase of height of fall.
- **Lungs:** Contusions of the lungs can be found in almost all fatal falls. With greater falling heights, pulmonary ruptures or complete hilus rupture can be found. Penetrating rib fractures with associated pulmonary injury are common.
- **Diaphragm:** Diaphragm rupture is relatively rare.

Abdominal Injuries

- **Liver:** Liver ruptures are more frequent in falls from height than in other mechanism of blunt abdominal trauma. The right lobe of the liver is involved more often than the left lobe. Tears are often irregular in nature, but have been shown to be almost parallel in many cases.
- **Spleen:** Multiple splenic rupture is common.
- **GIT:** Ruptures or bruises of the intestinal root are a common finding in greater falling heights, but traumatic ruptures of the esophagus, stomach and bowel are relatively rare—due to their compliance and relative mobility within the abdominal cavity.
- **Retroperitoneal organs:** Rupture of the abdominal aorta, in contrast to thoracic aortic rupture, is relatively rare. Psoas muscle bleeding may result from inguinal stretching especially in feet-first impacts. Renal injuries are seen rarely.

Cause of Death

- The majority of victims die instantaneously at the scene or within minutes, the cause of it is polytrauma, followed by head trauma and blood loss.
- In free-fall victims who survive for few hours to days, head trauma is most common cause of death.

- In victims who survive for few days, causes of death include septicemia, multiple organ failure and pulmonary embolism.

Medico-legal Aspects

The questions of medico-legal importance in fatal falls concern the manner of death and the toxicology. The determination of manner of death is quite difficult in some cases, and it may remain 'undetermined' even after complete autopsy.
- Most cases of fatal falls from height are suicidal.
- Accidents may occur at work, domestic settings and during recreational sports activity.
- Homicide is rare. There may be additional injuries that cannot be explained by the fall alone like defense or offense injuries. However, injuries inflicted prior to the fall might well be masked by the impact injuries.
- In cases of custodial deaths, where the detainee was later found below a high rise building's window, the allegation has always been that he was pushed, while the legal authorities maintaining that the person jumped when left unattended.

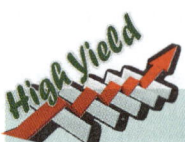

- Incendiary bombs primarily cause burns (contains phosphorus, magnesium, gasoline).
- **Molotov cocktail:** Incendiary bomb thrown by hand.
- **Blast injury:** Physical trauma resulting from direct or indirect exposure to an explosion due to change in atmospheric pressure.
- If force of explosion transmitted through air—*air blast*; if through water—*'immersion blast'*, if through solids—*'solid blast'*.
- **Air blast** produces compression of body towards the side of explosion.
- In **immersion blast**, body is compressed from all direction.
- In **solid blasts**, force is transmitted through part of the body in contact with vibrating solid structure.
- Blast injuries are divided into four categories—primary, secondary, tertiary and quaternary.
- **Primary injury** is due to blast wave injury; presence of internal injuries and absence of external injuries.
- **Secondary injury** is due to flying debris and shrapnel and bomb fragments.
- **Tertiary injury** is caused when thrown by blast wind against solid objects.
- **Quaternary injuries** are those not included in above categories.
- **Most common organs affected by primary injury:** Ears (tympanic membrane) → Lungs → GIT.
- **Most common cause of death who survives an explosion:** Blast lung (hemorrhage in lungs, pulmonary contusion, air embolism, thrombosis and DIC).
- GIT injury more common in underwater explosions than in air blasts. *Colon is most commonly affected*.
- **Marshall's triad** indicates bomb explosion (triad of bruises, abrasions and punctate lacerations with tattooing).
- **In feet-first impacts** during fall from height, longitudinal tears of inguinal regions, plantar injuries, fractures of ankle joint/calcaneus and ring fracture of skull are characteristic.
- **Head-first impacts:** Comminuted skull and facial bone fractures and externalization of brain over wide areas, and rarely severe internal organ injuries.
- Rupture of thoracic aorta is common in falls from height and located in isthmus area (aortic arch).
- In falls from height, liver rupture is more frequent in right lobe than left.

CHAPTER 16 : Explosion Injuries and Fall from Height

Interesting case

Blast Injury (Case of Rajiv Gandhi, 1991)

Rajiv Gandhi, former Prime Minister of India was assassinated by a suicide bomber while on election campaign in Chennai, Tamil Nadu on 21 May 1991. When his motorcade reached Sriperumbudur, he got out of his car and began to walk towards the dais for a speech. Along the way, he was garlanded by many well-wishers and school children. The assassin also approached and greeted him. She then bent down to touch his feet and detonated an RDX explosive-laden belt tucked below her dress. The assassination was caught on film by a local photographer whose camera and film was found intact at the site despite him also dying in the blast.

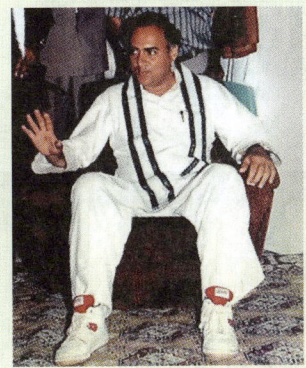

Of the 18 bodies including Rajiv Gandhi's, there was one which was just an ensemble of dismembered parts. Only the head, left forearm and two lower limbs were there, including some skin torn portions. The entire right hand and trunk of the body were missing. From the facial features, hair and smooth skin, the absence of body hair, nail paint on finger and toenails, it was evident that it was a female body and was the suicide bomber. Along with it, a Velcro fastenings denim vest (with concealed electrical wires) and tattered white bra were found indicating that the bomb might have been carried in an abdominal belt. The final conclusion was a belt-bomb carried by a woman. The missing body parts also acted like deadly shrapnel and can be considered as 'human bomb' (i.e., human body parts form part of the bomb).

At the crime scene, the bodies were all lying in a geometrical fashion or in lotus petal arrangement; the feet pointing towards the center. Normally, when human beings are knocked about above their center of gravity, say in the chest, they fall flat. It was concluded that the explosion occurred at a height of about 3½ feet above the ground level. Further examination revealed that the woman's face was intact, but back of scalp was avulsed, exposing her skull neatly. This indicated that the explosives were worn on the back of her belt only. If they had been all around her waist, then the tangential force would have also stripped off her face beyond recognition. It is common that if someone bends to touch feet, the other person will reflexively try to stop him/her from doing so. This is what Rajiv Gandhi was doing, so his face was exactly above her back and was completely blown off. His frontal face bones were thrown few meters away, but his back was intact. The body of Rajiv Gandhi could be identified from the Lotto shoes that he was wearing.

CHAPTER 17

Medico-legal Aspects of Injuries

LEARNING OBJECTIVES

Must know
1. Assault, battery, manslaughter, murder, dowry death
2. Clauses of grievous hurt (Sec. 320 IPC)
3. Hurt (Sec. 319 IPC); simple, and dangerous injuries
4. Injuries sufficient to cause death in ordinary course of nature
5. Common weapons of offense, dangerous weapons
6. Punishments for various offenses
7. Cause of death due to mechanical injuries
8. Thrombosis and embolism
9. Antemortem and postmortem wounds (Diff.)
10. Lacerated, incised and stab wound (Diff.)

Desirable to know
1. Shock
2. Histochemical changes in injured tissue
3. Age of wounds
4. Relationship of trauma with natural disease

Define injury, assault and hurt. Describe IPC pertaining to injuries.

Definitions

- **Injury:** Any harm, whatever illegally, caused to any person in *body, mind, reputation or property* **(Sec. 44 IPC)**.
- **Trauma:** A body wound or shock produced by sudden physical injury; from violence or an accident.
- **Assault:** An offer of threat or attempt to apply force to the body of another in a hostile manner **(Sec. 351 IPC)**. It does not matter whether it injures him physically or not. Shaking of head or showing of fist at a person in hostile manner will constitute an assault.
- **Battery:** It is the *actual application of force* to the body. It is an assault brought to execution. Beating or wounding will constitute battery. Battery need not require body-to-body contact. Any volitional movement, such as throwing an object towards another can constitute battery. Additionally, an individual can consent to battery in some situations, e.g., in boxing.
- **Homicide:** Killing of a human being as a result of conduct of the other. It may be *lawful or unlawful*.
    - I. **Lawful homicide:** It can be justifiable or excusable.
        - a. **Justifiable:** Homicide which is justified by the circumstances that led to killing of the person, e.g.,
            - i. Judicial execution.
            - ii. Maintenance of justice, like suppressing riots or executing arrest.
            - iii. In self-defense.
            - iv. In preventing some forcible and atrocious act, such as rape, murder or burglary.
        - b. **Excusable:** Homicide caused unintentionally, e.g.,
            - i. In defense of one's home/family.
            - ii. Causing death by accident/misadventure.
            - iii. Death following lawful operation.
            - iv. Homicide committed by an insane person.
            - v. In sports, such as boxing.
    - II. **Unlawful homicide:** Implies both, the fact of death and an accompanying state of mind known as '*malice aforethought*' on the part of the killer. *Without such a state of mind*, the act is known as *culpable homicide not amounting to murder*.
- **Culpable homicide (Sec. 299 IPC, '*manslaughter*'):** It is an offense wherein an individual by his act intentionally or knowingly causes death or causes such bodily injury which is *likely to cause death*.
  A person is liable under this section if he causes such injury to another person who is laboring under a disorder, disease or bodily infirmity, and thereby accelerating his death; or if he causes such injury which results in his death, although proper remedies and treatment might have been prevented his death.
- **Murder (Sec. 300 IPC):** Killing of a person with malice aforethought.
  If *the act by which death is caused*:
    - i. With the intention of causing death.

ii. With the intention of causing such bodily injury which is *likely to cause death* of the person or *sufficient in ordinary course of nature to cause death.*
- All 'murder' is 'culpable homicide', but not vice-versa. It does not include acts by which death is caused:
  i. Under grave and sudden provocation.
  ii. When there is no intention to kill, but death results from unlawful conduct by the person responsible.
  iii. Without premeditation.
  iv. In a person >18 years of age, suffers death or takes the risk of death with his own consent.
- **Punishment for culpable homicide not amounting to murder (Sec. 304 IPC):** If an individual commits culpable homicide not amounting to murder then he is punished with imprisonment from 10 years to life imprisonment and fine; and if the act was done with the knowledge of possibility to cause death, but without any intention to cause death, then punishment is imprisonment for 10 years and/or fine.
- **Attempt to murder (Sec. 307 IPC):** Any individual who does any act with intention or knowledge and under such circumstances that it (might have) caused death, he would be guilty of murder, and he is punished with imprisonment for up to 10 years and fine; and if hurt is (actually) caused to any person by such act, then punishment is imprisonment from 10 years to life imprisonment and fine.

For example, 'X' with the intention to kill 'Z' buys a gun and shoots and injures him, or 'Y' with the intention of causing death of a child leaves him in a deserted place (although the child is saved), then X and Y will be guilty under this section.

NOTA BENE
- **Honor killing:** Murder of a person by one or more fellow family members when they believe the victim brought dishonor upon the family. Victims are usually females who may marry someone from different caste. The cases are tried under Sec. 302 IPC.
- **Capital murder** is murder which is punishable by death.
- The law of India, differing from the law of the UK, does not regard every case of homicide as prima facie murder; it throws on the prosecution the burden of proving a certain intent or knowledge.
- In the US, murder or 'homicide' is normally a crime only under State law and a murder suspect will be arrested and held by local officials and tried in a local court on behalf of the State. For murders that are federal crimes (e.g., killing of a federal official or on federal property), the trial would occur in a federal court.
- In the UK, homicide can be divided into several offenses, including:
  i. *Murder*—Killing of another person whilst having either the intention to kill or to cause grievous bodily harm.
  ii. *Manslaughter*—Unintentional and unlawful killing of another person.
  iii. *Infanticide*—Intentional killing of an infant under 1 year, by a mother.

- **Dowry death:** Where the death of a woman is caused by any burn or bodily injury, or occurs in a manner other than under normal circumstances within 7 years of her marriage, and it is shown that she was subjected to cruelty or harassment by her husband or any relative of her husband for, or in connection with any demand for dowry, such death is called dowry death (**Sec. 304-B IPC**).
  - It is a cognizable and non-bailable offense and punished with imprisonment from 7 years to life imprisonment.
- **Sec. 498-A IPC:** Whoever, being the husband or the relative of the husband of a woman, subjects her to cruelty, is punished with imprisonment for a term which may extend to 3 years and also fine. The offense is non-bailable and non-compoundable.
  - 'Cruelty' is any conduct likely to drive the woman to commit suicide or to cause injury or danger to life, limb or health (mental or physical); or harassment with a view to coercing her or any person related to her to meet any unlawful demand for any property or valuable security.
  - To prevent the misuse of Sec. 498-A IPC, Supreme Court directed the State governments to ensure that the police would have to give reasons and proof to Magistrate before making an arrest in dowry harassment cases.
- **Hurt:** Hurt means any bodily pain, disease or infirmity caused to any person (**Sec. 319 IPC**).
  It is of two types:
  i. Simple
  ii. Grievous.

> **FM 3.5, 3.8**
> - Describe simple, grievous and dangerous injuries.
> - Describe and discuss different types of weapons including dangerous weapons and their examination.

Simple Hurt

Simple hurt is not defined in law. However, an injury which is neither extensive nor serious, and which heals rapidly without leaving any permanent deformity or disfiguration is considered as simple hurt.

GRIEVOUS HURT

Sec. 320 IPC defines the grievous hurt and comprises of eight clauses (**Table 17.1**):
1. **Emasculation:** Deprivation of a male of his masculine vigor by cutting of penis, castration, or by causing injury to testes or spinal cord at the level of L2–L4 vertebrae resulting in erectile dysfunction (ED) (**Fig. 17.1**). It covers both sterility and potency in a male. ED caused must be permanent (whether treatable or untreatable is immaterial) for the injury to be called grievous.

TABLE 17.1: Clauses of grievous hurt

Clause	Kinds of hurt
First	Emasculation
Second	Permanent privation of the sight of either eye
Third	Permanent privation of the hearing of either ear
Fourth	Privation of any member or joint
Fifth	Destruction or permanent impairing of the powers of any member or joint
Sixth	Permanent disfiguration of the head or face
Seventh	Fracture or dislocation of a bone or tooth
Eighth	Any hurt which endangers life, or which causes the sufferer to be during the space of 20 days in severe bodily pain or unable to follow his ordinary pursuits

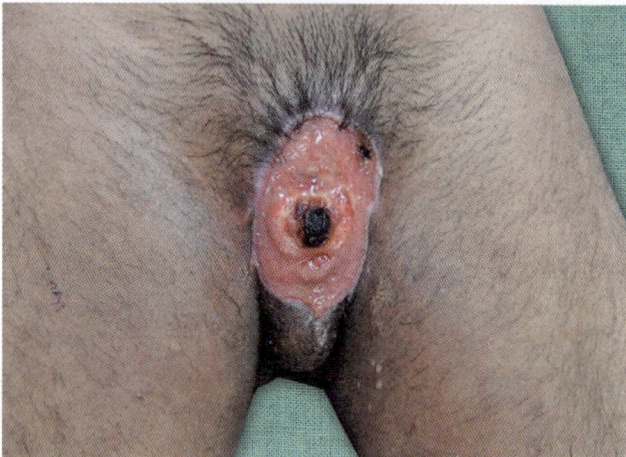

Fig. 17.1: Chopping off of male genitalia

- Only male castration comes under this clause. Female castration can however be a grievous hurt under clause 4 or 8.
- If only one testis gets damaged or removed and the other testis with intact male organ is present, then it is not considered as emasculation. However, it is still a grievous hurt under clause 4, which is privation of any member or joint.
- ED may occur following treatment for lower limb fractures (due to perineal neurovascular traction injury) and spinal cord injury with complete upper/lower motor lesions.

2. **Permanent privation of sight of either eye:** Gravity lies in its *permanency* as it deprives the use of organ of sight and also disfigures him.
    - It includes deep abrasions (involving the corneal stromal layer) within the central visual axis, dislocation of lens, breaking of zonules, retinal or choroidal tears and optic disc lacerations **(Fig. 17.2A)**.
    - The nature and extent of permanent impairment are typically measured in cases of loss of visual acuity and impairment of visual field.
    - It is not necessarily both eyes to be affected; only one is sufficient.

3. **Permanent privation of hearing of either ear:** It should be *permanent* deafness.
    - It can be due to blow on the head or ears, or blows which injure the tympanum, ear ossicles or auditory nerves, or injury by foreign body **(Fig. 17.2B)**.
    - It may be noted that tympanic membrane perforations may heal spontaneously (especially central perforations).
    - Audiometric assessment should be done to document hearing loss.
    - If needed, patient may be reviewed after 2 weeks to see permanency of hearing loss.

4. **Privation of any member or joint:** Privation is an act, condition or result of deprivation or loss. It is a state of being deprived.
    - '*Member*' means any organ or limb of a subject responsible for performance of distinct function. It includes eyes, ears, nostrils, mouth, hands or feet **(Fig. 17.3)**.
    - 'Joint' may be both small or big ones.
    - Loss of hair/nails would not come under this clause.

5. **Destruction or permanent impairing of the powers of any member or joint:** Use of limbs and joints are vital for discharge of normal functions of the body.
    - It includes cutting (severing) of any tendon, anywhere along its route—at its origin, in between or at its insertion. If it is not repaired, its function is

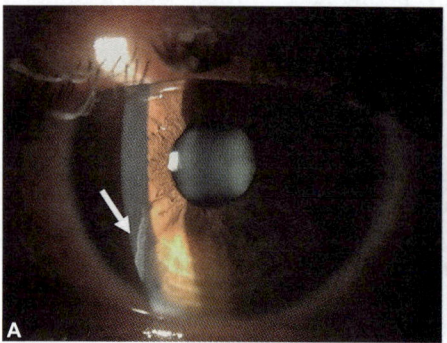 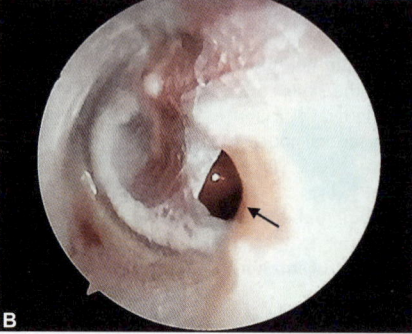 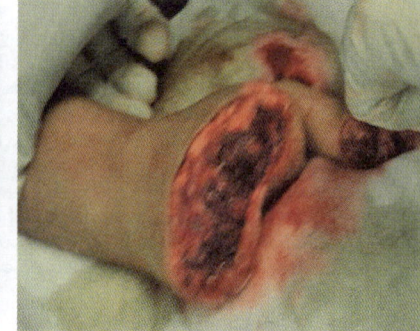

Figs. 17.2A and B: (A) Partial thickness corneal tear; (B) Perforation of tympanic membrane
[*Courtesy*: (A) Dr Ritesh Verma and (B) Dr Manish Munjal, DMCH, Ludhiana]

Fig. 17.3: Chopping off of hands

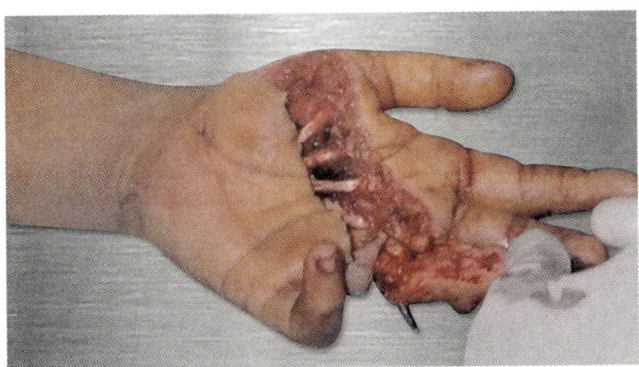

Fig. 17.4: Severing of tendons and muscles

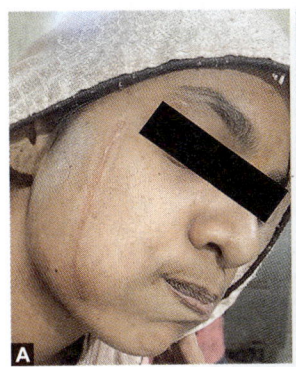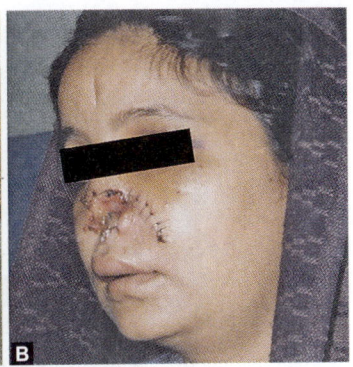

Figs. 17.5A and B: Permanent disfiguration
[*Courtesy:* (A) Dr Ashok Moondra, GMC, Kota and (B) Dr Shivrattan Kochar, SKMC, Sikar]

permanently lost. This may cause deformity, loss of movement and weakness **(Fig. 17.4)**.
- It is not necessary that destruction or loss of power should be 100%, e.g., contracture caused by burns involving joint.

6. **Permanent disfiguration of the head or face:** '*Disfiguration*' means change of configuration and personal appearance of the subject by some external injury which does not weaken him/her. A person is 'disfigured' when a reasonable observer would find the altered appearance distressing or objectionable **(Figs. 17.5A and B)**.
    - For example, chopping off an individual's ear or nose which would cause disfigurement, without consequential disability, so as to constitute grievous hurt under this clause.
    - A large cut on the face or branding may leave a permanent scar causing disfigurement.
    - Permanent disfiguration is seen when injuries to the eyes leave residual defects after healing like ptosis, entropion or squint.
    - Opinion of disfigurement should be given after complete healing, since the doctor can judge whether disability is permanent or not.

7. **Fracture or dislocation of a bone or tooth:** If there is a break by cutting or splintering of the bone, or there is a rupture or fissure in it, then it would amount to a fracture **(Fig. 17.6A)**.

- For the meaning of 'fracture' under this clause it is not necessary that a bone should be cut through and through or that the crack must extend from the outer to the inner surface or there should be displacement of any fragment of the bone.
- It should be seen whether the cuts in the bones noticed are only superficial or have affected a break in them.
- Even if the extent of the cut is not mentioned, it would amount to grievous hurt, if there has been a break in the bone.
- Fractures are possible without trauma when osteoporosis is present.

Dislocation implies traumatic displacement of the position of the members of the joint along with injury of tissues.
- Mere looseness of a tooth due to disease or old age will not amount to dislocation.
- Signs of inflammation should be searched for in cases where trauma is alleged **(Fig. 17.6B)**.
- Some people have tendency of dislocation, especially shoulder which they can do it by themselves too. Some people can reduce it too without difficulty.

8. **Any hurt which:**
    a. **Endangers life (Fig. 17.7).**
    b. **Causes the victim to be in severe bodily pain for 20 days.**

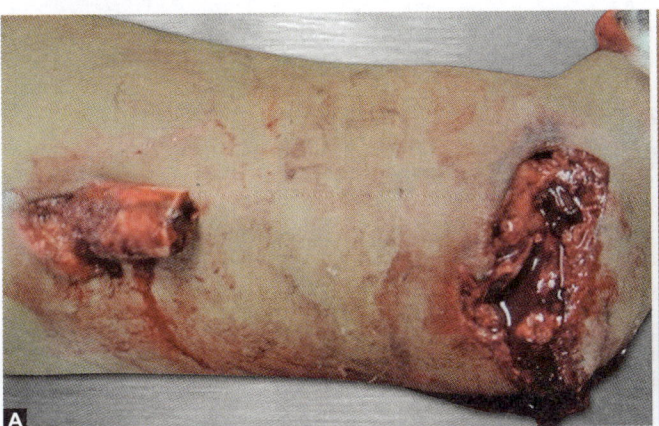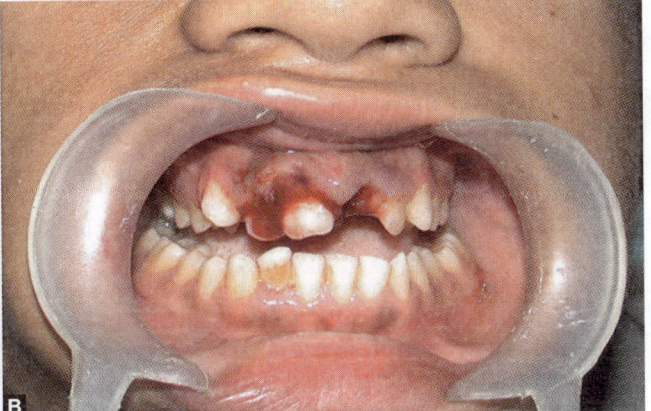

Figs. 17.6A and B: (A) Fracture of femur; (B) Traumatic dislodgement and dislocation of teeth

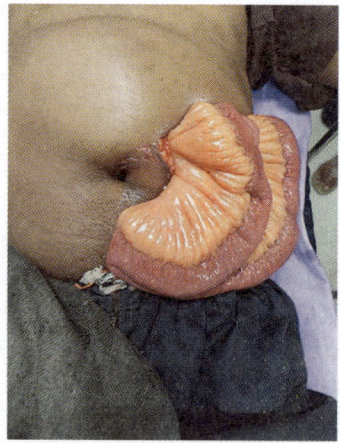

Fig. 17.7: Stab wound with protrusion of the gut and mesentery
(*Courtesy:* Dr Raghvendra Kumar Vidua, AIIMS, Bhopal)

to receive into the blood or by means of any animal (**Sec. 324 and 326 IPC**).

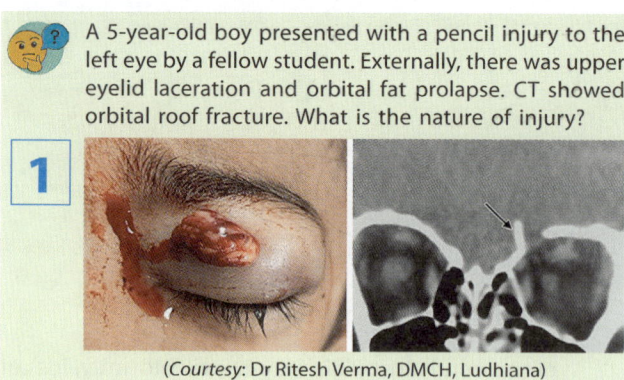

A 5-year-old boy presented with a pencil injury to the left eye by a fellow student. Externally, there was upper eyelid laceration and orbital fat prolapse. CT showed orbital roof fracture. What is the nature of injury?

(*Courtesy:* Dr Ritesh Verma, DMCH, Ludhiana)

  c. **Unable the victim to follow his ordinary pursuits for a period of 20 days.**
     - Any hurt which endangers life' means that the life is only endangered and not taken away, i.e., placing a person in danger of death.
     - A mere stay in hospital for 20 days will not constitute grievous hurt.
     - *Ordinary pursuits* signify day-to-day personal acts of an individual, like going to the toilet, having food or taking bath or wearing clothes. It does not include going to work, running, jumping or driving a vehicle.
- **Dangerous injury** has not been defined in the IPC. Medically, dangerous injuries are those which cause imminent danger to life by its direct or immediate effects because of being extensive in nature, involving important structures or organs of the body, and also being likely to prove fatal in absence of medical/surgical aid. Any tear in dura mater, intracerebral hemorrhages, cerebral edema, laceration of lungs resulting in hemothorax, rupture/perforation of GIT, any rupture of large arteries/veins are examples of dangerous injuries.
- **Injuries endangering life and dangerous injuries:** Medically, it is difficult to categorize injuries into injuries endangering life and dangerous injuries as the distinction is nonexistent, and doctors are using both the terms synonymously. The courts have held that whenever the doctor mentions 'dangerous injury' then such injury has to be treated under *clause eight of grievous hurt* (endangers life).
- It is recommended that the medical expert should desist from differentiating injuries endangering life and dangerous injuries.
- **Dangerous weapon or means:** Any instrument used for shooting, stabbing or cutting, or any instrument which if used as a weapon of offense is likely to cause death; or by means of fire or any heated substance, poison or any corrosive substance, explosive or any substance which is harmful to the human body to inhale, to swallow or

Common Weapons of Offense (Fig. 17.8)

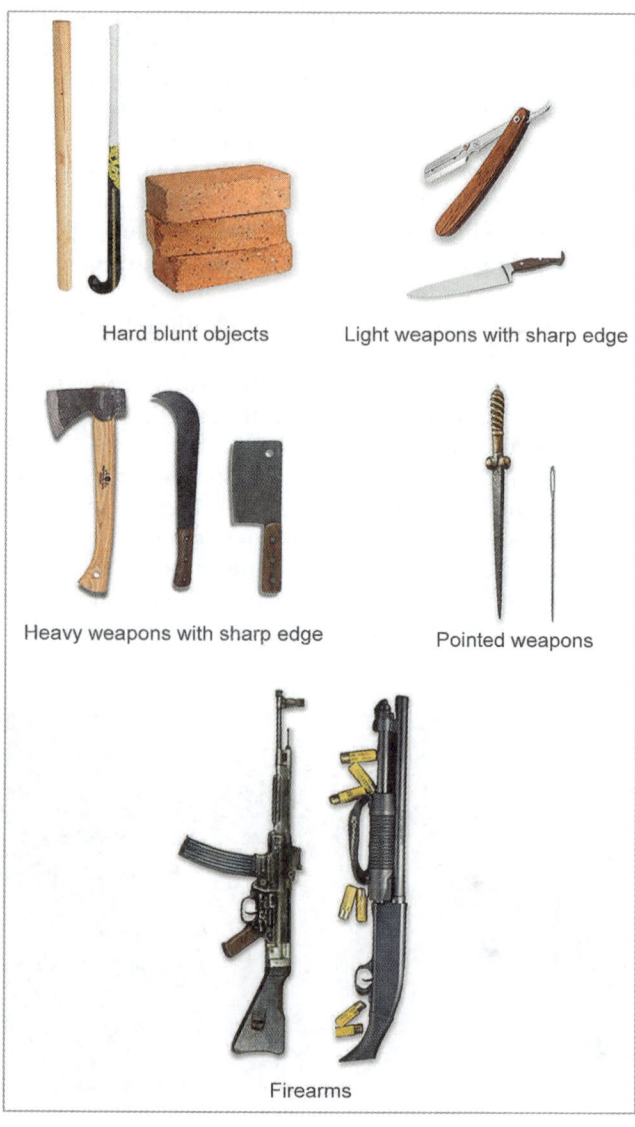

Fig. 17.8: Common weapons of offense

These weapons are grouped into:
 i. *Hard blunt* objects, e.g., sticks, stones or cricket bat.
 ii. *Light weapons* with a sharp cutting edge, e.g., knife or razor.
 iii. *Heavy weapons* with a sharp cutting edge, e.g., hatchet or axe.
 iv. *Pointed weapons*, e.g., dagger or needle.
 v. *Firearms*, e.g., shotgun or rifle.

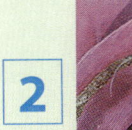

Identify the grievous hurt (and specific clause) and give explanation.

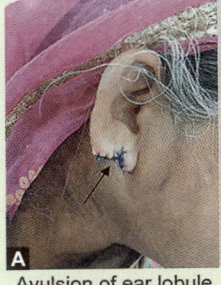
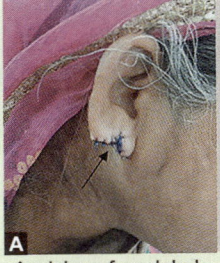
A Avulsion of ear lobule

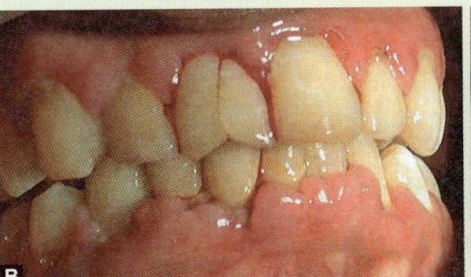
B Fracture of tooth

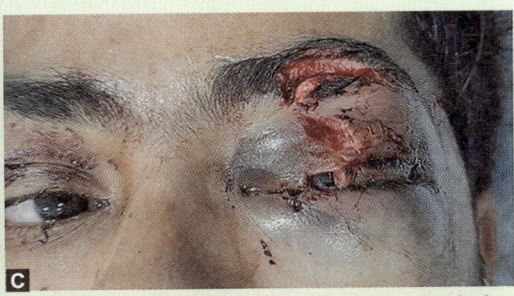
C Lid and brow laceration with ecchymoses, surgical repair done to restore vision

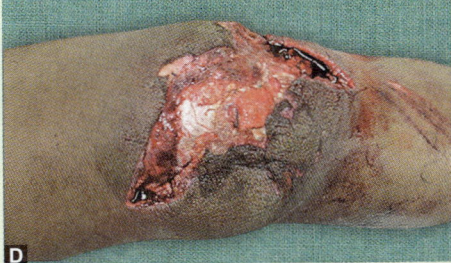
D Laceration on knee without any underlying fracture

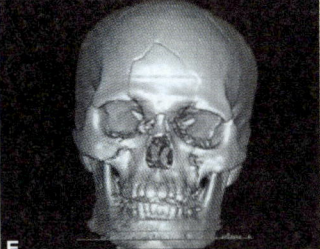
E Comminuted fracture of skull without any intracranial hemorrhage (CT face)

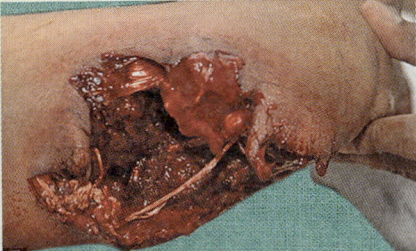
F Shotgun injury on the elbow joint with rupture of tendons, muscles and major vessels

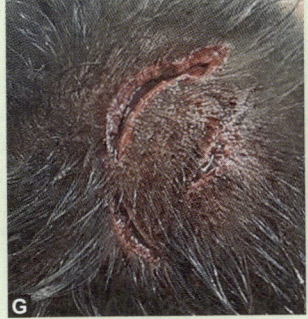
G Laceration with depressed fracture of skull

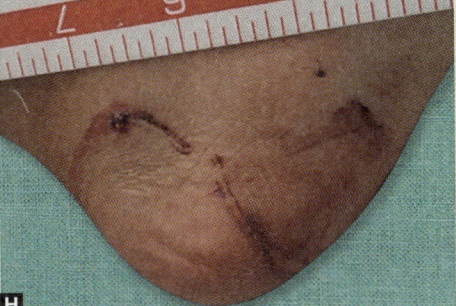
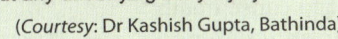
H Shotgun pellet injury to ankle without any underlying bony injury

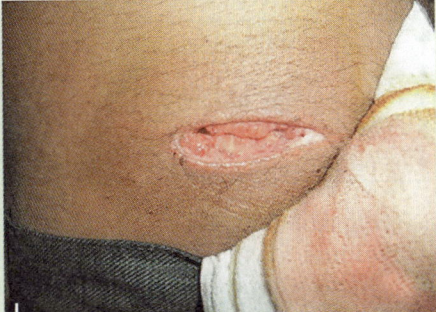
I Superficial stab wound of back of abdomen

(*Courtesy*: Dr Kashish Gupta, Bathinda)

Injuries Sufficient to Cause Death in Ordinary Course of Nature

 i. Injuries to the brain (intracranial hemorrhages) and spinal cord.
 ii. Injuries to heart or large blood vessels.
 iii. Injuries to respiratory organs.
 iv. Injuries involving GIT, e.g., rupture of liver, spleen, perforation of intestines, etc.
 v. Injuries (wounds) to highly vascular organs, like liver/spleen.
 vi. Extensive burns or scalds (affecting >1/3rd of the body surface area).
 vii. Combined effect of number of injuries, none of which by itself may be sufficient to cause death, but together may cause it.
 viii. Squeezing of testes.

PUNISHMENTS

Punishment for some of the offenses is given in **Table 17.2**.

TABLE 17.2: Punishment for some offenses committed by any individual

S.No.	Section of IPC	Offense	Punishment (Imprisonment)	Fine
1.	302	Murder	Death or life imprisonment	Yes
2.	304	Culpable homicide not amounting to murder	Up to 10 years to life imprisonment	Yes
3.	304-A	Death by rash and negligent act	Up to 2 years	With/without fine
4.	304-B	Dowry death	7 years to life imprisonment	—
5.	307	Attempt to murder	10 years to life imprisonment	Yes
6.	323	Voluntarily causing simple hurt	Up to 1 year	With/without fine (up to ₹1000)
7.	324	Voluntarily causing simple hurt by dangerous weapons/means	Up to 3 years	With/without fine
8.	325	Voluntarily causing grievous hurt	Up to 7 years	Yes
9.	326	Voluntarily causing grievous hurt by dangerous weapons/means	Up to 10 years	Yes
10.	326-A	Voluntarily causing grievous hurt by use of acids	10 years to life imprisonment	Yes (paid to the victim)
11.	326-B	Voluntarily throwing or attempting to throw acid	5–7 years	Yes (-do-)

> **FM 3.7, 3.12**
> - Describe factors influencing infliction of injuries and healing, and wound as a cause of death.
> - Describe and discuss crush syndrome.

CAUSES OF DEATH FROM WOUNDS

Immediate Causes

1. **Shock:** Types of shock

   - Hypovolemic
   - Vasovagal
   - Neurogenic
   - Burns
   - Anaphylactic
   - Traumatic
   - Cardiogenic
   - Septic
   - Psychogenic

   i. **Hypovolemic shock:** It is due to loss of intravascular volume by hemorrhage (*external bleeding—most common cause;* dehydration, vomiting and diarrhea are other causes of hypovolemic shock).
   - Rapid loss of 1.5–2 liters of blood (25–30% or 1/3rd of blood in an adult) is sufficient to cause death due to irreversible hypovolemic shock (blood volume in normal adult is 8–8.5% of body weight or 65–75 mL/kg).
   - *Methods to determine blood loss:* A clot, the size of a clenched fist is roughly equal to 500 mL. Loss of blood in closed fractures of long bones are given in **Table 17.3**.
   - *External blood loss:* Each 1 square feet of blood (on clothing or floor) represents approximately 100 mL of blood.
   - Men resist hemorrhage better than women, although the latter can sustain enormous loss of blood during childbirth without a fatal result.

TABLE 17.3: Blood loss in fractures

Fracture	Blood loss
Humerus	200–500 mL
Tibia with/without fibula	500–700 mL
Femur	1000–1500 mL
Pelvis	>2000 mL
Ribs	Variable, may be major

- Features of hypovolemic shock—body pallor, pituitary infarction and hypoxic-ischemic neuronal necrosis in the brain. All the viscera are mostly pale after acute death, often without the involvement of the brain and/or renal medulla.

> **NOTA BENE**
> - *Petechiae* are minute hemorrhage spots, usually of capillary origin.
> - *Ecchymoses* are larger areas of extravasated blood.
> - *Traumatic hemorrhage:* Bleeding occurring due to wounds.
> - *Spontaneous hemorrhage:* Bleeding occurring in the absence of trauma.
> - *Primary hemorrhage:* Hemorrhage occurring at the time of injury.
> - *Reactionary hemorrhage* occurs from the same site as primary hemorrhage, but is seen within 24 hours (h) (usually 4–6 h) after injury. It may occur due to:
>   i. Rise in blood pressure (which accompanies the recovery from shock).
>   ii. Muscular movements, which may dislodge the blood clot or cause 'slippage' of the ligature from the vessel.
> - *Secondary hemorrhage* may occur as a result of erosion of vessel wall due to infection (7–14th day).
> - *External hemorrhage:* If large vessels are involved, death is rapid. Sudden loss of blood is more dangerous than the same quantity lost slowly.
> - *Internal hemorrhage:* The amount of blood loss can be judged accurately and can often be measured at autopsy.

> **NOTA BENE**
>
> Hemorrhagic shock promotes the endovascular recruitment of activated neutrophils which lead to dysfunction of the organs. The expression of activated neutrophils in the organs (heart, lung, liver and kidney) might be useful as a morphological marker of hemorrhagic shock. These are elevated significantly during middle and long antemortem interval (2–8 h) which can be measured by immunohistochemical staining.

ii. **Traumatic shock:** It occurs due to hypovolemia from bleeding externally (open wounds), from bleeding internally (torn vessels in the mediastinal or peritoneal cavities, ruptured liver, spleen or fractured bones), or loss of fluid into contused tissue or into distended bowel. Traumatic contusion of heart itself may cause pump failure and shock.

iii. **Vasovagal shock:** Pooling of blood in the larger vascular reservoirs (limb or muscles) and dilatation of the splanchnic vascular bed cause reduced venous return to the heart, low cardiac output and reflex bradycardia. Consequently, the reduced cerebral perfusion causes cerebral hypoxia and unconsciousness. Cause of death is arrived at from negative findings.

iv. **Neurogenic shock:** It is caused by traumatic or pharmacological blockade of the sympathetic nervous system, producing dilatation of resistance arterioles and capacitance veins leading to hypovolemia, bradycardia and hypotension.
   - Spinal injury is the most common cause of neurogenic shock (sometimes referred to as *spinal shock*).
   - Neurogenic shock is a complication of acute complete spinal cord injury above thoracic T6 level.

v. **Burn shock:** Secondary shock results from rapid plasma loss from the area of burn causing hypovolemia. When >25% of the body surface is burnt, a generalized capillary leakage may cause hypovolemia in the first 24 h.

vi. **Anaphylactic shock:** Penicillin administration is a common cause. Other causes include serum injections, anesthetics, dextrans, stings and consumption of shellfish. The antigen combines with IgE with the release of histamine and substance of anaphylaxis (SRA-A) causing bronchospasm, laryngeal edema, respiratory distress, vasodilatation, hypotension and shock (mortality is about 10%).

vii. **Cardiogenic shock:** It results from interference in the action of the heart as in the case of:
   a. *Deficiency of filling*, e.g., cardiac tamponade.
   b. *Deficiency of emptying*, e.g., myocardial infarction (when >50% of left ventricle is involved).
   c. *Acute pulmonary embolism* from a thrombus originating in a deep vein or due to air emboli (>50 mL) causing obstruction of more than 50% of the pulmonary vasculature, resulting in right ventricular failure and sudden death or shock.
   d. Fluid overload, particularly with colloids can lead to overdistension of the left ventricle and pump failure.
      - The term 'obstructive shock' is used when blood flow in the great vessels becomes blocked, e.g., pericardial tamponade, obstruction of superior of inferior vena cava or pulmonary embolus or tension pneumothorax causing inadequate venous return.

viii. **Psychogenic shock:** It immediately follows sudden fright or severe pain, like blow to the testes.

ix. **Septic (endotoxic) shock:** Septic shock usually takes some time to develop following onset of infection, except meningococcal infection where death may occur within few hours.
   - *Hyperdynamic (warm) septic shock*: It occurs usually in the case of gram-negative infections. Initially, there is an increased cardiac output with tachycardia and warm skin, but the blood is shunted past tissues which become damaged by anaerobic metabolism. The capillary membranes start to leak, and endotoxin is absorbed into the bloodstream cause generalized systemic inflammatory state.
   - *Hypovolemic hypodynamic (cold) septic shock*: It develops in the presence of sepsis or endotoxemia which may produce circulatory failure from generalized increased vascular permeability and peripheral vasodilatation. The systemic infection induces cardiac depression, pulmonary edema, hypoxia and decreased cardiac output. The patient becomes cold, clammy, drowsy and tachypneic.

Pallor is seen in most types of shock, except spinal and sepsis. Neurogenic shock is not associated with cold peripheries, which are instead warm and well perfused.

2. **Death due to injury of an organ:** Extensive damage to vital organs, like brain, heart and lungs may be sufficient by itself to cause rapid death when even the quantity of blood loss may not be so important.

Remote Causes

i. **Infection:** Wound infection may be caused by:
   - Organisms present on body surface, e.g., *Streptococcus, Staphylococcus* or *Proteus*.
   - Organisms may invade the injured area from the environment, e.g., *Streptococcus, Staphylococcus, Clostridium perfringens* or *Clostridium tetani*.

Infection may be:
   a. *Primary*: Caused by organisms which are carried into the wounds at the time of injury, e.g., from skin, clothing or dirt.
   b. *Secondary*: Caused by organisms which invade the wound after injury, e.g., airborne droplet infection or contaminated dressings.
   c. *Direct*: Infection at the site of an open wound, such as a stab or gunshot wound with exposure to outside contamination.

d. *Remote*: Local sepsis can cause septicemia or pyemia; septic endometritis following criminal abortion can cause meningitis.
e. *Traumatic*: Trauma over an area of pre-existing infected lesion can cause dissemination of infection.
f. *Debilitating*: In case of poor vitality and debilitating disease, infection easily occurs in form of hypostatic pneumonia or ulcers.

ii. **Crush syndrome:** Systemic manifestation of crushing of muscles (rhabdomyolysis), especially those that involve the lower limbs, e.g., under fallen masonry, industrial and vehicular accidents. For such injury to occur there must be continuous prolonged pressure on the muscles. This syndrome is associated with myoglobinuria and acute renal failure. After 3–5 days of injury, death is due to renal failure, coagulopathy and hemorrhage (DIC) and sepsis.
Cause: Disturbance of renal blood flow and ischemia.
Other causes of rhabdomyolysis: Heat stroke, electrical burns, cocaine, amphetamine, snakebites.

iii. **Gangrene or necrosis:** It implies death, often with putrefaction of macroscopic portions of tissue.
- Traumatic gangrene may have a *direct cause* (crushes, pressure sores and constriction groove of strangulated bowel) or *indirect cause* from injury of vessels at some distance from the site of gangrene, e.g., pressure on popliteal artery by the lower end of a fractured femur.
- A gangrenous part lacks arterial pulsation, venous return, capillary response to pressure, sensation, warmth and function.
- *Signs and symptoms* include severe pain and tenderness, edema, skin discoloration with hemorrhagic blebs and bullae, nonodorous or sweet mousy odor, crepitus, fever, tachycardia, and altered mental status.
- It is usually dark brown, greenish black or black in appearance due to disintegration of hemoglobin and formation of iron sulfide.

iv. **Neglect of injured person:** Death may occur from complications arising from a simple injury due to improper treatment/negligence on part of doctor/nurse.

v. **Surgical operation:** Assaulted person is not bound to submit himself for operation. If death occurs due to this omission, assailant becomes responsible. If death follows surgical operation for the treatment of injury, the assailant is responsible for the result, if it is proved that the victim would have died even without the operation.

vi. **Natural disease:** Some natural disease may be present which was the cause of death, but death was accelerated by assault, e.g., person with fatty degeneration of heart may die with slight violence.

vii. **Supervening of disease from traumatic lesion**
- Head injury followed by meningitis may result in death.
- Abdominal injury on healing may be followed by strangulated hernia/stricture and obstruction.

viii. **Acute respiratory distress syndrome (ARDS)** occurs due to heavy impact on the thorax, blast injuries, injections, toxins, shock, irritant gases, aspiration of gastric contents or near drowning, in which there may be diffuse alveolar damage. Lungs become stiff, edematous and retain their shape after removal and may be double their weight.

ix. **Disseminated intravascular coagulation (DIC):** It occurs due to trauma, infection and other acute events. It is a consumption coagulopathy associated with blood clotting mechanism. There is an abnormal activation of the coagulation process within the blood vessels. Fibrin is consumed and precipitated in vessels, causing both vascular obstructive effects and a hemorrhagic diathesis from depletion of coagulative system.
Complications are microvascular destruction leading to infarction and bleeding.

> **NOTA BENE**
> **Martius Scarlet Blue (MSB) stain:** This trichrome stain is useful for examining thrombi and emboli and for seeking fibrin in DIC.

x. **Thrombosis and embolism (thromboembolism)**
- It is a common complication of traumatic lesions of lower extremities.
- *Most common sites of thrombosis are*: Deep femoral, popliteal and posterior tibial veins.
- Factors which predispose to leg vein thrombosis after injury are:
  a. Local tissue damage causing injury to veins.
  b. An increase in clotting time, which is maximum at about 2 weeks after injury.
  c. Immobility and bed rest.
  d. General debility, especially in old age, leading to poor general circulation and cardiac output.

Thrombus usually develops in 10–20 days after injury, gets detached in part or whole and can cause pulmonary embolism (*saddle embolism*).

> **NOTA BENE**
> **Embolism** means partial or complete obstruction of some part of the vascular system by any mass transported through circulation. The transported mass is known as *embolus* which can be:
> i. Solid, e.g., detached thrombi (pulmonary embolism)
> ii. Liquid, e.g., fat globules
> iii. Gaseous, e.g., air
> The embolus can be bland or septic; venous, arterial or lymphatic.

Pulmonary Embolism

- **Cause:** Pulmonary embolism is a complication of venous thromboembolism, *most commonly* deep venous thrombosis (DVT) of the legs. Less common causes include air, fat droplets, amniotic fluid, clumps of parasites or tumor cells and talc in drugs of IV drug abusers.
- It is present in 60–80% of patients with DVT.
- As a cause of sudden death, it is 2nd only to sudden cardiac death. Most patients die within the first few hours of the event.
- **Risk factors:** Venous stasis, hypercoagulable states, immobilization, surgery and trauma, pregnancy, oral contraceptives and estrogen replacement, malignancy, hereditary factors and acute medical illness.
- **Types**
  - *Acute*: If the embolus is situated centrally within the vascular lumen and occludes a vessel.
  - *Chronic*: If it is eccentric and contiguous with the vessel wall, and reduces the arterial diameter >50%.
- **Signs and symptoms**
  - *Classical presentation* includes abrupt onset of pleuritic chest pain, shortness of breath and palpitation. Severe cases can lead to collapse, hypotension and sudden death.
  - *Signs*: Tachypnea, tachycardia, fever, accentuated second heart sound, diaphoresis, lower extremity edema, cyanosis and signs of thrombophlebitis.
- **Diagnosis:** Pulmonary angiography is diagnostic, but with the improved sensitivity and specificity of CT angiography, it is now rarely performed.
- **Autopsy:** The gross appearance of the classic saddle pulmonary embolism includes a tangled embolism bulging from the proximal pulmonary arteries that is slightly adherent to the blood vessel and has a heterogeneous red-blue-tan appearance **(Figs. 17.9A and B)**.
- **Microscopically**, there may be "lines of Zahn" (interdigitating areas of pale pink and red) and fibrin thromboemboli scattered in pulmonary vessels. These lines represent layers of red cells, platelets and fibrin, which are laid down in the vessel as the thrombus forms.

Fat Embolism

Causes

a. Fracture of pelvis and long bones, especially of femur.
b. Injury to adipose tissue which forces fat into damaged blood vessels.
c. Injecting oil into circulation, e.g., criminal abortion.
d. Natural disease without any trauma, as in sickle cell anemia, diabetes, blood transfusion or in chronic alcoholics.
e. Burns and septicemia.

- Fat emboli occur in all patients with long-bone fractures, but only few patients develop systemic dysfunction, particularly the *triad* of cutaneous, neurological and respiratory dysfunction known as the **fat embolism syndrome** (FES).
- Fat embolism is rare in children, since bone marrow fat is scanty.
- *About 12–120 mL of free fat* causes embolic death.
- **Signs and symptoms:** Cyanosis, precordial pain, rapid pulse and respiration, tachycardia, thrombocytopenia, hyperpyrexia, and petechial hemorrhages in the axillae and neck may develop in 8–20 h. Later, the patient will have respiratory distress with hypoxemia and bilateral patchy infiltrates on chest X-ray. Fat globulin may be seen in urine.
- Death usually occurs in about 10 days, but may be delayed up to 3 weeks. Cerebral fat embolism causes death in about 1–2 days.
- **Diagnosis** is confirmed by frozen section using Sudan dyes, oil red O and osmic acid.
- **Microscopically**, lungs show massive intravascular fat droplets, as well as free fat in the alveoli. In addition, lungs show hyperemia, edema, petechial hemorrhages and changes of ARDS. Fat globules may be seen in cerebral arteries and glomerular capillaries, as well as

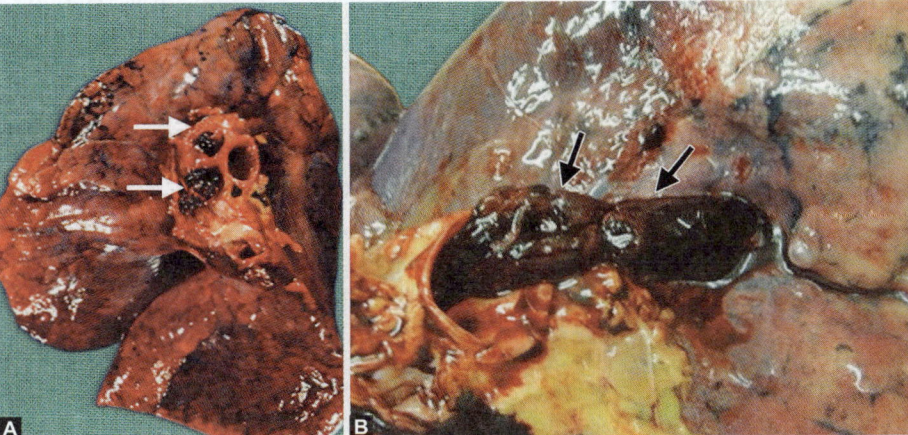

Figs. 17.9A and B: Pulmonary thromboembolism (arrows)

fibrin and platelet deposition around the apparently empty spaces in the blood vessels.
- CD61 and fibrinogen immunohistochemical study can be used to improve the postmortem diagnosis of FES.

Air Embolism

Causes

a. Incised wounds of lower cervical region involving jugular/subclavian vein. It may also happen when the subclavian vein is open to the air, e.g., in supraclavicular node biopsies, central venous line placement or lines that become disconnected.
b. Wounds of sagittal sinus inside the skull.
c. Injection of fluid mixed with soap and air into pregnant uterus for procuring abortion.
d. Cesarean section, version or manual extraction of placenta.
e. Injection of air under pressure in fallopian tube to test its patency.
f. Faulty technique in giving IV injection with gravity.
g. Crush injuries of chest.
h. Positive pressure ventilation in newborn infant.
i. Artificial pneumothorax and pneumo-peritoneum.
j. Air encephalography.
k. Caisson's disease.

- *About 100 mL of air* introduced under pressure produce fatal pulmonary air embolism.
- *Detection:* X-ray examination of whole body. Air bubbles in retinal arteries can be seen by ophthalmoscope.
- For systemic air embolism, *1–2 mL of air* may be enough to produce death.
- Death from air embolism occurs within few minutes, and usually not delayed beyond 45 minutes (min).

3 A 22-year-old male presented to the casualty after assault. He was diagnosed with fracture shaft of femur with respiratory distress and was admitted to ICU. Chest radiograph showed bilateral reticulonodular densities, and retinal examination revealed areas of arterial occlusion as multiple coin-shaped hemorrhages and cotton wool spots. What is your diagnosis?

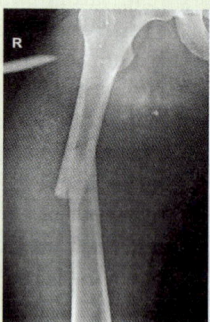
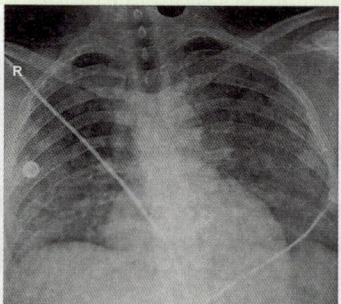
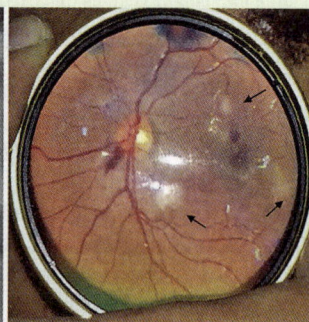

Fracture of femur   Chest X-ray   Fundus
(*Courtesy:* Dr Ritesh Verma, DMCH, Ludhiana)

Describe antemortem and postmortem injuries. Describe homicidal, suicidal and accidental injuries.

■ MEDICO-LEGAL QUESTIONS

Q. Whether the injuries are antemortem or postmortem in nature?

Refer to **Diff. 17.1**.

> **NOTA BENE**
>
> **Histochemical changes**
> In trauma to the living tissue, two zones are seen around the wound:
> i. **Central (superficial) zone:** Close to the edge of the wound, there is a zone, 0.2–0.5 mm wide which becomes necrotic and has decreased enzyme activity—zone of *negative vital reaction* **(Fig. 17.10)**.
> ii. **Peripheral zone:** Immediately beyond this layer, there is a 0.1–0.3 mm zone where enzymes become increased in concentration during reparative process—*zone of positive vital reaction*, compared to the normal level in the area outside the wound **(Fig. 17.10)**.
> - In postmortem wounds, positive vital reaction does not develop.
> - It is demonstrable as a diminishing stainability, and becomes visible in 1–4 h after wounding.
> - In the positive zone, the activity of adenosine triphosphatase and esterase increases within 1 h after injury, aminopeptidase by 2 h, acid phosphatase by 4 h and alkaline phosphatase by 8 h **(Fig. 17.11)**. These changes can be demonstrated for a few days after death, if autolysis is prevented by refrigeration.

Q. Whether the injuries are homicidal, suicidal or accidental in nature?

Opinion regarding the manner of injury is given after a detailed examination and investigation **(Diff. 17.2)**:
- Examination of crime scene
- Examination of the victim
- Examination of the suspected assailant (signs of struggle, blood group, fingerprint)
- Examination of the weapon
- Circumstantial evidence

DIFFERENTIATION 17.1: Antemortem and postmortem wounds

S.No.	Feature	Antemortem wounds	Postmortem wounds
1.	Hemorrhage	Abundant, copious	Slight or absent
2.	Nature	Arterial	Venous
3.	Signs of spurting	Present on body and clothes	No evidence
4.	Coagulation	Firmly coagulated blood	No clotting or soft clot
5.	Extravasated blood	Infiltrate in and around injured tissues and resist washing	Tissues are not deeply stained, can be easily washed with water
6.	Wound edges	Swollen, everted and retracted	Do not gape and edges are closely approximated
7.	Vital reaction	Present	Absent
8.	Histological examination	Evidence of infiltration by leukocytes, macrophages, formation of new capillaries, fibroblasts	No sign of cellular infiltration or proliferation
9.	Histochemical examination	Increased activity of adenosine triphosphatase, esterase, aminopeptidase, acid and alkaline phosphatase. Increase in serotonin and free histamine	No enzyme activity

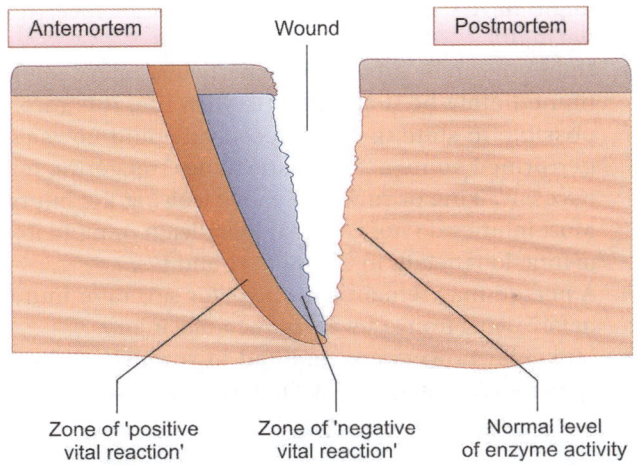

Fig. 17.10: Enzyme activity in antemortem and postmortem wound

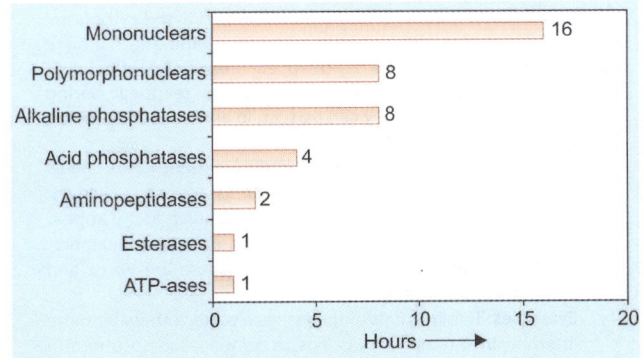

Fig. 17.11: Age of wounds

DIFFERENTIATION 17.2: Homicidal, suicidal and accidental wounds

S.No.	Feature	Homicide	Suicide	Accident
1.	Type	Laceration, incised, stab, chop	Incised or stab	Any type
2.	Number	May be multiple	Multiple, linear and parallel	Single or multiple (RTAs)
3.	Location	Usually head, face, neck and abdomen	Front of chest, neck, wrist	Anywhere
4.	Defense wounds	Present	Absent	Absent
5.	Hesitation cuts	Absent	Present	Absent
6.	Direction	Nothing particular, any direction	Left to right; above downwards	Nothing particular
7.	Severity	Severe, extensive, many deep wounds	Mostly superficial with 1–2 deep wounds	Varies
8.	Weapon at scene	Usually absent	Near the body	Present
9.	Clothes	Torn, cut	Not damaged	Damaged and cut
10.	Circumstantial evidence	Struggle, disturbance of scene	Secluded place, suicide note, locked room, no disturbance of scene	Rarely closed room, no suicide note, eye witness

Q. Whether the time of infliction of the injury can be determined?

It is not possible to determine the exact age of a wound by naked eye or histopathological examination. Only an approximate time can be determined **(Table 17.4)**. Moreover, the changes vary according to the size and type of wound, the tissue, and age and health of the patient.

NOTA BENE

Biochemical timing
- It depends upon the measurement of histamine and serotonin contents of the injured tissue.
- Serotonin becomes maximum in about 10 min and histamine in 20–30 min after wounding.
- To establish the antemortem nature of the wound, the level of histamine should be at least 50% greater and that of serotonin, at least twice the concentration of the control samples.
- Postmortem wounds do not show any increase.

Connective tissue histochemistry
- **Fibroblasts:** It shows increased RNA content in the cytoplasm, prominent glycogen and metachromatic granules.
- **Mucopolysaccharides:** They disappear immediately after injury (abrasion, bruises and electric marks), but reappear during healing process. But they can be seen in antemortem hanging and strangulation marks.
- **Fibrin:** In 4–12 h: network of fine fibrils are seen; >24 h: coarse fibrils; >4 days: small concentrated areas appear; >2 weeks: solid areas predominate; >1 month: granular areas appear amid solid areas; and at >4 months: only granular appearance.
- **Elastic tissue:** In antemortem wounds these are wavy, and straight in postmortem wounds.
- **Esterases:** Two fractions of the esterase pattern show up more intensely in antemortem wounds, as compared to postmortem wounds or undamaged skin using disc electrophoresis.

Q. Can a fatal internal injury be present without any external injury?

- Yes, sometimes the weight of the individual applied on the upper abdomen of another may cause laceration of the liver and death without leaving any visible injury mark.
- Manual strangulation and smothering may not leave any external signs of trauma.
- Fractures of ribs, vertebrae or pelvis with accompanying fatal visceral injuries can occur without external indications of serious violence.

Q. Which of the injuries caused death?

When there is more than one wound, it is necessary to determine which one of them caused death, since the wounds may not have been made by the same assailant or at the same time.

Q. How long did the victim survive, and could he have carried out any voluntary acts after receiving the injury?

- It is usually not possible to opine from an examination of wounds in a dead body as to how long the person might have lived or how much voluntary activity he might have performed before death, after receiving the injury.
- Unless, it can be proved that a particular injury would immediately be incompatible with life, it is rarely possible to state that the deceased could not have performed some activity (speaking, staggering few paces, walking or running) after receiving the injury. Most injuries do not cause sudden death or rapid loss of function (details in Chapters 11 and 12).
- A person may remain conscious for several minutes before dying from a severe intracranial injury.
- Muscular powers are retained in ruptures of liver, spleen or kidneys, unless there is marked immediate blood loss.

Q. Would the victim have survived, had he been given immediate medical care?

It depends on the nature and extent of injuries, as there is individual variation.

TABLE 17.4: Age of the wounds

S.No.	Age	Gross appearance	Microscopic
1.	4 h	Reddish with clotted blood	Nothing specific, but some extravascular emigration of leukocytes may be seen
2.	12 h	Edges of wound are gaping, reddish and swollen	Margination of leukocytes (neutrophils); lymphocytes and monocytes appear
3.	12–24 h	Small wound may show scab	Macrophages and mononuclear cells increases
4.	48 h	Scab, pus may form	Maximum leukocytic infiltration, fibroblasts and elastic fibers are seen
5.	72 h	Epithelial growth clearly visible	New capillary buds seen, granulation tissue forms
6.	4–5 days	Epithelialization of small wounds complete	Profuse growth of capillaries, hemosiderin, new collagen fibrils and giant cells appear
7.	6–7 days	Fibrous scar may be seen in small wounds	Lymphocytes are maximum, epithelium grows on the surface
8.	10–14 days	Vascular scar is formed, later it becomes dense and avascular	Fibroblasts are active, collagen fibers are laid, vascularity decreases, cellular reaction subsides

Q. Can the wounds be altered from their original appearance?

The wounds may be altered in many ways.
- In the living, the wound may be altered by surgical procedures and healing.
- In the dead person, the wound might have been deliberately altered by the assailant to mislead the investigators or by resuscitative measures applied or by insects, animals and decomposition.

Q. Whether the injuries can be produced by more than one type of weapon?

Several persons with different types of weapon may attack the victim producing diverse types of injuries.

Q. What is the relationship of trauma and natural disease?

Relationship of trauma and disease is important mainly for two reasons: compensation and insurance.

i. **Trauma and myocardial infarction:** Heart attack may occur while working, either incidentally (normal progression of chronic disease) or due to unusual physical/mental strain.
- Physical effort can damage a diseased heart due to unusual work or doing unfamiliar or un-accustomed work or accidents.
- Causal connection can be established with certainty only in direct trauma to the heart during work. A blow or physical trauma may precipitate myocardial infarction or arrhythmia.
- If the attack occurs within minutes after unusual effort, the causal connection can be established. It may occur few days later, due to subintimal hemorrhage in coronary artery leading to coronary thrombosis.

ii. **Trauma and neoplasia:** In some cases, there is apparent relationship between tumor and some preceding trauma to the part, e.g., development of osteogenic sarcoma and osteoclastoma after injury, malignancy in burn scars or on the skin adjacent to a chronic osteomyelitis sinus.
- Since, trauma disrupts tissue, it might activate a pre-existing tumor to grow and spread more rapidly.
- In accepting a relationship between trauma and malignancy, following **Ewing's postulates** should be satisfied:
  a. The tumor site prior to injury was normal.
  b. Undeniable and adequate trauma to disrupt the continuity must be proved.
  c. The tumor followed the injury within a reasonable time interval (between a minimum of 3–4 weeks and maximum of 3 years after receipt of injury).
  d. The tumor must have originated in the part of the body that has sustained the injury.
  e. The tumor must be of histological type that could originate from the cells that have been disrupted by the trauma.

iii. **Trauma and nervous system:** Some instances are there wherein trauma (head injury) was subsequently followed by meningitis, epilepsy, psychosis and rupture of congenital cerebral aneurysm.
Traumatic epilepsy: Sometimes, it is a late effect of a depressed fracture of the skull. Traumatic epilepsy usually manifests as a tonic and clonic fits which may be difficult to differentiate from idiopathic epilepsy, if injury occurred in early life. When fits begin within weeks to up to 2 years of a major head injury (depressed fracture impinging on the underlying cortex, often in the parietotemporal area) in a person who never had fits before, the diagnosis is easier.

> FM 1.9, 3.7, 3.8
> - Describe the importance of documentation in medical practice (medico-legal register and reports).
> - Describe examination and certification of wounds.
> - Describe the examination of various weapons.

INJURY REPORT

An injury report is a form of medico-legal report (MLR) giving the details of the condition of a patient, solicited for legal purposes. Casualty medical officer or any other medical officer may be called upon to examine the injured person.

Salient Features

- Medico-legal injury cases should be examined without delay at any time of the day or night and are prepared immediately after the examination is done.
- The medical practitioner should enter all details of examination of the injured person in a **Medico-legal Register** in his own handwriting with a ball-point-pen. It should be prepared in duplicate, one copy of which is given to the IO in a sealed cover and the other retained for future reference. This register is a confidential record and should be in safe custody of the medical officer. It has to be produced in the court of law, if summoned.
- The report should be written legibly and in understandable English. Cutting/overwriting should be avoided, and all corrections should be properly initialed.
- Medical terminology, jargon, abbreviations ('#' for 'fracture' or 'c.l.w' for 'contused lacerated wound') and an unduly technical description should be avoided.
- The doctor should ensure that the report contains both the patient's history and examination findings.
- A complete list of the injuries or conditions complained of by the patient along with line diagrams (pictograph) showing the location of the injury should be present. Color photographs of injuries are recommended.

- Details of all sample and specimens should appear in the report to establish the chain of custody. Failure to collect, destruction or loss of such an exhibit is punishable under **Sec. 201 of IPC**.
- The report should be impartial and unbiased, comprehensible and easy to read. Further, it should be clear about the opinion regarding the nature, cause and duration of injury.
- Whenever possible, a senior faculty should be asked to review and comment upon the report, particularly in complicated cases. It is difficult to alter the report once it has been issued.
- The report should always be signed by the medical practitioner along with date, full name, registration number, qualifications, designation and current employment.

An injury report comprises of three parts as given in **Flowchart 17.1**.

Preliminary Particulars

i. Serial number, admission number.
ii. Name, age, sex, address, and father's/guardian's name.
iii. Date, time, and place of examination.
iv. Name and number of the accompanying police constable and police station to which he belongs. A police case reference number where appropriate, if already reported (DDR/FIR No.).
v. Name of the person who accompanied the injured person with address and relation.
vi. If an unconscious patient is brought for examination, the name and address of the person bringing that patient is noted.
vii. Brief statement of the injured, as to how he was injured.
viii. Two identification marks.
ix. Size of the victim, i.e., stature, weight and development.
x. Informed consent of the person for examination.
xi. If the condition of the patient is serious, dying declaration should be recorded.

Findings/Observations

General physical examination: Consciousness, orientation, GCS (in head injury), pulse, temperature, blood pressure and reaction of pupils to light are to be noted.

Following are the various entries in the injury report

i. **Type of each injury:** All injuries observed, even insignificant should be noted. Type of injuries, i.e., abrasion, contusion, laceration, incised wound, firearm wound, etc., should be noted. Multiple injuries can be grouped anatomically, e.g., injuries of the head, of the trunk or of limb. A magnifying lens should be used to get an accurate idea of the nature of edges, ends and floor of the wound. Presence of any foreign material in wound, e.g., glass, hair or dirt should be noted and preserved.

   Features that may help in differentiating the common injuries are given in **Diff. 17.3**.

ii. **Size, shape and direction of each injury:** All injuries should be measured with a measuring tape and never guessed and amount of blood extravasated should be measured, and photographs (wherever possible) or sketches showing the position and size of the wound are desirable.
   - Shape of the wound, e.g., circular, oval or triangular should be noted and also the beveling of the edges.
   - Direction of the wound, i.e., horizontal, vertical or oblique should be noted with regard to anatomical position of the body.

iii. **Location:** Exact situation of wound with reference to some anatomical landmark, e.g., midline, bony structure or umbilicus should be mentioned. Technical terms should be avoided as far as possible.

Flowchart 17.1: Contents of an injury report

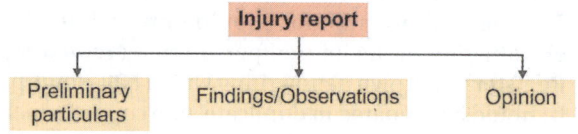

DIFFERENTIATION 17.3: Lacerated, incised and stab wound

S.No.	Feature	Lacerated wound	Incised wound	Stab wound
1.	Causative object	Blunt	Sharp edged	Pointed sharp
2.	Site	Usually over bony prominences	Anywhere	Usually over chest, abdomen or neck
3.	Shape	Irregular	Spindle shaped	Spindle shaped, but depends on the weapon
4.	Margins	Irregular	Clean cut and everted	Clean cut
5.	Dimensions	Variable	Length greater than depth, gaping	Depth greater than length
6.	Hair and blood vessels	Crushed	Clean cut	Variable
7.	Hemorrhage	Not pronounced, except in scalp	Profuse	Variable, may be concealed internally
8.	Surrounding abrasion and bruise	Usually present	Absent	May be seen (hilt mark)
9.	Foreign bodies	Present	Absent	May or may not be present

Opinion

i. **Nature of each injury:** Against each injury, it should be noted whether it is simple or grievous. Injured person must be kept 'under observation', if nature of particular injury cannot be made out at the time of examination, e.g., head injury or abdominal injury. In all injuries, when fracture of a bone is suspected, an X-ray should be done for confirmation.
   - Whether an injury is simple or grievous, is decided on the basis of *status of injury at the time of infliction*, and not after medical/surgical intervention. When deciding the question, one has to only regard the nature of the injury itself. If left untreated, would the injury have led to the defined result?

ii. **Weapon used to inflict the injury:** In many cases, examination of the wound and clothing give fairly definite information about the kind of weapon. With stab and incised wound, there is not much difficulty.
   - Clothes should be examined for the presence of cuts, tears or burns, and it should be seen whether these correspond to the injuries on the body.
   - Any weapon sent by the police allegedly used in producing injuries should be examined as given in **Box 17.1**.

iii. **Duration of injuries:** Opinion is based on the state of healing of the injuries as was recorded in the column of examination of the injuries.* However, the Supreme Court has stated that a doctor can never be absolutely certain on the point of the time of infliction of injuries.

iv. **Cause of the patient's condition:** The court usually wants to know whether the injury for which damages are claimed or punishment sought was caused, aggravated or accelerated by the accident or events complained of. Opinion on the precipitation factor or cause of the patient's condition is based on the history and the nature of injuries on his person.

v. **Whether the weapon was dangerous or not?** Doctor is guided by **Sec. 324 and 326 IPC**.

> **Box 17.1** Examination of a weapon
> - **Extraneous material:** The weapon should be examined for the presence or absence of extraneous material, such as bloodstains, hair, fibers or pieces of cloth adherent to it.
> - A tracing of the weapon is made and various dimensions like length, width and thickness of the blade must be mentioned. Presence or absence of hilt guard, sharpness of the tip (whether pinpoint or rounded), condition of the edges (whether serrated or not), any grooving, serration or forking of the blade should be mentioned.
> - In case of heavy blunt weapon, weight of the weapon must be recorded.
> - **Opinion:** The doctor should give opinion on whether the given injuries could have been produced by the said weapon or not.
> - After the examination, the doctor should affix his signature and date over some suitable spot on the weapon with a permanent marker and then seal it back. Signature on the weapon will help him to identify the weapon in the court.

Handing Over the Report

The initial or provisional report should be made available immediately. A subsequent report (supplementary report) may be given, once the investigation results (reports of blood examination, X-rays and CT scans) become available which reflects the final conclusions drawn from the examination findings that was available at the time of the initial consultation.

---

* When opining on the duration of the injuries, undue and complete dependence is placed on the history given by the patient or his/her relatives; while the doctor's own observations regarding the features of the injuries are often not taken into consideration or overlooked.

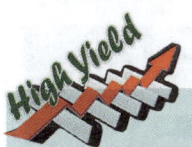

- Injury is defined under Sec. 44 IPC.
- In case of fight, even if there is no injury, the person can be booked under Sec. 351 IPC (assault).
- Justifiable homicides include judicial execution, for self-defense, or preventing rape.
- Culpable homicide is charged under Sec. 299 IPC.
- Attempt to murder is charged under Sec. 307 IPC and punished with imprisonment up to 10 years and fine and life imprisonment (if hurt is caused).
- **Dowry death:** Death of a woman caused under unnatural circumstances within 7 years of her marriage (Sec. 304-B IPC). Punishment is 7 years to life imprisonment
- **Hurt:** Any bodily pain, disease or infirmity caused to any person (Sec. 319 IPC).
- Grievous hurt is defined under Sec. 320 IPC.
- Dangerous injury has not been defined in the IPC.
- Medico-legally, injury causing corneal opacity followed by corneoplasty will be considered as grievous injury.
- Sec 320 IPC, Sec 325 IPC, Sec 326 IPC and Sec 331 IPC are all related to grievous hurt.
- Punishment for voluntarily causing simple hurt: Imprisonment up to 1 year ± fine (Sec. 323 IPC).

- Punishment for voluntarily causing grievous hurt with dangerous weapons: Imprisonment up to 10 years + fine (Sec. 326 IPC).
- **Most common cause of hypovolemic shock:** External bleeding.
- Rapid loss of 1.5–2 L of blood (1/3rd of blood in an adult) is sufficient to cause death.
- Size of clenched fist clot is about 500 mL of blood.
- Loss of blood in closed fracture of femur is about 1000–1500 mL.
- **Reactionary hemorrhage:** Hemorrhage from same site as primary hemorrhage within 24 h after injury.
- **Secondary hemorrhage** results from erosion of vessel wall due to infection (7–14th day).
- **Most common cause of neurogenic shock:** Spinal injury (*spinal shock*).
- Pallor is seen in most types of shock, *except* spinal and septic shock.
- Neurogenic shock is characterized by decreased peripheral vascular resistance.
- Neurogenic shock is not associated with cold peripheries, but warm and well perfused.
- **Features of neurogenic shock:** Hypovolemia, bradycardia and hypotension.
- **Features of septic shock:** Tachycardia, warm skin, decreased cardiac output, caused by gram-negative bacteria.
- Crepitus over skin of the swollen limb may indicate gas gangrene.
- **Crush syndrome:** Traumatic myoglobinuria and acute renal failure following crushing of muscles (e.g., industrial and vehicular accidents), especially of the lower limbs.
- **Most common sites of development of thromboembolism:** Deep femoral, popliteal and posterior tibial veins.
- **Most common cause of pulmonary embolism:** Deep venous thrombosis of legs.
- Thrombus develops in 10–20 days after injury, gets detached and can cause pulmonary embolism (*saddle embolism*).
- **Microscopic findings in pulmonary embolism:** 'Lines of Zahn' and fibrin thromboemboli scattered in pulmonary vessels.
- **Most common cause of fat embolism:** Fracture of pelvis and femur.
- **Triad of fat embolism syndrome:** Cutaneous, neurological and respiratory dysfunction.
- About 12–120 mL of free fat causes embolic death.
- About 100 mL of air produces fatal pulmonary air embolism.
- Thrombi, emboli and fibrin are stained by Martius Scarlet Blue stain.
- Fats are stained by Oil red O, Sudan dyes and osmic acid stain.
- In postmortem wounds, positive vital reaction does not develop.
- Ewing's postulates are related to causal relationship between trauma and malignancy.
- Traumatic epilepsy is a late effect of a *depressed fracture of the skull*.

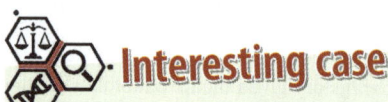

Interesting case

Simple or Grievous Injury (Case of the Alleged 'Fabrication' of Injury Report, 2008)

Tej Pal Singh and the complainant, both divorcees, had married in March 2008. After few months, Singh was accused of misappropriating dowry articles and beating up his wife. The woman lodged an FIR for dowry harassment against her estranged husband and in-laws after allegedly being beaten up by them. She was brought for medico-legal examination.

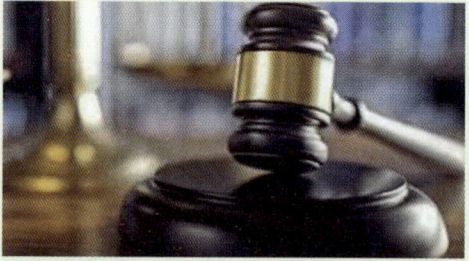

The case was examined by a board of three doctors. After examination and going through the medical reports of the patient, the board opined that the injury was 'grievous' in nature. The ENT report showed that there is mild conductive hearing loss to the patient. This could be due to physical injury or other medical reasons like infection, etc., but in this case the woman did not have any other medical problem.

However, Additional Sessions Judge (ASJ) considered the doctors on duty have acted either under pressure or in connivance with the complainant (woman) or at the behest of senior doctors or senior police officers and have knowingly and willingly fabricated medical records. He was of the opinion that the injury is simple in nature. Allowing the anticipatory bail plea of the accused Singh, the ASJ ordered that notices be issued against all three doctors under Sec. 340 of the CrPC for 'fabrication' of medical reports.

During the trial, the doctors were able to convince the Judge that they had purely gone by medical books, while terming the injury grievous in nature and had not fabricated records. 'Any physical damage which is partial can be termed grievous injury'. She was suffering from partial hearing loss, but could not convince him that it was actually 'grievous' in nature.

ASJ held that it was a 'bonafide mistake' in interpreting legal provisions and have been guided by their own medical literature in giving the opinion on injuries sustained by the woman, and directed that no further proceedings be initiated against them.

CHAPTER 18

Neglect and Starvation Deaths

LEARNING OBJECTIVES

Desirable to know
1. Death due to acute and chronic starvation (including PM findings)

Describe and discuss clinical features, postmortem findings and medico-legal aspects of death due to starvation and neglect.

Definitions

- **Starvation** is the result of irregular or continuous deprivation of nutrients (food alone, or food and drink both) necessary for the maintenance of the body.
- **Inanition:** It refers to the exhausted state due to prolonged undernutrition caused by lack of assimilation of food by the tissues.
- **Neglect:** Failure by person responsible to provide for the individual's basic needs like food, care, shelter or medical attention. It can be a form of child abuse. In general, neglect is an act of omission.

Starvation can be:
- **Acute starvation or total fasting** which results from sudden and total withholding of food, or food and drink.
- **Chronic starvation or malnutrition** which results from prolonged, but gradual and continuous deficiency in the intake of food and nutrients.

MODE OF STARVATION

Failure of Taking Food

i. *Ignorance:* Lack of knowledge of gross nutrition value of foodstuff, particularly among uneducated masses.
ii. *Diseased conditions:* Low intake (e.g., diabetes), loss of appetite (e.g., major depressive disorder), deficient absorption (e.g., celiac disease) or inability to eat (e.g., carcinoma esophagus).
iii. *Deliberate (neglect):* Deliberate improper feeding, or withholding of food in case of unwanted baby, old, invalid or diseased family member.
iv. *Circumstantial:* Accidents (e.g., shipwreck, air crash or colliery entombment) or famine.

Refusal to Take Food

i. In observance of religious rituals which is common in India.
ii. Intentional fasting as a form of protest against some alleged injustice—hunger strike or fast-unto-death.
iii. Mental illnesses, like schizophrenia or anorexia nervosa.

NOTA BENE

- Historically, starvation has been used as a death sentence. From the beginning of civilization to the Middle Ages, people were immured or walled in, and would die for want of food. In ancient Greco-Roman societies, starvation was sometimes used to dispose of guilty upper class citizens, especially erring female members of patrician families.
- Force-feeding of hunger strikers is considered to be a form of torture. The WMA's Tokyo Declaration prohibits doctors' involvement in force-feeding. Due to some untoward incidents in which hunger strikers died in several countries, like in Ireland, Turkey and South Africa, the WMA formulated the Declaration of Malta, dedicated in its entirety to the role and responsibility of doctors caring for hunger strikers.
- As long as the hunger striker is capable of decision making and refuses any medical examination, the doctors should respect his decision. Food or treatment refusal is the individual's voluntary choice. All kinds of interventions for enteral or parenteral feeding against the will of the mentally competent hunger striker are considered as "forced feeding", which is ethically unacceptable.
- Artificial feeding is acceptable if competent hunger strikers agree to it or if incompetent individuals have left no advance instructions refusing it.

PATHOPHYSIOLOGY

Individuals experiencing starvation lose adipose tissue and muscle mass as the body breaks down these tissues for energy. Initially, the body's glycogen stores are used up in about 24 hours (h). After that, the main means of energy production is lipolysis. Adipose tissue releases free fatty acids in starvation and these are used by many as fuel. Furthermore, in the liver they are the substrate for synthesis of ketone bodies (which are major metabolic fuels for skeletal and heart muscle, and the brain). There is an increase in plasma free fatty acids and ketone bodies as starvation progresses which can be detected in urine.

Constituent	Starvation	
	40 h (mmol/L)	7 days (mmol/L)
Glucose	3.6	3.5
Free fatty acids	1.15	1.19
Ketone bodies	2.9	4.5

SIGNS AND SYMPTOMS

Acute Starvation

In the beginning, there is initial feeling of hunger and hunger pains for first 2 days with craving for food wearing off very rapidly. Intense thirst is felt along with epigastric pain and subsequent loss of sense of thirst. This is followed by both mental and physical lethargy, fatigue, irritability, loss of libido and progressive loss of weight. Later, emaciation sets in and the body emits an offensive odor. As the starvation continues, the lethargy becomes extreme, with mental impairment, loss of self-respect and interest in everything.

Characteristic Findings (Fig. 18.1)

- *Skin:* Dry, dirty, lusterless, loose, cracked and inelastic with increase of pigmentation, creases and wrinkles.
- *Face:* Eyes—shrunken, pupils—dilated, lips—dry and cracked, cheek—shallow with prominent malar bones (loss of Bichat's fat of pad is among the last subcutaneous adipose depots to disappear).
- *Tongue:* Dry, furred and coated, foul smelling breath.
- *Temperature:* Hypothermia with sensitivity to cold.

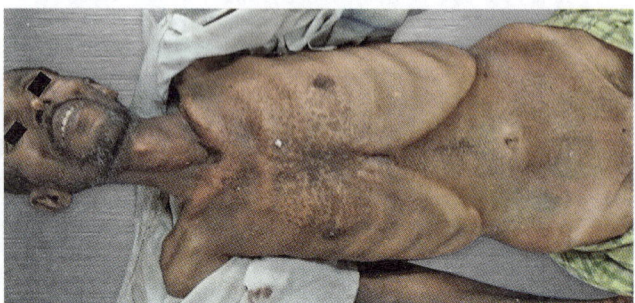

Fig. 18.1: Characteristic external features of starvation

- *Blood pressure:* Hypotension.
- *Pulse:* Quick, weak and feeble.
- *Abdomen:* Concave, prominent ribs and hip bones.
- *Bowel:* Constipated in early phase, followed by diarrhea and dysentery.
- *Renal:* Oliguria with concentrated, highly acidic urine.
- *Muscle:* Atrophy leading to weakness.
- All bony joints and bones look prominent.

Cause of death: Dehydration with progressive cardiac insufficiency. Loss of 40–50% of original body weight usually leads to death.

Chronic Starvation

- Anemia (first sign), hypoproteinemia, emaciation, weak pulse and blood pressure, cyanosis, and edema of feet, legs and face with ascites, hepatitis, diarrhea or dysentery.
- Reduced resistance to infections in general, and development of bronchopneumonia, tuberculosis and enteritis along with poor wound healing.
- In females, irregular menstruation can occur.
- Loss of weight is very rapid in the first place, but becomes slower after 3 months.
- In the terminal stages, adults may experience a variety of neurological and psychiatric symptoms, including hallucinations and convulsions, as well as severe muscle pain and disturbances in heart rhythm.

Cause of death: Prolonged caloric deficiency with subsequent complications, such as multiple organ failure, severe sepsis and ventricular fibrillation are major causes of death.

Fatal Period

- Total withholding of food and water: 14–21 days.
- With total deprivation of food only: 3–6 weeks (8–12 weeks in some cases).

> **NOTA BENE**
>
> **Factors influencing the fatality**
> i. *Age:* Children and infants are most vulnerable. Old person stands starvation better.
> ii. *Sex:* Women stand starvation better than men due to their body fat.
> iii. *Body condition:* Fatty and healthy individual stands starvation better.
> iv. *Environmental factors:* Exposure to cold and extreme heat shortens life.
> v. *Intercurrent infection:* It may cause early death.
> vi. *Physical exertion:* It will enhance the effects of starvation.

> **NOTA BENE**
>
> **Refeeding syndrome:** A potentially fatal condition wherein there is a severe electrolyte and fluid shift associated with metabolic abnormalities in long-term starvation patients undergoing refeeding, whether orally, enterally or parenterally. The hallmark biochemical feature is hypophosphatemia, but may also have abnormal sodium and fluid balance, changes in glucose, protein and fat metabolism, thiamine deficiency, hypokalemia and hypomagnesemia.

CHAPTER 18: Neglect and Starvation Deaths

■ POSTMORTEM FINDINGS

Typical picture of emaciation with loss of body weight and organ weights and exclusion of any other coexisting cause of death are prerequisite for a definite diagnosis of death due to of starvation.

i. Complete lack of fat in the subcutaneous and deep fat depots.
ii. *Skin* is pale and cadaverous in most of the cases, and dark brown in few.
iii. There is severe atrophy of skeletal muscles, lungs, heart, liver, spleen, kidneys, endocrine and reproductive organs (ovaries or testes), **except for the brain**. In infants, complete atrophy of thymus is pathognomonic of starvation.
iv. *Gastrointestinal tract (GIT):* Stomach and small bowel are empty along with presence of dry stools in the colon. Even foreign bodies may be found in the colon (starving person may try to eat everything accessible prior to death).
    - There is atrophy of the GIT with thin parchment-like translucent walls and loss of mucosal folds.
    - Gallbladder bigger in size and distended with bile (food acts as the natural stimulant of bile excretion) **(Fig. 18.2)**.
    - The small intestinal wall appears swollen with reddish discolored mucosa and ulcerations of the mucosa of the colon, described as '*pseudo-dysentery*'.
v. Edema and peritoneal effusions may occur.
vi. *Liver:* It may show centrilobular necrosis due to protein deficiency.
vii. *Kidneys:* It may show atrophy of nephrons.

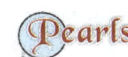

Typical autopsy findings in starvation (Fig. 18.1)
- Emaciation with sunken eyes and loss of Bichat's fat pad.
- Complete disappearance of body fat with pronounced rib cage.
- Loss of adipose tissue of the mesentery.
- Disuse atrophy of the GIT with translucent small intestinal walls.
- Distension of the gallbladder.

■ MEDICO-LEGAL QUESTIONS

Q. Whether the death was caused by neglect and starvation?

The diagnosis of neglect and starvation is done on the basis of history and postmortem findings.

Before opining on starvation as cause of death, the doctor should rule out tuberculosis, carcinoma, stricture of esophagus, anorexia nervosa, radiation sickness, pernicious anemia, inflammatory bowel disease and Addison's disease (chronic adrenocortical insufficiency).

Q. Whether it was suicidal/homicidal/accidental starvation?

If the diagnosis of death as a result of starvation is established, the underlying cause of starvation has to be determined: any pre-existing disease or deliberate withholding of food or neglect.

- **Suicidal:** Some individuals starve voluntarily for the fulfillment of their grievances. Sometimes, prisoners, mentally-ill or hysterical women may refuse to take food. Fasting may also be undertaken to attract public attention.
- **Homicidal:** These cases are related to elderly person or victims of child abuse. It is mostly seen in illegitimate children who are starved to death, by depriving them of food and exposing to severe cold.
- **Accidental:** It may occur during famine, shipwreck or trapped in mines or landslides during earthquakes.
- Deaths caused by starvation are mostly natural deaths in India, accidental cases are also common.
- It relatively rare in the US/industrialized countries. For the most part, they occur either as a result of child abuse, fasting or in mentally-ill person.

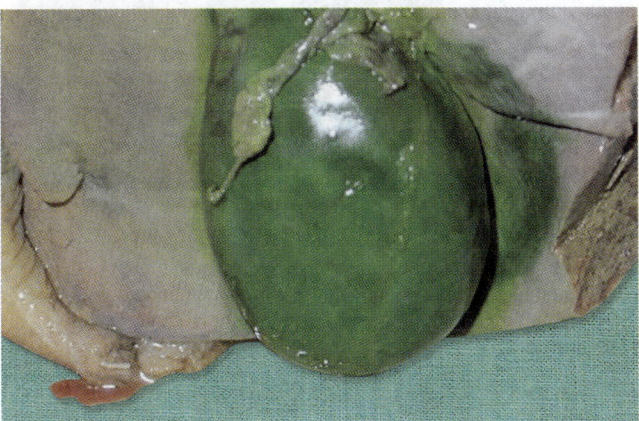

Fig. 18.2: Distended gallbladder in starvation

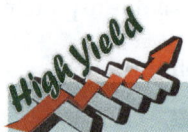

- **Acute starvation:** Results from sudden and total withholding of food and/or drink.
- **Chronic starvation:** Results from prolonged, but gradual and continuous deficiency in the intake of food and nutrients.
- In acute starvation, the source of energy is free fatty acids (acetone).
- In acute starvation, brain uses ketone bodies for metabolic fuels.
- In starvation, there is an **i**ncrease in plasma free fatty acids and ketone bodies which can be detected in urine.
- **Last subcutaneous adipose depot to disappear in acute starvation:** Buccal fat pad.
- **Cause of death in acute starvation:** Dehydration with progressive cardiac insufficiency.
- **Cause of death in chronic starvation:** Multiple organ failure, severe sepsis or ventricular fibrillation.
- If both water and food is completely stopped, the person will die in 14–21 days.
- **Refeeding syndrome** is seen in starvation patients undergoing refeeding wherein there is a severe electrolyte imbalance and metabolic abnormalities.
- In infants, complete atrophy of thymus is pathognomonic of starvation.
- Atrophy of all organs, *except brain* is seen in chronic starvation.
- Gallbladder is *distended* in chronic starvation deaths.

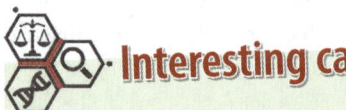

Starvation Death (Case of Kurt Gödel, 1977)

Kurt Gödel born in Brünn, Czech Republic in 1906 was a logician, philosopher and one of the 20th century's most brilliant mathematicians. His *incompleteness theorems* made him internationally famous, and he began giving mathematical lectures around the world starting in 1933. He gave his first lecture in the US that year, where he met Albert Einstein. The two struck up a close friendship that continued until Einstein died in 1955. In 1951, Gödel was awarded the first Albert Einstein Award, and was also awarded the National Medal of Science in 1974.

He also suffered from poor health, beginning with an episode of rheumatic fever at the age of six. He remained convinced that he had never fully recovered and was known for being paranoid, anxious and depressed. He suffered several mental breakdowns during his life. He spent several months in a psychiatric clinic in 1935.

Since the assassination of his close friend Moritz Schlick by one of his own students in 1936, Gödel lived in persecutory delusions of being poisoned. He became very suspicious of all food and was convinced that someone was trying to poison him. He trusted only his wife, Adele, and would eat the food she prepared by her (she would taste any provided food before he ate it). In 1977, when she was hospitalized for a few months after a stroke, Gödel refused to eat, and eventually died of starvation in 1978 at the age of 71. When he died, he weighed only 30 kg. Given his height of ~5′6″, he had a BMI of 10.6 (<18.5 is considered underweight, and potentially dangerous). His death certificate reported 'malnutrition and inanition caused by personality disorder.'

CHAPTER 19

Radiation Sickness, Anesthetic and Operative Deaths

LEARNING OBJECTIVES

Desirable to know
1. Acute radiation syndrome
2. Radiation sickness
3. Causes of death due to anesthesia
4. Postmortem in case of death due to anesthesia
5. Preservation and dispatch of samples in relation to anesthetic deaths

FM 2.25
Describe types of injuries, clinical features, pathophysiology, postmortem findings and medico-legal aspects in cases of radiations.

IONIZING RADIATION REACTIONS

The extent of damage due to radiation exposure depends on the quantity of radiation delivered to the body, dose rate, organs exposed, type of radiation (X-rays, neutrons, γ rays, α or β particles), duration of exposure and energy transfer from the radioactive wave to the exposed tissue.

In the US, the National Committee on Radiation Protection has established the maximum permissible radiation exposure for occupationally exposed workers (≥18 years) as 0.1 rad/week for the whole body (but not to exceed 5 rad/year) and 1.5 rad/week for the hands (routine chest X-rays deliver 0.1–0.2 rad).

The **acute radiation syndrome** may be dominated by CNS, GIT or hematologic manifestations depending on dose and survival.

- Fatigue, weakness and anorexia can occur following exposures exceeding 50 cGy [1 rad = 0.01 gray (Gy) = 1 cGy].
- Hematopoietic effects consisting of anemia, platelet loss and bone marrow suppression can occur 1–3 weeks after exposures exceeding 100 cGy.
- Whole body exposure levels of 1000–3000 cGy destroy GIT mucosa which may lead to toxemia, and death within 2 weeks.
- Total body doses >3000 cGy cause widespread vascular damage, cerebral anoxia, hypotensive shock and death within 48 hours.

Acute (Immediate) Ionizing Radiation Effects

System	Signs and symptoms
Skin and mucous membranes	Erythema, epilation, destruction of fingernails or epidermolysis
Hematopoietic tissues	Bone marrow suppression
Cardiovascular system	Pericarditis with effusion
Reproductive system	Aspermatogenesis, sterility, cessation of menses or abortion
Respiratory system	Pneumonitis
Gastrointestinal tract	Mucositis
Liver	Hepatitis
Renal	Nephritis

Systemic Reactions (Radiation Sickness)

Radiation sickness occurs when X-ray therapy is given over the abdomen, less often with thorax, and rarely when given on the extremities. The basic mechanism is not known.

Symptoms include anorexia, nausea, vomiting, weakness, exhaustion, lassitude, and in some cases, prostration may occur. Dehydration, anemia and infection may follow.

Death after whole body acute lethal radiation exposure is usually due to hematopoietic failure, GIT mucosal damage, CNS damage, widespread vascular injury or secondary infection may occur.

Prevention: Persons handling radiation sources can minimize exposure to radiation by decreasing the time of exposure, maintaining distance and shielding. Special protective clothing is necessary to protect against contamination with radioisotopes.

Nuclear Terrorism

The proliferation of radiation equipment and nuclear energy plants, terrorism and the increasing need for transportation of radioactive materials have made necessary hospital plans for managing patients who are accidentally exposed to ionizing radiation or are contaminated with radioisotopes. The threat of nuclear terrorism is raising the level of awareness about medical aspects of ionizing radiation exposure.

Treatment

The success of treatment of local radiation effects depends on the extent, degree and location of tissue injury.

i. Particulate or radioisotope exposures should be decontaminated in designated confined areas.
ii. Ondansetron, 8 mg orally twice or thrice daily, is given for nausea and vomiting.
iii. Blood and platelet transfusions, blood stem cell transplantation, bone marrow transplants, antibiotics, fluid and electrolyte maintenance, and other supportive measures may be useful.
iv. Newly developed therapy using a patient's own stem cells is safe and effective.
v. In severe and irreversible injury, surgical debridement, skin grafting and free-vascularized flaps are widely used.
vi. Recombinant hematopoietic growth factors have been effective in accelerating hematopoietic recovery.

> **FM 2.19**
> Describe and discuss special protocols for conduction of autopsy and for collection, preservation and dispatch of related material evidences in relation to investigation of anesthetic, operative deaths.

ANESTHETIC AND OPERATIVE DEATHS

Definition

Anesthetic death is defined as death occurring within 24 hours (h) of administration of anesthesia due to causes related to anesthesia. However, death may occur even afterward due to its complications.

Few examples of deaths in operation theater setting:
- A patient dies on table during anesthesia (the cause of death, i.e., whether it is related to the pathology itself, to the surgery or the anesthesia, is left to be determined by the investigation).
- A patient has not fully recovered from effects of general anesthesia, develops upper airway obstruction in recovery room, has a hypoxic arrest and dies.
- A patient aspirates on table, develops pneumonia and dies 2 weeks later from subsequent complications.

Deaths during anesthesia may be broadly classified into two groups:
1. Death during administration of anesthesia, but not due to anesthesia.
2. Deaths which are the direct result of administration of an anesthetic.

Death during Administration of Anesthesia (Not due to Anesthesia)

i. The injury or disease process which necessitated surgical intervention is serious enough, the anesthetic may have only precipitated the death.
ii. Patient may be suffering from a severe systemic illness, e.g., valvular heart disease or severe coronary disease and undergoes surgery for another disease or problem—the operation or anesthetic may have precipitated death.
iii. Patient may be having some undiagnosed serious lesions, e.g., major vascular aneurysm or severe coronary artery disease which could have been an important contributory factor in causing death.
iv. *Surgical shock and exhaustion:* When surgery has been unduly delayed and preoperative condition of patient is poor, shock and exhaustion may be major factors responsible for causing the death of the patient, or the patient has been unable to bear the stress of anesthesia and surgery.

Deaths Directly Related to Administration of an Anesthetic

i. **Inexperience:** Lack of adequate experience is the most common cause of death. Inability to take precautions and corrective measures when required is commonly observed, e.g., death during endotracheal intubation is due to:
   - Inability to place the tube in the trachea.
   - Esophageal intubation.
   - Inability to protect the airway against aspiration of foreign bodies, including regurgitant gastric content, tooth and blood.
   - Disconnection of circuit.
ii. **Equipment/device failure** due to:
   - Faulty connections or mislabeling of anesthetic gases and drugs.
   - Explosion and fire in operation theater. This problem is now rare due to advent of newer anesthetic agents which do not form explosive mixtures.
iii. **Respiratory failure:** Death occurs due to an inadequate supply of oxygen to tissues. It may be due to:
   - Depression of respiratory center by overdose of drugs used for pre-medication and pain relief, or overdose of anesthetic agent used.
   - Inadequate reversal of muscle relaxant leading to inefficient ventilation of lungs.
   - Obstruction of the respiratory tract from laryngeal spasm, impaction of loose material, like swabs or dentures in larynx, trachea and bronchi, or tongue falling back leading to airway obstruction. Regurgitant matter aspirated into lungs may affect gaseous exchange in the lungs.

- Large tidal volumes used during intermittent positive pressure ventilation may result in lung trauma leading to pneumothorax or tension pneumothorax. Nitrous oxide used during general anesthesia leads to a rapid expansion of the pneumothorax. If pneumothorax is significant, gaseous exchange is affected leading to hypoxic injury and death.

iv. **Neurogenic cardiovascular failure:** It is the *most common cause of sudden death* under general anesthesia. It usually occurs when some intervention is done at a time when the depth of anesthesia is still inadequate, e.g., traction on viscera or peritoneum, laryngoscopy and endotracheal intubation, and dilatation.

v. **Malignant hyperthermia:** When it occurs, it is usually seen with halogenated anesthetics and succinylcholine.
   - Individual involved usually has a genetic predisposition to the syndrome.
   - *Signs and symptoms:* Rapid rise in body temperature and a two-to three-fold increase in total body oxygen consumption, arrhythmias, tachycardia and skeletal muscle rigidity.
   - May be fulminant or insidious; may or may not occur every time anesthesia is administered.
   - *Complications:* Rhabdomyolysis, electrolyte abnormalities (especially hyperkalemia) and disseminated intravascular coagulopathy (DIC).

vi. **Local anesthetics:** Toxicity results from overdose or allergic reactions, hypersensitivity and idiosyncrasy. Important factors influencing toxicity are:
   - General condition and susceptibility of the patient.
   - Total dose administered.
   - Rate of administration of anesthetic agent.
   - Vascularity of the area injected.
   - Accidental intravascular injection.
   - Concomitant use of adrenaline: Adrenaline used along with local anesthetic agent can cause tachycardia, palpitation, sweating, hypertension and ventricular fibrillation.

   There may be general effect on CNS which can be:
   a. **Excitatory:** Causing convulsions, or
   b. **Depressive:** Causing respiratory paralysis.

   Very rarely, the heart may be affected directly, or when an abnormally high concentration is injected into a nerve, permanent loss of function may occur.

vii. **Spinal anesthesia:** During spinal anesthesia (block), sympathetic blockade occurs along with sensory and motor blockade. This sympathetic blockade leads to varying degrees of hypotension which may be fatal, if not detected and corrected early.
   - Marked hypotension is observed in elderly, in fluid deficit states like hemorrhage and dehydration, and whenever there is a pre-existing decompensating heart disease.
   - Cardiac activity may be inhibited leading to death due to vagus stimulation.
   - The vital centers in the brainstem may be affected by diffusion of drug upward. Cardiac or respiratory arrest may occur.
   - Post-lumbar puncture headache occurs when a large bore needle is used for lumbar puncture.
   - Contamination of the needle, syringe and ampoules with sterilizing and cleansing agent may lead to arachnoiditis, and may cause bladder-bowel dysfunction and paraplegia. Sepsis can also occur.

Complications of Anesthesia

Minor complications are not uncommon in anesthesia. These include—hypoxemia, atelectasis of lungs, pneumonia, pulmonary edema, pneumothorax, bronchospasm, oxygen toxicity and aspiration of gastric contents, blood or foreign bodies.

Neurological sequelae of these complications can be blindness, paraplegia, paresthesia, vegetative state and death.

Medico-legal Issues of Death in Operation Theater

♦ The death of a person whilst under the influence of a general anesthetic or local anesthetic, or of which the administration of an anesthetic has been a contributory cause, is considered to be an unnatural death. Hence in all such deaths, the surgical team must inform the hospital authorities, who in turn, should inform the police and must insist on an autopsy, for their own safety and defense. The attending clinicians should refrain from issuing a death certificate in these cases.

♦ The Karnataka High Court has held that in case of death on operation table, in the absence of postmortem and/or histopathology reports, the possibility of other causes of death cannot be ruled out. The death on the operation table by itself is not sufficient to prove rashness or negligence against the accused.

Anesthetists per se are likely to experience intraoperative death more than surgeons, the consequences of which can be extremely stressful. It is reasonable for medical staff not to take part in operations for 24 h after an intraoperative death. Moreover, when a death occurs on the operating table, the anesthetist may become inclined to hypercritical self-examination and subjected to prolonged, judgmental investigation by their peers.

Documentation of pre-anesthetic evaluation and assessment of the patient, and preoperative record of the events are of vital importance and can prove to be a tool for retrospective analysis of the information.

■ POSTMORTEM EXAMINATION

The most common causes of anesthesia-related deaths are:
♦ Circulatory failure due to hypovolemia and overdose of anesthetic agents such as thiopentone, opioids, benzodiazepines or regional anesthesia.

- Hypoxia and hypoventilation following undetected esophageal intubation, difficult intubation, technical failure in the anesthetic equipment or aspiration of gastric content.
- Anaphylactic reactions including malignant hyperthermia.
- Negligence such as lack of vigilance or errors in the administration of drugs and in the maintenance and control of the anesthetic equipment.

Most deaths concerning anesthesia are unlikely to be evident at autopsy. Surgical mistakes being anatomical, may be observable at the postmortem, and anesthetic mistakes being physiological are usually not appreciable after death, except where overdose with specific drug is involved. Findings of the autopsy surgeon alone will not be sufficient to explain death and therefore, it is advisable to hold a discussion across the autopsy table involving forensic expert, anesthetist and the surgeon/clinician concerned.

In case of death following anesthesia/surgery, the forensic pathologist must answer the following questions:
 i. Was the death due to the effects of the operation or anesthesia or is it due to the disease for which operation was being carried out?
 ii. Would the patient have died, if he has not undergone through the anesthesia or operation?
 iii. Was there any defect in anesthetic or surgical technique?
 iv. Was the patient suffering from any predisposing condition that made him more susceptible to death from anesthetic or operative procedure?
 v. Was the death due to some unsuspected natural disease, directly unrelated to the disease for which surgery was being performed?

During postmortem examination, the following are to be taken into consideration:
 i. Detailed hospital record of the patient, including full clinical and pre-anesthetic checkup.
 ii. Surgical intervention and its sequelae, like sepsis, hemorrhage or edema.
 iii. Postmortem changes need to be differentiated from abnormalities existing during life (e.g., resuscitative artifacts and agonal regurgitation).
 iv. Instances of surgical mishap which may not be negligence, if the operating conditions were difficult, like ligation of arteries and veins, ureters, bile ducts and perforation of large blood vessels, should be looked for.
 v. Presence of pre-existing natural disease, such as heart disease or respiratory insufficiency and their contribution to the cause of death must be evaluated.
 vi. Pneumothorax, air embolism or surgical emphysema should be clearly evaluated.
 vii. Surgical and anesthetic devices, such as airways, endotracheal tubes, needles or catheters should not be removed prior to autopsy. In esophageal intubation, a radiograph will show a ring of edema of esophageal mucosa at the level of the tube along with distention of stomach and intestines.
 viii. All the organs should be dissected, and surgical sutures should be inspected.
 ix. Chloroform and halothane are hepatotoxic, and chloroform may cause ventricular fibrillation sometimes. Halogenated hydrocarbons cause cardiac irritability.
 x. A full range of specimens for histological, toxicological and bacteriological examinations, and those required to exclude hazards associated with blood or fluid transfusions must be collected.

Histological examination of the brain is vital which is primarily intended to demonstrate the effects of hypoxia, particularly in the region of Sommer's area of the hippocampal gyrus and the cerebellum where changes are expected, even if the victim suffers hypoxia for a short period.

Toxicological examination: Following samples should be collected:

- Blood 10 mL (under liquid paraffin)
- One lung sealed in nylon bag
- Liver 100 g
- Skeletal muscle 10 g
- Fat from mesentery 2 g
- Cerebrum 100 g
- Kidney 100 g or half of each kidney
- Urine

In case of inhaled anesthetic, specimens should be kept in containers of appropriate size to avoid empty space, and are sealed and refrigerated/frozen. Alveolar air should be collected with needle and syringe by puncturing the lung underwater before the chest is opened.

Anesthetic Drugs and Suicide

- Mostly doctors and paramedics misuse anesthetic drugs. There are instances when these have been used for suicidal purpose.
- Opioids, like morphine, pethidine and pentazocine are administered along with muscle relaxants for painless death. While opioids produce analgesia, muscle relaxants cause paralysis of muscles including those of the diaphragm. Due to failure of ventilation of lungs, hypoxia results, leading to death.
- Death can be averted, if detected early, by instituting positive pressure ventilation of lungs till there is recovery from effects of muscle relaxants and opioids.

CHAPTER 19 : Radiation Sickness, Anesthetic and Operative Deaths

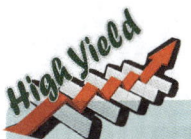

- Acute radiation syndrome mainly causes CNS, GIT or hematologic manifestations.
- Radiation sickness occurs when X-ray therapy is given over the abdomen, less often with thorax.
- Lack of adequate experience is the most common cause of anesthetic deaths.
- **Neurogenic cardiovascular failure** is the most common cause of sudden death under general anesthesia.
- Malignant hyperthermia occurs with halogenated anesthetics and succinylcholine.
- The police must be informed in cases of deaths during anesthesia or in the OT must be informed and autopsy should be conducted.

Interesting case

Propofol Toxicity (Case of Michael Jackson, 2009)

Michael Jackson, one of the greatest performers in pop music history, died in Los Angeles, US in June, 2009 due to drug overdose administered by his personal physician Dr Conrad Murray. He hired the doctor while preparing for a series of 'comeback' concerts. The autopsy report revealed that Jackson was otherwise healthy for his age, weighing 136 pounds, his BMI was in the normal range and his heart was in good condition. The most significant pathology was in his left lung. There was widespread respiratory bronchiolitis and chronic lung inflammation, but that did not contribute to his death. Toxicological analysis was done of his blood samples, vitreous, liver, stomach contents and urine. In addition, tests were performed on the 10 mL syringes and IV fluid setup and tubing (found at his home). Propofol (called 'milk' by addicts), a powerful anesthetic was detected in all samples. The levels of propofol found were within the therapeutic range. In addition to propofol, his blood contained anxiety sedatives lidocaine, diazepam, nordiazepam, lorazepam and midazolam, as well as ephedrine.

Based on toxicology findings, the cause of his death was determined to be acute propofol intoxication with a contributory benzodiazepine effect. The manner of death was homicide. Jackson's doctor admitted to have given sedatives and propofol for insomnia via IV drip. He was charged with involuntary manslaughter (unlawful killing of a human being without malice).

Jackson had a long history of substance abuse, addiction to medications and sleep disturbance but no cardiovascular problems. Murray was an interventional cardiologist and not trained to treat his specific needs. The prosecutor established that the level of propofol found in Jackson's body was consistent with major surgery anesthesia. Propofol is typically administered in a hospital setting by anesthetists with continuous pulse oximetry, ECG and BP monitoring and supplemental oxygen. An oxygen tank was found near his bed, but it was empty. Lorazepam found in Jackson's body would have accentuated the respiratory and cardiovascular depression from propofol. Moreover, use of propofol for insomnia was also disputed.

Murray pleaded not guilty to causing Jackson's death. The defense argued that Jackson's death was an accidental death caused by his own actions. He took the fatal dose of drug in the 2-minute time period that the doctor claimed was away to the washroom, which failed to convince the jury. It was more likely that the doctor accidentally overdosed Jackson. He was irresponsible, medically negligent and did not follow the standard of care. The doctor was convicted of involuntary manslaughter for improperly administering the anesthetic drug that led to his death and served two years prison sentence.

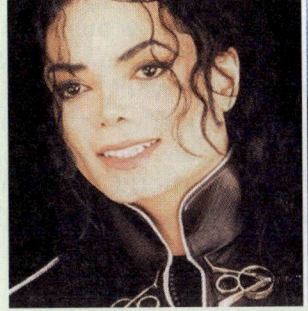 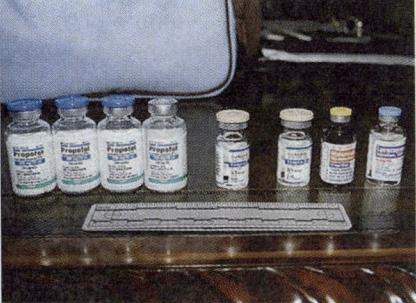

Medication found in Michael Jackson's home.

CHAPTER 20

Infanticide and Child Abuse

LEARNING OBJECTIVES

Must know
1. Infanticide, feticide, legal and medico-legal issues
2. Estimation of age of fetus from its features
3. Appearance of center of ossification—calcaneum, talus, femur, tibia
4. Rule of Hasse
5. Features of dead-born fetus, Spalding's sign, maceration
6. Age of viability
7. Vagitus vaginalis and vagitus uterinus
8. Signs of live birth
9. Hydrostatic test
10. Wreden's test, Breslau's second life test
11. Precipitate labor (medico-legal aspects)
12. Battered baby syndrome
13. Sudden infant death syndrome
14. Stillborn and dead-born (Diff.)
15. Stillborn and liveborn infant (Diff.)
16. Cephalhematoma and caput succedaneum (Diff.)

Desirable to know
1. Postmortem examination of infanticide cases
2. Changes in umbilical cord after birth
3. Causes of infant death
4. Munchausen syndrome by proxy
5. Head injury due to precipitate labor and blunt force (Diff.)

FM 2.27
Define and discuss infanticide, feticide and stillbirth.

Definitions

- **Infanticide** is killing of an infant at any time from birth up to the age of 12 months.
- **Feticide** is the killing of fetus at any time prior to birth.
- **Stillborn:** Fetus born after 28 weeks of pregnancy (24 weeks in the UK) and did not breath or show any other signs of life at any time after being completely born (as per WHO).
- **Neonaticide:** The act of killing of an infant within the first 24 hours (h) of life.
- **Neonatal death:** Death of a live born infant within the first 28 days of life.
- **Female feticide:** It is the act of aborting a fetus because it is female.
- **Perinatal mortality:** Stillbirths plus early neonatal deaths (death at 7 days or less).
- **Intrapartum death:** Death occurring during labor and delivery.

Legal Aspects

- Infanticide is charged under **Sec. 302 IPC** which is punishable by death or imprisonment for life and fine.
- The causing of the death of living child in the mother's womb may amount to culpable homicide, if any part of that child has been brought forth, though the child may not have breathed or completely born **(Sec. 299 IPC)**.
- Any person who does an act with intent to prevent the child being born alive or to cause it to die after birth (except done in good faith for the purpose of saving the life of mother) is punished with imprisonment up to 10 years with/without fine **(Sec. 315 IPC)**.
- Any person who does an act causing death of quick unborn child would be guilty of culpable homicide, and punished with imprisonment up to 10 years and fine **(Sec. 316 IPC)**. For example, a person knowingly injures a pregnant woman that causes the death of an unborn quick child; he is guilty of the offense defined in this section.

Infanticide does not include the death of fetus during labor, when it is destroyed by craniotomy or decapitation.

> **NOTA BENE**
>
> ♦ In Canada, Italy, UK and Australia, murder of a child <1 year of age by his/her own mother is not considered homicide. Instead, the mother is charged with the offense of *infanticide*, for which the punishment is lesser. This is because such murders could be due to '*postpartum depression*' or '*baby-blues*'.
> ♦ In India, there is no such special Act and there is no distinction between the murder of a newborn infant and that of any other individual.

Medico-legal Issues

The fetus/neonate may be brought for the examination so as to settle some of the matters cited below:
a. Questions pertaining to identification of the fetus/neonate and mother
b. Questions pertaining to artificial or induced abortion (willful termination of pregnancy before viability)
   ▪ Whether it is legal or justifiable abortion?
   ▪ Whether this is a case of criminal abortion?
c. Questions on viability
   ▪ Whether the baby was born alive or stillborn?
   ▪ Whether it is a case of infanticide?
   ▪ What is the cause of its death?
d. Questions on negligence
   Charges may be framed and a case for wrongful or negligent act may be brought against the doctor, if the act results in a miscarriage or stillbirth of the fetus. The doctor become liable to pay damages, if the harm suffered is the result of his tortious conduct.
e. Questions on trauma resulting in abortion
   It may be a case of a mother who is the victim of an assault, which results in premature labor, delivery of an extremely premature infant who survives a few hours, but then dies because of prematurity. Such a case could be considered an infanticide, and criminal charges could well be pursued.

POSTMORTEM EXAMINATION OF INFANTS

The relatives should identify the body, and radiological examination should be done prior to autopsy.
- Whole-body radiographs (anteroposterior and lateral) are taken.
- Photographs of the external features—frontal pictures of the entire body and close-ups of the face and side of the head, as well as any other unusual aspects are taken.
  The procedure for autopsy is nearly the same as in adults, except for certain variations. The presence of malformations is often the major consideration, and the dissection should be made to preserve anatomic relationships in order to define the abnormal anatomy.

External Examination

- **Clothings and wrappings** should be examined and retained for identification of the mother.
- **Measurements:** Head, chest and abdominal circumferences, length (crown-rump, crown-heel, and foot for fetuses) and weight of the body helps to assess the gestational age.
- **General features:** The presence of dysmorphic features should be documented, and karyotyping should be considered, if significant abnormal features are noted.
- **Head:** The distribution and quality of hair over the head and rest of the body are noted. Abnormalities of the shape of the head related to molding, trauma, soft tissue edema, hemorrhage or autolysis are noted.
- **Face:** The facial features are examined and abnormalities recorded. Configuration of the ear is examined, and plasticity (indicating amount of cartilage) evaluated as an index to developmental stage. By late intrauterine development, the crest of the external ear should be superior to the level of the lateral canthus.
- **Extremities:** The position of the hands and feet, as well as the fingers and nails must be noted.
- **Genital area:** The perineal area is inspected and checked for the patency of anal opening. In males, position of meatus, and scrotal sac and its contents are palpated. In females, the position of the meatus, and configuration and relative size of the labia and clitoris are observed.
- **Changes of putrefaction:** It helps in ascertaining the time since death. Bodies of the newborn infants are normally sterile. When they breathe and swallow, microorganisms enter into the body. Therefore, in the stillborn, putrefaction occurs from outside to inwards, and in liveborn infants, from within to outwards. Decomposition must be differentiated from maceration, as the latter is a sure sign of a dead-born fetus. If the fetus is decomposed, it will almost certainly be impossible to determine whether live birth had occurred.
- **Presence or absence of vernix caseosa:** Presence of vernix caseosa is not as useful a sign as its absence, as it indicates that the child had been washed, suggesting that it survived for sometime after birth **(Fig. 20.1)**.
- **Injuries:** All the injuries and bruises (particularly around nose, mouth and frenulum) should be noted and photographed. Inflicted injuries should be carefully distinguished from injuries owing to birth trauma, normal anatomical features and postmortem damage.
- **Placenta:** Placenta should be weighed to evaluate maturity, and any abnormality should also be observed (about 15–20 cm in diameter, central thickness 2.5 cm, weighs 500 g at term). Various placental conditions may result in the stillbirth of otherwise completely normal infants. *Abruptio placenta* may be associated with extensive retroplacental bleeding and compromise placental and fetal oxygenation. *Placenta previa* may lead to massive hemorrhage once labor is initiated, with death of both mother and infant, unless urgent medical intervention has occurred.

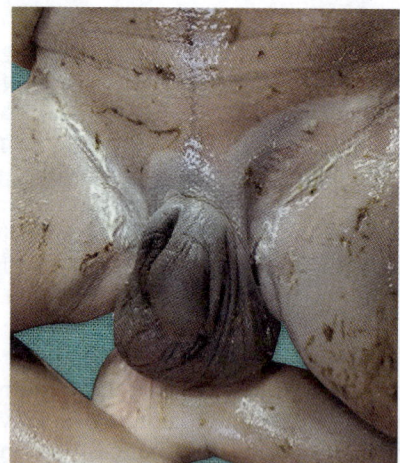

Fig. 20.1: Presence of vernix caseosa in the inguinal region and thighs

- **Umbilical cord:** The cord length is 54–61 cm with short cords measuring <30 cm and long cords measuring >100 cm. Long cords may cause blood flow obstruction if prolapse, torsion or knotting occurs, and may also wrap around the neck causing asphyxia. True knots are tight, with congestion of vessels on one side and pallor on the other. Conversely, blood flow in short cords may also be compromised, if there is excessive traction during delivery.
- **Preservation of sample:** Blood and tissue samples should be taken for matching with maternal blood groups and DNA, if these become available. Full microbiological workup of both the fetus/infant and the placenta should be undertaken, along with histological examination of all major organ/tissues and specialized testing for metabolic abnormalities. Swabs should be taken of every orifice, like that of a case of sexual assault.

Internal Examination

The *modified Y-shaped incision* from both mastoid to the top of the sternum is used, extending down the midline to the pubis. The *ear-to-ear incision* is used for reflecting the scalp.

Brain: While reflecting the scalp, note whether there is any subaponeurotic hemorrhage to exclude asphyxia or deep bruises.

Procedure: In fetuses and infants, **Beneke's technique** is used to open the skull. The cranium and dura on both the sides are cut with blunt scissors starting at the lateral edge of the anterior fontanelle extending the incisions along the midline and the lateral sides of the skull. The midline strip about 1 cm wide containing the superior sagittal sinus and the falx is left, and also an intact area in the temporal squama on either side, which serves as a hinge when the bone is reflected in a '*butterfly*' manner **(Fig. 20.2A)**.

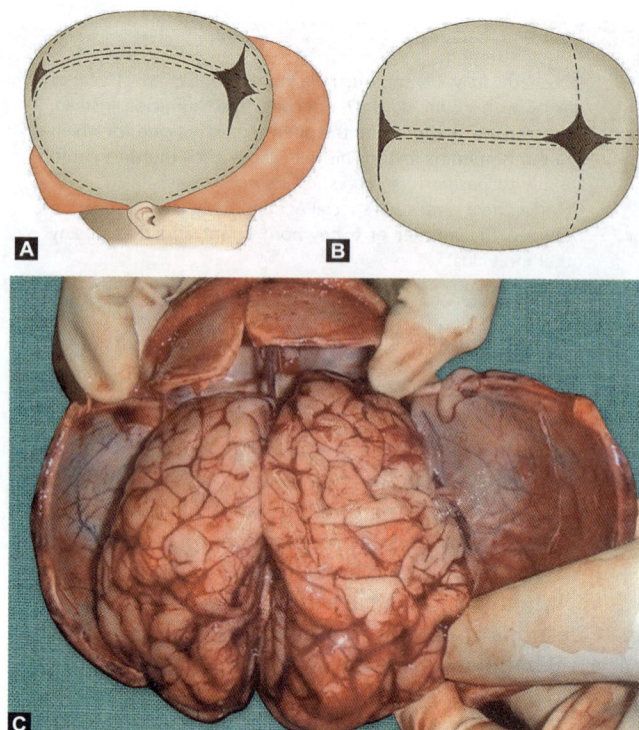

Figs. 20.2A to C: Two methods of opening the calvarium in fetus and neonate: (A) Beneke's technique; (B) Reflection of cranial bones along the suture lines; (C) Removal of brain in infants

- **Modified Beneke's technique:** An alternative method of cutting through the cranial suture lines (sometimes referred to as **Baar technique**) **(Figs. 20.2B and C)** which opens the skull in '*rose petal*' manner **(Figs. 20.2B and C)**.
- After carefully inspecting the hemispheres, falx cerebri and tentorium cerebelli through the openings, the midline bone and sinus are removed. Injuries to fontanelles (e.g., punctured wounds through anterior fontanelle) and subdural/subarachnoid hemorrhages are looked for.

Neck: This is examined for internal injuries, and the trachea for foreign body, froth, mucus or amniotic fluid.

Thorax: *Before opening the thorax, the abdomen is opened first* and position of diaphragm is noted by passing a finger.
- The whole chest cavity can be opened under water in order to demonstrate a pneumothorax.
- In infants and fetuses, **Letulle's technique** of *en masse* removal is the preferred in most cases so that certain rare malformations can be properly preserved, e.g., pulmonary venous connections.
- It should be noted whether there is free blood or fluid, pus or stomach contents present in the thoracic or abdominal cavity, or whether the diaphragm is ruptured or not. If there is any fracture of the ribs, it should be noted.

- Any evidence for malformations or birth-injuries should be meticulously searched which may reveal obvious incompatibility with the continuation of life.
- The lungs, stomach, heart, genitalia and other viscera are examined for different parameters as outlined below.

Limbs and sternum: They are examined for presence of ossification centers to determine the age of the fetus. Center of ossification for the calcaneum appears by the 5th month, four divisions of sternum by the 7th month, talus by the 7th month and lower end of femur by the 9th month (36th week). At birth, a center of ossification is usually present for the cuboid and upper end of tibia.

- The time of appearance of ossification centers is also no longer regarded uniform, as once thought.

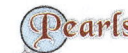

Salient features to determine maturity:
a. General body appearance
b. Distribution of vernix caseosa
c. Skin development
d. External genitalia development
e. Creases on the plantar surfaces of the feet
f. Presence of lanugo
g. Nipple bud development
h. Ear cartilage development
i. Fingernail and toenail length

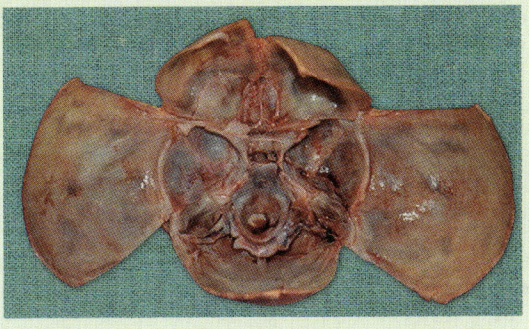

Name the technique of opening the fetal skull.

FM 2.28 — Describe and discuss age determination of fetus.

NOTA BENE

- **Conceptus:** Any product of conception at any stage of development from fertilization until birth including extraembryonic membranes, as well as the embryo or fetus.
- **Pre-embryo:** Fertilized ovum up to 14 days after conception, until the implantation occurs.
- **Embryo:** Prefetal product of conception from implantation to the end of 8th week (2nd month or 56 days).
- **Fetus:** Unborn young from the end of 8th week after conception till delivery.
- **Infant:** Child from the time of birth to 1 year of age.
- **Neonate:** Infant in the first 28 days of extrauterine life.
- **Meconium:** Mixture of bile, mucus and shredded-off mucosa.
- **Vernix caseosa:** White, cheesy substance composed of sebum and desquamated epithelial cells which covers the skin of the fetus.
- **Lanugo hair:** Fine, soft, downy, usually unpigmented hair on the body of the fetus and newborn.

AGE OF FETUS

- Human gestation lasts for 40 weeks or 280 days (10 lunar months) after the onset of last menstrual period (LMP).
- The field of embryology uses 38 weeks or 266 days as the total length of gestation, beginning from the day of oocyte fertilization and zygote formation, rather than from the first day of LMP. Thus, the embryonic calculation more accurately reflects the duration of human gestation.

However, the following discussion uses the obstetrical standard of 40 weeks for easy understanding and universal acceptance.
- Examination of various organs and its development can also assist an autopsy surgeon in estimating the gestational age of a fetus/infant **(Table 20.1)**.
- However, it must be understood that at any time of life, morphological measurements are by no means infallible indicators of chronological age.

RULE OF HASSE

Rule of Hasse* is a rough method of calculating the age of fetus.
- The length of fetus is measured from **crown to heel** in centimeters.
- During first 5 months of pregnancy—square root of length gives approximate age of fetus in months.
- During the last 5 months—length in centimeters divided by 5 gives age in months.
- For example, if the length of fetus is 40 cm and has crossed 5 months of gestation, then fetal age: 40 ÷ 5 = 8 months.

Nonosseous method of estimating maturity: Progressive development of surfactant-producing alveolar Type-II cells in fetal lungs.

After birth, increase in the length of the child is given in **Table 20.2.** Length is measured in children before they are able to stand; height is measured once the child can stand. Birth weight doubles by about 5–6 months of age, triples by about 1 year.

---

* Rule of Morrison mentioned in some books is not authentic and verifiable from any standard textbook/journal.

TABLE 20.1: Determination of age of fetus

Weeks of gestation	Features
4 weeks	Length: 1 cm, weight: 2.5 g Eyes are seen as 2 dark spots and mouth as cleft
8 weeks	Length: 4 cm, weight: 10 g Eyes and nose recognizable, hands and feet are webbed. Anus is seen as dark spot. Placenta is formed
12 weeks	Length: 9 cm, weight: 30 g Eyes are closed and pupillary membrane appears, nails appear, neck is formed
16 weeks (Fig. 20.3)	Length: 16 cm, weight: 120 g **Sex can be recognized**; lanugo hair is visible on body; pupillary membrane is visible and meconium is seen in the upper part of small intestine. Fingerprints are formed. Buds for all 20 temporary teeth laid down
20 weeks (Figs. 20.4A and B)	Length: 25 cm, weight: 400 g Nails are distinct and soft, vernix caseosa appears on the body. Fine hair on scalp, meconium at the beginning of large intestine. In females, ovaries differentiate and contain primordial follicles. Uterus is formed in females and canalization of the vagina begins **Center of ossification for calcaneum appears (Fig. 20.5A)**
24 weeks (Fig. 20.6)	Length: 30 cm, weight: 700 g, foot length: 4.5 cm Scalp and lanugo hair are visible. Eyebrow and eyelashes appear, eyelids are adherent and pupillary membrane is still present; skin is red and wrinkled for want of fat; testes are close to kidneys and scrotum is empty; meconium is seen in upper part of large intestine
28 weeks	Length: 35 cm, weight: 900–1200 g, crown-rump: 23–25 cm, foot length: 5.4 cm Eyelids are open, pupillary membrane disappears; pinna is soft and remains folded; nails are thick, but do not extend to the tips of fingers and toes; skin is dusky-red, thick and fibrous; meconium present in entire large intestine. Testes undescended and smooth scrotum (in males), and prominent clitoris, small widely separated labia (in females) Center of ossification for talus appears **(Fig. 20.5A)**
32 weeks (Fig. 20.7)	Length: 40 cm, weight: 1–1.5 kg, foot length: 6.4 cm Scalp hair is thick; nails reach the tips of fingers; pinna slightly harder but remains folded; skin is not wrinkled; lanugo hair on face; testes in inguinal canal and few scrotal rugae (in males), prominent clitoris and larger widely separated labia (in females), and 1–2 anterior creases on planter surface (32 weeks)
36 weeks	Length: 45 cm, weight: 2.5–3 kg, foot length: 7 cm Scalp is covered with dark hair; pinna harder, springs back; breast nodule 1–2 mm; lanugo hair is seen only in shoulders; vernix caseosa is present over the flexures of joints and neck folds; testes high in scrotum and more scrotal rugae (in males), clitoris less prominent and labia majora covers labia minora (in females); 2–3 anterior creases on plantar surface Meconium is near the end of large intestine **Ossification centers for lower end of femur** (36–37 weeks), **cuboid and capitate appear (Figs. 20.5A and B)**
40 weeks (Fig. 20.8) (Full term)	Length: 50–53 cm, weight: 3–3.5 kg, crown-rump: 28–32 cm, foot length: 8.25 cm Lanugo hair is seen only in shoulders; nails project beyond finger tips, but reach only the tip of toes; pinna firm and stand erect from head; breasts buds protrude in both in sexes (6–7 mm nodule); rectum contains dark green or black meconium; six fontanelles are present. Umbilicus is midway between xiphisternum and symphysis pubis **Center of ossification for upper end of tibia appears** (38–40 weeks) **(Fig. 20.5B)**

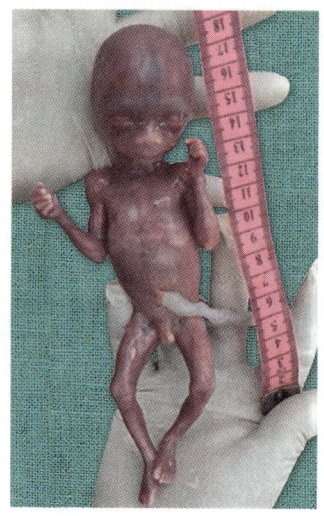

Fig. 20.3: Fetus of 16 weeks of gestation. Sex can be recognized

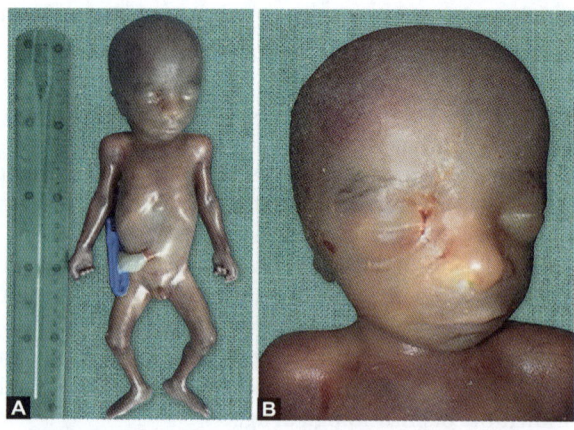

Figs. 20.4A and B: Fetus of 21–22 weeks of gestation. Scalp hair and eyebrows have appeared, eyelashes absent, skin transparent, neck well defined, limbs developed
(*Courtesy:* Dr Rajinder Gulati, SMO, Civil Hospital, Khanna)

CHAPTER 20 : Infanticide and Child Abuse

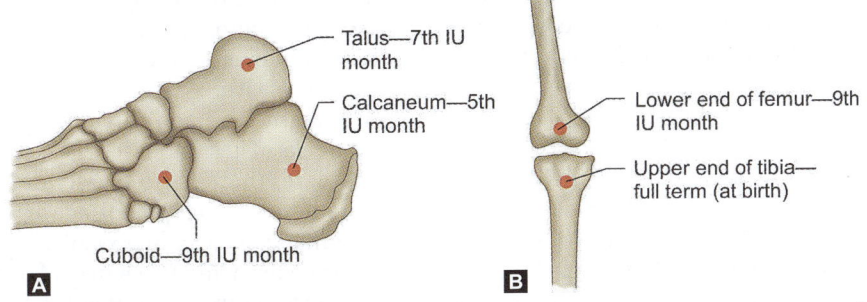

Figs. 20.5A and B: Ossification centers in: (A) Tarsal bones; (B) Lower end of femur and upper end of tibia

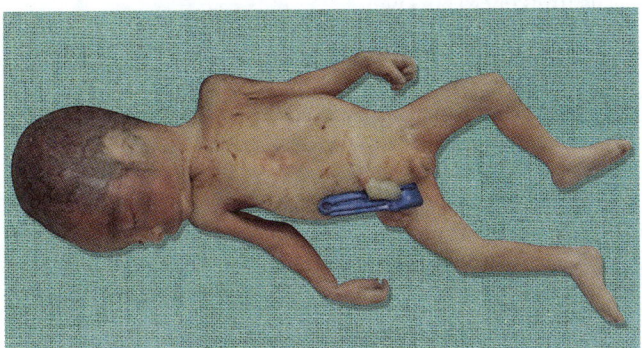

Fig. 20.6: Fetus of 24 weeks of gestation. Scalp hair, eyebrow and eyelashes appeared. Vernix caseosa and lanugo hair can be seen
(*Courtesy:* Dr Rajinder Gulati, Civil Hospital, Khanna)

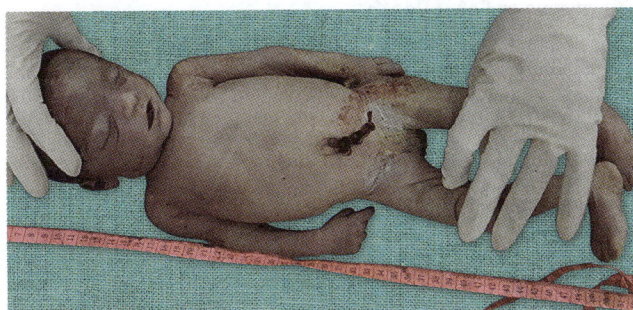

Fig. 20.8: Full term baby: Crown heel length 50 cm, scalp covered with dark hair, circumference of the abdomen greater than head, umbilical cord is dry, shriveled and mummified (tied with cotton thread)

TABLE 20.2: Length/height of infant/child

Age	Length (cm)
At birth	50
6 months	68
1 year	75
4 years	100

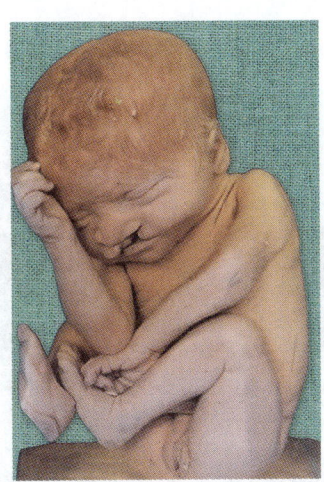

Fig. 20.7: Fetus of 32 weeks of gestation. Scalp hair is thick and non-pigmented; pinna remains folded; skin is not wrinkled, widely separated labia

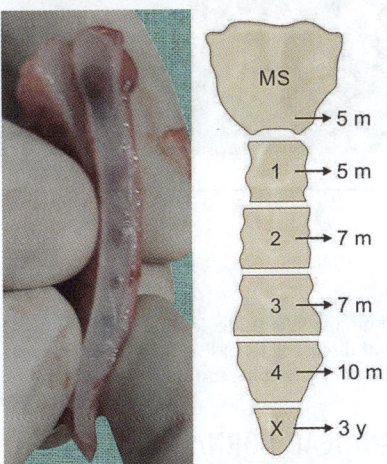

Fig. 20.9: Ossification centers in sternum and gestational age
(MS: Manubrium sternum; X: Xiphisternum)

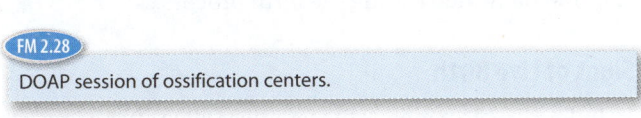

DOAP session of ossification centers.

DEMONSTRATION OF CENTERS OF OSSIFICATION

- **Sternum:** The bone is placed on a wooden board and sectioned in its long axis with a cartilage knife which exposes the centers of ossification **(Fig. 20.9)**.

- **Lower end of the femur and the upper end of tibia:** The leg is flexed against the thigh and a horizontal incision made into the knee joint and the patella is removed. A number of cross-sections are made through the epiphysis starting from the articular surface and continuing until the largest cross-section of the ossification center is reached. In the lower end of the femur, this is seen as brownish-red nucleus which is surrounded by a bluish-white cartilage.

- **Bones of the foot:** The heel of the foot is held by one hand and with the other hand an incision is made through the interspace between the 3rd–4th toes and carried downwards through the sole of the foot and heel.

Diagnosis of Fetal Death

Ultrasonography: On ultrasonography, absence of all fetal movements for 10 minutes (min) is taken as evidence of fetal death.

FM 2.28
Describe and discuss viability of fetus.

VIABILITY OF FETUS/INFANT

Viability of infant: It means physical ability of fetus to lead a separate existence after birth, apart from its mother by virtue of a certain degree of development which depends on biological, physiological and extrinsic factors.

- The age of viability varies among countries with 24 and 28 weeks being cited as the lower limits of potential survival. Fetuses weighing less than 500 g at birth usually do not survive.
- Medically, the age of viability in India is taken as 28 weeks of gestation.
- Till date, there is no legally defined cut-off limit of intrauterine development, age or weight at which a baby automatically becomes viable.
- Any newborn infant, whatever is the length of gestation, can be a victim of infanticide, if born alive.
- A premature baby in a rural area in a developing country is unlikely to survive.

NOTA BENE

- The UK has laid down the limit of 24 weeks of gestation, while the US has enacted 20 weeks for the age of viability regardless of body weight at birth.
- In the UK, a baby is stillborn, if after 24 weeks of gestation it did not at anytime after being completely expelled from its mother, breathe or show any other sign of life. Hence, a period of 24 weeks is fixed for the legal age of viability. However, there is no law or Section of IPC or CrPC in India which stipulates the age of viability.
- In other developed countries, fetal death occurring ≥20 weeks of fetal life or a birth weight of at least 400–500 g is considered as 'stillbirth.'

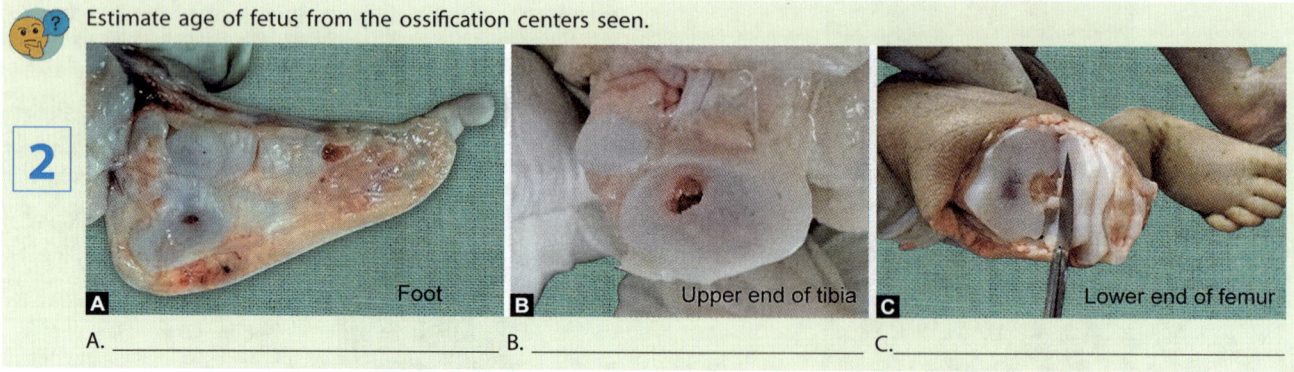

Estimate age of fetus from the ossification centers seen.

A. _____ Foot   B. _____ Upper end of tibia   C. _____ Lower end of femur

FM 2.27, 2.28
- Define and discuss infanticide, feticide and stillbirth.
- Describe and discuss signs of live birth.
- DOAP session of hydrostatic test.

LIVE-BORN/DEAD-BORN/STILLBORN

The question as to whether or not a fetus/infant was born alive is a contentious issue. When decomposition is not present, a variety of features are taken into consideration in attempting to answer this question.

There are essentially three possibilities:
i. the baby was born alive.
ii. the baby died in utero.
iii. the baby died during the birth process.

Signs of Live Birth

In India, live birth means the fetus was alive after complete birth or when at least one part of its body comes out of mother's womb. In the UK, it means the baby should be alive after complete birth.

Any sign of life after complete birth of child is accepted as proof of live birth. Following are considered as **signs of live birth:**
- Baby's cry—strong evidence in favor of live birth and respiration having taken place. Fetus may inhale air and cry when the head is inside the vagina—*vagitus vaginalis*, or inside the uterus—*vagitus uterinus*.
- Muscle twitching/movements of limbs.
- Sneezing and yawning.

POSTMORTEM FINDINGS

Assessment of the case involves determination of viability, and if viability is established, the considerations of factors in the determination of live birth. If determination of live birth is established, then a cause of death is assigned.

External Findings
- General findings.
- Changes in the chest, umbilical cord and skin.
- Caput succedaneum and cephalhematoma.
  i. **General findings:** Presence of clothing and absence of vernix caseosa—suggestive of live birth.
  ii. **Changes in the chest:** Chest is more flat anteroposteriorly in still/dead born. The circumference of the chest is about 2–3 cm less than that of the abdomen at the level of the umbilicus. After respiration, the chest expands and becomes drum-shaped.
  iii. **Changes in umbilical cord:** The appearance of the cut end of the umbilical cord may help to decide whether the birth was one where medical, nursing or midwife, or only amateur person was available. The cut end of the cord should be looked for vital reaction. Even where early putrefaction renders evaluation of breathing impossible, vital signs in the cord may indicate live birth, if survival reached 24–48 h **(Table 20.3)**.
  iv. **Changes in skin:** Vernix caseosa is present in axilla, inguinal region, folds of neck and buttocks. It is either cleaned or gets removed in 1–2 days. Skin of abdomen exfoliates during the first 3 days after birth **(Table 20.4)**.
  v. **Cephalhematoma and caput succedaneum (Diff. 20.1, Figs. 20.10A and B).**

TABLE 20.3: Time since birth by umbilical cord changes

Changes observed	Time since birth
Drying up of cut margin	2 h
Drying up of cord	1 day
Inflammatory line at the base of stump	2 days
Obliteration and mummification changes	3 days
Detach (falls off)	5–6 days
Complete healing (scar)	10–12 days

TABLE 20.4: Changes in skin color

Color of skin	Time since birth
Bright red	Just born
Darker	2–3 days
Brick red → yellow → normal	1 week

DIFFERENTIATION 20.1: Cephalhematoma and caput succedaneum

S.No.	Feature	Cephalhematoma	Caput succedaneum
1.	Definition	Collection of blood in between the periosteum and the skull due to rupture of a small emissary vein from the skull, and may be caused by forceps delivery	Swelling due to stagnation of fluid between the layers of scalp beneath the girdle of contact (dilated cervix or vulval ring)
2.	Situation	Usually unilateral, and present over parietal bone	May be bilateral
3.	Limitation by suture line	Yes	Not limited
4.	Underlying pathology	May be associated with fracture of skull bone	Not pathological
5.	Occurrence	It is never present at birth	It is present at birth
6.	Development and disappearance	Develops 12–24 h after birth and decreases in 6–8 weeks	Disappears spontaneously within 24 h
7.	Medico-legal importance	Regression process help to conclude about the separate existence and how many days the infant survived after birth	Definite evidence of fetus being alive in uterus. But in prolonged labor, the fetus may die before birth

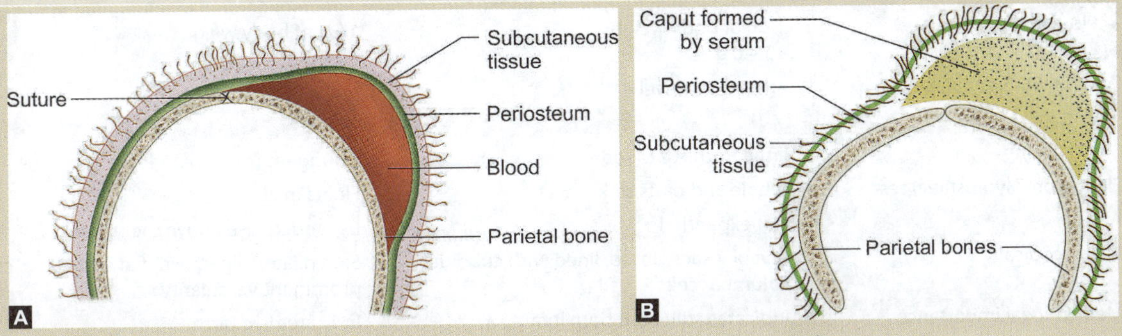

Figs. 20.10A and B: (A) Cephalhematoma; (B) Caput succedaneum

Internal Findings

i. **Changes in the lungs:** They are considered with reference to volume, consistence, color and weight **(Diff. 20.2)**.
   - *Volume:* Before respiration, the lungs lie in the back of the chest on either side of the vertebral column and are hardly seen on opening the chest, as the cavity is filled up by the heart and thymus **(Fig. 20.11)**. After respiration, the lungs occupy the cavity, the medial edges overlapping the mediastinum and part of the pericardium, though not as fully as in the older neonate.
   - **Ear crepitance test:** If on rubbing a small piece of lung gently between the fingers close to ear, no crepitation is heard—*non-crepitant lungs (stillborn)*, and if crepitance is heard—*crepitant lungs (live-born)*.
   - *Surface:* Before respiration, the surface of the lobules is marked with shallow furrows, but without a mottled appearance. On section, it is uniform in texture, being moist and resembling stiff strawberry jelly. After respiration, the air cells are mottled/marbled in appearance with circumscribed rose-colored patches. This is due to the blood vessels being filled with blood, and is characteristic of the lungs that have breathed.
   - *Weight*
     - **Fodere's/Static test:** The blood flow in lung beds increases after breathing, weight becomes double after respiration, but it is not constant.

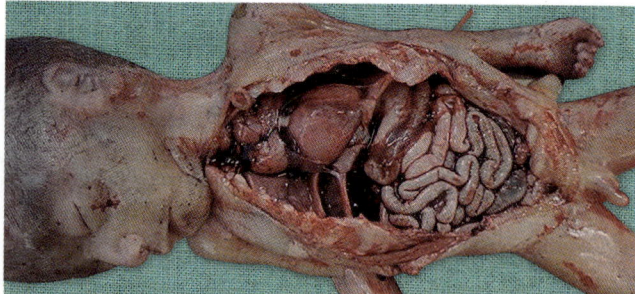

Fig. 20.11: Lungs are collapsed and heart and thymus fills up the thoracic cavity

Weight of the lungs may increase in the stillborn due to:
   a. Edema of lungs.
   b. Congenital pneumonitis.
   c. Inhalation of amniotic fluid.

- **Plocquet's test:** This test helps to demonstrate establishment of respiration. The ratio of the weight of the lungs and the whole body is reduced to half (1/35 of body weight) as compared to the said ratio before respiration (1/70 of body weight).

ii. **Position of the diaphragm:** The arch becomes flattened and depressed, and descends to 6th–7th rib after respiration. The position of the diaphragm may be affected by pressure of the gases of putrefaction.

iii. **Hydrostatic test**
Hydrostatic test is also called **lung floatation test or Raygat's test.***

DIFFERENTIATION 20.2: Unrespired and respired lung (stillborn and live-born)

S.No.	Feature	Unrespired lung	Respired lung
A. Gross			
1.	Color	Uniformly bluish red	Mottled salmon-pink
2.	Volume	Small	Large, covers heart
3.	Thoracic cavity	Not full	Occupies fully
4.	Pleura	Loose, wrinkled	Taut, stretched
5.	Margins	Sharp	Rounded
6.	Surface	Smooth	Uneven
7.	Consistency	Dense, firm, non-crepitant (liver-like)	Soft, spongy, elastic, crepitant
8.	Weight ♦ Ploucquet's test ♦ Fodere's (static) test	 1/70 of body weight 30–40 g	 1/35 of body weight 60–70 g
9.	Position of diaphragm	4th–5th rib level	6th–7th rib level
B. Cut section			
10.	Blood oozing	Little frothless blood	Abundant frothy blood
11.	Floatation (Hydrostatic) test	Whole and parts sink in water	Floats in water
12.	Alveoli	Not expanded	Expanded, rise above the surface
13.	Microscopically	Alveolar sacs closed, lined with cuboidal/columnar cells	Sacs dilated, lined with flat squamous cells with prominent vascularity
14.	Medico-legal importance	Indicates still/dead born infant	Indicates live birth

* Sometimes, this test is referred to as 'Breslau's first life test'.

Principle: It is based on the fact that specific gravity of lung before respiration is 1040–1050 and becomes 940-950 after respiration, which is less than that of water. This makes the respired lung to float.

Procedure: Dissect out the fetal lungs. Put both the lungs (tied at their hilar region) into a trough of water and observe. A small piece of liver serves as control. If the liver floats, the test is of no value.

Inference **(Fig. 20.12)**
- If they sink—unrespired lung.
- If they float—remove them from water, cut into small pieces and then squeeze or compress firmly between sponges (to remove the expiratory reserve volume and tidal air) and again put into water.
- If they sink—unrespired lung.
- If they float—respired lung.

Explanation: Floatation observed for second time is because of *residual air* that remains in the lungs which cannot be squeezed out by pressing, if the fetus has breathed after birth.
- The test is of limited value and it can at best be a suggestive pointer, but never a definitive test in itself.
- The slightest degree of putrefaction immediately negates any interpretation of this test. In such cases, the lungs will float in water, but so are the solid organs, such as the liver.
- However, assuming body is fresh, the floating of lungs and heart *en bloc* increases the sensitivity of the test.

Fallacies
- False positive is seen in accumulation of putrefying gases or artificial inflation (by intubation and forced air insufflation expanding the lungs with air after delivery).
- False negative is seen in atelectasis (non-expansion of lungs), obstruction by alveolar duct membrane, edema, feeble respiration, pneumonia and congenital syphilis.

Pearls

Hydrostatic test is not necessary if
i. Fetus shows congenital anomaly, like anencephaly.
ii. Fetus is macerated or mummified.
iii. Umbilical cord has separated and a scar has formed.
iv. Stomach contains milk **(Fig. 20.13)**.
v. Bruises on lungs indicating efforts to artificially respirate the child.
vi. Fetus is born before 180 days of gestation.*

iv. **Histology**
- Unrespired lung looks like the parotid gland with closed alveolar sacs lined with cuboidal/columnar cells, and less vascularity.
- Respired lung cells get flattened with dilatation—pavement (squamous) epithelium with increased vascularization.

v. **Changes in middle ear (Wreden's test):** Absence of gelatinous embryonic connective tissue which was present during fetal life and presence of air in middle ear is seen after live birth. It is also called *Wreden-Wendt tympanic cavity or middle ear test.*

vi. **Changes in stomach and intestines:** Live born infant swallows air into the stomach during respiration, and if present in small intestine it further confirms live birth. But air may be present in the stomach after decomposition, or in the stillborn attempting to free the air passages of fluid obstruction.

Demonstration: The stomach and intestines are removed after tying double ligatures at each end. They are kept under water and incision is given between the ligatures. Air bubbles will come out, if respiration has taken place—**Breslau's second life test or stomach bowel test**.

If milk is present in the stomach, it is a positive evidence of live birth **(Fig. 20.13)**.

vii. **Meconium:** In case of live birth, the large intestine is completely free of meconium within 24 h after birth,

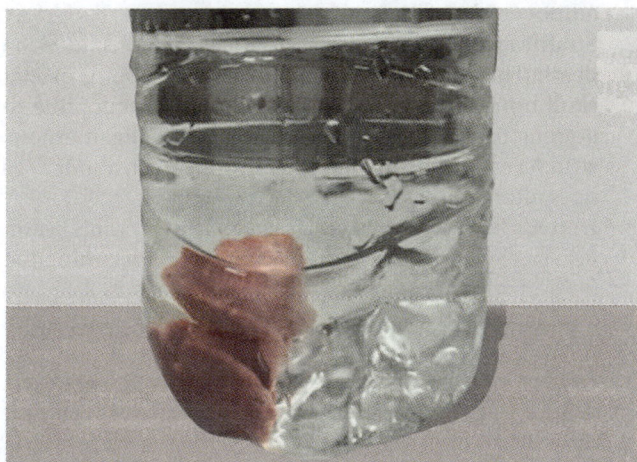

Fig. 20.12: Negative hydrostatic test: Sinking fetal lungs

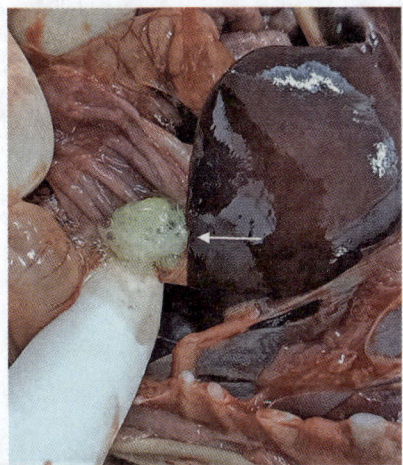

Fig. 20.13: Milk in stomach in a newborn infant (arrow)

---
* Not a criteria in India, since there is no legally defined cut-off limit of viability.

but in stillbirths it will be present in the intestine. In case of breech presentation and hypoxia, meconium may be completely expelled before birth, and thus may be absent even in such stillborn fetuses.

viii. **Changes in the blood vessels:** Umbilical arteries are obliterated within 12 h to 3 days. Obliteration of umbilical vein and ductus venosus is complete by 4th day. The ductus arteriosus obliterates in about 10 days.

ix. **Changes in heart:** Closure of foramen ovale occurs by 2–3 months after birth. In few cases, the foramen may not completely close.

x. **Changes in the blood:** Nucleated RBCs are absent in peripheral circulation within 24 h after live birth. Fetal hemoglobin may be present in the blood up to 6 months or more.

xi. **Incremental line in enamel of teeth:** Neonatal incremental line in the enamel of the teeth is formed at birth which is one of the surest sign of live birth.

xii. **Ossification centers:** Presence of ossification centers at the lower end of radius, heads of humerus and femur and capitulum of humerus may also be taken as signs of separate existence for few months.

xiii. **Closure of fontanelle:** Closure of different fontanelle occurs at different periods after birth. Closure of posterior fontanelle may occur at birth.

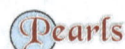

Possible determinants of live birth
a. Gestational age compatible with life (viability)
b. No signs of maceration
c. No determinable reason for intrapartum death
d. Air in lungs, middle ear, stomach or GIT
e. Food in the stomach or extrauterine materials
f. Inflation of the lungs—grossly or microscopically
g. Positive hydrostatic test with no signs of putrefaction
h. Positive ear crepitance test
i. Vital reaction of umbilical cord

 A 19-year-old woman was admitted following a suicidal attempt with allegation of killing her newborn baby by smothering, this occurred 2 days after birth. She denied the same and told the police that she had given birth to a premature baby who died subsequently. Can you comment on its viability?

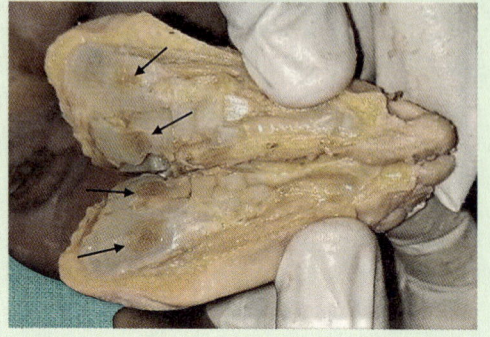

FM 2.28 Describe and discuss signs of intrauterine death.

SIGNS OF DEAD-BORN FETUS

In our Indian text of Forensic Medicine, the term "dead born" is used to indicate that the fetus has died in utero. But in Western textbooks, the term "stillborn" is used, whether the infant has died in the process of delivery or already dead in the uterus.

1. **Maceration:** It is a process of aseptic autolysis. This occurs when the dead child remains in the uterus for about 3–4 days surrounded with liquor amnii with exclusion of air.
   - *Earliest sign of maceration is skin slippage* of face, back or abdomen, and may be seen in 12 h after death in utero. By 24 h, skin is brown or purplish in color **(Fig. 20.14A)**.
   - The dead fetus is soft, flaccid with emission of sweetish disagreeable smell, but no gases are formed.
   - Internal organs show autolytic decomposition, but the lungs and uterus remain unchanged for a long time.
   - Cranial compression is seen in >36 h, desquamation over 75% of body surface is seen in 72 h, overlapping of cranial sutures in >96 h and the mouth is widely open in >1 week.
   - A rough index indicating the degree of autolysis should be given in context of the postmortem examination: mild (skin sloughing only), moderate (skin sloughing and organ softening) and marked (skin sloughing, organ softening and joint laxity) maceration.

   Putrefaction is characterized by an unpleasant odor, greenish discoloration of skin and formation of foul smelling gases **(Fig. 20.14B)**. Rarely, the fetus may show adipocere formation.

2. **Spalding's sign:** A pathogonomic sign of intrauterine death. There is loss of alignment and overlapping of fetal skull bones on X-ray/ultrasonography, occurs due to liquefaction of cerebrum and softening of ligamentous structures supporting the vault. It appears in about 7–10 days after death.

3. **Deuel's halo sign:*** A halo is seen around cranial vault due to elevation of pericranial fat by the accumulated fluid in subaponeurotic space. It develops in 2–3 days after fetal death. This sign can be seen on USG scan and X-ray, but not a reliable sign.

4. **Robert's sign:** Appearance of gas shadow in chambers of heart and great vessels, may appear by 12 h, but difficult to interpret.

5. **Ball sign:** Hyperflexion of spine is more common.

6. **Helix sign:** Presence of gas in two umbilical arteries which forms double or single helix.

---
* Halo sign is also a test done to determine whether the bloody discharge from the ears and nose contains CSF in head injury patients.

CHAPTER 20 : Infanticide and Child Abuse

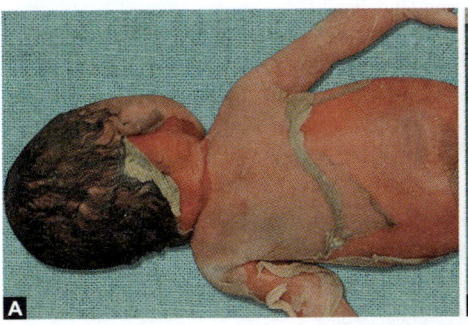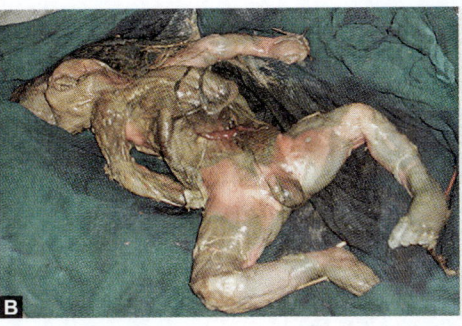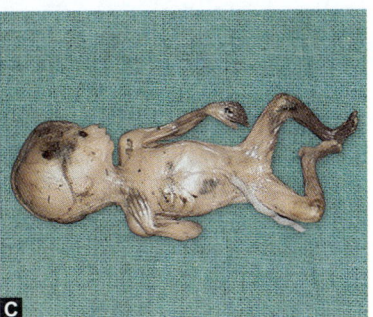

Figs. 20.14A to C: (A) Maceration; (B) Putrefaction; (C) Mummification

7. **Crowding of the ribs shadow** with loss of normal parallelism.
8. **Rigor mortis:** It may be seen in dead-born fetus.
9. **Mummification:** It results from deficient supply of blood or scanty liquor amnii. Fetus is dried up and shriveled in ≥2 weeks **(Fig. 20.14C)**.

♦ Cardinal signs to identify a dead born fetus are the presence of maceration, red-brown discoloration (normally yellow-tan color) of the umbilical cord stump along with lack of lung aeration ('primary atelectasis').
♦ The earliest reliable histological feature of fetal death is the loss of nuclear basophilia in renal cortical tubular cells.

 A 25-year-old, primigravida woman with a history of 32 weeks gestation presented with complaints of lower abdominal pain and pedal edema for two weeks. USG image was done. What is your diagnosis?

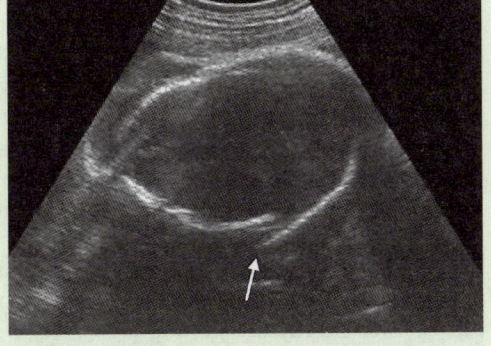

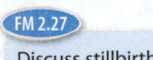
Discuss stillbirth.

SIGNS OF STILLBORN FETUS

Another possibility for deaths occurring in infants whose births are unattended or complicated is that the fetus/infant died during the birth process. It includes stillborn whose death occurs while the mother is undergoing monitoring in labor.

♦ The findings which suggest that a death is an intrapartum death are lack of maceration and lack of lung aeration.
♦ The difference between stillborn and dead-born fetus is given in **Diff. 20.3**.
♦ In most instances, it is not possible by autopsy alone to differentiate these cases from deaths that occur prior to birth but have not yet developed maceration or from deaths that occur after birth where there is little or no aeration of the lungs.
♦ When a precipitate birth occurs, air can enter the lungs, via the chest compression followed by rapid chest expansion that occurs during passage through the birth canal, even if the infant does not actively inhale.
♦ **Iatrogenic deaths** may result from improper body positioning of the mother, use of medications (such as epidurals), use of various maneuvers, instrumentation, and surgical interventions which can result in prolongation of the labor and birth process. Prolongation of labor might contribute to birth asphyxia.

DIFFERENTIATION 20.3: Stillborn and dead-born fetus

S.No.	Feature	Stillborn fetus	Dead-born fetus
1.	Gestational age	Fetus is born after 28 weeks of pregnancy	Any duration
2.	Condition in utero	Fetus was alive in utero, but dies during the process of delivery	Dead in utero
3.	Predominance	Seen mostly among illegitimate and immature male children in primiparae	No such predominance
4.	Findings	Signs of prolonged labor, like edema, bleeding into scalp, caput succedaneum and severe molding of head may be seen	Maceration Spalding's sign Robert's sign Rigor mortis at delivery Mummification
5.	Cause	Asphyxia, prematurity, infections, birth trauma or toxemia	Congenital anomaly, ABO and Rh incompatibility

SECTION 1: Jurisprudence and Forensic Medicine

> **NOTA BENE**
> - Evidence of acute asphyxia at autopsy includes thymic, pleural and epicardial petechiae with intra-alveolar hemorrhage, interstitial hemorrhage, and meconium, blood, liquor amnii, vernix caseosa and shed fetal skin (squames) in the bronchial tubes. Typical **"starry sky" pattern** with loss of cortical lymphocytes are seen in thymus in stress of short duration.
> - The law in the US and the UK presumes that every newborn child found dead was born dead, until the contrary is proved. When a woman is charged with infanticide, the burden of proof is upon the prosecution to demonstrate that the child had a separate existence. Unless the autopsy surgeon has absolute reasons to document postnatal survival, e.g., well-expanded lungs or food in the stomach, he is legally bound not to diagnose live birth.

A dead body of newborn was brought by the police found dumped in the garbage collecting box. Can you opine whether the infant was live-born or stillborn by external observations? Give reasons.

5

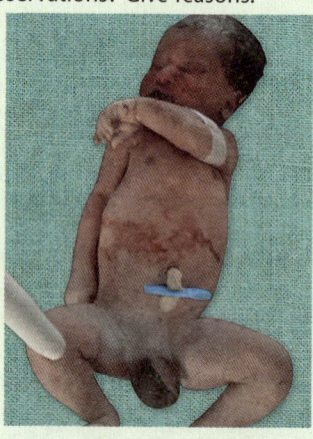

Identify the condition seen immediately after delivery. Give reasons.

6

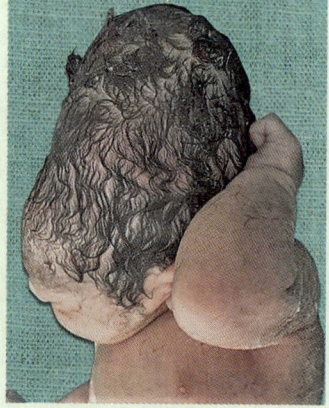

(*Courtesy:* Dr Deepak Bhat, DMCH, Ludhiana)

FM 3.19
Discuss precipitate labor.

INFANT DEATH (FLOWCHART 20.1)

Natural Causes

- Prematurity
- Congenital malformation
- Birth trauma
- Intrapartum asphyxia
- Neonatal infection
- ABO and Rh-incompatibility
- Post-maturity
- Early separation of placenta
- Preeclamptic toxemia
- Sudden infant death syndrome (SIDS)

Some common causes are:

- **Immaturity:** A prematurely born child generally dies immediately after birth. In the case of the premature birth of a child, the question may arise as to whether the birth was criminally induced or not, for under the IPC, the criminal induction of premature labor is an offense.
- **Debility:** Due to lack of general development, even a full term child may die after birth from debility. In these cases, no disease, except atelectasis of some portions of the lungs due to feeble respiration is detected.
- **Congenital diseases and malformations:** Syphilis and some fevers may cause death from the toxemic condition. Of the diseases of the internal organs, pulmonary infections and hyaline membrane of the lungs are seen. Certain conditions such as anencephaly, spina bifida and congenital diaphragmatic hernia are readily identifiable, although subtle cardiovascular or metabolic abnormalities may be difficult to diagnose **(Figs. 20.15A to D)**. It is however, unsafe to assume that actual live birth could not have taken place. Moreover, monstrosity or malformation is no justification for taking the life of an infant.
- **Spasm of the larynx** may occur from mucus or meconium being aspirated into the larynx, or from the enlargement of thymus gland.

Flowchart 20.1: Causes of infant death

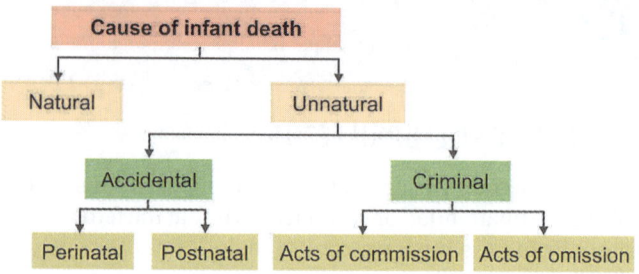

- **Erythroblastosis fetalis** due to iso-immunization, when an Rh-negative woman is carrying an Rh-positive fetus may result in death of the fetus **(Fig. 20.15E)**.
- **Birth asphyxia** can occur in preeclampsia/eclampsia, placenta abruption, cephalopelvic disproportion and shoulder dystocia. Evidence of asphyxia at autopsy includes thymic, pleural and epicardial petechiae with intra-alveolar hemorrhage, and meconium on the skin, and shed fetal skin within distal air passages.

Unnatural Causes

I. Accidental causes

Perinatal

i. **Injuries to the mother:** It may cause premature separation of the placenta or injury to the fetus (concussion of brain/fracture/rupture of blood vessels) and lead to death of the baby.
ii. **Prolonged labor:** It causes death of the fetus due to injury to the brain because of compression of the head or due to asphyxia.
iii. **Prolapsed cord or pressure on cord:** It may cause stoppage of fetal circulation during birth, and death of the newborn may occur during or just after birth.
iv. **Twisting of cord around the neck or knots of the cord:** It causes death of the fetus during birth or immediately after birth from asphyxia due to strangulation **(Fig. 20.15F)**.
v. **Death of the mother:** When the mother dies during the delivery, the question arises as to how long a child may live in utero after her death. The time depends upon the cause of the mother's death. If death occurs slowly from hemorrhage, there is little chance of saving the child, but it may be saved if an attempt is made to extract it within 25 min after sudden death from accident of the previously healthy mother.

Postnatal

i. **Suffocation:** Due to non-availability of nursing care, the neonate may die due to smothering or choking as a result of inhalation of amniotic fluid or blood immediately after birth.
ii. **Precipitate labor** (in this condition, all the three stages of labor occur in very quick succession so that delivery occurs suddenly, commonly seen in multipara): It may cause death of the newborn due to head injury **(Diff. 20.4)**, suffocation or drowning, or occasionally

DIFFERENTIATION 20.4: Head injury due to precipitate labor and blunt force

S.No.	Feature	Precipitate labor	Blunt force
1.	Contusion	Present on presenting part of scalp	Present anywhere on the scalp
2.	Laceration	Absent	May be present
3.	Fracture	Fissured fracture involving the parietal bones	Comminuted/depressed fracture, may involve all the bones
4.	Brain	Usually not injured	Contusions, lacerations and hemorrhage may be seen

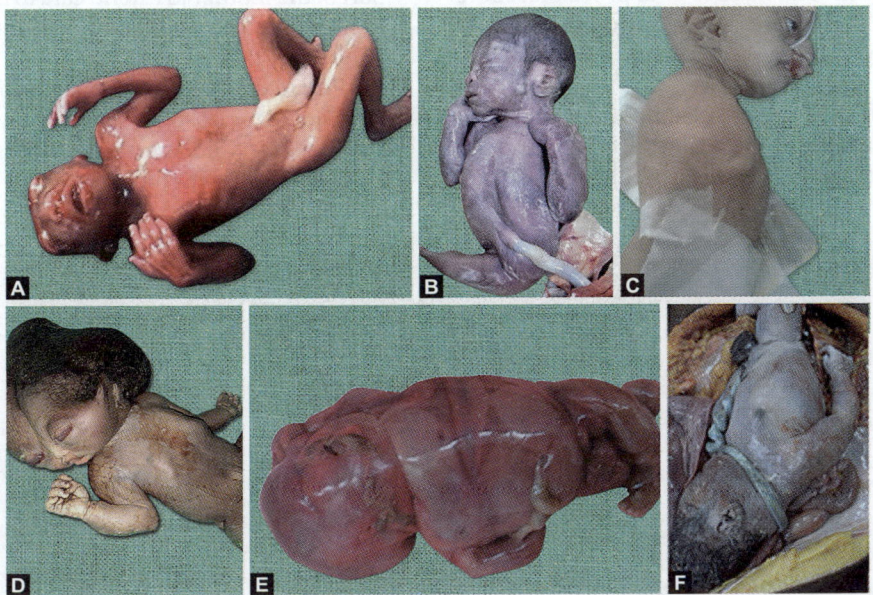

Figs. 20.15A to F: Natural and accidental causes of fetal/infant death: (A) Anencephaly (18 weeks of gestation); (B) Sirenomelia (mermaid syndrome); (C) Cleft lip and palate with amelia; (D) Hydrocephalus (full term IUD); (E) Non-immune hydrops fetalis; (F) Cord around neck

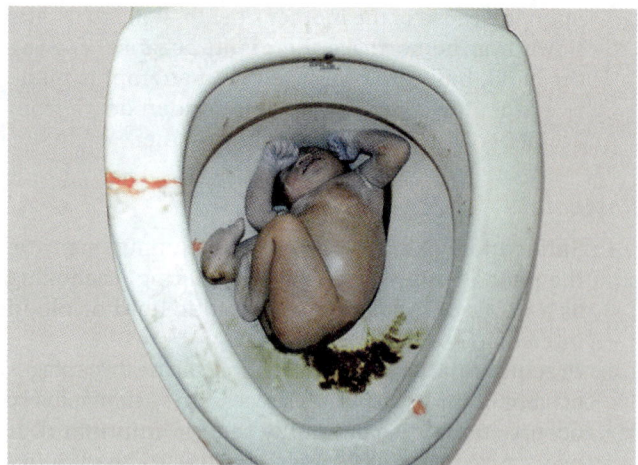

Fig. 20.16: Fetal death due to precipitate labor

due to bleeding from torn end of attached umbilical cord **(Fig. 20.16)**.

Medico-legal aspects
- Death of the newborn due to precipitate labor may be taken as a case of deliberate infanticide.
- The mother may claim infanticide (negligence on part of the doctor), but death of the newborn is due to precipitate labor.

II. Criminal causes

Where the autopsy surgeon proves separate existence and live birth, he has an additional burden to document that death occurred from an act of commission or omission. The 'willful' aspect is a matter for the prosecution, but it is for the autopsy surgeon to demonstrate fatal injuries or to prove that some lack of care led to the death which is often an impossible task.

a. **Acts of commission:** These acts are done positively to cause death of infant.
   i. **Strangulation** by a ligature material or the umbilical cord (to simulate natural twisting of cord round the neck) or by throttling **(Figs. 20.17A and B)**.
   ii. **Poisoning:** Earlier, opium was used for the purpose (*ideal infanticidal poison*). Nowadays, acids and insecticides are used.
   iii. **Smothering** the baby to death with the help of hand or clothes.
   iv. **Head injury:** The head of the fetus may be struck against a wall or on the floor by holding its legs, this may leave an impression on the legs also.
   v. **Concealed punctured wound** may be caused by a nail or a needle through the fontanelle, nape of the neck or inner canthus of eye.
   vi. **Twisting the neck:** Death occurs due fracture dislocation of the cervical vertebrae and injury to the medulla.
   vii. **Burning** the newborn alive or disposing the living newborn inside an oven.
   viii. **Drowning** which also serves the purpose of disposal of the unwanted child **(Fig. 20.17C)**.
   ix. **Cut throat injury.**

- Deaths are mostly due to airway obstruction from smothering or strangulation.
- **Injuries:** Strangulation marks around the neck with bruising from hands, or parchmented abrasions from ligatures that may have been left in situ **(Figs. 20.17A and B)**; bruising with subgaleal, extradural and subdural hemorrhages, skull fractures and cerebral lacerations, and contusions from blows to the head with blunt objects may be seen.
- Drowning and smothering may leave minimal findings.

b. **Act of omission or neglect:** Intentional failure on the part of the mother to extend care to the newborn leading to its death; this may amount to infanticide. It may be failure to:
   - Provide proper assistance during labor.
   - Clear air passages which may be obstructed by amniotic fluid/mucus.
   - Tie the cord after it is cut.

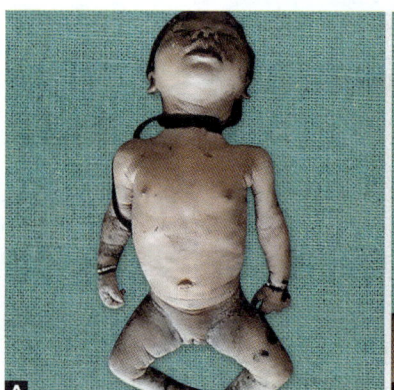 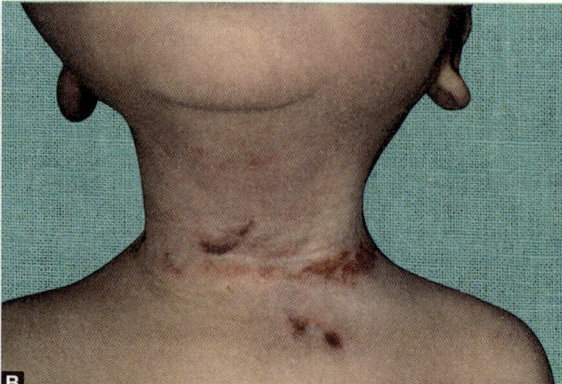 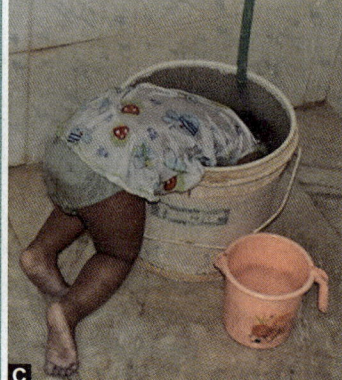

Figs. 20.17A and C: (A) Ligature strangulation; (B) Throttling with ligature mark; (C) Homicidal drowning
[*Courtesy:* (B) Sandeep Haridas, Swami Ramanand Teerth Rural GMCH, Maharashtra]

- Protect the child from exposure to heat/cold. Failure to adequately clothe or place the infant in a warm environment may result in fatal hypothermia.
- Supply the child with proper food.

Abandoning of Children

Sec. 317 IPC deals with abandoning by the father or mother of the child under the age of 12 years with imprisonment up to 7 years with/without fine.

Concealment of Birth by Secret Disposal of Dead Body

Any person who secretly buries or disposes of the dead body of a child and intentionally conceals the birth of such child is punished with imprisonment of 2 years with/without fine **(Sec. 318 IPC)**. It does not matter whether the child died before or after or during its birth. In a case where infanticide is not proved, the person is usually charged under this section.

> **FM 3.29**
> Describe and discuss battered baby syndrome and child abuse.

■ BATTERED BABY SYNDROME

Definition: A battered child is one who has received repetitive physical injuries as a result of non-accidental violence produced by a parent or a guardian.
- It is also called *Caffey syndrome, Caffey-Kempe syndrome,* or *maltreatment syndrome*—one of the important and usual missed causes of pediatric traumas.

Features

Related to the Child
i. **Age:** The majority is below 3 years of age.
ii. **Sex:** More common with male child (M:F ratio 2:1).
iii. **Status of the child:** Usually, illegitimate and unwanted child—pregnancy before marriage or failure of contraception.
iv. **Position in family:** Commonly, the eldest or the youngest. The child may be a mentally subnormal one.

Related to the parent/guardian
i. **Marital status:** Unmarried couple, commonly seen in some Western societies.
ii. **Age of parents:** Usually, the parents are young.
iii. **Educational status:** Lower level of education.
iv. **Addiction:** Reckless lifestyle, often indulging in drugs.
v. **Childhood history:** Often the parents themselves were the victims of battering during their childhood.
vi. **Psychological factors:** Low tolerance threshold, impulsive nature, aggressive personality and imbalanced temperament.

Socio-familial Factors
i. Low social background.
ii. Lack of equality between members of the family with lack of family harmony.
iii. Long-standing emotional problem.
iv. Financial hardship.
v. Trouble at the place of work.

Precipitating Factors
i. Act of disobedience by the child.
ii. Frequent crying may create annoyance.
iii. Refusal to take food.
iv. Soiling of napkin or bedclothes.
v. At times, any trifle act of the child may annoy the mentally challenged father or mother.

Features Arising Suspicion of Abuse

- Parents give vague history of accident to be the cause of the injuries like fall from stairs or cot, which does not appear consistent with the type of injuries or time narrated by the parents **(Fig. 20.18)**. Often the parents' gives a history of tendency of the child to bruise easily.
- The parents of the child seek medical aid rather late or when the condition of the children becomes serious.
- Often injuries in different stages of healing are found in the child.
- In many cases, the parents later admit to have assaulted their children, but 'only mildly' for punishment.

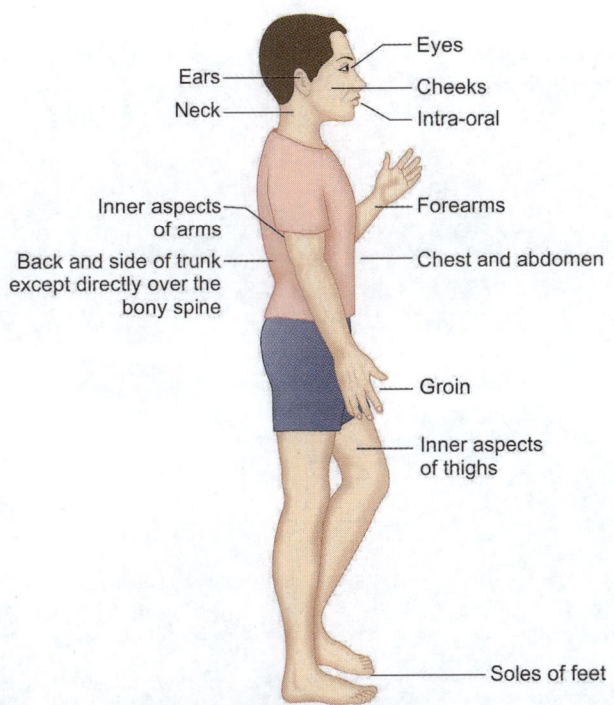

Fig. 20.18: Sites of non-accidental injury

> **NOTA BENE**
>
> *Accidental injuries* typically involve bony prominences [head (forehead, occipital or parietal region), nose, chin, palm, elbows, knees and shin], match the history given by the parents and are keeping with the development of the child.

Injuries

The injuries may be caused by hand, foot, teeth, stick, belt, shoe, hot water, lighted cigarette, hot frying pan or any household article.

i. **Surface injuries:** Bruises, abrasions and lacerations may be seen. Laceration of the oral mucosa along with labial frenulum of the lower lip is a characteristic lesion. Slap marks, lash mark, knuckle punches, pinch mark [*butterfly-shaped bruise* with one wing (caused by thumb) larger than other], bald patches on scalp due to pulling out the hair (*traumatic alopecia*) may be seen **(Figs. 20.19A to C)**.

ii. **CNS:** Injuries are inflicted by throwing the child, striking the child with fist or object or against a wall, dropping the child or vigorous shaking of the infant (**shaken baby syndrome or infantile whiplash syndrome**) leading to intracranial hemorrhage **(Fig. 20.20)**.
   - A strong suspicion of child abuse should be made in a child presenting with altered mental status, unresponsiveness, coma, convulsions or with focal neurologic deficit.
   - Shaken baby syndrome can occur from as little as 5 seconds of shaking.
   - The *triad of injuries* includes encephalopathy, retinal hemorrhages and SDH **(Figs. 20.19D)**. SDH is the most consistent component of the triad and may be the first clinical sign identified on CT scan. Additional traumatic injuries of the cord, brainstem and even skull may be produced **(Fig. 20.19E)**.

iii. **Eyes:** Retinal hemorrhages and lens displacement may be seen.

iv. **Visceral injuries:** Injury to spleen, liver or hollow viscera can occur resulting in massive hemorrhage, shock and death of the child.

v. **Burns:** Small circular pitted burns may indicate deliberate stubbing of cigarette ends on skin. Scalds are also common.

vi. **Skeletal injuries:** Bony injuries include transverse fractures, impacted fractures, spiral fractures, metaphyseal chip fractures, subperiosteal hematoma, and multiple deformities of the long bones and rib cage of the body due to multiple healed fractures and callus formation.
   - Fractures of long bones, ribs, skull and vertebral bodies are highly suggestive of abuse.
   - Anteroposterior compression of chest causes fractures in midaxillary line **(Fig. 20.20)**.

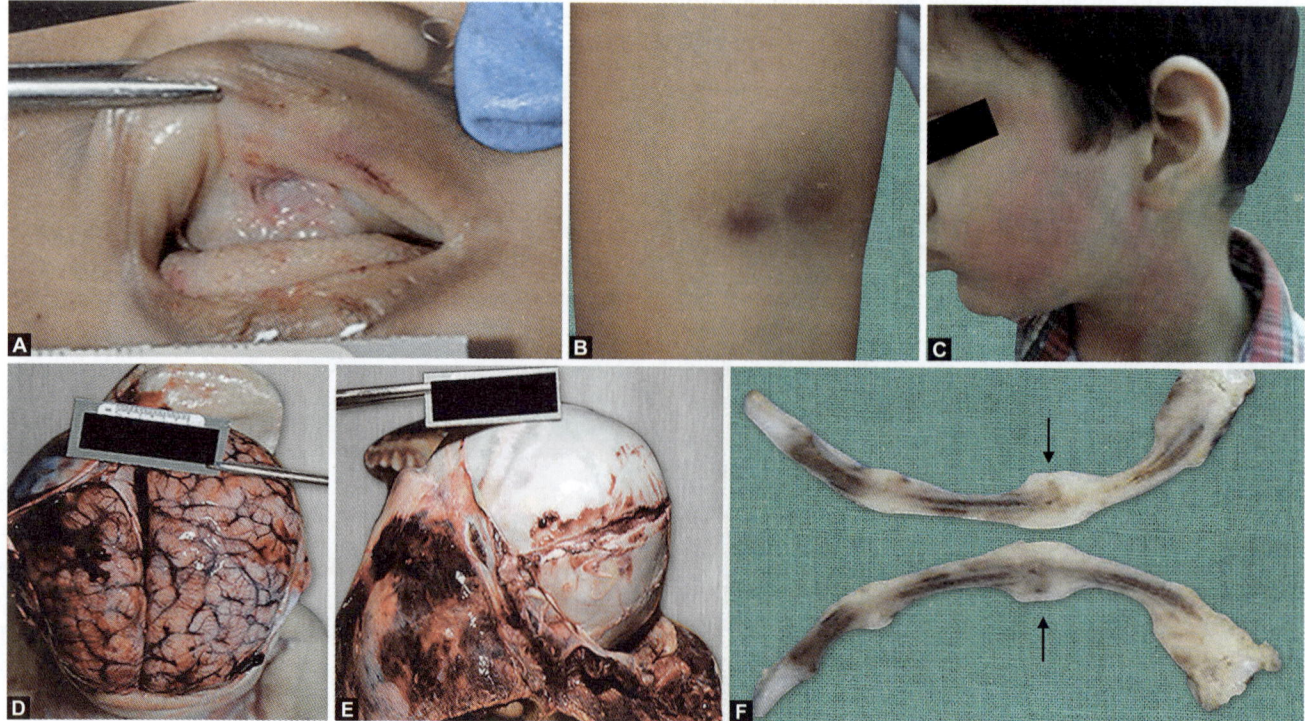

Figs. 20.19A to F: External and internal injuries in battered baby syndrome: (A) Torn frenulum and bruising; (B) Pinch mark; (C) Slap mark; (D) Subdural hematoma; (E) Subgaleal hematoma with linear fracture of skull; (F) Knob fractures of ribs (arrows)

CHILD ABUSE

Child abuse can be defined as causing or permitting of any harmful or offensive contact to a child's body and/or any communication or transaction which humiliates, shames, or frightens a child.

Major Types of Abuse

i. Physical abuse
ii. Sexual abuse
iii. Emotional abuse
iv. Neglect

i. *Physical abuse* of children includes any non-accidental physical injury caused by the child's caretaker. It can be beating or battering of a child, and has been described above.
ii. *Sexual abuse* refers to inappropriate sexual behavior with a child. It includes fondling a child's genitals, making the child fondle the adult's genitals, intercourse, incest, rape, sodomy, exhibitionism, indecent exposure and commercial exploitation through prostitution or the production of pornographic materials.
iii. *Emotional abuse (verbal/mental abuse or psychological maltreatment):* Acts of commission and omission which can be potentially damaging psychologically. This can include parents/caretakers using extreme and/or bizarre forms of punishment, such as confinement in a closet or dark room or being tied to a chair for long periods.
iv. *Neglect* is the failure to provide for the child's basic needs. Neglect can be physical, educational or emotional. In general, neglect is an act of omission.

Differential diagnosis of childhood fractures should be made from the several 'brittle bone diseases' that can cause abnormal skeletal fragility—congenital syphilis, rickets, scurvy, leukemia, osteogenesis imperfecta, copper deficiency, Menke's syndrome, infantile cortical hyperostosis (Caffey's disease) and juvenile osteoporosis.

It can be defense in a criminal trial of alleged child abuse on the grounds that such fractures can be observed within normal parental handling or spontaneous movements of the child.

Reporting of suspected child abuse: It is mandatory to report any suspected child abuse case in the US, Argentina, Finland, Israel, Korea and Spain. In other countries such as Croatia, Japan, Netherlands and Romania reporting is voluntary.

- In India, it is mandatory to report to the police about sexual abuse under the Protection of Children from Sexual Offenses Act (POCSO), 2012.
- In order to protect the child, the diagnosis of child abuse must be reported irrespective of the context of such battery. The confidentiality of the physician patient

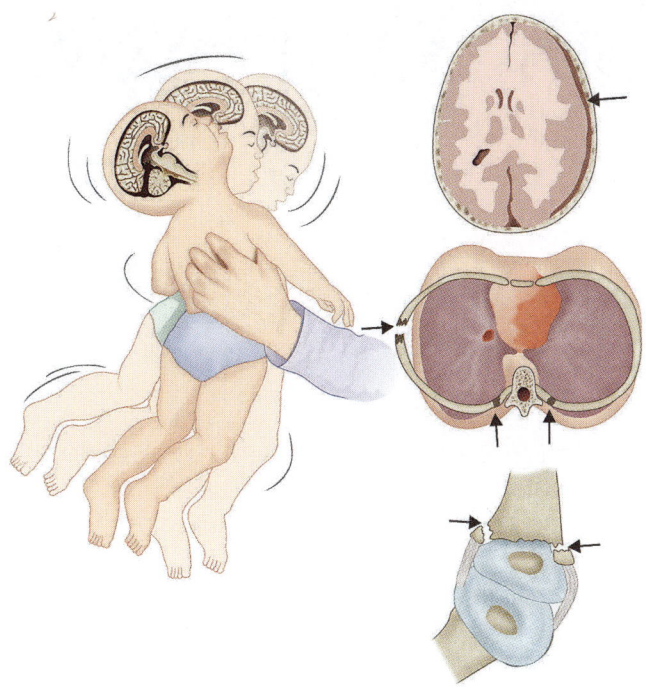

Fig. 20.20: Shaken infant syndrome: Internal injuries (arrows)

- Multiple rib fractures also occur along posterior angle of ribs on side-to-side squeezing **(Fig. 20.20)**. The fractured ribs heal by callus formation in 1–2 weeks, giving characteristic appearance of a knob (*knob fractures*) **(Fig. 20.19F)**, and on X-ray '*string of beads*' appearance is seen in paravertebral gutter.
- In whiplash movement of arms and legs, typical '*corner*' or '*bucket-handle*' *fractures* in the metaphyseal region may be seen **(Fig. 20.20)**.

vii. **CVS:** Blunt trauma to chest may cause multiple rib fractures leading to lung and heart contusions, pneumothorax, hemothorax, rupture of diaphragm and cardiac tamponade.
viii. **Genitourinary system:** Physical and sexual abuse should be considered in a child presenting with hematuria, dysuria, increased frequency of urination and enuresis.

Diagnosis

i. Nature of injuries.
ii. Delay in seeking medical treatment.
iii. Recurrent injuries.
iv. Radiological manifestations, especially those involving the ribs, metaphyseal-epiphyseal injuries, and avulsive fractures of the clavicle and acromium process.

Cause of death: Head injury with or without skull fracture is the leading cause of death in child abuse followed by rupture of an abdominal viscus.

relationship no longer holds in cases of abuse and cruelty to child.

> **NOTA BENE**
>
> **Shaken baby syndrome:** Infants are susceptible to subdural/subarachnoid hematoma and retinal hemorrhages due to vigorous shaking of the baby as a method of punishment.
> - *Predisposing factors:* Infant's relatively large head, weak neck muscles and delicate subarachnoid bridging vessels.
> - *Signs and symptoms:* Seizures, irritability, meningismus and focal or general neurologic deficit.
> - *Diagnosis:* Confirmation by CT/MRI scan, bloody spinal or subdural fluid and normal skull X-rays. β-amyloid precursor protein immunohistochemical staining is used to detect axonal injuries.

Describe and discuss Sudden Infant Death syndrome and Munchausen's syndrome by proxy.

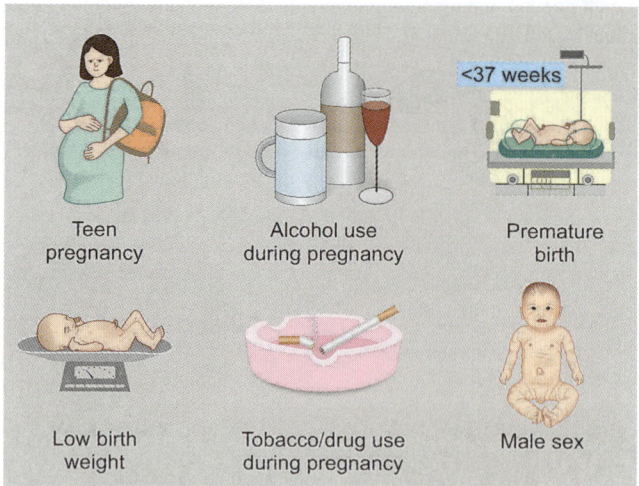

Fig. 20.21: Predisposing factors for SIDS

SUDDEN INFANT DEATH SYNDROME (SIDS)

Definition: Sudden and unexpected death of seemingly healthy infant (usually <12 months) whose death remains unexplained even after complete autopsy.
- It is also called *cot death or crib death.*
- SIDS is an autopsy diagnosis, and not a clinical or emergency department diagnosis.
- It is more accurate to use "Sudden Unexpected Infant Death (SUID)" if there is no external evidence of injury to the infant and no scene information to suggest another cause of death.
- After a thorough case investigation, some of these SUIDs may be due to poisoning, metabolic disorders, hyper- or hypothermia, child abuse and neglect resulting in homicide and suffocation (but much less common).

Features and Risks Factors (Fig. 20.21)

i. **Incidence:** 0.2–0.4% of all live births.
ii. **Geographical distribution:** Worldwide.
iii. **Age:** Between 2 weeks to 2 years. Mid infancy is the most vulnerable age (peak 2–4 months).
iv. **Sex:** Male infants have a proportionately higher death rate (M:F ratio 3:2).
v. **Socio-economic status:** Low and middle class family with poor housing condition, large family and lack of health consciousness.
vi. **Time of death:** In most cases, the infant is discovered dead either in the early morning (death possibly occurring at late night) or sometime after first feed in the morning.
vii. **Season:** In most occasions, deaths are seen to occur commonly in rainy and winter seasons in temperate zones, but no clear pattern in tropical zones.
viii. **Twins:** More among twins (two-fold) as opposed to singletons. Prematurity and low birth weights which are often present in twins increases the risk of SIDS.
ix. **Addiction:** Smoking (pre-or postnatal) and drug abuse by pregnant women increases risk.

Cause

No definite cause is known.
i. **Prolonged sleep apnea** is presently accepted as the most acceptable of the suggested causes. A periodic failure to breath during sleep makes them susceptible to hypoxia. Hypoxic state may be promoted by many allied factors, e.g., some infective condition of the respiratory tract.
ii. **Respiratory infection** may cause viremia which leads to sleep depression of respiratory center and death.
iii. **Nasal edema and mucus secretion** may narrow upper respiratory passages, a flaccid pharynx and neck posture may reduce airway.
iv. Local **hypersensitivity of the respiratory tract** lumen to cow's milk was thought to cause laryngeal spasm.
v. **Bedclothes and pillow falling accidentally** over the nose and mouth by the movement of the child.
vi. **Overlying** of the baby by a sleeping or intoxicated mother. Infants placed to sleep prone or on their side increases the risk of SIDS.
vii. **Miscellaneous causes:** Conduction system anomalies; hypoparathyroidism; deficiency of selenium, antibodies, calcium, magnesium and vitamins B, C, D and E; house-mite allergy; sodium overload in feeds and hypothermia.

There is an increased risk of SIDS, as well as other causes of death in families that have one SIDS death.

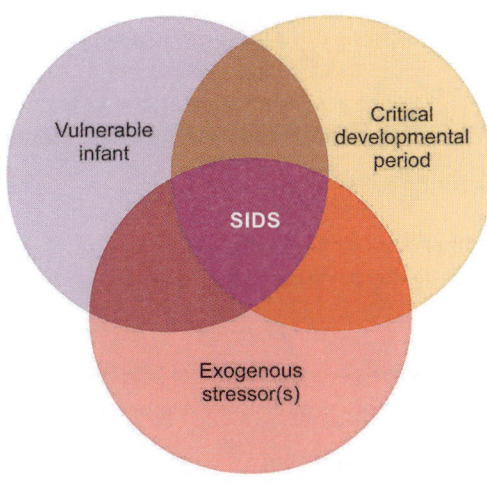

Fig. 20.22: Triple-risk model

Triple-risk Model

A triple-risk model has been proposed by Filiano and Kinney. SIDS occurs when three conditions exist simultaneously **(Fig. 20.22):**

a. The infant has an underlying (e.g., brainstem) abnormality that makes him unable to respond to low O_2 or high CO_2 blood levels
b. The infant is exposed to a triggering event, such as prone sleeping position
c. These events occur during a vulnerable stage in the infant's development, i.e., the first six months of life.

Postmortem Findings

To confirm the diagnosis of SIDS, a complete autopsy needs to be performed, using information gathered from the scene investigation, interview of caregivers and review of medical and social history—diagnosis of SIDS is one of exclusion.

External
- Well-cared-for appearance, with no significant skin trauma.
- Serosanguineous watery, frothy or mucoid discharge from mouth or nose.
- Reddish-blue mottling on the face and dependent portions of the body.
- Marks on pressure points of the body.
- Hands are clenched around fibers from bedclothes.

Internal
- Trachea contains milky vomit, sometimes blood-stained with shed epithelial cells.
- Multiple petechial hemorrhages on heart (posterior epicardial surface), lungs and thymus—agonal in nature.
- Pulmonary edema is common.

Medico-legal Aspects

- SIDS is a natural death in which the parents may be wrongfully linked for having criminal involvement or negligence.
- Some infanticide cases may be presented as cot death cases.

MUNCHAUSEN SYNDROME BY PROXY

Munchausen syndrome by proxy (MSBP), a factitious disorder is a form of child abuse in which parent or guardian fabricates or produces symptoms of an illness in a child in order to gain sympathy or attention for themselves.

- The parents frequently have abnormal or borderline personality disorder.
- Since vulnerable people are the victims, MSBP can be a form of elder abuse too.
- Diagnosis may require a high level of suspicion and may be met with considerable resistance from family.

Features

i. The child may be brought with vague complaints such as vomiting, diarrhea, fever or seizures inflicted by the parent intentionally and repetitively, e.g., bleeding may be caused by anticoagulants and simulated by exogenous blood, seizures can be caused by suffocations, shaking or intoxications, vomiting can be caused by giving ipecac syrup and fever triggered by injecting contaminants into IV lines while the child is in the hospital.
ii. The parent or guardian derives some non-economic benefit at the expense of the victim.
iii. Some perpetrators 'doctor shop' while some maintain a constant relationship with one or more healthcare providers.
iv. When confronted, the parent or guardian usually denies any allegations of causing the victim's condition.

Diagnosis

i. The illness does not conform to the expected presentation or follow the usual course.
ii. Signs and symptoms are not substantiated by laboratory or imaging findings.
iii. Failure of wounds to heal.
iv. The child becomes ill or worsens when the parent or guardian is present, with recovery when separated.
v. Positive drug or toxicological analysis for something not prescribed for the patient.
vi. Finding that the child has been admitted to multiple hospitals and has been seen by multiple physicians.

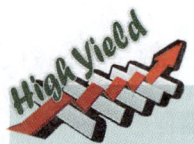

- **Infanticide:** Killing of an infant ≤1 year of age.
- Infanticide is punishable under Sec. 302 IPC.
- **Live born:** Fetus was alive after complete birth or when any part of its body comes out of mother's womb.
- **Stillborn:** Fetus born after 28 weeks of pregnancy and did not show any signs of life after being completely born.
- **Neonaticide:** Killing of an infant within first 24 h of life.
- **Neonatal death:** Death of an infant within first 28 days of life.
- Causing of death of living child in mother's womb may amount to culpable homicide irrespective of viability of fetus (Sec. 299 IPC).
- **Cephalhematoma:** Collection of *blood* in between periosteum and skull due to rupture of a small emissary vein; develops 12–24 h after birth.
- **Caput succedaneum:** Swelling due to accumulation of *fluid* between layers of scalp; present at birth.
- Absence of vernix caseosa indicates that the child had been washed, suggesting that it survived for sometime after birth.
- **Method to open infant's skull during autopsy:** Beneke's technique.
- Letulle's technique of *en masse* removal is used in fetus and infant.
- During autopsy of fetus, the abdomen is opened first before thorax to note the position of diaphragm.
- **Characteristic features seen in fetus:** Differentiated external genitalia (16 weeks); fingerprints formation, lanugo hair, wrinkled and red skin (24 weeks); fingernails reach fingertips, skin smooth (32 weeks); breasts protrude, testes palpable, fingernails beyond fingertips (40 weeks).
- **Characteristic features seen at 28 weeks (fetal viability):** Weight: 1000 g, meconium in entire intestine, eyelids open and pupillary membrane absent.
- **Appearance of center of ossification:** Calcaneum—5th month, talus—7th month *(determines fetal viability)* and lower femoral epiphysis—9th month (36th week) and upper tibial epiphysis—full term (38–40 weeks).
- **Rule of Hasse:** Method to calculate age of fetus from length.
- Medically, age of viability is 28 weeks of gestation (no legal section is there).
- Fetus may inhale air and cry when the head is inside vagina—*vagitus vaginalis*, or inside uterus—*vagitus uterus*.
- Unrespired lung (stillborn) is dense, firm consistency and non-crepitant (liver-like).
- Respired lung (live born) is soft, spongy, elastic and crepitant.
- **Signs of live birth**
  - *Ear crepitance test:* Crepitance is heard if piece of lung is rubbed between the fingers close to ear.
  - *Hydrostatic/Raygat's test:* Respired lung floats in water (specific gravity decreases after respiration).
  - *Wreden's test:* Absence of gelatinous embryonic connective tissue and presence of air in middle ear.
  - *Breslau's second life test:* Stomach and intestines are incised under water—air bubbles will come out if respiration has taken place *(stomach bowel test).*
- **Fodere's test** is used to determine live birth based on weight of the lungs (doubles after respiration).
- **Ploucquet's test** is based on increase in weight of lungs in relation to body weight after respiration.
- In hydrostatic test, residual air cannot be squeezed out by pressing.
- Milk present in stomach—*positive evidence of live birth*.
- Neonatal incremental line in the enamel of teeth—*surest sign of live birth*.
- Closure of foramen ovale occurs 2–3 months after birth.
- **Surest sign of dead-born fetus:** Maceration.
- **Earliest sign of maceration:** Slippage of skin of face, back or abdomen.
- **X-ray, USG signs of fetal death (dead born)**
  - *Spalding's sign:* Overlapping of fetal skull bones.
  - *Robert's sign:* Gas shadow in chambers of heart and great vessels.
  - *Halo sign:* Elevation of scalp due to edema.
  - *Ball sign:* Hyperflexion of spine.
  - *Helix sign:* Gas in umbilical arteries.
- **Findings of intrapartum (stillborn) death:** Lack of maceration and lack of lung aeration.
- **Ideal infanticidal poison:** Opium.
- Concealment of birth is punishable under Sec. 318 IPC (imprisonment for 2 years ± fine).

CHAPTER 20 : Infanticide and Child Abuse

- **Caffey syndrome:** Repetitive non-accidental violence produced by a parent or a guardian.
- **Shaken baby/infantile whiplash syndrome:** Vigorous shaking of the infant causing subdural hemorrhage (SDH).
- **Triad of injuries seen in shaken baby syndrome:** Encephalopathy, retinal hemorrhages and SDH.
- Multiple rib fractures along posterior angle of ribs give rise to *knob fractures* on healing, and *'string of beads'* appearance on X-ray (SDH).
- In child abuse, whiplash movement of arms and legs causes *'corner'*/*'bucket-handle' fractures*.
- **SIDS:** Sudden and unexpected death of an apparently healthy infant whose death remains unexplained even after autopsy.
- Triple-risk model for SIDS includes a vulnerable infant, critical developmental period in homeostatic control and exogenous stressor(s).
- SIDS is an autopsy diagnosis and not a clinical diagnosis. No definite cause is known.
- **Munchausen syndrome by proxy:** Form of child abuse in which parent fabricates symptoms of an illness in a child in order to gain sympathy/attention for themselves.

Interesting case

Munchausen Syndrome by Proxy (Case of Marybeth Tinning, 1985)

Marybeth Tinning, a US resident was convicted for the murder of her ninth child, 4-month-old daughter Tami Lynne in 1985. The autopsy indicated her death was from asphyxia by suffocation. What made the case unique and gained considerable attention was that all the nine of children died young between 1971 and 1985, eight of them under suspicious circumstances. The time line of events are given below:

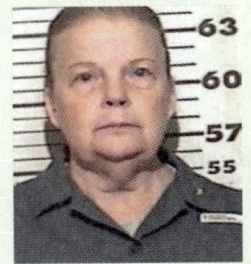

1965	Marybeth and Joseph Tinning got married.
1967	First child Barbara was born followed by their second child Joseph Jr in 1970.
1971	Jennifer, the third child was born but died 8-days later from hemorrhagic meningitis and multiple brain abscesses.
1972	Joseph Jr died due to cardiopulmonary arrest. Several weeks later, Barbara had convulsions and died after being in a comatose state; her death was attributed to Reye syndrome.
1973	Fourth child Timothy was born but was found lifeless in his crib; his death was attributed to SIDS.
1974	Joseph Tinning (her husband) was admitted to the hospital with a near-fatal dosage of barbiturate poisoning administered by Marybeth in juice.
1975	Fifth child Nathan was born and died in the car while out with her.
1978	The Tinnings adopted Michael; and Marybeth gave birth to her sixth child, Mary Frances.
1979	Mary Frances was brought to the hospital with cardiac arrest; she was revived, but had irreversible brain damage. She died two days later.
1980	Eighth child Jonathan died after being kept on life support.
1981	Michael, the adopted child fell down the stairs and died later.
1985	Ninth child Tami Lynne was born and died from being smothered.

The cause of death for the first eight children was initially thought to be genetic defect and was listed diversely between natural, undetermined and SIDS. Even when their adopted child Michael died, the authorities failed to open an investigation into his death. However, friends and family suspected something more sinister as the children seemed healthy and active before they died. Family members also noticed how Marybeth would get upset if she was not receiving enough attention at the children's funerals and other family events. Her pattern of behavior aligned perfectly with Munchausen syndrome by proxy (MSBP).

During the police interrogation after Tami Lynne's death, Marybeth confessed that she had murdered Tami Lynne, Timothy and Nathan (which she later retracted). According to her statement, she killed Tami Lynne because she would not stop crying. She was arrested and charged with Tami Lynne's murder. The investigators could not find enough evidence to charge her with murdering the other children. Two prosecution expert witnesses gave evidence that Tami Lynne was smothered to death with a soft object. In 1987, after a six-week trial, the jury convicted Marybeth of second-degree murder and sentenced her to 20 years imprisonment.

Criminal Abortion

LEARNING OBJECTIVES

Must know
1. Abortion, classification, causes of natural abortion
2. Methods of criminal abortion
3. Abortifacients drugs, cupping, abortion stick
4. Complications of criminal abortion
5. Natural and criminal abortion (Diff.)
6. Duties of a doctor in suspected case of criminal abortion

Desirable to know
1. Postmortem examination in case of criminal abortion
2. Relation of trauma and abortion

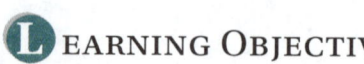

Define, classify and discuss abortion.

Definitions

- **Abortion:** *Medically*, abortion is expulsion or extraction from its mother of an embryo or fetus weighing 500 g or less, when it is not capable of independent survival (WHO). This 500 g of fetal development is attained at about 22 weeks of gestation.
  Legally, abortion is defined as expulsion of products of conception from the uterus at any period before full term **(Fig. 21.1)**.
- **Criminal abortion:** It is the termination of a pregnancy in violation of the legal regulations in force.
- **Unsafe abortion:** A procedure for terminating an unintended pregnancy either by individuals without the necessary skills or in an environment that does not conform to minimum medical standards, or both (WHO).

- **Abortus:** The non-viable product of abortion.
- **Abortifacient:** Any agent that induces abortion.

Some authors use the term *abortion* as expulsion of ovum within first 3 months of pregnancy; *miscarriage* for the expulsion of fetus from 4th–7th months; and *premature delivery* as the delivery of baby after 7 months of pregnancy and before full-term **(Fig. 21.1)**. The term miscarriage is synonymous with spontaneous abortion.

CLASSIFICATION OF ABORTION (FLOWCHART 21.1)

Natural or Spontaneous Abortion

- **Incidence:** 10–20% of all pregnancies (approx).
- Most frequent within first 3 months, owing to weak attachment of ovum to uterine wall (75% abortions occur before 16th week, and out of these, 75% before 8th week of gestation).
- Abortion occurs without any induction procedures and usually coincides with menstrual flow.

Causes

i. Genetic (50%)	iv. Infections (15%)
ii. Anatomic (10–15%)	v. Immunological (5–10%)
iii. Endocrine (10–15%)	vi. Others

i. **Genetic:** Majority of early abortions are due to chromosomal abnormality.
   - Autosomal trisomy is the commonest cause (50%) and most common is trisomy 16 (30%).

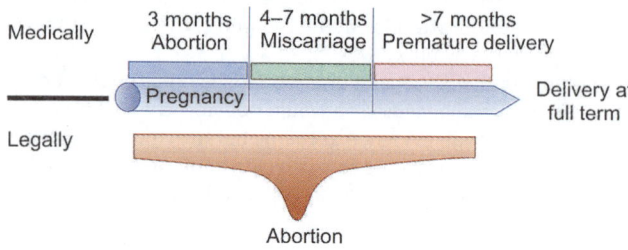

Fig. 21.1: Definition of abortion

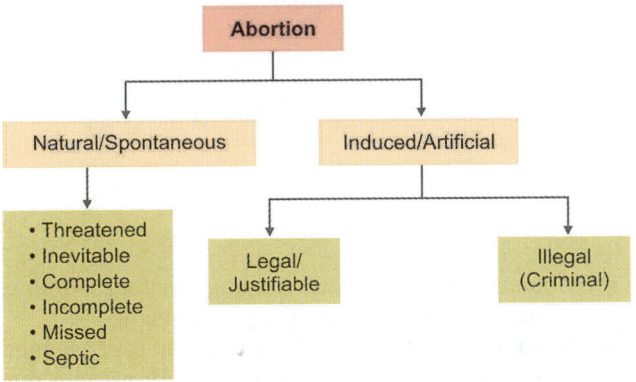

Flowchart 21.1: Classification of abortion

- Monosomy and chromosomal aberration (including deletion, duplication, translocation and inversion) constitutes 20% and 2–4% of all abortions respectively.

ii. **Anatomic:** Cervicouterine factors usually cause second trimester abortions.
   - Cervical incompetence.
   - Congenital malformation of uterus, e.g., hypoplasia, bicornuate/septate uterus or duplication of upper part of uterus.
   - Uterine fibroid.

iii. **Endocrine and metabolic abnormalities**
   - Diabetes mellitus.
   - Hypo- or hyperthyroidism.
   - Luteal phase defect.
   - Deficient progesterone secretion from corpus luteum.

iv. **Infections**
   - *Viral:* Rubella, cytomegalovirus, vaccinia, variola or HIV.
   - *Bacterial:* Ureaplasma, *Chlamydia* or *Brucella*.
   - *Parasitic: Toxoplasma* or malaria.

v. **Immunological:** Both autoimmune and alloimmune factors can cause miscarriage.

vi. **Others**
   - *Maternal illness:* Cyanotic heart disease or hemoglobinopathies.
   - Antifetal antibodies.
   - *Blood group incompatibility:* Incompatible ABO and Rh group.
   - Premature rupture of the membranes.
   - *Environmental factors:* Cigarette smoking, drugs, chemicals, noxious agents, *in-situ* contraceptive agents, X-ray exposure and antineoplastic drugs.

Unexplained (40%): In spite of the numerous factors mentioned, it is sometimes difficult to pinpoint exact cause of abortion.

Pearls

Common causes of abortion
- *First trimester:* Genetic factors, endocrine disorders, immunological disorders, infections and unexplained.
- *Second trimester:* Anatomic abnormalities, maternal medical illness and unexplained.

Artificial or Induced Abortion

It means willful termination of pregnancy before viability. It can be:
- *Legal or justifiable*: When it is done in good faith to save the life of the woman, and performed within the legal provisions of the MTP Act (details in Chapter 4).
- *Criminal or illegal*: Induced destruction and expulsion of fetus from womb unlawfully. It is usually induced before the 3rd month, and causes infection and inflammation of the endometrium.

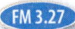

Discuss methods of procuring criminal abortion.

CRIMINAL ABORTION

Legal aspects: Dealt under **Section 312–316 IPC**.
- **Sec. 312 IPC:** Whoever (including the pregnant women herself) voluntarily causes criminal abortion *with the consent* of the patient is liable for imprisonment up to 3 years and with/without fine, and if the woman is quick with child, then imprisonment may extend up to 7 years and fine.
- **Sec. 313 IPC:** If miscarriage is caused *without the consent* of the woman, whether the woman is quick or not, then the person is punished with life imprisonment or imprisonment up to 10 years and fine.
- **Sec. 314 IPC:** If pregnant woman *dies from the act* done with the intent to cause miscarriage, then imprisonment is up to 10 years and fine. If the act is done without the consent of the woman, then the person is punished with life imprisonment or up to 10 years and fine.
- Sec. 315 and Sec. 316 have already been discussed in Chapter 20.

Methods for Inducing Criminal Abortion (Fig. 21.2)

i. Abortifacient drugs
ii. General violence
iii. Local violence

Abortifacient Drugs

- Most of the abortifacient drugs have no effect on the uterus or fetus, unless given in toxic doses, and often sold to exploit distressed woman.
- Usually used in the 2nd month of pregnancy.
   i. *Ecbolics*: They increase uterine contractions, e.g., ergot preparations, synthetic estrogens, pituitary extract, strychnine or quinine.

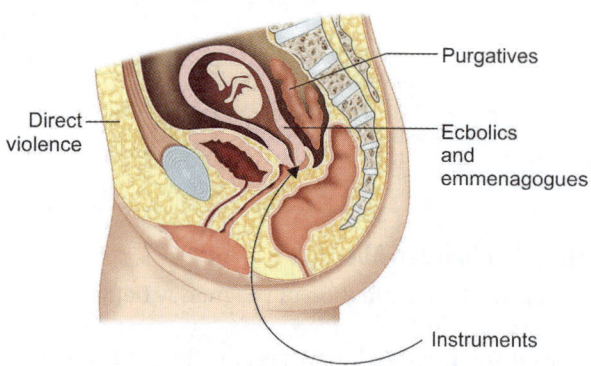

Fig. 21.2: Various sites of action of methods designed to induce an abortion

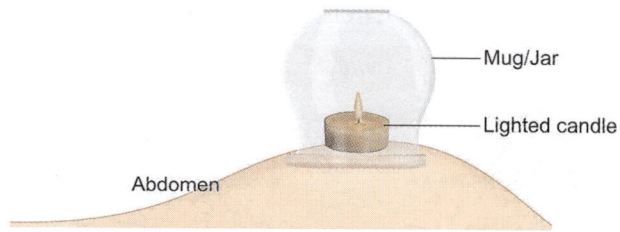

Fig. 21.3: Cupping

ii. *Emmenagogues*: These drugs initiate or increase menstrual flow, e.g., estrogen, savin, borax or sanguinarin.
iii. *GIT irritants*: These causes irritation of uterus, e.g., purgatives, like castor or croton oil, julap, senna or $MgSO_4$.
iv. *Genitourinary irritants*: They produce reflex uterine contraction, e.g., cantharides, oil of turpentine or tansy or pennyroyal.
v. *Drugs having systemic toxicity*
  - Inorganic irritants, e.g., lead, copper, iron or mercury.
  - Organic irritants, e.g., *Abrus precatorius, Calotropis,* seeds of custard apple and carrots, and unripe fruit of papaya or pineapple.*
vi. Abortion pills made of lead (diachylon) or diphenylethylene.

> **NOTA BENE**
> In *De Materia Medica Libri Quinque*, the Greek pharmacologist Dioscorides listed the ingredients of a drink called **'abortion wine'**—hellebore, squirting cucumber and scammony. Hellebore (*'Christmas rose'*), in particular, is known to be abortifacient.

General Violence

- Any act directly on the uterus or indirectly to produce congestion of pelvic organs or hemorrhages between uterus and membranes.
- Resorted to up to end of 1st month.
- It is more likely to cause injury than abortion.
- It can be **intentional or accidental**.

Intentional
i. Severe pressure on abdomen by kneading, blows, kick, tight bandage and massage of uterus through abdominal wall.
ii. Violent exercise, like horse riding, cycling, skipping, rolling downstairs, or jumping from height.
iii. **Cupping:** A mug is turned upside down over a lighted wick and placed on the hypogastria. Air escapes due to heat and the mug sets tightly on the abdomen. The mug is then pulled which may result in partial separation of placenta (**Fig. 21.3**).
iv. Very hot and cold hip bath alternately.

Accidental: A general shake-up in advanced pregnancy can produce abortion, but if the fetus is healthy, abortion will not occur.

Local Violence

- Usually employed in 3rd–4th month when other methods have failed.
- Interference may be skilled, semi-skilled or unskilled (**Table 21.1 and Fig. 21.4**).

Various methods are:
i. **Syringing:** Ordinary enema syringe with a hand bulb is commonly used to inject fluid into uterus, the hard nozzle being inserted into cervix. Higginson's syringe can also be used. Soap water is often used as injection material. Irritating substances are added to water, such as lysol, cresol, alum, $KMnO_4$ or formalin.
ii. **Syringe aspiration:** Large syringe with a plastic cannula is inserted into cervix; develops suction which

TABLE 21.1: Different methods of interference

Unskilled interference	Semi-skilled interference	Skilled interference
Self-instrumentation	Instrumentation	Dilatation and evacuation
Abortion stick	Abortion paste—Utus paste	Vacuum aspiration
	Slippery elm bark	Laminaria tent
	Syringing	Prostaglandins
		Electric current
		Intrauterine instillation of hyperosmotic solution

---

*Unripe papaya contains papain (in the latex) that may produce uterine contractions and pineapple contains bromelain which may soften cervix—early labor.

CHAPTER 21: Criminal Abortion

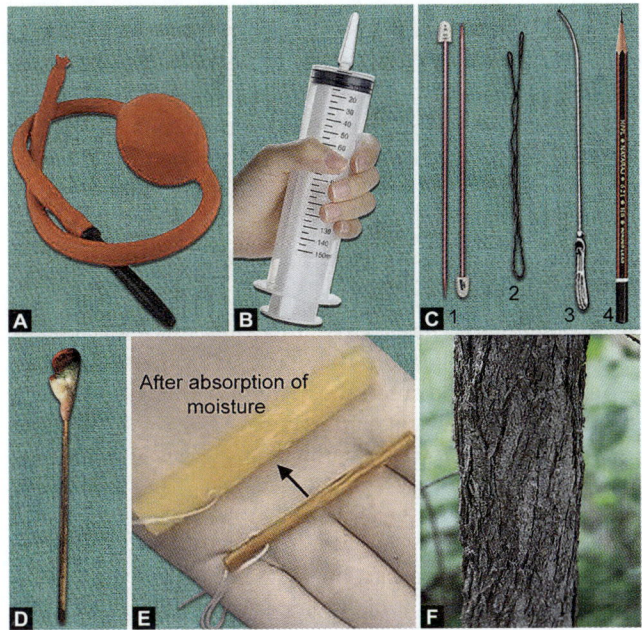

Figs. 21.4A to F: Common methods used to procure criminal abortion: (A) Higginson's syringe; (B) Syringe; (C) 1. Knitting needle, 2. Hairpin, 3. Uterine sound, 4. Pencil; (D) Abortion stick; (E) Laminaria; (F) Slippery elm bark

- It is introduced into the vagina or os by *dais* (traditional birth attendants) and retain there, till contraction starts **(Fig. 21.5B)**.
- Instead of this stick, a twig of some irritant plant, like *Plumbago rosea*, *Calotropis* or *Nerium odorum* may be used.

vi. **Dilation of cervix:** Foreign bodies are introduced and left in cervical canal, like pessaries, laminaria (a dried seaweed) or sea tangle tent which dilate the cervix, irritate uterine mucosa and produce marked congestion and uterine contractions with expulsion of fetus.
- Cervical canal may be dilated by introducing a compressed sponge into the cervix and leaving it there. Sponge swells from moisture in the uterine segment with expulsion of fetus.
- *Slippery elm* bark (*Ulmus fulva*) obtained from tree in Central America, is inserted into cervical canal in portions of 1–3 inches long. It absorbs moisture, and on each side of the bark, a jelly like layer is produced that is as thick as the bark itself, due to which the cervical canal is dilated.

vii. **Air insufflations:** Air is introduced into vagina and uterus by various means, like pumps or syringes leading to abortion.

viii. **Electric current:** An electric current of 110 V with negative pole applied to posterior vaginal cul-de-sac and positive pole to lumbosacral region, leads to contraction of uterus and expulsion of contents.

ix. **Pastes:** Utus paste (semi-solid soap mixed with potassium iodide, thymol and mercury) or Fetex paste is introduced in the extra-ovular space for abortion.

ruptures early gestational sac, and leads to aspiration and expulsion of contents.

iii. **Vacuum aspiration:** The cervix is dilated and a tube attached to a suction pump extracts the fetus **(Fig. 21.5A)**.

iv. **Rupturing of membranes:** The membranes are ruptured by introduction of an instrument, like probe, stick, uterine sound, umbrella ribs, catheter, pencil, pen holder, knitting needle or hairpin.

v. **Abortion stick:** It is a wooden or bamboo stick, 12–18 cm long, wrapped at one end with cotton, wool or piece of cloth and soaked with juice of marking nut, calotropis or paste made of arsenious oxide or lead.

> **NOTA BENE**
> - Other orally ingested abortifacients include indigenous and homeopathic medicines, chloroquine tablets, prostaglandins, high dose progesterones and estrogens and liquor before distillation.
> - Chloroquine is given intramuscularly as an abortifacient.

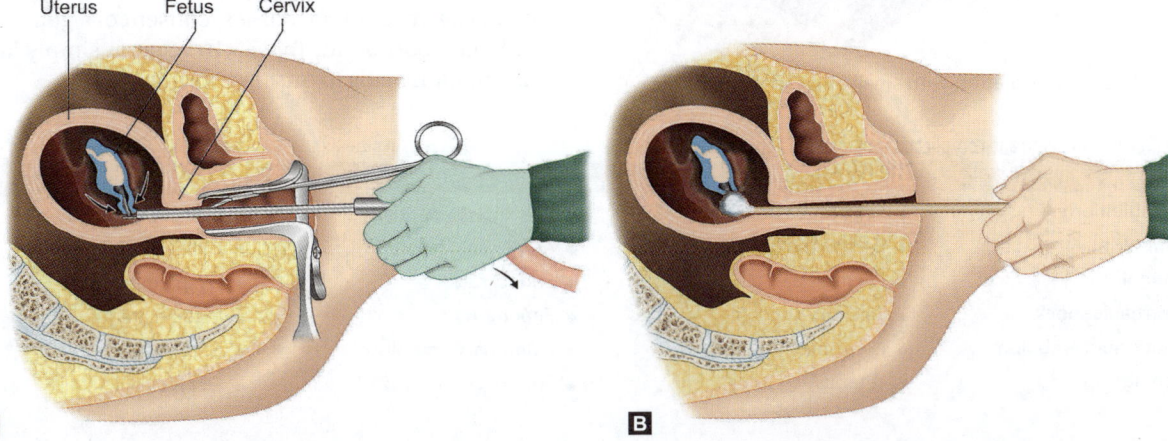

Figs. 21.5A and B: Methods to bring about abortion: (A) Vacuum aspiration; (B) Abortion stick

> **FM 3.27**
> Discuss complications of abortion.

COMPLICATIONS OF CRIMINAL ABORTION

Most of the complications develop as a result of incomplete evacuation (retained products of conception) of the uterus, infection and injury due to instruments used during the procedure, which may cause cervical laceration, uterine perforation with associated bowel and bladder injury **(Fig. 21.6)**. Complications that may occur due to criminal abortion are given in **Table 21.2**.

Septic Abortion

- **Definition:** It is defined as a type of abortion associated with sepsis of the products of conception and the uterus.
- Infection usually involves the endometrium and may spread into the myometrium and parametrium. Parametritis may progress into peritonitis.
- Pelvic inflammatory disease is the most common complication of septic abortion.
- Microorganisms causing uterine sepsis (mixed infection is more common):
    - **Anaerobic:** *Bacteroides* group (*fragilis*), anaerobic *Streptococci*, *Clostridium perfringens* and tetanus bacilli.
    - **Aerobic:** *E. coli*, *Klebsiella*, *Staphylococcus aureus*, *Pseudomonas* and hemolytic *Streptococcus*.

Cause of sepsis:
- Proper antiseptic and asepsis is not maintained
- Incomplete evacuation
- Inadvertent injury to the genital organs and adjacent structures, particularly the gut.

Amniotic Fluid Embolism

- Amniotic fluid embolism (AFE) is a rare, unforeseeable and dreadful complication. This occurs when massive amount of amniotic fluid enters the maternal venous system.
- Most of the cases occur during:
    - 1st and 2nd trimester abortion
    - Active labor
    - Amniocentesis
    - Abdominal trauma
- **Signs and symptoms:** There may be cough, hypotension, encephalopathy, tonic-clonic seizures, breathlessness, uterine atony and loss of consciousness. In half the cases, death occurs in the first hour.
- It causes DIC and fibrin deposition in many organs.
- *Diagnosis* is established by demonstration of mucin, lanugo hair, vernix caseosa, fat globules, meconium and fetal squamous cells in cut sections of the lung.*

> **NOTA BENE**
> - **Lendrum's stain (Phloxine-Tartrazine):** This stain is useful to detect amniotic fluid embolism deaths, since keratin of amniotic squames is stained red, nuclei blue and cytoplasm yellow.
> - **The 'WHO' method:** It is helpful to demonstrate keratin and mucin-like substances in amniotic fluid embolism.

Medico-legal Aspects

- Nearly all criminal abortion take place at about 2nd and 3rd month of pregnancy, when the woman in certain about her condition.
- It is resorted mostly by widows and unmarried girls. Stigma against premarital sex, consent of a guardian to undergo abortion for those <18 years or simply lack of information leads to unsafe abortions.

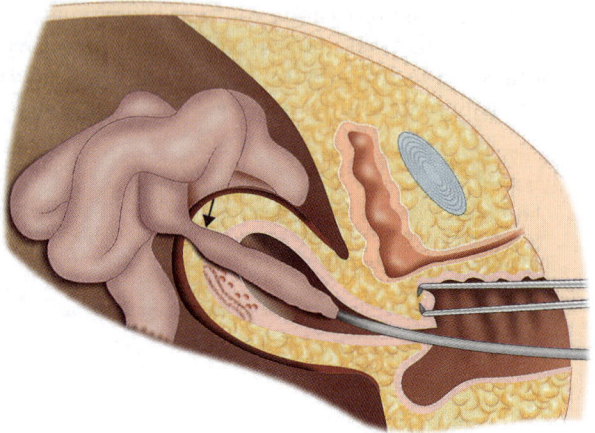

Fig. 21.6: Uterine perforation with small bowel prolapse (arrow)

TABLE 21.2: Cause of death and complications of criminal abortion

Immediate	Delayed	Systemic complications	Remote complications
◆ Vagal inhibition	◆ Septicemia	◆ Jaundice, hepatitis	◆ Chronic debility
◆ Air embolism	◆ Generalized peritonitis	◆ Acute renal failure	◆ Chronic pelvic pain
◆ Fat embolism	◆ Pyemia	◆ Endocarditis	◆ Dyspareunia
◆ Hemorrhagic shock	◆ Toxemia	◆ Pneumonitis	◆ Ectopic pregnancy
◆ Amniotic fluid embolism	◆ Local infection	◆ Pulmonary embolism	◆ Secondary infertility
◆ Poisoning (rare)	◆ Tetanus	◆ Endotoxic shock	◆ Depression

---

* Four criteria to make the diagnosis of AFE—acute hypotension or cardiac arrest, acute hypoxia, coagulopathy or severe hemorrhage, and these occurring during labor, cesarean delivery, dilation and evacuation, or within 30 min postpartum with no other explanation of findings.

- **Fabricated abortion:** Rarely, when a woman is assaulted, she may try to exaggerate the offense by alleging that it caused her to abort. She may acquire a human or an animal fetus to support the charge.

Medico-legal Importance of Placenta

- Gives an idea of the length of gestation.
- Transfer of poisons, bacteria and antibodies across the placenta may result in death, disease or abnormalities of fetus.
- In criminal abortion, pieces are often retained in the uterus.

NOTA BENE

- Second trimester abortion (rate is among the highest in the world) increases the risk in women—they are more likely to go to an uncertified provider, and the risk of complications is higher for physiological reasons.
- Most common reasons for second trimester abortions—sex selective abortions and delay of accessing abortion services for an unwanted pregnancy.
- Legal abortion is not an option for most Indian women from lower socioeconomic classes, hence these women gets the abortion done from less trained, but more accessible providers.

Describe duties of doctor in cases of abortion.

DUTIES OF A DOCTOR IN SUSPECTED CASE OF CRIMINAL ABORTION

i. He should ask the patient to make a statement about the induction of criminal abortion. If she refuses, he should not pursue the matter, but inform the police.
ii. Doctor should keep all the information obtained by him as professional secret.
iii. He must consult a professional colleague.
iv. If the woman's condition is serious, he must arrange to record the dying declaration.
v. If the woman dies, he should not issue a death certificate, but should inform the police for postmortem examination.

FM 3.28
Describe evidences of abortion—living and dead, and investigations of death due to criminal abortion.

EXAMINATION OF A WOMAN WITH ALLEGED HISTORY OF ABORTION

The doctor may have to examine a living subject, or sometimes, a dead body may be sent for postmortem examination for alleged abortion. The findings are similar to those found in the recent delivery and will depend upon the period of gestation, the mode of abortion procured and the time elapsed between abortion and examination. The major differentiating features between natural abortion and criminal interference are given in **Diff. 21.1**.

Examination of a Living Individual

It includes:
- Requisition from the concerned authority
- Identification of the female
- Written informed consent of the female
- A female nurse (if the doctor is male)
- Brief history—date time, place of abortion, method used to procure abortion. History of illegal termination by an unauthorized person is mostly concealed. The behavior of the woman may also be indicative, e.g., if she refuses medical help or if there is evidence of contradictory statements.

Clothing must be examined, especially the undergarments for bloodstains, stains from abortifacients (fluid, soapy materials)—preserved and sent to CFSL.

Clinical Examination

- Since, most of the abortifacients are irritants, the woman may show signs of ill health, GIT disturbances and exhaustion.
- In case of sepsis, there will be pyrexia with chills and rigor, pain abdomen and increased pulse rate (100–120/min).

DIFFERENTIATION 21.1: Natural and criminal abortion

S.No.	Feature	Natural abortion	Criminal abortion
1.	Cause	Predisposing diseases	Pregnancy in unmarried woman or widow
2.	Injuries on genital organs	Absent	Contusions and lacerations may be present
3.	Marks of violence on abdomen	Absent	May be present
4.	Foreign bodies in genital tract	Absent	May be present
5.	Fetal injuries	Absent	May be present
6.	Toxic effect of drugs	Absent	Inflammation of vagina, cervix, GIT or urinary tract may be present
7.	Infection	Rare	Frequent

Local Examination

- Appearance of perineum, vulva and vagina is noted.
- Presence/absence of injuries (abrasions/contusions/lacerations) is noted.
- Condition of os is noted. It remains dilated for few days and may also show some injuries due to instrumentation.
- Presence of recent tears, the marks of forceps or other instruments in and around genitalia should be noted.
- Character and amount of discharge is noted. In case of sepsis, offensive purulent vaginal discharge or a tender uterus with patulous os may be found.

Laboratory investigations: Serum and urine gives positive result for the test for hCG up to 7–10 days.

In abortion during early months of gestation, the signs will be ill-defined, whereas signs persist for a longer time if sepsis has taken place and if abortion has been carried out in late months of gestation.

Examination of a Dead Body

The conviction of a person for criminal abortion should be based on autopsy, laboratory and circumstantial findings.

a. Sudden death of a woman of child-bearing age should give rise to the suspicion of criminal abortion if:
   - The deceased was pregnant and deeply cyanosed.
   - Instruments to procure an abortion or abortifacient drugs are found at scene of death.
   - Underclothing appears to be disturbed after death.
   - Fluid, soapy material or blood coming out of vagina.

b. Following point should be proved to convict the abortionist:
   - The dead woman was pregnant.
   - The accused was responsible for the act which resulted in the interruption of pregnancy.
   - The accused acted for the purpose of procuring an illegal abortion.
   - Death occurred as a result of attempt to interrupt the pregnancy.

Moreover, any criminal charge must be substantiated not only by positive evidence of interference relating to the deceased's death, but also to exclude the possibility of self-induced abortion.

Postmortem Examination

The autopsy involves identification of fetal remains and association with the alleged mother.

- Autopsy examination should include absolute identification of the victim and careful examination of the clothing including undergarments which must be preserved for any traces of foreign solutions.
- External features of pregnancy should be looked for. If death is due to hemorrhage, body will look pale.
- Presence of injuries (general or local) is noted. If abortifacient drug was injected, then the injection mark(s) can be detected over usual sites.
- *Local examination*: Labia majora, minora, vagina and cervix may show injuries and may be congested. It may be stained by locally used abortifacient agents.
- *To confirm or exclude air embolism*, the body must be opened after radiological examination as it may show translucency of the right ventricle and pulmonary artery (details in Chapter 7). Evidence of air embolism in pregnancies of <24 weeks duration is also an indication of death due to criminal abortion.
- The *abdominal cavity* is opened and may be full of blood, if there is perforation of uterus. Uterine and adnexal tissues are assessed for crepitation due to gas formation in the uterine wall, and venous channels and the inferior vena cava is inspected for air or soap embolism bubbles.
- The *skull vault* must then be carefully removed, avoiding puncture of the meninges and vessels over the brain surface which allows air to enter these vessels; a detailed examination of the basal sinuses, veins and arteries is made for the presence of air embolism.
- Following removal of the thoracic and abdominal organs in the usual manner, the pelvic organs are excised *en-masse* after separation of the symphysis pubis and a circular dissection to include vagina, vulva and rectum with adjacent skin, taking care to collect any foreign fluid or material for chemical and bacteriological examination. The vagina and uterus are opened along their anterior surface because injuries are more likely to occur on the posterior vaginal wall following criminal interference.
- *Findings in the uterus*: Cavity may show presence of products of conception (in full or in parts), clots, hemorrhages, pus, etc. **(Fig. 21.7)**. It may be enlarged, soft and congested. Wall may show thickening in longitudinal section. Examination of fetal remains

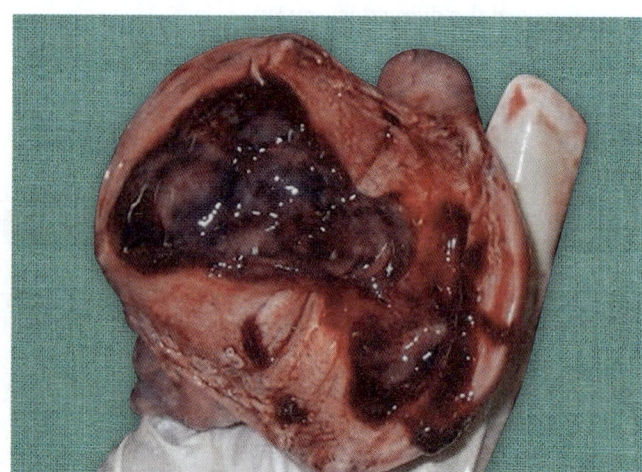

Fig. 21.7: Multiple hemorrhagic contusions in uterus caused by abortion stick

Box 21.1 Samples to be collected in criminal abortion.
♦ Vaginal contents pipetted in a clean sterile container for chemicals, drugs or soap
♦ Pubic hair
♦ Blood, urine and stomach contents
♦ Blood from the inferior vena cava and both cardiac ventricles
♦ Any fluid from the uterine cavity
♦ Swabs of the uterine wall
♦ Tissues for histology from all organs

consists of physical and histological examination of the fetus and organs.
- Samples to be collected are given in **Box 21.1**.

TRAUMA AND ABORTION

Allegation may be leveled against a person that because of the alleged assault, the pregnant female suffered an abortion. It may be a case of a mother who is the victim of an assault or domestic abuse, which results in premature labor, delivery of an extremely premature infant who survives a few hours, but then dies because of prematurity. Such a case could be considered a homicide, and criminal charges could well be pursued. In similar cases, where the fetus dies in-utero, criminal charges are framed under various sections of IPC.
- Travel, in the absence of trauma, does not increase the incidence of abortion.
- Trauma may rarely cause an abortion, in the absence of serious or life-threatening injury to mother.
- General violence does not appear to cause abortion during first trimester of pregnancy as the gravid uterus is an intrapelvic structure, well protected by the pelvic bones and the strong attachment of embryo with the uterine wall.
- Following *criteria suggests a causal relationship between trauma and abortion:*
  a. The traumatic event was followed within 24 h by processes that ultimately lead to abortion.
  b. Appearance of the fetus and placenta should be compatible with the period of pregnancy at which the traumatic event occurred.
  c. The fetus and placenta should be normal.
  d. Factors known to cause abortion should be absent, such as:
     i. History of repeated abortion without any cause or exposure to abortifacients, e.g., X-ray or lead.
     ii. Chronic infections in mother, e.g., syphilis, toxoplasmosis or tuberculosis.
     iii. Abnormalities of uterus including congenital defect of uterine development, leiomyomas, endometrial polyps and incompetent os.
     iv. Physical attempt to induce abortion.

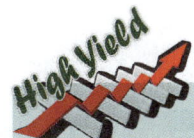

- **Abortion:** Expulsion of products of conception from the uterus *at any period before full term* (legally).
- **Criminal abortion:** Termination of a pregnancy in violation of the MTP Act.
- **Abortus:** Non-viable product of abortion.
- **Abortifacient:** Any agent that induces abortion.
- **Most common cause of first trimester abortion:** Genetic factors (chromosomal abnormality).
- **Most common cause of second trimester abortion:** Anatomic abnormalities (cervical incompetence).
- Legal aspects of criminal abortion are dealt under sections 312–316 IPC.
- Abortion with woman's consent is punishable under Sec. 312 IPC; without consent under Sec. 313 IPC.
- **Ecbolics** increase uterine contractions, e.g., ergot preparations, strychnine or quinine.
- **Emmenagogues** increase menstrual flow, e.g., borax, savin, sanguinarin
- **Cupping:** An intentional method to bring about abortion using lighted wick.
- **Abortion stick**: Bamboo stick with cotton wrapped at one end and soaked with juice of marking nut/calotropis used for criminal abortion.
- Complications of abortion are due to incomplete evacuation of uterus, infection and injury.
- **Most common complication of septic abortion:** Pelvic inflammatory disease.
- Amniotic fluid embolism occurs during 1st and 2nd trimester abortion, active labor and amniocentesis.
- **Lendrum's stain:** Useful to detect amniotic fluid embolism deaths.
- Air embolism in pregnancies of <24 weeks duration is an indication of death due to criminal abortion.

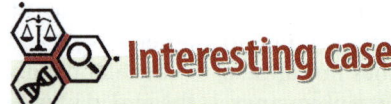

Denial of MTP (Case of Savita Halappanavar, 2012)

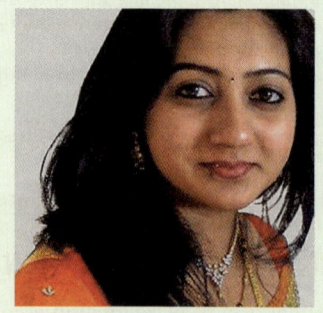

In 2012, 17-weeks pregnant Savita Halappanavar visited the hospital with complaints of a sensation of 'something coming down'. On examination, the gestational sac was seen protruding out. She was admitted to hospital, as it was determined that miscarriage was inevitable. Several hours later, she had a spontaneous rupture of membranes but did not expel the fetus. The following day, she and her husband discussed the possibility of using medication to induce labor with the consulting doctor but her request was promptly refused. Under Irish law, an abortion is illegal since there was 'not a real and substantial risk to her life at that stage and there is a fetal heart'. It treated 'the right to life of the unborn' child as equal to the right of life to the mother, allowing terminations only when there was a risk of suicide or harm to the health of the mother (but not in the event of rape/incest). By the time her life was at risk, it was too late to save her with a termination. She developed sepsis and her condition rapidly deteriorated, and despite doctors' best efforts she had a cardiac arrest and died after one week of admission.

The cause of her death was septic shock (*E. coli* in her bloodstream) and a miscarriage at 17-weeks. A Coroner's inquest held that she died of medical misadventure. An independent inquiry found out an 'over-emphasis on the need not to intervene until the fetal heart had stopped', as well as not diagnosing the sepsis soon enough, poor patient monitoring and risk assessment.

Her unexpected death became a catalyst for groundbreaking social change in Ireland. Voters agreed to remove the Ireland's constitutional ban on abortion. This followed a constitutional amendment which was signed into law as the Health (Regulation of Termination of Pregnancy) Act, 2018. Abortion is now permitted during the first 12 weeks of pregnancy, and later in cases where the pregnant woman's life or health is at risk, or in the cases of a fatal fetal abnormality.

Erectile Dysfunction and Sterility

LEARNING OBJECTIVES

Must know
1. Marriage, divorce, erectile dysfunction, sterility, frigidity, quod, premature ejaculation, vaginismus
2. Causes of erectile dysfunction and sterility in males, and impotence and sterilty in females
3. Sterilization, classification, methods, medico-legal aspects
4. Artificial insemination, medico-legal aspects
5. Surrogate mother
6. AIH and AID (Diff.)

Desirable to know
1. Examination of a person with erectile dysfunction
2. Nullity of marriage and divorce
3. Assisted reproductive technology including various types

Define and discuss the impotence, sterility, frigidity, sexual dysfunction, and premature ejaculation.

Definitions

- **Marriage** is a state of being united to a person of the opposite sex as husband and wife in a consensual and contractual relationship recognized by law (marriage between same-sex couple is not legal in India).
- **Divorce** is the legal cessation of a matrimonial bond.
- **Sexual potency** is the ability to carry out and consummate sexual intercourse, usually referring to the male.
- **Sexual dysfunction** refers to a person's inability to participate in a sexual relationship as he/she would wish. Sexual dysfunction can be categorized into:
   a. Decreased libido
   b. Erectile dysfunction
   c. Ejaculatory disorder
      - Premature ejaculation
      - Retarded ejaculation
- **Erectile dysfunction*** (**impotence**) is the consistent or recurrent inability to attain and/or maintain a penile erection sufficient for sexual intercourse.
- **Premature ejaculation**: Persistent or recurrent problem in which a male experiences orgasm or ejaculation in the early phases of sexual contact and before he and his partner wish it.
- **Quod** *(impotence quod hanc, 'as regards')*: A male may be impotent with one particular female, but not with another.
- **Frigidity** (Latin, coldness): It is the inability to initiate or maintain the sexual arousal pattern in female (absence of desire for sexual intercourse or incapacity to achieve orgasm).
- **Sterility:** It is the absolute inability of either a male or a female to procreate. In male, it is inability to make a female conceive, and in females, it is inability to conceive a child.
- **Fertility:** Capacity to reproduce or the state of being fertile.
- **Infertility:** Failure to conceive (regardless of cause) after 1 year of unprotected and regular intercourse.

Discuss the causes of impotence and sterility in male and female.

CAUSES OF ERECTILE DYSFUNCTION AND STERILITY IN MALES

Some of the important causes of erectile dysfunction (ED) are given in **Table 22.1 and Figure 22.1**.

---

* Term was coined by Kaplan in 1974. Before 1970s, the preferred term for erectile dysfunction was 'impotence'.

i. **Psychological:** Earlier, psychogenic causes were supposed to be the most common cause of ED, but recently organic diseases (causes)* are found to be the most common. Absence of desire for sexual intercourse may result from dislike of partner, fear of failure, anxiety or mood disorder, guilt, aversion, low self-esteem, hypochondriacs, childhood sexual abuse, masturbatory anxiety ('*dhat syndrome*'—passage of whitish discharge in urine and believed to be semen), widower syndrome, or post-traumatic stress disorder. Excessive masturbation may also lead to ED.
ii. **Age:** Before puberty, boys are usually impotent and sterile with certain exceptions, like precocious puberty. Poor physical development of penis is common cause of ED—examination depends more on its development than the age. In advanced age, libido diminishes, but they are not impotent or sterile. As long as live spermatozoa are present in seminal fluid, individual is presumed to be fertile.
iii. **Developmental and acquired abnormalities:** Absence of penis, intersexuality, malformations, e.g., hypospadias, epispadias, absence of testicles, Klinefelter syndrome, retrograde ejaculation and cryptorchidism **(Fig. 22.2)**.
iv. **Local diseases:** Priapism, hydrocele, elephantiasis, phimosis, Peyronie disease, adherent prepuce, orchitis following mumps, syphilis and tuberculosis **(Fig. 22.2)**. Mumps may cause sterility, not ED. Exposure to X-rays may cause sterility.
v. **General diseases:** ED is common during acute illness and in any severe or debilitating illnesses.
   - *Neurological conditions*, like tabes dorsalis, multiple sclerosis, paraplegia, hemiplegia, syringomyelia, temporal lobe damage and 3rd ventricle tumors; *endocrine disorders*, e.g., diabetes, hypothyroidism, hyperprolactinemia and testicular atrophy following renal failure, hemochromatosis or cirrhosis; *blood vessel and nerve trauma* (e.g., long-distance bicycle riding),

TABLE 22.1: Causes of erectile dysfunction (ED)

S.No.	Cause		Examples
1.	**Congenital anomalies**		
		Penile	Hypospadius, epispadius, non-development of penis, maldevelopment of penis, hermaphroditism, Peyronie's disease, micropenis
		Testicular	Absence of both testes, cryptorchidism (undescended testes), pseudo-hermaphroditism, Klinefelter syndrome
2.	**Local diseases/causes**		
		Penile	Phimosis, paraphimosis, ulcer on penis due to syphilis or tuberculosis, malignancy, elephantiasis, adherent prepuce, balanitis
		Testicular	Local diseases affecting testicles, epididymis, elephantiasis, large hydrocele, scrotal hernia, acute/chronic inflammation of the testis, atrophy of testis, malignancy
		Traumatic/Surgical	Accidental injury to testicles resulting in hematocele, blows on head or spine at level of lumbar 4 or 5 vertebrae, previous surgeries like abdominoperineal resection, radiation therapy and surgeries done for malignancies
		Constitutional/Hormonal	Acute illness, fever, endocrine disorder, sexual infantilism. Major and chronic diseases such as diabetes mellitus, hypertension, atherosclerosis, pulmonary tuberculosis, hyperlipidemia, Addison's disease, hypopituitarism, thyrotoxicosis, uremia, myxedema, paraplegia, hemiplegia, hyperprolactinemia, syringomyelia, tabes dorsalis, transverse myelitis, schizophrenia, bipolar disorder
3.	Neurological		Traumatic brain or spine, Parkinsonism, Alzheimer's disease, cerebrovascular disease, multiple sclerosis, brain tumors, peripheral neuropathies (*e.g.,* diabetic), cauda equina syndrome, pelvic and pudendal nerve lesions due to pelvic surgery, tumors of spine involving lumbar segments
4.	Overindulgence of habit forming drugs		Barbiturates, alcohol, opium, cannabis, cocaine, heroin, LSD, tobacco (smoking)
5.	Medicinal drugs		Beta blockers, digoxin, clonidine, methyl-dopa, luteinizing hormone-releasing hormone (LHRH) analogs, antidepressants (selective serotonin reuptake inhibitors/tricyclics), H_2-receptor antagonists (cimetidine/ranitidine), spironolactone, chemotherapy and hormonal medications
6.	Age		Erectile dysfunction is usually observed at the extremes of ages
7.	Psychological		Temporary ED may result from absence of desire, fear, guilt, anxiety, hypochondriasis, timidity and aversion, fear of inability to complete the act especially when the opposite partner is very virile. Sexual overindulgence may result in premature ejaculation or temporary ED

---
* Includes vascular, neurogenic, endocrinologic and drug induced.

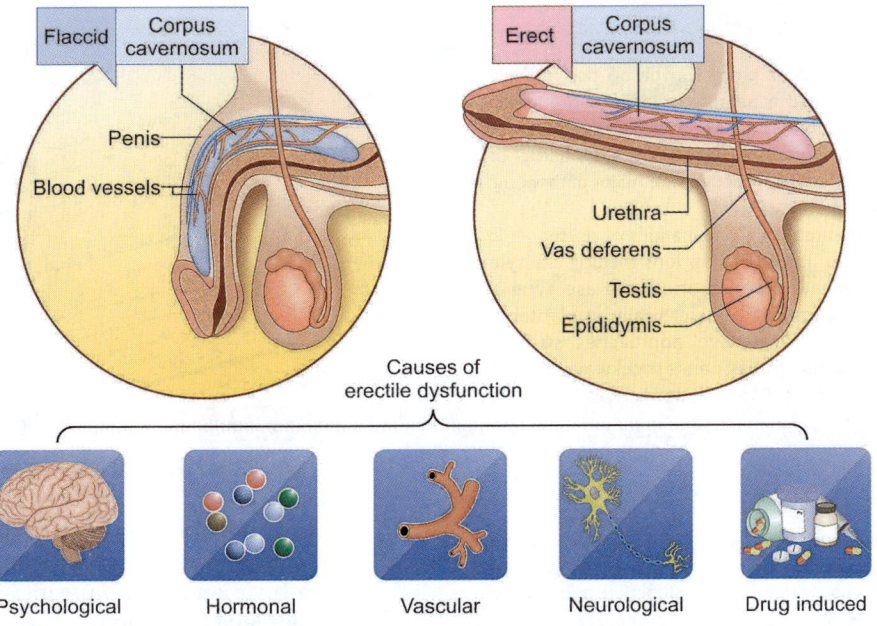

Fig. 22.1: Major causes of erectile dysfunction

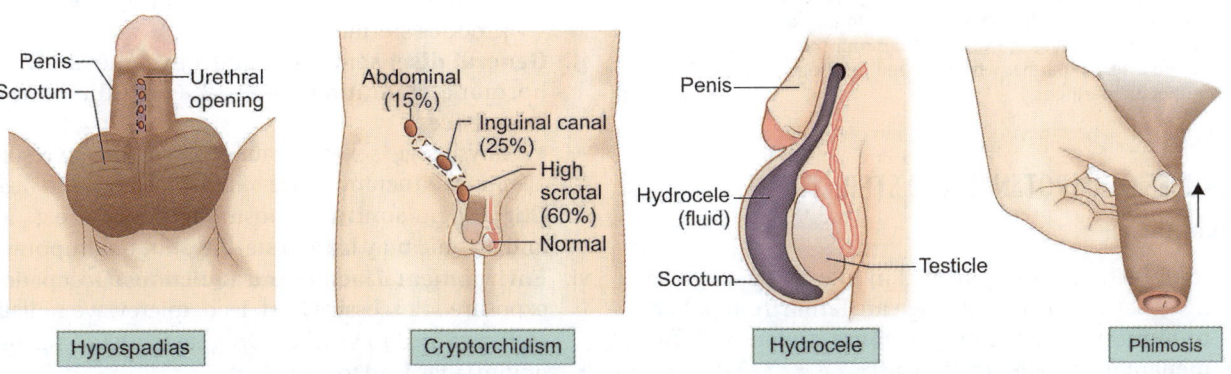

Fig. 22.2: Causes of erectile dysfunction and sterility in males

    CVS disorders, e.g., Leriche syndrome, and diseases like tuberculosis and nephritis may cause ED and sterility.
- Malnutrition, vitamin C and zinc deficiency may cause ED.

vi. **Injuries:** Infertility is a significant problem after spinal cord injury. The two major causes are poor semen quality and ejaculatory dysfunction.
- ED may occur following treatment for lower limb fractures due to perineal neurovascular traction injury acquired during surgery.
- Fracture of the penis (rupture of both corpora cavernosa with urethral rupture) may result in ED. The commonest causes of fracture of penis are coitus and penile manipulations, especially masturbation.

vii. **Chronic poisoning:** Exposure to poisons, e.g., lead, arsenic, pesticides or aphrodisiac agents may lead to ED and/or sterility.

viii. **Medications:** Antidepressants (e.g., selective serotonin reuptake inhibitors), antipsychotics, antihypertensives, antiulcer agents (e.g., cimetidine), cholesterol-lowering agents and finasteride may cause ED.

ix. **Behavioral factors:** Lifestyle choices—chronic alcoholism, smoking, being overweight and avoiding exercise are possible causes of ED. Tight-fitting underwear causes increase in scrotal temperature that may result in decreased sperm count.

x. **Addictions:** Certain drugs, e.g., morphine, heroin, opium, cannabis, cocaine and tobacco (smoking) may cause ED, and sometimes sterility.

NOTA BENE

♦ Penile erection is a complex process involving psychogenic and hormonal input, and a neurovascular nonadrenergic, noncholinergic mechanism. Nitric oxide (NO) is considered as the main vasoactive neurotransmitter and chemical mediator of penile erection. Impaired NO bioactivity is a major pathogenic mechanism of ED.

♦ Treatment of ED often requires combinations of psychogenic and medical therapies. Treatment options include lifestyle changes, oral medications (phosphodiesterase type 5 inhibitors), penile injections, and surgically implantable penile prostheses as well as novel approaches, such as belted external penile prostheses, penile shockwave therapy and the injection of stem cells or platelet-rich plasma (PRP).

NOTA BENE

♦ **Honeymoon impotence** is the inability to perform successful sexual intercourse during first few nights of marriage—considered as psychogenic erectile dysfunction and related to performance anxiety.

♦ **Madonna–whore complex** (Madonna–mistress complex) is the inability to maintain sexual arousal within a committed, loving relationship. In the early 1900s, Sigmund Freud identified a psychological dichotomy in his male patients wherein men saw women as either saints (the Madonna) or prostitutes (the whore), loving the first and desiring the second. They desire a sexual partner who has been degraded and not the respected partner.

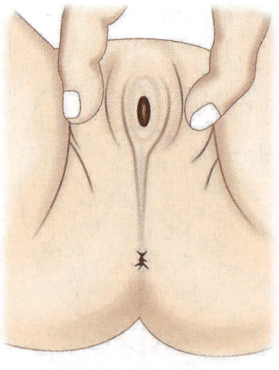 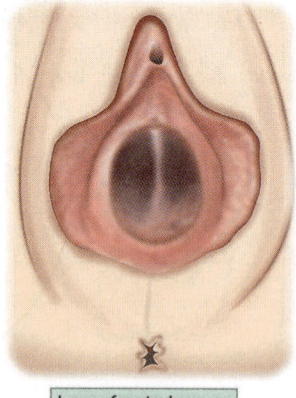

Labial adhesion | Imperforate hymen

Fig. 22.3: Causes of impotence in females

CAUSES OF IMPOTENCE AND STERILITY IN FEMALES

i. **Age:** Being passive partners in intercourse, age has no effect on potency. Women are fertile from puberty to menopause, but may become pregnant before menarche and after menopause.
   ▪ Kraurosis vulvae in old women may cause narrowing of the vagina.
   ▪ The occurrence of infertility rises significantly as age increases.

ii. **Developmental and acquired abnormalities**
   ▪ Impotence* may result from total occlusion of vagina, adhesion of labia, imperforate hymen—can be cured by surgery **(Fig. 22.3)**.
   ▪ Injury or operation of vagina may cause stricture which can lead to impotence.
   ▪ Absence/abnormal uterus, ovaries or fallopian tubes produces sterility, but not impotence.

iii. **Local diseases**
   ▪ Bartholin cyst, chancre of vulva, stricture due to perineal tear during previous pregnancy, prolapse of uterus/urinary bladder and dyspareunia causes impotence, but not sterility.
   ▪ Pelvic inflammatory disease, peritoneal adhesions secondary to previous pelvic surgery, endometriosis, and ovarian cyst rupture may produce blockage of fallopian tubes and sterility.
   ▪ Diseases of the genital organs (e.g., gonorrhea), leukorrhea, acidic vaginal secretions and recto-vaginal fistula do not cause impotence but may produce sterility.

iv. **General disease:** General infective, metabolic and hormonal conditions may cause sterility, but not impotence.
   ▪ Physiologic sexual dysfunction can be the result of impaired neurovascular tone to the clitoris and vagina.

v. **Chronic poisoning:** Exposure to poisons, e.g., lead and arsenic may lead to sterility, but not impotence.

vi. **Environmental factors and addictions:** Occupational exposure to excessive heat, lead, microwave radiation or X-rays lead to sterility. Drug dependence (alcohol, opium) may lead to sterility.

vii. **Medications:** Chemotherapy, cessation of oral contraceptives—hormonal imbalance may remain for some time after stopping the pill.

viii. **Psychological:** In males, psychological factors lead to non-erection (passive), but in females it is active in nature.
   ▪ Fear, pain, disgust or apprehension for intercourse may give rise to *vaginismus* [severe spasm of the lower one-third of vagina involving the paravaginal muscles (levator ani and adductor femoris muscle) **(Table 22.2 and Fig. 22.4)**].
   ▪ The spastic contraction of vaginal outlet is an involuntary reflex which replaces the rhythmic contraction associated with anticipated or actual attempt of vaginal penetration.
   ▪ It may occur with equal severity in the women who has borne children, as in virgins.

---

* Impotence indicates 'sexual dysfunction' which can be *sexual desire disorder* (lack of interest or aversion in sex); *sexual arousal disorder* (failure to get sexually aroused to engage in or sustain sexual intercourse); *sexual pain disorder* (persistent or recurring pain during coitus); or *orgasmic disorder* (difficulty in reaching orgasm or reaching orgasms more rapidly than one would like).

CHAPTER 22: Erectile Dysfunction and Sterility

TABLE 22.2: Types of vaginismus

Type	Condition
Primary (lifelong)	Inability to ever experience vaginal penetration
Secondary (acquired)	Female who previously experienced vaginal penetration, but now unable to
Complete	Inability to tolerate any vaginal penetration
Partial	Ability to tolerate some degree of vaginal penetration
Situational	Inability to tolerate certain forms of vaginal penetration, yet is able to tolerate some, like tampons or fingers
Spasmodic	Spasm of the vagina

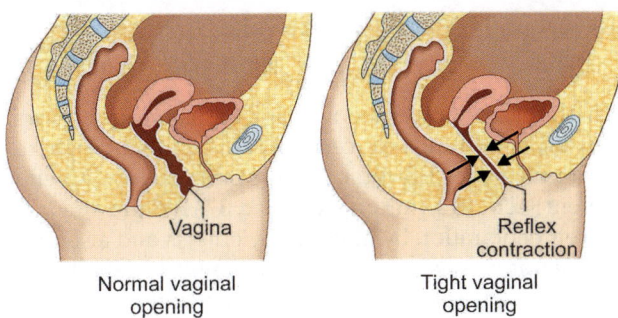

Fig. 22.4: Vaginismus

- *Etiological factors:* Male sexual dysfunction, psychosexually inhibiting influence due to religious orthodoxy, incidents of prior sexual trauma, secondary to dyspareunia or personal dislike/disgust for coitus.

EXAMINATION OF A PERSON IN AN ALLEGED CASE OF ERECTILE DYSFUNCTION AND STERILITY

- A sterile person may or may not have ED, and a person with ED may or may not be sterile.
- A simple way to distinguish between organic and psychological ED is to determine whether the patient 'ever' had an erection. If never, the problem is likely to be organic; if sometimes, it could be organic or psychological.
- The person is examined only when asked by the court or by the police. Informed consent of the person should be taken and the consequences of the examination should be explained.

History: Complete history of previous illness (including surgery), mental condition and sexual history is taken. History of smoking, dietary habits, obesity and the use of various medications are also evaluated.

Psychosocial examination: A psychosocial examination using an interview and a questionnaire reveals psychological factors. A man's sexual partner may also be interviewed to determine expectations and perceptions during sexual intercourse.

Examination of a Male

- Complete medical examination including CNS is done, especially if there is history of CNS illness, peripheral neuropathy, diabetes or penile sensory deficit.
- It includes pulse, blood pressure, any abnormal secondary sexual characteristics (hair pattern or breast enlargement), site of urethral meatus, urethral stenosis, sensitivity of the penis to touch or if there is any deformity in the penis itself—whether it is bent or curved when erect, or any other congenital anomalies of the genitalia.
- Presence of gynecomastia, sparse facial and body hair, soft and small testicles, increased abdominal fat and poor masculine development may indicate long-standing hypogonadism.
- Testicular size, epididymis, spermatic cord and presence of varicocele are also noted. Abnormal position, size and consistency of testes may also suggest hypogonadism.
- Detection of deformity in penis, such as micropenis, congenital chordee, fibrous plaques in the corpora cavernosa and abnormal curvature suggests Peyronie's disease which may indicate physical barrier to sexual intercourse.
- **Bulbocavernosus reflex test** is done to determine if there is adequate nerve sensation in the penis. The doctor squeezes the glans of the penis which immediately causes the anus to contract, if nerve function is intact.

Laboratory Investigations

It will vary depending upon the history and clinical findings.
- Examination of semen is essential in cases of infertility.
- Tests for systemic diseases include blood counts, blood sugar (evaluation of diabetes), urinalysis, lipid and thyroid profiles, creatinine, liver enzymes and prostate-specific antigen.
- Serum testosterone, LH and serum prolactin.

> **NOTA BENE**
>
> **Other tests**
> - *Erectile capacity (intracavernosal injection):* Evaluation of penile function can be done by direct injection of PGE1 into the corpora. If the penile vasculature is adequate, an erection will develop.
> - *Duplex ultrasonography:* Vascular function within the penis including signs of atherosclerosis and scarring or calcification can be evaluated.
> - *Ultrasonography of testes:* Detect abnormalities in testes and epididymides. Transrectal ultrasonography can disclose abnormalities in the prostate and pelvis.
> - *Nocturnal penile tumescence testing:* Normally, a man has 5–6 erections during sleep, especially during REM—their absence may indicate defect in nerve function or blood supply in the penis. It may be useful in distinguishing psychogenic from organic impotence.
> - *Penile biothesiometry:* This test uses electromagnetic vibration to evaluate sensitivity and nerve function in the glans and shaft of the penis.

Examination of a Female

- Gynecologic examination should include an evaluation of hair distribution, clitoris size, Bartholin glands, labia majora and minora, and any lesion that could indicate the existence of venereal disease.
- In case of impotency in females, the defect usually lies in vagina and can be clearly observed. The inspection of the vaginal mucosa may also indicate a deficiency of estrogens or the presence of infection.
- The evaluation of the cervix should include a Papanicolaou test and cultures for sexually transmitted diseases.
- The postcoital test (*Sims-Huhner test*) consists of evaluating the amount of spermatozoa and its motility within the cervical mucus during the pre-ovulatory period.
- *Bimanual examination* should be performed to establish the direction of the cervix, and the size and position of the uterus to exclude the presence of uterine fibroids, adnexal masses, tenderness or pelvic nodules indicative of infection or endometriosis.

Laboratory Investigations

Besides routine blood and urine analysis, hysterosalpingogram (HSG), pelvic ultrasonography, hysterosonogram and MRI are required.

Opinion

- An opinion of ED (in males) cannot be given, because of the difficulty in ruling out all the causes, particularly the psychological component, unless there is gross deviation from normal.
- The opinion should be given in *double negative form*—stating that from examination of the male, there is nothing to suggest that the person is incapable of sexual intercourse.
- In case of infertility, opinion can be given with certainty depending on clinical and laboratory findings.

Medico-legal Issues

ED may form the basis of medico-legal investigation both in civil and criminal cases.

Civil Cases

The *civil court* may call upon a medical man to determine this point in suits of:

♦ Nullity of marriage	♦ Divorce
♦ Contested paternity	♦ Legitimacy
♦ Inheritance	♦ Claims for damages in ED due to assault

- Under the Indian law, permanent ED is a ground for nullity of marriage as he is incapable of fulfilling the rights of consummation of marriage (physical union by coitus), but sterility is not. The development of ED subsequent to consummation of marriage is not a valid ground for granting a decree of divorce.
- Under the IEA, there is presumption in favor of legitimacy of a child born during the continuance of a valid marriage between his mother and any man, or within 280 days after its dissolution, the mother remaining unmarried. The presumption can only be rebutted if it is shown by competent evidence that the parties to the marriage had no access to each other at any time when the child could have been begotten.

Criminal Cases

The *criminal court* may have to decide this question with the aid of medical man in accusation of alleged:

♦ Sodomy	♦ Bestiality
♦ Rape	♦ ED due to assault

- In the cases of rape, sodomy, and bestiality, the accused try to put forward the defense of ED, i.e., he is incapable to commit the act. However, after the Criminal Law (Amendment) Act, 2013, the amended Sec. 375 IPC provides that even penetration by finger or by objects and also non-penetrative acts come under the ambit of definition of rape/sexual assault. Thus, doing a potency examination of the accused in such cases appears irrelevant.
- In assault cases, an injured individual may assert that he has developed ED from wounds or injuries received, especially if they happen to have been inflicted on the head, neck, or loins (fracture of spine with cord injury).

NULLITY OF MARRIAGE AND DIVORCE

Sec. 11, 12 and 13 of the Hindu Marriage Act, 1955 deals with grounds for void and voidable marriages, and grounds for divorce respectively.

Grounds for Void and Voidable Marriage

a. **Void marriage**, i.e., null from the time of inception
   - Bigamy (another marriage without dissolution of earlier marriage)
   - Prohibited degree of relationship (related by blood) unless custom permits such marriage
   - Sapinda relationship (relationship extending to 3rd generation in the line of ascent through mother and 5th generation through father).
b. **Voidable marriage**, i.e., it remains valid until annulled by the court
   - Impotence
   - Unsoundness of mind of either party at the time of marriage
   - Consent of either party was obtained by force, fraud or misconception of facts
   - Pregnancy of the female by someone else, and the husband was ignorant of the fact at the time of marriage.

Grounds for Divorce

- *Adultery*: Voluntary sexual intercourse with any person other than his/her spouse.
- *Cruelty*: Willful and unjustifiable conduct so as to cause danger to life, limb or health of another (including mental health).
- *Desertion*: Abandonment of one spouse without reasonable cause and without consent or against the wish of other.
- *Apostasy*: Change of religion.
- *Unsoundness of mind.*
- *Virulent leprosy and sexually transmitted diseases* including AIDS.
- *Renouncing the world.*
- *Additional grounds for woman*: Husband convicted of rape, sodomy or bestiality.

NOTA BENE

- Impotence is inability to consummate the marriage (and not merely incapacity for procreation), and to be a ground for nullity, such inability must exist at the time of marriage and continue to exist at the time of the institution of the suit. For this purpose, sexual intercourse has been defined as ordinary and complete intercourse, not partial and imperfect intercourse.
- The birth of a child is not conclusive evidence that the marriage has been consummated, since **fecundation ab extra** (a rare occurrence) can take place. *Fecundatio ab extra* means pregnancy that occurs by mere deposition of semen on the vulva and there is no penile penetration into the vagina.

FM 3.23, 3.24
- Discuss sterilization of male and female.
- Discuss the relative importance of surgical methods of contraception (vasectomy and tubectomy) as methods of contraception in the National Family Planning Programme.

STERILIZATION

Definition: It is the process to cause a person sterile without affecting his/her potency or sexual functions.

Classification

Sterilization can be classified as given in **Flowchart 22.1**.

- **Compulsory:** It is performed on a person, compulsorily by an order of the State, carried out on mentally or physically defective person, or as punishment to sexual criminals, or for the purpose of eugenics. It is not done in India.
- **Voluntary:** It is carried on married persons with consent of both the husband and wife (preferable to have consent of both). It can be:
  i. *Therapeutic:* It is done to prevent danger to health or life of women due to future pregnancy.
  ii. *Eugenic:* It is carried out to prevent conception of the children who are likely to be physically or mentally defective.
  iii. *Contraceptive:* It is done as a family planning measure.

NOTA BENE

Chemical castration involves the administration of antiandrogen cyproterone acetate, contraceptive Depo-Provera or antipsychotic Benperidol. Unlike surgical castration, where the testicles are removed, chemical castration does not remove organs, nor is it a form of sterilization. These patients experience reductions in frequency and intensity of sexual drive, frequency of masturbation and sexual fantasies. This may be a treatment strategy for sex offenders and can be an alternative to life imprisonment or death penalty. The Justice Verma committee set up after the Delhi gang rape rejected the Government's proposal of chemical castration, since it considered such punishments as violation of human rights.

Contraception: The term contraception includes all measures (temporary or permanent) designed to prevent pregnancy due to coital act.

Methods (Flowchart 22.2)

Permanent

- **In males:** Vasectomy (dividing the vas deferens). Newer technique uses chemical sclerosing agents, like ethanol, formaldehyde and $AgNO_3$ that can eliminate the need of surgery.

Flowchart 22.1: Classification of sterilization

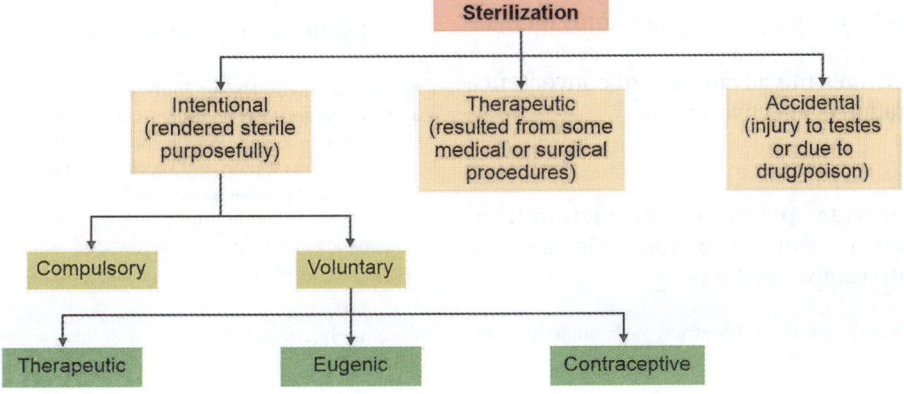

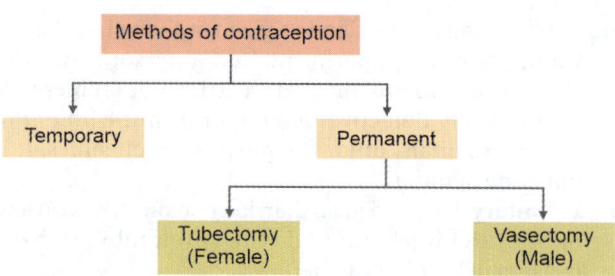

Flowchart 22.2: Methods of contraception

- **In females:** Tubectomy (fallopian tubes are ligated), hysteroscopy using electrocoagulation/cauterization, laparotomy or minilap (Pomeroy, Madelener, Aldridge methods, cornual resection, and fimbrectomy), and laparoscopy using clips.

Temporary

- Natural contraception—rhythm method, coitus interruptus and breastfeeding.
  - Rhythm period: Observing safe period—abstinence during fertile period of a cycle.
  - Coitus interruptus—withdrawal of penis shortly before ejaculation.
- Barrier contraceptives (spermicidal agents, diaphragm in females, condom in males).
- Intrauterine devices (IUD) or hormone containing IUD (Copper T 200, Cu T 380A, Multiload 250/375, levonorgestrel intrauterine system, progestasert and Lippes loop).
- Steroidal contraception
  - *Oral contraceptive pills*: Commonly used progestins are levonorgestrel, norethisterone or desogestrel; and estrogens are ethinyl-estradiol or mestranol.
  - *Injectable steroids*: Depo medroxy progesterone acetate (DMPA), norethisterone enanthate (NET-EN).
  - *Implants*: Norplant (levonorgestrel), Implanon (desogestrel).

Importance of Surgical Methods of Contraception

- Surgical procedures for contraception include tubal ligation for female sterilization and vasectomy for male sterilization.
- Sterilization provides the advantages of convenience and longer duration of effective action.

Advantages

- Sterilization provides permanent protection from unwanted pregnancy with no potential side effects of temporary contraceptive methods.
- It eliminates the need for continuous involvement in family planning activities.
- It spares couples from common worries associated with temporary methods, including partner compliance, domestic violence (arising from disagreements between partners about fertility goals), inconvenience, supply needs, and the consequences of forgetfulness.
- Vasectomy is generally more effective and safer than tubal ligation—it is performed under a local anesthetic and does not require as much technical expertise as tubal ligation.

Disadvantages

- Risk of surgery—infection, bleeding, damage to internal organs, anesthetic complications (tubal ligation)
- Permanent form of birth control—some may regret their decision because of unpredictable life events such as change in marital status or death of a child
- Do not protect against HIV and other STDs.

Medico-legal Aspects

i. There is no absolute guarantee to sterility after the operation, and the procedure may prove irreversible.*
   - A man is not sterilized immediately after vasectomy. Additional protection is needed for about 2–3 months following this operation. Condom should be advised for at least 20 ejaculations. ED may occur which is mostly psychological.
   - Overall failure rate in tubal sterilization is about 0.7%—failure due to fistula formation or due to spontaneous reanastomosis.
ii. Doctor may be implicated, if he performs sterilization without consent and proper indication. *Legally, the consent of the spouse is not required for sterilization.*
iii. Clients should be married; age of males should be <50 years and females >22 and <50 years of age. The couple should have at least one child whose age is >1 year unless the sterilization is medically indicated.
iv. Healthy unmarried or married persons without any issue should not be permanently sterilized, even if they volunteer for the same.
v. Failure of contraceptive measure adopted by males may lead to suspicion of wife having sexual relationship with another man who may initiate litigation—divorce, illegitimacy or disputed paternity.

Recent Advances: Newer contraceptives
- *Percutaneous vas occlusion* is an effective and reversible method, popular in China. Polyurethane elastomere is injected into vas which forms a plug and blocks the sperm passage. This plug can be removed under local anesthesia.
- *Gossypol*, an extract from cotton seed (discovered in China) and gonadotropin-releasing hormone (GnRH) analogs are other male contraceptives.

---

* According to Munro Kerr's Operative Obstetrics, 'no method of sterilization is entirely safe and complete, and there are possibilities of failure of operation due to many natural reason'.

- In females, centchroman, transdermal delivery system (nestorone), vaginal rings containing levonorgestrel, levonorgestrel (LNG) rod, uniplant (nomegestral), biodegradable injectable contraceptives, luteinizing hormone-releasing hormone (LHRH) agonist, quinacrine pellet, frameless intrauterine device (IUD) (GyneFix) and anti-hCG vaccine are being tested.
- The MoHFW has launched 'Antara' (DMPA) an injectable reversible contraceptive and the 'Chayya' (centchroman) pill.
- Phexxi, a nonhormonal gel is placed inside the vagina just before intercourse. The gel keeps the pH of the vagina in more acidic range, making it inhospitable to sperm.
- A new copper IUD—IUB Ballerine has been designed in Israel which is hormone-free, but it comes in a round shape.
- Other newly available contraceptives are Nextstellis (drospirenone and estetrol tablets), Annovera (segesterone acetate and ethinyl estradiol vaginal system), Slynd (drospirenone, a progestin-only pill) and Twirla (levonorgestrel and ethinyl estradiol transdermal system, a patch).

Discuss artificial insemination, test tube baby, surrogate mother, hormonal replacement therapy with respect to appropriate national and state laws.

ARTIFICIAL INSEMINATION (AI)

Definition: It is the process of introduction of semen from the husband or a donor by instruments into the vagina or uterus of a female to bring about pregnancy, which is not attainable by sexual intercourse.

- Semen can be introduced into the vagina (intra-vaginal insemination—IVI), cervix (intracervical—ICI), fallopian tube (intratubal—ITI) or uterine cavity (intrauterine—IUI) of the recipient.
- IUI is the most commonly used method of AI (higher success rate); and IVI (low success rate) and ITI (more invasive, greater risk of infection and higher costs) are the least commonly done AI.

Female infertility accounts for one-third of infertility cases, male infertility for another third, combined male and female infertility for another 15%, and the remainder of cases is 'unexplained'.

Types (Diff. 22.1)

i. AIH (artificial insemination homologous/husband)
ii. AID (artificial insemination donor)
iii. AIHD: 'Pooled' donor semen to which semen from husband has been added. There is a technical possibility of husband being father of the child.

Procedure: Semen is obtained by masturbation after a week's abstinence and 1 mL is deposited by means of a sterile needleless syringe just above the internal os, at the time of ovulation (14th day after menstruation) **(Fig. 22.5)**.

- The semen to be implanted is 'washed' in a laboratory and concentrated in Hams F10 media without L-glutamine, warmed to 37°C. This 'washing' increases the chances of fertilization while removing mucus and non-motile sperms in the semen.

- A more efficient method of AI is to insert semen directly into the woman's uterus. When this method is employed, it is important that only 'washed' semen is used and inserted by means of a catheter.

The success rate of AI vary depending on the type of insemination used, but typically the success rate varies between 5% and 30%. The success rate can be affected by factors such as stress, and quality of the egg and sperm.

Medico-legal Aspects

i. **Danger of litigation:** The doctor may be sued following the birth of a defective child. To avoid this, the donor must be screened for any genetic defects.
ii. **Nullity of marriage and divorce:** It is not a ground for divorce, if AI is done for sterility. If AI is due to erectile dysfunction, it is a ground for decree of nullity in favor of the wife due to non-consummation of marriage. If AID is done without the consent of the husband, then he can file for divorce and sue the doctor (regarded as an act of cruelty for the purpose of divorce).
iii. **Legitimacy of the child:** A child born through AID shall be presumed to be legitimate, born within wedlock, with consent of both the spouses, and with all the rights of parentage, support and inheritance.
iv. **Adultery or rape:** AID used for married woman with the consent of the husband does not amount to adultery on part of the wife or rape on part of the donor because there is no physical union by coitus.
v. **Incest:** Risk of incestuous relationship between the offspring born by AI and children of donor is possible.
vi. **Unmarried woman or widow:** A divorcee who is currently not married or a widow can opt for AID. Unmarried single woman (both Indian and foreign) or foreign couples, LGBTQIA+ and other third gender are not allowed to avail ART services.
vii. **Posthumous AID through a sperm bank:** A child born through AIH with the stored sperms of her deceased husband is considered to be legitimate, despite the existing law of presumptions under the Indian Evidence Act.
viii. **Psychosocial aspect:** If it is known that the husband consented to AID and the husband was not capable of consummating the marriage, difficulties may arise. The identity of the donor is kept secret; nevertheless, it is not uncommon for such secrets to be leaked out with adverse consequences.
ix. **Rights of sperm donors** are debatable issue nowadays.

For details of the ART Act, 2021 refer to Chapter 4.

Hormone replacement therapy (HRT) or hormone therapy involves the administration of synthetic estrogen and progesterone to replace a female's depleting hormone

DIFFERENTIATION 22.1: Artificial insemination by husband (AIH) and artificial insemination by donor (AID)

S.No.	Feature	AIH	AID
1.	Principle	Semen used is derived from woman's husband	Semen of person other than husband is used
2.	Indications	*Male factor* ♦ Erectile dysfunction ♦ Defects of the penis, e.g., hypospadias ♦ Retrograde ejaculation ♦ Decreased sperm counts, motility or quality *Female factor* ♦ Scant/unreceptive mucus ♦ Persistent cervicitis ♦ Cervical stenosis	♦ Husband sterile ♦ Husband suffering from hereditary disease ♦ Widows/unmarried women desiring children ♦ Rh incompatibility/Rh isoimmunization ♦ Multiple failures at in vitro fertilization (IVF) and intracytoplasmic sperm injection (ICSI)
3.	Pre-condition	None	Any healthy married or unmarried male Indian can donate sperms
4.	Consent	Needed from both husband and wife	Needed from husband, wife, donor and donor's wife (only donor, if single)
5.	Relation with recipient	Husband	Must not be a related to either spouses
6.	Donor characteristics	Nothing specific	Must be 21-55 years, should resemble closely to the husband in race
7.	Medical tests	Routine tests	Tuberculosis, diabetes, epilepsy, blood and Rh grouping, psychosis, endocrine dysfunction, hereditary or familial disorders (thalassemia), Venereal Disease Research Laboratory (VDRL), HbsAg B and C, and HIV are ruled out
8.	Disclosure of identity	Not a problem, wife knows	Donor and recipient should not know
9.	Outcome of AI	Known to the husband	Donor should not know
10.	Confidentiality	None	Strictly maintained*
11.	Doctor's role	May deliver the child who administered the AI	Should avoid delivering the child, as it would lead disclosing the identity of father in birth record
12.	Legal problems	No legal complications, except for divorce	Legal problems, like litigation against the doctor, illegitimacy, inheritance claims, divorce, incest and mental trauma may arise

*Disclosure of the donor's identity is to be made only when the court asks for it. In some countries, donor's identity is disclosed when the child attains 18 years of age.

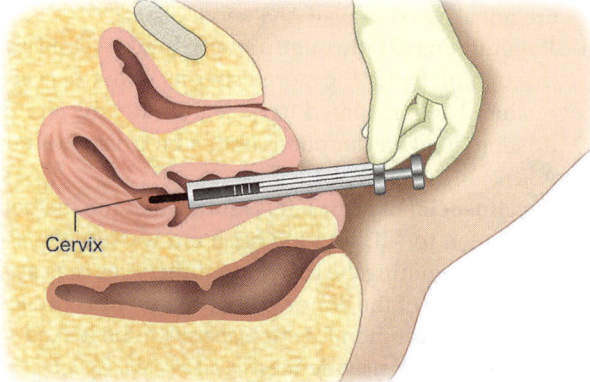

Fig. 22.5: Artificial insemination (intracervical)

levels and thus alleviate menopausal symptoms (like hot flashes, sweating, palpitations, irregular menstrual cycles, dyspareunia, etc.)

In ART procedures, HRT for a variable duration prior to the egg donation cycle enhances uterine (endometrial) receptivity during and after embryo transfer.

> **NOTA BENE**
>
> **Test tube baby:** Any child born from an embryo created by means of medical intervention that directly manipulates the sperm and egg cells.
>
> **Assisted reproductive technology (ART)**
> ♦ Surgical removal of eggs is known as *egg retrieval*.
> ♦ In vitro fertilization is the most common ART procedure.
>
> *Types of ART procedures*
> 1. **In vitro fertilization:** IVF involves controlled ovarian hyperstimulation with exogenous gonadotropins, oocyte retrieval via transvaginal ultrasonographic-guided aspiration, fertilization of oocytes with sperm in culture (or intracytoplasmic injection of sperm into the oocyte), and subsequent transfer of the resultant zygotes (3–5 days later) transcervically under ultrasound guidance into the uterine cavity.

CHAPTER 22 : Erectile Dysfunction and Sterility

Indications: Irreversible pathology of the fallopian tubes, infertility due to a subnormal male factor or immunological origin, idiopathic infertility and endometriosis.

2. **Gamete intrafallopian transfer (GIFT):** This involves ovarian stimulation; egg retrieval, followed by laparoscopically guided transfer of a mixture of unfertilized eggs and sperms into the fallopian tube (fertilization takes place inside the female's body).
3. **Zygote intrafallopian transfer (ZIFT):** Eggs are removed, day 1 fertilized eggs (zygotes) are laparoscopically transferred into the fallopian tube, rather than uterus.
4. **Intracytoplasmic sperm injection (ICSI):** Indicated in male factor infertility. One sperm is directly injected into an egg prior to intrauterine transfer of the fertilized eggs.
5. **Ovum donation:** Donor egg IVF is used for patients with poor egg numbers or quality. After inducing super-ovulation in an egg donor and followed by egg retrieval; eggs are fertilized by the sperms of the patient's husband and the embryos transferred to the patient's uterus.
6. Micromanipulation techniques include zona drilling and partial zona drilling.

Oocyte cryopreservation (egg freezing): This is a technique wherein the ovum from a healthy woman is taken and preserved at –196°C for future use. The process takes 2–4 weeks from injecting hormones to stimulate ovulation and egg retrieval. This is being used by working women—both single and married, who wants to delay pregnancy and focus on their careers. Initially, egg freezing was used for medical reasons where women suffering from diseases like cancer used to freeze their eggs before chemotherapy.

SURROGATE MOTHER

Definition: Surrogacy (surrogate pregnancy) is a legal agreement in which a woman agrees to carry a pregnancy that is genetically unrelated to her and her husband, with the intention to hand over the child to the genetic parents for whom she is acting as a surrogate (also called surrogate mother).

The surrogate mother may be the baby's biological mother (*traditional surrogacy*) or she may be implanted with someone else's fertilized egg (*gestational surrogacy*). She accepts pregnancy either by AI or by implantation of *in vitro* fertilized ova at the blastocyst stage, till delivery, for the woman who is incapable to bear child.

For details of the Surrogacy Act, 2021 refer to Chapter 4.

NOTA BENE

- **Surrogate parenting** involves a woman bearing the child of another woman, who is not in a position to bear children as a result of blocked Fallopian tubes or lack of a uterus. It is the reverse of donor insemination.
- The most common reason for using a surrogate mother is infertility. Gay male couples have also used surrogate mothers in order to have children that at least one partner is biologically related to.
- Surrogacy and posthumous reproduction are the extensions and ramifications arising out of ART. However ethical, legal, religious and social issues surrounding these procedures need to be clarified and understood. These are gray areas to be cautious about.

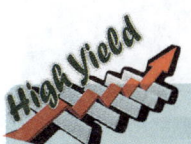

- **Marriage:** Contract between a man and a woman which implies physical union by coitus (legally).
- Same sex marriage is not legalized in India.
- **Divorce:** Legal cessation of a matrimonial bond.
- **Erectile dysfunction (impotence):** Consistent or recurrent inability to attain and/or maintain a penile erection sufficient for sexual intercourse.
- **Most common cause of erectile dysfunction:** Organic diseases.
- **Quod:** A male may be impotent with one particular female, but not with another.
- **Frigidity:** Inability to initiate or maintain the sexual arousal pattern (sexual coldness) in females (*feminine equivalent of impotence*).
- **Vaginismus:** Spastic contraction of vaginal outlet (involuntary reflex) in females due to fear, pain, disgust or apprehension for intercourse (may lead to impotency in females).
- **Test to determine nerve sensation in penis:** Bulbocavernosus reflex test.
- **Test to distinguish psychogenic from organic impotence:** Nocturnal penile tumescence test.
- **Grounds for nullity of marriage (divorce):** Impotency, pre-existing mental illness.
- **Fecundatio ab extra**: Pregnancy by deposition of semen on the vulva and there is no penile penetration into the vagina.
- **Sterility:** Absolute inability of either a male or a female to procreate.
- **Infertility:** Failure to conceive after 1 year of unprotected and regular intercourse.
- **Sterilization:** Process to make a person sterile without affecting his/her potency.
- In artificial insemination, semen from husband/donor is introduced by instruments into vagina or uterus of a female.

- **Indications for husband insemination:** Erectile dysfunction, defects of penis, retrograde ejaculation, oligospermia, unreceptive mucus, persistent cervicitis.
- **Indications for donor insemination:** Husband sterile, hereditary disease, widows/unmarried women, Rh incompatibility.
- In AID, donor can be single or married, must not be a related to either spouses, must be 21-55 years and strict confidentiality is maintained.
- If AI is done for sterility, it is not a ground for divorce; but if AI is due to ED, it is a ground.
- **Assisted reproductive technology:** Any infertility treatment in which gametes are manipulated outside the body and are replaced back to establish pregnancy.
- **Surrogate mother:** A woman who under a legal agreement carries a child for a couple/single person with the intention of giving up the child, once it is born.
- **Most common reason for using a surrogate mother:** Infertility.
- **Adoption of child:** Permits single female to adopt a child of any gender, whereas single male person is allowed to adopt only male child and not a girl child.

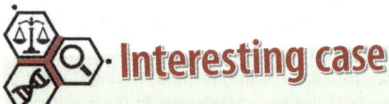

Potency Test (Case of Asaram Bapu, 2013)

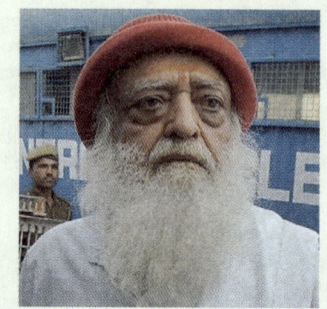

In 2013, a 16-year-old girl lodged a police complaint accusing the 72-year-old godman Asaram Bapu of sexually assaulting her at his ashram on the pretext of exorcism. He was arrested under various sections of the POCSO Act and the IPC after the medical examination of the girl confirmed sexual assault. Asaram denied the charge, and his son claimed that the girl was 'mentally unstable'. The preacher was made to undergo a potency test after he told the police that he is suffering from erectile dysfunction and incapable of committing the crime for which he has been charged with.

The potency test is done to determine whether an accused is physically capable of the act of penetration. Asaram consented for the potency test. His potency was established in the first stage of the examination—visual examination and physical stimulation. The doctor ruled out any sort gross damage or deformity from visual examination. Then manual stimulation was administered to his private parts by the medical staff that resulted in erection. If manual stimulation does not work, then drugs like papaverine is injected to check potency which was not required in his case. Penile Color Doppler or Nocturnal Penile Tumescence tests were also not done.

The potency report stated that 'there is no evidence to suggest that he is incapable of performing a sexual act'. The positive test gave prosecutors the circumstantial medical evidence against Asaram. The law recognizes these tests that clearly indicated that the septuagenarian did not suffer from erectile dysfunction. In 2018, the court found him guilty of raping the minor girl and awarded life imprisonment, along with a fine of ₹500,000 which was to be paid to the victim.

CHAPTER 23

Virginity, Pregnancy and Delivery

LEARNING OBJECTIVES

Must know
1. Virgin, defloration, pregnancy, delivery, legitimate and illegitimate child
2. Normal female genitalia anatomy
3. Causes of rupture of hymen, signs of virginity and why 'virginity testing' is unscientific, inhuman and derogatory
4. Presumptive, probable and positive (conclusive) signs of pregnancy
5. Medico-legal aspects of pregnancy
6. Pseudocyesis
7. Superfetation and superfecundation
8. Supposititious child, posthumous birth, atavism
9. Signs and symptoms of recent delivery in living
10. Signs and symptoms of remote delivery in dead
11. Lochia
12. True and false virgin (Diff.)
13. Nulliparous and parous uterus (Diff.)

Desirable to know
1. Types of hymen
2. Medico-legal aspects of delivery, legitimacy
3. Fetus compressus

FM 3.18
- Describe and discuss how 'signs' of virginity (so called 'virginity test', including two finger tests on female genitalia) are unscientific, inhuman and discriminatory.
- Describe and discuss how to appraise the courts about unscientific basis of these tests if court orders it.

Definitions

- **Virgin** (Latin *virgo*: maiden, *intacta*: untouched): A female who has not experienced sexual intercourse.
- **Defloration:** The act of depriving a woman of her virginity.
- **Pregnancy:** It is a condition which occurs in the female when she carries a fertilized ovum within the uterus.
- **Delivery:** Expulsion or extraction of the child at birth.

NORMAL FEMALE GENITALIA (FIG. 23.1)

- **Vulva** includes female genitalia visible externally—the *mons veneris* (pad of fat lying in front of the pubis), labia majora and minora, clitoris, vestibule, hymen and urethral opening.
- **Perineum** is the wedge-shaped area between the lower end of posterior wall of vagina and the anterior anal wall.
- **Labia majora** are the two elongated folds of skin projecting downwards and backwards from the mons

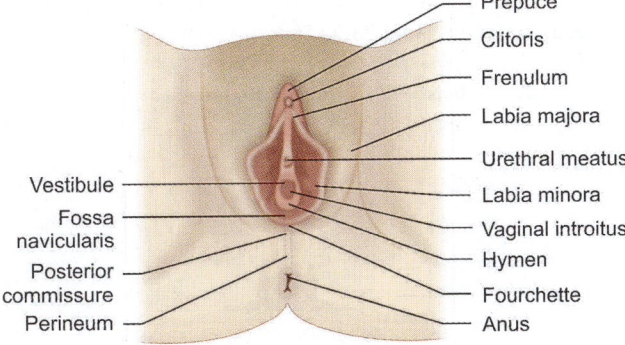

Fig. 23.1: Normal female genitalia (vulva)

veneris—homologous with the scrotum in males. They meet in front to form the *anterior commissure,* and in back, the *posterior commissure,* in front of the anus.

- **Labia minora** are two pinkish, thin folds of skin just within the labia majora. Anteriorly, they divide to enclose the clitoris, and unite with each other in front and behind the clitoris to form the *prepuce* and *frenulum* respectively. The lower portions of labia minora fuse in midline to form a fold called *fourchette*. The depression between fourchette and the vaginal orifice is called *fossa navicularis*.

- **Vestibule** is the triangular space bounded anteriorly by clitoris, posteriorly by fourchette and laterally by labia minora. The clitoris is small, and the vestibule is narrow in virgins.
- **Vagina** is narrow and tight, the mucosa is rugose, reddish in color and its walls are approximated. After frequent sexual intercourse, the rugae become less marked, and the vagina lengthens into the posterior fornix.

Hymen: The hymen is a fold of mucous membrane, about 1 mm thick, situated at the vaginal outlet.
- It is usually a thin transparent membrane, but it may be tough, fleshy or cartilaginous.
- In infants, a small swab can be passed through the hymenal orifice into the vagina.
- At 10 years of age, the tip of the small finger and at puberty, one finger may be passed into the vagina.

Types of Hymen (Fig. 23.2)

i. **Annular:** Opening is situated centrally.
ii. **Semilunar or crescentic:** Opening is placed anteriorly.
iii. **Cribriform:** Multiple openings.
iv. **Septate:** Two openings occur side by side, separated by thin hymenal tissue.
v. **Infantile:** Small linear opening in the middle.
vi. **Vertical:** Opening is vertical.
vii. **Imperforate:** No opening.
- The margin of the hymen is sometimes *fimbriated* and shows multiple notches which may be mistaken for artificial tears **(Fig. 23.2)**.*

- After the birth of a child, hymen is completely lost and the remnants are represented by cicatrized nodules of varying sizes called *the carunculae hymenales or myrtiformes*. On both sides, it is lined by stratified squamous epithelium.

Causes of Rupture of Hymen

i. **Sexual intercourse:** Most common cause of defloration.
ii. **Masturbation**, especially with some large foreign body. Hymen is not injured in most cases, as manipulation is usually limited to parts anterior to the hymen.
iii. An **accident**, like fall on a projecting substance or by slipping on the furniture or fence. It does not rupture by jumping, riding, vigorous exercise and dancing.
iv. **Gynecological examination** or **surgical operation**.
v. **Foreign body insertion** for rendering minors fit for sexual intercourse.
vi. **Sanitary tampons**.

When a virgin is placed in lithotomy position with legs wide apart, the vagina remains closed and only the edges of labia minora are seen slightly protruding from between the closed labia majora. A single intercourse does not alter the parts much, except rupture of the hymen.

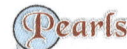

Principal signs of virginity
i. An intact hymen
ii. Normal condition of fourchette and posterior commissure
iii. Narrow vagina with rugose walls

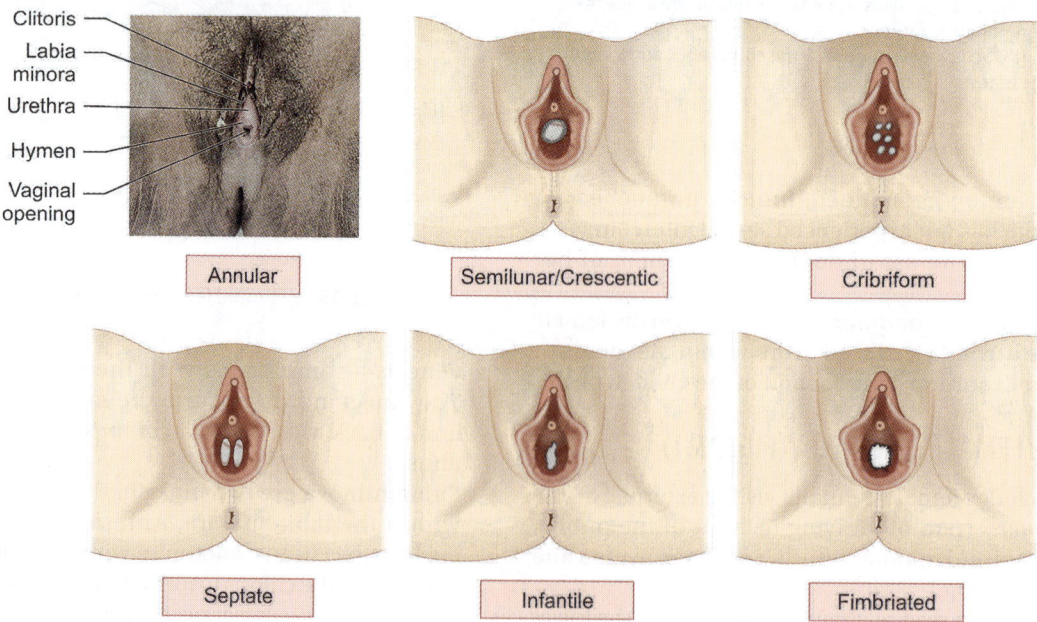

Fig. 23.2: Types of hymen

---
* The notches are usually symmetrical, occur anteriorly, do not extend to the vaginal wall, mucous membrane over the notches is intact, and with no signs of inflammation.

CHAPTER 23 : Virginity, Pregnancy and Delivery

Match the following hymen:

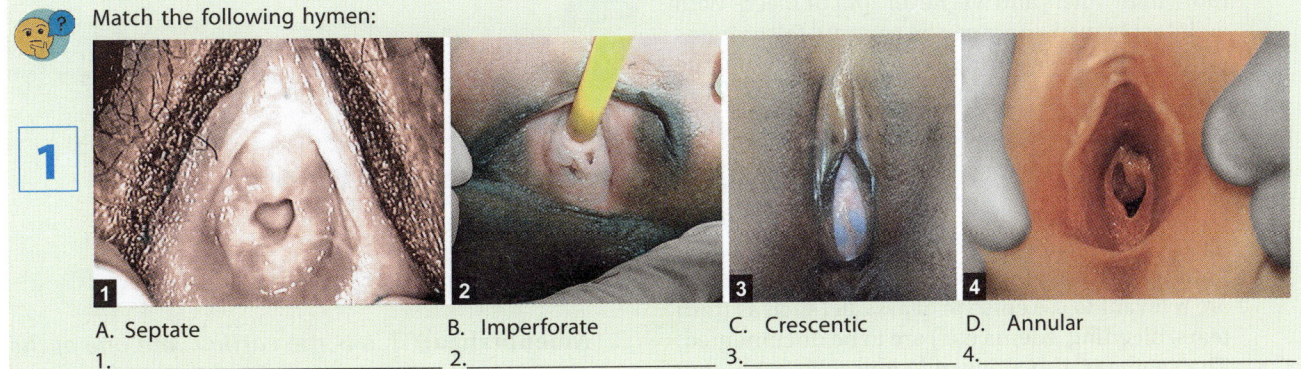

A. Septate B. Imperforate C. Crescentic D. Annular
1._____ 2._____ 3._____ 4._____

MEDICO-LEGAL ASPECTS

'Virginity test' or 'two-finger test' is an explicitly intrusive physical examination wherein a doctor inserts two fingers inside the vagina (*per vaginal* examination)* to check if the hymen is intact or torn, assess the size of a vaginal opening and determine the laxity and rugosity of vaginal muscles.

Reasons for Two-Finger Testing

Two-finger testing is/was performed on women/girls:
- To determine a bride's virginity before she is married (still being used in many countries).
- Accused of moral crimes or have run away from home.
- During medical examinations of female applicants in military and police (in Indonesia).
- To refute claims that the women had been raped while in detention (Egyptian revolution, 2011).
- To deter pre-marital sexual activity and reduce HIV prevalence (among school girls in rural South Africa and Swaziland).
- In nullity of marriage and divorce cases.
- To assess rape survivors.

NOTA BENE
- In rape survivor, if the fingers are inserted too easily and there is still room for more fingers, the doctor would write that the woman is 'habitual to sexual intercourse'.
- The test is often used by defendant's lawyer to label rape survivors as 'loose women', and identified as being 'habituated to sex'.
- The medical evidence of past intercourse is used to cast doubt on the rape allegation and weaken her case—either to
  - Suggest a survivor lied about the sexual assault
  - Imply that the sexual assault wasn't harmful
  - Suggest the moral impropriety of the survivor and therefore her lack of entitlement to justice.

Current Status

In 2022, the Supreme Court again reiterated the ban (earlier done in 2003 and 2013) on the 'two-finger test' in rape cases.

Two-finger test is against the ethical principles, medical indications and legal status.

- Forcibly conducting a two-finger examination without the patient's consent is a form of sexual assault (like any genital examination without consent)—against autonomy. In many situations, even when requested by a patient (for virginity certificate), 'virginity testing' is not voluntary.
- Virginity is not a medical condition requiring diagnosis and treatment. This test does not provide any clinical benefit to a patient, and have several harms associated with it, such as the risks of physical discomfort and pain. It may mimic the original act of sexual violence, aggravating survivors' sense of disempowerment and cause revictimization. This can also cause anxiety, depression and PTSD, especially if it is done against the patient's will and without her consent.
- Virginity testing is, in most cases, for the benefit of other parties (usually family, intended spouses or State). Being put in a position to 'prove' to third parties that one is a 'virgin', may result in experiencing a sense of powerlessness, fear, humiliation, worthlessness and lack of the right to self-determination.
- 'Two-finger testing' is an example of gender-based oppression and discrimination, and it puts doctors in a morally and professionally complex position of acting as 'the morality police'. Doctors should resist pressure from any source to use medical skills in ways that attempt to legitimize violations of human rights.
- Even if a doctor agrees to do the 'two-finger examination,' their ability to determine whether a woman has ever had intercourse (with or without consent) from the physical examination alone is extremely limited, if non-existent. Published literature has proven that physical examination of the hymen and vagina is an extremely poor predictor and unreliable in determining if prior sexual intercourse has occurred.
  - The hymen is a flexible piece of mucosal tissue that may be thick, thin or even absent in some women. Hymenal injuries may heal rapidly with little or no evidence of previous trauma. Some hymens stretch

---
* Most commonly done to assess status of vagina, cervix, and progress of descent of fetus through birth canal.

more than others and will never split or bleed. With an intact hymen, there can be true and false virgins **(Diff. 23.1)**. The features will be same for a deflorate woman and a false virgin with the exception of presence of hymen in the latter. Hence, an intact hymen does not rule out sexual violence, and a torn hymen does not prove previous sexual intercourse.

- Hymen should therefore be treated like any other part of the genitals while documenting examination findings in cases of sexual violence. Only those that are relevant to the episode of assault (such as fresh tears, bleeding, edema etc.) are to be documented.
- The vagina is also a dynamic muscular canal that varies in size and shape depending on individual, developmental stage, physical position, and various hormonal factors such as sexual arousal and stress, etc. Vaginal mucosal barrier is also resistant to abrasion from friction.
- Moreover, determining the laxity is also dependent on the observer variations. If an examiner has slender fingers it may be loose, and if thick fingers, then it may be tight.

Hence, two-finger test is not prescribed as one of the procedures to be adopted while examining survivors of sexual assault and rape. For civil cases of nullity of marriage/divorce or defamation, examination should to be done with consent and not to rely on 'two-finger examination' only. The fallacies/drawbacks of the examination should be to be informed to all the stakeholders.

Discuss the signs of pregnancy.

PREGNANCY

Diagnosis of Pregnancy in the Living

See **Flowchart 23.1**.

PRESUMPTIVE SIGNS/SYMPTOMS

i. **Amenorrhea:** This is the *earliest and one of the most important symptoms of pregnancy.* Cessation of menstruation may result from ill-health, intense desire for pregnancy or fear of pregnancy after illicit intercourse. Women who have never menstruated may become pregnant, and pregnancy may also occur in a woman during lactational amenorrhea.

ii. **Changes in breasts:** Changes are quite characteristic in primigravidas, but are of lesser value in multiparas. Tenseness and tingling in the breasts is evident by 6–8th week. The nipples become deeply pigmented and more erectile, and the areola becomes dark-brown.

- Around the nipple, the sebaceous glands become enlarged *(Montgomery's tubercles)* by the end of 3rd month **(Fig. 23.3A)**. *Colostrum* (thin, yellowish fluid) is secreted as early as 12th week, which becomes thick and yellow by 16th week.

DIFFERENTIATION 23.1: True and false virgins

S.No.	Feature	True virgin	False virgin
1.	Basic difference	Woman has not experienced sexual intercourse	Woman has experienced sexual intercourse
Genital signs			
2.	Hymen	◆ Intact, rigid, inelastic ◆ Admits tip of little finger through orifice painfully	◆ Intact, but loose, elastic or thick, tough and fleshy ◆ Easily admits two fingers through orifice
3.	Labia majora	Thick, fleshy, completely close the vaginal orifice	Less fleshy, not apposed to each other, not prominent, vaginal orifice may be seen
4.	Labia minora	Small, pinkish, covered by majora and are in close contact with it	Enlarged, pigmented, not in contact, exposed and separated from majora
5.	Vagina	◆ Narrow ◆ Marked rugosity of wall ◆ Full length of finger cannot be admitted	◆ Capacious ◆ Rugae less obvious ◆ Full length can be admitted
6.	Fossa navicularis	Present	Disappears
7.	Fourchette	Intact	Torn, may show healed scar
8.	Vestibule	Narrow	Gaping, wide, spacious
9.	Clitoris	Small	Enlarged
10.	Posterior commissure	Intact	May be torn
Extragenital signs (in breasts)			
11.	Size, shape and consistency	Small, hemispherical, firm	Large, pendulous, flabby
12.	Areola	Pink	Pigmented
13.	Nipples	Small, pink	Enlarged, pigmented

Flowchart 23.1: Signs of pregnancy

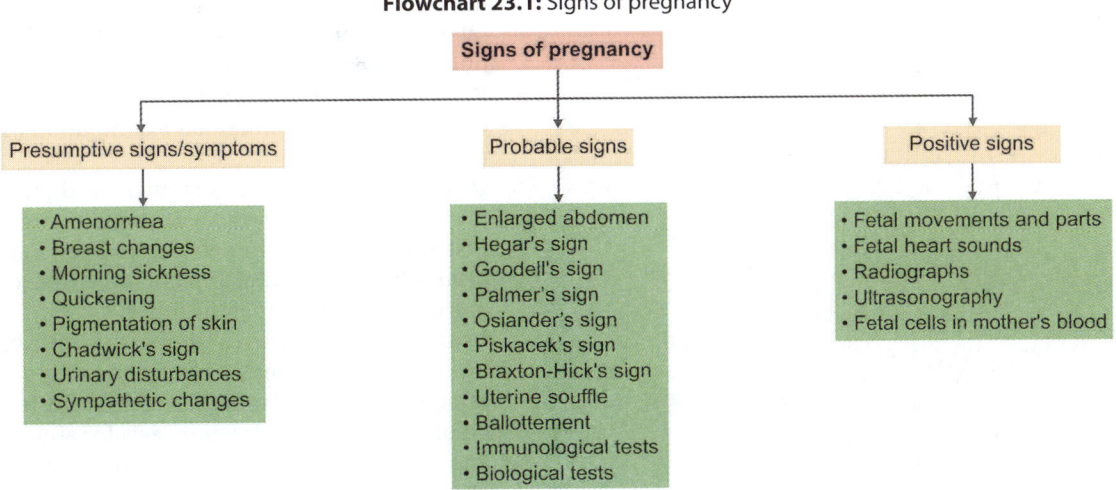

- Secondary areola, especially in primigravida usually appears by 20th week.
- After 6th month, *silvery lines or striae gravidarum* (stretch marks) are seen, especially in primiparae due to the stretching of the skin **(Fig. 23.3B)**.

iii. **Morning sickness:** It usually appears about the end of the 1st month and disappears by end of 3rd month. Nausea and vomiting are usually present in the morning and pass off in a few hours. It more prominent in primigravidas.

iv. **Quickening:** Near about 18th week (16th week in multipara), the pregnant woman feels slight fetal movements in her abdomen (their first appearance is known as '*quickening*'), which gradually increase in intensity.

v. **Pigmentation of the skin:** The vulva, abdomen and axillae become darker due to the deposition of pigment, and a dark line extends from the pubis to beyond the umbilicus which is called the *linea nigra* (Latin, black line; seen by 20th week) **(Fig. 23.3B)**.

vi. **Melasma/Chloasma:** Pigmentation over forehead and cheek (pregnancy mask) may appear at about 24th week **(Fig. 23.3C)**.

vii. **Jacquemier's or Chadwick's sign:** The mucous membrane of the vagina changes from pink to violet, deepening to blue as a result of venous obstruction at about 8th week of pregnancy.

viii. **Urinary disturbances:** During 8–12th week of pregnancy, the enlarging uterus exerts pressure on the bladder and produces frequent micturition. This gradually disappears after 12th week as the uterus straightens up into the abdomen, and reappears a few weeks before term when the head descends into the pelvis.

ix. **Fatigue:** Easy fatigue is very frequent.

x. **Sympathetic disturbances:** Salivation, altered appetite and irritable temper are common.

> **NOTA BENE**
> Mnemonic for presumptive signs of pregnancy: **ABCDEF**
> A: Amenorrhea; B: Breast changes; C: Chadwick's sign, chloasma; D: Diuresis; E: Emesis; F: Fatigue

PROBABLE SIGNS OF PREGNANCY

i. **Enlargement of the abdomen (fundal height):** During pregnancy, abdomen gradually enlarges in size

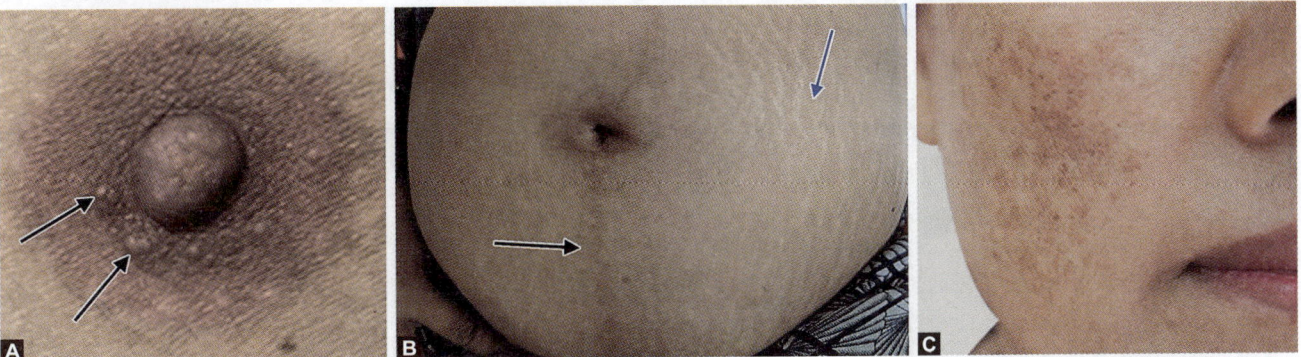

Figs. 23.3A to C: Presumptive signs of pregnancy: (A) Montgomery's tubercles; (B) Linea nigra (black arrow) and striae gravidarum (blue arrow); (C) Melasma

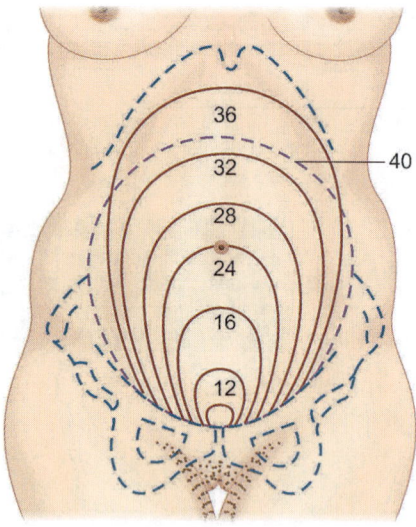

Fig. 23.4: The level of fundus uteri at different weeks

after the 12th week as shown in **Figure 23.4**. During the last two months, the uterus sinks into the pelvis and tends to fall forward due to its weight.
- Uterus feels soft and elastic, and becomes ovoid in shape, which changes to spherical shape beyond 36th week.
- The umbilicus becomes level with the skin by about the 7th month.

ii. **Hegar's sign** is positive between 6–10th week.
Demonstration: If one hand is placed on the abdomen and two fingers of other hand in the vagina, the firm hard cervix is felt and above it the elastic body of the uterus, while between the two, the isthmus is felt as a soft compressible area **(Fig. 23.5)**. This is the most valuable physical sign of early pregnancy.

iii. **Goodell's sign:** As early as 6th week, the cervix progressively softens from below upward. Pregnant woman's cervix feels like lips and non-pregnant woman's like the tip of the nose. The cervical orifice, during the last months of pregnancy, becomes circular instead of being transverse and admits the point of finger to a greater depth.

iv. **Palmer's sign:** Regular rhythmic contractions of uterus can be elicited by bimanual examination as early as 4–8th week.

v. **Osiander's sign:** There is an increased pulsation felt through the lateral fornices at about 8th week.

vi. **Piskacek's sign:** Asymmetrical enlargement of uterus occurs, if there is lateral implantation. Here one half of uterus is more firm that the other.

vii. **Braxton-Hick's contractions:** Intermittent, spasmodic, painless uterine contractions are observed rarely before the 3rd month, but are easily felt after the 4th month. Each contraction lasts for about a minute and relaxation for about 2–3 minutes (min). *They are present even when the fetus is dead.*

viii. **Ballottement** (toss up like a ball): This is positive during the 4th–5th month of pregnancy as the fetus is small in relation to the amount of amniotic fluid present.

Demonstration
- *Vaginal/internal ballottement:* Two fingers are inserted into the anterior fornix and a sudden upward motion given. This causes the fetus to move up in the liquor amnii and after a moment, the fetus drops down on the fingers, like a ball bouncing back—can be elicited between 16th to 28th weeks **(Fig. 23.5)**.
- *External ballottement:* A sudden motion is given to the abdominal wall covering the uterus, in a few seconds the rebound of the fetus can be felt **(Fig. 23.5)**.

ix. **Uterine souffle:** It is a soft blowing murmur, which is synchronous with the mother's pulse. It is heard towards the end of 4th month by auscultation, on either side of the uterus (due to passage of blood through the uterine vessels) just above inguinal ligament.

x. **Biological tests:** These are based on the reaction of test animals to human chorionic gonadotropins (hCG) in

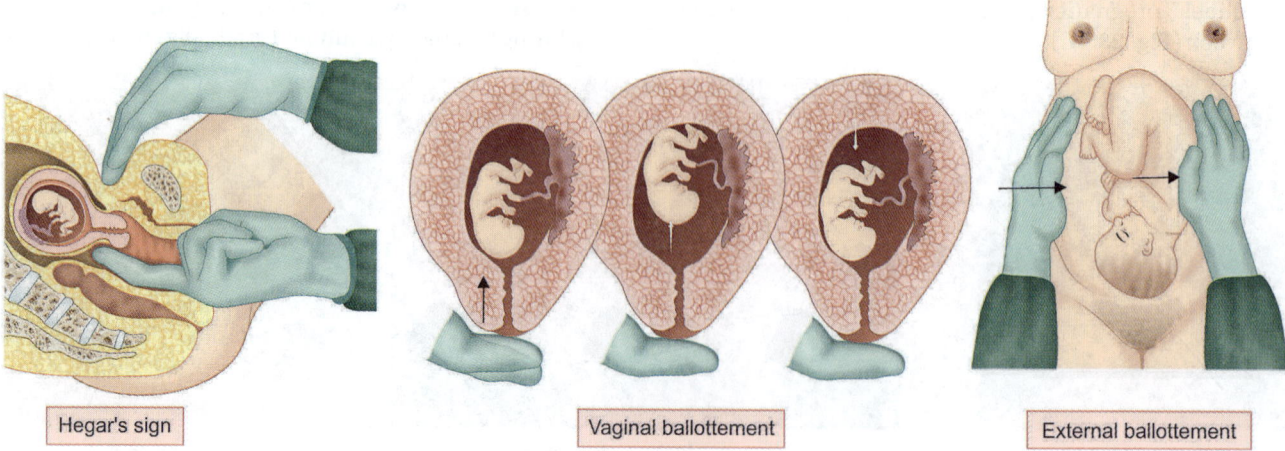

Fig. 23.5: Probable signs of pregnancy

the pregnant woman's serum or urine. These tests are rarely done nowadays.

xi. **Immunological tests**
- Human chorionic gonadotropin (hCG) appear in the maternal urine/serum about 1 week after implantation as the placenta begins to develop and produce increasing amounts of hCG. It has been detected in urine on day 16 of the cycle, and in serum 6–8 days after the presumed day of conception.
- By the first missed menstrual period, the hCG level may exceed 100 mIU/mL and by 10–12th week of pregnancy, the level is >100,000 mIU/mL.
- Level begins to decline about the 3rd month of pregnancy and is not detectable within a few days after delivery.
- Many tests are designed to detect hCG levels as low as 25 mIU/mL in urine and often positive before menstrual period is missed.
- Immunological tests have replaced biological tests for routine screening. The first voided urine in the morning contains the highest level of hCG and is preferable for testing.
- *Limitations*: It will give positive test with ectopic pregnancy, hydatidiform mole, choriocarcinoma and breast or ovarian tumors.

1. **Immunoassays without radioisotopes**
   a. *Indirect agglutination inhibition test* (**Gravindex test**): A simple rapid test using latex particles coated with a purified preparation of hCG as the antigen and an antiserum to hCG. A drop of antiserum is mixed with a drop of urine on a glass slide for 30 seconds. Then, 2 drops of the sensitized latex particles are added and the slide shaken for 2 min (**Flowchart 23.2**).
   b. *Direct agglutination test:* The latex particles are coated with anti-hCG antibodies. This reagent is mixed directly with the urine. If hCG is present in the urine, it will combine with the antibodies and cause agglutination of the latex particles (**positive test**). If no hCG is present in the urine, there will be no agglutination of the latex particles (**negative test**).
   c. *Enzyme-linked immunosorbent assay (ELISA):* Icon II test is based on beta-hCG monoclonal antibody detection.
   d. *Fluoroimmunoassay.*
2. **Immunoassays with radioisotopes**
   a. *Radioimmunoassay (RIA):* The test detects levels of beta-hCG as low as 2–4 mIU/mL.
   b. *Immunoradiometric assay (IRMA).*

POSITIVE/CONCLUSIVE SIGNS OF PREGNANCY

i. **Fetal movements and parts:** Fetal movements and fetal parts can be identified distinctly by 20th–22nd week on abdominal palpation.

ii. **Fetal heart sounds:** *Definite sign of pregnancy.* They are heard between 18–20th week with an ordinary stethoscope. The sounds are like the ticking of a watch placed under a pillow. The rate is usually about 160/min at 5th month and 140/min at 9th month (normal range 110–160 beat/min), and is not synchronous with the mother's pulse.
   - Uterine souffle and fetal souffle (due to inrush of blood through umbilical arteries) may be confused with fetal heart sound.

Pearls
Fetal heart sounds are not audible
- Before 18 weeks of pregnancy
- When the fetus is dead
- Hydramnios (excessive quantity of liquor amnii)
- Obese patient
- Fetal position in the uterus is such which prevents transmission of sounds

iii. **Radiographic imaging:** The earliest fetal skeletal shadow of vertebral dots is visible at about 16th week of pregnancy. The shadows to be searched in the pelvis of the mother are:
   - Series of small dots in a linear arrangement of the vertebral column.
   - Crescentic or annular shadows of the skull.

Flowchart 23.2: Indirect agglutination inhibition test

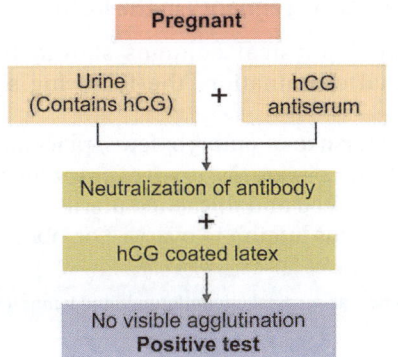 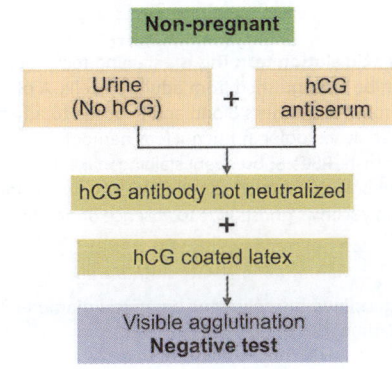

- Series of fine curved parallel lines of the ribs.
- Linear shadows of the limbs.

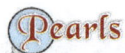

Radiological signs of fetal death
- **Spalding's sign** (loss of alignment and overriding of skull bones)
- **Robert's sign** (presence of gas in the heart and great vessels)
- **Ball sign** (excessive flexion of the spinal column due to absence of muscle tone)
- **Deuel's halo sign** (elevation of the subcutaneous fat of fetal scalp from cranial bones)
- **Helix sign** (presence of gas in umbilical arteries)

iv. **Ultrasonography***: Gestational sac and yolk sac can be identified by 4–5th menstrual week (after first day of last menstrual period), fetal pole and embryonic movements by 7th week.
  - *Transvaginal sonography* (TVS) is the most accurate means and can detect cardiac activity by 5th week and transabdominal sonography by 6th week.
  - A real-time scanner can detect cardiac activity by 8th week. Doppler ultrasound can pick up the fetal heart rate reliably by 10th week (average 8–10 weeks).
  - Fetal sex can be determined by ultrasound by 11 weeks of pregnancy, but reliable assessment is not possible until 12–13 weeks of gestation (those with normal external genitalia).
  - Magnetic resonance imaging (MRI) can also be used to determine fetal anatomy.

v. **Fetal cells and fetal DNA in maternal blood:** Some fetal cells also make their way into the maternal bloodstream. These cells can be detected in the mother's peripheral blood.
  - Fetal sex can be determined as early as 6 weeks of gestation by using molecular diagnostic methods that analyze the free fetal DNA (acellular fetal DNA shed from placental cells) from maternal blood using real-time PCR.

Mnemonic for positive signs of pregnancy: RUFFF
R: Radiological signs; **U:** Ultrasound; **F:** Fetal heart sounds; **F:** Fetal movements; **F:** Fetal cells in mother's blood.

NOTA BENE

Kleihauer-Betke or acid elution test: This is a staining technique in which fetal cells can be distinguished from adult red cells. A blood smear is prepared from the mother's blood and exposed to an acid bath.† This removes adult hemoglobin, but not fetal hemoglobin (HbF is resistant to acid) from the RBCs. Subsequent staining makes fetal cells (containing fetal hemoglobin) appear rose-pink in color, while adult red blood cells are only seen as 'ghosts' due to absence of staining.

Sequential appearance of signs and symptoms of pregnancy are highlighted in **Table 23.1**.

TABLE 23.1: Signs and symptoms of pregnancy

Duration	Signs and symptoms
At 6–8 weeks	
Symptoms	Amenorrhea, morning sickness, frequent micturition, fatigue and breast discomfort
Signs	Breast enlargement. Signs—Jacquemier's, Osiander's, Goodell's, Hegar's and Palmer's. Immunological tests positive Sonography: Cardiac activity and embryonic movements
At 16–18 weeks	
Symptoms	Amenorrhea, quickening, other symptoms disappear
Signs	Breast—pigmentation of areola, prominence of Montgomery's tubercles, colostrum. Uterus—midway between pubis and umbilicus, Braxton-Hick's contractions, uterine souffle and internal ballottement. X-ray: Fetal shadow
At 20 weeks	
Symptoms	Amenorrhea, quickening
Signs	Breast—appearance of secondary areola, linea nigra. Uterus—at level of umbilicus (24 weeks), Braxton-Hick's contractions, external ballottement and internal ballottement (16–28 weeks). Fetus—parts, movements and heart sounds

Maximum and Minimum Period of Gestation

- The usually accepted average is 280 days from the first day of the last menstrual period, so that the actual period of gestation is about 266 days or less.
- The woman may over-carry the fetus to post-maturity up to a period of 320 days or even up to 350 days.
- Expulsion of fetus may occur at any period before full term. Medically, for a fetus to be viable, it should be ≥28 weeks of gestation.
- A fetus born after 180 days of gestation may survive, if proper care is taken.

Diagnosis of Pregnancy in the Dead

External physical changes should be noted. In the internal examination, the following should be looked for:
  i. Presence of embryo, fetus, placental tissue or membranes—*positive proof of pregnancy*
  ii. Enlarged and thickened uterus
  iii. Corpus luteum in ovary—corroborative evidence.

---

* Gestational age is determined by measuring biparietal diameter, head circumference, abdominal circumference and femur length. Absence of fetal cardiac motion in real-time USG confirms fetal death.
† In Apt test, alkali is used as HbF is also resistant to it.

CHAPTER 23 : Virginity, Pregnancy and Delivery

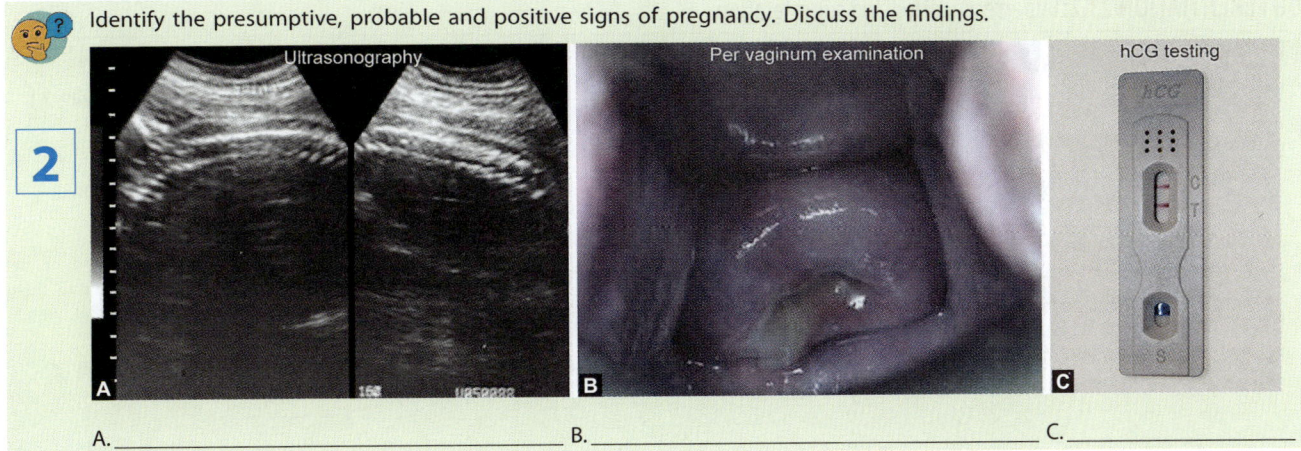

Identify the presumptive, probable and positive signs of pregnancy. Discuss the findings.

A. _____ B. _____ C. _____

PSEUDOCYESIS (SPURIOUS/FALSE/PHANTOM PREGNANCY)

Definition: It is a psychological disorder where the woman has a false but firm belief that she is pregnant, although no pregnancy exists.
- It is generally observed in infertile females or women nearing menopause, who desire a child intensely.
- Most of these women suffer from some form of psychic or hormonal disorder.
- Such patients may present with all the subjective symptoms of pregnancy including cessation of menstruation and associated with a considerable increase in the size of the abdomen which may be due to abnormal deposition of fat or due to pathological conditions, like ovarian tumor or ascites.
- The woman may have secretions from the breasts and intestinal movements, which she imagines as fetal movements and may have false labor pains.
- Obstetrical examination along with ultrasonography and/or immunological tests for pregnancy will clear the patient of her imagination.

Medico-legal importance: The patient may sue the doctor for causing miscarriage or aborting the fetus. He should disclose the information in the presence of a witness such as a nurse or her relative. It is also essential to collect and preserve any evidence confirming pseudocyesis, e.g., urine pregnancy test and ultrasound scan.

FM 3.19
Discuss superfetation and superfecundation.

SUPERFECUNDATION

Definition: Fertilization of two ova discharged from the ovary *at the same period of ovulation* by two different acts of coitus committed at short intervals.

- The term is also used to refer to instances of two different males fathering fraternal twins, though this is more accurately known as *heteropaternal superfecundation*. This leads to the possibility of twin conception with two different partners (twin of different color or racial phenotypes), classic example being one baby is white and the other black.
- **Medico-legal importance:** Gross variations may occur in the complexion and features of the two babies and may give rise to the doubt of adultery and infidelity.

SUPERFETATION

Definition: Fertilization of two ova discharged from ovary *at different periods of ovulation*.
- It is fertilization of second ovum in an already pregnant woman.
- In this, one fetus always remains more developed than the other, and may be born either at the same time showing different maturation or may born at different periods, varying from 1–3 months.
- Possibility is more with septate or double uterus.

The differences between superfecundation and superfetation are highlighted in **Diff. 23.2**.

Fetus compressus or papyraceus: In a twin pregnancy, one fetus may grow at the cost of the other. The latter may die, flattened by pressure into a 'mummified' parchment-like state known as *fetus papyraceus* and may not be recognizable. It is retained till labor expels it **(Fig. 23.6)**.

NOTA BENE
- **Fraternal twins** (non-identical twins) occur when two fertilized eggs are implanted in the uterine wall at the same time and form two zygotes. They are also known as *dizygotic twins*.
- **Identical twins** occur when a single egg is fertilized to form one zygote (*monozygotic*), but the zygote then divides into two separate embryos which develop into fetuses sharing the same womb.

DIFFERENTIATION 23.2: Superfecundation and superfetation

S.No.	Feature	Superfecundation	Superfetation
1.	Definition	Fertilization of two ova discharged from the ovary at the same period of ovulation	Fertilization of two ova discharged from ovary at different periods of ovulation
2.	Menstrual cycle	Same cycle	Different cycle
3.	Interval between two acts of coitus	Few days	Weeks or months apart; interval longer than an ovulatory cycle
4.	Development stage of initial conceptus	Pre-embryo stage	Embryo or fetus stage
5.	Consequences on fetuses	Not much differences in development	Fetal growth disorder, interval delivery or sonographic error
6.	Legal issues	Gross variation in features may lead to allegation of adultery → divorce	Allegation of adultery→divorce; negligence of sonologist

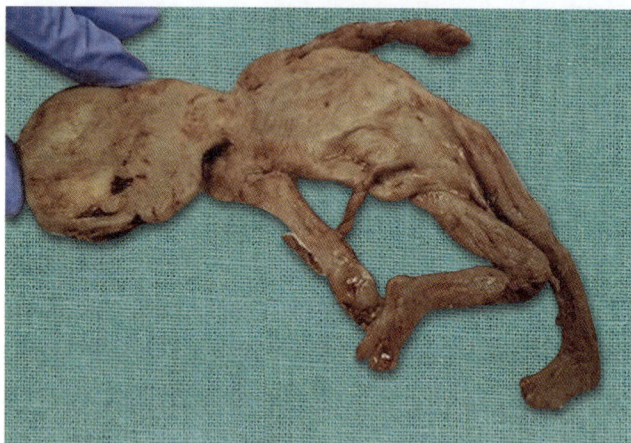

Fig. 23.6: Fetus papyraceus

- **Fraternal twins** (non-identical twins) occur when two fertilized eggs are implanted in the uterine wall at the same time and form two zygotes. They are also known as *dizygotic twins*.
- **Identical twins** occur when a single egg is fertilized to form one zygote (*monozygotic*), but the zygote then divides into two separate embryos which develop into fetuses sharing the same womb.
- **Vanishing twin syndrome** (*twin embolization syndrome/ fetal resorption*) is the presence of a multifetal gestation with subsequent disappearance of one or more fetuses. This syndrome has been diagnosed more frequently since the use of sonography in early pregnancy. In this, there may be complete resorption of a fetus or formation of a fetus papyraceus or development of a subtle abnormality on the placenta such as a cyst, subchorionic fibrin or amorphous material.
- **Lithopedion or 'stone baby':** In rare instances, an extrauterine pregnancy is retained within the mother's abdomen for years, with the fetus becoming calcified. Usually, a lithopedion occurs after a fetus dies during an ectopic abdominal pregnancy and is too large to be reabsorbed by the body. To shield itself from the degenerating tissue of the fetal foreign body, the woman's body will encase the fetus and/or covering membranes in a calciferous substance.

FM 3.18, 3.20

- Define legitimacy and its medico-legal importance.
- Discuss disputed paternity and maternity.

LEGITIMACY AND PATERNITY

Definitions

- **Legitimacy:** It is the legal state of a person born in a lawful marriage.
- **Paternity:** The state of being someone's father.
- **Legitimate child:** Person who is born during the continuance of a legal marriage or within 280 days after the dissolution of the marriage by divorce or death of the husband and the mother remaining unmarried **(Sec. 112 IEA)**.
- **Illegitimate child or bastard:** Child born out of lawful wedlock or not within a competent time after dissolution of marriage, or if it can be proved that the alleged father is:
   i. Under the age of puberty.
   ii. Physically incapable to beget children, because of illness, impotence or sterility.
   iii. Not having access sexually to his wife during the time that the child was begotten.
   iv. Having incompatibility of blood groups.

Questions of legitimacy and paternity arise in:
   i. **Inheritance claims:** A legitimate child born during lawful wedlock can inherit the property of his father.
   ii. **Affiliation cases:** A woman may allege a particular man to be the father of her child and file a case in the court for fixing the paternity.
   iii. **Supposititious child (fictitious child):** A woman may pretend pregnancy and delivery, and later produce a living child as her own, or she may substitute a male child for female child born of her, or after an abortion. This is done for obtaining money or for the purpose of claiming property (although, currently as per the Hindu Succession Act, 2005 a woman has equal rights as men in the parent's property).

iv. **Posthumous births:** Birth of a child after the father has died.
v. **Nullity of marriage and divorce.**
vi. **Atavism** (Latin *atavus*: ancestor; atta: father + avus: grandfather): The child may not resemble his parents, but resembles his grandparents. The reappearance of a characteristic in an individual after several generations of absence, usually caused by the chance recombination of genes.

Discuss the signs of recent and remote delivery in living and dead.

SIGNS AND SYMPTOMS OF RECENT DELIVERY IN LIVING

Symptoms

- Indisposition, fatigue and loss of weight
- Diuresis: 2–5 days
- Intermittent contraction of uterus—*after pains*
- Rise in temperature (100–101°F)—first 24 hours (h)
- Transient depression—puerperal psychosis.

Signs

i. **Breast changes:** Voluminous and pendulous. Colostrum or milk may be expressed. Areola is dark, nipples are enlarged and superficial veins are prominent. Montgomery's tubercles are present.
ii. **Abdomen:** Walls are pendulous, wrinkled with striae gravidarum and linea nigra.
iii. **Perineum:** Rupture of fourchette and posterior commissure with/without a sutured incision of episiotomy may be seen **(Fig. 23.7)**.
iv. **Vagina:** Purple hue, loss of rugosity, relaxed, spacious and may show recent tears.
v. **Labia majora and minora:** Tender, swollen, gaping and congested.
vi. **Cervix:** Soft, collapsed and congested; external os shows transverse laceration of its outer margins and admits 2 fingers easily. At the end of 1 week, the cervix admits 1 finger with difficulty and comes back to normal within 2 weeks.
vii. **Uterus:** The size of uterus decreases over the first few weeks which is called involution (apoptosis). This can be observed by palpating the height of the uterine fundus **(Fig. 23.8)**.
- Fundus is midway between the umbilicus and symphysis pubis: Immediately after delivery.
- Fundus at the level of umbilicus: About 1–12 h after delivery.
- Upper border lies 1 cm below umbilicus: 1st day after delivery.
- Fundus midway between umbilicus and symphysis pubis: 6th day (steady decrease in height by one fingerbreadth or 1 cm/day).
- At the level of symphysis pubis: 10th day.
- Descends within true pelvis: 2 weeks.
- Returns to parous size (normal size): 5–6 weeks.
viii. **Laboratory investigations:** Immunological tests are positive for about 7–10 days after delivery.
ix. **Lochia:** It is an alkaline discharge from uterus, cervix and vagina with peculiar, disagreeable fishy odor.
- It results from involution, during which the superficial layer of the decidua basalis becomes necrotic and is sloughed off.
- The amount is considered moderate for a vaginal delivery and scanty for a cesarean section (never absent).
- It lasts for 2–3 weeks after delivery.
- In women who breastfed, lochia resolves more rapidly because of rapid involution of the uterus caused by uterine contractions associated with breastfeeding.

Various types and its composition are given in **Table 23.2**.

> **NOTA BENE**
> **Significance of lochia:** The average amount of discharge for first 4–5 days is about 250 mL. If it smells offensive, then it indicates infection. If scanty or absent or excessive—infection; persistence of red color beyond normal—subinvolution or retained bits of conceptus; and duration beyond 3 weeks suggest local genital lesion.

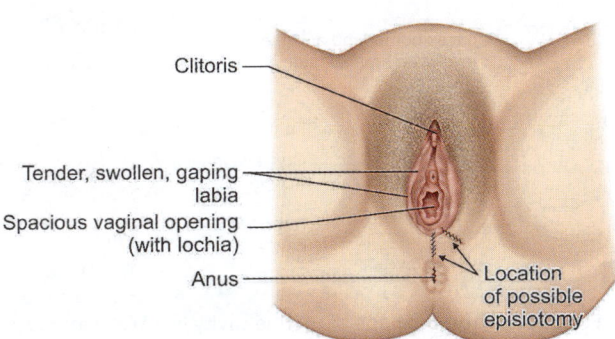

Fig. 23.7: Signs of recent delivery

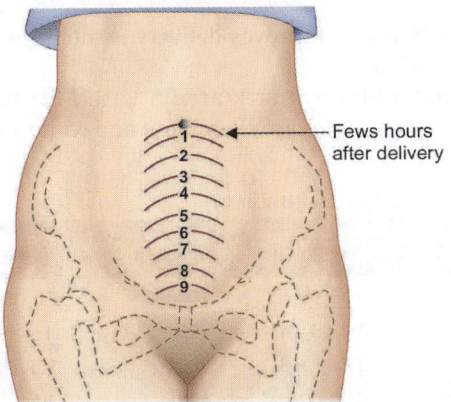

Fig. 23.8: Level of upper border of uterus (in days) post-delivery

TABLE 23.2: Types of lochia and its composition

Type	Color	Composition
Lochia rubra (1–4 days postpartum)	Bright red	Blood, fragments of deciduas, vernix caseosa, mucus
Lochia serosa (5–9 days postpartum)	Pink, watery	Blood, WBCs, wound exudates, mucus, microorganisms (anaerobic Streptococci and Staphylococci)
Lochia alba (10–14 days postpartum)	Yellowish-white	Decidual cells, cholesterol crystals, leukocytes, mucus, fatty and granular epithelial cells

Signs of Recent Delivery in Dead

All the local signs mentioned above may be present.
- The size of uterus will vary with the time after delivery at which death occurred **(Table 23.3)**.
- The size of the area where the placenta has been attached to the uterus is about 3–4 inches (8–10 cm) in diameter. A tissue layer remains attached from placenta.
- The ovaries and fallopian tubes are congested and become normal in few days. A large corpus luteum is present in one of the ovaries.

Pearls

Signs of recent delivery (both living and dead)
- Engorged breasts
- Pink striae on the abdomen
- Enlarged uterus
- Fresh tears of the vulva, vagina or cervix
- Lochia from the uterus

SIGNS OF REMOTE DELIVERY IN LIVING

The only sign which proves delivery is the *appearance of the external os*.
- **Breasts:** Flabby, dark areola with Montgomery's tubercles, nipples are prominent and white striae.

TABLE 23.3: Size of uterus after delivery

Time after delivery	Dimension (cm)	Weight (g)	Placental site diameter (cm)
Immediate	20 × 15 × 5	1000	10–15
1st week	14 × 8 × 4	500	4
2nd week	12 × 7 × 3	300	2.5
3rd week	9 × 5 × 2	100	1.5

- **Abdominal wall:** Lax, loose, presence of striae gravidarum and linea alba.
- **Perineum:** Lax, old scarring from previous perineal laceration or episiotomy may be seen.
- **Introitus:** Gaping; labia majora are not in close apposition, and labia minora is pigmented and protrude out; presence of carunculae myrtiformes.
- **Uterine wall:** Less rigid, contour of uterus is broad and round rather than ovoid.
- **Vagina:** Roomy with loss of rugosity.
- **Cervix:** Cylindrical, external os is transverse, patulous slit and may admit tip of finger **(Figs. 23.9A and B)**.

Signs of Remote Delivery in Dead

In addition to the signs seen in the living subjects, there will be findings in the uterus as mentioned in **Diff. 23.3** and shown in **Figures 23.9A and B**.

Discuss the medico-legal aspects of pregnancy and delivery.

MEDICO-LEGAL ASPECTS OF PREGNANCY AND DELIVERY

Questions of pregnancy and/or delivery may arise in the following cases:

i. **Execution of judicial death sentence:** When a woman sentenced to death, pleads that she is pregnant to avoid execution. If a woman sentenced to death is found to be pregnant, the High Court should commute the sentence to life imprisonment [Sec. 416 CrPC and CrPC (Amendment) Act, 2008]. Post-delivery, if the mother is

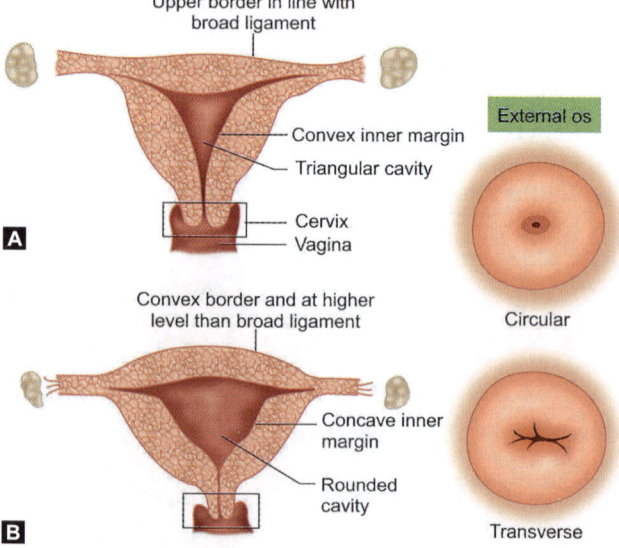

Figs. 23.9A and B: Shape of uterine cavity in: (A) Nulliparous; (B) Parous woman

DIFFERENTIATION 23.3: Nulliparous and parous uterus (Figs. 23.9A and B)

S.No.	Feature	Nulliparous uterus	Parous uterus
1.	Size	Small ($7 \times 5 \times 2$ cm^3)	Large ($10 \times 6 \times 2.5$ cm^3)
2.	Weight	40–50 g	80–100 g
3.	Length	Body and cervix have same length	Body twice the length of cervix
4.	External os	Circular, dimple like	Transverse patulous slit
5.	Internal os	Circular, well defined	Ill-defined, margin wrinkled
6.	Shape of cervix	Conical	Cylindrical
7.	Upper surface of fundus	Less convex and in same line as broad ligament	More convex and at higher level than the line of broad ligament
8.	Uterine cavity	Inner walls convex, smaller and triangular cavity	Inner walls concave, spacious and rounded cavity
9.	Arbor vitae*	Present	Disappears (absent)
10.	Scar for placental attachment	Absent	Present

* Mucosal folds in the cervical canal which extends from internal to external os.

put to death, the child will be orphaned and punished for no fault of his/her.

ii. **Deferring trial of a case:** When a woman pleads pregnancy (delivery is imminent) to avoid attendance as witness in the court.

iii. **Feigned pregnancy and delivery:** When a woman feigns pregnancy soon after death of her husband, and later produces a child to claim greater share of property and compensation.

iv. **Criminal breach of trust/rape:** When pregnancy is claimed to be the result of rape, kidnapping and seduction or breach of promise of marriage.

v. **Blackmail:** When a woman blackmails a man and claim's that she is pregnant by him to compel marriage. She may produce a suppositious child to extort money.

vi. **Disputed chastity:** In allegations of an unmarried woman, widow or a wife living apart from her husband that she is pregnant or delivered a child.

vii. **Homicide or suicide:** When pregnancy is alleged to be the motive for murder or suicide of an unmarried woman or widow.

viii. **Affiliation cases:** The woman may claim a child fathered by her husband who has subsequently divorced her or by a person who is not her legally wedded spouse and force him to adopt the child as his own and pay maintenance allowance.

ix. **Concealment of birth:** In cases of alleged concealment of birth or pregnancy in an unmarried woman or widow or out of wedlock.

x. **Criminal abortion and infanticide:** When there is an allegation of sex selective abortion or killing of an infant.

xi. **Nullity of marriage and divorce:** When there is allegation of the woman becoming pregnant when the husband was not having access physically, or delivery occurring before the minimum period of gestation, the issue may be brought to the court for nullity of marriage.

xii. **Maternity/Paternity leave:** For claiming benefit of leave facility for working women or men.

xiii. **Legitimacy:** For such claims, it must be proved that the woman indeed delivered a child at the time claimed by her.

Written informed consent needs to be taken before examination after explaining reasons and possible consequences.

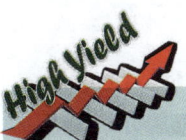

- **Virgin:** Female has not experienced sexual intercourse.
- **False virgin:** Female has experienced sexual intercourse but the *hymen is intact*.
- **Defloration:** Act of depriving a woman of her virginity.
- **Most common cause of rupture of hymen:** Sexual intercourse.
- **Principal signs of virginity:** Intact hymen, normal condition of fourchette and posterior commissure, narrow vagina with rugose walls—although there is no absolute certainty in determining the same.
- Traumatic rupture of hymen is seen on posterolateral aspect.
- **Most important symptom of pregnancy:** Amenorrhea.
- **Chadwick's/Jacquemier's sign:** Mucous membrane of vagina changes from pink to bluish due to venous obstruction (8th week).

- **Quickening:** Felt by 18th week (16th week in multipara).
- **Most valuable physical sign of early pregnancy:** Hegar's sign (6–10th week).
- **Goodell's sign:** Cervix softens from below upward (6th week).
- **Palmer's sign:** Regular rhythmic contractions of uterus (4–8th week).
- **Braxton-Hick's contractions:** Intermittent, spasmodic, painless uterine contractions (felt after 16th week). *Present even when the fetus is dead.*
- In a normal pregnancy, maternal hCG level is maximum at gestational age of 8 to 10 weeks.
- **Definite sign of pregnancy:** Fetal heart sound.
- Gravindrex test can detect pregnancy in 2 weeks.
- **Positive or conclusive signs of pregnancy:** Fetal movements and fetal parts, fetal heart sounds, X-ray of fetal skeleton, USG of gestational sac and yolk sac, fetal cells in maternal blood.
- Transvaginal USG can detect fetal cardiac activity in 5 weeks.
- **Most accurate method of diagnosis of pregnancy at 6 weeks:** Fetal heart sound by USG.
- **Staining technique to distinguish fetal from adult RBCs:** Kleihauer-Betke or acid elution test.
- No death sentence is given to a pregnant woman; the High Court will commute it to life imprisonment [Sec. 416 CrPC and CrPC (Amendment) Act, 2008].
- **Pseudocyesis (phantom pregnancy):** Psychological disorder where the woman has a false but firm belief that she is pregnant, although no pregnancy exists.
- **Superfecundation:** Fertilization of two ova discharged from the ovary *at the same period of ovulation* by two different acts of coitus committed at short intervals.
- **Superfetation:** Fertilization of two ova discharged from ovary *at different periods of ovulation*.
- **Fetus compressus/fetus papyraceus:** In a twin pregnancy, one fetus may die, flattened by pressure into a 'mummified' parchment-like state.
- **Vanishing twin syndrome:** Presence of multifetal gestation with subsequent disappearance of one or more fetuses.
- **Identical twins** *(monozygotic twins):* Zygote from single fertilized egg divides into two separate embryos which develop into fetuses sharing the same womb.
- **Fraternal twins** *(non-identical twins/dizygotic twins):* Two fertilized eggs are implanted in the uterine wall at the same time and form two zygotes.
- **Legitimacy:** Legal state of a person born in a lawful marriage.
- **Paternity:** State of being someone's father.
- **Supposititious child (fictitious child):** A woman may pretend pregnancy and delivery, and later produce a living child as her own.
- **Legitimate child:** A child born within 280 days after dissolved marriage (divorce or death of husband); the mother remaining unmarried.
- **Illegitimate child or bastard:** Child born out of lawful wedlock or not within a competent time after dissolution of marriage, or if it can be proved that the alleged father is: (a) Under the age of puberty. (b) Physically incapable to beget children, because of illness, impotence or sterility. (c) Not having access sexually to his wife during the time that the child was begotten. (d) Having incompatibility of blood groups.
- Affiliation cases are related to paternity dispute.
- **Atavism:** Child resembles grandparents; not the parents.
- **Delivery:** Expulsion/extraction of the child at birth.
- **Posthumous births:** Birth of a child after the father has died.
- Immediately after delivery, the uterus is midway between the umbilicus and symphysis pubis, but ascends up to umbilicus in 1 h.
- **Fundus of uterus midway between umbilicus and symphysis pubis:** 6th day
- **Uterus descends within true pelvis:** 2 weeks.
- **Order of lochia:** Rubra → Serosa → Alba.
- **Sign of remote delivery in living:** External os is transverse, patulous slit and may admit tip of finger.
- **Findings of remote delivery in dead:** Body of uterus twice the length of cervix with external os showing transverse patulous slit.

CHAPTER 23 : Virginity, Pregnancy and Delivery

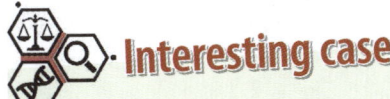

Superfecundation (Case of Charlotte Kallehauge, 2005)

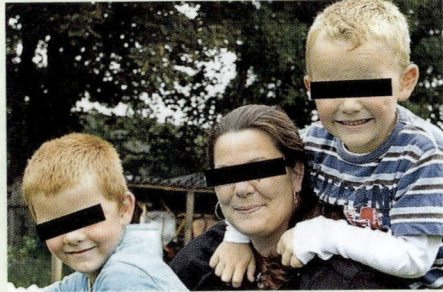

Charlotte Kallehauge, a 38-year-old woman and a mother of two boys from her husband Michael Nielsen filed for divorce in August 2004. She began dating Tommy even as Michael still hoped to get back together with her. In the heat of the moment, she ended up in having sexual intercourse with Michael. In less than 48 h, she had intercourse with Tommy too. Charlotte kept quiet about the incident. After few weeks, doctor confirmed that she was pregnant and was expecting twins. She decided—to inform both men as either could be father of the twins.

Charlotte lived alone and gave birth in 2005 to twin boys Marcus and Lucas. Michael took care of her while she was carrying the twins, and was there for the delivery. Charlotte got back with Tommy and after 6 months they decided to stay together. In couple of weeks after delivery, it was evident that the boys were not alike exactly. Marcus's face was round with red hair, while Lucas was fair, with a long face. Marcus looked like Michael, and Lucas like Tommy.

Tommy and Michael took a DNA test to find out for certain that the boys had different fathers. Blood samples were collected from the twins, the mother and two fathers. DNA was extracted from whole blood and dried blood stains samples. The report based on the paternity test showed that there is a 99.999% chance that the twins are fathered by different men. Marcus and Lucas are twins with two different fathers and are genetic half-brothers. Interestingly, both Michael and Tommy got on well later and have accepted the kids.

CHAPTER 24

Sexual Offenses

Learning Objectives

Must know
1. Sexual violence, sexual assault, sexual abuse, sexual harassment, sexual offense
2. Classification of sexual offenses
3. Rape, gang rape, statutory rape, custodial rape, invalid consent, punishment for rape (Sec. 375 and 376 IPC)
4. Duties of a doctor in a case of sexual assault (rape)
5. Procedure and examination findings of a rape survivor (in virgins)
6. Examination of rape accused
7. Specimen collection of rape survivor and accused
8. Incest and adultery

Desirable to know
1. Carnal knowledge
2. Medico-legal aspects of definition of rape
3. Contents of a 'SAFE kit'
4. Examination findings of SAFE in a deflorate woman and in a child
5. Rape trauma syndrome
6. Marital rape
7. Battered wife syndrome

Definitions

- **Sexual violence:** Any sexual act, attempt to obtain a sexual act, unwanted sexual comments or advances or acts to traffic, or otherwise directed against a person's sexuality, using coercion, by any person regardless of their relationship to the victim, in any setting, including but not limited to home and work (WHO).
- **Sexual assault:** Any unwanted sexual act or behavior which is threatening, violent, forced, or coercive and to which a person has not given consent to or was not able to give consent.
    - The term *'sexual assault'* is often used synonymously with forced/non-consensual vaginal intercourse (rape). However, sexual assault could include anything from touching another person's body in a sexual way without the person's consent to forced sexual intercourse—oral and anal sexual acts, child molestation, fondling or unwanted touching above or under clothes and attempted rape.
- **Sexual abuse:** Any act of sexual contact that a person suffers, submits to, participates in, or performs as a result of force or violence, threats, fear, or deception or without having legally consented to the act—most frequently the term is used in relation to the involvement of children and adolescents in sexual activities with an adult.
- **Sexual harassment:** Physical contact and advances involving unwanted and explicit sexual overtures, or demanding sexual favors, showing pornography against her will or making sexually colored remarks, or any other unwelcome physical, verbal or non-verbal conduct of sexual nature.
- **Sexual offenses** are legal constructs involving sexual behavior that are defined and proscribed by society and its laws as criminal offenses due to the harm they cause and/or their impact on public order. Such legal definitions vary over time and between countries.

Sexual violence is a broad term that includes sexual assault, sexual offense, sexual abuse and sexual harassment **(Fig. 24.1)**. The word violence does not refer only to physical violence but includes emotional and psychological harm.

Classification

Sexual offense can be classified into:
1. **Forced/non-consensual* vaginal intercourse:** Physically forced or otherwise coerced penetration, even if slight, of the vulva with a penis.

---
* Forced—no will, no consent; non-consensual—will present, but no consent.

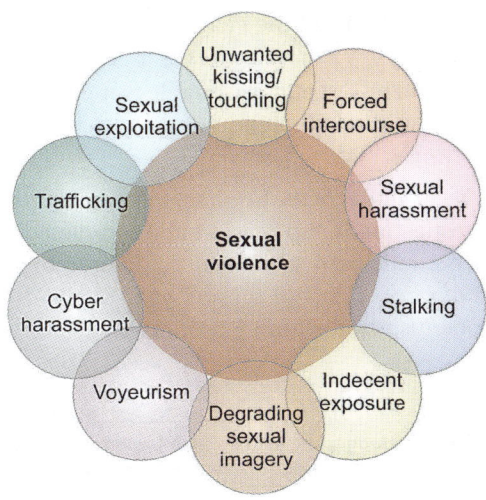

Fig. 24.1: Sexual violence

2. **Forced/non-consensual anal intercourse** between two males or between a male and a female.
3. **Forced/non-consensual oral intercourse** between two males or between a male and a female.
4. **Forced/non-consensual insertion of fingers or foreign bodies** into vagina, urethra or anus.
5. **Sexual acts with animals** (bestiality/zoophilia—sexual attraction to animals).
6. **Paraphilias** are conditions in which sexual excitement or orgasm is associated with acts or imagery that are considered unusual, abnormal or deviant within the culture, e.g., voyeurism, frotteurism, exhibitionism, etc.*
7. **Other sex-linked acts:** Forced/non-consensual touching or groping or disrobing ('indecent assault'), sexual harassment, stalking.
    - **Indecent assault:** Any unwanted sexual behavior or touching of a female without her consent, with the intention or knowledge to outrage her modesty. A sexual assault that does not meet the legal definition of rape may constitute indecent assault.
    - **Sexual harassment:** Physical contact and advances involving unwelcome and explicit sexual overtures, or demanding sexual favors, showing pornography against her will or making sexually colored remarks. It is punishable with (rigorous) imprisonment for 1–3 years with/without fine **(Sec. 354-A IPC)**. The offense is cognizable and bailable.
- As per the **Criminal Law Amendment Act, 2013**, legal definition of rape is no longer considered as forceful/non-consensual vaginal intercourse only. It has expanded the definition of rape to include all forms of sexual violence—oral, anal, vaginal including by objects/weapons/fingers/mouth and has addressed the previous limitations of rape laws.

- The law also recognized the right to treatment for all survivors of sexual violence by the public and private healthcare facilities. Failure to treat is now an offense under the law.
- The law further disallows any reference to past sexual practices of the survivor.

> **FM 3.13, 3.16**
> - Describe various sections of IPC & CrPC related to definition of rape and sexual assault, medical examination of rape victim and accused of rape, police information by the doctors and medical care with recent amendments notified till date (i.e., Section 375 IPC, 166 B IPC, 357 C & 164 A, 53 A of CrPC).
> - Describe and discuss informed consent in sexual intercourse.

RAPE

Definition: Rape is an unlawful sexual intercourse by a man with a woman, and is defined under **Sec. 375 IPC**.

A man is said to commit 'rape' if he himself or makes a woman to do so with him or any other person the following:
a. penetrates his penis into the vagina, mouth, urethra or anus; or
b. inserts any object or any part of his body (not being his penis) into the vagina, urethra or anus; or
c. manipulates any part of her body so as to cause penetration into the vagina, urethra, anus or any part of her body;** or
d. applies his mouth to the vagina, anus, urethra of a woman;** and under the following circumstances:
   i. Against her will
   ii. Without her consent
   iii. With her consent, when:
       - It has been obtained by putting her or any person in whom she is interested, in fear of death or hurt.
       - The man knows that he is not her husband, but she consents believing him as the man to whom she is lawfully married (*impersonation*).
       - At the time of giving such consent by reason of unsoundness of mind or intoxication or the administration by him or through another of any stupefying substance, she is unable to understand the nature of consequences of that to which she gives consent.
   iv. With or without her consent, when she is under 18 years of age–**statutory rape**.
   v. When she is unable to communicate consent.

Exceptions

i. Medical intervention or procedure will not constitute rape.
ii. Sexual intercourse by a man with his wife not being under 15 years of age is not rape.

---
* Not all paraphilias are sexual offense, unless done publicly or comes under any of the sections of IPC.
** Insertion of finger or any object in the mouth or kissing (mouth to mouth) will not amount to the offense of rape.

> The Supreme Court has held that sexual intercourse by a man with his minor wife aged between 15–18 years is *rape*. It ruled that a man can be prosecuted if his underage wife registers a complaint within a year of the offense.

Explanations

- 'Penetration' or 'insertion' can be any extent.
- 'Vagina' is labia majora.
- 'Consent' is voluntary agreement by the woman by words, gestures or any form of verbal or non-verbal communication—communicates willingness to participate in the specific sexual act.
- **Custodial rape:** Rape of a woman by persons who are in position of authority, e.g., police officers, jail warden or hospital staff and who abuse their position to commit the offense, when the woman is under their custody/care.
- **Gang rape (pack rape):** When more than one person constituting a group or acting in furtherance of a common intention rapes a woman, each one is deemed to have committed rape.
- **Statutory rape:** It is the crime of having sexual intercourse with a girl under the age of consent. In India, the age of consent for sexual intercourse is 18 years.

Punishment for Rape

Death penalty to those convicted of raping children <12 years came into effect as per the Criminal law (Amendment) Act, 2018 **(Table 24.1)**.

- All the offenses are cognizable and non-bailable, except under **Sec 376-B** which is cognizable but bailable (only on the complaint of the victim), and tried in Session Court.
- Fine should be just and reasonable to meet the medical expenses and rehabilitation of the victim and paid to the victim.

Other salient features of the Criminal law (Amendment) Act, 2018: Investigation in rape cases to be completed within 2 months; no anticipatory bail can be granted to a person accused of rape of girls of age <16 years; appeals in rape cases to be disposed within 6 months.

> **NOTA BENE**
>
> - **Carnal knowledge:** The act of a man having sexual relation with a woman and includes even 'slight penile penetration of the labia minora'.
> - **Sexual battery:** It means non-consensual oral, anal or vaginal penetration by or union with the sexual organ of another, or the anal or vaginal penetration of another by any other object; however, sexual battery shall not include acts done for bonafide medical purposes.
> - **Drug-facilitated rape:** Drugs, such as flunitrazepam (Rohypnol) and gamma-hydroxybutyrate are referred to as *'date rape drugs'* have been used by people to render the victims unconscious, before raping them.

Consent

A woman of 18 years and above can give valid consent for sexual intercourse. The consent must be free and voluntary, and given while she is of sound mind and not intoxicated. The consent should be obtained prior to the act.

TABLE 24.1: Punishment for rape

IPC	Criteria	Punishment
Sec. 376 (1)	Raping a female ≥18 years	≥10 years to life imprisonment and fine
Sec. 376 (2)	Custodial rape, rape on pregnant female, by relative, guardian or teacher, during communal violence, physically/ mentally disable, repeatedly on same woman, rape causing grievous injury, mutilating or disfiguring or endangering her life	≥10 years to life imprisonment (remainder of natural life) and fine
Sec. 376 (3)	Raping a girl <16 years	≥20 years to life imprisonment (remainder of natural life) and fine
Sec. 376-A	Rape causing death or persistent vegetative state	≥20 years to life imprisonment (remainder of natural life) or *death*
Sec. 376-AB	Raping a girl <12 years	≥20 years to life imprisonment (remainder of natural life) and fine or *death*
Sec. 376-B	Sexual intercourse by husband during separation without her consent	2–7 years and fine
Sec. 376-C	Sexual intercourse by a person of authority/fiduciary relationship (not amounting to the offense of rape)	5–10 years and fine
Sec. 376-D	Gang rape	≥20 years to life imprisonment (remainder of natural life) and fine
Sec. 376-DA	Gang rape of a girl <16 years	Imprisonment for life (remainder of natural life) and fine
Sec. 376-DB	Gang rape of a girl <12 years	Imprisonment for life (remainder of natural life) and fine or *death*
Sec. 376-E	Repeat offenders	Imprisonment for remainder of his natural life or *death*

Presumption and Absence of Consent

Absence of consent can be presumed from the attendant circumstances of each case.
- The foremost circumstance is the evidence of resistance (tearing of clothes or infliction of personal injuries on the body and even on the genitalia) from a woman unwilling to yield to sexual intercourse forced upon her.
- The resistance offered depends upon the type of woman, her age, development and on her social status.
- The absence of signs of struggle or injuries does not mean the victim has consented to sexual activity. As per law, resistance was not offered does not mean the person has consented.
- The woman may yield from fear or exhaustion in which case it is regarded as rape. A woman may faint due to fear and suddenness of the situation or may have been drugged or may get unconscious from any cause, and children may not be able to resist.

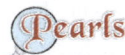

Consent is invalid when:
i. Obtained by fraud as by impersonation of the husband or by misrepresentation of facts.
ii. Obtained by putting her or any person whom she is close, in fear of death or hurt.
iii. Obtained from a woman who is of unsound mind, insensible, asleep, unconscious or in a state of drunkenness.
iv. The woman is <18 years of age.
v. Obtained after the act.

The age at which individuals are considered competent to give consent for sexual intercourse is called the **age of consent**. The age set by each country/State vary in accordance with local standards.

Medico-legal Aspects of Definition of Rape

Will and consent are different: Every act done *against the will* is done *without her consent*, but an act done *without the consent* of a person is *not necessarily against her will*. Sexual intercourse with an unconscious woman cannot be said to be against her 'will', but it will be 'without her consent'. But an act against her will is necessarily 'without her consent'.
- A woman may have the will for sexual intercourse, but she may not give consent for shyness, fear of detection and social stigma of getting pregnant.
- Women may be raped during sleep, thus being unable to give prior consent. But sexual intercourse is usually not possible without waking up the lady.
- A man can impersonate as the husband of the victim in the darkness, or in case of twins one may impersonate the other.
- A woman may give her consent suppressing her unwillingness due to some other factor, e.g., for monetary benefit, for getting good grades or for promotion.
- Sometimes, a girl may give her consent for intercourse, and then later deny that she agreed and accuses the man of rape. This may be due to fear of pregnancy, venereal disease or breakdown of relationship where motive of revenge is present.
- **False promise of marriage:** Intercourse under promise of marriage constitutes rape only if from initial stage accused had no intention to keep promise (*misconception of fact*). However, SC has ruled that every breach of promise to marry is not rape.
- Ordinarily, the burden to prove unwillingness and absence of consent lies with the prosecution. But in rape case, under **Sec. 376 IPC**, if the victim states in the court of trial that she did not give consent, it then lies with the accused to prove that she consented for the intercourse.
- The law provides the same protection to a prostitute against sexual assault, as it does for chaste woman (i.e., consent is required for intercourse). But when a prostitute makes a charge of rape, the case must be more closely scrutinized, something more than medical evidence would be required to establish such a charge.
- **Medical proof of intercourse is not legal proof of rape.** In short, rape is not a medical diagnosis, but a legal definition.

By a man: *In India, the law does not presume any limit of age* under which a boy is considered physically incapable of committing rape. In a charge of rape brought against a boy, the court decides the question of his potency from evidence of the case and is guided by **Sec. 82** and **83 IPC** in awarding punishment. Likewise, there is no upper limit and even old people have committed rape.

In England and Wales, a boy under 14 years of age cannot be charged of rape.

Of a woman: Only a man can rape a woman as per law on rape in most countries, *except in France* where just like a man, a woman can be charged for committing rape on a man.
- In India, a woman may be charged for committing an indecent assault on a man.
- There is no age limit of a female, below or above which a man cannot commit rape.

What Constitutes Rape?
- *The slightest penetration of penis within the vulva* (passage of glans between the labia) with or without emission of semen or rupture of hymen constitutes rape. There need not be intercourse and the act may not be completed.
- Rape can be committed even when there is inability to produce an erection or ejaculation.
- As per the law, even penetration (or applying mouth) of vagina, anus, or urethra by finger or any other object constitutes the offense of rape.

SECTION 1: Jurisprudence and Forensic Medicine

> **NOTA BENE**
>
> **Legal sections related to rape**
>
> - *Treatment and information to police:* All hospitals, public or private, should immediately provide first-aid or medical treatment, free of cost, to the survivor/victim of rape or acid attack, and should immediately inform the police [**Sec. 357-C CrPC** (Criminal Law Amendment Act, 2013)]. Denial of treatment of such victims is punishable under **Sec. 166-B IPC** with imprisonment up to 1 year and with/without fine. The offense is non-cognizable and bailable.
> - *Punishment of revealing the identity of rape victim:* If anyone prints or publishes the name or any matter which may reveal the identity of victim of rape, then he is punished with imprisonment for a term up to 2 years and fine (**Sec. 228-A IPC**).
> - *Presumption of consent:* In a prosecution for rape under **Sec. 376 IPC** when sexual intercourse by the accused is proved, and the question is whether it was without the consent of the woman and she states in her evidence before the court that she did not consent, *the court shall presume that she did not consent* (**Sec. 114 IEA**).
> - *Cross-examination in rape trial:* It is not permissible to put questions in cross-examination of victim about her general immoral character, and court should not describe her to be of loose character (**Sec. 146 IEA**).
> - *Courts in which rape offenses to be tried:* The offense under **Sec. 376** should be tried as far as practicable by a court presided over by a woman [**Sec. 26 (a) CrPC**].
> - *Recording of statement:* The statement of the survivor/victim should be recorded and video-graphed by a woman police officer, and the officer should get the statement recorded by a Judicial Magistrate as soon as possible (**Sec. 154 CrPC**).
> - *Time period of trial of rape cases:* The inquiry/trial of an offense under **Sec. 376** should be completed within a period of 2 months from the date of commencement of the examination of witnesses and without any adjournment on frivolous grounds (**Sec. 309 CrPC**).
> - *Trial of rape cases* are to be held in-camera by a woman Judge/Magistrate if available, and allowed the printing or publication of proceedings in rape cases subject to maintaining anonymity of the parties [**Sec. 327 (2) & (3) CrPC**].
> - **In-camera:** 'In a room'. Proceedings are heard in a Judge's private chamber or in a courtroom which has been cleared of all spectators.
> - The Supreme Court has held that there is no need for corroborating evidence, if the victim's version inspires confidence and appears credible since Indian girls will not lie about sexual assault. At the same time, the Court has stated that rape victim's testimony cannot be considered to be the gospel truth. Although, the statement of victim must be given primary consideration, there can be no presumption that she is telling the ultimate truth as the charge has to be proved beyond reasonable doubt as in any other criminal case.

- Rape can occur without causing any injury, and hence, negative evidence does not exclude rape. The doctor should mention only the negative facts, but *should not give his opinion that rape has not been committed.*

DUTIES OF A DOCTOR IN CASE OF A SURVIVOR OF SEXUAL ASSAULT (RAPE)

> - **Survivor:** The term 'survivor' is preferably used instead of 'victim' since it recognizes that the person is capable of taking decisions despite being victimized, humiliated and traumatized due to the assault.*
> - **Victim:** A person suffering harm including those who are subjected to non-consensual sexual act which could be sexual assault. It also means a person in need of compassion, care, validation and support, and is not fully capable of comprehending situation at hand because of the victimhood faced.

i. Any female of any age (including any child) who claims to be a survivor of sexual assault should always be treated as a possible rape victim. She must be treated as a priority case by all staff and doctors (although life-threatening cases may be given priority over a rape survivor who is not in immediate danger).

ii. Survivor should be seen within all health facilities, such as clinics, nursing homes and hospitals. The doctor should not refuse to examine a rape survivor on the ground that she was not brought by the police or she came on her own.

iii. Under **Sec. 164-A CrPC** (*medical examination of the victim of rape*), the examination should be conducted without delay by a registered medical practitioner (RMP) employed in a Govt. hospital or any other RMP with the consent of the survivor or person competent to give consent on her behalf, and she should be sent to the RMP within 24 hours (h) from the time of receiving the information relating to the commission of such offense.

iv. Senior medical staff, if possible, should examine the sexual assault case. This is especially necessary to ensure that the doctor is seen as a reliable expert witness.

v. Parents/guardians can request medico-legal examination and treatment on behalf of a rape/sexual abuse survivor, if she is:

> - under 12 years
> - mentally retarded
> - under the influence of alcohol
> - unconscious

vi. Survivors should at all times be treated with dignity and respect by the medical staff. The examiner must

---

* Although in the text, the words 'victim' or 'survivor' have been used liberally, it is recommended to use the terminology "the patient who experienced sexual assault" or "the patient who is a victim/survivor of sexual assault" during documentation, as the word 'victim/survivor' indicates that the doctor is confirming that the patient has been raped or sexually assaulted (advocacy). They are not 'victim' or 'perpetrator' until they go to court and are found innocent or guilty by the judge.

be reassuring, empathetic and nonjudgmental and should not rush the patient.
vii. Privacy should be ensured, like by allowing her to be brought into the examining room through a separate entrance. The history taking and examination should be carried out in privacy in a special room in the hospital.
viii. Forensic evidence should be collected, as soon as possible during the process of examination. However, the serious injuries of the victim must be treated and are more important than forensic needs.
ix. The doctor should prepare a detailed report and describe the material taken from the person of the woman for DNA profiling.
x. The RMP should give a provisional opinion based on basis of history and findings of clinical examination, and hand over the report without delay to the investigation officer who shall forward it to the Magistrate.
xi. Even if the sexual assault occurred outside the jurisdiction of the hospital, the survivor must first be examined and treated, before referring her to the hospital in the appropriate area.

FM 3.14
Describe and discuss the examination of the victim of an alleged case of rape, and the preparation of report, framing the opinion and preservation and dispatch of trace evidences in such cases.

EXAMINATION OF SEXUAL ASSAULT SURVIVOR

Doctors are legally bound to examine and provide treatment to survivors of sexual assault. The timely reporting, documentation and collection of forensic evidence may assist the investigation of this crime. The Ministry of Health and Family Welfare (MoHFW) has issued a uniform protocol and guidelines for medical practitioners that highlight the medical and forensic responsibilities including collecting relevant evidence, so that the culprit could be brought to the book. The guidelines describe in detail the stepwise approach to be used for a comprehensive response to the sexual violence survivor **(Flowchart 24.1)**:
i. Initial resuscitation/first aid.
ii. Establish a rapport with the survivor and informed consent.
iii. Detailed history taking.
iv. Medical examination—general physical and local.
v. Age estimation (physical/dental/radiological)—if requested by the investigating agency.
vi. Documentation.
vii. Treatment of injuries.
viii. Evidence collection.
ix. Packing, sealing and handing over the collected evidence to the police.
x. Testing/prophylaxis for sexually transmitted disease, HIV, hepatitis B and pregnancy.
xi. Psychological support and counseling.

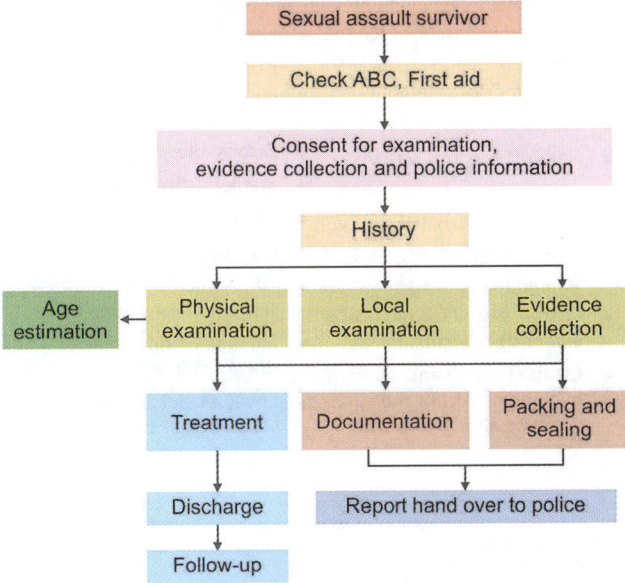

Flowchart 24.1: Stepwise approach to a sexual assault survivor

The purpose is:
- Establish a uniform method of examination and evidence collection by following the protocols using the Sexual Assault Forensic Evidence (SAFE) kit.
- Search for physical signs that will corroborate the history given by the victim.
- Search for, collect and preserve all trace evidence for laboratory examination.
- Treat the victim for injuries, to prevent/treat venereal disease (STDs) or pregnancy, and to prevent or alleviate psychological damage.
- Maintain a clear and fool-proof chain of custody of medical evidence collected.

This will help in forming an opinion on:
- Whether a sexual act has been attempted or completed?
- Whether such a sexual act is recent, and whether any harm has been caused to the survivor's body?
- The age of the survivor needs to be verified in the case of adolescent girls/boys.
- Whether alcohol or drugs have been administered to the survivor?

SAFE Kit

Sexual assault forensic evidence (SAFE) kit is a set of items used by medical personnel for gathering and preserving physical evidence following an allegation of sexual assault. It is also called physical evidence recovery kit (PERK). The kit was developed by *Louis Vitullo* and was referred to as the *Vitullo kit*. The MoHFW guidelines strongly advocate the use of SAFE kit for collecting and preserving physical evidence **(Box 24.1 and Fig. 24.2)**.

Box 24.1 Sexual assault forensic evidence (SAFE) kit

- Detailed instructions for the examiner
- Forms for documentation
- Catchment paper
- Nail cutter, comb, scissors
- Glass slides
- Sealing wax, labels
- Wooden stick for fingernail scrapings
- Cotton swabs for biological evidence collection
- Clean clothing and shower/hygiene items (for the survivor's use after examination)
- Large sheet of paper for patient to undress over
- Paper bags for clothing collection
- Disposable gloves
- Sterile/distilled water
- Urine sample container
- Unwaxed dental floss
- Tubes/vacutainers for blood sample (EDTA, plain, NaF)
- Syringes and needles for drawing blood
- Envelopes or boxes for individual evidence samples

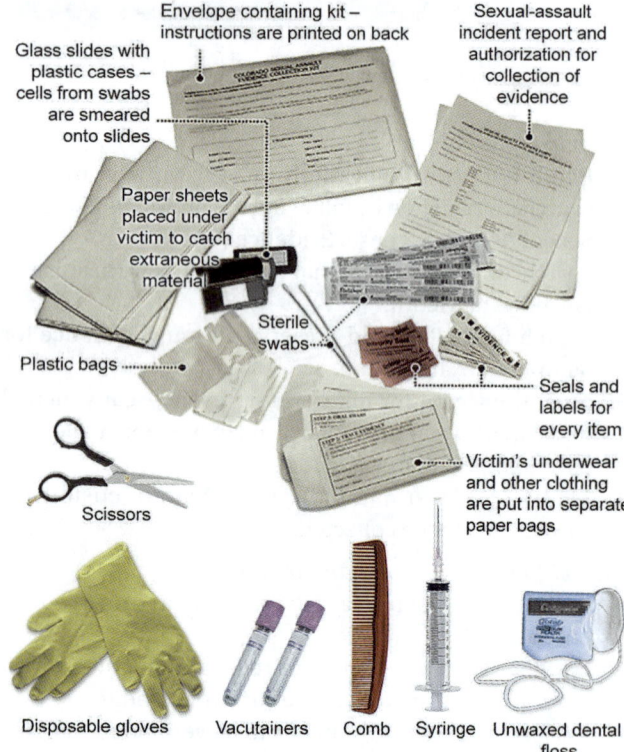

Fig. 24.2: Contents of SAFE kit

Facilitating Procedures

- The police should advise the survivor not to change clothes or have a bath—to prevent the loss of physical evidence and to ensure that medical attention is not delayed.
- A visit to the scene of alleged offense may be desirable.
- It is important that the RMP should be sensitive to the survivor as she has experienced a traumatic episode and she may not be able to provide all the details. An environment of trust should be created so that she is able to speak out.
- The doctor should explain to the survivor in simple and understandable language the rationale for history taking and various procedures, and details of how they will be performed.
- Specific steps when dealing with a survivor from marginalized groups such as children, persons with disability, LGBTQIA (lesbian, gay, bisexual, transsexual, queer, intersex and allied) persons, sex workers or persons from minority community, may be required.
- Ensure confidentiality and explain to the survivor that she must reveal the entire history to health professional without fear.
- The survivor should be informed about the need to carry out additional procedures, such as X-rays which may require her to visit others departments.

NOTA BENE

Caste and religion: One should not pass any explicit or implicit comments about the person's caste or religion while medically treating them, except if relevant to the nature of injuries or for treatment purposes.

Examination Procedure

i. A requisition for examination of the survivor should come from an authorized person, either a Magistrate or in-charge of a police station. If she has approached the doctor herself to have a medical examination, the doctor is bound to conduct her medico-legal examination without any delay. A police requisition is not required for this. Information is sent to the police for recording her statement and lodging of complaint.

ii. **Informed consent:** The survivor being examined should be informed about the nature and purpose of examination **(Box 24.2)**. Only in life-threatening

Box 24.2 Information given to the survivor

- The medico-legal examination may involve an examination of the mouth, breasts, vagina, anus and rectum depending on the particular circumstances.
- Forensic evidence may be collected which may include removing and isolating clothing, scalp hair, foreign substances from the body, saliva, pubic hair, samples from the vagina, anus, rectum, mouth and collecting a blood sample.
- She has the right to refuse either a medico-legal examination or collection of evidence or both, but that refusal will not be used to deny treatment. The court or the police have no power to compel a woman for medico-legal examination against her will **[Sec. 164-A (7) CrPC]**. She has a right for partial examination—she may also decide on whether she wants to undergo a physical examination and/or genital examination, and allow collection of bodily evidence.
- The hospital/examining doctor is required/duty bound to inform the police about the incidence. However, if she does not wish to participate in the police investigation, she has the right to refuse to file FIR and it would not result in denial of medical examination and treatment.
- Any evidence obtained may be used in court, and that she will then be exposed to publicity and cross-examination.

situation, the doctor may initiate treatment without consent **(Sec. 92 IPC)**.
- The consent form should be signed by the survivor if she is ≥12 years of age, and the guardian/parent if she is <12 years.
- In case of persons with mental disability, their informed consent (assent) should be sought and obtained after providing the necessary information and adequate time. Assistance of a friend/colleague/caregiver can be taken in forming the decision.
- Consent should be obtained before the examination, collection of specimens, release of information to authorities and taking of photographs. The form should be signed by the survivor, a witness and the examining doctor. Any major 'disinterested', person may be considered a witness.
- The survivor may refuse to give consent for any part of examination, particularly genital examination. In this case the doctor should explain the importance of examination and evidence collection for legal purposes; however, the refusal should be respected and documented. Even if there is informed refusal for police intimation, the doctor is bound to inform the police. At the time of intimation being sent to the police, a clear note stating '*informed refusal for police intimation*' should be made.

iii. The survivor should be identified by the escorting police constable (whose name and number should be recorded), relatives or attendants accompanying her. Police officers, regardless of their sex, should never be in the examining room.

iv. If possible, the survivor is examined by or under the supervision of a female doctor. If a board of doctors is examining her, at least one doctor must be a female. Otherwise, a female nurse/attendant should be there, if she is examined by a male doctor. If the survivor requests, her relative may be present while the examination is done.

v. The examination should be carried out without delay. Minor degrees of injury may fade rapidly, and swelling and tenderness of vulva may disappear in few hours. Chances of detection of spermatozoa from the genital tract diminish with delay.

vi. Statement of the survivor and others accompanying her are recorded separately. This is particularly important in cases of children wherein she may be accompanied by the abuser. In such situations, a female person appointed by the head of the hospital may be present during the examination.

vii. The inadvertent discovery during history or examination that a person is transgender/intersex should not be treated with ridicule, surprise or shock. There should be no judgment on the person's sexual orientation in general or as a cause of the assault. In the case of a transgender/intersex person, the survivor should be given a choice as to whether she/he wants to be examined by a female or male doctor. Transgender male individuals who still have ovaries and uterus or intersex women can become pregnant.

viii. The Supreme Court has acknowledged that a woman who is a sex worker has the right to decide with whom she will have sex, and so any non-consensual intercourse with her would therefore amount to rape. Only information of the current episode of violence that the survivor is reporting must be documented. Any information of past sexual encounters is irrelevant to the current incident of sexual violence and should not be noted.

ix. Persons with disability include those who have long-term physical, mental, intellectual or sensory impairments. Women and children with disability are particularly vulnerable to sexual violence. Since, abuse by near and dear ones is common, it is important not to let the history be dictated by the person accompanying the survivor. History must be sought independently, directly from the survivor.

Preliminary Data

Following details should be noted (Sec. 164-A CrPC):

i. Name of the survivor, age, height, marital status, residence, occupation and social status.

ii. Date, time (commencement and completion) and place of examination. Date and time are important, because the interval between the alleged incident and the examination is important. If there was any undue delay, the reason for such a delay.

iii. Two identification marks such as moles, scars or tattoos, preferably from the exposed parts of the body should be documented. Left thumb impression is to be taken in the space provided.

History of Chief Complaints (Flowchart 24.2)

- The details of history will guide the examination, treatment and evidence collection, and therefore seeking a complete history is critical to the medical examination process, sample collection, treatment and police intimation. A clear differentiation should be made between a 'negative' and 'not sure' history. If the survivor does not know if a particular act occurred, it should be recorded as 'did not know'.
- It is noted who is narrating the incident—survivor or an informant. If history is narrated by a person other than the survivor herself, his/her name should be noted. Especially, if the identity of assailants is revealed it is better to have a countersignature of the informant. The doctor should record the complete history of the incident, in survivor's own words as it has evidentiary value in the court of law.

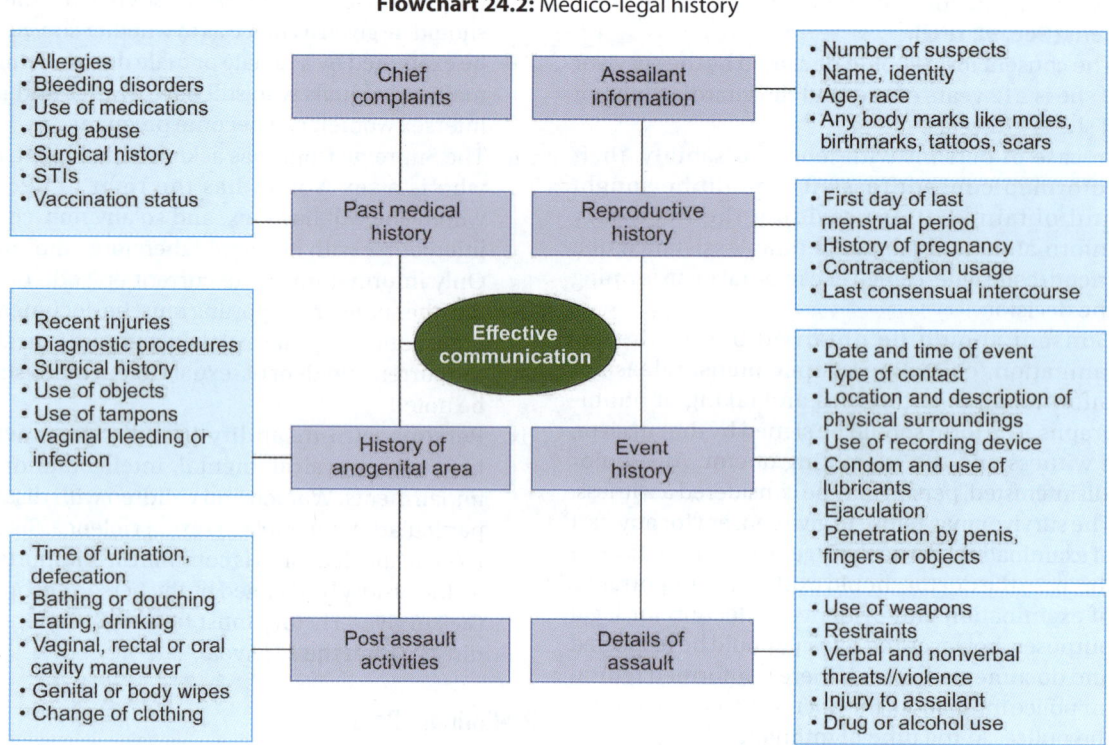

Flowchart 24.2: Medico-legal history

Circumstances of Attack

- It should include date, time and place of alleged offense, description of the perpetrator(s) [name (if known) and number of persons], use of threats or restraints, exact relative positions of the partners, details of struggle or resistance, calls for help, sensation as to penetration and emission (whether emission was within the vagina or outside), any condom used during the act, and any bleeding or pain during or after the incident.
    - Other nongenital acts, such as kissing, touching, licking, and biting, and where on the body.
    - Information about emission of semen outside the orifices should be elicited as swabs taken from such sites can have evidentiary value.
    - Information regarding use of condom during the assault is relevant because in such cases, vaginal swabs and smears would be negative for sperm/semen.
    - Information regarding attempted or completed penetration by penis/finger/object in vagina/anus/mouth should be recorded.
- Whether any drug or alcohol was taken (it may help establish lack of consent).

Physical Violence

- Use of any physical violence is recorded with description of the type of violence and its location on the body (e.g., beating on the legs, biting cheeks, pulling hair, or kicking the abdomen).

- History of injury inflicted by the survivor on the assailant's body is noted so that it can be matched eventually with the findings of the assailant's examination.
- Whether consciousness was lost at any time during the attack?

Post-assault Activities

Details of the events after the alleged assault, such as douching or bathing, cleaning or changing clothes, using tampon or sanitary napkin, urination or defecation, eating or drinking, and use of toothpaste, mouthwash, enemas or drugs.

Sexual History

- Date and time of the last consensual intercourse (because sperm from this encounter may still be present in the vaginal canal and cervix, and confuse the issue).
- While seeking such history, explain to the survivor why this information is being sought, because the survivor may not want to disclose such history as it may seem intrusive.

Menstrual and Obstetric History

History of menarche, last menstrual period, gravidity, parity and the method of contraception. If the survivor is menstruating at the time of examination, then a second examination is required on a later date in order to record the injuries clearly. Some amount of evidence is lost because of menstruation.

Medical and Surgical History

- Relevant medical history in relation to sexually transmitted infections (gonorrhea, HIV or HBV) can be elicited by asking about discharge per urethra, warts, ulcers, burning micturition and lower abdominal pain.
- History in relation to treatment of fissures/injuries/scars of ano-genital area should be noted.
- Vaccination history with regard to tetanus and hepatitis B, so as to ascertain if prophylaxis is required.

EXAMINATION

Physical Examination

Before beginning, the examiner should ask for the survivor's permission. When feasible and consent is forthcoming, photographs of injuries are taken.
- Orientation in time and space, pulse, blood pressure, respiration, temperature and state of pupils are noted.
- **General:** Stature and weight (for children) and nutritional status. Whether the survivor is anxious, fearful, tearful, happy or withdrawn is noted. Any signs of intoxication by ingestion/injection of drug/alcohol are noted. Oral cavity should also be examined for any evidence of bleeding, discharge, tear, edema or tenderness.
- **Clothes:** It should be ascertained whether the clothes are those which were worn at the time of the attack or changed. The survivor, in the presence of the doctor, should remove each item of clothing herself. She should be standing on a clean sheet of paper and anything that falls, e.g., mud, buttons, hair and fibers should be preserved.
    - Clothing should be examined for stains (blood, seminal, sand or grass), soiling, tears and loss of buttons, and the site and type of damage.
    - It should be air dried at room temperature and stored in a clean paper bag and sent to the laboratory. Clothes are very important in corroborating or contradicting her story.
    - If the offense has been committed outdoors, corroboration can sometimes be obtained by finding grass, leaves or mud on the buttock or on the back.
- **Breasts:** Sexual maturation (described by Tanner stage 1–5 or as 'pre-pubertal,' 'pubertal,' 'mature') is noted.
- **Examination with Wood's lamp** (filtered UV light): Examination using a Wood's lamp may detect semen or foreign debris on the skin. Dried seminal stains on the skin appear as pale yellow glistening areas, and will fluoresce under a Wood's lamp.

> **Sexual assault may result in the following:**
> - Extragenital injury
> - Genital injury
> - Psychologic symptoms
> - Sexually transmitted diseases (STDs)
> - Pregnancy

Extragenital Injury

Frequent sites for extragenital trauma include breasts, extremities, neck, buttocks and oropharynx. They represent residual features to the use of force and restraint. Ligature marks over wrists and ankles, and traction alopecia are additional signs of use of restraint and force.

The survivor's entire body must be thoroughly examined for areas of tenderness, soft-tissue swelling, abrasions, contusions, bite marks, lacerations, fractures and other evidence of violence—their appearance, extent, situation and approximate age (whether they correspond to the alleged time of infliction) should be noted **(Fig. 24.3)**.

Injuries are best represented on body charts. They must be numbered on the body charts and each must be described in detail.
- The back of the head may be banged against the ground resulting in soft tissue swelling and lacerations.
- Facial injuries including fracture of mandible and nose, and broken or loose teeth are often present.
- If the assailant pulls and twists the survivor's clothing, petechial hemorrhages or a line of punctuate bruising may occur on the skin, commonly in the area of the bra-strap or near the axilla.
- Marks of violence, especially contusions and abrasions, particularly fingernail abrasions may be found **(Fig. 24.3)**:
    i. Around the mouth and throat, inflicted while preventing her from calling for help **(Figs. 24.4A and B)**. Contusion of the lips and even tearing of the inner aspect may be found due to blows or rough handling.
    ii. About the wrists and arms where the man gripped her in restraint.
    iii. Around the medial aspects of thighs and knees caused by forcing her thighs wide apart.
    iv. On the back from pressure on gravel or hard ground on being held down on rough surface.
    v. On the breasts because of manual squeezing and manipulation.
    vi. True bite marks and love bites (*suction petechiae* result from rupture of small vessels due to reduced pressure) may be found on the breasts, neck, chest wall and also on the lower abdomen and upper part of the thighs **(Fig. 24.4C)**. The nipples may be bitten off.

The extent and nature of the general injuries should correspond to the survivor's description of the assault. If the throat has been gripped or if a severe blow is struck on the head, her capacity for resistance becomes greatly impaired. Injuries found on the body must be described specially with reference to the possibility of self-infliction or corroboration of survivor's tale.

Local Examination

- **Genitals:** The survivor is laid in the lithotomy position on the examination table, in good light with the parts

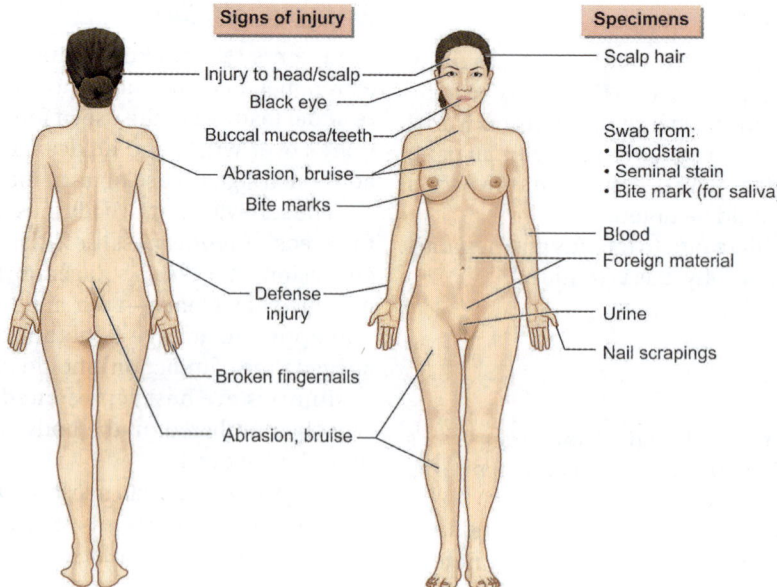

Fig. 24.3: General physical examination and specimens to be preserved in a survivor of rape

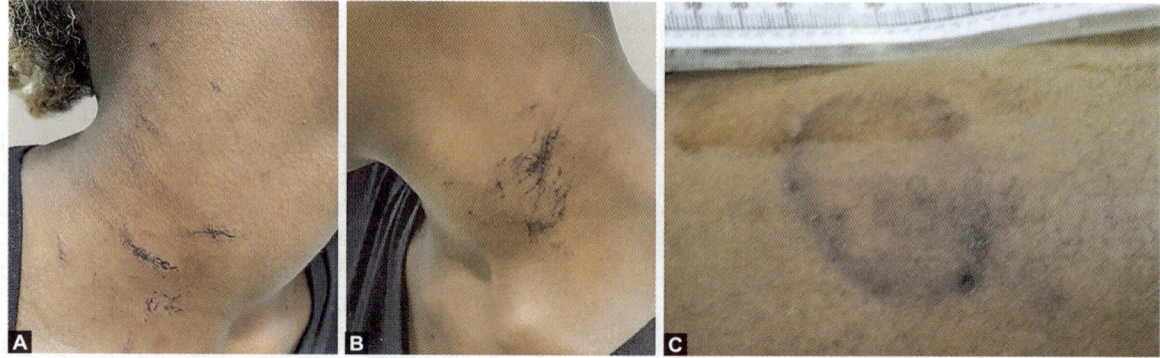

Figs. 24.4A to C: Extragenital injuries: (A and B) Nail scratches on both sides of neck in an attempted sexual assault; (C) Bite mark on thigh

fully exposed. The examination of genitalia is done using a speculum or a glass globe (*Glaister-keen globe*), sometimes transilluminated to stretch the hymen around for inspection of the edges.

- **Stains:** The presence or absence of bloodstains about the legs or vagina should be looked for and preserved.
- **Pubic hair:** The pubic hair should be examined for matting from seminal fluid or blood and for foreign hair. If the hair are matted together, a portion must be cut off and kept for examination. The pubic hair should also be combed out to collect loose foreign pubic hair and a comparison sample of cut/plucked hair (15–20 hair) is preserved. A catchment paper is used to collect and preserve the specimens. If pubic hair is shaved, it should be noted.

Genital Injury

- Acute findings of injury, whether in the genital or anal area include abrasions, bruising, edema and lacerations [acronym is TEARS: tears (T), ecchymosis (E), abrasions (A), redness (R) and swelling (S)].
- In case of sexual assault, the survivor's vagina is not lubricated, physical constraints may place the pelvis in an awkward position and insertion of penis into the vagina is usually by excessive force, which results in injuries to the vulva, hymen, vagina and the perineum (**Fig. 24.5**). Genital findings must also be marked on body charts and numbered accordingly.
  i. **Vulva:** The vulva is inspected systematically for any signs of recent injury such as bleeding, TEARS, or discharge and infection. Women with unclean habits often have superficial areas of erythema, irritation, and occasionally abrasions on their genital region. Therefore, any superficial injuries found in this area must be carefully assessed.
  ii. **Labia:** Injury to labia is not common, but fingernail scratches may be present on the labia, particularly the labia minora. Swelling and tenderness of the labia minora may be indicative of sexual activity. Swelling and engorgement of the vulva at the introitus, clitoris and labia minora are caused by penile stimulation,

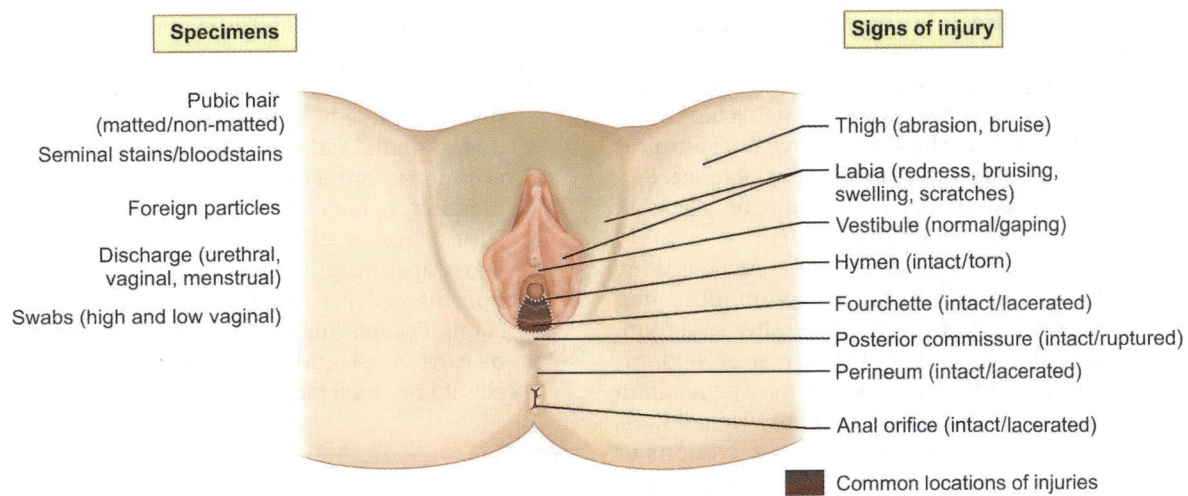

Fig. 24.5: Local examination and specimens to be preserved in a survivor of rape

but they may be caused by digital stimulation or masturbation. These signs normally fade in 1–2 h.

iii. **Hymen:** *Laceration of hymen occurs with the first intercourse, and in a virgin, this is the principal evidence of the same.* Tearing of hymen usually occurs postero-laterally or in the middle (5 to 7 O'clock position) (**Figs. 24.6 and 24.7**).
- The semilunar hymen often ruptures on both sides. The annular hymen, which nearly closes the vaginal orifice may suffer several tears.
- Soon after the act, the torn margins are sharp, red and bleed on touch (**Fig. 24.8**). Even when examined after 3–4 days of the act, the edges are swollen, congested and smaller.
- *Signs of recent rupture of hymen* are ragged tears in the hymen with lack of epithelial healing, edema and hemorrhage.
- The status of hymen is irrelevant because it can be torn due to cycling, riding or masturbation. An intact hymen does not rule out sexual violence, and a torn hymen does not prove previous sexual intercourse. Only those that are relevant to the episode of assault (such as fresh tears, bleeding or edema) are to be documented.

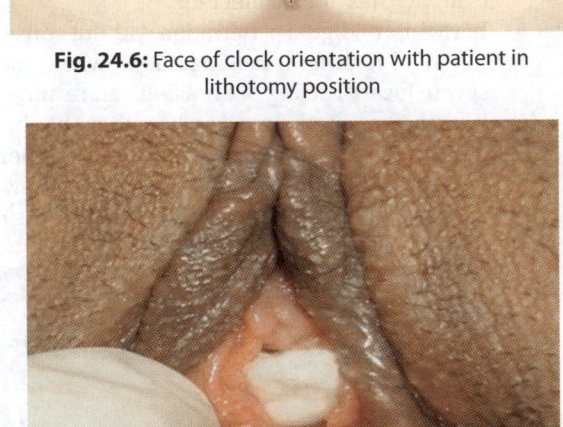

Fig. 24.6: Face of clock orientation with patient in lithotomy position

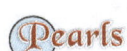

Pearls

| Hymen may not rupture after sexual intercourse if: |
- Penetration was not full
- Hymen is tough, fleshy and elastic
- In young child, full penetration may not occur
- In deflorated woman

iv. **Posterior commissure:** The posterior commissure may be ruptured, especially if there is disparity in size between the male and the female organs (**Fig. 24.8A**).

v. **Fourchette:** The fourchette is fragile and often tears during first intercourse (**Fig. 24.8A**).

Fig. 24.7: Sexual intercourse in 16-year-old girl, one year back; fimbriated hymen got torn at 5–6 O'clock position and subsequently healed (cotton has been kept to highlight the tear)

(*Courtesy:* Dr Promila Jindal, Ex-Professor & Head, DMCH, Ludhiana)

vi. **Fossa navicularis:** Fossa navicularis is obliterated.
vii. **Vagina**
- Per-vaginum examination, or the **'two-finger test',** *must not be conducted* for establishing rape/sexual violence. The size of the vaginal introitus has no bearing on a case of sexual violence. Per-vaginum examination can be done only in adult women when medically indicated.
- Vaginal examination of an adult female is done with the help of a sterile speculum lubricated with warm saline/sterile water. Per speculum examination is not a must in the case of children/young girls when there is no history of penetration and no visible injuries. The cervix, vaginal walls and vault is inspected, and any secretions or injury is noted. If there is vaginal discharge, note its texture, color and odor.
- Contusions of the vagina are seen as dark red areas against the overall redness of the vaginal mucosa, and within 24 h the color becomes deep red or purple. They are more frequently seen on the anterior vaginal wall in lower third and posterior vaginal wall in upper third.
- In case injuries are not visible, suspected injuries are looked for using a magnifying glass/colposcope (whatever is available). If 1% toluidine blue is available, it is sprayed and excess is wiped out. Subtle injuries will stand out in blue **(Fig. 24.8B)**. Care should be taken that this test is done only after swabs for trace evidence has been collected.
- In vaginal or digital penetration without consent, initial lubrication is lacking due to which more severe local bruising or abrasion can result.
- With violent intercourse or where there has been considerable disproportion between the penis and the vagina, laceration of the vaginal wall occurs posteriorly **(Fig. 24.8C)**. The gait is broad based and painful. The examination may have to be performed under general anesthesia.

viii. **Cervix:** Abrasion of the cervix occurs almost invariably due to vaginal penetration, and usually due to digital rather than penile penetration. The abrasion is found away from the external os and the margins are not clearly defined.

ix. Bleeding/swelling/tears/discharge/stains/warts around the anus and anal orifice must be documented. Per-rectal examination to detect tears/stains/fissures/hemorrhoids in the anal canal must be carried out, and relevant swabs from these sites should be collected.

> **NOTA BENE**
>
> **Colposcopic examination:** Colposcopy is particularly sensitive for subtle genital injuries. Some colposcopes have cameras attached, making it possible to detect and photograph injuries simultaneously. Using colposcopy, it has been found that the injury to the posterior fourchette is the most commonly seen in women after sexual assault.
>
> **Hymeneal examination**
> - The hymen is examined by application of gentle traction outwards and downwards at posterior edge of labia majora. The patient is asked to 'push against' the fingers which will open up the hymeneal orifice if not visible on traction. A cotton swab inserted through the hymeneal orifice may also be used to look at the hymeneal rim. It can then be used as a specimen for laboratory examination.
> - *Glaister-keen globes* are glass rods (diameter of 0.6 mm with one end of the rod being expanded into globe from 1–2.5 cm in diameter) which can be inserted gently behind the hymen to display its edges over the glass. In this way, apparent folds and indentations smooth out and small nicks and tears can be easily identified.
> - Hymeneal swelling is often difficult to document at the time of initial examination.
> - A statement about the state of the hymen should be made: words such as *intact or nonviolated, remnants, parous* and *old scarring* are preferable; *marital* should be avoided.

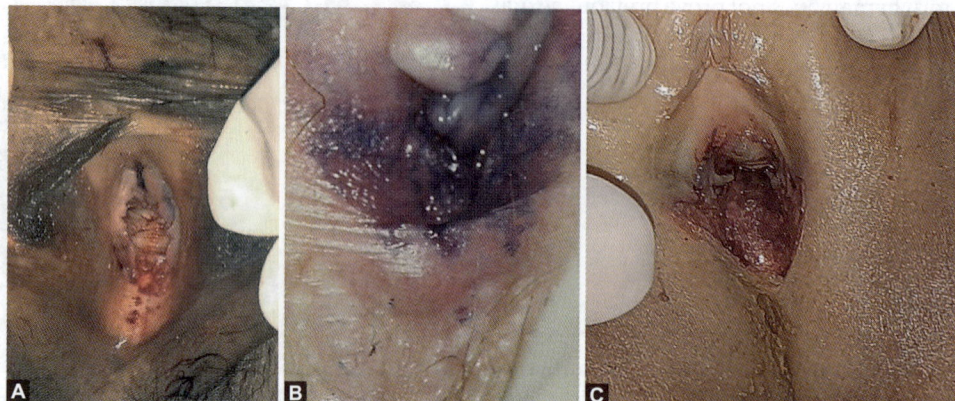

Figs. 24.8A to C: (A) Rupture of hymen (6 O'clock), tearing of fourchette and posterior commissure; (B) Toluidine blue test to showing subtle abrasions in perineum; (C) Laceration of vaginal wall
[*Courtesy:* (A) Dr Promila Jindal, Ex-Professor & Head, DMCH, Ludhiana; (C) Dr Mahender Singh, PGI Rohtak)]

SPECIMENS FOR LABORATORY EXAMINATION

Investigations and Collection of Samples for Hospital Laboratory

- *Age estimation:* If requested by the police, radiographs of wrist, elbow, shoulders and pelvis along with dental examination can be advised for age estimation.
- For any suspected fracture, X-rays for the relevant part of the body is advised.
- Urine pregnancy test should be done.
- Blood is collected for evidence of baseline HIV status, VDRL and HbsAg.

Collection of Samples for Forensic Science Laboratory (FSL)

After assessment of the case, evidence is collected and preserved **(Box 24.3, Figs. 24.3, 24.5 and 24.9)**. The nature of swabs and samples is determined by the history, nature of assault, and time lapse between incident and examination, and if she has bathed/washed herself since the assault. The likelihood of finding evidence after 72 h (3 days) is greatly reduced; however, it is better to collect evidence up to 96 h in case the survivor may be unsure of the number of hours lapsed since the assault. Evidence on the outside of the body and on materials such as clothing can be collected even after 96 h.

- *Clothes* that the survivor was wearing at the time of the incident. Pack each piece of clothing in a separate bag, seal and label it duly. The sheet of paper on which she removed her clothes is folded carefully and preserved in a bag for trace evidence detection.
- *Swabs* are used to collect bloodstains on the body, foreign material on the body surfaces, seminal stains on the skin surfaces and other stains.
- *Hair:* Detection of scalp hair and pubic hair of the accused on the survivor's body (and vice-versa) has evidentiary value. All hair must be collected in the catchment paper which is then folded and sealed.
- *Nail scrapings:* Nail clippings and scrapings are taken from both hands, and packed separately. In case of struggle, the accused and the survivor may have scratched each other, and epithelial cells of one may be present under the nails of the other that can be used for DNA detection.
- *Blood sample* is collected for grouping and also helps in comparing and matching bloodstains at the scene of crime. Venous blood is collected with a sterile syringe and needle and transferred to 3 sterile vials/vacutainers for the following purposes: plain vial/vacutainer—blood grouping and drug estimation, sodium fluoride—alcohol estimation, EDTA—DNA analysis.
- *Urine sample* is collected to test for drugs and alcohol levels as required.
  If drug/alcohol is found in the blood/urine, the validity of consent is called into question. There may not be any physical or genital injuries, since this may have affected the survivor's ability to offer resistance.
- *Oral swab* is collected for detection of semen and spermatozoa. Oral swabs are taken from the posterior parts of the buccal cavity, behind the last molars where the chances of finding any evidence are highest.

Genital and Anal Evidence

If a woman reports within 96 h (4 days) of the assault, all swabs based on the nature of assault are collected. For example, if the survivor is certain that there is no anal intercourse; anal swabs need not be taken. The spermatozoa can be identified till 72 h after assault. If she reports after 3 days, swabs for spermatozoa are useless. In such cases, swabs should only be sent for identifying semen.

- Take two swabs from the vulva, vagina and anal opening for anogenital evidence depending on the history and examination **(Figs. 24.10A and B)**. Swabs from orifices should be collected only if there is a history of penetration.
- Two vaginal smears are to be prepared on the glass slides provided, air-dried in the shade and sent for seminal fluid/spermatozoa examination **(Fig. 24.10C)**.
- Often lubricants are used in penetration with finger or object, so swabs must be taken for detection of lubricant. Other pieces of evidence such as tampons (may be available as well), which should be preserved.
- Vaginal washing is collected using a syringe and a small rubber catheter. Two millilitre of normal saline is instilled into the posterior fornix of vagina and fluid is aspirated. Fluid filled syringe is sent to FSL for motile sperms after putting a knot over the rubber catheter. Spermatozoa are best recovered from the posterior fornix. Detection of spermatozoa is thus possible in cases where a speculum examination is denied. The presence of spermatozoa serves as proof of sexual intercourse and may give the identity of the alleged perpetrator through DNA-profiling.
- Oral and rectal smears and swabs should be kept in all autopsy cases.

> **Box 24.3** Specimens preserved for laboratory examination
>
> i. Clothing: Stained, torn, foreign material.
> ii. Scraping of dried bloodstains: Grouping, DNA characteristics.
> iii. Scraping of dried seminal stains: Grouping, sperms, acid phosphatase, semen specific glycoprotein (p30), DNA profiling.
> iv. Hair: Matted pubic hair, foreign hair, plucked/cut hair from pubis and scalp.
> v. Broken nails and scraping from under the nails.
> vi. Bite mark examination: Bite marks can be as individual as fingerprints.
> vii. Blood: Grouping, alcohol, drugs, VDRL, HIV, DNA profiling.
> viii. Saliva: Secretor status.
> ix. Swabs from any soiled area of skin, bite marks and swabs from mouth, pharynx, vagina and anus for spermatozoa, microorganisms, p30 glycoprotein and sexually transmitted diseases.

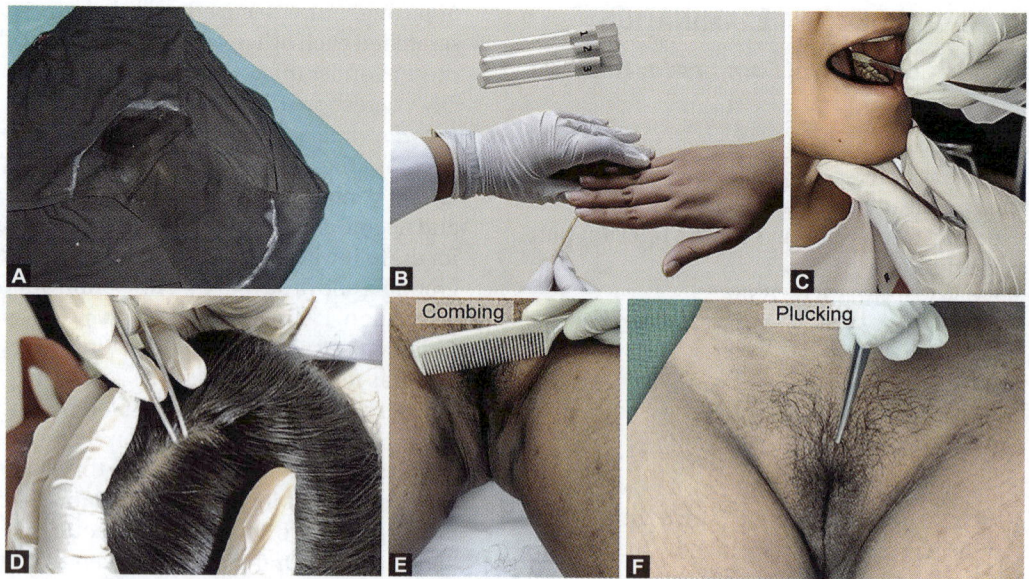

Figs. 24.9A to F: Collection of evidences and samples: (A) Stained undergarments; (B) Nail scrapings; (C) Oral swab; (D) Scalp hair; (E and F) Pubic hair

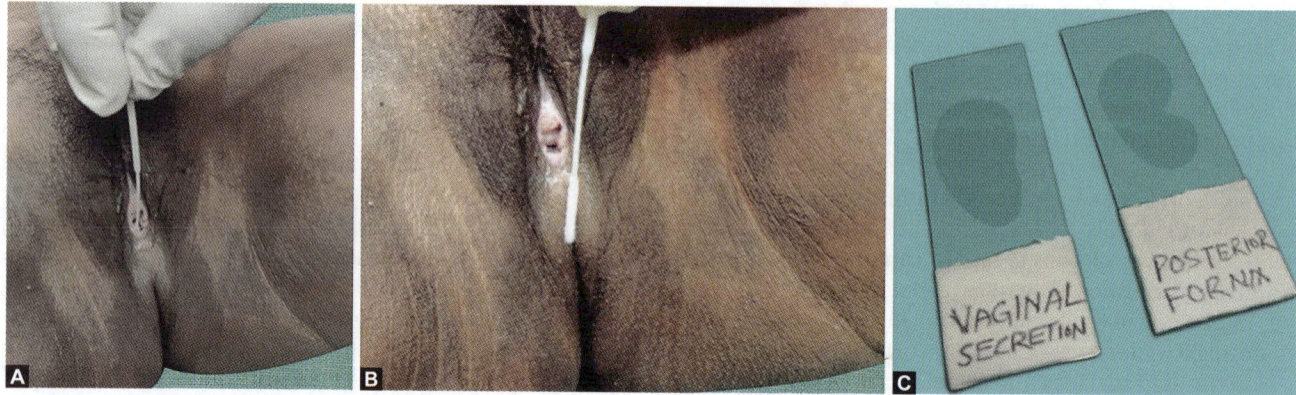

Figs. 24.10A to C: Genital evidence collection: (A) Vaginal swab; (B) Perineal swab; (C) Swabs on glass slides

Swab sticks for collecting samples should be moistened with distilled water provided. Swabs must be air dried, but not dried in direct sunlight. Drying of swabs is absolutely mandatory as there may be decomposition/degradation of evidence which can render it unusable.

The collected samples for evidence are preserved in the hospital till such time that police are able to complete their paper work for dispatch to FSL. Vaginal swab samples need to be refrigerated if not sent immediately for testing. While handing over the samples, a requisition letter addressed to the FSL, stating what all samples are being sent and what each sample needs to be tested for should be stated. This form must be signed by the examining doctor, as well as the officer to whom the evidence is handed over. A chain of custody must be maintained.

- After completion of examination, she is allowed to wash-up using the toiletries provided by the hospital, change clothing, use mouthwash, and urinate or defecate, if needed.
- Survivors should receive all services free of cost. This includes OPD/inpatient registration, laboratory and radiology investigations, urine pregnancy test and medicines.
- A copy of all documentation (including that pertaining to medico-legal examination and treatment) must be provided to her free of cost.

OPINION

- The medical practitioner should write the report and forward it without delay to the IO who in turn forwards it to the Magistrate. The report must state precisely the reasons for each conclusion arrived at **(Sec. 164-A CrPC)**.
- The provisional opinion must, in brief, mention relevant aspects of the history of sexual violence, clinical findings and samples which are sent for analysis to FSL. The report should contain negative, as well as

positive findings. An inference must be drawn in the opinion, correlating the history and clinical findings **(Table 24.2)**.

- The final opinion of whether sexual intercourse has taken place or not is based on a consideration of **(Table 24.2)**:
    i. Signs of struggle.
    ii. Presence of blood and/or seminal stains on clothes and body.
    iii. Presence of seminal matter in the vagina.
    iv. Transmission of venereal disease.
    v. FSL reports.
- It should be always kept in mind that normal examination findings neither refute nor confirm the forceful sexual intercourse. Hence circumstantial/other evidence may be taken into consideration.
- Doctors must not entertain questions from the police such as 'whether rape has occurred?', or 'whether survivor is capable of sexual intercourse?' They should explain the nature of medico-legal evidence and its limitations.
- The doctor should never make a diagnosis of 'rape' because it is a legal term. He may give opinion that there are signs of recent vaginal penetration, general physical injury and/or intoxication and that the signs are consistent with the history given. In short, the opinion should be regarding sexual intercourse and not regarding rape which will be decided in the court. *Rape is an allegation easy to make, hard to prove and still harder to disprove.*

Follow-up: It involves:
  i. Treatment of injuries.
  ii. Tetanus prophylaxis.
  iii. Prevention and termination of pregnancy.
  iv. Prevention and treatment of any venereal disease.
  v. Psychiatric consultation to regain dignity and self-respect, and prevention of development of post-traumatic stress disorder (PTSD).

CORROBORATIVE SIGNS OF SEXUAL ASSAULT

Based on **Locard's exchange principle** 'every contact leaves a trace'; evidence is collected during and soon after the examination is completed.

Evidence from Seminal Fluid

The thighs, pubic hair and vagina of the survivor should be examined. The presence of spermatozoa in the vagina is proof of connection, but not of rape; *their absence is no proof that connection has not taken place.*

Sometimes, the history and examination suggests sexual intercourse, but evidence is often absent or inconclusive. There may be number of explanations besides the obvious suggestion of a false complaint (**Table 24.3**). Evidence becomes weaker or disappears as time passes, particularly after >36 h; mechanical elimination (drainage, hygiene), biological degradation and physiologic dilution.

Swabbing of mouth, vagina and anus for sperm detection should always be performed on rape survivors. The presence of smegma bacilli is suggestive of coitus. Its absence is without any significance.

Evidence from Vaginal Discharge

Vaginal discharge may arise from local infection, worms or uncleanliness. If the assailant is suffering from venereal disease such as hepatitis, syphilis, gonorrhea, chlamydial

TABLE 24.2: Drafting of opinion based on examination findings and FSL report

Genital injuries	Physical injuries	Provisional opinion	FSL report	Final opinion
Present	Present	There are signs suggestive of recent forceful penetration of vagina/anus. Sexual violence cannot be ruled out	Positive for presence of semen	There are signs suggestive of forceful vaginal/anal intercourse
			Negative for presence of semen/lubricant	There are no signs suggestive vaginal/anal intercourse, but evidence of physical and genital assault present
Present	Absent	There are signs suggestive of recent forceful penetration of vagina/anus	Positive for presence of semen	There are signs suggestive of forceful vaginal/anal intercourse
			Negative for presence of semen/lubricant	There are no signs suggestive of vaginal/anal intercourse, but there is evidence of genital assault
Absent	Present	There are signs of use of force, however, vaginal/anal/oral penetration cannot be ruled out	Positive for semen	There are signs suggestive of forceful vaginal/anal intercourse
			Negative for semen/lubricant	There are no signs suggestive of vaginal/anal intercourse, but there is evidence of physical assault
Absent	Absent	There are no signs of use of force; however, final opinion is reserved pending availability of FSL reports. Sexual violence cannot be ruled out	Positive for semen	There are signs suggestive of vaginal/anal intercourse
			Positive for semen and alcohol	There are signs suggestive of vaginal/anal intercourse under the influence of alcohol
			Positive for lubricant	There is a possibility of vaginal/anal penetration by lubricated object
			Negative for semen/alcohol/lubricant	There are no signs suggestive of penetration of vagina/anus

TABLE 24.3: Factors resulting in failure to detect semen from the victim

No seminal constituents recovered	No spermatozoa recovered
♦ Time delay between assault and examination (drainage and degradation)	♦ Impaired delivery (vasectomy, trauma, congenital anomalies)
♦ Victim's hygiene (douching, bathing, gargling)	♦ Depleted stores (due to frequent ejaculation)
♦ Condom use	♦ Very old age
♦ Physiologic activity (urination, defecation, menstruation)	♦ Impaired spermatogenesis (azoospermia)
♦ Sexual dysfunction in the assailant	
♦ Poor technique of the examining doctor	

infection, trichomoniasis or HIV infection, he may transmit it to his victim, which is a strong corroborative evidence of intercourse.

- In gonorrhea, an inflammation with abundant micropurulent discharge will be seen in 2–4 days (occasionally a week), while in syphilis, an indurated ulcer on the external genitals may appear in about 3 weeks.
- An initial negative smear may be of value, if a positive smear is obtained within a few days of the assault.
- A blood sample should be taken for serological examination for syphilis. An initial negative reaction may be of value, if a positive reaction is obtained after 6 weeks.
- Sometimes, the sores on the genitals may be due to chancroid. Smears from sores or bubo fluid, when stained show the Ducerey's bacillus.

Evidence of Struggle

Signs of active resistance may be present. The fingernails may be broken due to scratching the accused. Under the nails, debris may be present, e.g., blood, fibers, hair and skin fragment from the accused. Other signs of defense may also be present.

Time of Assault

i. **Wounds:** Age of abrasions and contusions should corroborate with the alleged time of assault.
ii. **Seminal fluid:** Survival time of spermatozoa in vagina of living individual is quite variable.
    - Normally, sperms remain motile in the vagina for about 6–8 h, and occasionally up to 12 h, and very rarely up to 24 h. In the later case, it is probable that the specimen was obtained from cervical mucus.
    - Non-motile forms are detectable for about 24 h with occasional reports of 48–72 h.
    - If motile sperms were seen in wet smears on a slide, it would mean that intercourse has taken place within about 12 h. If the sperms are not motile, it is not possible to say exactly when intercourse took place, except that it may be over 12 h and within about 24–48 h and occasionally up to 72 h.
iii. **Venereal disease:** Development of venereal disease may be helpful in estimating the time of assault.

> **NOTA BENE**
>
> ♦ **Motile sperms:** The technique requires the preparation of a 'wet mount' slide (vaginal or cervical swab sample placed with a drop of saline plus cover slip) and examined with a phase-contrast microscope.
> ♦ Swabs should be taken from the vaginal pool and not the cervix because sperm can survive in cervical mucus much longer than in the vagina. It is important when searching for motile sperms in an individual allegedly raped only few hours before, to obtain the specimen from the vaginal pool and not from the cervix, since sperm seen on a cervical swab may not be caused by the rape, but by sexual intercourse 2–3 days before (if history of consensual intercourse is present).
> ♦ Sperms have been identified in the vagina of dead individuals 1–2 weeks after death. In dead, the sperm are destroyed by decomposition and not by drainage or by the action of vaginal secretions. Sperms that are deposited on materials like cotton, cloth or paper and air dried can be identified years after the event.
> ♦ When no sperm are observed, part of each of the swabs from the vagina, rectum and mouth can be used for presumptive tests for acid phosphatase. If however, sexual intercourse is still strongly suspected or if acid phosphatase test was weakly positive, an assay for prostate specific antigen (p30) should be performed. Occasionally, p30 is positive in the face of a negative acid phosphatase.
> ♦ **Acid phosphatase:** It is usually present in the vagina for up to 18–24 h after sexual intercourse and occasionally up to 72 h. The highest levels are within the first 12 h with gradual disappearance by 48–72 h. Because it usually disappears in the first 24 h after intercourse, it is most useful as an indicator of recent intercourse, compared with non-motile sperm which can be identified up to 2–3 days after intercourse.

RAPE ON DEFLORATE/SEXUALLY ACTIVE WOMAN

- In deflorate women, even without childbirth, the hymen is completely destroyed, the vaginal orifice is dilated and the mucous membrane wrinkled and thickened with complete loss of rugosity. Complete penetration can occur in such women and leaves no evidence, except for semen. *The only proof that the penetration has occurred is presence of spermatozoa in the vagina.*
- The absence of injury under certain circumstances, therefore, does not exclude even complete penetration. However, mark of genital injury should be looked for, as rape is generally associated with greater violence than consensual sexual intercourse.
- The majority of adult rapes are associated with a sudden forcible dilation of vagina resulting in some degree of local or general injury. Bruising, abrasion or lacerations are at all times consistent with forcible intercourse with a consenting woman, and do not necessarily indicate sexual assault.

- A second examination of the victim would be made, for bruising may take a little time to come to the surface, especially in the lower vagina.
- The vagina may show laceration or bruising with effusion of blood, and swelling and inflammation of the vulva, even when no marks of violence indicating a struggle may be found externally. Tearing or perforation of the vagina may occur when it is thin or friable.
- In case of older women, senile atrophy and friability of their genitalia results in extensive vaginal lacerations and perineal trauma.
- In women who have been used to sexual intercourse, injuries from rape normally disappear or become obscure in 3–4 days. When there has been much violence, the signs may persist longer. The presence of violence in other parts of the body is the chief evidence of the crime.
- All injuries of the labia and vagina found in cases of sexual assault are not due to rough manual and penile contact. Tears in the deeper part of vagina and gross lacerating wounds of the vault are not likely to occur during sexual intercourse, but are often caused by sexual perverts using instruments (*impalement*). The acts may be separate incidents or they may follow coitus.

RAPE ON CHILDREN

Medical examination and treatment for children is similar as that for adults. However, it is important to follow some specific rules:

- In case the child is <12 years of age, consent for examination is taken from the parent/guardian.
- In case the parent or legal guardian is suspected of possible sexual abuse, the superintendent/in-charge of the hospital can give the necessary permission and appoint a female person to be present during the examination. Otherwise, a police officer can apply for legal consent from a Magistrate for the child to be examined.
- It should not be assumed that because of tender age, the child will not be able to provide a history. History seeking can be facilitated by assuring confidentiality and providing privacy, and use of dolls and body charts.
- What the child is reporting should be believed. There is mistaken belief that children lie or that they are tutored by parents to make false complaints against others.
- A few indicators for routine enquiry are pain on urination and/or defecation, abdominal pain, inability to sleep, sudden withdrawal from peers/adults, feelings of anxiety, nervousness, helplessness, weight loss, and feelings of ending one's life.

Examination

Lubricants, child's 'cooperation' and delayed disclosure of the events—all reduce the possibility of identifying acute findings of sexual contact.

A small child must never be held down during examination of the genital area, this is equivalent to sexually assaulting the child and will intensify the trauma. When indicated, the child should be taken to the operating room and anesthetized so that proper assessment and treatment can be done.

- In a young child, there are few or no signs of general violence, for the child usually has no idea of what is happening and also incapable of resisting.
- As the hymen is deeply situated and the vagina is less capacious, it is impossible for penetration of the penis to take place. Usually, the penis is placed either within the vulva or between the thighs. As such, the hymen is usually intact, and there may be little redness and tenderness of the vulva.
- During forceful penetration, the penis can compress the labia both anteriorly and laterally, producing bruising of both the labia majora and minora. Further penetration forces the penis backwards (symphysis pubis prevents its anterior movement) and the hymen is torn posteriorly. If the penis advances into the vagina, the hymenal tear extends into or through the perineal body and often involves the anterior wall of the anorectal canal.
- The younger the child, the more widespread are the injuries. Full penile penetration produces bruising of the vaginal walls and frequently tears of the anterior and posterior vaginal walls. Anterior tears can involve the bladder and posteriorly the anorectal canal. Vaginal vault may rupture and there may be vaginal herniation of abdominal viscera.
- Any attempt to separate the thighs for examination causes great pain because of the local inflammation. The child walks with difficulty due to pain.
- The absence of marks of violence on the genitals of the child when an early examination is made, is strong evidence that sexual intercourse has not taken place.
- In **digital penetration** of the infant vagina, there is frequently some scratching or bruising of the labia and vestibule, but circumferential tears are absent. The hymen shows a linear tear in the posterior or posterolateral quadrant which may extend into the posterior vagina and on to the skin of the perineum. Anorectal canal is rarely torn.
- In **fondling of genitals**, the findings will depend on the degree of force applied. In most of the cases, force is not used and thus findings are nonspecific. In cases of excessive force being used, there may be erythema of the fondled area, edema, superficial abrasions and contusions. In case of rubbing of penis during fondling, the child may experience superficial trauma to the urethra and the mucosa of the vestibule. Dysuria is common symptom.

MEDICO-LEGAL QUESTIONS

Q. Whether resistance was offered by the victim?

- In ordinary conditions, it is not possible for a male to have sexual intercourse with a healthy adult female in full possession of her senses and against her will.

- The victim may not be able to offer marked resistance from terror or from an overwhelming feeling of helplessness or when her movements may have been obstructed by her clothing.
- The social status, physical development and type of woman should also be considered—a woman used to look after herself is less likely to be terrified than a woman who has led a sheltered life.
- When a woman is overpowered by two or more men, she cannot resist much, and marks of violence may not be marked.
- Absence of injuries may be due to inability of survivor to offer resistance to the assailant because of intoxication or threats, or delay in reporting for examination.

Q. Whether any drug/narcotic was given before the act?

- Rape may be committed without the knowledge of the woman while she is under the influence of drugs, such as opium, cocaine, hyoscine, alcohol, anesthetic or in a coma and in a hypnotic trance.
- When a woman takes alcohol voluntarily in order to encourage caressing or increase sexual feeling and becomes a victim of sexual assault, the question of consent depends on the extent to which she had become affected. If she is conscious, she can refuse consent. In such cases, complete history should be taken, and blood and urine should be preserved for examination.
- The use of anesthetic agent for surgical or dental operations may result in a charge of rape, especially in neurotic women, who in their anesthetic flights of imagination believe themselves to have been sexually assaulted.
- It is difficult to put a woman under the influence of chloroform, ether or halothane by force so as to rape her. There is no drug which can produce immediate unconsciousness when placed in front of the nostrils.

False Allegations

The possibility of accusation and false allegation must be suspected when:
i. Statement of the victim which is neither convincing nor consistent with relation to the description of assailant, time of assault, scene, consent, clothing and circumstances.
ii. Injuries—the dating of which does not correspond to the time of the alleged incident.
iii. Doubtful story about administration of drugs.
iv. Injuries are not serious and are made either by fingernails, instruments or irritants.
v. Injuries do not involve sensitive areas, such as face, genitals, nipples and lips.
vi. Confirmatory laboratory findings are absent.

INDICATORS OF SEXUAL ABUSE

Sometimes, survivors may not reveal a history of sexual violence; the following signs and symptoms may lead to suspect the possibility of sexual abuse/assault:
- **Physical health consequences:** Abdominal pain, burning micturition, sexual dysfunction, dyspareunia, menstrual disorders, urinary tract infections, unwanted pregnancy, miscarriage of an existing fetus, exposure to sexually transmitted infections (including HIV/AIDS), pelvic inflammatory disease, infertility, and mutilated genitalia.
- **Psychological health consequences**
  - *Short-term psychological effects*: Fear and shock, physical and emotional pain, intense self-disgust, powerlessness, worthlessness, apathy, denial, numbing, withdrawal, inability to function normally in their daily lives.
  - *Long-term psychological effects*: Depression and chronic anxiety, feelings of vulnerability, loss of control/self-esteem, emotional distress, nightmares, self-blame, mistrust, avoidance and post-traumatic stress disorder, chronic mental disorders, attempting suicide or endangering their lives.

Rape Trauma Syndrome

It is a psychological trauma and is regarded as post-traumatic stress disorder (PTSD). PTSD is an anxiety disorder marked by biological changes, as well as psychological symptoms.

It is characterized by two phases:
i. *Phase of disorganization* where there is headache, GIT complaints, immune system problems, dizziness, chest pain, discomfort, emotional imbalance, depression and feeling of guilt.
It is followed by:
ii. *Phase of reorganization* in which there is gradual adjustment with occasional phobia and fear state (nightmares), avoidance of thoughts, feelings and situations related to the assault, and increased arousal (e.g., difficulty in sleeping and concentrating, jumpiness, and irritability).

Symptoms last for >1 month, and significantly impair social and occupational functioning.

Treatment: PTSD is treated by psychotherapy and drug therapy (selective serotonin reuptake inhibitors). At present, cognitive-behavioral therapy appears to be somewhat more effective than drug therapy.

Marital Rape

Legally, it is assumed that consent for sexual intercourse is implicit in the contract of marriage. So, it has been assumed that husband cannot rape his wife. But now, the concept of marital rape is being considered in modern law.

The common law must take prevailing social attitudes into account. Marriage is regarded as a partnership of equals, and females are no longer considered as a weaker sex and subordinate to the husband. Husband has got no extra privilege or an absolute right to enjoy his wife's body even against her will and less so, by the use of force causing pain or injury.

Husband may be charged with cruelty and assault on wife. On the other hand, if the wife continuously and unreasonably refuses sexual intercourse, he may plead for divorce.

Findings: Anal and rectal injuries are known as markers for marital rape. In married couples, the most frequent type of forced sex is vaginal intercourse followed by forced anal intercourse. Rectal penetration can also be associated with an increased risk of genitorectal injury.

Battered Wife Syndrome

Battered wife syndrome is a symptom complex of repeated unwanted violent acts of physical, sexual and psychological abuse of a woman (partner) by her husband.

- *Presenting complaints*: They often present with vague somatic complaints, such as headache, insomnia, lower back pain, abdominal pain and dyspareunia **(Box 24.4)**. The diagnosis is usually made by asking nonthreatening open-ended questions.
- *Characteristics*: Battering men and battered women are found in all levels of society, although younger, lower income, less-educated men who have observed parental violence in their own home are at higher risk of abusing their spouses. Additionally, antisocial personality disorder, depression, and/or alcohol and drug abuse increases the risk.
- This violence is usually motivated by his need to control her by inducing fear and pain.
- In most cases, battering occurs in cycles comprising of a tension building phase of unpredictable length, a violent explosion, and then calm and loving respite. These contradictory behaviors cause confusion and ambivalence in battered woman; they develop a pattern of 'learned helplessness'.

Box 24.4 Symptoms of battered wife syndrome

- Intrusive recollections of the trauma event(s)
- Hyperarousal and high levels of anxiety
- Avoidance behavior and emotional numbing (usually expressed as depression, dissociation, minimization, repression, and denial)
- Disrupted interpersonal relationships from batterer's power and control measures
- Body image distortion and/or somatic or physical complaints
- Sexual intimacy issues

EXAMINATION OF RAPE ACCUSED

It is better to examine the accused after the survivor, and to look specifically for any injuries which she says, she has inflicted. The procedure of examination of the accused is similar to the survivor.

The medical practitioner should without delay, examine and prepare the report giving the following particulars **(Sec. 53-A CrPC)**:

Preliminary Data

i. Name, age, occupation, address, brought by whom, identification marks, date, place and time of examination should be noted.
ii. Consent should be asked for. But if refused, then he can be examined without consent and necessary evidence, e.g., blood, swabs, etc. can be collected with application of reasonable force.
iii. Presence of attendant is not necessary.
iv. History of his version of the case is recorded.
v. Mental state and behavior should be noted.

Clothes should be examined for tears, loss of buttons, foreign matter, stains—blood, seminal, mud and cosmetic stains.

General examination: General physical examination including development of genital organs, secondary sexual characters and physical built of the accused is noted.

Marks of injury (bruises, scratches or bite marks) on the body should be noted. A thorough examination should be done of fingers and nails, as well as knees and elbows for any abrasions. Age of the injuries should be determined.

Local Examination

Genitals

1. *Pubic hair:* Any foreign/matted/female pubic hair to be preserved. The person's pubic hair is also preserved.
2. *Development of genital organs* with special reference to the potency. Any injury to the genital organs is to be noted. Forceful penetration against the resistance into a hymen may produce tears or bruising of the frenulum of the prepuce in uncircumcised penis, and abrasion of the glans in both the uncircumcised and circumcised penis.
3. The penis should be examined for:
   i. **Smegma** (thick cheesy secretion along with desquamated epithelial cells and smegma bacilli), if present under the prepuce and corona glandis is inconsistent with recent sexual intercourse. The smegma is rubbed off during intercourse which takes about 24 h for re-deposition.
   ii. **Lugol's iodine test:** It is now redundant. Iodine solution painted on the glans would reveal the presence vaginal epithelial cells by turning brown due to the glycogen present in them. Alternatively,

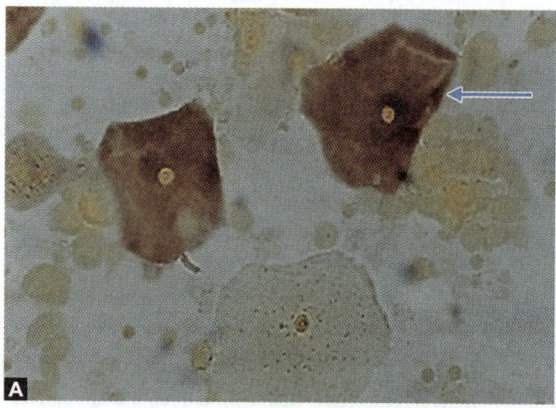
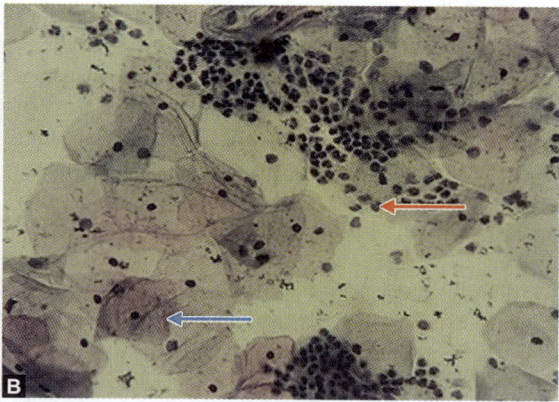

Figs. 24.11A and B: Smear showing mature vaginal squamous cells (blue arrows): (A) Lugol iodine; (B) PAP stain [showing neutrophils also (red arrow)]

air-dried penile swabs can be preserved from glans of the penis and then staining can be done with Lugol's solution **(Fig. 24.11A)**.

iii. Suspect penis is washed with saline and the material is stained with Papanicolaou's stain. Vaginal and cervical cells, and Barr body identification suggest recent intercourse, unless the assailant has used a condom **(Fig. 24.11B)**.

iv. Presence of venereal discharge or syphilitic chancre.

Specimens to be collected and preserved are given in **Box 24.5**.

If samples from both the victim and the suspect are packed on the same table or surface, contamination of the samples can occur. Therefore, care must be taken to ensure that accidental contamination of samples does not occur.

> **Box 24.5** Specimens to be preserved.
> i. Clothing: Stained, torn, missing buttons, foreign matter
> ii. Scrapings of blood and seminal stains: Grouping, DNA characteristics
> iii. Hair: Matted pubic hair, foreign hair and control hair sample from the scalp (minimum of 20 hair)
> iv. Saliva: Secretor status
> v. Debris under the nail
> vi. Blood: Grouping, alcohol, drugs, VDRL, ELISA for HIV

> **NOTA BENE**
>
> **Examination of rape accused (Sec. 53-A CrPC)**
> - If a person is arrested on a charge of committing rape and an examination may afford evidence, then a RMP working in a Govt. hospital or local authority or any other RMP (in the absence of such a doctor) within the radius of 16 kms from the place where the offense has been committed, at the request of a police officer (not below S.I.) may examine the person using reasonable force as necessary.
> - The doctor should prepare a report without delay, giving reasons for each conclusion arrived at, and document the specimens taken from the accused.
> - This may include the examination of blood, bloodstains, semen, swabs, sputum and sweat, hair samples and fingernail clippings by use of modern techniques including DNA profiling.
> - The report is handed over to the IO who then forwards it to the Magistrate.

INCEST

Definition: Sexual intercourse by a man with a woman who is closely related to him by blood or by marriage (prohibited degrees of relationship), e.g., a daughter, grand-daughter, sister, stepsister or aunt.

Examples are:
- Between father and daughter (e.g., the Electra complex).
- Between mother and son (e.g., Oedipus complex).
- Between brother and sister (e.g., Pharaonic incest).

Circumstances of incest can be both social and environmental:
i. Family strife and disorganization.
ii. In low socioeconomic groups.
iii. Overcrowding.
iv. Lack of parental supervision.
v. Low morality and delinquency.
vi. Where alcohol removes natural inhibitions.
vii. In case of cerebral diseases—general paralysis or senile degeneration.
viii. Where brother and sister have been separated in childhood and meet later as strangers.

Medico-legal Aspects

- It may lead to progression of genetic defects arising from mating of close relations.
- In India and many Asian countries, incest is not an offense (unless it amounts to rape or adultery) because of social acceptability of intra-caste marriage.
- It is punishable by legislation and constitutes a valid ground for divorce, and is prohibited by religious laws in many developed countries. In the UK, the law forbids marriage between a man and his close relatives. In

Romania, all forms of incest are punishable by up to 7 years of imprisonment.
- Three European Union nations—France, Spain and Portugal—do not prosecute consenting adults for incest.

A 16-year-old boy was accused of raping of a 12-year-old girl 10 h back and brought for medico-legal examination. Following was observed during examination of his genitals. What are your observations and opinion? The age of the boy is 16 years; can he be charged of rape?

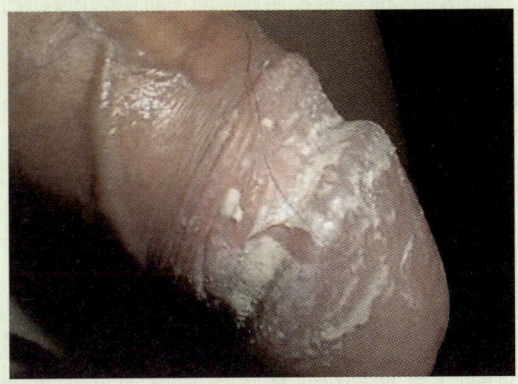

FM 3.16

Describe history of decriminalization of adultery.

ADULTERY

Definition: Consensual sexual intercourse between a married person and a person of the opposite sex, not being the spouse, during the continuation of marriage.

Legal Aspects

- Adultery was a criminal offense under **Sec. 497 IPC**. *Recently, Supreme Court has decriminalized adultery* **(Table 24.4)**. However, adultery is a valid ground for civil offense (dissolution of marriage or divorce).
- Adultery is considered illegal in 21 American states, including New York.

TABLE 24.4: Timeline of decriminalization of adultery

Year	Development
1951	The adultery law was first challenged in the case of Yusuf Aziz vs. State of Bombay wherein the petitioner contended that the law violates the fundamental right of equality guaranteed under the Constitution.
1954	After losing the case in Bombay, the petitioner approached Supreme Court (SC). The SC observed that the Section is not ultra vires under the Constitution as it is only the man, who is held liable for adultery and not the wife with whom adultery is committed—wife is not punished as an abetter.
1985	In Sowmithri Vishnu vs. Union of India, the SC held that the section is not discriminatory between man and woman or offend the Constitution.
1988	In V Revathi vs. Union of India, the SC held that not including women in prosecution of adultery cases promoted social good and adultery law was a shield rather than a sword.
1971 & 1994	The Law Commission of India reports argued to make Sec. 497 IPC gender neutral (i.e., wife, who has sexual relations with a person other than her husband, should be punishable for adultery). It was not given effect.
2017	Joseph Shine filed public interest litigation (Joseph Shine vs. Union of India) which challenged the constitutionality of the offense of adultery read with Sec. 198(2) CrPC.
2018	The SC acknowledged the 150 years old law on adultery as unconstitutional and repealed it, thus eliminating it as an offense. Sec. 198 CrPC also declared unconstitutional thereby decriminalizing the offense of adultery.

- Many Muslim nations practicing Sharia Islamic law (Iran, Saudi Arabia, Afghanistan, Pakistan and Bangladesh) retain the death penalty for adultery.

NOTA BENE
- Sec. 497 IPC stated 'whoever has sexual intercourse (not amounting to the offense of rape) with a person knowingly or believing to be the wife of another man, without the consent or connivance of that man, is guilty of the offense of adultery.' It was punishable [only man (adulterer) and not the woman (adulteress)] with imprisonment up to 5 years with/without fine.
- Sec. 198 (2) CrPC allowed a husband to bring charges against the man with whom his wife has committed adultery.

High Yield

- **Sexual offense:** Any sexual act directed against another person, without the consent of that person, including instances when the person is unable to give consent.
- **Paraphilias** *(sexual perversions)*: Sexual excitement/orgasm is associated with acts or imagery that is considered unusual, abnormal or deviant within the culture.
- **Rape** is defined under Sec. 375 IPC (unlawful sexual intercourse by a man with a woman).
- **Custodial rape:** Rape of a woman by a person in position of authority, e.g., police officer, jail warden or hospital staff.
- **Gang rape:** Rape of a woman by two or more persons.
- **Statutory rape:** Sexual intercourse with any girl <18 years even with her consent is rape (Sec. 375 IPC).
- **Age of consent:** A woman of ≥18 years can give valid consent for sexual intercourse.

- It is considered rape if sexual intercourse is done with a girl <18 years of age even with her consent.
- Rape is not a medical diagnosis, but a legal definition.
- Only a man can rape a woman. There is no age limit under which a boy is considered incapable of committing rape.
- Punishment for rape under Sec. 376 IPC is ≥10 years and fine.
- Death sentence is awarded in case of rape resulting in PVS, age of survivor <12 years and in case of repeat offenders.
- Husband having sexual intercourse with wife during separation without her consent is punished under Sec. 376-B IPC.
- Hospitals should provide first-aid and medical treatment free of cost to the rape/acid attack survivor, and immediately inform the police (Sec. 357-C CrPC).
- **In-camera:** Proceedings are heard in a Judge's private chamber or in a courtroom which has been cleared of all spectators.
- Disclosure of name of the survivor is punishable under Sec. 228-A IPC.
- Sec. 164-A CrPC deals with medical examination of the victim of rape.
- Consent for medical examination should be signed by the survivor if she is ≥12 years, and the guardian/parent if she is <12 years, drunk, insane or unconscious.
- Examination using a Wood's lamp may detect semen or foreign debris on the skin.
- **Glaister-keen globe** is used to examine the hymen for inspection of edges.
- Laceration of hymen occurs with first intercourse; usually *postero-laterally*.
- **Two-finger test** must *not* be conducted for establishing sexual assault/rape.
- **Toluidine blue** is used to detect subtle injuries (microabrasions) in genitalia.
- In sexual assault of a child, the hymen is usually *not ruptured* as it is deeply seated.
- Spermatozoa can be identified till 72 h after assault.
- Presence of spermatozoa in vagina is proof of sexual intercourse, but not of rape; *their absence is no proof that connection has not taken place.*
- Presence of smegma bacilli is suggestive of coitus; absence is without any significance.
- Rape trauma syndrome is regarded as a form of post traumatic stress disorder (PTSD).
- Hallucination is not a feature of PTSD.
- Examination of rape accused is carried out under Sec. 53-A CrPC.
- Presence of smegma is inconsistent with recent sexual intercourse.
- **Test to detect presence vaginal epithelial cells on glans:** Lugol's iodine test.
- **Incest:** Sexual intercourse by a man with a woman who is closely related to him by blood or marriage.
- In India, incest is not a criminal offense (unless it amounts to rape).
- **Adultery:** Consensual sexual intercourse by a married person with someone other than his/her legally wedded spouse.
- Adultery has been decriminalized. It was a criminal offense and the man committing adultery was punishable under Sec. 497 IPC.

Interesting case

Rape and Punishment (Case of Shiney Ahuja, 2009)

In 2009, a house-maid lodged a FIR alleging that she was raped by Shiney Ahuja, a Bollywood actor at his residence. Medical reports confirmed that she was sexually assaulted which corroborated with the allegations against the actor in the FIR. The DNA tests showed male haplotypes in the vaginal smear a perfect match with his blood sample. Later, the maid backtracked from her allegation and told the court that she had filed the complaint at the behest of a woman who had secured her the job at his residence.

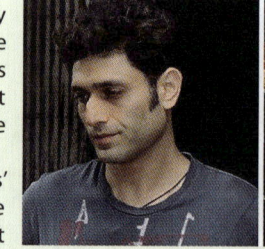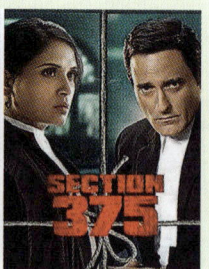

The Sessions Court convicted him of rape and sentenced him to 7 years' imprisonment. It held that the victim had 'purposefully' turned hostile to help the accused and action may be taken against her for giving false evidence. The court mainly relied on her statement given before the Magistrate, medical reports, forensic tests, including DNA, bloodstains on her clothes, traces of semen on bed sheet and curtains, and a nail injury on the actor's arm (indicating that force was used on the victim) while convicting him.

Ruling out consensual sex, the Judge did not accept his defence that the maid was in love with him and had made several phone calls to him the night before the incident. It also disagreed that the results of the Kalina Laboratory which had conducted DNA tests cannot be relied upon as it was not accredited by NABL.

The story of the movie Section 375 staring Akshaye Khanna and Richa Chadha is based on Shiney Ahuja rape case.

CHAPTER 25

Homosexuality

LEARNING OBJECTIVES

Must know
1. Homosexuality, buccal coitus, lesbianism, bestiality
2. Sodomy, examination findings of habitual and non-habitual passive patient, medico-legal importance

Desirable to know
1. Specimens to be preserved from active and passive patient involved in sodomy

Introduction

- 'Homosexual' is a term derived from the Greek word '*homos*', which means 'the same'.
- Homosexuality means sexual drive oriented towards members of same gender or sex.
- The term 'gay' is frequently used as a synonym for male homosexual; female homosexuality is often referred to as 'lesbianism'.
- The most frequent form of male homosexual activity is fellatio and masturbation; anal intercourse occurs much less often.
- Lesbian couples are conceiving and bearing children through various artificial methods like infertile heterosexual couples. Adoption is another means to parenthood for gay and lesbian couples.
- Rights affecting LGBTQIA+ (lesbian, gay, bisexual, transgender, queer, intersex and allied) people vary greatly by country or jurisdiction—from the legal recognition of same-sex marriage to the death penalty for homosexuality.
- Some countries only criminalize sexual intercourse between men but a growing number have recently expanded their laws to include bisexual and lesbian women.

NOTA BENE

National Medical Commission (NMC) has issued recommendations to include the LGBTQIA+ community and its issues in medical education.
- Medical institutions should not teach students in a way that is derogatory or insulting to the LGBTQIA+ people.
- Authors of medical textbooks should amend all unscientific and discriminatory information about the community.
- Medical universities, colleges, institutions should not approve books with such derogatory references.
- The NMC and the Indian Psychiatric Society should bring in necessary changes in the curriculum.
- Police are advised not to harass sexual minorities. Changes suggested to the police conduct rules to provide for punishing erring police personnel in this regard.
- It directed to remove the word 'unnatural' from the classification of sexual activities.

FM 3.15, 3.16
- Describe and discuss examination of victim and accused of sodomy and preparation of report, framing the opinion and preservation and dispatch of trace evidences in such cases.
- Describe history of decriminalization of consensual adult homosexual sexual behavior. Describe forced/non-consensual penetrative anal sex with its medico-legal significance.

SODOMY

Definition: Anal intercourse between two males (homosexual sodomy) or between a male and a female (heterosexual sodomy). It is also called **buggery**.

- **Pederasty** is intimate sexual relations, especially anal intercourse with a boy outside his immediate family as the passive partner (the boy is known as *catamite*, and the man as *pederast*).
- The Greeks of Golden Age were said to practice it and is also called '*Greek Love.*'
- It is frequently seen among sailors, prisoners and in military barracks, and prevails at all levels of society.

> **NOTA BENE**
>
> **Brief anatomy of anal canal**
> Normally, the anal orifice is slit-like and running anteroposteriorly with marked ridges (folds) due to the action of corrugator cutis ani muscle. The perianal skin is pigmented and keratinized and has skin appendages (e.g., hair, sweat glands and sebaceous glands). The external anal sphincter has the ability to dilate significantly without any obvious injury to the sphincter or anal canal.

EXAMINATION OF PASSIVE PARTNER OF SODOMY

Non-consensual sodomy is when someone is forced to have anal intercourse (passive victim and active accused) or passive partner forces someone to have anal intercourse (passive accused and active victim).

Pre-requisites and Preliminary Particulars

- Written authorization from Magistrate or in-charge of a police station is a must before undertaking an examination. The patient can also request for an examination, but the doctor should inform the police.
- General information—name, age, sex, address, occupation, time, date and place of examination.
- Two identification marks are noted.
- Written informed consent should be obtained in case of non-consenting victim. Consent in case of an accused is guided by **Sec. 53 (1) CrPC**.
- History, date and time of the incident, defecation, change of clothing, bathing or washing the anal area after the alleged act, use of lubricant and degree of penetration is specifically asked for.
- Any history of pain/burning sensation associated with defecation or walking is specifically asked for.
- Gait of the victim is noted.

Clothings: Clothings are examined for damage, loose pubic hair, stains of blood/semen/lubricant/feces.

General examination: General physical examination including development of secondary sexual characters is noted. Any injuries, like abrasions and bruises indicating resistance should be noted.

Local Examination

A number of variables may affect the possibility of finding physical evidence of anal intercourse:
- Frequency of the acts
- Time interval between intercourse and examination
- Age, built and size of the orifice in the individual
- Degree of force applied during the act
- Size of the penile organ
- Cooperativeness of the partner
- Use of lubricants

Non-habitual Passive Patient

- Examination is done in left lateral decubitus position (**Fig. 25.1A**).
- Lesions are marked in children because of great disproportion in size between anal orifice of victim and penis of the accused. A perianal and rectal swab should be taken first and any matted (anal/pubic) or foreign hair should be preserved for examination.

Following examination findings may be seen (**Fig. 25.2**):
  i. There is pain/tenderness during examination.
  ii. Smears of lubricant and loose foreign pubic hair around/in the anus.
  iii. Fresh/dried semen may be present around/in the anus.
  iv. **Injuries:** Superficial injuries include perianal abrasions, bruising, erythema, hematoma, edema and anal fissures. Deep injuries include anal lacerations/tears extending onto the perineum, complete transection of the external anal sphincter and perforation of the rectosigmoid (more common in children).
      - Linear abrasions may be seen around the anal opening—produced by frictional shearing of

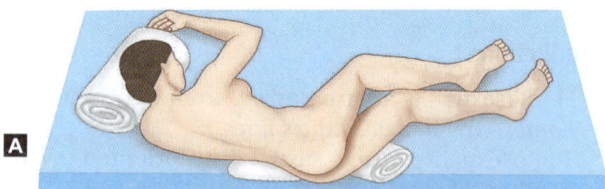

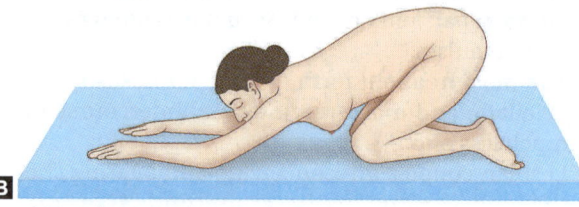

Figs. 25.1A and B: (A) Left lateral decubitus position; (B) Knee chest position

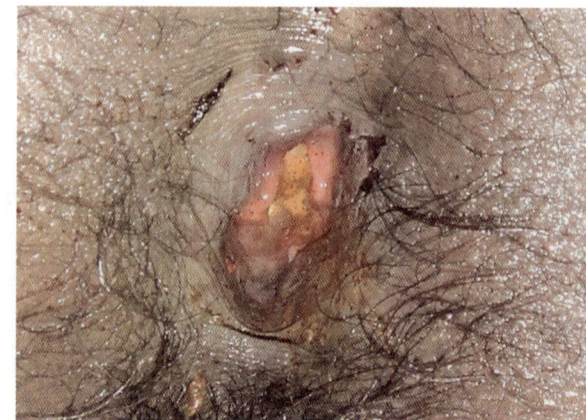

Fig. 25.2: Non-habitual passive patient: Perianal abrasions, tears, bleeding, lubricant and fecal matter seen

the penetrating penis, but may be caused by fingernails, severe constipation or due to poor hygiene. Extensive abrasions are seen when there is disproportion between anal orifice and the penis.
- Anal fissures (splits in the skin of anal margin) may involve the external skin or may extend within anal canal to mucocutaneous junction and are usually present in the posterior quadrant. It is generally wedged shaped (triangular), directed radially towards the anal canal (**Fig. 25.3**).
- Hematoma may be present, which is diffuse and present circumferentially around anal margin with obliteration of fine, symmetric rugal pattern giving an appearance of a tyre (**'tyre sign'**) or appears as localized swelling. The anus opening appears blue and there may be some edema around the anus which may last up to 2 days after the assault—this may be mistaken for hemorrhoids.
- There may be anal prolapse.
- First intercourse may result in overt tearing of anal skin and underlying sphincter muscle or splitting of skin and production of anal fissure or mere abrasion/contusion of the opening.

v. Digital examination is extremely painful, may show loss of elasticity and tone.
vi. At the end, anal canal and lower rectum is examined with the help of proctoscope (if there is spasm of the sphincter, it may be carried under anesthesia).

Habitual Passive Patient (Figs. 25.3 and 25.4)

- Sometimes, the patient may have been forcefully subjected to anal intercourse (non-consensual). She/he may then come for an examination.
- Examination is done in knee chest position (**Fig. 25.1B**).
- Injuries may not been seen in such cases.
  i. There may be shaving of anal hair.
  ii. Bloodstains are usually not observed.
  iii. Loose foreign hair and smears of lubricant may be present.
  iv. Perianal skin may be thickened and keratinized with mucocutaneous eversion. Shiny silvery hyperkeratinized skin may also be due to scratching from chronic irritation associated with hemorrhoids, threadworms or viral infections.
  v. Person does not experience any pain or tenderness during digital examination. Anal sphincter is lax, opening is patulous, canal is dilated and there may be loss of fine symmetric rugal pattern, along with congested or dilated veins.
  vi. *Lateral traction test:* External anal sphincter relaxes reflexly when bimanual traction is applied to the buttocks. Normally, gentle traction of the perianal area should elicit reflex contraction of the sphincter muscle.
  vii. *Anal opening* is more deeply situated than usual due to absorption of subcutaneous fat, giving

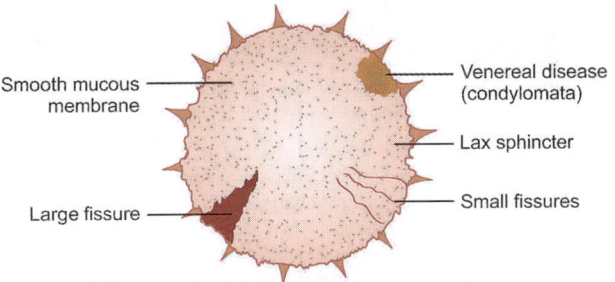

Fig. 25.3: Findings in a passive patient of sodomy

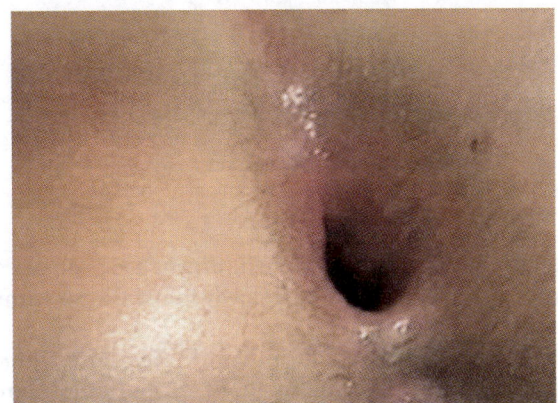

Fig. 25.4: Habitual passive patient: Shaving of anal hair, lax sphincter, patulous and dilated canal, loss of fine symmetric rugal pattern

a **funnel-shaped depression** of buttocks. The 'funnel shaped' anus is rarely seen.

viii. *Rectum:* Thickened, congested and prolapse of mucosa with disappearance of radial fold.
ix. *Other signs:* Venereal disease, cryptitis, piles, fissures, anal scars from healed injuries.

OPINION

Opinions should be restrained, but not vague, especially on matters where lack of experience makes it dangerous to be assertive.

- The opinion is based on (**Table 25.1**)
  - Presence of semen/seminal stains in and/or around the anus.
  - Soiling of the anal region with lubricants.
  - Smearing of clothes with semen, blood, lubricants or any other material.
  - Injuries in and around the anus.
  - Foreign hair.
  - Changes in the general anatomy of the anal opening and the surrounding area.
- There may or may not be any residual findings from either the single or repeated acts of anal intercourse, since anus is anatomically designed for passage of stools, it is able to expand to a large extent in both adults and children.

TABLE 25.1: Perianal signs of abuse

Signs	Findings
Non-specific acute signs	Erythema, perianal abrasions, edema, fissures, venous congestion, bruising
Signs supportive of abuse	◆ Anal laxity ◆ Reproducible reflex anal dilatation >15 mm ◆ Chronic changes, i.e., thickening of anal opening, increased elasticity and reduced anal sphincter tone, asymmetry of the rugal folds, changes in pigmentation ◆ Rectal discharge ◆ Dilation and tags ◆ Stigmata of STDs ◆ Signs of trauma including bite marks
Diagnostic signs	◆ Fresh laceration ◆ Transection of the anus ◆ Perforation of the rectosigmoid colon ◆ Healed scar extending beyond anal margin onto perianal skin ◆ Recovery of seminal products from the anorectal canal

- Signs may be minimal when lubricant has been used or the organ been introduced slowly into the anus without using undue force.
- It has a good blood supply and, the acute signs of penetration get healed in about 24–48 hours. Hence, time interval between alleged offense and examination is vital in documentation of the findings.
- The presence of semen, feces, soft paraffin and pubic hair on clothes is almost diagnostic of sodomy.
- The only absolute proof of sodomy is the presence of semen in the anus.

EXAMINATION OF ACTIVE PARTNER OF SODOMY

Pre-requisites and preliminary particulars
- Written authorization from police/magistrate is required.
- General information—name, age, sex, address, occupation, time, date and place of examination.
- Two identification marks are noted.
- Consent in this case is guided by **Sec. 53 (1) CrPC**.
- History of his version is noted.

Examination
i. Clothes are examined for the presence of stains—blood, fecal, seminal or mud.
ii. The patient is examined for abrasions and contusions on glans or tearing of the frenulum. Forceful penetration against resistance may produce tears or bruising of frenulum or prepuce, and abrasion of glans penis.
iii. There may be traces of feces and lubricant about his genitalia and the peculiar smell of anal glands.
iv. There may be presence of blood, seminal stains, venereal disease and foreign hair.
v. In habitual active individual, the penis is usually twisted with constriction at some distance from glans due to constriction force of the sphincter ani.

Specimens to be Preserved for Passive and Active Partners

Passive patient	Active patient
◆ Clothing	◆ Clothing
◆ Swab from anal canal	◆ Swab from glans
◆ Swab from bite mark	◆ Urethral discharge
◆ Blood	◆ Blood
◆ Nail scrapings	◆ Nail scrapings
◆ Matted and foreign pubic hair	◆ Pubic hair
	◆ Urine

FM 3.16
Describe history of decriminalization of consensual adult homosexual sexual behavior.

LEGAL ASPECTS

- In the 13th century, the term 'sodomites' became a common term to broadly refer to same-sex acts, prominently between men. The offense constituted in penetration per annum and it can be committed by a man with a man, or with a woman, or with an animal.
- In India, both active and passive partners were held guilty of the offense under Sec. 377 IPC, even if the act has been committed with consent.

> **NOTA BENE**
> - **Sec. 377 IPC** states that 'if an individual voluntarily has sexual intercourse against the order of nature with any man, woman or animal, he is punishable with imprisonment for life or with imprisonment up to 10 years and fine.' Penetration is sufficient to constitute offense under this section.
> - Furthermore, the offense is cognizable, non-bailable, non-compoundable, and tried by a Magistrate of First Class.

- Supreme Court (SC) has decriminalized anal sex between two consenting adults **(Table 25.2)**. Individuals are to be tried under Sec. 377 IPC if it is non-consensual sexual act, sex with minors and bestiality.
- The SC also observed that homosexuality is not a mental illness or mental disorder. Consensual penile-anal intercourse is viewed as sexual deviation (and not an offense) as judged by psychologists since it is closest to heterosexuality in offering sexual gratification.
- Same-sex marriages are not legally recognized in India. Marriage contract gives implied consent for sexual intercourse per vaginum, not per anum. Under **Sec. 13** of Hindu Marriage Act, conviction for sexual offenses is a valid ground for divorce.
- Penetrative anal sex is legal in the UK between consenting adults who are over the *age of consent*,

TABLE 25.2: Timeline of decriminalization of consenting adult homosexual behavior

Year	Developments
2001	Naaz Foundation, an NGO fighting for gay rights, filed PIL in Delhi HC seeking legalization of gay sex among consenting adults.
2004	HC dismissed the PIL; gay right activists filed review petition in SC.
2006	SC remanded the case back to HC, directed it to reconsider the matter on merit.
2008	The government said gay sex is immoral and a reflection of a perverse mind and its decriminalization would lead to moral degradation of society.
2008	HC pulled up the government for relying on religious texts to justify ban on gay sex and asked it to come up with scientific reports to justify it.
2009	Delhi HC decriminalized consensual homosexual activities between adults.
2013	SC set aside 2009 Delhi HC order and held that amending or repealing this section should be left to the Parliament, not the judiciary.
2014	Curative petition filed by gay rights activists against the SC's verdict criminalizing homosexuality.
2017	SC declared right to privacy a fundamental right under the Constitution, also observed that "sexual orientation is an essential attribute of privacy".
2018	The government left it to the wisdom of SC to decide the validity of Sec. 377 IPC.
2018	Constitution bench unanimously decriminalized part of Sec. 377 IPC (only consensual anal sex), since it violated the right to equality.
2023	SC ruled against legalizing same-sex marriage leaving it up to the legislature.

i.e., at least 16 years of age. The sexual act had to take place in private, and members of the Armed Forces and merchant seamen are excluded, whatever their age.

NOTA BENE

- The term **sodomy** is derived from the name of the ancient city of Sodom, which according to the Bible was destroyed by God for its misdeeds. Traditionally, the misdeeds of Sodom have been understood to be male homosexual anal intercourse.
- **Sin of Gomorrah:** According to the Bible, the men of Sodom and Gomorrah desired to perform homosexual gang rape on the angels. Homosexuality was the reason God poured fiery sulfur on the cities, completely destroying them and all of their inhabitants.
- At the extreme, homosexuality remains punishable by death in Afghanistan, Iran, Nigeria, Pakistan, Saudi Arabia, Sudan, United Arab Emirates and Yemen.
- Research has shown that anal sex is significantly associated with fecal incontinence, anal cancer (human papilloma virus), and STD including HIV infection.
- **Intragluteal coitus** occurs when the penis is placed between the gluteal fold which may result in edema, contusion and abrasions involving the natal cleft, perianal and anal tissues due to friction. There may be presence of seminal stains on the back or buttocks, and pubic hair and other trace elements (e.g., fibers) may also be found on the body.

LESBIANISM/TRIBADISM

Definition: Female homosexuality in which two women by mutual acts of sexual indulgence achieve gratification.

Features

- Active and passive partners are usually exchanged, although one partner may habitually play as active sex partner and the other as passive. A preferentially active lesbian is known as a **'butch' or 'dyke'**, while the passive partner is known as **'femme'** (these terms are not preferred).
- It is not possible to identify a lesbian based on her personality or characteristics.
- The predominant forms of sexual activity to achieve orgasm are oral-genital and manual genital stimulation. Self-stimulation of clitoris is frequently the preferred method. Use of artificial phallus, anal stimulation and other practices are infrequently used.
- The acts include lip kissing, massaging the breasts and private parts, generalized body contact and mutual rubbing of private parts.
- On examination, the external genitalia may show scratch marks and/or bite marks.

Medico-legal Issues

- Lesbianism is difficult to prove unless there are injuries to vagina due to forcible introduction of artificial phallus, or saliva or buccal mucosal cells are detected around the vagina.
- There may be bite marks (love bite), nail scratch marks, abrasions, teeth marks, etc., on genitalia, perineum, breasts, etc.

NOTA BENE

- The word '*tribadism*' is derived from the obsolete word *tribade*, meaning 'lesbian'.
- The word '*lesbian*' originally referred to an inhabitant of the island of Lesbos, in ancient Greece. The term has come to have its current meaning due to the ancient Greek poet *Sappho*, who lived on the island; some of her poems concerned love between women. This led to the term **'sapphism'** being used for lesbianism.
- **Bisexual:** Sexually attracted not exclusively to people of one particular sex; attracted to both men and women (*cisgender attraction*).
- **Transgender:** A person whose sense of identity does not correspond with his/her birth sex, e.g., a man who, despite having male genitalia, feels he is a woman.
- **Transsexual:** A person who feels he or she belongs to the opposite sex, and has a desire to assume the physical characteristics and gender role of the opposite sex (wants to/undergone sex reassignment surgery).
- **Nymphomania:** Abnormal, excessive, insatiable desire in a woman for sexual intercourse.
- **Satyriasis:** Morbid, insatiable sexual need or desire in a man.
- **Anilingus:** The practice of oral stimulation of the anus.
- **Urningism:** Sexual practice in which sexual desire is only for one of the same sex (obsolete word for male homosexuality).

FM 3.16
Describe sexual acts with animals/bestiality/zoophilia with its medico-legal significance.

BESTIALITY/ZOOPHILIA

Definition: Sexual intercourse with animal, either vaginal, anal or oral. This includes all animals, including birds, the usual victims being pets and farm animals.

Generally, sheep are used by males, and dogs or cats by females as they are easily available and relatively docile.

Medico-legal Issues

- Doctor may sometimes be asked to examine genital injuries or infections in a man acquired during such episodes.
- The surest evidence of bestiality is finding of human spermatozoa in the genital tract of the animal. The penis may be contaminated with fecal matter, vaginal secretion or hair of the animal. There may be injury to the penis, dung stains, general body injuries or bloodstains.
- **Other evidences:** Hair and tissue analysis can determine whether evidence is human or non-human. Fingerprinting techniques are useful, since animal paw-prints is as uniques as human's fingerprint.
- DNA can be found in semen, saliva, blood, urine and other body fluids.
- Bestiality is punishable under **Sec. 377 IPC** (imprisonment for life or up to 10 years and fine).

NOTA BENE

- **Formicophilia:** A subtype of zoophilia in which sexual arousal and orgasm occurs by being crawled upon or nibbled by small insects such as ants, mostly in the genitals or anal areas or around the nipples.
- In the UK, under the '*Sexual Offenses Act, 2003*', the sentence was reduced to a maximum of 2 years imprisonment for penile penetration of or by an animal.

FM 3.16
Describe forced/non-consensual oral sex with its medico-legal significance.

BUCCAL COITUS

Definition: It denotes penile or vaginal oral sexual intercourse, and can be performed by both males and females.

- It is also called the '*Sin of Gomorrah*', because it is alleged that buccal coitus was prevalent in Gomorrah, the Biblical twin city of Sodom.
- **Fellatio** (Latin, to suck) means oral stimulation of the penis either by the female or male.
- **Cunnilingus** means oral stimulation of female genitalia.
- Earlier buccal coitus was considered as a sexual deviation, but nowadays it is considered normal sexual foreplay.

Medico-legal Issues

- *Injuries:* A person who is forced to perform fellatio may have trauma in the oral cavity, such as petechiae of the palate and/or posterior pharynx. Abrasions, bite marks to the genitalia, and tears to the labial frenulum may result from forceful traction on the upper lip. If a fellator's scalp hair is grasped forcibly during the act, traction alopecia may be seen. Seminal stains may be seen on victim's face, mouth, etc.
- Death may result from aspiration of semen or impaction of penis in the hypopharynx. Semen may be found in respiratory tract and stomach.
- The only material evidence of buccal coitus is the presence of seminal products including spermatozoa in oral cavity and nasopharynx of the fellator (dependent upon time since contact and a history of ejaculation) and buccal mucosal cells on the external genitalia of the subject.
- The mouth and pharynx should be swabbed with nonabsorbent cotton swabs and a smear should be made similar to that made of the vaginal material. Positive amylase testing will indicate the presence of saliva. A culture for gonorrhea should be taken from the nasopharynx.
- In India, under the Hindu Marriage Act, insistence on buccal coitus, if it is non-consensual and repetitive, constitutes a valid ground for divorce.
- Buccal coitus performed by consenting adults over 21 years of age is permitted by law in the UK.

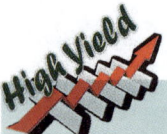

- **Sodomy:** Anal intercourse between two males or between a male and a female.
- **Pederasty:** Anal intercourse with a boy as the passive partner (boy is called *catamite* and the man as *pederast*).
- **Tyre sign:** Diffuse hematoma around the anal margin seen in non-habitual passive victim of sodomy.
- **Test done to check habitual passive patient of sodomy:** Lateral traction test.
- In habitual passive victim, anal opening is situated deeply giving a *funnel-shaped depression* of buttocks.

- **Diagnostic of sodomy:** Presence of semen, soft paraffin and pubic hair on clothes.
- **Absolute proof of sodomy:** Presence of semen in anus.
- In habitual active individual, penis is twisted with constriction at some distance from glans due to constriction force of the sphincter ani.
- SC has decriminalized consensual sodomy between two consenting adults.
- Punishment for nonconsensual sodomy is under Sec. 377 IPC (imprisonment for life or up to 10 years and fine).
- Under Hindu Marriage Act, conviction for sexual offense is a ground for divorce.
- **Tribadism/lesbianism:** Female homosexuality in which two women by mutual acts of sexual indulgence achieve gratification.
- Active lesbian is known as *butch/dyke*, while the passive partner is known as *femme*.
- **Nymphomania:** Excessive, insatiable desire in a woman for sexual intercourse.
- **Bestiality/zoophilia:** Sexual intercourse with animal—vaginal, anal or oral.
- **Surest evidence of bestiality:** Finding of human spermatozoa in genitalia of the animal.
- **Buccal coitus/sin of Gomorrah:** Penile or vaginal oral sexual intercourse; can be performed by both males and females.
- **Fellatio:** Oral stimulation of penis (by female or male).
- **Cunnilingus:** Oral stimulation of female genitalia.
- **Surest evidence of buccal coitus:** Presence of seminal products including spermatozoa in oral cavity of fellator and buccal mucosal cells on external genitalia of the subject.
- Under the Hindu Marriage Act, non-consensual and repetitive insistence on buccal coitus constitutes a ground for divorce.

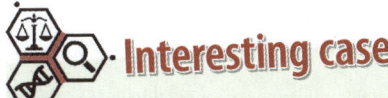

Interesting case

Consensual Sodomy (Case of Srinivas Ramachandra Siras, 2010)

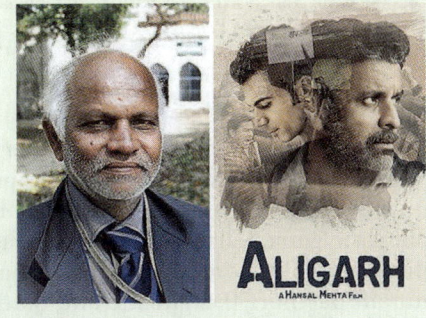

Dr Shrinivas Ramchandra Siras, 62-year-old, Reader and Chair of Modern Indian Languages had been teaching in Aligarh Muslim University for the last 22 years. In 2010, three men from a local TV channel did a sting operation of him having consensual sex with a rickshaw puller. They then barged into his house inside the campus to confront him, who repeatedly pleaded the men to stop filming. As soon as the news broke, the university administration suspended him on charges of homosexuality and evicted him from his varsity premises for 'gross misconduct'.

Supported by gay rights activists, he challenged the university action in the Allahabad High Court as being violative of his civil liberties. He argued that the university action violated the Delhi High Court order decriminalizing homosexuality. The High Court revoked the suspension and ordered his reinstatement. Less than a week after the judgment he died mysteriously in his rented home in Aligarh. The body was found lying on the bed and police broke open the door which was locked from inside. Siras was due to retire officially in 6 months, and the letter revoking his suspension arrived at his office the day after his death.

The autopsy showed no external injury marks on the body. There was discharge from his nose, mouth and other body parts, and maggots had covered his body. He apparently died 2–3 days before his body was found. The doctors could not find any definite signs of heart attack (although traces of poison was found in his body). The report could not ascertain the cause of death. His heart and viscera had been preserved and sent to the forensic science laboratory. The results are still awaited.

Police suspected suicide and ruled out murder, since the door was locked from inside. The suspension of Siras, as well as the intrusion and filming in the privacy of his home prompted a nationwide outrage. Many saw it as yet another case which highlighted the difficult lives of homosexuals in India. Actor Manoj Bajpayee portrayed him in his biopic titled 'Aligarh'.

CHAPTER 26

Paraphilia

LEARNING OBJECTIVES

Must know
1. Paraphilia, sadism, masochism, fetishism, exhibitionism, transvestic fetishism, voyeurism, frotteurism, masturbation
2. Paraphilia vs paraphilic disorder (Diff.), indecent assault

Desirable to know
1. Lust murder
2. Troilism, pedophilia, urolagnia, coprophilia
3. Stalking

- Describe the difference between paraphilia and paraphilic disorder.
- Describe paraphilic disorder as per the latest guidelines of DSM and ICD and describe medico-legal implications of paraphilic disorder by referring scientific literature and legal justification (if any).
- Describe and discuss the various paraphilias in the context of informed consent during any sexual interaction.

Definitions

Paraphilia (previously known as *sexual perversion/sexual deviation*) is anomalous sexual activity preference. It is any intense and persistent sexual interest other than sexual interest in genital stimulation or preparatory fondling with phenotypically normal, physically mature, consenting human partners [Diagnostic and Statistical Manual of Mental Disorders, Fifth Edition (DSM-5)]

- If a paraphilia causes distress or impairment to the individual or if its satisfaction entails personal harm (or the risk of such harm) to others, it is considered a **paraphilic disorder**. The addition of the word "disorder" to the classification of paraphilias is new to DSM-5 **(Diff. 26.1)**.
- In DSM-5, eight specific paraphilic disorders are described **(Table 26.1)**.

NOTA BENE

As per ICD-11, *paraphilic disorders* include five specific categories:
1. Exhibitionistic disorder
2. Voyeuristic disorder
3. Pedophilic disorder
4. Coercive sexual sadism disorder*
5. Frotteuristic disorder
6. Other paraphilic disorder involving non-consenting individuals

It has removed three categories from ICD-10: fetishism, fetishistic transvestism, and sadomasochism. These conditions involved consensual or solitary sexual activity that do not involve inherent harm to self or others and are not necessarily distressing to the individual or associated with functional impairment.

SADISM (ALGOLAGNIA)

Definition: Person gets sexual gratification by infliction of pain or physical cruelty, such as beating, biting, whipping, cigarette burns or humiliating the partner.

- Multiple injuries are inflicted on any body parts, but breasts and external genitalia are generally selected. In extreme cases, even a murder is committed (*lust murder*).
- Sexual arousal is focused on the infliction of physical or psychological suffering on a non-consenting partner.
- This paraphilia is more common in males.
- Incidence is low (2–5% of sexual offenders).
- The name **sadism** is derived from the French writer *Marquis de Sade* (1740–1814) who regarded sexually deviant acts as being natural, which was apparent in both his writings and actions. His life consisted of numerous acts of extremely violent physical and sexual abuse; most of his victims were female prostitutes, and male and female employees of his estate. He wrote pornographic and erotic books in which characters enjoyed being cruel.

---

* Coercive sexual sadism disorder is a sustained, focused and intense pattern of sexual arousal manifested by persistent sexual thoughts, fantasies, urges or behaviors that involves the infliction of physical or psychological suffering on a non-consenting person.

DIFFERENTIATION 26.1: Paraphilia and paraphilic disorder

S.No.	Feature	Paraphilia	Paraphilic disorder
1.	Basic difference	Sexually arousing fantasies or behaviors that involve inanimate objects, children or nonconsenting adults, or suffering or humiliation of the person or a partner.	Paraphilia that causes harm, distress, or functional impairment of the affected individual or may harm another person
2.	Patient's experience	The urge may not necessarily classify as 'intense and persistent'	Patient experience intense and recurrent sexual arousal and must have acted on these impulses
3.	Interview	Clinicians can *ascertain* when talking about paraphilia (according to actions and self-report, e.g., sexual attractions to inanimate objects)	Clinicians can *diagnose* when talking about paraphilia (on the basis of distress and impairment)
4.	Diagnosis	Not ipso facto psychiatric disorders	Psychiatric and pathological condition
5.	Management	Paraphilia by itself does not necessitate clinical intervention as long as it is not a disorder	Medication and psychotherapy is needed
6.	Complications	Anxiety, depression, substance use, mental health issues which may progress to paraphilic disorder	Harm, distress, functional impairment and legal ramifications

- Common features in sexually sadistic crime scenes include torture, use of weapon, humiliation, victim confinement, bondage, expressive violence, post-death physical and sexual mutilation and object insertion into the vagina.

Lust Murder

Definition: It is a homicide in which the offender stabs, pierces, slashes or otherwise mutilates the sexual organs or areas of the victim's body. With torturing the partner, sexual arousal starts, and with death of the partner, full gratification is obtained.

TABLE 26.1: Types of paraphilic disorders*

S.No.	Disorder	Summary definitions
1.	Sexual sadism disorder	Inflicting pain or humiliation of a person is sexually pleasing
2.	Sexual masochism disorder	Receiving pain or humiliation for sexual pleasure
3.	Transvestic disorder	Arousal from clothing associated with members of the opposite sex
4.	Voyeuristic disorder	Urges to observe an unsuspecting person who is naked, undressing or engaging in sexual activities, or in activities deemed to be of a private nature
5.	Exhibitionistic disorder	Exposing one's genitals to an unsuspecting person or performing sexual acts that can be watched by others
6.	Fetishistic disorder	Use of inanimate objects to gain sexual excitement
7.	Frotteuristic disorder	Touching or rubbing against a non-consenting person
8.	Pedophilic disorder	Sexual preference for prepubescent children
9.	Other specified paraphilic disorder	These include partialism, zoophilia, necrophilia, klismaphilia, coprophilia, urophilia, infantilism, telephone scatologia

*All these should be recurrent and cause intense sexual arousal.

- The mutilation of the victim may include evisceration and/or displacement of the genitalia.
- After murder, the sadist may have sexual intercourse with her (**necrophilia**). He may tear out the genitalia or other organs, may suck or lick the wounds or eat the flesh of his victim to derive sexual pleasure (**necrophagia/anthropophagy**).
- It is the consequence of extreme sadist practice.
- A lust murder begins with the obsessive compulsions of the offender. Generally, they have a sexual obsession with their victims, and organized lust murderers may stalk their victims for months or weeks before the actual killing.
- The *signature component* of the crime that which names it a 'lust murder' is the killer acting out their fantasies with their victims and the bodies of those victims.
- **Legal aspect:** Necrophagia is punishable under **Sec. 297 IPC** (trespassing on burial places; indignity to any human corpse). Imprisonment is up to 1 year with/without fine.

MASOCHISM (PASSIVE ALGOLAGNIA)

Definition: Sexual gratification is obtained only when they receive painful stimulus from opposite partner.
- It is the *reverse of sadism*.
- The acts performed on the masochist including being humiliated, beaten, bound, and any other act aimed at experiencing suffering.
- Sexual masochism is more common in males, but the incidence in females is on the rise.
- Women prefer less intense forms of masochism usually related to a relationship (e.g., light spanking); men prefer acts that reduce their status as a man (e.g., being forced to kiss a partner's feet or being cuckolded).
- The term is derived from the 19th century author *Leopold von Sacher-Masoch,* an Austrian novelist who portrayed his principle male character suffering from this paraphilia. His story appeared to parallel his

relationship with his wife as he used to plead her to treat him as a slave and whip him, and his eccentric requests gradually became more demeaning to satisfy his sexual appetite.

- Masochistic asphyxial death may occur due to accidental hanging or strangulation *(autoerotic death)*.

Sadism and masochism are rarely found in pure state (combined entity is known as *sadomasochism*). They are usually found together with one type dominant over the other. The combination is known as **bondage**.

BDSM sexual practices (bondage and discipline, dominance and submission, and sadism and masochism) is characterized by consensual sexual preferences and activities.

This is found in all age groups and among all socio-economic strata. These acts of cruelty may completely substitute the sexual intercourse.

> **NOTA BENE**
>
> **Asphyxiophilia** *(autoerotic asphyxia, hypoxyphilia, erotic asphyxiation or breath control play)*: Sexual paraphilia where a person seeks to achieve the level of oxygen depletion to the brain up to the point of loss of consciousness to enhance sexual arousal.

TRANSVESTIC FETISHISM (EONISM)

Definition: It is a disorder characterized by recurrent, intense, sexually arousing fantasies, sexual urges or behaviors involving cross-dressing.

- Sexual gratification is obtained by wearing the dress of opposite sex. In contrast, trans-sexuals wear clothes of other sex because they feel a part of the other sex and *not* for sexual excitement.
- It is usually seen in males. They collect items of distinct feminine look and feel, like nightgowns, slips, bras, lingerie, stockings and pantyhose, and may dress in these feminine garments and take photographs of themselves while living out their secret fantasies **(Fig. 26.1)**.

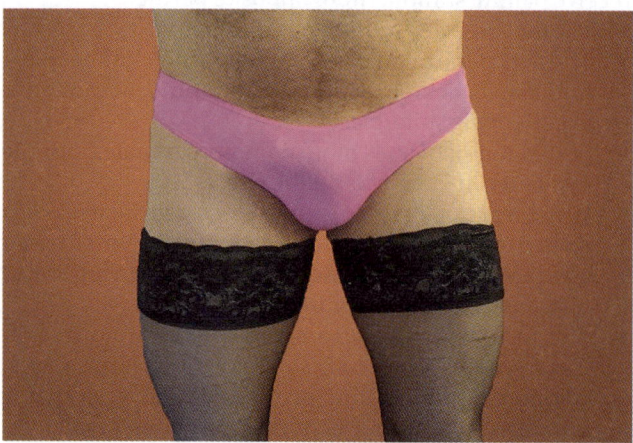

Fig. 26.1: Eonism

- *Magnus Hirschfeld* coined the term **'transvestism'** (Latin *trans*: across, over; *vestitus*: dressed) to refer to the sexual interest in cross-dressing. The term has undergone several changes of meaning since it was first coined. Hirschfeld's group of transvestites consisted of both males and females with heterosexual, homosexual, bisexual and asexual orientations.
- The term 'eonism' is derived from the Frenchman, *Chevalier d'Eon de Beaumont,* who practiced this paraphilia.

> **NOTA BENE**
>
> - **Cisvestism:** It is a disorder characterized by obtaining sexual pleasure from dressing up in clothes typical of one's own sex but inappropriate to the individual's position or status, e.g., biker's 'leathers' or cowboy's outfit.
> - **Infantilism** *(autonepiophilia, Adult Baby Syndrome)*: Paraphilia in which a person obtains sexual arousal and gratification by acting and dressing like an infant or being treated as an infant by one's sexual partner. Behaviors may include drinking from a bottle or wearing diapers *(diaper fetishism)*.
> - **Autogynephilia** Male's propensity to be sexually aroused by the thought of himself as a female. It is the paraphilia that is theorized to underlie transvestism and some forms of male-to-female (MtF) trans-sexualism.

> **NOTA BENE**
>
> **Gender dysphoria (Gender identity disorder)**
> - Strong persistent feelings of identification with another gender and discomfort with one's own assigned gender and sex, causing significant distress or impairment (being uncomfortable with their body).
> - For example, a person with female sex characteristics may privately identify as a man, but continue to publicly present as a woman.
>
> **Conversion therapy**
> - Conversion therapies (or "reparative therapies") are interventions purported to alter same-sex attractions or an individual's gender expression with the specific aim to promote heterosexuality as a preferable outcome.
> - From psychiatric treatment, electroshock therapy to exorcism and violence or the use of psychosomatic drugs, conversion therapy can comprise any of these which can lead to trauma, depression, anxiety, drug use or even suicide.
> - There is no evidence to support the application of any "therapeutic intervention" operating under the premise that a specific sexual orientation, gender identity, and/or gender expression is pathological.
> - Based on the scientific evidence, "conversion therapies" (or other interventions imposed with the intent of promoting a particular sexual orientation and/or gender as a preferred outcome) lack scientific credibility and clinical utility. The practice has been banned in several countries.
> - The NMC has banned the conversion therapy under the IMC (Professional Conduct, Etiquette and Ethics) Regulations, 2002. The Commission has warned doctors that offering conversion therapy to any individual belonging to the LGBTQIA+ will amount to **"professional misconduct"**. These individuals are often subjected to conversion therapy, especially the youth.

CHAPTER 26 : Paraphilia

■ VOYEURISM (SCOPTOPHILIA)

Definition: There is a morbid desire of the individual to observe unsuspecting people undress or naked, taking bath, see the genitalia or watch intercourse to get erotic excitement and sexual gratification **(Fig. 26.2)**.

♦ It is commonly seen in males.
♦ Voyeurs frequently peep into the bedrooms of others, and are called as '*Peeping Toms*' or '*Jags*'.
♦ Some voyeurs prefer to observe their own wives being seduced by other men. The act of observation may be accompanied by exhibitionism or masturbation.
♦ It occurs in case of sociopathic personality disorder, and such individuals may commit sexual crimes.
♦ Psychoanalysts postulate that voyeurism may be attributed to a child witnessing episodes of his/her parents engaged in sexual intercourse.
♦ **Legal aspect:** Under **Sec. 354-C IPC**, voyeurism is a punishable offense. It states that any man who watches or captures the images of a woman engaged in a private act (changing clothes, using lavatory or doing a sexual act) in circumstances where it is expected of not being observed, or circulate such image is punishable with imprisonment from 1–3 years and fine (cognizable and bailable), and for 2nd offense, imprisonment is for 3–7 years and fine (cognizable and non-bailable).
♦ In the UK, non-consensual voyeurism is a criminal offense, and in the US video voyeurism is criminalized in many states.

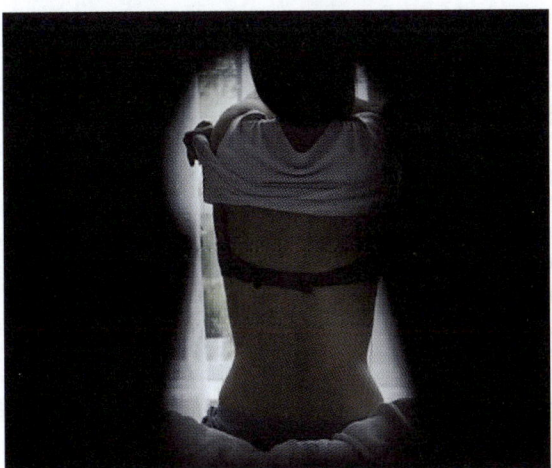

Fig. 26.2: Voyeurism

> **NOTA BENE**
> ♦ **Video voyeurism:** Act of secretly recording someone in an intimate state, typically for purposes of sexual interest or gratification.
> ♦ **Troilism:** The paraphiliac gets sexual gratification by inducing his wife to have sexual intercourse with another man and by observing the same.
> ♦ **Stalking** involves following a woman or contacting such woman in spite of her clear disinterest, or monitors her through internet, e-mail or any other form of electronic communication. It is punishable under **Sec. 354-D IPC** with imprisonment for up to 3 years and fine (cognizable and bailable) and imprisonment up to 5 years and fine for subsequent offense (cognizable and non-bailable).

■ EXHIBITIONISM

Definition: It is a desire and intentional exposure of genitalia in public places while in presence of others (mostly in front of unsuspecting children or females) to obtain sexual pleasure **(Fig. 26.3)**.

♦ This paraphilia is mostly seen in males, and are called **flashers**. Occasionally, women may expose themselves in public.
♦ Most of them are psychopathic or suffer from compulsive neurosis.

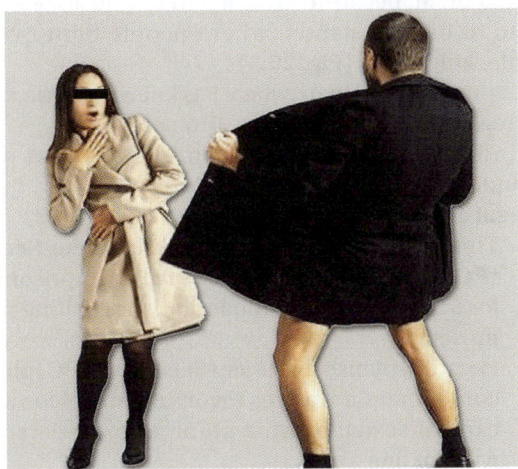

Fig. 26.3: Exhibitionism

♦ *Narcissism,* the extreme form of self-admiration is also believed to contribute to exhibitionism.
♦ **Legal aspect:** It is an obscene act punishable under **Sec. 294 IPC** with imprisonment up to 3 months with/without fine.

> **NOTA BENE**
> ♦ **Flashing:** Momentarily exposing (indecent exposure) to unsuspecting strangers in public.
> ♦ **Streaking:** Running naked through a public place.
> ♦ **Mooning:** Displaying one's bare buttocks by removing clothing.

■ FETISHISM

Definition: It is a fixation on an inanimate object or body part that is not primarily sexual in nature and the compulsive need for its use in order to obtain sexual gratification **(Fig. 26.4)**.

♦ *Alfred Binet,* the French psychologist coined the term 'erotic fetishism'.
♦ It is mostly seen in males.

- **Fetish objects:** Although, the list of objects is inexhaustible, more commonly fetish objects are handkerchief, dress, particularly the undergarments—panties, bras, slips, stockings, pantyhose or negligees.
- **Essential feature** is recurrent intense sexual urges and sexually arousing fantasies involving specific objects. They cannot suppress their desire to steal the fetish object.
- **Diagnosis** is made if an individual has acted on these urges and is markedly distressed by them or the fetish object is required for gratification.

FROTTEURISM (TOUCHERISM)

Definition: It is the act of obtaining sexual arousal and gratification by rubbing of one's genitals against a non-consenting person in public places.
- It is usually seen in males.
- Frotteurism occurs in crowded trains, buses, elevators and at bicycle stands (where people bent over for unlocking locks) **(Fig. 26.5)**.
- It is prevalent in Japan, where it is known as *chikan* and is regarded as a public safety problem.
- Fondling (groping) the victim may be part of the condition and is called *toucherism*.
- **Legal aspect**
  - This is an offense and punishable under **Sec. 290 IPC** (fine of ₹ 200) and **Sec. 291 IPC** (imprisonment for 6 months with/without fine) for creating public nuisance.
  - He is also punishable under **Sec. 354-A IPC** (physical contact and advances involving unwelcome and explicit sexual overtures) for up to 3 years with/without fine.

PEDOPHILIA

Definition: It is the recurrent, intense sexual fantasies, urges or behaviors involving sexual activity with a prepubescent child or children (≤13 years) by a person who is ≥16 years old and at least 5 years older than the child.
- Pedophiles are usually men and can be attracted to either or both sexes.
- Typical activities vary from just looking at a child undressing and fondling, to acts like oral-genital contact, rubbing the penis between orifice or thighs and actual penetration.
- Usually, the child is not able to understand the nature and consequences of the act, and the perpetrator is influential (elder), i.e., having parental or other position of authority with respect to the child (incestuous or non-incestuous relationship).
- It is one of the few psychiatric diagnoses for which the symptom behavior constitutes a criminal act. If a person is having pedophilia, it is not illegal but an adult having sexual contact with a child (≤18 years) is illegal. Identification and treatment of this disorder is important to reduce future risk.

> **NOTA BENE**
> - **Infantophilia** (subcategory of pedophilia): Sexual preference for children under the age of 5 (especially infants and toddlers).
> - **Ephebophilia (hebephilia):** Sexual attraction of an adult to pubescent or post-pubescent adolescents.
> - **Gerontophilia:** Sexual preference for the elderly.

MASTURBATION (ONANISM)

Definition: Deliberate self-stimulation which results in sexual arousal.
- Masturbation is common in both men and women.
- *In males,* methods are mostly manual—by moving the penis with hand or against a bed or other object. Anal stimulation and insertions are rare. Hollow articles, like bottles or test tubes or articles made of rubber and plastic, which stimulate female genitalia are sometimes used.
- *In females,* a finger or a hand is gently and rhythmically moved over clitoris or labia minora. The genitalia may be rubbed against a pillow, bed or some other object. She may insert fingers, wooden rods, test tubes, metallic bars, bananas or artificial phallus made of rubber or plastic into the vagina.
- It is an offense when practiced openly, e.g., in telephone booths, bus, metros or toilets.

> **NOTA BENE**
> The word **onanism** was formerly used as a synonym because in biblical times under Jewish law, a brother was required to procreate with his brother's widow. Onan of Judah refused, and ejaculated on the ground instead. This is the origin of the term onanism (*The Sin of Onan*) which is incorrectly used in place of masturbation.

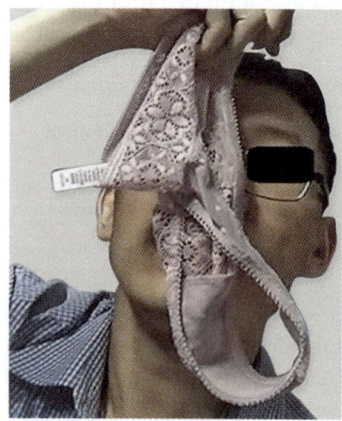
Fig. 26.4: Fetishism

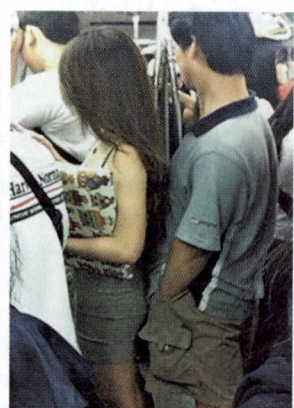
Fig. 26.5: Frotteurism

Uranism

The paraphiliac gets sexual gratification by fingering, fondling or licking (homosexuality in males).

Urolagnia (Urophilia, Undinism)

- The paraphiliac gets sexual gratification by sight or odor of urine and/or by urination.
- Those who enjoy urolagnia (Greek *ouron*: urine, *lagneia*: lust) may enjoy urinating on another person or being urinated upon (**golden showers**).
- In New Zealand, publishing anything promoting or supporting urolagnia, whether in print or online, is punishable with imprisonment up to 10 years.

Coprophilia

Coprophilia (Greek *koprós*: excrement, *filía*: fondness) is a morbid attraction to, and sexual gratification obtained from feces (liking the smell, taste or feel). Eating of feces is known as **coprophagia**.

> **NOTA BENE**
>
> - **Telephone scatologia (telephonicophilia):** Paraphilia that comprises overt or covert repetitive telephone calls with sexual and/or obscene content to an unsuspecting victim. This behavior has a high association with other paraphilic disorders, such as voyeurism and exhibitionism.
> - **Partialism:** Sexual interest exclusively focused on a particular body part.
> - **Klismaphilia:** Sexual activity involving enemas.

Identify and match the following paraphilic disorders with their punishments:

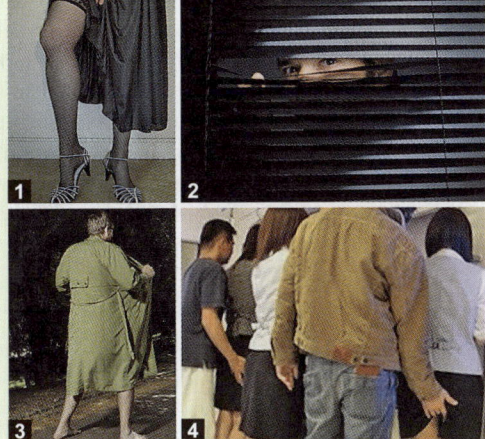

A. Punishable under Sec. 354-C IPC
B. Punishable under Sec. 294 IPC
C. Punishable under Sec. 354 and 354-A IPC
D. Not punishable

1._____ 2._____ 3._____ 4._____

FM 3.16
Describe forced/non-consensual insertion of fingers or objects with its medico-legal significance.

INSERTION OF FOREIGN OBJECTS/FINGERS

- **Definition:** Foreign object/finger (digit) insertion in a sexual assault refers to when the offender has inserted an object/finger into the vagina, anus or mouth of the victim.
    - Object may include sexual objects such as vibrators or other 'sex-toys' or non-sexual objects such as sticks, rods, umbrellas or clothing **(Figs. 26.6A and B)**.
    - Sexual sadism may also play a role in foreign object insertion. The sadist enjoys seeing the suffering he inflicts on the victim. Sometimes, sexual murders may result.
- When an item is inserted into the mouth of the victim it is necessary to determine whether the insertion had a practical function, such as to gag/suffocate/silence a victim (insertion is not for sexual purposes), or if it served a psychological function for the offender (sexual or pseudosexual, and not practical purposes).

> **NOTA BENE**
>
> - Inserting foreign bodies into orifices (**polyembolokoilamania**) is a rare disorder, and rectal insertions happen mostly due to erotic activity and psychiatric disorders, e.g., schizophrenia. Various objects that have been inserted into the rectum include bottle, bones, seeds, carrots, vessel jar, and thermometer.
> - Sometimes, drug packets may be inserted in an attempt to conceal them from police, may be introduced intentionally but become lodged unintentionally; occasionally perforation may occur during insertion.

Medico-legal Aspects

- Non-consensual vaginal, anal or oral penetration by foreign objects is considered as sexual assault (rape).
- **Injuries:** There may or may not be any residual findings depending on the force applied. Only superficial and nonspecific mucosal injury may be seen. Superficial injuries may include abrasions, fissures, chafing and erythema. Rubbing an object over the anal verge may result in abrasion or ulcerative-like lesions between the buttocks.
    - Significant acute injuries include bruising, lacerations, bowel obstruction, perforations, severe hemorrhage, edema, abscess formation, septicemia; or undergo distant embolization.
- Victim specific blood group substance and recovery of large numbers of glycogenated epithelial cells from the

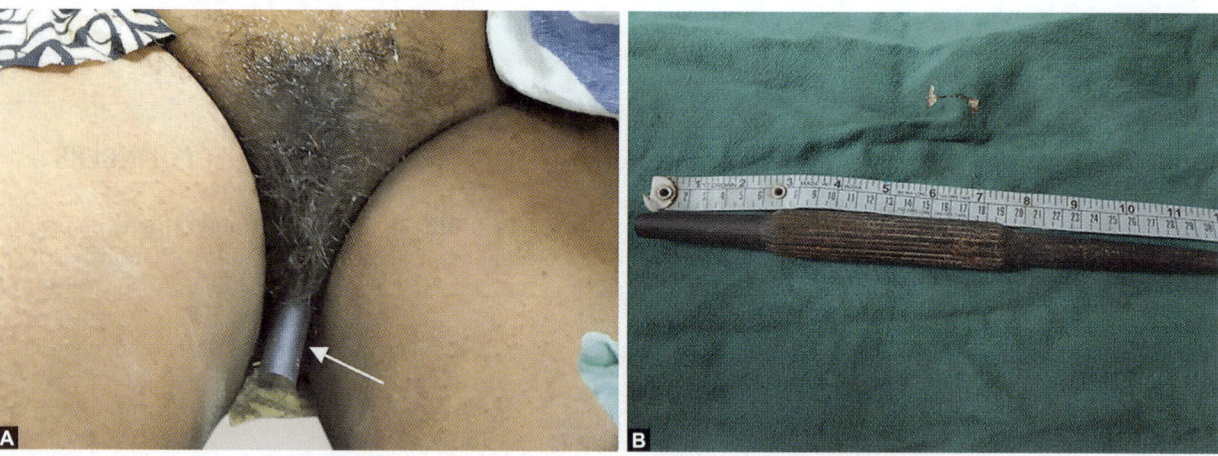

Figs. 26.6A and B: (A) Foreign body *in situ* in vagina in a case of sexual assault (arrow); (B) Recovered foreign body from the patient
(*Courtesy:* Dr Manas Sahoo, AIIMS, Bhubaneswar and Dr Mukul Sharma, AIIMS, Raebareli)

foreign body is strongly suggestive of vaginal or anal penetration.
- Fecal matter and amylase recovery from an object may suggest anal or oral origin of deposited secretions.

FM 3.16
Describe forced/non-consensual touching or groping or disrobing ('indecent assault') with its medico-legal significance.

INDECENT ASSAULT

Definition: Any unwanted sexual behavior or touching of a female without her consent, with the intention or knowledge to outrage her modesty.
- Males usually do it often to females or adolescents.
- The meaning of indecency depends upon prevailing views of what is unacceptable behavior.
- This can mean many things, from an unproven rape to merely touching the buttocks in a crowded bus.
- Forcing someone to watch pornography or masturbation, disrobing or compelling a female to get naked in public place, or fondling the breasts, thighs, perineum, or kissing a woman forcefully, or putting a hand up a woman's skirt constitute indecent assault.

Allegations Against Doctors

One particular risk in medical practice is the vulnerability of male doctors to the allegations by women patients of indecent assault during consultation or treatment session which may vary from intimate touching, to kissing, fondling the breasts or pudenda and even actual intercourse (which may amount to rape). Stripping naked a female patient for medical examination (without her consent) is regarded as an assault.

Legal Aspect

- It is a punished under **Sec. 354 IPC** with 1–5 years imprisonment with/without fine. The offense is cognizable, non-bailable, non-compoundable and can be tried by any Magistrate.
- Any man who assaults or uses criminal force on any woman or abets such act with the intention of disrobing or compelling her to be naked is punishable with imprisonment for 3–7 years and fine **(Sec. 354-B IPC)**. It is a cognizable and non-bailable offense.
- Any person with their word, gesture or act intended to insult the modesty of a woman is punished with simple imprisonment up to 3 years with fine **(Sec. 509 IPC)**.
- In the UK, indecent assault is an offense under **Sec. 3** of Sexual Offenses Act, 2003.

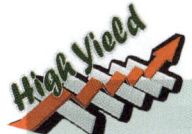

- **Paraphilia:** Any intense and persistent sexual interest other than sexual interest in genital stimulation.
- **Paraphilic disorder:** Paraphilia which causes significant distress and impairment of functioning to the individual or if the paraphilia involves personal harm or risk of harm to others.
- Most common of paraphilic disorders—frotteurism, voyeurism and exhibitionism.
- **Sadism:** Inflicting pain on a person for sexual pleasure.
- Term *sadism* is derived from French writer *Marquis de Sade*.
- In extreme cases of sadism, lust murder may be committed.
- **Lust murder:** Sadist stabs, pierces or mutilates the sexual organs or other areas of victim's body to obtain sexual gratification.
- **Necrophilia:** Sexual intercourse after her murder.
- **Necrophagia:** Sadist may tear out the genitalia or eat the flesh of his victim to derive sexual pleasure.
- **Masochism:** Receiving pain for sexual pleasure.
- Term *masochism* is derived from Austrian novelist *Leopold von Sacher-Masoch*.
- Sexual asphyxia is seen in cases of masochism.
- **Transvestism/eonism:** Arousal from wearing clothing associated with members of opposite sex. Not punishable.
- Term transvestism was coined by *Magnus Hirschfeld*.
- **Voyeurism/scoptophilia:** Urges to observe an unsuspecting person who is naked, undressing or engaging in sexual activities. Punishable under Sec. 354-C IPC.
- **Peeping Toms:** Voyeurs who frequently peep into the bedrooms of others.
- **Stalking:** Following or contacting a disinterested woman or monitoring her through internet, e-mail or any other form of electronic communication. Punishable under Sec. 354-D IPC.
- **Exhibitionism:** Exposing one's genitals or performing sexual acts to non-consenting people, particularly strangers. Punishable under Sec. 294 IPC.
- **Fetishism:** Use of inanimate objects to gain sexual excitement.
- **Frotteurism:** Touching or rubbing against a non-consenting person. Punishable under Sec. 290, 291 and 354-A IPC.
- **Pedophilia:** Sexual preference for prepubescent children, where the offender/patient is at least 16 years of age, and the victim is at least five years younger.
- Punishment for outraging the modesty of women is under Sec. 354 IPC and Sec. 509 IPC.

Section	Offense	Punishment (Imprisonment)
354	Indecent assault	1–5 years ± Fine
354-A	Frotteurism	up to 3 years ± Fine
354-B	Disrobing	3–7 years ± Fine
354-C	Voyeurism	1–3 years ± Fine –1st offense; 3–7 years ± Fine—2nd offense
354-D	Stalking	up to 3 years ± Fine –1st offense; up to 5 years ± Fine—2nd offense

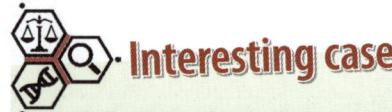

Interesting case

Necrophilia and Pedophilia (Nithari Serial Murders, 2006)

The case came to light after a continued series of disappearances of the children (both boys and girls) and one adult in the year 2005-2006 with subsequent discovery of eight skeletal remains from the drain of a house in Nithari, Noida. Two suspects, the owner of the house Moninder Singh Pandher and his domestic help Surinder Koli were arrested. More skeletons tumbled out of the drainage and the crime scene was dubbed India's 'house of horrors'. This case involved the commission of heinous crimes like sexual abuse, pedophilia, murder, cannibalism and attempted necrophilia.

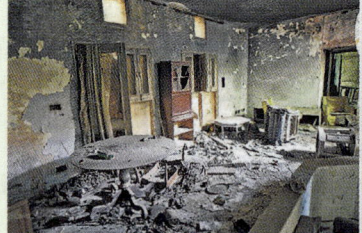
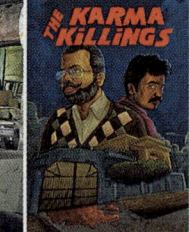

House of horrors

The police determined that out of the 17 confirmed people killed, 10 were girls (there were at least 31 victims). The DNA samples from the remains were sent to a forensic laboratory in Hyderabad for the identification of the victims while forensic samples were sent to the laboratory in Agra for determining the age, cause of death and other details. It was determined that one girl 'Payal' was the only adult victim, with 11 victims below the age of 10.

The investigation revealed that several children from the slums had been lured to their deaths by the domestic help, who invited them to the house after offering them sweets and chocolates. He confessed that he had raped the children, strangled them and had sex with the corpses of victims. He would then disembowel them, eat their body parts (in the belief that cannibalism cures impotency), dismembered their body parts and dump it in an open drain nearby. The confession made it clear that he is a psychopath. During the trial, he retracted his confession, saying he had been tortured and coerced into making his statement. Mr Pandher denied all the charges against him from day one. The investigating agencies ruled out the possibility of organ trade as the motive for the killings or child pornography.

The accused duo underwent brain mapping, polygraph and narco-analysis tests. Koli had confessed to the crimes and gave his employer a clean chit saying that he was unaware of his actions. It is very hard to believe that not once in any of the murder, neither Pandher nor any other person employed by him noticed all these things.

Koli was found guilty of five homicides and sentenced to death, but commuted to life imprisonment by the Allahabad High Court on the ground of 'inordinate delay' in deciding his mercy petition. However, Pandher spent 7 years in prison and walked out of jail in 2014. Allahabad High Court granted him bail for the pending cases against him. In 2017, both were sentenced to death for serial rape and murder by the CBI court. Recently, they were acquitted by High Court over lack of evidence.

It is considered a serial killing since no type and pattern of choice in the selection of the victim which is the hallmark of a serial killer. The postmortem reports revealed that there had been a pattern in the killings. The bodies had been cut into three pieces before being disposed off by the servant. Moreover, the modus operandi and motive of the murders were not clear.

A documentary based on the infamous Nithari serial murders titled 'The Karma Killings' by Indian American filmmaker Ram Devineni premiered exclusively in Netflix.

27 CHAPTER

Postmortem Artifacts

LEARNING OBJECTIVES

Desirable to know
1. Postmortem artifacts
2. Undertaker's fracture

Definition: Postmortem artifacts (Latin *arte*: art, *factum*: something made) are any changes caused or features introduced in a body after death which may lead to misinterpretation of findings.

Ignorance and misinterpretation of such postmortem artifacts leads to:
- Wrong cause/manner of death
- Undue suspicion of criminal offense
- A halt in the investigation of criminal death
- Unnecessary wastage of time and effort, as a result of misleading findings
- Miscarriage of justice

The artifacts can be those introduced in the period between death and autopsy, and those introduced during autopsy **(Table 27.1)**.

 FM 2.14
Describe and discuss examination postmortem artifacts.

ARTIFACTS DUE TO POSTMORTEM CHANGES

These artifacts are due to rigor mortis, postmortem (PM) staining, autolysis and putrefaction.
  i. **Rigor mortis:** Existing rigor mortis may be broken down while removing the body from the scene of crime to the mortuary, which may cause error in interpretation of time since death. Rigor affecting the heart may simulate hypertrophy of the heart.
 ii. **Postmortem staining:** Isolated patches of postmortem lividity may be mistaken for bruises **(Fig. 27.1)**. Such patches on the front and sides of the neck may be mistaken for bruising due to throttling. Lividity of the

TABLE 27.1: Postmortem artifacts

Artifacts due to PM changes	Third party artifacts	Environmental artifacts	Miscellaneous
Rigor mortis	Animal or insect activity	Heat effects	Refrigeration induced
Postmortem staining	Pathologist induced	Postmortem corrosion	Mishandling of the body
Autolysis	Deliberate mutilation	Postmortem maceration	Delay in autopsy
Putrefaction	Embalming		Exhumation
	Therapeutic		

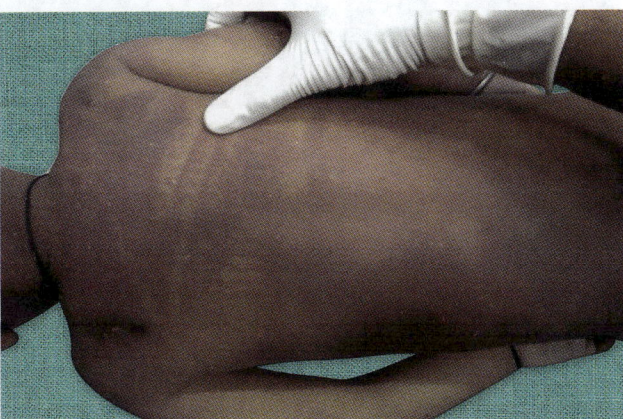

Fig. 27.1: Artifacts of PM staining: Simulation of abuse (tramline bruise)

internal organs may be mistaken for congestion due to disease.
- Postmortem staining in the posterior left ventricle of the heart in an individual lying supine after

death may cause confusion of ischemic myocardial damage, in the lungs—pneumonia, and in the GIT—irritation due to poisoning.
- Certain poisons like CO, HCN or nitrites may change the color of the hypostatic area.

> **NOTA BENE**
>
> **Prinsloo Gordon artifact:** A common artifact seen in all types of autopsy. It represents hemorrhage on the anterior aspect of the cervical spine, posterior to the trachea and esophagus which happens due to PM staining. Hence, caution must be used in interpreting bleeding into the posterior neck tissues.

iii. **Autolysis:** Autolysis leads to discoloration of skin and viscera, such as gallbladder, pancreas, liver, kidney, GIT mucosa and brain, where it may simulate injury or disease. Pancreas is one of the first organs to undergo autolysis because of proteolytic enzymes within it, which can be mistaken for acute hemorrhagic pancreatitis. Perforation of the stomach due to autolysis should be distinguished from that due to corrosive acid or peptic ulceration (**Fig. 27.2**).

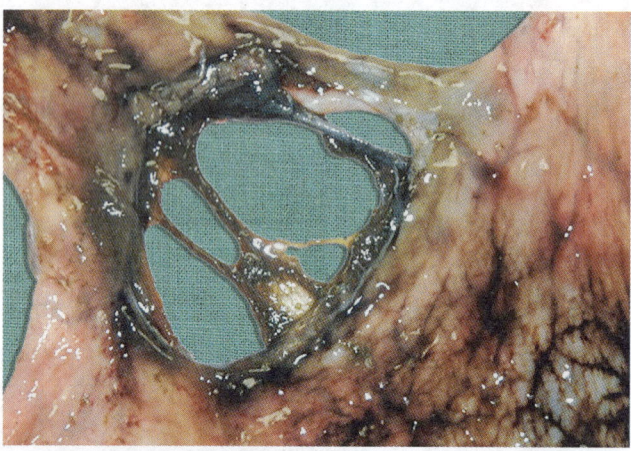

Fig. 27.2: Perforation of the stomach due to autolysis

iv. **Putrefaction**
External
- Swelling of lips, nose, eyelids and extremities, distension of the chest and the abdomen may occur, giving a false impression of antemortem obesity.
- Large quantities of sanguineous fluid may escape from the mouth and nose in case of pulmonary edema, giving the impression of hemorrhage.
- A deep groove simulating ligature mark of strangulation may be seen around the neck, if the deceased has been wearing buttoned shirt or beaded threads or ornaments around the neck.
- The bulging of eyes, protrusion of tongue and discharge of red stained froth from mouth and nose may be mistaken for signs of throttling (**Fig. 27.3A**).
- Owing to pressure effects of putrefactive gases, postmortem staining may be displaced in any direction and may simulate antemortem bruises.
- Putrefactive blisters may be confused with blisters from burns and contact with petroleum products (**Fig. 27.3B**). The skin from the hand may peel like a glove as in burns.
- Splitting of skin may give a false impression of antemortem lacerations, incised wounds or thermal injuries.
- The female genitalia appear pendulous and may simulate antemortem sexual assault.

Internal
- Softening of 'synchondrosis' between the body and greater cornu of the hyoid bone may produce abnormal mobility which may be confused as a fracture.
- Gas bubbles in the blood and air in the right side of the heart may be mistaken for air embolism. Oxygen in right heart will indicate antemortem air embolism.
- The blood becomes darker, and the brain, heart and lungs appear congested which may be mistaken for asphyxia.

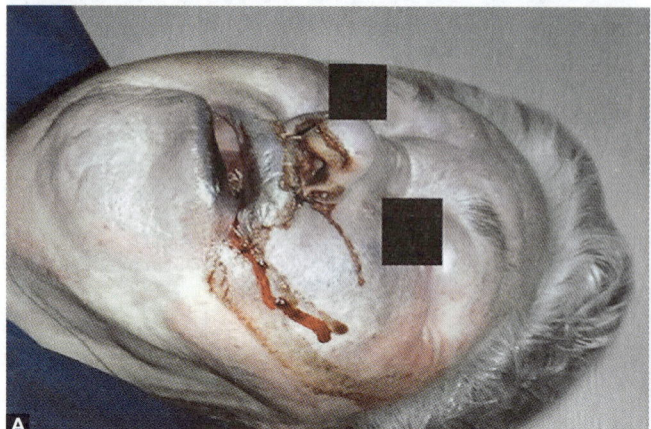
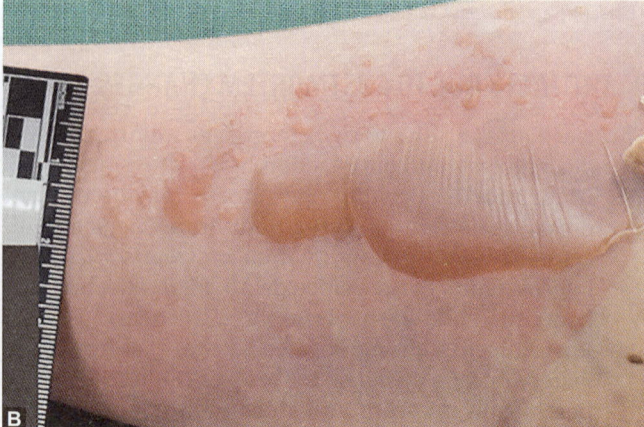

Figs. 27.3A and B: Artifacts of putrefaction: (A) Serosanguineous discharge of fluid from mouth and nose; (B) Postmortem blisters

- Bluish discoloration of the loop of bowels, especially in the pelvic cavity may be confused as an infarcted bowel.
- If a body lies on its back, blood gets accumulated in the posterior part of the scalp due to gravity. Lysis of red blood cells and breakdown of vessels cause the blood to seep into the soft tissues of the scalp giving the appearance of a bruise.
- Postmortem separation of the sutures of child's skull and bursting of the abdomen with protrusion of the abdominal viscera due to advanced decomposition may be mistaken for trauma.

THIRD PARTY ARTIFACTS

Artifacts due to Animal and Insect Activity

- The bites by dogs are clear-cut, with deep impression of teeth in a small area. Individual punctures may resemble stab wounds.
- Insect bites (ants or roaches) are dry, brown with irregular margins, and usually seen in moist parts of the body, e.g., armpits, groin, scrotum and anus, these may resemble antemortem abrasions **(Fig. 27.4)**.
- Rodents gnaw away the tissue over localized areas. They produce shallow craters with irregular borders and leave long grooves **(Fig. 27.5)**.
- Flies, maggots and larvae may alter the wounds.

Insects can also cause misinterpretation of blood spatter pattern analysis. Roaches walking through pooled and splattered blood will produce trailing. Specks of blood in unique and unusual areas (such as on ceilings) may mislead forensic scientists.

Therapeutic Artifacts

- External cardiac massage, especially in elderly patients is associated with the fracture of ribs (3rd–5th) and sometime fracture of the sternum along with laceration of the lungs, liver, spleen and diaphragm which can create an impression of a crushing force applied to the chest.
- Use of defibrillator may leave an impression of circular contusion over the pericardium **(Fig. 27.6)**. Multiple intra-cardiac injections may result in bruising of heart and hemopericardium.
- Gastric contents are aspirated in the trachea due to the handling of the body or as a terminal agonal event in natural deaths or due to resuscitation.
- Investigative procedures, like carotid angiography may result in bruising of the neck muscles giving a false impression of throttling.
- Surgeons may often take laparatomy incision through incised or stab wounds leading to misinterpretation of wounds.
- Endotracheal intubation, positive pressure and artificial respiration may lead to surgical emphysema and pneumothorax.

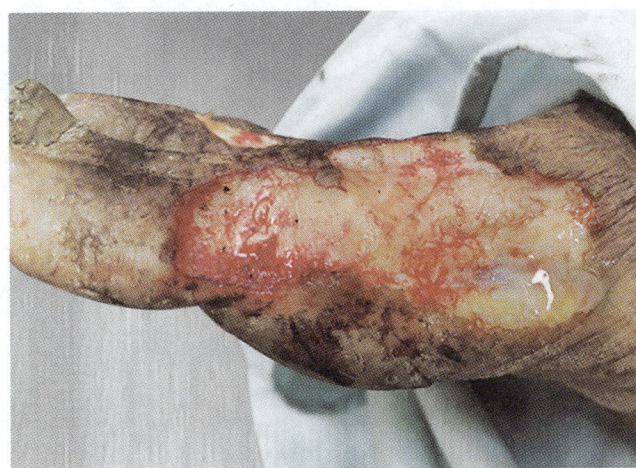

Fig. 27.5: Postmortem nibbling of foot by rats

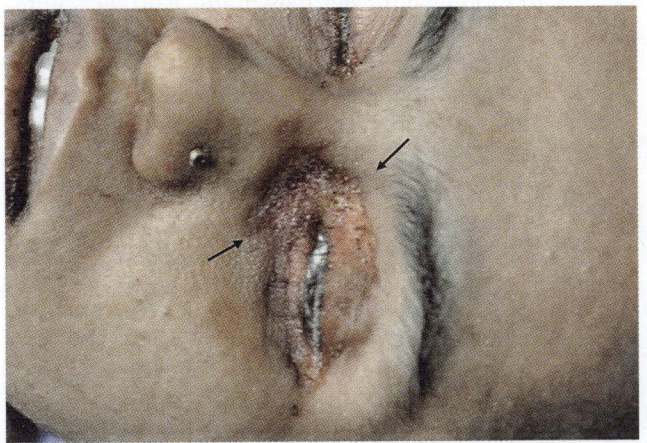

Fig. 27.4: Postmortem ant bites (arrows)

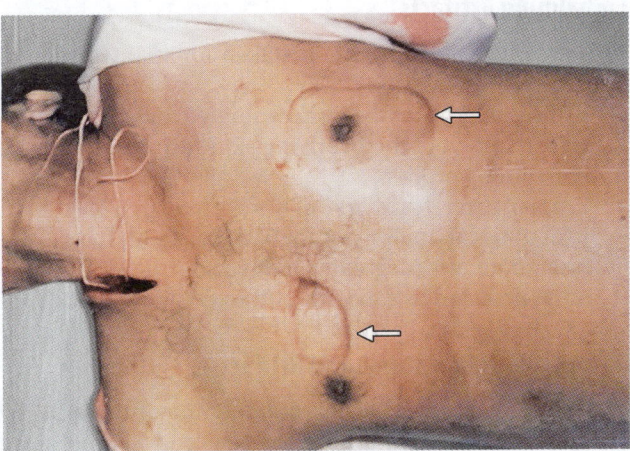

Fig. 27.6: Defibrillator marks (arrows)

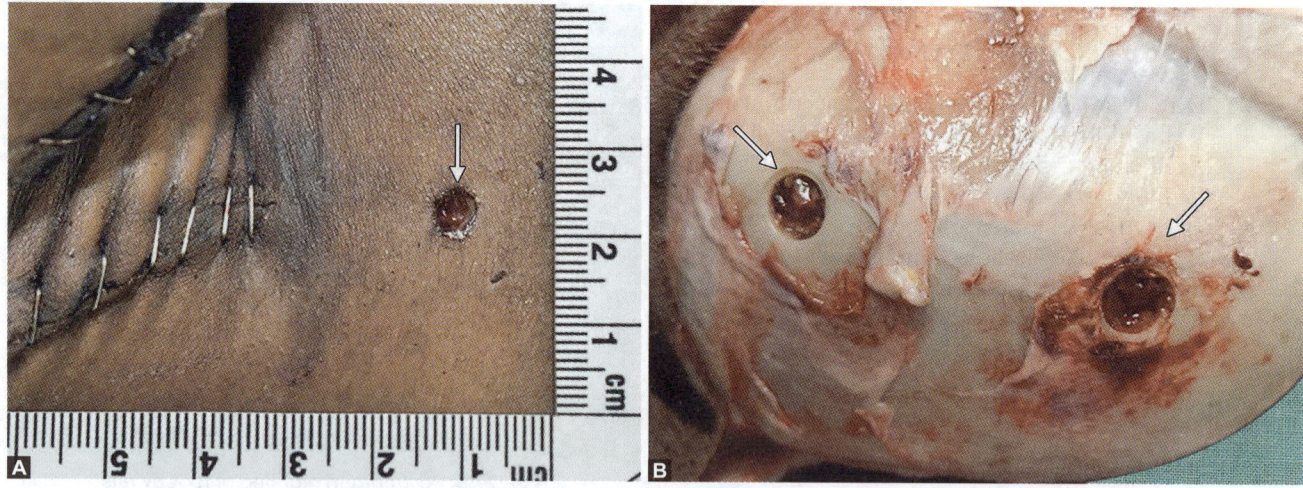

Figs. 27.7A and B: Gunshot entry wound mimic: (A) Surgical drain site (arrow); (B) Burr holes in skull (arrows)

- Drainage wounds or burr hole surgery for draining subdural hematoma in skull may be mistaken for firearm wounds **(Figs. 27.7A and B)**.

Deliberate Mutilation, Dismemberment

- Sometimes, criminals may inflict injuries, mutilate or dismember the body after death to mislead the investigation.
- Some mutilations are produced in a ritualistic sense displaying significant psychopathology of the assailant. It may include removal of the breasts, genital mutilation, such as removal of the penis, and scarification type injuries.
- Persons may be killed and thrown into water or set on fire. Careful examination for violence will help in the correct diagnosis of the cause of death. Chemical analysis of the viscera for poisons may be necessary.
- Occasionally, a person may be beaten to death or poisoned and then hanged to mislead people.

Embalming Artifacts

- Trocar wounds may be mistaken for stab wounds or bullet wounds.
- Bruises may be markedly accentuated due to increased transparency of the overlying skin resulting from the embalming process.
- Embalming fluid used may pose problems in toxicological analysis of the viscera, as high levels of methanol, anticoagulants and various other dyes are often detected by sophisticated screening methods.

Autopsy Pathologist-induced Artifacts

i. **Skull fractures:** During the opening of the skull by forceful sawing or by using a chisel and a hammer, an existing fracture of the skull may become extensive or fresh fractures may be caused.

ii. **Air in blood vessels:** During pulling of the dura, air may enter the blood vessels. This may lead to an erroneous diagnosis of air embolism. When neck structures are pulled forcefully, air may enter the neck vessels or there may be seepage of blood around the neck structures leading to erroneous traumatic neck pathology.

iii. **Visceral damage:** The liver, if pulled instead of being dissected out, may cause tears in the diaphragm and laceration in the bare area of the liver. While the abdomen and the peritoneum are being cut open, bowel coils may be cut.

iv. **Extravasation of blood**
   - When viscera are pulled apart in toto, as in evisceration (*en masse* removal), there would be profuse bleeding into the pleural and peritoneal cavities that may be mistaken as antemortem hemorrhage.
   - The removal of the neck structures en block as in routine autopsies may produce artifacts in the neck tissues which resemble bruises (as seen in throttling).
   - Rough handling of the brain during removal may damage the dura and the dural venous sinuses that may lead to an escape of blood into the subdural space, simulating an antemortem subdural hemorrhage.

v. **Fracture of hyoid bone:** While removing neck structures, the hyoid bone and thyroid cartilage may be fractured, especially in old persons which may be mistaken for being antemortem in origin.

vi. **Toxicological artifacts**
   - Faulty technique in collecting a sample or faulty storage or use of preservatives.

- While collecting blood from the heart, the blood may get diluted due to pericardial fluid. Use of anticoagulants, e.g., EDTA, formalin, heparin or methenamine may give a false positive result for alcohol or methanol.
- Use of contaminated bottles/instruments/preservatives may result in wrong analysis of poisons.
- Decomposition of the tissues after death produces ethyl alcohol and significant amounts of cyanide. Decomposition also causes an increase in concentration of CO in the blood.
- In cases of death due to burns, significant amounts of cyanide may be found in blood, possibly due to inhalation of hydrogen cyanide.
- In buried bodies, arsenic may be imbibed from the surrounding earth.

ENVIRONMENTAL ARTIFACTS

Heat Effects

- Heat applied to the skin of a dead body may loosen the epidermis from the dermis and produce a postmortem blister.
- Heat hematoma may simulate extradural hemorrhage.
- An unburnt groove around the neck due to a tight collar may resemble a ligature mark.
- Fat droplets may be found in the pulmonary vessels which may be mistaken for antemortem pulmonary fat embolism.
- Heat ruptures may resemble lacerated or incised wounds **(Fig. 27.8)**.

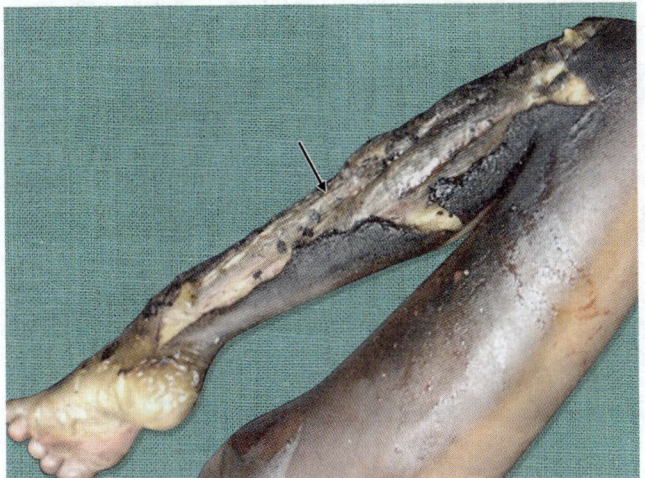

Fig. 27.8: Artifacts due to heat (heat ruptures): Postmortem lacerated wound (arrow)

Postmortem Corrosion

Dead bodies exposed or lying in kerosene, water or gasoline show chemical injuries. The epithelium detaches while handling the body, and then the underlying dermis turns yellow to brown which may be misinterpreted as antemortem chemical injury or abrasion or burns.

Postmortem Maceration

Physical contact of the body with water, soil or air may cause marked changes, depending upon the chemical constituents of earth, water and the duration of contact. The body may be totally skeletonized leaving decalcified and deformed bones.

MISCELLANEOUS ARTIFACTS

Artifacts due to Refrigeration

Pink postmortem staining is seen in bodies kept in cold storage. If the bodies are kept in a cold storage immediately after death, goose skin may develop.

Artifacts due to Mishandling of the Body

- During the process of transfer of the body from the scene of crime to the mortuary, abrasions may be produced over the back or bony prominences, clothes may get bloodstained or torn.
- Sometimes, fractures of the ribs or long bones or cervical spine may occur by rough handling of the bodies, especially in the elderly or debilitated, during attempts to straighten limbs which are contracted due to rigor mortis.
- Contusion may occur over occiput due to bumping of the head on hard surface.
- **Undertaker's fracture** may be seen which is a subluxation of the lower cervical spine due to tearing of the intervertebral disc at about C6-C7.

Exhumation Artifacts

- Gravedigger's tools can produce postmortem fracture, abrasions and lacerations.
- The discoloration of the skin beneath fungus growth simulates contusion.
- Postmortem imbibition of toxicological elements from the earth may result in inaccurate toxicological analysis.

Artifacts due to Delay in Autopsy

Uncle grooving, seen in cerebral edema, tends to be more prominent when there is a delay in removing the brain.

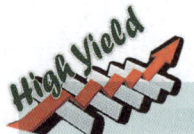

- **PM artifacts:** Changes caused or features introduced in a body after death which may lead to misinterpretation of findings.
- **Prinsloo Gordon artifact:** Hemorrhage on anterior aspect of cervical spine, posterior to the trachea and esophagus due to PM staining.
- First organ to undergo autolysis is pancreas.
- External cardiac massage may cause fracture of ribs (3rd–5th) and sternum.
- **Undertaker's fracture:** Subluxation of lower cervical spine due to tearing of the intervertebral disc at about C6–C7.

Interesting case

Resuscitation Artifact Confirmed by PM Angiography

A 23-year-old woman attempted suicide by taking drugs in the toilet of the hospital. Empty packs of sotalol and flecainide were found and she was found in comatose condition. After 2 h, she suffered a cardiac arrest and given cardiopulmonary resuscitation, but could not be revived.

During autopsy, external examination showed bruises due to defibrillation in the middle of the chest and inferior of the left lower chest. Fractures of 1–6th left ribs and 3rd right rib in the midclavicular line were found along with 80 mL of blood in the right pleural cavity. Right and left lung weighed 787 g and 765 g, respectively and edematous. On opening the abdominal cavity, about 1300 mL of blood was found. Liver was ruptured in the left posterior lobe **(Fig. A)**. No pathologic features were observed in the other abdominal organs.

To determine that the bleeding originated from liver rupture and to confirm that there was no other bleeding sources, an abdominal angiography was performed. The aorta was clamped just above the diaphragm. Barium sulfate (radiopaque contrast) was injected towards the aorta from the iliac bifurcation; abdominal aorta and the other abdominal arteries were screened under fluoroscopy **(Fig. B)**. A similar process was applied to the inferior vena cava and iliac veins after the arterial phase. No leakage was observed during the examination. Intra-abdominal vessels were intact suggesting that bleeding was caused by the liver rupture. Toxicological analysis found atropine—1441 ng/mL, midazolam—8941 ng/mL, lidocaine—57213 ng/mL, sotalol—4090 ng/mL, flecainide—4350 ng/mL (lethal dose).

Since there was history of trauma (no traumatic lesions observed in the autopsy except for the lesions associated with medical interventions), it was concluded that the liver rupture, the resulting bleeding along with the rib fractures were a result of resuscitation efforts and the cause of death was given as drug overdose.

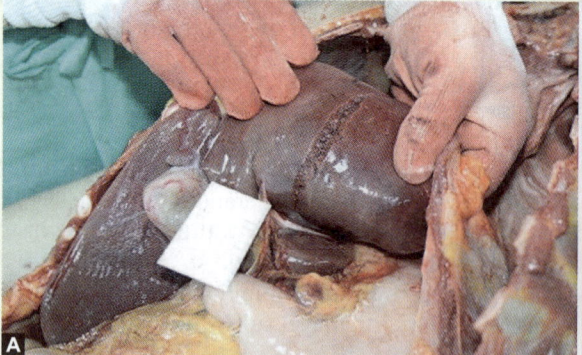
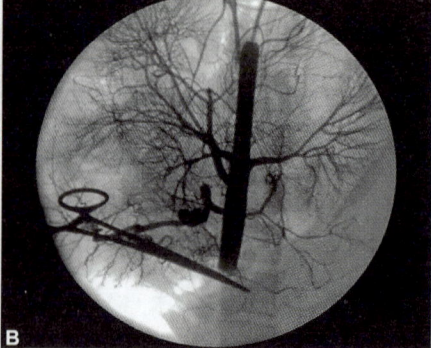

Rupture in left posterior lobe of the liver   Abdominal aorta and its branches

Hüseyin Eş et al. Resuscitation artefact confirmed by postmortem angiography. [Case report. Rom J Leg Med 24: 2016:14–16.] (*Courtesy:* Dr Abdurrahman Emir; Bitlis Branch Directorate, Council of Forensic Medicine, Bitlis, Turkey)

28 CHAPTER

Forensic Psychiatry

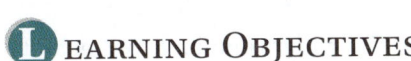

Must know
1. Forensic psychiatry, delusion, hallucination, illusion, obsession, impulse (including types)
2. Lucid interval, delirium, dementia, fugue, twilight state, insight
3. Classification and Medico-legal issues related to insanity
4. Schizophrenia
5. Phobic disorder
6. Obsessive compulsive disorder (OCD)
7. Somnambulism and somnolentia, narcolepsy, cataplexy
8. Civil and criminal responsibility (Sec. 84 IPC) of an insane
9. McNaughten's rule (legal test of insanity)
10. Illusion and hallucination (Diff.)
11. Psychosis and neurosis (Diff.)
12. True and feigned insanity (Diff.)

Desirable to know
1. Lucid interval of head injury and insanity (Diff.)
2. Hallucination and illusion (Diff.)
3. Psychiatric assessment of a patient
4. First rank symptoms of schizophrenia
5. Mood disorders (manic and depressive episode)

Definitions

- **Psychiatry:** It is that branch of medical science, which deals with the study, diagnosis, treatment and prevention of mental illness and behavioral disorders.
- **Forensic psychiatry:** It deals with the application of knowledge of psychiatry to aid in the administration of justice.
- **Insanity or unsoundness of mind:** Disease of the mind, which affects the personality, mental status, critical faculties, emotional processes and interaction with the social environment.
- **Mentally ill person:** Any person who is in need of treatment by reason of any mental disorder other than mental retardation [as per Persons with Disabilities (Equal Opportunities, Protection of Rights and Full Participation) Act, 1995].
- **Mental retardation:** A condition of arrested or incomplete development of mind of a person which is specially characterized by sub-normality of intelligence (Sec. 2(r) of the Act).

FM 5.2
Define, classify and describe delusions, hallucinations, illusion and obsessions with exemplification, lucid interval.

Some of the *important symptoms* commonly associated with psychiatric disorders are:
- Delusion
- Hallucination
- Illusion
- Impulse
- Obsession-compulsion

DELUSION

Definition: False personal belief, based on incorrect inference about external reality that is *firmly held*, despite objective and obvious contradictory proof or evidence.
- A thought disorder is not unusual in normal persons, but he is capable of correcting it by reasoning power, arguments or when convinced by others.
- Delusion is a symptom of schizophrenia. Delusions are not seen in neurotic illnesses, such as anxiety neurosis or obsessive compulsive disorder (OCD).

Types (Table 28.1)

Medico-legal importance: The *doctrine of diminished responsibility* is applicable to an insane person who does an unlawful act due to delusion, which reduces his power of reasoning and understanding capacity, e.g., if he commits some act which is not directly related with the effect of the delusion, but has an indirect bearing, such person cannot be regarded as fully responsible for his illegal acts.

HALLUCINATION

Definition: Hallucination (Latin, to wander in mind) is false perception by senses *without any external object or stimulus*. They are seen in insanity and in conditions, like high fever, drug intoxication and during withdrawal from drug addiction.

Types (Table 28.2)

i. In visual hallucination, the person observes something without anything being present. A person may see a plane flying in the sky or an oasis at a distance in a desert when there is none are quite common experience.
   - In a mentally ill person, hallucinations experienced may be located outside the field of vision (e.g., behind the head) or beyond the sensory range (e.g., able to look out of the window and see someone in distant city).
   - Visual hallucinations are seen in dissociation and conversion disorder, severe affective disorder, organic mental conditions, substance abuse and schizophrenia.
- Auditory hallucinations are the *most common*, followed by visual.
- Hallucinations are not under voluntary control and a person suffering from unpleasant hallucinations may be incited to commit suicide or homicide.
- Auditory hallucinations may occur in the context of a clear sensorium (especially when tired); those that occur while falling asleep (*hypnagogic*) or waking up (*hypnopompic*) are considered to be within the range

TABLE 28.1: Common types of delusions **(Fig. 28.1)**

S.No.	Type	Delusional belief
1.	Delusion of grandeur/exaltation	False belief about one's power, wealth, talents, and other traits. For e.g., the patient may imagine being very rich, while in reality he is poor. Seen in mania, and associated with delusion of persecution
2.	Delusion of persecution	False belief that someone is mistreating, conspiring against, or planning to harm the patient. For e.g., the patient imagines to be poisoned by his relatives (wife, son) or they are going to rob his property (*most common type*)
3.	Delusion of poverty	Patient is convinced that he is deprived of all material possessions
4.	Delusion of infidelity/jealousy (Othello syndrome) **(Fig. 28.2)**	Patient believes that his spouse is unfaithful. *Males more affected*
5.	Delusion of reference	Patient believes that he is referred to by all agencies, media and persons (usually of negative nature)
6.	Delusion of influence/control	Patient complains that his thought processes, actions are being influenced and controlled by some external power, such as radio or telepathy
7.	Hypochondriacal delusion	Patient believes of having serious disease (such as cancer) based on patient's own unrealistic interpretations of signs and symptoms
8.	Delusion of self-reproach/self-criticism	Patient criticizes himself for some imaginary offense or misdeed committed in the past
9.	Nihilistic delusion*	Patient does not believe in his existence or the world. Seen in depression
10.	Erotomania (*de Clérambault's syndrome*)	Patient believes that a person of higher social status is in love with him/her. *Common in women*. Seen in psychosis (schizophrenia, delusional disorders and bipolar mania)
11.	Delusion of doubles (*doppelganger*)	Patient believes that another person has been physically transformed into themselves
12.	Capgras syndrome	Patient believes that someone close to him has been replaced by an exact double
13.	Delusion of disguise (*Fregoli's phenomenon*)	Strangers are identified as familiar people in his life
14.	Delusion of parasitosis (*Ekbom syndrome*) **(Fig. 28.3)**	Patient believes that he is infested with parasites or insects crawling on or under the skin (*formication*) and try to remove it with tweezers
15.	Folie á deux	Mental illness shared by two persons, usually involving a common delusional system

* **Cotard's syndrome (walking corpse syndrome)** is characterized by the presence of nihilistic delusions in which the person thinks that one has lost his soul, blood, organs and body parts to the belief that one is dead.

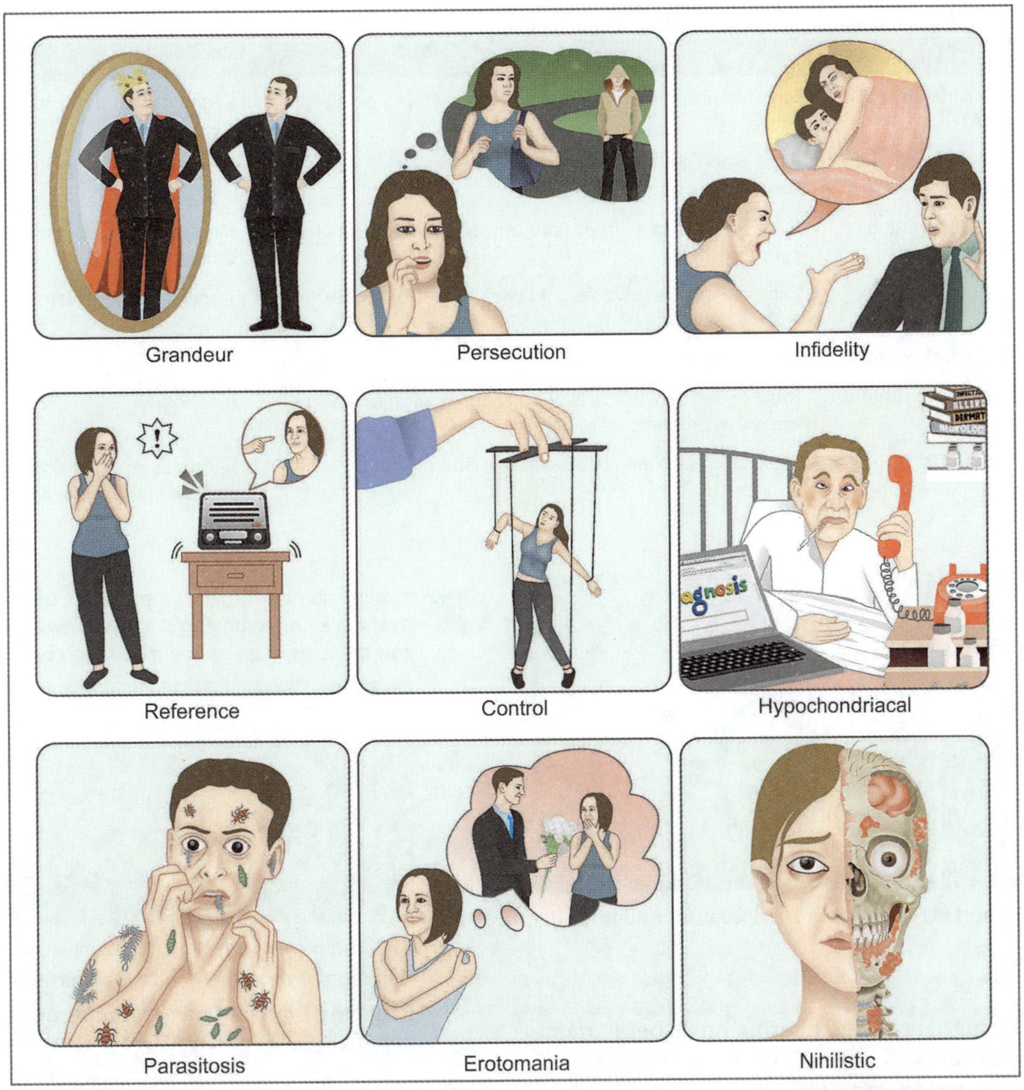

CHAPTER 28 : Forensic Psychiatry

Fig. 28.1: Various types of delusions

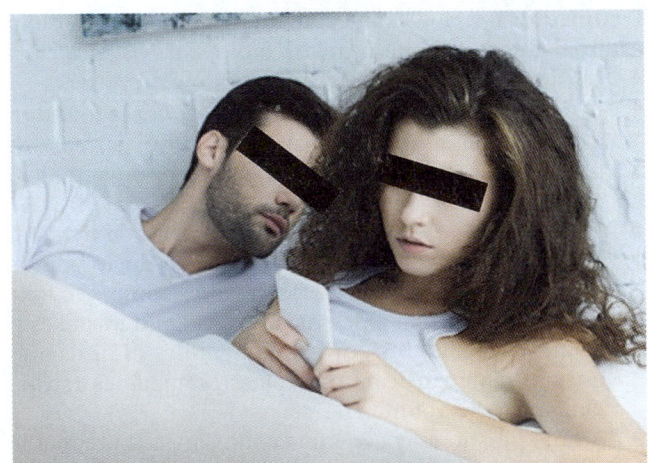

Fig. 28.2: Delusion of infidelity: Othello syndrome

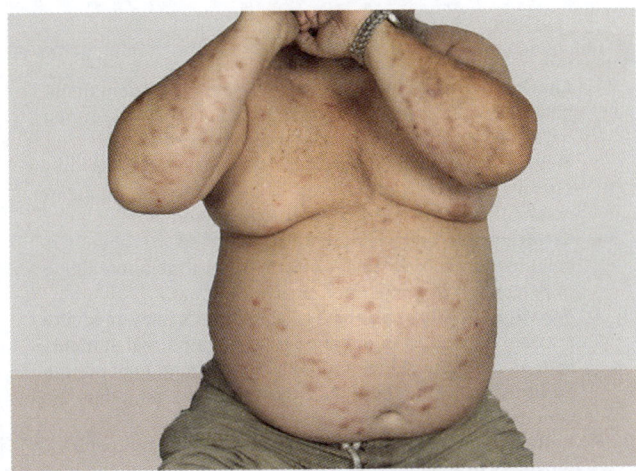

Fig. 28.3: Delusion of parasitosis: Ekbom syndrome. Lesion produced while attempting to remove 'bugs' from under his skin
(*Courtesy:* Dr Nancy Hinkle, Professor, Department of Entomology, University of Georgia, Athens, GA)

TABLE 28.2: Types of hallucinations

S.No.	Type	Experience	Seen in
1.	Visual hallucination **(Fig. 28.4A)**	Patient observes something without anything being present	Organic mental disorders (delirium tremens)
2.	Auditory hallucination **(Fig. 28.4B)**	False perception of sound (noises, music) without any source	Functional disorders (schizophrenia)
3.	Olfactory hallucination	False sense of smell (pleasant/ unpleasant) without any source	Medical disorders (temporal lobe), schizophrenia
4.	Gustatory hallucination	Patient experiences different tastes (sweet/bitter/sour) without any food or drink	Temporal lobe epilepsy
5.	Tactile hallucination (touch)	Patient experiences crawling of insects/rats over his body	Cocainism, schizophrenia
6.	Psychomotor hallucination	False sensation that parts of body are moving or being moved to different areas of body	Alcoholism
7.	Lilliputian hallucination *(micropsia)*	Persons/objects are reduced in size *(sort of illusion)*	Migraine, lesion of right temporo-parietal cortex, epilepsy, cannabis

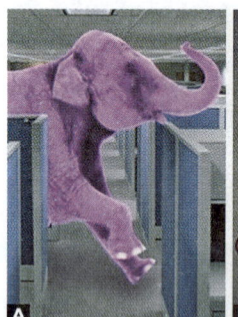
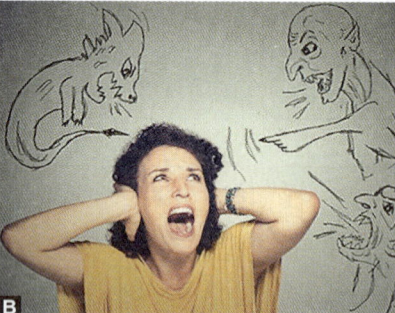

Figs. 28.4A and B: Hallucination: (A) Visual; (B) Auditory

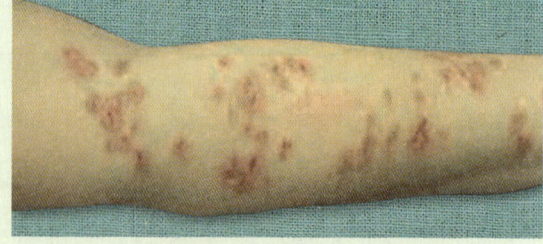

Patient came with the complaints of spending hours every evening removing scabs with tweezers. The lesions can be seen in all of the following conditions, *except:*

A. Ekbom syndrome　　B. Cocaine addicts
C. Fregoli syndrome　　D. Magnan syndrome

(*Courtesy:* Dr Nancy Hinkle, Professor, Department of Entomology, University of Georgia, Athens, GA)

of normal experience, e.g., hearing one's being name called when there was none. They are sometimes seen in narcolepsy and affective illnesses.

NOTA BENE

- **Charles Bonnet syndrome:** Healthy elderly patients with bilaterally decreased vision may experience vivid, formed hallucinations in the absence of a psychiatric disorder.
- **Elemental hallucinations:** Hallucinatory experience of simple sensory elements, such as flashes of light or unstructured noises. They are associated with organic disorders.
- **Extracampine hallucinations:** False perceptions where the hallucination is of external object beyond the normal range of perception of the sensory organs.
- **Functional hallucinations:** Hallucinations of any modality that are experience simultaneously with a normal stimulus in that modality. For example, a person may experiences auditory hallucinations when he hears the sound of air conditioning.
- **Reflex hallucination:** Hallucinations in one modality of sensation experienced after experiencing a normal stimulus in another modality of sensation.

ILLUSION

Definition: It is a false interpretation by the senses of an external object or stimulus *which has a real existence*.

- Illusions can be **universal** and **personal**.
- *Universal illusions or permanent illusions* are found in all individuals as they do not change with experience or practice, e.g., the rail tracks appear to be converging to all of us **(Fig. 28.5A)**.
- *Personal illusions* differ from individual to individual. For example, when a person mistakes his doctor/nurse for his father or mother or for the devil coming to take him away, or when a person sees a cat and mistakes it for tiger **(Fig. 28.5B)**, or hears the notes of birds and imagines them to be human voices, or imagines a string hanging in his room to be snake.
- A sane person may experience illusion, but is capable of correcting the false impressions. An insane person continues to believe in the illusions, even though the real facts are clearly pointed out.

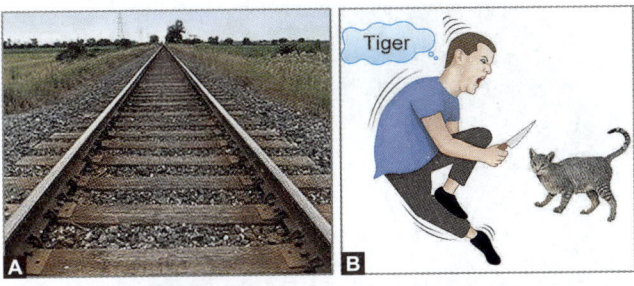

Figs. 28.5A and B: (A) Universal illusion: Rail tracks appear to be converging to all; (B) Personal illusion

- Illusions are a feature of psychoses, particularly of the organic type.

Types

a. **Completion illusion:** The brain's tendency to fill the missing part of the object to produce a meaningful percept. It can be resolved by closer attention.
b. **Affective illusion:** Occurs at times of heightened emotion (depressed or manic state). For example, a person walking through a dark alley late at night may see a tree blowing in the wind as an attacker.
c. **Pareidolic illusion:** Experiencing intense imagery of a poorly defined stimulus that persists even the subject looks at a real object in the external environment (e.g., seeing a face when looking at the cloud or fire).
d. **Jamais vu:** Illusion of unfamiliarity—reacting to everything as though it is seen for the first time; everything is unfamiliar, fresh or incomprehensible.
e. **Déjà vu:** Illusion of familiarity. The patient reacts as though everything seen has been seen and experienced before in exactly the same way—down to the last detail, when that cannot actually be the case.
f. **Macropsia:** Illusion of exaggeration of size.
g. **Micropsia:** Illusion of reduction in size.

Difference between illusion and hallucination is given in Diff. 28.1.

■ IMPULSE

Definition: This is a sudden and irresistible force compelling a person to the conscious performance of some act without motive or forethought.

Types (Table 28.3)

Some other types of impulses are:
a. **Pathological gambling:** Recurrent gambling behavior that is maladaptive (e.g., loss of judgment, excessive gambling) and in which personal, family or vocational endeavors are disrupted.
b. **Suicidal impulse:** Often intoxication (e.g., LSD) may lead to suicidal impulse.
c. **Homicidal impulse:** With certain chronic intoxications, e.g., cannabis, a man may go on a sudden killing spree.
- A sane person is capable of controlling an impulse. An insane person having no judgment and no reasoning power may do things on impulse.
- These are usually seen in dementia, acute mania and epilepsy.

TABLE 28.3: Common impulses

S.No.	Type	Compulsion
1.	Kleptomania (Fig. 28.6A)	Compulsion to steal articles which may be useless or of little value
2.	Dipsomania	Compulsion to drink alcoholic beverages
3.	Pyromania	Irresistible desire to set things on fire without motive
4.	Mutilomania	Irresistible desire to injure and mutilate domestic animals (pets)
5.	Oniomania	Compulsive desire to shop (*shopping addiction*)
6.	Trichotillomania (Fig. 28.6B)	Irresistible desire to pullout hair resulting in hair loss

■ OBSESSION–COMPULSION

Obsession: Persistent and recurrent idea, image, thought, or emotion that cannot be eliminated from consciousness by logic or reasoning and are usually associated with anxiety. The individual attempts to ignore or suppress obsessions or neutralize them by performing compulsions.

Compulsion: Repetitive behavior or mental acts that the person feels driven to perform in response to an obsession.
- It is a *disorder of content of thought* and is regarded as senseless by the patient (insight is present). This is a sort

DIFFERENTIATION 28.1: Illusion and hallucination

S.No.	Feature	Illusion	Hallucination
1.	Basic difference	Wrong interpretation by senses	False perception by senses
2.	Stimulus	External, explicit, and distinct	Internal, not clear, and within the person
3.	Situation	It happens in normal state of mind	It happens in abnormal condition (insanity, intoxicated, addiction)
4.	Nature	Universal, experienced by all	Personal experience
5.	Character	Experience is identical, same situation arouses the same type of interpretation	Experience is not identical, differs in situations and with people
6.	Remedy	Corrected by individual himself	Treated appropriately

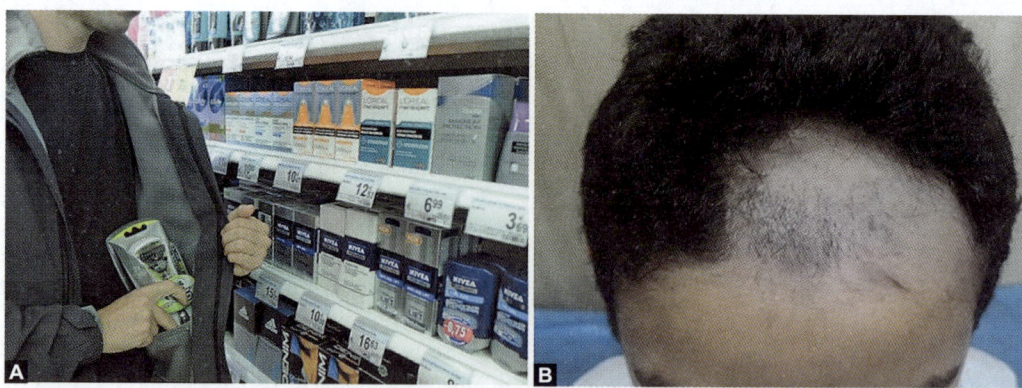

Figs. 28.6A and B: Impulse disorder: (A) Kleptomania; (B) Trichotillomania. Alopecia involving large area of the scalp due to the habit of pulling of hair occurred in 6 months

[*Courtesy:* (B) Dr Nameer Al-Sudany, Professor of Dermatology, Ibn Sina University, Iraq]

of compulsive phenomenon which is involuntary and ego-dystonic (foreign to one's personality).
- For example, a person while going to sleep, bolts the door from inside, but after going to the bed he needs to verify and does so, to see if he has bolted the door or not. He repeats this act again and again, in spite of his conscious desire to stop the act. A sane person will stop after repeating the act of verification once, but an insane person may continue the act all through the night without sleeping.*

Neurosis and Psychosis

- *Neurosis* is when a patient suffers from emotional or intellectual disorders which causes subjective distress, but does not lose touch with reality.
- *Psychosis* is characterized by gross impairment in reality-testing (withdrawal from reality), as if living in a world of fantasy **(Diff. 28.2)**.

LUCID INTERVAL

Definition: It is a period in insanity during which all the signs and symptoms of insanity disappear, and behavior is like that of a normal person.

- Lucid interval is common in mania and melancholia. A first manic attack is almost always followed by a lucid interval, seldom by a depressive attack.
- During lucid interval, the individual may have the minimal abilities to fulfill the legal criteria for testamentary capacity.
- The person is responsible for all his acts performed during the period of lucid interval.
- If he commits a crime, then he may take the plea of previous insanity. Moreover, it is difficult to know whether he was suffering from some mental illness at the time of committing the crime.
- Lucid interval is also seen in head injuries (e.g., extradural hemorrhage) **(Diff. 28.3)**.

DIFFERENTIATION 28.3: Lucid interval in insanity and head injury

S.No.	Feature	Insanity	Head injury
1.	History	Of insanity	Of trauma
2.	Preceding symptoms	Of insanity	Of concussion
3.	Following symptoms	Of insanity	Of cerebral compression
4.	Occurrence	Repeated	Once

DIFFERENTIATION 28.2: Psychosis and neurosis

S.No.	Feature	Psychosis	Neurosis
1.	Contact with reality	Lost	Preserved
2.	Interpersonal behavior	Marked disturbance in personality and behavior	Preserved
3.	Empathy	Absent	Present
4.	Insight	Absence of understanding of current symptoms (insight absent)	Symptoms are recognized as undesirable (insight present)
5.	Organic causative factor	Present	Absent
6.	Symptoms	Delusions, illusions and hallucinations	Usually physical or psychic symptoms
7.	Dealing with reality	Capacity is grossly impaired	Preserved
8.	Examples	Dementia, schizophrenia	Anxiety, phobia, depression, conversion disorder

---

*A few patients with brain trauma and dementia may develop a compulsive urge to crack facetious jokes or tell inappropriate jokes in socially inappropriate situations called *witzelsucht* (German for 'joke addiction') and *moria*, or inappropriate cheerfulness.

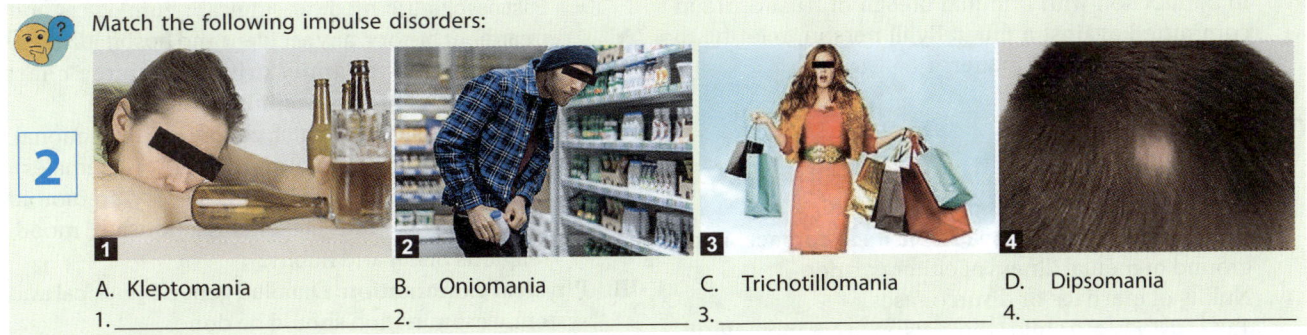

2 Match the following impulse disorders:

A. Kleptomania B. Oniomania C. Trichotillomania D. Dipsomania

1. _____ 2. _____ 3. _____ 4. _____

Some More Definitions

- **Abreaction:** Process by which repressed material, particularly a painful experience or a conflict is brought back to consciousness.
- **Ambivalence:** Coexistence of two opposing impulses toward the same thing in the same person at the same time.
- **Aphasia:** Any disturbance in the understanding or expression of language caused by a brain lesion.
- **Cognition:** Mental process of knowing and becoming aware.
- **Confabulation:** Unconscious filling of gaps in memory by imagining experiences or events that have no basis in fact, commonly seen in amnestic syndromes; should be differentiated from lying.
- **Echopraxia:** Repeating the act of another.
- **Empathy:** The degree to which the observer is able to enter into the thoughts and feelings of the patient and establish good contact.
- **Negativism:** Doing just the opposite of what he is asked to do.
- **Neurasthenia:** A condition arising out of physical or mental exhaustion.
- **Paranoia:** Rare psychiatric syndrome marked by the gradual development of a highly elaborate and complex delusional system, generally involving persecutory or grandiose delusions, with few other signs of personality disorganization or thought disorder.
- **Parasuicide** (*attempted suicide*), a term coined by *Norman Kreitman*, is a conscious often impulsive, manipulative act, undertaken to get rid of an intolerable situation. It is a non-fatal act in which a person deliberately causes injury to himself or ingests any drug in excess. The *most common method* is taking an overdose of drugs.
- **Stupor:** Used synonymously with mutism and does not necessarily imply a disturbance of consciousness; in catatonic stupor, patients are ordinarily aware of their surroundings.
- **Twilight state:** Disturbed consciousness of short duration with hallucinations during which the patient may carry out actions of which he has little or no subsequent memory.
- **Vegetative signs:** In depression, denoting characteristic symptoms, such as sleep disturbance (especially early morning awakening), decreased appetite, constipation, weight loss and loss of sexual response.

FM 5.4
Differentiate between true insanity and feigned insanity.

ROLE OF FORENSIC PSYCHIATRIST

Forensic psychiatrists are often called upon to produce legally binding documents, which are presented before the courts that can determine the course of an individual's life and liberty, and his/her life choices.

An individual with a mental disorder should be assumed to have mental capacity to decide on various matters unless the contrary can be shown. The criterion for incapacity is based upon the following when it is proved that the person is:

i. Unable to comprehend and retain information relevant to the decision and its consequences
ii. Incapable of believing the information
iii. Incapable of weighing up information to reach a decision.

Feigned insanity: With some motive, a person may pose to be insane, or a sane person may be presented as an insane person.

The process of deciding fitness or otherwise is of vital importance, and 'opinions' are regularly issued by forensic psychiatrists in the following situations:

Criminal Cases

i. When an accused on the ground of mental illness, expresses his inability to stand trial and plead his defense.
ii. When a defense is attempted on the ground that an act has been committed by a mentally ill person.
iii. When the individual after being convicted in a court of law pleas insanity so as to defer the execution of the punishment or to send him in a mental asylum.
iv. When it is claimed that a person has committed suicide due to mental illness.
v. In connection with abetment of suicide of a mentally ill person.

vi. In connection with criminal breach of trust or fraud committed against a mentally ill person, relating to business or property matter.

Civil Cases

i. Validity of consent given by a mentally ill person.
ii. Competency as a witness.
iii. Continuance/dissolution of a business contact on the ground of mental illness of either partner.
iv. Nullity of marriage or divorce cases.
v. Take custody of a child whose parents are mentally ill.
vi. Certain eventuality, like appointment of a caretaker to a mentally ill person who is unable to look after his property.
vii. Capacity to make a valid will (**testamentary capacity**).

In Western countries, legal incapacity decisions are done under very high statutory prescription, ethical dialogue and technical development of tools of assessments. In India, the opinion regarding 'fitness' is often a personal judgment based on clinical assessment, and hence should be undertaken diligently.

To differentiate feigned insanity from true insanity, guiding principles are given in **Diff. 28.4**.

PSYCHIATRIC ASSESSMENT

I. **Identification data,** informants (if any) and their relationship with patient.
II. **History:** It should be done confidentially. Interview should be taken with maximum patience and should include:
   - Presenting chief complaints and history of present illness.
   - Past psychiatric, medical, surgical, neurological, and treatment history, any accident and hospitalization.
   - *Family history*: Family origin, pedigree chart (family tree), history of similar illnesses.
   - *Personal history*: Perinatal, childhood, educational, play, puberty, menstrual and obstetric (in females), occupational, sexual and marital history, premorbid personality like interpersonal relationship, mood, religious belief and habits.

III. **Physical examination:** Detailed general physical and systemic examination should be done.

IV. **Mental status examination (MSE):** It is done using a standardized protocol:
   i. *General appearance and behavior* along with his gait, posture, motor activity, social manner, attitude and rapport towards the examiner.
   ii. *Speech*: Its volume, tone, rate, quantity, flow and rhythm.
   iii. *Affect and mood*
      - **Affect** is the subjective and immediate experience of emotion attached to ideas or mental representations of objects. Quality, range, depth or intensity and appropriateness of affect are assessed.
      - **Mood** is pervasive and sustained feeling tone that is experienced internally, and that can markedly influence all aspects of a person's behavior and perception of the world. Quality, stability, reactivity and persistence of mood are assessed.
   iv. *Thought*: Stream, form, content and possession of thought is assessed. There can be thought insertion, latency, broadcasting or withdrawal.

DIFFERENTIATION 28.4: True and feigned insanity

S.No.	Feature	True insanity	Feigned insanity
1.	Onset	Gradual	Sudden
2.	Motive	Absent	Present, e.g., commission of crime
3.	Predisposing factors	Usually present, such as history of insanity in parents	Absent
4.	Signs and symptoms	Uniform, specific for some type of insanity	Not directed to any particular type of insanity
5.	Activity	Careless, present whether the patient is being observed or not	Present only when conscious of being observed; variable and always exaggerated
6.	Mood	Excited, depressed or fluctuating	May overact to show abnormality in mood
7.	Facial expression	Peculiar vacant/agitated/worried look	No peculiarity; frequently changing, exaggerated and voluntary
8.	Insomnia	Present	Cannot persist, patient sleeps soundly after a day or two
9.	Exertion	Can withstand exertion of fatigue, hunger and sleep for several days	Cannot stand exertion for few days and breaks down
10.	Habits	Dirty and filthy	Not dirty and filthy
11.	Dressing up	Carelessly dressed	Dressed reasonably properly
12.	Skin and lips	Dry, harsh and dirty	Normal
13.	Tongue	Coated	Clean
14.	Repeated examination	Does not mind	Resents for fear of detection

Match the following phobias:

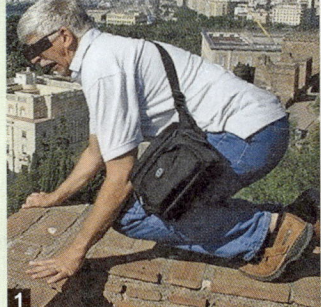
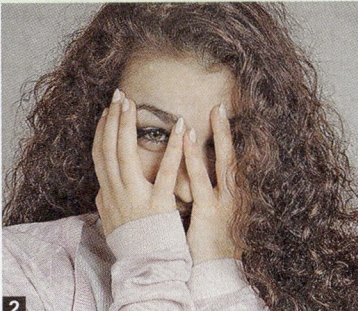
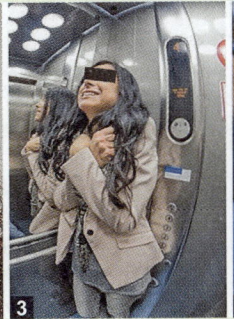
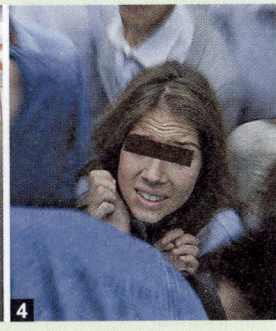

A. Erythrophobia   B. Claustrophobia   C. Acrophobia   D. Agoraphobia
1. _____   2. _____   3. _____   4. _____

v. *Perception:* Mental process by which all kinds of data—intellectual, emotional and sensory are meaningfully organized.
   - Perception is assessed by presence or absence of hallucinations, illusions, depersonalization/derealization and somatic passivity phenomenon.
vi. *Cognition (neuropsychiatric)/higher mental function assessment*: Mental process of knowing and becoming aware, and is closely associated with judgment. It is assessed under:
   - **Consciousness:** State of awareness with response to external stimuli. Grading the level of consciousness is done.
   - **Orientation:** State of awareness of oneself and one's surrounding. Whether he is well oriented in time, place and to person is noted.
   - **Attention:** Patient is asked to repeat digits forwards and backwards.
   - **Concentration:** Simple test, such as counting backwards from 20 is given.
   - **Memory:** Process whereby what is experienced or learned is established as a record in the CNS. It can be immediate retention, recall or remote.
   - **Intelligence:** Capacity to learn and ability to recall, to integrate constructively and to apply what one has learnt. Tests for reading, writing and calculation are given depending on patient's educational background.
   - **Abstract thinking:** Thinking characterized by the ability to grasp the essentials of a whole (situation or concept), to break a whole into its parts and to discern common properties.
vii. *Insight:* Conscious recognition of one's own condition. Attitude towards the illness, its causation and need for treatment is assessed.
viii. *Judgment:* Ability to assess a situation correctly and act appropriately within that situation. Judgment is assessed by social (assessed during the interview) and test situation (certain situation is given, such as house on fire).

FM 5.1
Classify common mental illnesses including post-traumatic stress disorder (PTSD).

CLASSIFICATION OF MENTAL, BEHAVIORAL OR NEURODEVELOPMENTAL DISORDERS (ICD-11)

- Mental, behavioral or neurodevelopmental disorders are characterized by clinically significant disturbance in an individual's cognition*, emotional regulation or behavior that reflects a dysfunction in the psychological, biological or developmental processes.
- Currently, there are two widely established systems for classifying mental disorders:
  1. Chapter 6 of ICD-11 by the WHO (2022) **(Table 28.4)**
  2. Diagnostic and Statistical Manual of Mental Disorders (DSM-5) by the American Psychiatric Association (2013)

Some important disorders are discussed below:

NEURODEVELOPMENTAL DISORDERS

Neurodevelopmental disorders are behavioral and cognitive disorders arising during the developmental period that involve significant difficulties in the acquisition and execution of specific intellectual, motor or social functions.

Disorders of intellectual development are a group of diverse conditions occurring during the developmental period characterized by significantly below average intellectual functioning and adaptive behavior (as confirmed by the clinical assessment and standardized tests), and is associated with impaired maturation, learning and social maladjustment.

---
* Cognition includes all of the conscious and unconscious processes involved in thinking, perceiving, and reasoning.

TABLE 28.4: Classification of mental, behavioral or neurodevelopmental disorders (ICD-11)

S.No.	Classification	Types (Major)
1.	Neurodevelopmental disorders	Disorders of intellectual development, Autism spectrum disorder, Attention deficit hyperactivity disorder, Stereotyped movement disorder, etc.
2.	Schizophrenia or other primary psychotic disorders	Schizophrenia, Schizoaffective disorder, Acute and transient psychotic disorder, Delusional disorder
3.	Catatonia	—
4.	Mood disorders	*Bipolar and related disorders*—Bipolar I disorder, Bipolar II disorder and Cyclothymic disorder *Depressive disorders* (major depressive disorder, dysthymia, recurrent depressive disorder, premenstrual dysphoric disorder, disruptive mood regulation)
5.	Anxiety or fear-related disorders	Panic disorder, Agoraphobia, Specific phobia, Social anxiety disorder (social phobia), Generalized anxiety disorder, Separation anxiety disorder, Selective mutism
6.	Obsessive-compulsive or related disorders	Obsessive-compulsive disorder (OCD), Body dysmorphic disorder, Hoarding disorder, Body focused repetitive behavior (e.g., trichotillomania), Hypochondriasis
7.	Disorders specifically associated with stress	Post-traumatic stress disorder, Acute stress disorder, Adjustment disorder, Prolonged grief disorder, Reactive attachment disorder (in children)
8.	Dissociative disorders	Dissociative identity disorder, Dissociative amnesia, Trance disorder, Possession trance disorder, Depersonalization disorder
9.	Feeding and eating disorders	Anorexia nervosa, Bulimia nervosa, Binge eating disorder, Purging disorder, Avoidant restrictive food intake disorder
10.	Elimination disorders	Nocturnal enuresis, daytime urinary incontinence, and encopresis or fecal incontinence
11.	Disorders of bodily distress	Bodily distress disorder (Somatic symptom disorder), Conversion disorder, Factitious disorders
12.	Disorders due to substance use or addictive behaviors	Acute substance intoxication, Harmful use of substances, Substance dependence, Substance withdrawal syndrome, Substance-induced mental disorders, Behavioral addictions (gambling and gaming disorder)
13.	Impulse control disorders	Intermittent explosive disorder, Kleptomania, pyromania, compulsive sexual behavior
14.	Disruptive behavior and dissocial disorders	Oppositional defiant disorder, Conduct-dissocial disorder
15.	Personality disorders and related traits	Personality disorder (mild, moderate and severe) Negative affectivity/ Detachment/ Dissociality/ Disinhibition/Anankastia in personality disorder
16.	Paraphilic disorders	Exhibitionistic disorder, Voyeuristic disorder, Pedophilic disorder, Coercive sexual sadism disorder, Frotteuristic disorder
17.	Factitious disorder	Munchhausen syndrome
18.	Neurocognitive disorders	Delirium, Dementia, Amnestic disorders
19.	Mental or behavioral disorders associated with pregnancy, childbirth, and the puerperium	Postnatal blues (mild depression and irritability) postpartum depression and postpartum psychosis (severe psychiatric symptoms including depressive episode, schizophrenia, manic episode or delirium).
20.	Secondary mental or behavioral syndromes associated with disorders or diseases classified elsewhere	Sleep-wake disorders, Sexual dysfunctions

- Intellectual functioning is commonly defined in terms of IQ (intelligence quotient). IQ testing is used to certify the range of disability for children.
- Disorder of intellectual development can be:
    i. **Mild (IQ: 50–70):** *Commonest type*, 85–90% of all cases, can achieve vocational and social self-sufficiency with little support.
    ii. **Moderate (IQ: 35–50):** 10% of all cases, can learn to speak, drop out of school after 2nd grade, can be trained to perform semi-skilled or unskilled work under supervision.
    iii. **Severe (IQ: 20–35):** Recognized early in life with poor motor development (delayed milestones) and absent speech. Later in life, elementary training in personal health care can be given and taught to talk.
    iv. **Profound (IQ: <20):** 1–2% of cases, developmental milestones markedly delayed, associated physical disorders are present, and often need nursing care or life-support.

SCHIZOPHRENIA

- Schizophrenia is characterized by significant impairments in reality testing and alterations in behavior.
- Prognosis is best with acute onset. Common age group affected is late adolescence and early second decade.

Clinical Features

i. **Disorders of thought and speech** (*hallmark feature*)
   - **Autistic thinking:** Thoughts are narcissistic (all source of pleasure are recognized as coming from within self), egocentric (self-centered, lacking interest in others) and without regard for reality.
   - **Thought blocking** (sudden interruption of stream of speech before the thought is completed) to loosening of association and incoherence—disorganized speech.
   - **Neologisms:** New word or phrase whose derivation cannot be understood (e.g., headshoe for hat).
   - **Delusions** (persecution, reference, grandeur, influence and hypochondriacal are common), *mutism* (absence of the faculty of speech), *poverty of speech* (restriction of amount of speech), *echolalia* (repeating of words or phrases of the examiner), *perseveration* (persistent repetition of specific words or concepts in speech), *verbigeration* (meaningless or stereotype repetition of words or phrases) are other features of schizophrenia.

ii. **Disorders of perception:** Hallucinations (commonest—auditory) are frequent. Visual hallucination can also occur, usually along with auditory hallucinations.

iii. **Disorders of affect** includes apathy, emotional blunting, *anhedonia* (loss of interest and withdrawal from all regular and pleasurable activities), and inappropriate emotion.

iv. **Disorders of motor behavior:** There may be decrease (inertia or stupor) or increase (excitement, restlessness or agitation) in psychomotor activity. *Stereotypy* (continuous mechanical repetition of speech or physical activity) and grimacing may be seen.

v. **Negative symptoms** include attention impairment, anhedonia, avolition, alogia (inability to speak) and affective flattening.

Symptom Specifier (Fig. 28.7)

The following symptoms are assessed individually on a scale from zero (absent) to 4 (severe). ICD-11 does not emphasize Schneider's first-rank symptoms.

1. Positive symptoms*
2. Negative symptoms¥
3. Depressive symptoms
4. Manic symptoms
5. Psychomotor symptoms
6. Cognitive impairments

♦ Persistent delusions, persistent hallucinations, thought disorder, and experiences of influence, passivity or control are considered '*core symptoms*'.

♦ Symptoms must have persisted for at least 1 month and presence of two of the symptom categories, including one 'core' symptom for diagnosis of schizophrenia (ICD-11).

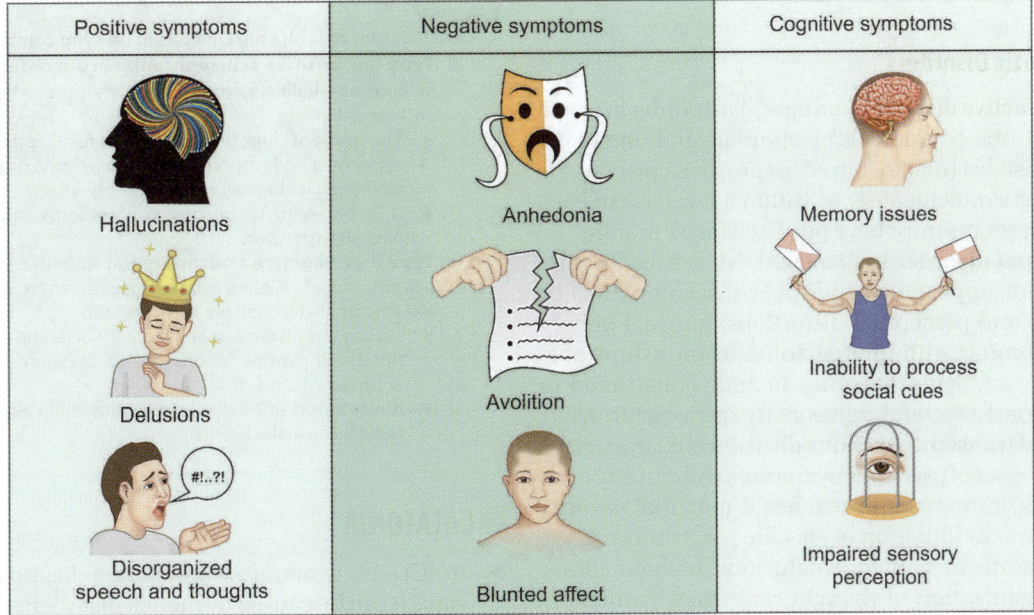

Fig. 28.7: Symptoms of schizophrenia

---

* The term 'positive' means there is an *addition of new experiences* due to disease process of schizophrenia.
¥ 'Negative' represent *loss of normal functions* of the brain.

> **NOTA BENE**
>
> **Positive symptoms** include persistent delusions, persistent hallucinations (most commonly verbal auditory hallucinations), disorganized thinking (formal thought disorder such as loose associations, thought derailment, or incoherence), grossly disorganized behavior (behavior that appears bizarre, purposeless and not goal-directed) and experiences of passivity and control (the experience that one's feelings, impulses, or thoughts are under the control of an external force).
>
> **Negative symptoms** include constricted, blunted or flat affect, alogia or paucity of speech, avolition (general lack of drive, or lack of motivation to pursue meaningful goals), asociality (reduced or absent engagement with others and interest in social interaction) and anhedonia.

Classification (Course Specifier)

ICD-11 classifies schizophrenia according to the course of illness. Both DSM-5 and ICD-11 have removed subtypes (e.g., paranoid, hebephrenic, catatonic, etc.) based on symptoms.

1. **Schizophrenia, first episode** should be used to identify individuals experiencing symptoms that meet the diagnostic requirements for schizophrenia (including duration) but who have never before experienced an episode earlier.
2. **Schizophrenia, multiple episodes** should be used to identify individuals experiencing symptoms that meet the diagnostic requirements (including duration) and who have also previously experienced episodes.
3. **Schizophrenia, continuous:** Symptoms fulfilling all definitional requirements of schizophrenia present for ≥1 year.

Other Psychotic Disorders

1. **Schizoaffective disorder** is an episodic disorder in which the diagnostic criteria of schizophrenia and one of the mood episodes (manic, mixed, depressive episode) are met either simultaneously or within a few days of each other. Symptoms must have persisted for >1 month.
2. **Schizotypal disorder** is characterized by eccentricities in behavior, appearance and speech, accompanied by cognitive and perceptual distortions, unusual beliefs, and discomfort with interpersonal relationships over several years. Symptoms may include constricted or inappropriate affect and anhedonia (negative schizotypy).
3. **Acute and transient psychotic disorder** is characterized by acute onset of psychotic symptoms without any early signs or symptoms, and reaches it maximal severity within 2 weeks (duration of episode is < 3 months).
    - Symptoms may include delusions, hallucinations, disorganization of thought processes, confusion, and disturbances of affect and mood. Catatonia-like psychomotor disturbances may be present.
4. **Delusional disorder** is characterized by presence of one or more delusions for > 3 months. Other psychotic symptoms (depressive, manic, or mixed mood episode) are usually absent.

> **NOTA BENE**
>
> - **Pfropf schizophrenia:** Schizophrenia occurring in presence of mental retardation. There is poverty of ideations, and delusions are usually not well systematized.
> - **Van Gogh syndrome:** Repetitive self-mutilation under the influence of hallucination may be seen in schizophrenia. It is named after the famous painter who cut off his ear to dedicate it to his beloved one.
> - The term 'schizophrenia' (Greek *schizo*: split, *phren*: mind) was coined by *Eugene Bleuler* (1911) to refer to the lack of interaction between thought processes and perception. Bleuler described the *fundamental symptoms* of schizophrenia as 4 A's—Ambivalence, Autism, Affect disturbances and Association disturbances.
> - Despite its etymology, schizophrenia is not synonymous with dissociative identity disorder, also known as multiple personality disorder or '*split personality*'; the two are often confused and misunderstood.
> - First rank symptoms were given by *Kurt Schneider* for diagnosis of schizopherina.* It includes:
>   i. Auditory hallucinations (thought echo—patient hears his thoughts spoken aloud)
>   ii. Thought broadcasting
>   iii. Somatic passivity
>   iv. Thought withdrawal
>   v. Voices heard arguing
>   vi. Delusional perception
>   vii. Thought insertion
>   viii. Voices commenting on one's action
>   ix. 'Made' feelings, impulses and acts (delusion of being controlled).

> **NOTA BENE**
>
> **Classification of schizophrenia based on symptoms:**
> a. **Type I or positive schizophrenia:** Acute onset of positive symptoms—hallucinations, delusions, bizarre behavior and confused thinking.
>   - The patient functioned well before appearance of symptoms and responds to anti-psychotic drugs. During clarity, social behavior is reasonably intact.
>   - It is believed to be due to problems in dopamine neurotransmission.
> b. **Type II or negative schizophrenia:** Negative symptoms—poverty of speech, emotional unresponsiveness, seclusiveness and impaired attention are predominant.
>   - Usually, they have a poor history of social and educational functioning prior to onset, and are unresponsive to antipsychotic drugs.
>   - It is believed to be due to structural brain abnormalities, but CT is usually normal.

CATATONIA

- In ICD-11, catatonia is a separate diagnostic category since it can be caused by mental disorders, psychoactive substances (including medications) and by medical conditions.

---
* Mnemonic is ABCD: Auditory hallucinations, Broadcasting of thought, Controlled thought (delusions of control), Delusional perception.

- **Clinical features:** There is marked disturbance in the voluntary control of movements characterized by extreme slowing or absence of motor activity, mutism, purposeless motor activity unrelated to external stimuli, assumption and maintenance of rigid, unusual or bizarre postures, resistance to instructions or attempts to be moved, or automatic compliance with instructions.
- **Diagnosis:** Presence of significant motor or catatonic symptoms.

MOOD DISORDERS

Mood disorders are defined according to particular types of mood episodes and their pattern over time. It includes bipolar and depressive disorders.

Clinical Features

Manic Episode

It is characterized by (**Fig. 28.8A**):
- *Elevated or irritable mood:* Usually pass through 4 stages—euphoria (exaggerated sense of wellbeing), elation, exaltation and ecstasy. Sometimes, irritable mood may predominant.
- *Psychomotor activity:* Increased psychomotor activity (overactiveness, restlessness and excitement).
- *Speech and thought:* More talkative (joking, teasing or rhyming), flight of ideas (rapid speech with shift in topics), delusions (grandeur) and distractible.
- *Goal-directed activity:* Patient is unusually alert and tries to do many things at one time.
- *Other features:* Insomnia and increase appetite may be present. Insight is absent (in mania).
  - In **hypomania** (mood abnormality of lesser intensity than mania), ability to perform becomes better, and there is marked increase in productivity and creativity.
  - In **mania**, there is striking increase in activity and execution of multiple activities with distractibility and decrease in functioning ability. Patient may become hypersexual, impulsive, drive recklessly and be involved in buying sprees.

Depressive Episode

It is characterized by following features (**Fig. 28.8B**):
- *Depressed mood:* Sadness of mood or loss of interest in all activities and throughout the day which results in social withdrawal, impaired occupational activity and interpersonal relationship.
- *Depressive ideation/cognition:* Patient becomes pessimistic and feels hopeless, helpless and worthless. He may have guilt feelings, indecisiveness, poor memory, lack of initiation and suicidal ideation.
- *Psychomotor activity:* In young patients (< 40 years), retardation is seen (decreased energy, slowed thinking and stuporous), but in older patients, agitation is common (hand-wriggling or inability to sit still). Anxiety, irritability and frustration are common.

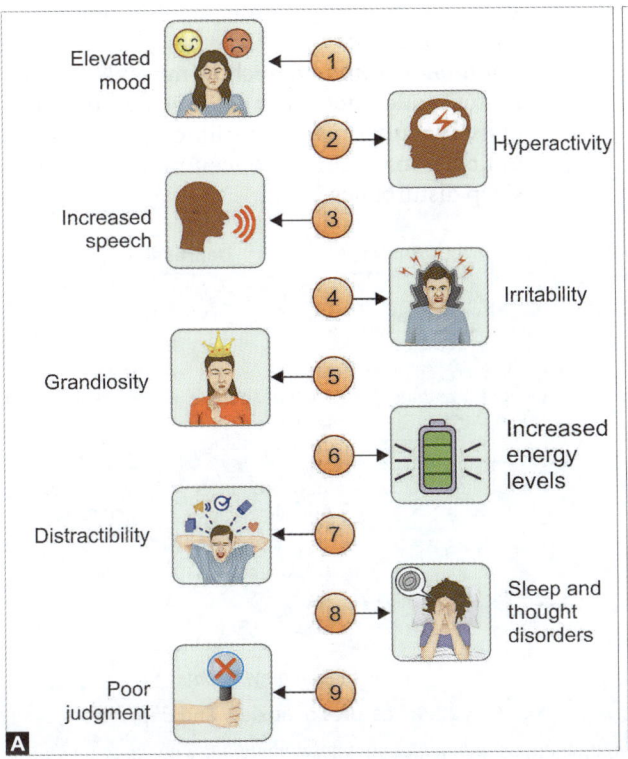
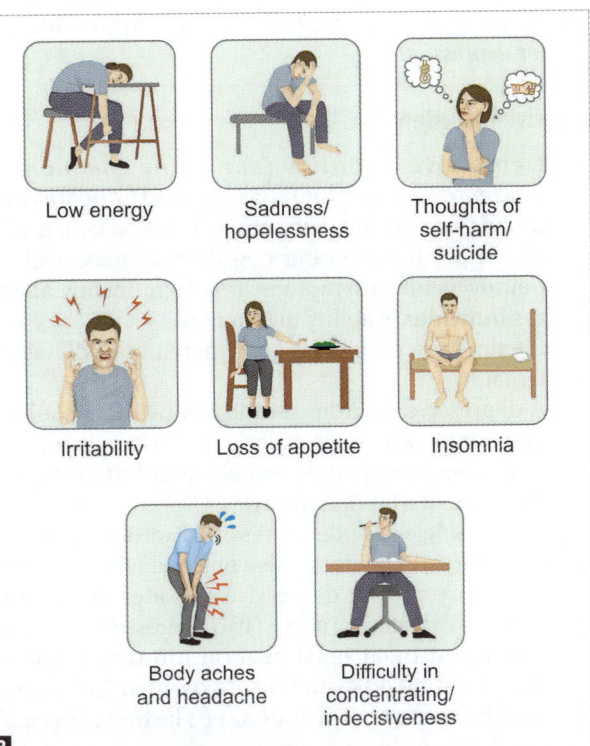

Figs. 28.8A and B: Symptoms of (A) Mania; (B) Depression

- *Physical symptoms:* Headache, heaviness of head, bodyache, easy fatigability and decreased energy are common.
- *Disturbance of biological functions:* Insomnia, loss of appetite and weight, and loss of sexual drive.
- *Psychotic features:* Delusions (nihilistic, poverty or guilt), hallucinations, inappropriate behavior and stupor may be seen.

Bipolar or Related Disorders

These are episodic mood disorders with manic, mixed or hypomanic episodes. The episodes alternate with depressive episodes/symptoms.

a. **Bipolar type I disorder** is an episodic mood disorder defined by the occurrence of one or more manic or mixed episodes *(presence of both manic and depressive episodes)*. Symptoms should last for >1 week for its diagnosis (usually last 3–4 months), and cause disruption in social and occupational activities.
b. **Bipolar type II disorder** is an episodic mood disorder defined by the occurrence of one or more hypomanic episodes and at least one depressive episode *(presence of depressive episodes and hypomanic episodes but never mania)*.
c. **Cyclothymic disorder** is characterized by a persistent instability of mood over a period of at least 2 years, involving numerous periods of hypomanic and depressive symptoms that are present during more of the time than not *(presence subsyndromal hypomanic and depressive symptoms but no mania, hypomania or major depression)*.

Depressive Disorders

- Depressive disorders *(one of the commonest psychiatric disorder)* are characterized by depressive mood (e.g., sad, irritable, empty) or loss of pleasure accompanied by other cognitive, behavioral or neurovegetative symptoms that significantly affect the individual's ability to function.
- Lifetime risk of depression is more in middle-aged females.
- A depressive disorder should not be diagnosed in individuals who have experienced a manic, mixed or hypomanic episode, which would indicate the presence of a bipolar disorder.
- **Types:** Single episode depressive disorder (presence or history of one depressive episode when there is no history of prior depressive episodes), recurrent depressive disorder (at least two depressive episodes separated by at least several months without significant mood disturbance), dysthymic disorder [persistent depressive mood (i.e., lasting ≥ 2 years) for most of the days] and mixed depressive and anxiety disorder (symptoms of both anxiety and depression for ≥ 2 weeks, most of the days).

ANXIETY OR FEAR-RELATED DISORDERS

- These disorders are characterized by excessive fear and anxiety and behavioral disturbances that are severe enough to result in significant distress or significant impairment in personal, family, social, educational, and occupational functioning.
- Differentiating feature among the anxiety and fear-related disorders are disorder-specific foci of apprehension (stimulus or situation) that triggers the fear or anxiety*.
- **Phobic disorder:** Persistent, pathological, unrealistic and intense fear of an object or situation. The phobic person (usually seen in women) may realize that the fear is irrational (insight present) but, nonetheless, cannot dispel it.

Clinical Features (Fig. 28.9)

- *Physical:* Restlessness, tremors, muscle twitchings, palpitations, sweating, dyspnea, dry mouth, diarrhea and dizziness.
- *Psychological:* Apprehension, fearfulness, insomnia, irritability, depersonalization and poor concentration.
1. **Generalized anxiety disorder** manifests by either general apprehension (i.e., 'free-floating anxiety') or excessive worry focused on multiple everyday events, most often concerning family, health, finances, and school or work.
    - *Additional symptoms* such as muscular tension or motor restlessness, sympathetic autonomic over-activity, subjective experience of nervousness, difficulty maintaining concentration, irritability or sleep disturbance.

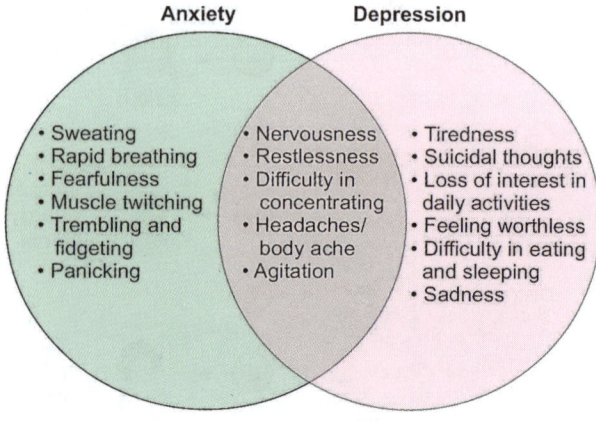

Fig. 28.9: Features of anxiety and depression

---

* Fear represents a reaction to and external, well-defined and perceived imminent threat in the present; anxiety is response to perceived anticipated internal, vague threat.

- Insidious onset in the third decade, usually chronic, which may or may not be punctuated by repeated panic attacks* (episodes of acute anxiety).
2. **Panic disorder** is characterized by discrete episodes of acute anxiety *(panic attacks)*; onset is usually in third decade, seen more often in females. The symptoms are usually sudden in onset, unexpected or out-of-the-blue, last for few minutes and characterized by very severe anxiety.
3. **Agoraphobia** is characterized by excessive fear/anxiety of places from where *escape may be difficult*, such as using public transportation, being in crowds, outside the home alone (e.g., in shops, theatres, standing in line).
4. **Specific phobia** is characterized by a marked and excessive fear/anxiety that consistently occurs when exposed to one or more specific objects/situations (e.g., proximity to certain animals, flying, heights, closed spaces, sight of blood or injury, etc.) and that is out of proportion to actual danger **(Table 28.6)**.
5. **Social anxiety disorder** is characterized by excessive fear/anxiety of humiliation/embarrassment in social situations such as social interactions (e.g., having a conversation), being observed (e.g., eating or drinking), or performing in front of others (e.g., giving a speech).
    - *Symptoms* include blushing (hallmark symptom), trembling, dryness of mouth, sweating, stumbling over words, etc.

OBSESSIVE-COMPULSIVE OR RELATED DISORDERS

♦ This group of disorders is characterized by repetitive thoughts and behaviors.

TABLE 28.6: Common types of phobias

S.No.	Type	Description
1.	Agoraphobia	Fear of open places, public places, crowded places (*commonest type; common in women*)
2.	Acrophobia	Dread of high places
3.	Acarophobia	Abnormal fear of mites or insects
4.	Algophobia	Dread of pain
5.	Claustrophobia	Abnormal fear of closed or confining spaces
6.	Social phobia	Fear of social activities and interaction (public speaking, stage performance, etc.)
7.	Erythrophobia	Fear of blushing
8.	Gamophobia	Fear of getting married or being in a relationship
9.	Xenophobia	Fear of strangers
10.	Zoophobia**	Fear of animals
11.	Hydrophobia	Fear of water
12.	Arachnophobia	Fear of spiders
13.	Hemophobia	Fear of blood

♦ Cognitive phenomena such as obsessions, intrusive thoughts and preoccupations are central to obsessive-compulsive disorder, body dysmorphic disorder, and hypochondriasis and are accompanied by related repetitive behaviors.

♦ Hoarding disorder is not associated with intrusive unwanted thoughts but there is a compulsive need to accumulate possessions, and distress related to discarding them.

1. **Obsessive-compulsive disorder (OCD)** can be predominantly obsessive thoughts or compulsive acts or mixed. Depression is common, and insight is present. *OCD has four major symptom patterns:*
    a. **Contamination:** Most common pattern is obsession of contamination followed by washing (repeated many times in a day) or accompanied by compulsive avoidance of the presumably contaminated object **(Figs. 28.10A and B)**.
    b. **Pathological doubt:** Next to contamination, is the obsession of doubt (whether the door has been locked or proper counting of money), followed by compulsion of checking repeatedly to remove the doubt **(Fig. 28.11)**.

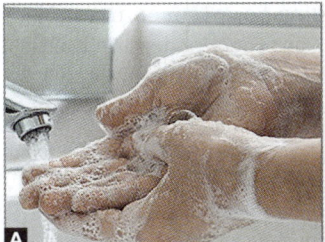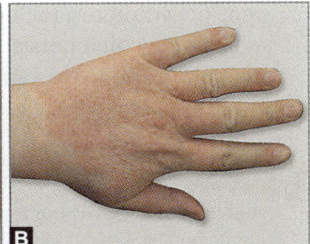

Figs. 28.10A and B: Obsessive-compulsive disorder: (A) Repetitive hand washing (contamination); (B) Contact dermatitis following it

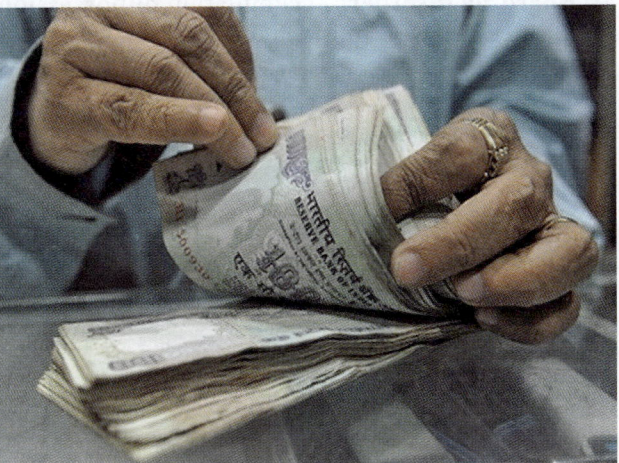

Fig. 28.11: Obsessive-compulsive disorder: Repetitive counting to check the money (pathological doubt)

---

* Panic attacks are episodes of intense fear or apprehension with a feeling of impending doom which is accompanied by the rapid onset of symptoms (e.g., palpitations, sweating, trembling, shortness of breath, chest pain, dizziness or lightheadedness, chills, hot flushes, fear of imminent death).
** Not to confuse with 'zoophilia' which is sexual intercourse with an animal.

c. **Intrusive thoughts:** There are intrusive obsessional thoughts (usually sexual or aggressive in nature) without any associated compulsive acts.
d. **Symmetry:** Another common pattern is the need for symmetry or precision, which will lead to compulsion of slowness. Patients may take hours to eat meals or shave.
   Other symptom patterns: Religious obsession or masturbation may be compulsive.
   These repetitive and unwanted thoughts are time consuming (at least 1 h a day) and cause distress or significant impairment.
2. **Body dysmorphic disorder:** Persistent preoccupation with imagined defects or flaws in appearance that is either unnoticeable/slightly noticeable to others. Individuals experience excessive self-consciousness, often with ideas of reference (i.e., the conviction that people are taking notice, judging or talking about it) with presence of repetitive behaviors (e.g., mirror gazing, excessive grooming) and reassurance seeking from others about the appearance.
3. **Hypochondriasis:** Persistent preoccupation with or fear about the possibility of having serious or life-threatening diseases. This is secondary to misinterpretation of bodily signs or symptoms, including normal or commonplace sensations which persists or reoccurs despite medical evaluation and reassurance. For e.g., a patient may misinterpret cough or pain in the chest as that of lung cancer.

> **NOTA BENE**
> **Cyberchondria:** Searching for medical information online for information about particular real or imagined symptoms or illness. It overlaps anxiety and OCD.

4. **Hoarding disorder:** Accumulation of possessions due to excessive acquisition of or difficulty discarding possessions, regardless of their actual value. *Excessive acquisition* is characterized by repetitive urges or behaviors related to amassing or buying items. *Difficulty discarding* possessions is characterized by a perceived need to save items and distress associated with discarding them.
5. **Body-focused repetitive behavior disorders:** Recurrent and habitual actions directed at the integument (e.g., hair-pulling, skin-picking or lip-biting). For e.g., **trichotillomania** is characterized by recurrent pulling of one's own hair leading to significant hair loss, accompanied by unsuccessful attempts to decrease or stop the behavior (**Fig. 28.6B**).

STRESS DISORDERS

These disorders are related to exposure to a stressful or traumatic event, or a series of such events or adverse experiences. For each of the disorders, an identifiable stressor (stressful event) is a necessary causal factor.

1. **Post-traumatic stress disorder (PTSD)** is a psychiatric disorder that can occur in people who have experienced or witnessed a traumatic event, such as a natural disaster, terrorist act, an accident, sexual assault or other violent personal assault.
   Symptoms of PTSD fall into four categories (**Fig. 28.12**):
   a. **Intrusive thoughts:** Repeated, involuntary memories of the traumatic event, nightmares or distressing dreams or dissociation (including flashbacks) and intense, negative emotional or physiological reaction on exposure to reminders (traumatic triggers).
   b. **Avoiding reminders of the traumatic event:** Avoiding people, places, activities, objects and situations that bring on distressing memories. Patient may try to avoid remembering or thinking about the traumatic event.

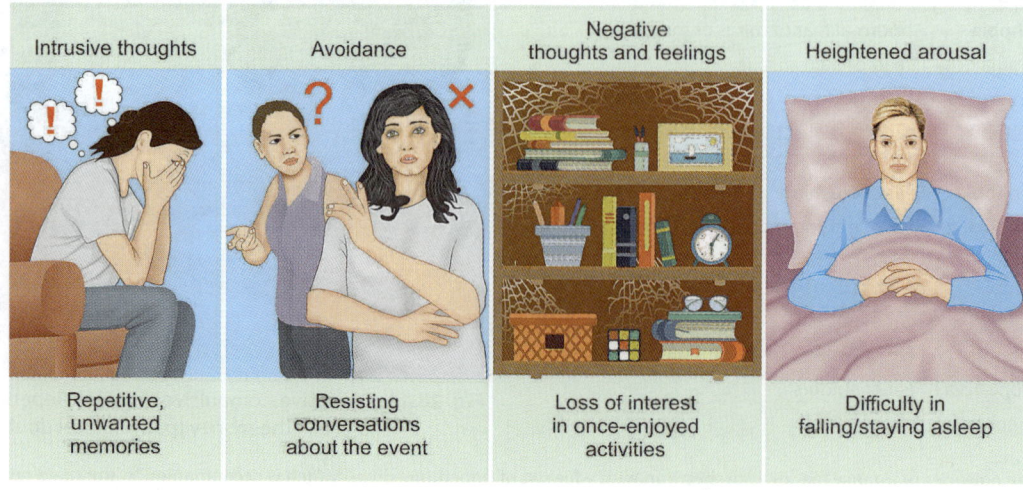

Fig. 28.12: Post-traumatic stress disorder symptoms

c. **Negative alterations in cognition and mood:** Ongoing and distorted beliefs about oneself or others; inappropriate blaming of oneself for the trauma, persistent negative emotional state (sadness, horror, guilt or shame), less interest in activities previously enjoyed, or feeling detachment from others.
d. **Arousal and reactive symptoms:** Difficulty in falling or staying asleep, difficulty in concentration, increased startle reaction, irritability or angry outbursts, increased vigilance for potential danger, self-harming acts or recklessness.

The symptoms must persist for several weeks and cause significant impairment in personal, family, social, educational, or occupational functioning.

2. **Prolonged grief disorder** is a disturbance in which, following the death of a spouse/parent/child or a close person, there is persistent grief characterized by longing for the deceased or persistent preoccupation with the deceased accompanied by intense emotional pain.
   - **Symptoms** include sadness, guilt, anger, denial, blame, difficulty accepting the death, feeling one has lost a part of one's self, inability to experience positive mood, emotional numbness, difficulty in engaging with social or other activities.
   - **Diagnosis:** Grief should persist for ≥ 6 months.

DISSOCIATIVE DISORDERS

Dissociative disorders are characterized by involuntary disruption or discontinuity in the normal integration of one or more of the following: identity, sensations, perceptions, affects, thoughts, memories, control over bodily movements or behavior.

1. **Dissociative amnesia:** Inability to recall important personal information/memories, typically of recent traumatic or stressful event that is inconsistent with ordinary forgetting.

> **NOTA BENE**
>
> **Dissociative fugue** is feature of dissociative amnesia characterized by a period of almost complete amnesia during which a person actually flees from an immediate life situation (usually from home) and begins a different life pattern with a completely new identity for period of time. There is amnesia for the period of travel and the patient may find it difficult to recall most of the past.

2. **Trance disorder** is characterized by trance states. In this state, there is a marked alteration in the state of consciousness (not fully alert and may be confused) and narrowing of awareness of immediate surroundings (can focus on limited things in his surroundings). There is loss of normal sense of personal identity (may not behave like his usual self) and the patient's movements, postures and speech may be restricted. He may repeat certain movements and words and may experience being outside of one's control.

3. **Dissociative identity disorder** *(Multiple personality disorder)*: Disruption of identity in which the patient is dominated by two or more personalities, and one is manifest at a time and the other is not aware of its existence (takes control of the individual's consciousness and functioning in interacting with others or with the environment). There are typically episodes of amnesia, which may be severe.

4. **Depersonalization-derealization disorder:** Persistent or recurrent experiences of depersonalization, derealization or both.
   - Depersonalization is characterized by experiencing the self as strange or unreal, or feeling detached from one's thoughts, feelings, sensations, body or actions.
   - Derealization is characterized by experiencing other persons, objects or the world as strange or unreal (e.g., dreamlike, colorless, distant, foggy or visually distorted) or feeling detached from one's surroundings.
   - During experiences of depersonalization or derealization, *reality testing* remains intact.

FEEDING OR EATING DISORDERS

- They are abnormal eating or feeding behaviors that are not explained by another health condition and are not developmentally appropriate or culturally sanctioned.
- **Feeding disorders** involve behavioral disturbances that are not related to body weight and shape concerns, such as eating of non-edible substances or voluntary regurgitation of foods.
- **Eating disorders** include abnormal eating behavior and preoccupation with food, as well as prominent body weight and shape concerns.

1. **Anorexia nervosa** is intense fear of becoming obese. Appetite may be preserved, but the patient refuses to eat **(Figs. 28.13A and B)**. They have significantly low body weight for the individual's height, age and developmental stage (BMI < 18.5 kg/m² in adults).
2. **Bulimia nervosa** is frequent, recurrent episodes of binge eating* (overeating) with attempts to counteract it by self-induced vomiting, strenuous exercise or purgatives **(Fig. 28.13C)**. The individual is not significantly underweight and therefore does not meet the diagnostic requirements of anorexia nervosa.
3. **Pica:** Regular consumption of non-nutritive substances (e.g., clay, soil, chalk, plaster, plastic, metal and paper, large quantities of salt or corn flour) causing damage to health and impairment in functioning in children (diagnosed only if they are >2 years).

---

*Large amount of food is consumed in short period due to individual's loss of control over eating, followed by severe discomfort.

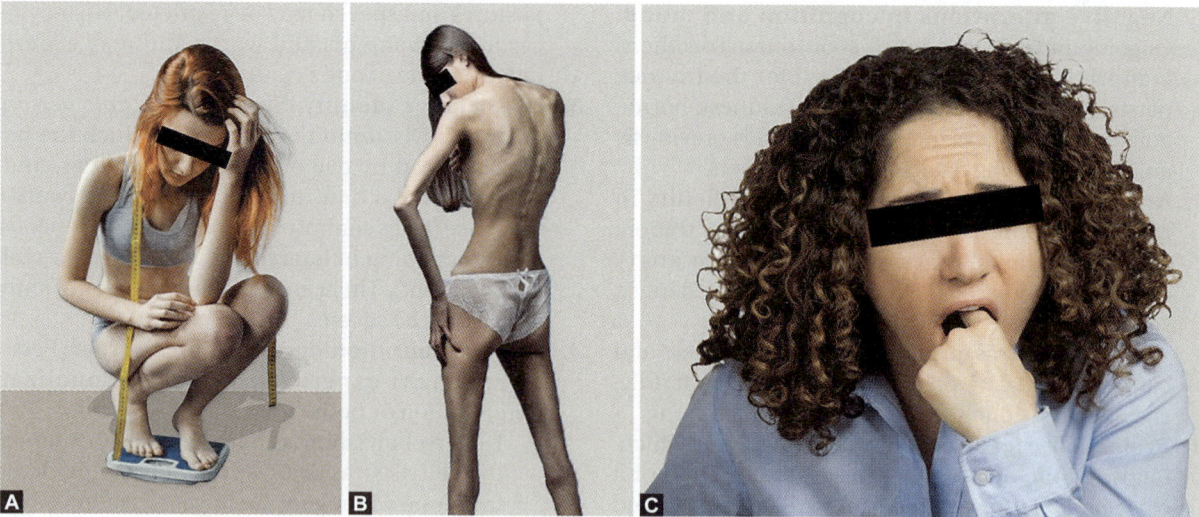

Figs. 28.13A to C: (A and B) Anorexia nervosa; (C) Bulimia nervosa

BODILY DISTRESS OR BODILY EXPERIENCE DISORDERS

In these disorders, there is a disturbance in the person's experience of his or her body.

1. **Bodily distress disorder:** Bodily symptoms that the individual finds distressing and to which excessive attention is directed, which may be manifest by repeated contact with healthcare providers. Occasionally, there is a single symptom—usually pain or fatigue—that is associated with the other features of the disorder.
2. **Body integrity dysphoria:** Disturbance in the person's experience of the body manifested by the persistent desire to have a specific physical disability (e.g., amputation of one or more healthy limbs) accompanied by persistent discomfort, or intense feelings of inappropriateness concerning current non-disabled body configuration.

SUBSTANCE USE OR ADDICTIVE BEHAVIORS DISORDERS

Disorders due to substance use and addictive behaviors are mental and behavioral disorders that develop as a result of the use of psychoactive substances, including medications, or specific repetitive rewarding and reinforcing behaviors.

1. **Disorders due to substance use** include single episodes of harmful substance use, substance use disorders (harmful substance use and substance dependence), and substance-induced disorders such as substance intoxication, substance withdrawal and substance-induced mental disorders, sexual dysfunctions and sleep-wake disorders.
2. **Disorders due to addictive behaviors:** Recognizable and clinically significant syndromes associated with distress or interference with personal functions that develop as a result of repetitive rewarding behaviors other than the use of dependence-producing substances.
   - These include *gambling and gaming disorder*, which can be both online and offline.
   - It manifests by—impaired control; increased priority over other life interests and daily activities; and continuation or escalation despite negative consequences.
   - *Diagnosis:* This should be present for ≥ 12 months.

IMPULSE CONTROL DISORDERS

- Impulse control disorders is characterized by repeated failure to resist an impulse, drive or urge to perform an act that is short-term rewarding to the person, despite longer-term harm either to the individual or to others causing marked distress or significant impairment in functioning.
- There is an increasing sense of tension or affective arousal prior to instances of *the impulsive act*, and a sense of pleasure, excitement, relief or gratification during and immediately after the act.

1. **Pyromania:** Recurrent failure to control strong impulses to set fires to property, in the absence of an intelligible motive (e.g., monetary gain, revenge, sabotage, political statement).
2. **Kleptomania:** Recurrent failure to control strong impulses to steal objects in the absence of an intelligible motive (e.g., objects are not acquired for personal use or monetary gain) **(Fig. 28.6A)**.
3. **Compulsive sexual behavior disorder:** Persistent pattern of failure to control intense, repetitive sexual impulses or urges resulting in repetitive sexual behavior. This should be manifested > 6 months for a diagnosis.

DISRUPTIVE BEHAVIOR OR DISSOCIAL DISORDERS

Disruptive behavior and dissocial disorders are characterized by persistent behavior problems that range from markedly and persistently defiant, disobedient, provocative or spiteful (i.e., disruptive) behaviors that persistently violate the basic rights of others or major age-appropriate societal norms, rules or laws. Onset is commonly during childhood.

PERSONALITY DISORDERS AND RELATED TRAITS

- Personality disorder is characterized by problems in functioning of aspects of the self (e.g., identity, self-worth, accuracy of self-view, self-direction), and/or interpersonal dysfunction (e.g., ability to develop and maintain close and mutually satisfying relationships, ability to understand others' perspectives and to manage conflict in relationships) that have persisted over an extended period of time (e.g., 2 years or more).
- The disturbance is manifest in patterns of cognition, emotional expression, and behavior that are maladaptive (e.g., inflexible or poorly regulated) and is manifest across a range of personal and social situations (i.e., is not limited to specific relationships or social roles).
- The patterns of behavior characterizing the disturbance are not developmentally appropriate and cannot be explained primarily by social or cultural factors, including socio-political conflict.

FACTITIOUS DISORDERS

- Factitious disorders are characterized by intentionally feigning, falsifying, inducing, or aggravating medical, psychological or behavioral signs and symptoms or injury in oneself or in another person (most commonly a child), associated with identified deception.
- A pre-existing disorder or disease may be present, but the individual intentionally aggravates existing symptoms or falsifies or induces additional symptoms.
- Individuals with this disorder seek treatment or present themselves or another person as ill, injured or impaired based on these signs, symptoms or injuries (e.g., Munchausen syndrome).
- The deceptive behavior is not solely motivated by external rewards or incentives (e.g., obtaining disability payments or evading criminal prosecution).
- This is in contrast to *malingering*, in which external rewards or incentives are the goal.

NEUROCOGNITIVE DISORDERS

- Neurocognitive disorders are characterized by primary clinical deficits in cognitive functioning that are acquired rather than developmental.
- They do not include disorders with cognitive deficits that are present from birth or that arise during the developmental period, which are classified as neurodevelopmental disorders.
- These disorders are associated with transient or permanent brain dysfunction and include those with demonstrable cerebral disease, which may be either primary brain pathology or secondary to systemic diseases.

1. **Delirium:** Acute reversible mental disorder characterized by confusion and impairment of consciousness, disorientation (most commonly in time), emotional lability, hallucination or illusion, disturbance of the sleep-wake cycle, and inappropriate, impulsive, irrational or violent behavior.
    - It usually occurs in physical diseases like high fever or due to overwork, mental stress, acute poisoning (*Datura*), chronic alcoholics or drug intoxication.
    - A delirious person may become impulsive and violent, and may commit suicide. Such person is not responsible for his criminal acts.

2. **Dementia** is an acquired brain syndrome characterized by a decline from a previous level of cognitive functioning with impairment in two or more cognitive domains (such as memory, executive functions, attention, language, social cognition and judgment, psychomotor speed, visuoperceptual or visuospatial abilities).
    - Dementia due to Alzheimer disease is the *most common* form of dementia.
    - Onset is insidious with memory impairment as the initial presenting complaint.
    - **Clinical features**
        i. Impairment in intellectual functioning
        ii. Disturbance of orientation (late)
        iii. Failing memory
        iv. Reduced facility with language
        v. Alterations in mood and affect
        vi. Impaired judgment and abstraction
        vii. Distractibility
        viii. No impairment of consciousness.

    Usually irreversible, and impairment of all functions occurs globally, causing interference of day-to-day activities and interpersonal relationships. The sufferer may lead a vegetative life. At some phase, the person may become agitated, aggressive and violent.

3. **Amnestic disorder:** Severe memory impairment relative to the individual's age and general level of intellectual functioning that is disproportionate to impairment in other cognitive domains.
    - It manifests by a severe deficit in acquiring memories (recent) or learning new information or the inability to recall previously learned information, without disturbance of consciousness or generalized cognitive impairment.

> **NOTA BENE**
> - Earlier, the neurocognitive disorders were called 'organic mental disorders' as these were caused by a demonstrable disturbance (e.g., infarcts, infections, etc.) of cerebral functioning (*disorders of brain*). In contrast, the disorders with no disturbance of the brain were called 'functional disorders' (*disorders of mind*), e.g., schizophrenia, mood disorders.
> - Currently, it is understood that the so-called 'functional disorders' too are caused by demonstrable disturbances of brain (using advanced structural and functional imaging). Hence, the classification of *organic vs. functional* has been discarded.

SLEEP-WAKE DISORDERS

Sleep-wake disorders involve problems with the quality, timing, and amount of sleep, which result in daytime distress and impairment in functioning.

1. **Insomnia disorders:** Difficulty in falling asleep or difficulty in staying asleep, and includes frequent awakenings during night and early morning awakening, which results in some form of daytime impairment (like fatigue, decreased mood or irritability, general malaise and cognitive impairment), e.g., chronic insomnia, short-term insomnia.
2. **Hypersomnolence disorders:** Excessive time spent asleep.
   a. **Kleine-Levin syndrome or 'Sleeping Beauty syndrome'** is a rare sleep disorder characterized by persistent episodic hypersomnolence, behavioral and cognitive disturbances, hyperphagia, and in some cases hypersexuality.
   b. **Narcolepsy:** Common cause of hypersomnia; characterized by excessive daytime sleepiness, often diminished night-time sleep and disturbances in REM sleep. Hallmark is decreased REM latency.
   - **Types:** Narcolepsy type 1 (*Gelineau's syndrome*, formerly narcolepsy with cataplexy) and narcolepsy type 2 (formerly narcolepsy without cataplexy).
   - *Classical tetrad of symptoms seen in Type 1*
     i. **Sleep attacks** (*most common*) from which he awakens refreshed, and can occur at any time of day, even while driving.
     ii. **Cataplexy:** Temporary sudden loss of muscle tone causing weakness and immobilization which may result in a fall.
     iii. **Hypnagogic hallucinations:** Vivid perceptions, usually dream-like which occur at the onset of sleep (if occurring at awakening—*hypnopompic hallucinations*) and associated with fearfulness.
     iv. **Sleep paralysis** (least common) usually occurs at awakening in morning. The individual is conscious but unable to move his body for 30 seconds to few minutes.

> **NOTA BENE**
> - **Somnolentia or semisomnolence:** It is the condition when a person is in between sleep and wakefulness. The person needs much more time to awaken, and during this period, he is confused or disoriented. This is often termed as **sleep-drunkenness**.
> - When suddenly awaken from a deep sleep, such person may perform some violent act without awareness and understanding. He is not responsible for any criminal act performed by him during such a state of mind.

3. **Sleep-related movement disorders:** Restless legs syndrome, sleep-related **bruxism** *(tooth-grinding)*—patient forcefully and involuntarily grinds teeth during this phase, and is unaware of it on awakening.
4. **Parasomnia disorders:** Undesirable physical events or experiences occurring during sleep, sleep stages or partial arousals. It can be **stage IV sleep disorders** occurring during deep sleep (stage III and IV of NREM sleep).
   a. *Disorders of arousal from non-REM sleep*
      i. **Sleepwalking disorder (somnambulism):** A state of altered consciousness in which phenomena of sleep and wakefulness are combined. The patient walks during sleep and carries out automatic motor activity. He may get up from the bed, open the door, walk out a distance and return to his bed to sleep again, and remember nothing on awakening. During the whole episode, the subject is in a state of dissociated consciousness, and arousal is difficult.
      - If, in a fit of somnambulistic automatism, a person commits a criminal act, he will not be held responsible for the same.
      ii. **Sleep-terrors (pavor nocturnus):** Patient gets up screaming with tachycardia, sweating and hyperventilation during the first third of nocturnal sleep, but rarely recalls anything in the morning.
      iii. **Sleep-talking (somniloquy):** Patient talks during this stage, but does not remember about it in the morning on awakening.
   b. *Parasomnias related to REM sleep*
      i. **REM sleep behavior disorder:** REM sleep behavior disorder is characterized by a loss of normal muscle tone during REM sleep and motor activity associated with dream content.
      ii. **Nightmare disorder:** Dream experiences full of anxiety or fear. There is very detailed recall of the dream content which is related to threats to survival, security or self-esteem. Upon awakening, the individual rapidly becomes alert and oriented.

NOTA BENE

CHANGES IN THE ICD-11

The following are either added or deleted in the new ICD-11.

Added diagnoses
- **Complex PTSD** involves the three symptoms of PTSD (re-experiencing, avoiding reminders, and a heightened sense of threat/arousal) along with broader problems in emotion regulation, shame, guilt, and interpersonal conflict, such that it affects the person's entire life.
- **Compulsive sexual behavior disorder** is characterized by a persistent pattern of failure to control intense, repetitive sexual impulses or urges resulting in repetitive sexual behavior. It is classified as an impulse control disorder rather than an addictive disorder.
- **Gaming disorder** is persistent or recurrent gaming behavior ('digital gaming' or 'video-gaming').
- **Prolonged grief disorder** is defined as grief that extends beyond what most people would consider a reasonable or expected amount of time.

Deleted diagnoses
- **Acute stress disorder** is no longer included as a mental disorder and instead is now classified as a reaction to trauma (factor influencing health).
- **Gender incongruence** is no longer considered as a mental disorder but rather a sexual health condition to avoid stigma about it being a psychological rather than medical condition.
- **Personality disorders** have been completely overhauled. There is now one diagnosis of 'personality disorder' as it was found that there was much overlap in clinical practice.

FM 5.3
Describe civil and criminal responsibilities of a mentally ill person.

MENTAL DISORDER AND RESPONSIBILITY

Responsibility, in the legal sense, means the liability of a person for his acts or omissions, and if these are against the law, the liability to be punished for them. *The law presumes that every person of age of discretion is mentally sound (sane), until the contrary is proved (defense on ground of insanity needs to be proved).*

Civil Responsibility

The question of civil responsibility arises in the following conditions:

i. **Management of property:** The court may appoint a guardian to take care of the mentally ill, and may appoint a manager to manage the property. The court may order the sale of the mentally ill person's property for the payment of his debts and expenses. Only persons competent to contract are authorized to transfer property.

ii. **Contracts:** A contract is invalid, if one of the parties at the time of making it was, by reason of mental illness, incapable of understanding it and forming a rational judgment as to its effect upon his interests. However, a mentally ill person is liable for contracts entered into during lucid intervals.

iii. **Marriage and divorce:** As per *Hindu Marriage Act*, marriage can be declared null and void, if one of the parties, at the time of ceremony, was incapable of giving valid consent or was unfit for marriage due to unsoundness of mind. As per *Muslim Marriages Act,* a woman can obtain a divorce on ground of husband's insanity within 2 years of marriage, but a man could get divorce by pronouncing '*talak*' three times, without assigning any reason (oral, written or electronic forms).*

iv. **Adoption:** Under *Hindu Adoption and Maintenance Act,* taking/giving adoption of a child is not allowed, if either of the parents is mentally ill.

v. **Competency as a witness:** Under **Sec. 118 IEA**, a mentally ill person is not competent to give evidence, if he is prevented by his illness from understanding the questions put to him and giving rational answers to them.

vi. **Validity of consent:** The consent given by an insane or intoxicated person, who is unable to understand the nature and consequences of that to which he gives his consent is invalid (**Sec. 90 IPC**).

vii. **Testamentary capacity:** This means the capacity of a person to make a valid will. The law defines it as the possession of a sound disposing mind (*compos mentis*) which must be certified by a doctor.

NOTA BENE

- **Holograph will**: Will written by the testator in his own handwriting.
- Valid will must fulfill the following conditions:
  a. The testator must be a major, should understand the nature of the will, have knowledge of the property to be disposed and the ability to recognize those who have justifiable claims on his property.
  b. It should be executed voluntarily without any undue influence of any person.
  c. The testator must sign it in presence of two witnesses.
- Will is *valid* under special circumstances:
  a. Made by deaf, dumb or blind persons.
  b. Made during lucid intervals of mental illness.
  c. Suicide by testator immediately after making the will, in the absence of any mental illness.
- Will is *invalid* when made by imbecile or drunk persons or under insane delusions, because the testator was incapable of rational views and judgment.

---

* It has been declared unconstitutional by the Supreme Court. The government has formulated 'The Muslim Women (Protection of Rights on Marriage) Act, 2019' which makes 'triple talaq' illegal and void, with up to 3 years imprisonment for the husband.

Criminal Responsibility

Sec. 84 IPC deals with the criminal responsibility of insane persons.*

It states that:

"Nothing is an offense which is done by a person who, at the time of doing it, by reason of unsoundness of mind, is incapable of knowing the nature of the act, or what he is doing is either wrong or contrary to the law".

There is a minor difference between **Sec. 84 IPC** and the McNaughten's rule, which is the guideline followed in British Courts for consideration of the liability of a mentally ill person who commits a crime.

McNaughten Rule(s)

In 1843, Mr Edward Drummond, the private secretary of the then Prime Minister of England, Sir Robert Peel was shot dead by a young Scotsman Daniel McNaughten. McNaughten was suffering from delusion of persecution and believed that his life was in danger due to the acts of persecution by the Tory Party on him. He shot dead Mr Drummond on the belief that he was going to kill the Tory Party Prime Minister Mr Peel. It was established that McNaughten suffered from paranoid delusions and was acquitted on the ground of insanity. Upon this development, the Supreme Court Judges of the UK were summoned by the House of Lords to know the position of the law of England regarding crime and insanity. From the answers given by them, rules were framed for criminal responsibility of the insane, and they have been named after McNaughten.

The most important and relevant part of the McNaughten rules states: 'Every man is to be presumed to be sane, and to possess a sufficient degree of reason to be responsible for his crimes, until the contrary be proved; and that to establish a defense on the ground of insanity, it must be clearly proved that at the time of committing the act, the party accused was laboring under such a defect of reason from disease of the mind, so as not to know the nature and quality of the act he was doing, or if he did know it, that he did not know that what he was doing was wrong'.

These rules are given the status of 'legal test' for insanity.

The Legal Test of Insanity (The 'Right or Wrong' Test)

Under this test, a person is not criminally responsible, *if at the time of the crime, he did not know the nature of the act or that it was wrong.* It excludes responsibility of the insane for the commission of crime, and has the following requirements:
  i. There should be evidence of mental disease.
  ii. This mental disease or defect must exist at the time of commission of crime.
  iii. It should be of such degree that the person is unable to understand that the act is wrong and/or contrary to the law.

Comments

- The insanity must be directly related to the offense in such a way as to satisfy the court that the mental abnormality had a direct causative relationship to the offense, and that the offense would not have occurred, if there was no mental abnormality.
- The law recognizes as 'abnormality of the mind' as any disease which is capable of producing mental dysfunction. The law is not concerned with the brain, but with the mind, as the term means reason, memory and understanding. However, when mental dysfunction is attributable to external factors (e.g., alcohol and drugs consumed voluntarily), this is not called as the abnormality of the mind. It is usually assumed to mean one of the major functional or organic psychoses.
- It must be clearly established that the reasoning powers of the accused were not functioning normally due to defect in intellectual and cognitive faculties.
- The rule concerns itself with the ability of the accused to distinguish between 'right' and 'wrong' with reference to the particular crime. If at the time of the commission of the crime, the accused had the capacity to know that his act was wrong, he will be fully responsible, even if he was mentally ill and unable to refrain from doing the act at that time. If a person commits a crime under the influence of an insane delusion, he is judged as though the delusionary facts were real.

  Examples
  i. If under the influence of an insane delusion, a person thinks another man is attempting to kill him and he kills that man in self-defense, he will not be held criminally responsible.
  ii. If under the influence of an insane delusion, a person thinks another man to be a wild animal and kills him, he will not be held criminally responsible.
  iii. If under an insane delusion, a person thinks that another person has caused serious injury to his character, family or property and kills him, he becomes responsible because under the law, no one can kill a person in revenge.
- The defect of McNaughten rule is that, from deciding that a person is insane, only cognitive (intellectual) faculties are taken into consideration, whereas emotional factors, hallucinations and the ability of the individual to control the impulse (resistible impulse) are not considered.

---

* There is no definition of "unsoundness of mind" in the IPC. The courts have, however, mainly treated this expression as equivalent to insanity.

NOTA BENE

To assess the criminal responsibility of insane persons, certain other rules have come into use in subsequent periods in different countries at different times.

- **Durham's rule (1954):** An accused person is not criminally responsible, if his unlawful act is the product of mental disease or mental defect.
- **Curren's rule (1964):** This rule states that an accused person is not criminally responsible, if at the time of committing the act, he did not have the capacity to regulate his conduct to the requirements of the law as a result of mental disease or defect.
- **American Law Institute test (1970):** A person is not responsible for criminal conduct, if at the time of such conduct as a result of mental disease or defect, the person lacked adequate capacity either to appreciate the wrongfulness of his conduct or to conform his conduct to the requirements of law *(Model Penal Code test)*.
- **The Brawner rule (1972)** argues that insanity should be decided by a Jury. Under this proposal, Juries are allowed to decide the 'insanity question' as they see fit.
- **Guilty but mentally ill (1975):** Michigan introduced this as an alternative to the insanity defense. Some jurisdictions permit a defendant to plead guilty but mentally ill. A defendant who receives this verdict is still considered legally guilty of the crime in question, but since he is mentally ill, he is entitled to receive mental health treatment while institutionalized.
- **The Irresistible Impulse:** It argues that a person may have known an act was illegal, but because of a mental impairment, he could not control his actions. In 1994, *Lorena Bobbitt* was found not guilty of a crime, when her defense argued that an irresistible impulse led her to cut off her husband's penis.

NOTA BENE

Procedure of examination of a mentally ill person (Secs. 328 and 329 CrPC)
- If during trial, the Magistrate finds the accused to be of unsound mind and incapable of making his defense, then he should order such person to be examined by the civil surgeon or any medical officer as the State Government may direct, and postpone further proceedings in the case.
- If the civil surgeon finds the accused to be of unsound mind, he should refer such person to a psychiatrist/clinical psychologist for treatment and prognosis of the condition, and should inform the Magistrate regarding the same.
- If the accused is aggrieved by the report given to the Magistrate, he can make an appeal before the Medical Board consisting of:
  - i. Head of psychiatry unit in the nearest government hospital; and
  - ii. A faculty member in psychiatry in the nearest medical college.

Release of person of unsound mind pending investigation or trial (Sec. 330 CrPC): On the basis of medical opinion, whenever a person if found incapable of entering defense by reason of unsoundness of mind or mental retardation, the Magistrate may decide to order release of such person on bail or kept in such a place where regular psychiatric treatment can be provided.

Resumption of trial/inquiry (Sec. 331 CrPC): Whenever a trial is postponed under **Sec. 328 or 329**, the Magistrate may resume it at any time after the person concerned has ceased to be of unsound mind.

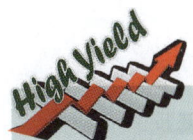

- **Mentally ill person:** Any person who is in need of treatment by reason of any mental disorder *other than mental retardation*.
- **Neurosis:** Patient suffers from emotional or intellectual disorders which causes subjective distress, but does not lose touch with reality, e.g., anxiety, phobia, depression.
- **Psychosis:** Gross impairment in reality-testing (withdrawal from reality), as if living in a world of fantasy, e.g., schizophrenia, dementia.
- **Delusion:** False, fixed, unshakeable and firm belief in something which is not a fact despite contradictory proof or evidence.
- **Delusion of grandeur:** Person imagines being very rich, while in reality he is poor.
- **Delusion of persecution:** Person imagines to be poisoned by his near relatives.
- **Delusion of infidelity:** Patient believes that his spouse is unfaithful.
- **Hypochondriacal delusion:** Patient believes of having serious disease (like cancer).
- **Nihilistic delusion:** Patient does not believe in his existence or the world.
- **Delusion of reference:** Patient believes that he is referred to by all agencies, media and persons.
- **Delusion of poverty:** Person is convinced that he is deprived of all material possessions.

- **Erotomania:** Delusional belief that a person of higher social status is in love with her/him.
- **Most common type of delusion:** Delusion of persecution.
- A person is not responsible if a person does an unlawful act due to delusion (doctrine of diminished responsibility).
- **Hallucination:** False perception by senses *without* any external object or stimulus.
- **Illusion:** False interpretation of an external object or stimulus *which* has a real existence.
- **Visual hallucination:** Visualizes non-existent sights.
- **Auditory hallucination:** Sound perception (noises, music) without any source.
- **Most common hallucination:** Auditory hallucination.
- **Impulse:** Sudden and irresistible force compelling to the conscious performance of some act without motive or forethought.
- **Kleptomania:** Compulsion to steal articles which may be of little value.
- **Obsession:** Persistent and recurrent idea, thought or emotion that cannot be eliminated from consciousness by logic or reasoning.
- **Compulsion:** Repetitive behavior or mental acts that the person feels driven to perform in response to an obsession.
- Delusion is a thought disorder.
- Hallucination is a disorder of perception and is not under voluntary control.
- Obsession-compulsion is a disorder of content of thought.
- **Lucid interval:** Period during which all the signs and symptoms of insanity disappear (also seen in head injury).
- **Feigned insanity:** With some motive, a person may pose to be insane or a sane person may be presented as an insane person.
- **Hallmark feature of schizophrenia:** Thought and speech disorders.
- Term 'schizophrenia' was coined by *Eugene Bleuler*.
- First rank symptoms of schizophrenia were given by *Kurt Schneider*.
- Prognosis is best with acute onset schizophrenia.
- **Schizophrenia with mental retardation:** Pfropf schizophrenia.
- **Agoraphobia:** Fear of open places, public places, crowded places (*commonest type*).
- **Acrophobia:** Dread of high places.
- **Claustrophobia:** Abnormal fear of closed or confining spaces.
- Agoraphobia is associated with panic disorder.
- Most common pattern in OCD is obsession of contamination followed by washing (repeated many times in a day).
- **Fugue:** Period of complete amnesia wherein a person flees from an immediate life situation and begins a different life pattern.
- **Anorexia nervosa:** Intense fear of becoming obese.
- **Postpartum psychosis:** Severe psychiatric symptoms including depressive episode, schizophrenia, manic episode or delirium seen after delivery.
- **Somnolentia:** Person is in between sleep and wakefulness.
- **Narcolepsy:** Common cause of hypersomnia; characterized by excessive daytime sleepiness.
- **Tetrad of narcolepsy:** Sleep attacks, cataplexy, hypnagogic hallucinations and sleep paralysis.
- **Somnambulism (sleep walking):** Patient walks during sleep and carries out automatic motor activity and remembers nothing on awakening.
- The law presumes that every person is mentally sound, until the opposite is proved.
- **Testamentary capacity:** Capacity to make a valid will. Mentally sound person (≥18 years) can make a valid will.
- A mentally ill person is not competent to give evidence.
- Consent is invalid if given by an insane/intoxicated person **(Sec. 90 IPC)**.
- An insane person cannot give valid consent for marriage.
- **Sec. 84 IPC** deals with the criminal responsibility of insane persons (act of a person of unsound mind).
- McNaughten rule is related to criminal responsibility of insane persons.
- **Legal test of insanity (Right or wrong test):** A person is not criminally responsible, if at the time of the crime, he did not know the nature of the act or that it was wrong.

Interesting case

Schizophrenia (Case of John Forbes Nash Jr, 1959)

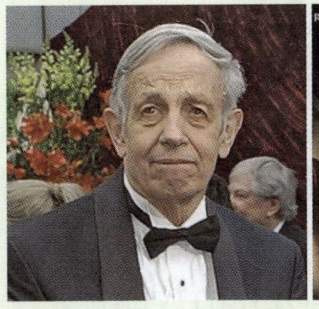 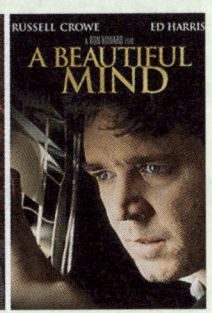

John Nash was one of the greatest thinkers in mathematics of the 20th century and best-known people with schizophrenia of the same period. He was an American mathematician who made fundamental contributions to game theory, differential geometry, and the study of partial differential equations. He is the only person to be awarded both the Nobel Memorial Prize in Economic Sciences and the Abel Prize.

His first signs of mental illness were evident by 1958 when he was 30 years of age. While teaching at Massachusetts Institute of Technology (MIT) he would disappear without warning for days, take long reveries in the midst of his lectures or make meaningless statements to colleagues and students. He became increasingly paranoid, such as not allowing visitors to his office to stand between him and the door and believed that he was being followed all the time. He believed that all men who wore red ties were part of a communist conspiracy against him. He was known as the 'Phantom of Fine Hall' as he would prowl the college halls at all hours scribing intricate and arcane formulae on blackboards. Although Nash continued to work, his behavior and conversations became increasingly disturbed. In 1959, Nash visited Columbia University for a lecture about the Riemann hypothesis, but he became incomprehensible. His colleagues in the audience realized that something was wrong and that he needed professional help. At this time, his wife Alicia was pregnant with their first child. He resigned from the MIT mathematics faculty and was admitted to a hospital for treatment. At first, he was offered voluntary admission, but on refusal, he was admitted involuntarily. The psychiatrists made a diagnosis of paranoid schizophrenia based on his very complex system of delusions which were both grandiose and persecutory. Nash responded well with chlorpromazine and began to show improvement within a short time. He was discharged after agreeing to OPD treatment after some 50 days of confinement.

In the next ten years or so, he was admitted to the hospital multiple times interspersed by periods of varying degrees of mental health and ill health. His relationship with his wife and child became strained and in 1963 they divorced. When he was released from hospital in 1970, he moved into Alicia's home, but as a lodger. After that, he was never admitted to psychiatric hospital again. Nash gradually got better over time with support from his ex-wife; without the use of psychotropics. They eventually remarried in 2001. He lived a stable life and was allowed to work on mathematics at Princeton, and doing some auditing of classes there. Eventually, he started doing some teaching.

Nash gradually found other methods for managing his illness. He stated that he did not experience any auditory hallucinations until around 1964. Later, he began a process of consciously rejecting them. He developed an 'insight' into his delusions and began to intellectually interrogate and demanded that they justify themselves. In this way, he was able to recognize over time that the delusions did not represent reality and could be allocated to a part of his mind that did not require urgent attention. In the end, he concluded that his delusional thinking was 'essentially a hopeless waste of intellectual effort'.

Nash further stated he was always taken to hospitals against his will. He felt psychotropic drugs were overrated and that the adverse effects were not given enough consideration once someone was deemed mentally ill. He also suggested hypotheses on mental illness. He has compared not thinking in an acceptable manner, or being 'insane' and not fitting into a usual social function, to being 'on strike' from an economic point of view. He advanced views in evolutionary psychology about the value of human diversity and the potential benefits of apparently nonstandard behaviors or roles.

'A Beautiful Mind' his biography by Sylvia Nasar's was published in 1998. A movie by the same name was released in 2001 with Russell Crowe playing Nash. It won four Academy Awards, including Best Picture. In 2015, Nash and his wife died in a car crash while returning home from the airport after a trip to Norway where he had received the Abel Prize from the Norwegian Academy of Science and Letters.

CHAPTER 29

Bloodstain Analysis

LEARNING OBJECTIVES

Must know
1. Chemical examination of blood
2. Microscopic examination of blood
3. ABO system
4. Secretors
5. Precipitin test
6. Medico-legal aspects and application of blood groups

Desirable to know
1. Source and origin of bleeding
2. Antemortem or postmortem bleeding
3. Sex determination from blood
4. Blood pattern analysis

Forensic serology involves the examination and analysis of a variety of body fluids which includes blood, saliva, semen and urine.

Analysis of Blood

Blood is a complex fluid with pH-7.4, cells about 45% and plasma about 55%. Legal requirements state that identification of the stain should be established to a scientific certainty, before it can be presented in the court.

The protocol applied to blood as regards forensic serology is given in **Flowchart 29.1**.

A visual observation of an untested stain, coupled with positive chemical presumptive and confirmatory tests will provide sound data to support the identification.

BLOODSTAIN PATTERN ANALYSIS

Interpreting bloodstain patterns can yield information on the manner in which a bloodstain was deposited and helps in the reconstruction of crime scenes.
- The distance from the impact origin, the object that may have been responsible for the impact, the direction of the impact, the number of impacts (e.g., shots, blows) or the movement of an individual after injury may be determined by studying blood deposition.
- Bloodstain shapes are determined by the angle of impact. When a drop of blood strikes a horizontal surface at an angle of 90°, the resulting bloodstain will be round with spiked edges giving a '*crown*' appearance.

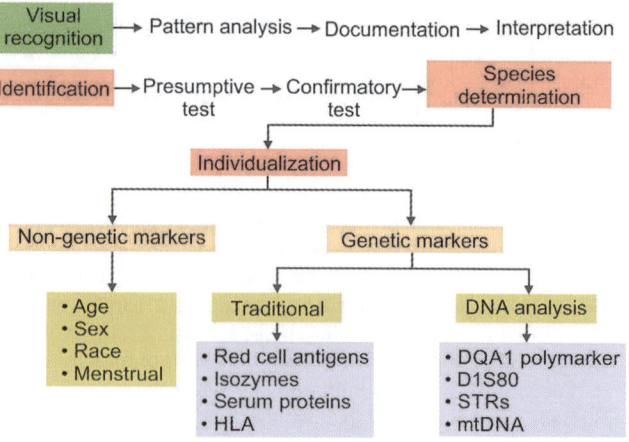

Flowchart 29.1: Approaches to bloodstain analysis

The bloodstain becomes longer and narrower as the angle decreases and a tapering or '*tear-drop*' stain is formed, the sharp end points to the direction the droplet was travelling in when it impacted on the surface **(Fig. 29.1)**. Sometimes, a small separate spot may be present in front of the sharp end of the stain resembling 'exclamation mark' (*lance-shaped*).
- Smearing indicates movement of the bloodstained object across the surface. Sometimes, a pattern may be left which may help to indicate the shape of a weapon, or fingerprints in blood may help in identification.

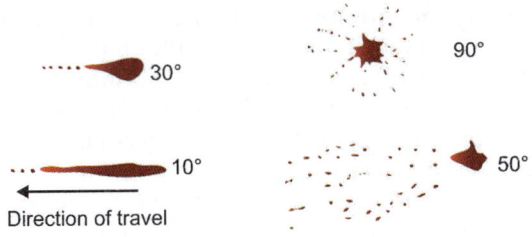

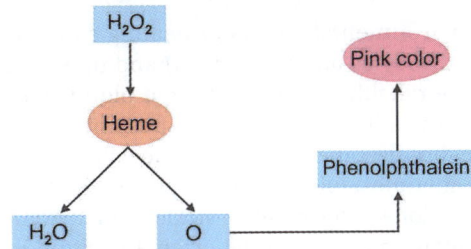

Flowchart 29.2: Kastle-Meyer test

Fig. 29.1: The angles of impact of bloodstains against a target surface

FM 14.7
Demonstrate and identify that a particular stain is blood and identify the species of its origin.

■ PRESUMPTIVE TESTS FOR BLOOD

Presumptive or screening test, when positive, leads to the conclusion that blood is present, and further tests are usually undertaken to confirm the presence of blood, since no single test is absolutely specific. When negative, stains need not receive further consideration. The screening tests are exceedingly sensitive (1:100,000), specificity is not very satisfactory.

Presumptive tests may be recognized as those that produce a *visible color reaction or result in release of light*. Both types rely on the catalytic properties of blood to drive the reaction.

Catalytic Color Tests

- Catalytic tests employ chemical oxidation of a chromogenic substance by an oxidizing agent (H_2O_2).
- The heme group of hemoglobin exhibit *peroxidase* activity which catalyzes the breakdown of hydrogen peroxide.
  H_2O_2 + reduced reagent (color 1) ↔ H_2O + oxidized reagent (color 2)
- Misleading results (false positive) may be given by other materials that can catalyze the peroxidase reaction, including pus, saliva, mucus, milk, infected CSF, formalin, plant juices (vegetable peroxidases are thermolabile and can be destroyed with heating), metallic salts (copper and nickel) and oxidizing agents.

Method: A questioned stain is sampled with a clean, moistened cotton swab. To it, one drop of the color reagent solution is added, followed by a like amount of hydrogen peroxide. Nascent oxygen is liberated by the action of peroxidase on hydrogen peroxide. The immediate development of the color, typical of particular reagent used, indicates the presence of blood in the sample.
  i. **Benzidine (Adler) test:** The reaction is carried out in ethanol/acetic acid solution and results in a characteristic *blue color*. The test is given by blood of almost any age, or even by blood that has been subjected to heat or cold. Benzidine is seldom used nowadays because of its *carcinogenic effect*.
  ii. **Phenolphthalein (Kastle-Meyer) test:** This test is commonly used. The reagent consists of reduced phenolphthalein in an alkaline solution that is oxidized by peroxide in the presence of hemoglobin in blood. The reaction shows phenolphthalein (colorless in alkaline solution) being oxidized to phenolphthalein (*bright pink* in an alkaline environment) (**Flowchart 29.2**). It is more specific than benzidine, but less sensitive.
  iii. **o-Tolidine (Kohn or O'kelly) test:** The reaction, similar to that of benzidine, is conducted under acidic conditions and produces a *green-blue color* reaction.
  iv. **Tetramethylbenzidine (TMB):** Color change is from *green to blue-green*.
  v. **Leucomalachite green (LMG)** produces a *green color*.

Tests using chemiluminescence and fluorescence: A washed drag/spatter pattern in large areas is tested with luminol and fluorescein tests. This involves spraying a chemical mixture on a suspected bloodstained area and observing the result, either in darkness or in reduced light. Luminol (3-aminophthal-hydrazide) gives *blue-white to yellowish-green glow* which indicates presence of blood (again a catalytic test).

Other Tests

Spectroscopic examination: It is a *delicate and reliable test* for detecting presence of blood in both recent and old stains, but seldom used. The blood is dissolved in water or normal saline and is placed in a small test tube which is then kept between the spectroscope and the source of the light. The solution has the property of absorbing some of the rays from the spectrum, producing characteristic dark absorption bands between Fraunhofer's lines C, D, E and F, which vary with the type of blood pigment present.

Thin layer chromatography (TLC): A thin layer of silica gel is prepared on a suitable glass plate. An appropriate quantity of sample extract, standard hematin chloride solution and control sample of blood are placed on the prepared gel. The plate is then placed in a chamber having a convenient solvent system. After the desired run of the solvent to a certain height (front), it is removed from the chamber. When the plate is dry, benzidine and hydrogen peroxide are sprayed on it. If the stain contains blood, the sample extract gives a blue spot at the same height.

Microscopic Examination

Aging, environmental factors or heating can alter blood cells (erythrocytes and leukocytes) and make it difficult to produce reliable results. Intact red blood cells (RBCs) are observed only when the stain is fresh or when a clot is available, but become unrecognizable when the stain has dried. Sometimes, microscopic appearance of RBCs may reveal additional information—sickle shaped erythrocytes may indicate that the sample originated from a person having sickle cell disease.

Procedure: The stained piece is cut and dipped and teased in a watch glass with 2–3 drops of Vibert's fluid (sodium chloride, mercuric chloride and distilled water or normal saline) for half an hour and then examined under a microscope.

- *Non-mammalian RBCs,* e.g., bird, fish, reptile and amphibian are oval, biconvex and nucleated **(Fig. 29.2A)**.
- *RBCs of humans and mammals* are circular, biconcave and non-nucleated with the *exception of camel and llama* which are oval and biconvex, but non-nucleated **(Fig. 29.2B)**. In primates, nucleated RBCs may be found.

CONFIRMATORY TESTS FOR BLOOD

Crystal Tests

Crystal tests are regarded as confirmatory tests. These tests involve the non-protein heme group of hemoglobin, called porphyrins.

i. **Teichmann or Hemin crystal test:** Place a sample of suspected blood on a glass slide, add few crystals of sodium chloride and a few drops of glacial acetic acid from the side of the cover slip and heat it to form a hematin derivative.
   - These hemin or hematin chloride crystals are *brownish rhombic shaped,* arranged singly or in clusters **(Fig. 29.3A)**.
   - The reaction is negative, if the stain is old, is washed or treated with chemicals, too much salt is added, if there is moisture in the acid or by overheating.

ii. **Takayama or hemochromogen crystal test:** Place a small stain sample under a coverslip and allow the Takayama reagent (sodium hydroxide, pyridine and glucose) to flow under and saturate the sample. After a brief heating, the crystals are viewed microscopically.
   - *Pink feathery crystals* of reduced alkaline hematin (hemochromogen—pyridine ferriprotoporphyrin) arranged in clusters are seen **(Fig. 29.3B)**.
   - It can be carried out on a small stain quantity, is effective on aged stains and is more dependable.

> **NOTA BENE**
>
> **Wagenaar test (acetone-chlor-hemin crystal test)**
> A few drops of acetone are added to the suspected bloodstain, followed by a drop of dilute mineral acid (HCl). Characteristic crystals are formed which can be observed under microscope. Crystals are formed even when the stains are old or the blood partially putrefied.

SPECIES IDENTIFICATION

A wide variety of tests is available for the determination of species origin of an identified bloodstain, and most use immunoprecipitation to effect a result.

Electrophoretic Methods

Two methods are usually used for identifying bloodstains:
i. Separation and identification of hemoglobin by electrophoresis.
ii. Separation and identification of serum proteins by immunoelectrophoresis.

Precipitin Methods

If host animal (e.g., a rabbit) is inoculated with a human serum protein, the immune system of the rabbit will normally recognize the protein as foreign and produce antibodies (γ globulins) against it. Harvesting the antibodies

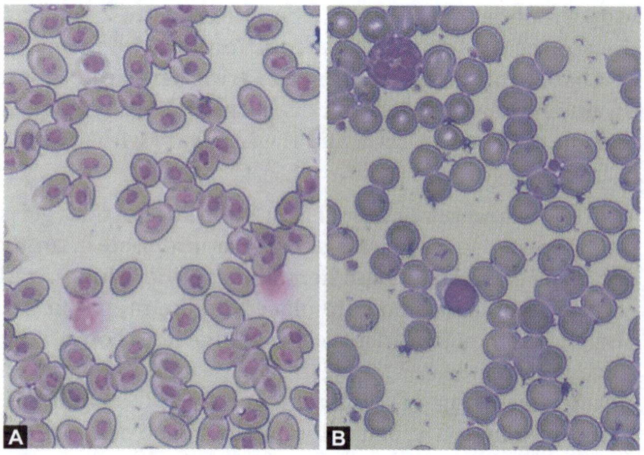

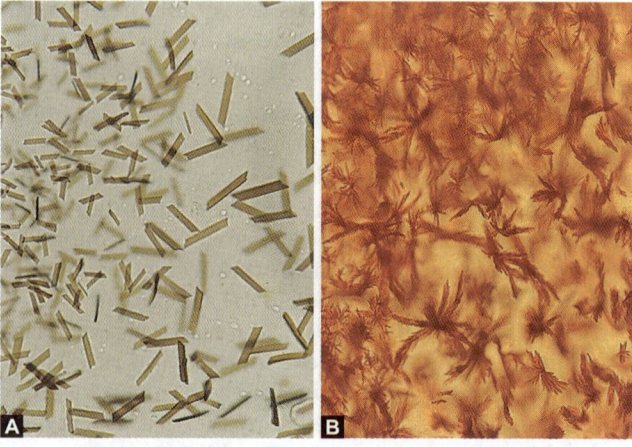

Figs. 29.2A and B: (A) Animal RBCs; (B) Human RBCs

Figs. 29.3A and B: (A) Teichmann test (hemin crystals); (B) Takayama test (hemochromogen crystals)

provides an antiserum to the protein (antigen), and when a sample of the antiserum and the antigen are brought in contact, a precipitin reaction normally occurs.

The various precipitation tests are:

- Ring precipitin test
- Antiglobulin consumption test
- Ouchterlony method
- Crossed-over electrophoresis
- Latex test
- Diffusion precipitation test
- Passive hemagglutination test

Some of the tests are described below:

i. **Ring precipitin test:** The ring precipitin test employs simple diffusion between two liquids in contact inside a test tube. The two liquids are the antiserum and an extract of the bloodstain in question. If the antiserum (anti-human) is placed in a small tube and a portion of the (human) bloodstain extract is carefully layered over the denser antiserum, dissolved antigens and antibodies from the respective layers will begin to diffuse into the other layer. The result will be a fine line of precipitate at the interface of the two solutions. In cases where the bloodstain extract is not human, no reaction will occur **(Figs. 29.4A and B)**.

ii. **Antiglobulin consumption test** (*Hemagglutination inhibition test*): When human globulin is mixed with antihuman globulin serum, the latter is absorbed and is no longer capable of agglutinating Rh positive red cells sensitized with incomplete anti-D. This detects globulins.

iii. **Ouchterlony method** (double diffusion in two directions): It involves the use of agar gel plates with wells for both antibodies and antigens. The two reactants diffuse into the gel, where the soluble antigens and antibodies form an insoluble complex—a precipitate.

iv. **Crossed-over electrophoresis:** It involves both quantitative and qualitative determination of blood sample—a variant of the Ouchterlony test. Under the influence of an electric field, the antigen and the antibody migrate toward each other and a precipitate is formed at the point of their interaction.

v. **Latex test:** A saline extract of bloodstain is mixed with dilute suspension of latex particles sensitized with antiserum. A positive reaction is shown by agglutination of the particles into clumps.

Other Methods

- **Nonserum protein analysis:** *Anti-human hemoglobin serum:* Highly specific anti-hemoglobin precipitin sera have been used for the identification of human bloodstains in a single procedure, i.e., it confirms the sample as blood of human origin.
- **Isoenzyme methods:** These are based on the electrophoretic demonstration of the existence of enzymes in blood of the same species in multiple molecular forms known as *isoenzymes*. These methods (commonly used methods are LDH and Px) are relatively less sensitive than immunological methods.
- **Rapid stain identification of human blood (RSID-Blood)** is a commercially available confirmatory test for human blood as it is highly sensitive and specific. No other human body fluids or animal blood samples cross-react. The RSID-blood immunochromatographic strip uses dual monoclonal antibodies specific for human glycophorin A found in RBCs membranes, not hemoglobin. Visible red lines at both control (C) and test (T) position indicate positive result. The test can detect 1 µL of human blood and the strip results are complete in 10 mins.
- **ABAcard HemaTrace test strips:** HemaTrace test strips are used to detect blood by identifying the presence of human hemoglobin. The test strip contains antihuman hemoglobin antibody which reacts with the antigens in the extract resulting in antigen-antibody complex where it reacts with dye particles to create visible reactions.
    - The presence of two pink lines, one in the 'T' area (test sample) and one in the 'C' area (control) indicate a positive result.
    - The presence of only one pink line in the 'C' area indicates a negative result. A negative result indicates there is no hemoglobin antigen present or is below the limit of detection of the test.
    - If there is no pink line in the 'C' area, the test is invalid **(Fig. 29.5)**.

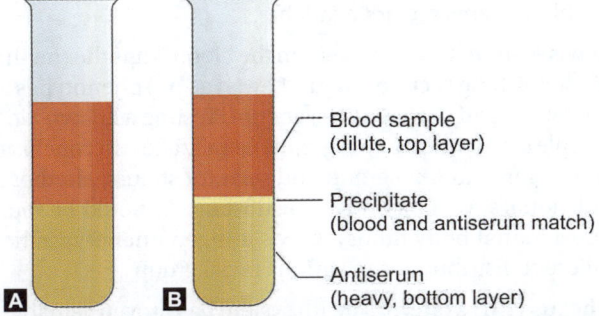

Figs. 29.4A and B: Ring precipitin test: (A) Non-human blood; (B) Human blood

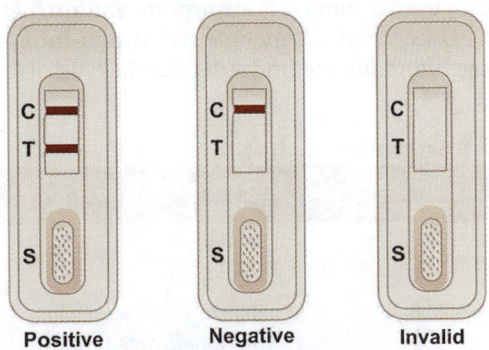

Fig. 29.5: ABAcard test

Once human origin of bloodstain is confirmed, its individualization is attempted (whose blood is it?).

> **FM 14.8**
> Demonstrate the correct technique to perform and identify ABO and Rh blood group of a person.

GENETIC MARKERS IN BLOOD

Antigen-based Markers: Blood Groups

ABO system: The first and best known blood grouping is the ABO system discovered by *Karl Landsteiner* in 1900. The types A, B, O and AB refer to the antigens on the surface of the red blood cells. The corresponding antibodies (agglutinins)—anti-A (α-A) and anti-B (α-B) are present in plasma.

A person of blood group A will have α-B in his plasma and if that plasma is mixed with group B cells, the two are said to be homologous, and agglutination is the result. The characteristics of the person with group O blood present a different picture. There are no antibodies in humans for red cell H antigens **(Table 29.1)**.

> **NOTA BENE**
>
> The tests are based on antigen-antibody agglutination test. Commonly used method is the *'slide method'*: In this method, a glass slide support is labeled into three parts. Then:
> - Place one drop of anti-A (blue), anti-B (yellow) and anti-D (colorless) reagent separately on the labeled slide.
> - Add 1 drop of blood to each drop of antiserum.
> - The cells and reagent are mixed using a clean stick.
> - The subject is blood group A if agglutination occurred with the Anti-A test serum; group B if agglutination occurred with the Anti-B test serum; group AB if agglutination occurred with both test serums, and O if there was no agglutination in either case.
> - If agglutination was present in 3rd column, then Rh positive; if no agglutination, Rh negative.
>
> **Other methods** are tube test, microplate technology and column/gel centrifugation.

Forensic testing for the ABO system in dried bloodstains centers on identifying the antigens and antibodies present. Different methods have been devised, but the most commonly used technique is **absorption elution** (described in 1930). Other methods include absorption-inhibition or mixed agglutination methods (detects the type of antigens on the RBC surface), or for antibodies by the *Lattes crust method*.

- Absorption elution technique involves the exposure of a portion of the stain bearing the blood (and antigen) to absorb the homologous antibody.
- Unreacted antibody is then washed away and the absorbed antibody is eluted and mixed with a known cell suspension to be identified.
- For example, a group A stain exposed to α-A, α-B, and α-H lectin in separate containers, will absorb the α-A and not the α-B or α-H. After allowing sufficient time for absorption, the unreacted antibodies (and lectin) are washed away and gentle heating is applied to release (elute) the absorbed α-A. This α-A is detected by addition of group A cells which agglutinates, and can be viewed microscopically. The other two containers exhibit no reaction, as no antibody or lectin was absorbed and eluted to react with the B and O cells added.

> **NOTA BENE**
>
> **Lattes crust test:** This method was developed in 1915 wherein red blood cells were added to dried bloodstains to determine the ABO blood type. Separate portions of a bloodstained crust are allowed to react with A, B and O red blood cell suspensions. Microscopical observation of agglutination indicates the presence of the similar antibody. This method is not useful for old stains and interpretation of results is difficult.

Secretors

- Some individuals secrete their ABO antigenic characteristics (A, B and H blood group substances) into body fluids, such as saliva, semen, gastric juice and vaginal fluid in a high concentration, and in a low concentration in sweat, tears and urine.
- This ability to secrete is under the control of a pair of genes, Se and se. With Se being dominant, homozygous (Se Se) and heterozygous (Se se) individuals are 'secretors' (80% of the general population) and homozygous (se se) are 'nonsecretors' (20% of the population).
- The secretor phenomenon is intimately related to the Lewis blood group antigens.
- It is of great value in medico-legal studies when bloodstains are not available.

Lewis system: Lewis antigens in the blood is another method of establishing secretor status. Lewis (a– b+) phenotypes are 'secretors' and Lewis (a+ b–) are not. Testing a known blood sample for ABO and Lewis groups usually allows a conclusion with regards to ABO group and secretor status (whether an individual's ABH blood group substances should be found in evidential body fluids). Lewis antigen phenotypes have different distributions in various racial groups.

Rhesus (Rh) system: The Rh system has proven valuable in forensic work in spite of the larger quantity of sample required

TABLE 29.1: ABO system

Blood group	Antigen present	Antibody present	Population (%)
A	A	Anti-B	23
B	B	Anti-A	32
AB	A, B	None	6.5
O	H	Anti-A and Anti-B	38.5

for dried stain analysis and the degree of sophistication of available techniques. The method used in grouping dried stains is an absorption elution technique. In cases of disputed paternity, five anti-Rh reagents are used, each defining different Rh specificity: anti-D, anti-C, anti-E, anti-c and anti-e.

Gm and Km systems: The Gm and Km systems present distinct advantages to the forensic serologist because of stability of the antigens and the variety of types possible (especially with Gm). The antigens are stable at moderate heat, may be stored at room temperature for extended periods, and can be frozen for years.

Medico-legal Aspects of Blood Groups

The application of blood groupings to medico-legal problems is based on the following principles:
  i. A blood group antigen cannot appear in a child, unless present in one or the other parent.
  ii. If an individual is homozygous for a blood group factor, it must appear in the blood of all his children.
  iii. If a child is homozygous for a blood group factor, the gene for the same must have been inherited by him/her from each of his/her parents.
  iv. The blood group characters are characteristic to the individual and are unchanged throughout life.

Many cases can be solved by means of the blood groups of the parent and the child. However, the tests have their limitations. They may exclude a certain person as the possible father of the child, but they cannot definitely establish paternity. They can only indicate its possibility. For example, a child with the blood type AB whose mother is type A could not have a father whose blood type is A or O. The father must have blood type B.

Exclusion of Paternity

> ♦ *First-order exclusion:* Where the child has a blood group gene that is absent in both the mother and the alleged father.
> ♦ *Second order exclusion:* Where the alleged father is homozygous for a blood group gene, but the gene is not present in the child.

- The ABO system can exclude paternity in 1/6th of all cases (17.6%). Addition of the MNS system can exclude paternity in about 44% of all cases. Addition of Rh subgroups can clear about 60% of wrongly accused men.
- The addition of blood protein and red cell enzyme variants, such as phosphoglucomutase can raise 'non-father' exclusion to about 90%.
- The HLA system alone can exclude non-paternity in 90% of cases, but in combination with other grouping systems, it can achieve exclusion rate up to 98%.
- DNA fingerprinting provides absolute certainty, rather than a probable exclusion as in other systems.

> **FM 14.6**
> Demonstrate and interpret medico-legal aspects from examination of blood.

MEDICO-LEGAL APPLICATION OF BLOOD (GROUPS)

Identification of blood and bloodstains has importance both in civil and criminal fields of investigation:

Civil Cases

1. **Disputed paternity:** The question of disputed paternity arises in the court in the following conditions:
   a. *Adultery and divorce:* When a child is born in lawful marriage, but the husband denies that he is the father of the child.
   b. *Blackmail:* When a child is born out of lawful marriage, and the mother accuses a certain man of being the father of the child, while the man denies the accusation.
   c. *Maintenance claims:* Under Sec. 125 CrPC, an individual must adopt his illegitimate child or support him up to certain age.
   d. *Share of property:* When a woman pretends pregnancy and delivery, and obtains a child claiming him/her as her own, in order to obtain a share in her husband's property.
2. **Disputed maternity:** The question of disputed maternity arises in the following circumstances:
   a. When the same child is claimed by two women.
   b. When there has been an allegation of interchange of a child with another in the maternity hospital, either purposely or accidentally.
   c. In case of a kidnapped child, when the woman who has kidnapped the child claims to be the mother.
   d. In case of a suppositious child, when a woman pretends pregnancy and delivery, and brings forth a child to pass it off as her own.
3. **Inheritance claims:** The question of legitimacy arises, since a legitimate child only can inherit the parent's property.
4. **Divorce and nullity of marriage cases**, e.g., question of intersex and some forbidden diseases.
5. **Civil negligence** cases arising in hospital or medical practices, e.g.,
   a. Incompatible blood transfusion.
   b. Neglect of expiry dates leading to transfusion reactions.
   c. Presence of pathogenic organisms, such as malaria, syphilis, hepatitis B and HIV in the transfused blood.
6. **Blood doping:** It is a method of increasing athletic performance by artificially increasing an athlete's RBC count. Several practices, such as autologous blood transfusions and microdoses of performance enhancing drugs like erythropoietin (EPO) are used to increase oxygen delivery to muscles. The use of blood doping is forbidden by the World Anti-Doping Agency (WADA).

The methods of total hemoglobin mass measurements and the detection of metabolites of blood bags plasticizers (caused by the leakage of plasticizers from the blood bags) in urine is useful for detecting blood transfusion. A blood screening is performed first, and a urine test is used to confirm possible use of EPO.

Criminal Cases

1. **Identification of victim or offenders** of crime in circumstances, such as murder, wounding, rape and vehicular accidents.
   - Bloodstains may be found on the clothing and person of the suspect. If the character of these stains is similar to that of blood of the victim, it establishes association.
   - Bloodstains may be present under the fingernails of assailant in a case of throttling.
   - If there has been a struggle, bloodstains derived from the accused may be found under the fingernails of the victim due to scratching.
   - Vehicles which have caused injury can be identified when they show bloodstains resembling that of the victim.
2. **Stains due to body fluids:** The blood group antigens can be demonstrated in stains on clothes due to semen, sweat or saliva ('secretors'). This may be a corroborative evidence of the accused.
3. **Crime scene reconstruction:** Blood spatter interpretation can be valuable in determining how blood was deposited on an item or at a scene.
4. **Corroborate or refute an individual's allegation:** It can substantiate a complainant's or suspect's account of alleged events of an assault, and can be critical in establishing guilt or innocence during criminal proceedings.
5. **Cases of malingering:** The specificity of various blood group combinations is like that of the fingerprints. When an individual has some rare blood group, he can be identified with certainty.
6. **Cause of death**, e.g., detection of poison in the blood.
7. **Time since death** can be estimated by use of different chemical or biochemical tests.

> **NOTA BENE**
>
> - **Sample collection for paternity testing:** In the case of the adults, 5 mL of venous blood is taken and placed in plain tube. Neither party should have had a blood transfusion within 3 months, before taking the sample. The infants should preferably be 6 months of age, but not <2 months before testing is performed; one mL of blood is obtained by a heel or ear prick or venepuncture into a plain tube. The same person should do the testing of mother, child and alleged father in the same laboratory, on the same day, and using the same batch of reagents and antisera.
> - The blood groups in current use in the investigation of cases of doubtful paternity are ABO, MNS, Rh, Kell, Lutheran, Duffy, and Kidd.
> - **Grouping based on white cell antigens:** The *human leukocyte Antigen (HLA)* system consists of protein substance on the surface of a wide variety of tissues and organs, tumors, white cells and platelets. They are reported to be present on spermatozoa, but not on ovum or trophoblast. They are found both on lymphocytes and granulocytes. The major human leukocyte antigens HLA-A, B, C, D, and DR are determined by a single chromosomal segment, the major histocompatibility complex (MHC), which is situated on the short arm of chromosome 6.
> - **Protein markers:** *Hemoglobin* exhibits 180 or more variants, but only four (Hb A, Hb F, Hb S and Hb C) are readily distinguished forensically with electrophoresis or IEF based on the positioning of bands.
> - **Enzyme markers:** *Phosphoglucomutase (PGM)* is found in many tissues of plants, animals, and microorganisms. In humans, the enzyme exists in significant concentrations in blood and semen, and in small amounts in vaginal secretion and cervical mucus. Electrophoresis of samples for PGM analysis using IEF methods can detect 10 phenotypes. With this, it is possible to place the subtypes of PGM in 10 different population groups, and thus presents the highest discrimination probability of any enzyme system used in forensic serology.
> - **Human DNA quantitation:** A sample can be determined to be blood of human origin with a probe specific for human DNA. Probes complementary to primate specific DNA sequences, such as those found at the locus D17Z1 are used primarily to determine the amount of human DNA extracted from the sample prior to DNA typing.

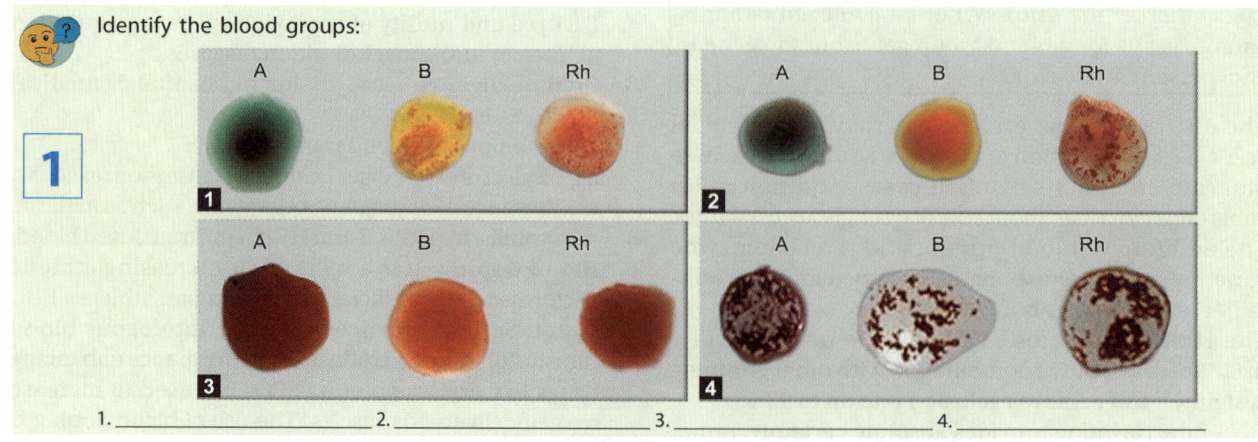

Identify the blood groups:

1. _____ 2. _____ 3. _____ 4. _____

MEDICO-LEGAL QUESTIONS

Q. Whether the stain is due to blood or some other material?

It is essential to establish positively that stain is in fact blood before conducting further analyses. Presumptive tests (color tests) and confirmatory tests, such as, chemical methods, spectrophotometric analysis are done for this purpose. Some substances that may resemble bloodstains are:
  i. *Rust stains*, tests are positive for iron.
  ii. *Synthetic dyes* stain changes to yellow with nitric acid, blood remains unchanged.
  iii. *Mineral stains* contain oxides of iron or red lead.
  iv. *Vegetable stains:* Fruits, such as mulberry, gooseberry and currant produce stains resembling bloodstains. Tests are negative for blood, and ammonia turns the vegetable stain green.
  v. *Other stains,* such as grease or tar on dark fabrics may resemble bloodstains.

Q. If it is blood, is it human?

In some cases, it may be necessary to confirm the presence of human blood in questioned stain before obtaining a known sample from a suspect or a victim. Confirmation is done by immunological methods.

Q. If it is human, what information towards individualization (victim or assailant) is possible?

- Blood groups (ABO) may be different. Stains on the inner side of the clothes usually belong to the victim, while those on the outer side may be of the victim or assailant. Bloodstains may bear marks of fingerprints or footprints of the assailant.
- Sometimes, there may be some disease, such as leukemia, filariasis or sickle cell anemia either in the victim or the assailant which may provide valuable information.
- Traces of blood may be found underneath the fingernails of the victim as a result of struggle or of the assailant in case of throttling; these can be typed and grouped.
- An individual bloodstain can also be identified by using DNA typing.

Q. Whether the sex of the person (male or female) can be determined from the bloodstain?

Sex can be determined from presence of sex chromatin in leukocytes.
- *Barr body* count in WBC can be done using orcein and acriflavine reagent.
- *Y chromosome* is fluorescent to quinacrine when examined under fluorescent microscope.
- *Fluorescent in situ hybridization (FISH)* technique can also be used for sex determination. Probes specific for X and Y chromosomes are applied.

Q. Whether the age of the person can be determined?

- *In infants,* the red blood cells exhibit more fragility, the hemoglobin is of the fetal type (fetus specific hemoglobin $\alpha_2\gamma_2$ detectable up to about 6 months), and the blood when shed forms a thin and soft coagulum.
- *In adults,* the red blood cells are non-nucleated, their fragility is within certain limits, hemoglobin is of the adult type, and the blood when shed forms a thick and firm coagulum.

Q. How long (recent or old) the stain has been on the object/surface?

- *Recent stains* on white cloth are at first red due to conversion of hemoglobin to methemoglobin and hematin.
- The color changes to dull red within hours, reddish brown within 24 h, dark brown or even blackish within *few days* and remains so for several years.

So, it is only possible to state that the stain is recent or not very recent.

Q. What could be the source of the blood?

Bleeding due to disease, accident, menstruation, parturition, abortion, hematemesis or hemoptysis may cause stains.
- Most common defense in cases of assault on females is that the stain is from *menstruation*. It has a disagreeable smell, being mixed with urine and vaginal mucus, it is more fluid and dark in color. Menstrual blood does not clot, due to extensive degradation of the clotting factor fibrinogen. Fibrinogen degradation products are present in high concentration that can be detected immunologically.
- *Hemoptysis* blood is bright red, frothy and alkaline in reaction.
- *Hematemesis* blood is dark in color, not frothy and is acidic in reaction.
- *Parturition and abortion* blood may have some clot or products of conception, like decidual tissue, fetal parts, chorionic villi, vernix caseosa or lanugo hair. Color may be yellowish or greenish from admixture with meconium.

Q. What could be the site of bleeding (arterial or venous)?

Damage to different types and sizes of blood vessels will result in different degrees of bleeding, but it is difficult to predict the exact type of flow of blood from an injury.

- *Arterial bleeding* has a spurting effect (jet-like ejection) from the wound. It is bright red in color when fresh **(Fig. 29.6A)**.
- *Venous bleeding* occurs passively in drops without any projectile force, has stellate appearance and dark in color **(Fig. 29.6B)**. It may ooze and produce a pool, if the victim falls down.

Q. Whether the bleeding was antemortem or postmortem?

- Blood which has effused during life can be peeled off in scales on drying due to presence of fibrin, and the clot can be taken *en masse*.
- Blood which has flowed after death tends to break up into powder on drying, and the clot cannot be taken *en masse*.

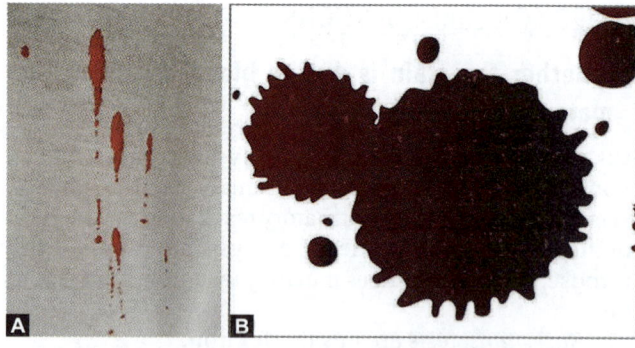

Figs. 29.6A and B: (A) Arterial bleeding; (B) Venous bleeding

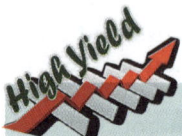

- Positive presumptive (screening) test → blood is present.
- Phenolphthalein (Kastle-Meyer) is a presumptive test for blood.
- Benzidine test for blood is not done because of its carcinogenic effect.
- Non-mammalian RBCs, e.g., bird, fish, reptile and amphibian are oval, biconvex and nucleated.
- RBCs of humans and mammals are circular, biconcave and non-nucleated, except camel and llama (oval and biconvex, non-nucleated).
- Crystal tests (Teichmann and Takayama) are confirmatory tests for blood.
- Crystal tests involve the non-protein heme group of hemoglobin (porphyrins).
- Teichmann test gives brownish rhombic–shaped (hemin/hematin chloride) crystals.
- Takayama test gives pink feathery crystals (hemochromogen).
- Confirmation of *human blood* is done by immunological methods.
- Immunoprecipitation is commonly used for species identification.
- **Confirmatory test for human blood:** RSID-blood with immunochromatographic test strip.
- First known blood grouping is the ABO system discovered by Karl Landsteiner.
- Commonly used technique for forensic testing for the ABO system in dried bloodstains is *absorption elution*.
- **Lattes crust method:** Used to detect ABO blood type.
- **Secretors:** Some individuals secrete their ABO antigens into body fluids, such as saliva, semen, gastric juice and vaginal fluid.
- ABO antigens are not found in CSF.
- Blood grouping may exclude a certain person as the possible father of the child, but they *cannot* definitely establish paternity.
- **Technique for absolute determination of paternity:** DNA fingerprinting.
- Under Sec. 125 CrPC, an individual must adopt his illegitimate child or support him.
- Sex can be determined from bloodstain by identifying Y chromosome, Barr body and using FISH technique.

Interesting case

Bloodstain Pattern Analysis (Case of Ronald Rudin, 1994)

Ronald Rudin was a prominent Las Vegas real estate developer and had been married to Margaret for 7 years (they got married in 1987)—fifth marriage for each **(Figs. A and B)**. He financed her dream of opening an antique store in Las Vegas. In 1994, the 64-year-old Ron mysteriously disappeared. Fishermen stumbled across a skull, charred dismembered bones and some metal strips a month later near Lake Mojave, Nevada. A distinctive bracelet with the name 'RON' was found at the scene. An autopsy determined the person was shot in the head at least four times with a .22 caliber gun.

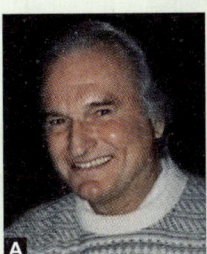 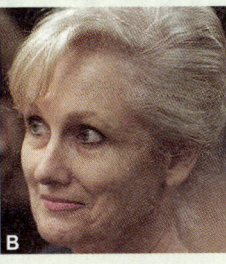

Investigation turned up a significant amount of circumstantial evidence pointing to Margaret. The police became suspicious of Margaret learning that she had accused him of affairs and had his phones tapped. He disappeared shortly after the couple argued over money, with Ron telling Margaret he planned to divorce her. She had not reported him missing until his co-workers insisted. The crime scene analysts also determined the metal strips found along with charred remains were the remnants of an antique trunk which they were able to trace back to Margaret.

Police later searched their residence and found blood spatter in the bedroom, as well as a blood-soaked mattress that had been removed from the home. The crime scene analysts found reddish-brown spots on the ceiling and wall of the couple's bedroom. Testing the spots with Hemastix proved that the substance is blood, which was followed up by spraying the room with Luminol. After applying it, patterns on the wall glowed florescent showing where the blood spatter had occurred.

One of the investigators reported that he has investigated a death in that very bedroom before. Ten years earlier, Ron Rudin's former wife, Peggy Rudin, committed suicide by shooting herself in the head in the same room. Now the challenge was to determine which blood spatter patterns belonged to which death. There were circular stains and stain with a tail. Analysts used trigonometry to calculate the angle of impact and lasers to show the path of each blood splatter (convergence of lasers showed the point of death). The analysis proved two separate deaths had occurred in the bedroom—Ron Rudin's in 1994 and Peggy Rudin's in 1984. It also mapped the two separate sets of blood splatter.

The subsequent discovery of a .22-caliber handgun with a silencer wrapped in plastic (murder weapon) in 1996 by divers in Lake Mead provided the last piece of evidence police needed to arrest Margaret. A ballistic expert determined it was Ron Rudin's gun and was used to kill him. It was reported missing in 1988, shortly after he got married.

Prosecutors proved he had been shot in the head in the couple's Las Vegas home as he slept and that his body was hauled in a trunk to the desert and burnt. Margaret was indicted on a murder charge in April 1997, but she vanished and spent two years as a fugitive ahead of her 2001 trial. During this time, the television show 'America's Most Wanted' featured her case relentlessly, describing her as the '*Black Widow of Las Vegas*'.

In 2001, she was convicted of first-degree murder and sentenced to life imprisonment with eligibility for parole. She has challenged her conviction several times over the year without success. In 2019, she was granted parole.

30 CHAPTER

Seminal Stains and Other Biological Samples

LEARNING OBJECTIVES

Must know
1. Chemical tests of seminal stain
2. Microscopic examination of seminal stain
3. Proof of semen
4. Medico-legal importance of seminal stain

Desirable to know
1. Non-cellular semen markers
2. Tests for salivary stains

Describe anatomy of male genitalia.

Introduction

- The male reproductive system comprises of the testes, sex accessory ducts and sex accessory glands. The testes reside within the scrotum. Spermatozoa are produced in the seminiferous tubules within the testes.
- The epididymis is the first section of the sex accessory ducts through which spermatozoa will travel to the outside of the body. The tail of the epididymis merges into the vas deferens, the second sex accessory duct.
- The seminal vesicles, the prostate and the bulbourethral glands are the sex accessory glands.
- Semen is the fluid discharged from the penis during ejaculation, usually at the time of orgasm.
- Like blood, semen consists of two compartments, the cellular compartment (spermatozoa) and noncellular compartment (seminal plasma), which is secreted from the prostate gland, seminal vesicles, Cowper's glands (bulbouretral gland) and the glands of Littre **(Fig. 30.1)**.
- The reference values for 'normal' ejaculate—volume of 1.6–5.5 mL, and contain 17–192 million sperm/mL of which atleast 60% should be motile.

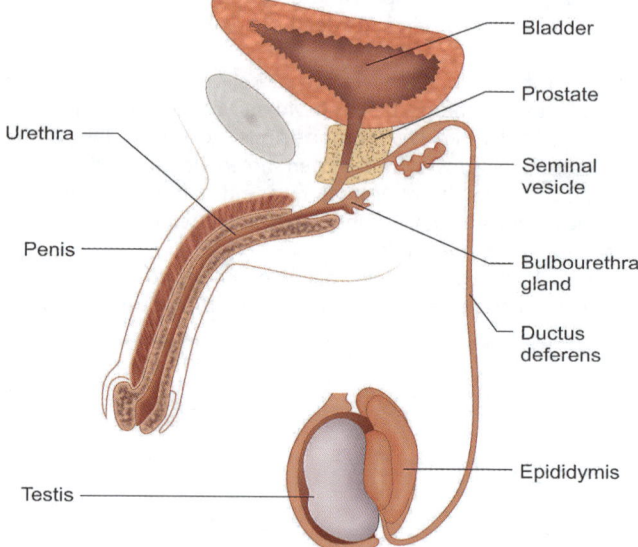

Fig. 30.1: Male reproductive system

- Spermatozoa constitute about 5% of the volume of the semen which contains water and small amounts of salt, protein and fructose.
- Prostatic secretions in humans contain high levels of citric acid, acid phosphatase and zinc. The secretion is alkaline with a pH of 7.4.

> **FM 14.6**
> Demonstrate and interpret medico-legal aspects from examination of semen and other biological fluids.

PURPOSE OF SEMINAL IDENTIFICATION

Seminal stains may have to be detected/examined in criminal and civil cases.

Criminal cases	Civil cases
Rape/attempted rape	Disputed paternity
Sodomy	Legitimacy
Bestiality	Artificial insemination
Sexual homicide of female	Compensation on grounds of acquired sterility/failure of vasectomy cases
	Divorce

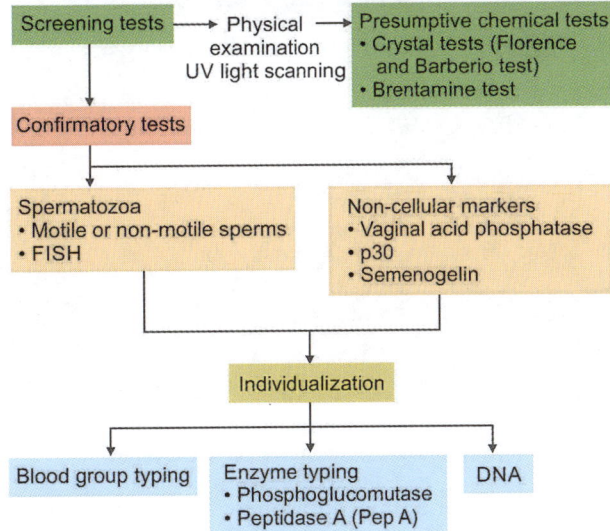

Flowchart 30.1: Evaluation of a suspected seminal stain in sexual assault

Collection of Material

The stains are usually found on the clothing, but may be found on the person of either the victim or the accused. They may also be found on bedclothes, furniture, vehicles, carpet, floor or grass, where the offense was committed or any item the victim may have used to clean up after the assault (tissue or washcloth). Seminal stains have to be differentiated from those due to starch, pus, leukorrheal discharge and egg albumen.

Before proceeding with the examination, stains may have to be collected and preserved from different sources:

i. **Clothing:** Portion of cloth with the stain is cut, dried in shade (not heated) and preserved.
ii. **Vaginal fluid:** Fluid from the vagina is collected with a pipette or vaginal washing is done which is concentrated by centrifugation. Swabs are taken with sterile gauze and smears are prepared on sterile slides.
iii. **Dried stains on other parts of body:** Dried seminal fluid on the perineum or thighs is collected with a wet swab.
iv. **Matted pubic hair:** It is plucked/cut and placed in a small container.
v. **Stains on smooth surface:** These are gently scraped off into a glass container and preserved.

Samples must be packed in paper bags that allow air circulation; never in plastic bags or sealed nonporous tubes, jars or boxes. Chain of custody must be documented and adhered to the prevailing policies.

EXAMINATION OF SEMINAL STAINS

The sequence of analyzing the evidence (as described above) is given in **Flowchart 30.1**.

Screening Tests

Physical Examination

- *When fresh*, semen is a whitish or yellowish-white in color, slightly viscous, jelly-like, sticky and has a characteristic odor. On standing, viscosity is lost due to prostatic fibrolysin, and it becomes thin.
- *Dried seminal stains* on clothes are grayish-white or yellowish-gray in color, show an irregular outline and starchy hard in feeling. When examined under filtered UV light (Wood's lamp), they fluoresce with a bluish-white color (due to flavin and choline-conjugated proteins in semen) which is not specific, as other albuminous materials, such as nasal or leukorrheal discharges and detergents also fluoresce.
- A fresh stain on a non-absorbent material appears translucent. After a month, it becomes yellow to brown.

Presumptive Chemical Examination

Presumptive tests for semen are based on colorimetry, and are qualitative in nature. Positive presumptive tests must be followed by a confirmatory test, such as microscopic examination, quantitative acid phosphatase test or detection of p30.

i. **Florence test:** The stain is extracted, dried on a glass slide and covered with a coverslip and a drop of Florence solution (8% w/v of iodine in water containing 5% w/v of potassium iodide) is allowed to run under the coverslip. If semen is present, *dark brown rhombic crystals* resembling hemin (but larger) arranged in clusters or rosettes of *choline periodide* appear immediately **(Fig. 30.2A)**. Choline originates from the seminal vesicles. A positive test is not proof of seminal fluid, but confirms the presence of some

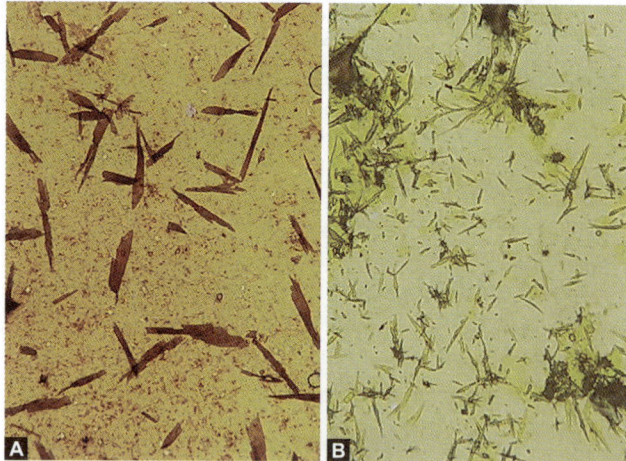

Figs. 30.2A and B: (A) Florence test (choline iodide crystals); (B) Barberio's test (spermine picrate crystals)

vegetable or animal substance. A negative reaction proves that the stain is not semen, but may occur if choline content is low or the stain is decomposed.

ii. **Barberio's test:** A saturated aqueous or alcoholic solution of picric acid when added to dried stain extract on a glass slide covered with a coverslip, produces *yellow needle-shaped crystals of spermine picrate* **(Fig. 30.2B)**. The reaction depends on the presence of spermine from prostatic secretions. This test is positive without the presence of spermatozoa.

iii. **Acid phosphatase test/Brentamine test/Walker test**
   - It is the most common presumptive test for seminal *acid phosphatase* which is secreted by the prostate gland. Acid phosphatase activity is 500–1000 times greater in human semen than in any other bodily fluid. The levels remain high till 40 years of age with gradual decrease thereafter; levels are not related to sperm count.
   - The reaction is based on the hydrolysis of phosphate esters and detection of the liberated organic moiety by production of a color complex. An enzyme substrate, sodium α-naphthyl phosphate is converted to sodium phosphate and naphthol by the acid phosphatase enzyme in the semen and a coupled reaction with brentamine fast blue dye takes place, forming a *purple color* **(Flowchart 30.2)**.
   - Acid phosphatase catalyzes the removal of the phosphate residue on the substrate 4-methylumbelliferone phosphate (MUP), which generates fluorescence under UV light.

Flowchart 30.2: Brentamine fast blue test

α-naphthyl acid phosphate monosodium salt — Acid phosphatase → Sodium phosphate + naphthol

Naphthol + Brentamine — Coupling reaction → Purple azo dye (Dark purple)

- It can produce false positives because similar enzyme activity is found in other body fluids (e.g., vaginal secretions and fecal stains), human red cells, semen of higher apes, as well as in presence of fungi, bacteria and even plants (juice of cauliflower). Moreover, pregnancy, menstruation, bacterial vaginosis may also elevate its level.
- Dried and old seminal stains, which have not undergone putrefaction give positive reaction.

CONFIRMATORY TESTS

- The presence of spermatozoa under light microscopy is considered as the '*gold standard*'.
- Confirmatory testing involves solubilization of sample followed by centrifugation, which yields a supernatant and a cell pellet. The cell pellet is used to detect spermatozoa and for DNA analysis, whereas the supernatant is useful to detect non-cellular markers when sperms are not detected, and for grouping or genetic profiling.
- Sometimes, the sample is contaminated by other bodily fluids (saliva, vaginal secretions), epithelial cells, cellular debris wherein selective degradation may be done by treating the cell extract with a mixture of proteinase K and sodium dodecyl sulfate before staining and microscopic examination.
- Most commonly used confirmatory test for semen is visualization of one or more intact spermatozoa after staining with dyes such as hematoxylin and eosin or '*Christmas tree*' stain.

Microscopic Examination

Procedure: A small piece of the stained fabric is moistened with a few drops of 1% HCl in a watch glass for half to one hour if the stain is fresh, or 2–4 hours (h) if it is old. Slides are prepared by dabbing the fabric gently on them. Films are dried in the air without heat fixed and then stained.
- Slide is stained either with Harris's hematoxylin for 2–5 minutes (min) and eosin for 3 min, or methylene blue for 15–30 min and counterstained with eosin for 2 min.
- Posterior half to one-third of head and the tail takes eosin and is stained deep red or pink, while anterior half to two-thirds takes very light or faint basic or blue stain or may appear unstained **(Fig. 30.3)**.
- Size of human spermatozoa is about 55 µ in length. Head is ovoid and flattened, 5 × 3.5 µ in dimensions. It has a short neck and a long filamentous tail (50 µ) which tapers to a fine point **(Fig. 30.4)**.
- Bacteria, fungi, trichomonas, yeast, monilia and naked nuclei from vaginal epithelial cells give false positive test.
- Older the stain, lesser is the chance of finding intact sperms.
- *Single photon fluorimetry* has been used to differentiate between different semen.

CHAPTER 30 : Seminal Stains and Other Biological Samples

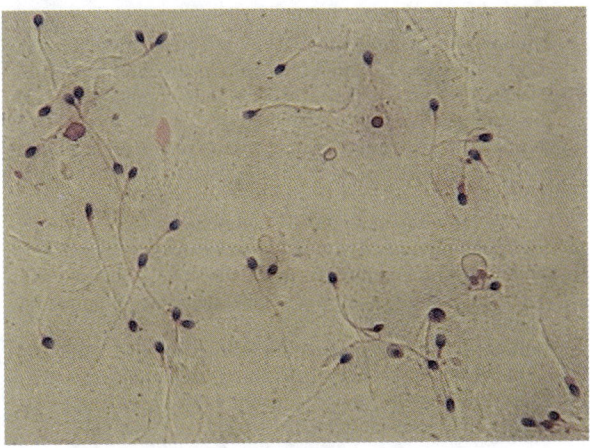

Fig. 30.3: Spermatozoa under light microscope

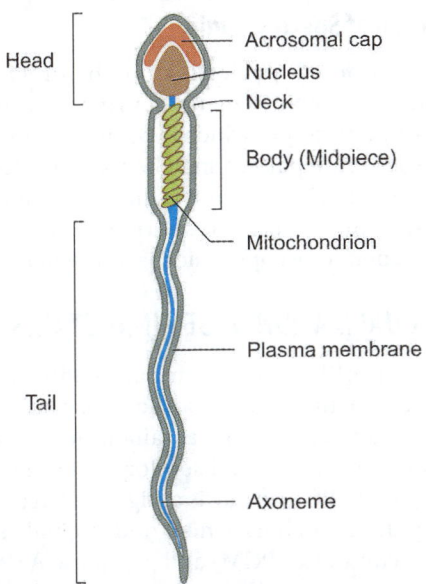

Fig. 30.4: Morphological appearance of spermatozoon

Motility of Sperms

- At room temperature, motility depends on time elapsed since ejaculation.
- At body temperature (in living victims), sperms retains full motility in vagina between 6–12 h. The sperms remain motile in the uterine cavity for 3–7 days. Later, the sperms disintegrate into head and tails which may be recovered from the vagina up to 7–10 days and 12–14 days in the cervix and uterus.
- Complete motile sperms may be seen up to 28 h in vagina after ejaculation (non-motile sperms may be found up to 10 days).
- Non-motile sperms may be seen in oral cavity from 2–31 h, in rectum from 4–113 h, and in anus from 2–44 h.

Fluorescence In Situ Hybridization (FISH)

- In situations where spermatozoa are not likely to be present, alternative staining methods, such as FISH is beneficial so as to consider other male cells within a sample. Epithelial cells can be deposited during penetration and/or ejaculation.
- This cytogenic analysis uses a Y chromosome specific DNA probe to identify Y-bearing (male) cells. This technique identifies cells of male origin and confirms male-female contact.

Non-cellular Semen Markers

Markers are specific and unique to seminal plasma, but independent of spermatozoa. The two most commonly employed constituents are acid phosphatase and the prostate-specific glycoprotein p30 (PSA). These tests are conclusive even in the absence of demonstrable sperms, azoospermia or vasectomized individuals.

i. **Acid phosphatase test (quantitative):** Finding a significantly elevated vaginal acid phosphatase level is consistent with the presence of semen. Undiluted semen has an acid phosphatase level of 340–360 Bodansky units/mL. A value of >100 Bodansky units with/without motile sperms indicate that ejaculation occurred within 12 h of examination. level decreases with time after intercourse, and there is little chance of identifying it after 48 hours.

ii. **Prostate specific antigen or PSA (p30):** The glycoprotein p30 is derived from prostrate and is found in seminal plasma, male urine and blood, and has not been found in any female body tissue or fluid.
    - p30 in sample reliably identifies semen regardless of whether acid phosphatase is elevated or spermatozoa are detected. Some laboratories even use p30 testing in place of microscopical examination for semen identification.
    - It is determined serologically using antiserum that is specific for the p30 antigen.

> **NOTA BENE**
>
> *Others staining methods*
> - **Christmas tree stain:** This staining technique consist of nuclear fast red (red stain for sperm head) and picroindigocarmine (green counter-stain for the tail and other cytoplasmic material) and are sometimes referred to as 'Christmas tree' stain because of the red-green combination.
> - **Papanicolaou staining:** In Pap smear, acrosome is stained pink, postacrosome—dark blue, and tail—pink.
> - **Baecchi stain** uses acid fuchsin and methyl blue. Sperm heads stain red and nuclei blue.
> - **Giemsa stain:** Acrosome stained pink, postacrosome—dark blue.
> - **Ziehl-Neelsen's method:** Smear is stained and examined for the presence of spermatozoa and smegma bacilli (*Mycobacterium smegmatis*). It is an acid fast, rod-shaped bacillus and thicker than the tubercle bacillus.
> - **Other stains:** Bryan-Leishman stain, May-Grunwald Giemsa stains (MGG), supravital stain, Shorr stain and alkaline fuchsin.

- Traditional detection tests utilize electrophoretic methods, such as crossover electrophoresis or diffusion methods, such as Ouchterlony double diffusion wherein a precipitation band is formed due to the formation of antibody-antigen complex.
- It can also be done using immunochromatographic strip test using antibodies raised against the human PSA and enzyme-linked immunoassay (ELISA).
- The currently accepted method of choice for identification of semen is detection of p30 using the *ABAcard test strips*. The strips work in the same way as described earlier for confirmation of blood (Chapter 29), except that they use anti-p30 monoclonal and polyclonal antisera, and a pink dye.
    - Its normal range in semen is 300–4200 µg/mL with mean of 1200 µg/mL, and is detectable in vaginal fluid up to 27 h (range 13–47 h) after intercourse as compared to 12–14 h for acid phosphatase.
    - p30 can be detected in dried and old stains (> 10 years in material stored at room temperature) and in cadavers.
  iii. **RSID test for semen:** *Semenogelin (Sg)*, a protein originating in the seminal vesicles and a substrate for PSA, is also a useful marker for the identification of semen.
    - This antigen is unique to human semen, hence no cross reactivity with other body fluids in males and females or with semen from other mammals.
    - Detection of Sg with immunochromatographic test strip is rapid and simple. It is useful for the identification of seminal plasma, an alternative to the method for PSA detection.
    - The test is useful even if the stain was stored in less favorable conditions.

Using these three tests together (acid phosphatase, PSA and spermatozoa detection) the presence of semen can be conclusively determined in vaginal swabs of the sexual assault victims. DNA laboratories now screen first with PSA and semenogelin (as there are false positive reports of both of these individually), before going further with DNA markers and profiling.

> **NOTA BENE**
>
> **Other tests**
> - **Creatine phosphokinase test:** Spermatozoa contain a high concentration of creatine phosphokinase, which is more than double than that found in any other body fluid. Values >400 units/mL are diagnostic of seminal stains. The enzyme is stable and can be demonstrated even in old stains. The test will be negative in case of azoospermia.
> - **Choline and spermine test:** Fresh and dried seminal stains can be identified by a thin layer chromatographic technique due to the combination of choline and spermine, which is present only in semen.
> - **Ammonium molybdate test:** It gives a yellow color (due to presence of phosphorus) when the reagent is added to the seminal stain extract.
> - **Lactate dehydrogenase (LDH) isoenzyme:** Polyacrylamide gel electrophoresis is used to separate the various isoenzymes. This method gives a specific biochemical detection of spermatozoa in semen in the presence of vaginal fluid, blood, urine and saliva.
> - **Monoclonal antibody mouse antihuman semen-5 (MHS-5)** is produced in the seminal vesicle, and is not found in any other bodily fluid besides semen. It is not widely used in forensic evaluation of seminal stain.

Identification of Species Origin

- Confirmation of species is done by precipitin test. Specific anti-human-semen serum may be used in place of anti-human serum which is commonly used.
- LDH isoenzyme pattern may be used for detection of human origin of semen as it is different in animals.
- Detection of Y bodies in spermatozoa heads using fluorescent microscope which is not seen in animals.

INDIVIDUALIZATION OF SEMINAL STAINS

The genetic profile can be compared with the genetic profiles of the victim and the suspect(s). The subject can thus be included as possible assailant or excluded from consideration. Conventional serology is limited to blood group antigens (ABO and Lewis antigens) that are secreted into bodily fluids such as semen and vaginal secretions; phosphoglucomutase (PGM) and peptidase A (Pep A).

a. **Blood group typing:** If the seminal stain is from secretor, absorption-elution method is used to determine the ABO blood group. In sexual assault cases, it requires the comparison of blood group substances recovered in the evidence material with those of the victim and the suspect **(Table 30.1)**.
   - Traditional grouping is cheap, fast and universally available.
   - ABO blood grouping is superior to DNA analysis for typing semen that contains few or no sperm.

TABLE 30.1: ABO blood types and antigens useful in forensic evaluation

Victim's phenotype	Expected antigens from the victim	Foreign antigens from the assailant
O	H	A and/or B
A	A and H	B
B	B and H	A
AB	A, B and H	None

- Seminal blood groups have been detected in the vagina up to 21 h after deposition.
b. **Enzyme typing:** PGM and Pep A are two enzyme markers commonly used in the genetic profiling of semen. These enzymes are found in semen and vaginal secretions regardless of ABO type or secretor status. Pep A is most commonly used as a discriminator in cases in which the perpetrator is thought to be black. PGM can be detected till 6 h and Pep A till 3 h.
c. **DNA profiling:** The primary advantage of DNA profiling is its ability to accurately individualize semen that contains only minimal numbers of spermatozoa. It has a high degree of sensitivity and discrimination.

Recent Advances
- **Messenger RNA:** Most of the new methods being developed to identify semen involve RNA markers. Core markers that have been used are protamines 1 and 2 for spermatozoa and transglutaminase 4 or semenogelin 1 for seminal fluid.
- **SPERM HY-LYTER™** is especially designed for the detection of human spermatozoa. It uses green fluorescein isothiocyanate tagged monoclonal antibody, which specifically targets an antigen on the nuclear membrane of spermatozoa.
- **Raman spectroscopy** is not a new technique, but currently being used for identification of semen. It is based on the application of a calculated spectroscopic signature. However, the resulting spectrum is complex and advanced statistical analysis is required. This method requires no sample preparation, no reagents, minimal sample requirement, is nondestructible and is portable.
- **DNA methylation profiling:** Recent advances in the field of epigenetics have determined that it is possible to differentiate DNA methylation profiles for different types of cells or tissue. DNA methylation typically involves the addition of a methyl group to the 5′ position of cytosine in CpG nucleotides. This DNA modification has been explored for identification of semen since epigenetic differences are found in various body fluids.

MEDICO-LEGAL QUESTIONS

Q. Did sexual assault occur?
- Positive recovery of any component of semen (especially intact spermatozoa) from the victim is considered conclusive proof of sexual contact.
- Recovery of spermatozoa from anal swabs of a male or a female sodomy victim is consistent with anal intercourse.
- However, many factors will influence the recovery of spermatozoa including but not limited to oligospermia, azoospermia, condom use, coitus interruptus, penetration with no ejaculation and vasectomy.

Q. When did the sexual contact occur?
The interval between semen deposition and sample collection may be estimated by comparing the specific findings in the case with the published normal and maximum recovery intervals.

Q. Can a specific suspect be included or excluded?
Genetic profiles (from the evidence material) of the victim and the suspect can be developed using conventional serology and DNA.

Q. Was the sexual contact consensual or nonconsensual?
If the victim is beyond the age of consent, finding of semen is not helpful, but if the victim is underage, then consent is invalid and the recovery of semen is consistent with the commission of the crime.

IDENTIFICATION OF BIOLOGICAL SAMPLES AND BODY FLUIDS

1. **Saliva:** Identification of saliva on bite marks, cigarette or 'bidi' ends and on clothes, and determination of secretor status is important in criminal offenses.

   The salivary stains are identified from the presence of enzyme α-amylase and buccal epithelial cells. The commonly used methods for α-amylase detection are:
   a. *Radial diffusion* utilizes agar gel containing starch. The α-amylase activity is detected by the classical starch-iodine reaction that gives a characteristic purple reaction.
   b. *Dyed starch substrates*: Starch is covalently linked to a dye, such as cibacron blue or procion red to form insoluble complex. Subsequently to α-amylase activity, the dye is released from the complex and becomes soluble causing change of color which can be measured by spectrophotometry. This forms the basis of the **Phadebas test** which uses starch-cibacron blue tablets as the substrate.
   c. *RSID test for human saliva* detects the α-amylase molecule itself from human saliva (in comparison to the testing for enzymatic activity seen in Phadebas test). Performing both these tests is considered a confirmatory test.
- Precipitin test is used for species identification and absorption-elution technique is preferred for blood grouping.

- As with blood, antibody tests using lateral flow strips have been developed that are specific for saliva. mRNA can also be isolated from saliva.
2. **Fecal matter:** Identification may be necessary in cases of sodomy and bestiality. The stains can be identified from odor, and presence of undigested muscle fibers, plant cells, starch, bacteria, stercobilin and urobilinogen.
   - **Urobilin:** Urobilinogen (a precursor of urobilin) is oxidized to urobilin by alcoholic mercuric chloride. Subsequent addition to alcoholic zinc chloride produces a green fluorescence which is due to the formation of a stable zinc-urobilin complex.
3. **Urine:** The stains may have to be identified in cases of homicide and sexual assault. It is identified from the presence of urea, uric acid and creatinine.
4. **Vaginal secretion:** It consists of white coagulated material consisting of shed vaginal epithelium and Doderlein's bacilli. Glycogen-rich squamous epithelial cells of the vaginal tract may be stained with Lugol's iodine.
5. **Dental tissue:** Absorption-elution technique is preferred for blood grouping of dental tissues including dentin, cementum and dental pulp. Results are most accurate with dental pulp.
6. **Hair:** With absorption-elution technique, a single hair shaft can determine blood group. Blood grouping is practicable with scalp hair from fetuses and newborn infants and also with gray scalp hair. If hair is heated at 250°C, it is impossible to detect blood groups.
7. **Nails:** The human nails contain mainly ABO blood group antigens. MN blood groups have been detected in some cases.

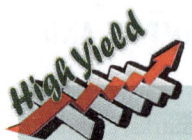

- Semen gives a bluish-white color under UV light (Wood's lamp).
- Presumptive tests for semen are based on colorimetry, and are qualitative in nature.
- At body temperature, sperms retain full motility in vagina for 6–12 h.
- **Florence test:** Presumptive test for semen; dark brown rhombic crystals of choline periodide are seen (choline from seminal vesicles).
- **Barberio's test:** Presumptive test for semen; yellow needle-shaped crystals of spermine picrate are seen (spermine from prostatic secretions).
- **Most common presumptive test for semen:** Acid phosphatase/Brentamine test (gives purple color).
- Acid phosphatase is an enzyme secreted by the prostate gland into seminal fluid.
- **Confirmatory test for semen:** Visualization of one intact spermatozoon.
- **Christmas tree stain:** Microscopic examination of semen (for sperms).
- **Technique to determine male cells in absence of spermatozoa:** Fluorescence in situ hybridization (FISH).
- **Method to detect prostate specific antigen (PSA/p30):** ABAcard test strips.
- **Alternative to the method for PSA detection:** Detection of semenogelin with immunochromatographic test strip.
- **Conclusive determination of semen in vaginal swabs:** Acid phosphatase + PSA + spermatozoa detection.
- **Confirmation of species of semen:** Precipitin test using anti-human serum.
- If the victim is <18 years, recovery of semen is consistent with the commission of the crime (consent is invalid if <18 years).
- If the seminal stain is from secretor, absorption-elution method is used to determine the ABO blood group.
- Phosphoglucomutase and peptidase A enzyme markers are used in genetic profiling of semen.
- DNA profiling can accurately individualize semen.
- **Phadebas test:** Identification of saliva (α-amylase detection).

Interesting case

Seminal Stain (Case of Clinton–Lewinsky Scandal, 1998)

In 1998, 49-year-old Bill Clinton, President of US and 22-year-old Monica Lewinsky, White House intern were involved in a political sex scandal. The sexual relationship took place during 1995-97 and came to light in 1998.

In 1997, Monica confided with co-worker about her relationship with the President and a blue GAP dress in her possession that still bore the semen stain that resulted from her administering fellatio. She persuaded Monica not to dry clean the semen-stained dress in order to keep it as an 'insurance policy' should Monica later be accused of lying about the affair. The co-worker secretly recorded their telephone conversations and gave the tapes to Independent Counsel Kenneth Starr, who was investigating the Paula Jones case.

Clinton had previously been confronted with allegations of sexual misconduct during his time as Governor of Arkansas. Former Arkansas state employee Paula Jones filed a civil lawsuit alleging sexual harassment against him. Monica's name surfaced during the discovery phase of Jones case, when her lawyers sought to show a pattern of behavior by Clinton which involved inappropriate sexual relationships with other employees. Under oath in the Jones suit, Clinton denied having any 'sexual affair' or 'sexual relationship' with Monica. He claimed that certain acts were performed on him, not by him, and therefore, he did not engage in sexual relations.

In July 1998, after a substantial delay since the scandal broke (Monica was unwilling to discuss the affair or testify about it), she received transactional immunity in exchange for grand jury testimony. According to her testimony, she had nine sexual encounters during that time that involved fellatio and other sexual acts, but not sexual intercourse. Her testimony contradicted Clinton's claim of being totally passive in their encounters.

She also turned over the semen-stained blue dress to the investigators. A blood sample was taken from Clinton, and the FBI reported its conclusion that Clinton was the source of the semen on the dress 'to a reasonable degree of scientific certainty' thereby providing unambiguous DNA evidence that could prove sexual relationship despite his official denials. Clinton admitted in grand jury testimony that he had engaged in an 'improper physical relationship' with Lewinsky. That evening he gave a nationally televised statement admitting that his relationship with Monica was 'not appropriate'.

Based on the evidence—the blue dress—Starr concluded that the President's sworn testimony was false which led to charges of perjury and to the impeachment of Clinton. He was subsequently acquitted on all impeachment charges of perjury and obstruction of justice in a 21-day Senate trial. However, Clinton was held in civil contempt of court for giving misleading testimony in the Paula Jones case and was also fined $90,000. In 2001, his license to practice law was suspended in Arkansas for 5 years and later by the United States Supreme Court. His wife, Hillary Clinton remained supportive of her husband throughout the scandal, despite the betrayal and public humiliation.

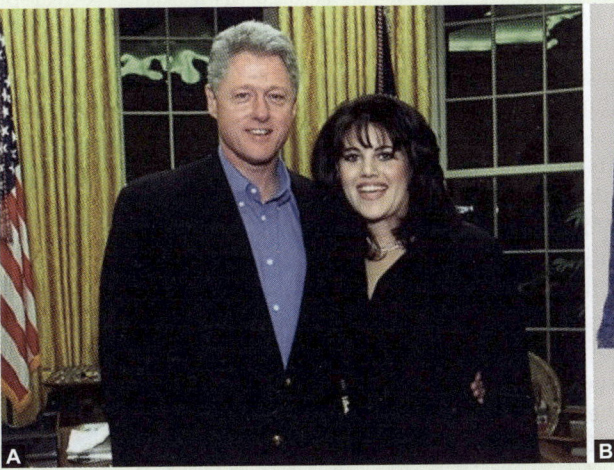
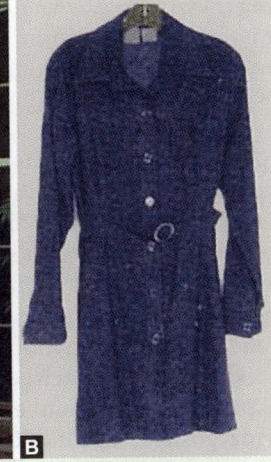

Bill Clinton with Monica Lewinsky   'The blue dress'

CHAPTER 31

DNA Fingerprinting

LEARNING OBJECTIVES

Must know
1. Restriction fragment length polymorphism technique
2. Polymerase chain reaction
3. Collection of samples for DNA fingerprinting
4. FTA card
5. Uses of DNA fingerprinting

Desirable to know
1. Limitations of DNA testing

Enumerate the indications and describe the principles and appropriate use for DNA profiling.

Definitions

- **DNA fingerprinting** *(DNA typing, DNA identification):* A laboratory technique used to determine the probable identity of a person based on the nucleotide sequences of certain regions of human DNA that are unique to individuals.
    - This technique is capable of distinguishing every individual, with the exception of *identical/monozygotic twins and clones.** DNA fingerprinting has become the primary method for identifying and distinguishing among individual human beings.
- **DNA or genetic profile:** It is an encrypted set of numbers reflecting the genetic make-up of an individual for the specific genetic markers analyzed. Each genetic marker analyzed can be expressed as two numbers (e.g., 8–10) in the case of heterozygosity or one number (e.g., 8) in the case of homozygosity.
- **DNA extraction method:** Any method used to purify DNA from a biological sample, such as blood, saliva, semen, hair, bone, used garments, etc.
- **Polymerase chain reaction (PCR):** An enzymatic process in which a specific DNA sequence is replicated or copied thousands of times.

Introduction

- DNA is a sturdy molecule which can tolerate wide range of temperature, pH and other factors. DNA mixed with detergents, oil, gasoline and other adulterants does not alter its typing characteristics.
- DNA fingerprint was first developed in England in 1985 by *Alec Jeffreys*, professor of genetics at the University of Leicester who made the discovery by accident while tracking genetic variations in myoglobin.
- Two methods of DNA analysis are in common use **(Diff. 31.1)**:
    i. Restriction fragment length polymorphism (RFLP)
    ii. Polymerase chain reaction (PCR)

RESTRICTION FRAGMENT LENGTH POLYMORPHISM

In the human genome, in between the active base pairs which code for a particular protein, there is large number of inactive base pairs forming 95% of DNA which is considered as '*junk DNA*' or '*filler DNA*' or '*nonsense DNA*'. Technically, these 'introns' separate the 'exons' which serve as protein patterns. DNA fingerprinters overlook the DNA in genes, in favor of 'junk DNA' between the genes.

In 'junk DNA' short sequences of base repeat themselves over and over again like a *stutter* (repetitive DNA), e.g., CGTA, CGTA, GACA, GACA, etc. The regions containing repetitive DNA demonstrating hypervariability from

---

* Ultra-deep next generation sequencing, also known as massively parallel sequencing, has made it possible to identify a number of genetic variations (such as copy number variations, single nucleotide polymorphisms and DNA methylation—methylation status of monozygotic twins change during their lifetime) that make it possible to solve paternity and forensic cases involving monozygotic twins as alleged fathers or originators of DNA traces.

DIFFERENTIATION 31.1: RFLP and PCR

S.No.	Feature	RFLP	PCR
1.	Amount of DNA sample required	Large (300–500 ng)	Small (25 ng)
2.	Sensitivity	Less	More
3.	DNA degradation	Useless when degradation is present	Useful
4.	Decomposed sample	Not useful	Useful
5.	Time required	More	Less
6.	Tedious	More	Less
7.	Labor intensive	More	Less
8.	Sensitivity to contamination with other samples	Less sensitive	More sensitive
9.	Result of the test	Non-discrete	Discrete (binary 'yes/no')

person to person are called '*satellite DNA*' which shows an extremely high degree of variability, and these variants are called 'variable number tandem repeats' (VNTR) or 'minisatellites'. Selected regions of VNTR are broken into fragments using special enzymes (restriction endonucleases). The resulting fragments are called *restriction fragments length polymorphisms (RFLP)*. Gel electrophoresis can be used to separate and determine the size of the RFLPs (fragments are of variable lengths). The exact number and size of fragments produced by a specific restriction enzyme digestion varies from individual to individual, i.e., they are individualistic in nature and establish 100% identity.

Procedure (Fig. 31.1)

The most common method of DNA typing is RFLP analysis of VNTR loci.

i. **Isolation/extraction of DNA:** DNA must be recovered from the cells or tissues of the body. Only a small amount of tissue—blood, hair or skin—is needed. For example, the amount of DNA found at the root of one hair is usually sufficient.

ii. **Cutting and sizing:** Special enzymes called *restriction enzymes* are used to cut the DNA at specific places. For example, an enzyme called EcoR1, found in bacteria, will cut DNA only when the sequence GAATTC occurs.

iii. **Sorting by gel electrophoresis:** The DNA pieces are sorted according to size by a sieving technique called electrophoresis. The DNA pieces are passed through an agarose gel. This results in separation of the DNA fragments based on their length (size).

iv. **Transfer of DNA to nylon (Southern blotting)**
   - It is possible to identify specific DNA fragments that hybridize with a complementary genetic probe. However, it is impossible to hybridize a probe to DNA fragments contained in a gel. For this reason, the DNA is usually denatured and then transferred to a nitrocellulose or nylon membrane which picks up the DNA like a blotter picks up ink. DNA is transferred to the membrane by capillary action and fixed by baking, making it accessible to a probe. The resulting blot formed is essentially a replica of the gel.
   - This method of detecting DNA fragments—separating them by gel electrophoresis and

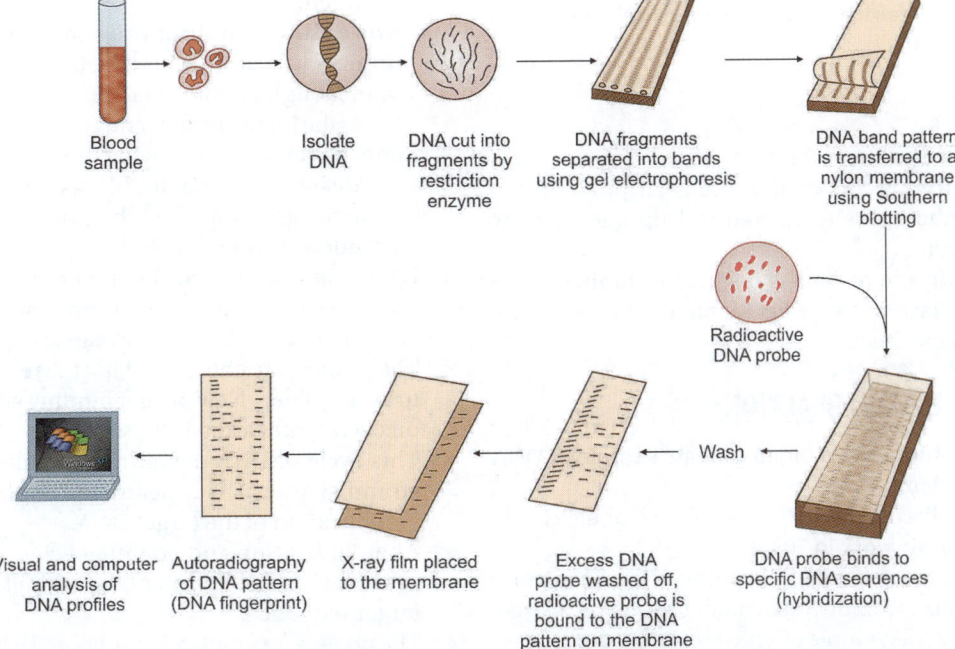

Fig. 31.1: Procedure of DNA profiling (RFLP)

then transferring them to a nitrocellulose/nylon membrane—is called *Southern blot*, named after its inventor, *Dr Edward Southern*. Similar blotting techniques are used to study RNA (*Northern blot*), and proteins or polypeptides (*Western blot*).

v. **Hybridization:** Adding known radioactive DNA-probes (short sequence probe, complementary to the region of DNA which one wishes to detect) to the nylon sheet leads to fragment location. The nylon membrane is immersed in a solution that contains DNA probe impregnated with radioactive P^{32}. Each probe typically sticks to only one or two specific/complementary sequences on the nylon sheet. This process is termed as *hybridization*.

vi. **Washing:** The membrane is washed to remove excess or unbound probe, and then exposed to an X-ray film.
  - The resulting spots on the X-ray film correspond to the locations of the fragments in the gel that are complementary to the probe (*autoradiography*).
  - Nowadays, many radioactive probes are detected by chemical luminescence which is analyzed by computer scanners, eliminating the need for autoradiography.

vii. **DNA fingerprint:** The final print is known as an autoradiograph or 'DNA fingerprint' which appears as lines on the film.

Current practice in use of DNA samples for crime investigations and paternity suits does not use multilocus DNA analysis, but utilizes highly polymorphic single locus genes such as the VNTR genes. Due to the large number of distinguishable alleles in most populations, it is possible to establish a '*DNA signature*' for almost any individual.

Limitations

- It takes few weeks to perform.
- For every probing, the membrane is stripped off the previous probe and rehybridized and autoradiography performed again.
- It is not useful where DNA is degraded—limited value in testing cadaveric tissue for identification of human remains, unless fresh.

POLYMERASE CHAIN REACTION

- PCR is a technique used for amplifying sample of DNA fragments *in vitro*.
- PCR won its discoverer *Kary B. Mullis*, a Nobel Prize in chemistry for his work in 1993.
- In this process, a particular DNA segment from a mixture of DNA chains is rapidly replicated, producing a large, readily analyzable sample of a piece of DNA; the process is also called **DNA amplification**.
- PCR itself does not accomplish DNA typing, but increases the amount of DNA available for typing.
- It is used to produce multiple copies of segments from a very limited amount of DNA. Once a sufficient sample has been produced, the pattern of the alleles from a limited number of genes is compared with the pattern from the reference sample.
- A nonmatch conclusively excludes a suspect, but the technique provides less certainty when a match occurs.

Procedure

The theory behind PCR is based on certain aspects of DNA replication. The enzyme *DNA polymerase* helps to expand a short sequence into a longer one or a polymer. But, DNA polymerase needs single stranded DNA that acts as a template for the synthesis of a new strand. It also requires a small portion of double stranded DNA to initiate synthesis (*primers*). Then, new DNA strands are synthesized and amplified behind the primer.

> **Pearls**
> **Requirements for PCR**
> - Heat resistant DNA polymerase (Taq polymerase)
> - Primers (short sequences of nucleotides designed to bind at the end of the desired DNA segment)
> - Deoxynucleoside triphosphates (equal amounts of dATPs, dTTPs, dCTPs, dGTPs)
> - DNA-fragments.

Three steps are involved in this process **(Fig. 31.2)**:

i. **Denaturation:** Heating the double stranded DNA to almost boiling will dissociate it and will become single stranded.

ii. **Annealing:** Cooling the reaction will cause the primers to pair up with the single-stranded template (annealing). On the small length of double-stranded DNA (the joined primer and template), the polymerase attaches and starts copying the template.

iii. **Extension:** DNA building blocks complementary to the template are coupled to the primer, making a double stranded DNA molecule.

- Each separated strand can serve as a template for synthesis as long as primer is provided for each strand, and the reaction is cooled to cause the primers to bind. The primers are chosen to flank the region of DNA that is to be amplified. New primer binding sites are generated on each synthesized DNA strand.
- This cycle of DNA denaturing, primer annealing and strand synthesis is repeated multiple times, thereby amplification of the target DNA.
- After 20 heating and cooling cycles, this exponential process yields 2^{20}, or more than a million copies of the target sequence.
- The process is completely automated with thermocyclers that contain a heating block and microprocessors. The

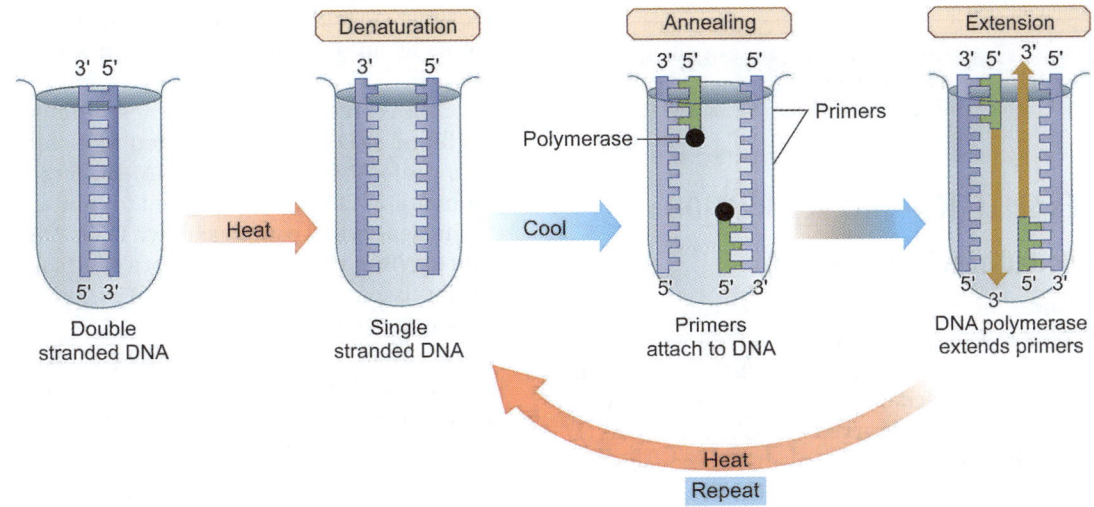

Fig. 31.2: Steps in PCR

time and temperature can be programmed for repetitive cycles of heating and cooling, alleviating manual intervention.

Other PCR based methods
- Dot blots, involving a series of DNA probes to detect target sequences such as the HLA DQa locus in chromosome 6, producing a pattern of colored dots.
- Amplified fragment length polymorphism (AmpFLP)
- Short tandem repeats (STRs) in which the core repeat unit are 2–6 bp length.
- System utilizing mitochondrial DNA.
- Digital DNA typing.

STR analyzes the DNA segments for the number of repeats at 13 core loci. STR analysis is less susceptible to DNA degradation than other AmpFLPs. The chance of misidentification in this procedure is one in several billion.

Applications: PCR technique has virtually limitless applications. It enables researchers to amplify and analyze tiny DNA samples from variety of sources—ranging from crimes scenes to archeological remains.

Limitation: It is too sensitive; a tiny amount of contaminant DNA in a sample may become amplified if it includes a DNA sequence complimentary to the primers, leading to an erroneous conclusion.

Current Technique of DNA Profiling

- Modern-day DNA profiling is also called STR analysis and relies on microsatellites rather than the minisatellites used in DNA fingerprinting.
- Unlike the original DNA fingerprinting method, DNA profiling does not use restriction enzymes to cut the DNA. Instead, it uses the PCR to produce many copies of specific STR sequences.
- In STR analysis, the primers used in the PCR are designed to attach to either end of the STR sequence of interest.
- The primer for each STR is labeled with a specific colored fluorescent tag. This makes it easier to identify and record the STR sequences after PCR.
- Once enough copies of the sequence have been produced by PCR, electrophoresis is used to separate the fragments according to size.
- Each fragment passes by a laser which causes the fragments with fluorescent tags to glow with a specific color. The output is displayed as a series of colored peaks highlighting the color and length of each STR sequence.
- The more STR sequences that are tested, the more accurate the test is at identifying someone.
- Other STRs used for forensic purposes are called Y-STRs, which are derived solely from the male Y chromosome. This is useful for identifying a male perpetrator from mixed DNA samples.

NOTA BENE

Criteria to determine the source

DNA testing laboratories use a two-step process to determine if two samples arose from one source. First, DNA-banding patterns are compared visually. If banding patterns of a sample in question do not match a known DNA sample, exclusion is declared and no further analysis is required. Second, a visualized match is verified by a technique called computer assisted allele sizing which is done by computer software. Basically, the calculated sizes of an apparent match should fall within 2.5% of each other. When samples fall outside of the 2.5% window, they should be considered 'nonmatching'. If the DNA-banding pattern of a sample cannot be positively determined due to technical problems, the results should be considered 'inconclusive'.

> FM 6.1, 6.2
> - Describe different types of specimen and tissues to be collected both in the living and dead for DNA fingerprinting.
> - Describe the methods of sample collection, preservation, labeling, dispatch, and interpretation of reports.

SPECIMEN SELECTION AND PRESERVATION

Samples Collected from Living Subjects

i. **Blood** (*most common sample*): 5 mL of venous blood is collected in a purple stoppered vacutainer (EDTA tube) and mixed thoroughly without shaking. Heparin is not used as an anticoagulant since it interferes with PCR. Sample can be preserved at 2–8°C (not frozen).

ii. **Buccal epithelial cells** (buccal swabs) are considered a convenient alternative for collecting genetic material, as they are relatively easy to collect, inexpensive and noninvasive. The swab is removed from the packing and without handling the tip, immediately swabbed the subject's mouth for 10 seconds. After swabbing, it placed directly into the receptacle (packaging) to dry.

iii. **Hair follicles with roots** (plucked hair), about 10–20, from the head is used as a reference standard. The root of the hair contains nuclear DNA, and the shaft contains mitochondrial DNA. The root contains *keratinocytes* which are ideal for the extraction of nuclear DNA. Cut or naturally shed hairs (without follicle) may not be entirely unhelpful, since some nucleated *corneocytes* (keratinocytes in their last stage of differentiation) are present which make it possible to extract a DNA profile.

Samples Collected from Dead Bodies (Flowchart 31.1)

DNA can be isolated and tested from practically any postmortem tissue, although after death it will undergo progressive degradation. DNA is broken down into fragments by autolytic and bacterial enzymes, especially DNases.

i. In relatively fresh dead bodies, unclotted 10 mL of blood (EDTA anticoagulated in a sterile tube) is the preferable source of DNA. Buffers (e.g., those containing EDTA) are designed to inhibit the activity of nucleases that can breakdown DNA. Due to settling out of WBCs, clotted blood is not a good source of DNA.

ii. Brain tissue is a good source of DNA in intermediate postmortem intervals.

iii. Hard tissue (bone and vascular pulp of teeth) is the best source of DNA in cases of advanced decomposition.

- Best material is said to be muscle or spleen if decomposition is establishing; bone marrow (from femur) and teeth (usually molars) are also recommended.
- Postmortem material is inferior to live blood and tissue for DNA testing. Any disturbance to nuclear chromatin due to putrefaction is dangerous.

Samples Encountered in Forensic Practice

- Blood (EDTA/heparinized/clotted/stain on cloth, newspaper, wood or tiles).
- Semen (stain on cloth/paper/floor).
- Hair (head/body/pubic).
- Tissue (bone marrow/muscle/spleen/fingernail scrapings).
- Mouth swabs, and saliva stain on cigarette buds/licked envelope/glass.

DNA Storage and FTA Card

In general, there are four broad strategies for long-term DNA preservation:
1. Room temperature on a 'dry' solid matrix
2. –20°C
3. –80°C
4. –196°C (storage in liquid nitrogen)

- In a laboratory setting, DNA is most commonly stored at 4°C, –20°C or –80°C.
- Blood and other biological samples can be stored on Whatman FTA® (Flinders Technology Associates) cards at room temperature with subsequent amplification by PCR (**Fig. 31.3**).
  - FTA is also an acronym for *fast technology for analysis* of nucleic acids, developed as a means of protecting nucleic acid samples from degradation by nucleases and other processes.
  - The concept was to apply a weak base, chelating agent, anionic surfactant or detergent, and uric acid (or a urate salt) to a cellulose based matrix (filter paper). A sample containing DNA could then be applied to the treated filter paper for preservation and long-term storage. The expected storage length is over 50 years.

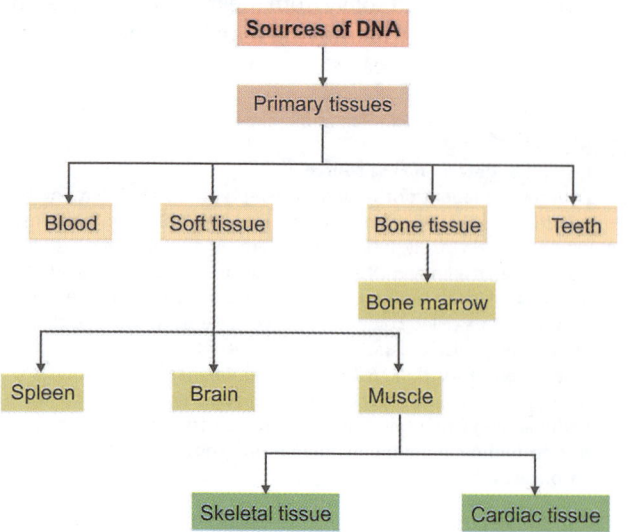

Flowchart 31.1: Sources of DNA

CHAPTER 31: DNA Fingerprinting

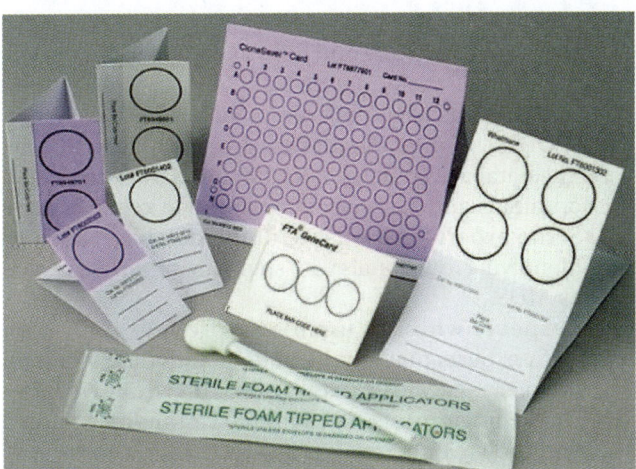

Fig. 31.3: Whatman FTA cards (colored cards are indicating cards which change color on using colorless samples to facilitate its handling)
(*Source:* www.sigma-aldrich.com)

- Biological samples adhere to the paper through the mechanism of entanglement, while the mixture of chemicals lyses cells and denatures proteins.
- Nucleic acid damage from nucleases, oxidation, UV damage, microbes and fungus is reduced when samples are stored on the FTA card. Since, nucleases are inactivated; DNA is essentially stable when the sample is properly dried and stored.
- For analysis, a small disc is punched from the card containing the DNA, washed, dried and used for PCR amplification, or restriction enzyme digestion can be performed directly on the treated paper without the need for extensive extraction procedures.
- Since, the cards are small in size (approximately 5" × 3.5"), they can be easily packaged, shipped and stored for data basing (**Box 31.1**).

Box 31.1 Features of the FTA card
- Rapid isolation of pure DNA
- Designed to kill pathogens and prevent future colonization by bacteria or fungi
- Protects DNA from microbial and environmental degradation
- Archive samples at room temperature
- Reduces potential for cross-contamination between samples
- Eliminates shearing forces associated with conventional extraction methods

FM 7.1
Enumerate the appropriate use for DNA profiling.

USES OF DNA FINGERPRINTING

i. **Identification:** It is used to link suspects to biological evidence—blood or semen stains, hair or items of clothing—found at the scene of a crime. It is used to establish identity of an assailant in sexual assaults, like rape, incest and bestiality.

ii. **Diagnosis of inherited disorders** in adults, children, newborn and prenatal babies. It includes cystic fibrosis, hemophilia, Huntington's disease, familial Alzheimer's, sickle cell anemia and thalassemia. Genetic counselors use DNA fingerprint information to help prospective parents understand the risk of having an affected child or decisions concerning affected pregnancies.

iii. **Developing cures for inherited disorders:** By studying the DNA fingerprints of relatives who have a history of some particular disorder or by comparing large groups of people with and without the disorder, it is possible to identify DNA patterns associated with the disease in question.

iv. **Establish paternity** in custody and child support litigation. Cases are resolved via parent-child VNTR prototype analysis. Additionally, immigration and inheritance proceedings may make use of this information.

NOTA BENE

In this, DNA from the child, mother and putative fathers is cut by the same restriction enzyme. The DNA fragment is separated by gel electrophoresis for each individual in a separate lane. The patterns of bands thus formed (DNA fingerprints) is then compared between the children and his/her parents (**Fig. 31.4**). It should be noted that each band present in the child is also found in at least one of the parents.

v. **Identifying the remains of soldiers:** In the US armed services, a program is there to collect DNA fingerprints from all personnel for use later, in case they are needed to identify casualties or persons missing in action.

vi. **Breeding program:** Breeders typically assess a plant or animal's genotype using its phenotype. Since

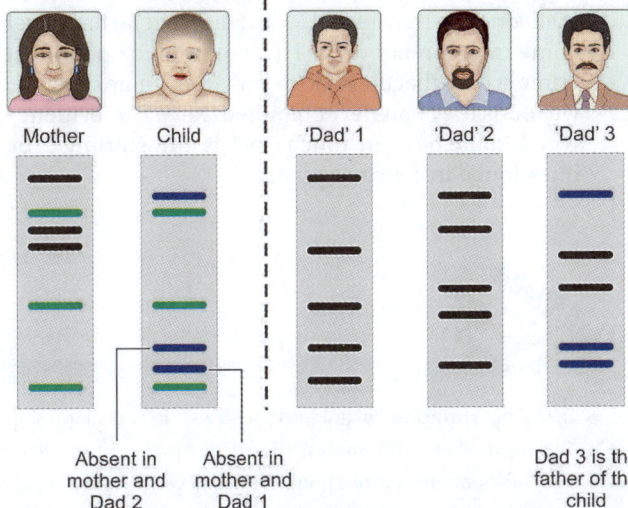

Fig. 31.4: DNA fingerprints of child, mother and putative fathers

homozygous or heterozygous dominance is difficult to distinguish from appearance, the genotype can be determined with accuracy using DNA fingerprinting. Hunting dogs and racehorses can both benefit from it.

vii. Accidents/mass disaster investigations and post-mortem identification of skeletal remains/mutilated bodies.

viii. **Detection of AIDS:** A person with AIDS can be diagnosed by comparing the HIV "RNA" band (converted to DNA via RTPCR) with the bands formed by the individual's blood.

LIMITATIONS OF DNA TESTING

Generally, the courts have accepted the reliability of DNA testing and admitted DNA test results into evidence. But, DNA fingerprinting is controversial in a number of areas:

i. **Uniqueness of DNA fingerprinting:** DNA segments rather than complete DNA strands are 'fingerprinted', a DNA fingerprint may not be unique.

ii. **Accuracy of the results:** Tests are often performed in private laboratories that may not follow uniform testing standards and quality controls. Ambiguity in interpretation of the bands may arise from scientist's own misinterpretation of band-pattern and on the other hand, it may occur from actual shifts, degradation, missing bands, extra bands—all due to technical problems.

Moreover, forensic specimens are often contaminated, making the extraction of pure DNA difficult, and cross contamination of DNA between two specimens, or aerosol DNA from previous reactions on one's hands at very small concentrations can alter results.

iii. **"Touch DNA":** People leave invisible genetic markers everywhere they go and on virtually everything they come into contact with. Current methods have reduced the number of cells recovered from a scene for a DNA print to be made to as little as 20 cells. It is relatively common for an innocent person's DNA to be inadvertently transferred to surfaces that he has never come into contact with. This could place people at crime scenes that they had never visited or link them to weapons they had never handled. Key DNA evidence which could be from 'touch DNA' is now starting to be questioned in courts regularly.

iv. **Cost:** Testing is expensive.

v. **Invasion of privacy and ethical concerns:** In the US, the FBI has created a national database of genetic information called the Combined DNA Index System (CODIS). Similar database is present in the UK also. The database contains DNA obtained from convicted criminals and from evidence found at crime scenes. Some experts fear misuse of the database, such as identifying individuals with stigmatizing illnesses such as AIDS.

vi. Suspects who are unable to provide their own DNA experts may not be able to adequately defend themselves against charges based on DNA evidence.

vii. Unlike fingerprints, DNA profile cannot be enlarged and shown in the court of law.

NOTA BENE

- In 1986, DNA fingerprinting was used by Jeffreys for the first time in the UK, clearing a suspect of two rapes and murders and helping convict the culprit Colin Pitchfork. The first criminal conviction based on DNA evidence in the US occurred in 1988. It was only in 1996 that the DNA evidence provided by *Lalji Singh* was accepted in a court in India (in the '*tandoor* murder case' reported in New Delhi).
- **Mitochondrial DNA (mtDNA)**, a small circular genome located in the mitochondria, has provided forensic scientists with a valuable tool for determining the source of DNA recovered from damaged, degraded or very small biological samples. Cells contain hundreds of copies of mtDNA genomes, as compared to two copies of the DNA located in the nucleus. This increases the likelihood of recovering sufficient DNA from compromised DNA samples, and for this reason mtDNA can play an important role in missing persons investigations, mass disasters and other investigations involving samples with limited biological material. Additionally, mtDNA is maternally inherited. Therefore, barring a mutation, an individual's mother, siblings, as well as all other maternally-related family members will have identical mtDNA sequences. As a result, comparisons can be made using a reference sample from any maternal relative, even if the unknown and reference sample are separated by many generations.
- *Nucleic acid sequence-based amplification* (NASBA), is used to amplify RNA sequences.
- *Ligase chain reaction:* Method of DNA amplification similar to PCR.
- *DNA sequencing:* Biochemical methods for determining the order of the nucleotide bases in a DNA oligonucleotide.

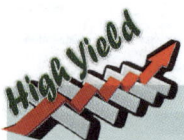

- ◆ **DNA fingerprinting:** Technique that is capable of distinguishing every individual, with the exception of identical twins and clones.
- ◆ **Two methods of DNA analysis:** Restriction fragment length polymorphism (RFLP) and polymerase chain reaction (PCR).
- ◆ In DNA fingerprint, introns (junk DNA) with variable number of tandem repeats (VNTR) are used for matching.
- ◆ DNA fingerprint was first developed by Alec Jeffreys in the UK.

CHAPTER 31 : DNA Fingerprinting

- PCR was discovered by Kary B Mullis (got Nobel Prize in chemistry).
- **Father of DNA fingerprinting in India:** Lalji Singh.
- **Technique used for restriction fragment length polymorphism:** Southern blot (Dr Edward Southern invented it).
- Blotting technique to study RNA is *Northern blot*, and blotting technique for proteins or polypeptides is *Western blot*.
- **Requirements for PCR:** Heat resistant DNA polymerase *(Taq polymerase)*, primers, deoxynucleoside triphosphates and DNA-fragments.
- PCR is done for replication of DNA *in vitro*.
- **Best sample for DNA fingerprinting:** Blood in EDTA tube (both in living and dead).
- **Best sample for DNA fingerprinting if decomposition is establishing:** Muscle or spleen.
- **Best sample for DNA fingerprinting in advanced decomposition:** Bone marrow (from femur) and teeth (usually molars).
- DNA fingerprinting is not possible with RBCs.
- In a laboratory setting, DNA is most commonly stored at 4°C, –20°C or –80°C.
- Blood and other biological samples can be stored on *FTA cards* at room temperature with subsequent amplification by PCR.

Interesting case

DNA Fingerprinting (Case of Colin Pitchfork, 1987)

Colin Pitchfork, who was 22 at the time of the first murder, was married with two sons **(Fig. A)**. He was a baker who grew up in rural Leicestershire and lived in Littlethorpe (UK). Before marriage, he had been convicted of indecent exposure and had been referred for therapy.

In 1983, a dead body of a 15-year-old schoolgirl was found near a footpath in the village Narborough. A postmortem revealed that she had been raped and strangled, and a semen sample was retrieved from her body. The semen belonged to a person with blood group A and an enzyme profile that matched only 10% of

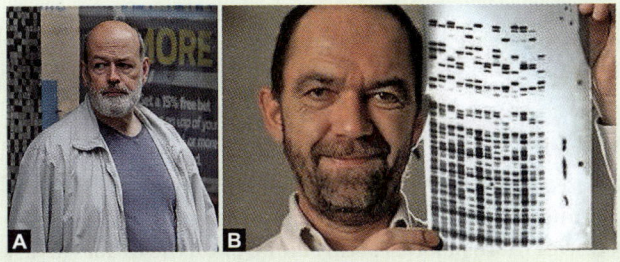

males. Although the case was left open, there were no remaining leads for investigators to follow. The case went cold.

A few years later, in 1986, the second victim—a 15-year-old girl's dead body was found in a field which was only a short distance from the site where the first victim was murdered. The pathologist established that she had put up a considerable struggle before being raped and strangled, and semen samples revealed the same blood type. The modus operandi matched that of the first attack—the clothes had been removed in the same manner, and both had been raped before being strangled with their scarf. The police soon realized that they were looking for a serial killer and a local man, someone who knew the area and the victims.

The police arrested a 17-year-old youth Richard Buckland with learning difficulties, who revealed knowledge of second victim's body, and admitted to the crime under questioning, but denied the first murder. The police, in their certainty that both girls' were strangled and raped by the same person, were convinced he was lying.

In 1985, at the University of Leicester, Alec Jeffreys and his team had developed a promising individualization technique which can produce a unique DNA 'fingerprint' from a sample **(Fig. B)**. The investigators requested him to use this technique in this case. Jeffreys compared semen samples from both murder victims against a blood sample from this youth and conclusively proved that both girls were killed by the same man but not by this accused. He became the first person to be exonerated by DNA fingerprinting.

With no further leads, the investigators started a project in which men were asked to give a blood or saliva sample for DNA testing for comparison with the suspect's DNA profile. After eight months and 5,511 sampling, there was no match with the semen samples. However, a break in the case was yet to come. In August 1987, one of Pitchfork's colleagues at the bakery revealed in a pub that he had taken the blood test while impersonating as Pitchfork. This information was conveyed to a local policeman. Subsequently in September 1987, Pitchfork was arrested. A DNA fingerprinting was done which matched the crime scene samples. He admitted to the rape and strangulation of the two girls, and went on to explain his paraphilia for flashing, an impulse that had soon led to sexual assault and finally murder. He was sentenced to life imprisonment in 1988, becoming the first person to be convicted of murder based on DNA fingerprinting evidence. In 1994, Alec Jeffreys was given the knighthood for services to genetics.

CHAPTER 32

Torture and Custodial Deaths

LEARNING OBJECTIVES

Must know
1. Torture, types
2. Falanga, dry submarino, wet submarine, telefono

Desirable to know
1. Findings in various physical torture
2. NHRC guidelines regarding torture and custodial deaths
3. Postmortem examination in custodial deaths

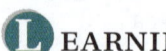
Describe and discuss issues relating to torture, identification of injuries caused by torture and its sequalae, management of torture survivors.

Definition

Torture (Latin *tortura*: act of twisting) is 'a deliberate, systemic or wanton infliction of physical or mental suffering by one or more persons acting alone or on the orders of any authority, to force another person to yield information, to make a confession, or for any other reason' (as per WMA's **Declaration of Tokyo**).

- The definition contains three collective elements (a) intentional infliction of severe mental or physical suffering; (b) by a public official, who is directly or indirectly involved; and (c) for a specific purpose.
- This declaration states that doctors should refuse to participate in, condone or give permission for torture, degradation or cruel treatment of prisoners or detainees.
- Throughout history, torture has often been used as a method of effecting political re-education. Nevertheless in the 21st century, torture is almost universally considered to be an extreme violation of human rights, as stated by the Universal Declaration of Human Rights.

Ethical Issue

Organizations, like Amnesty International argue that the universal legal prohibition is based on a universal philosophical consensus that torture and ill-treatment are repugnant, abhorrent and immoral. But, to obtain information from suspected terrorists by using torture methods to save innocent civilians, is debatable.

Reasons for Torture

The United Nations Convention identifies four reasons for torture:
i. To obtain a confession
ii. To obtain information
iii. To punish
iv. To coerce the sufferer or others to act in certain ways.

TYPES OF TORTURE

Four types
i. Physical
ii. Psychological
iii. Pharmacological
iv. Sexual

Physical Torture

Physical torture is the infliction of pain on the body **(Table 32.1)**.
- **Cold torture:** Icy water is poured over head or forced to strip naked and stand outside on a winter night or forced to stand in snow or on ice with bare feet or submersing in ice-cold water.
- **Force-feeding** of saturated salt-water, vinegar, liquor, pepper, mustard oil, boiling water, urine or feces.
- **Shooting** as means of execution or nonfatal punishment is carried out in some parts of the world.
  - Victims are sometimes shot either through knee joint or thigh *(knee-capping)*.

Determining bone lesion by scintigraphy is considered a valuable non-invasive diagnostic method to assess and document long term torture practices where beating was a common denominator with no detectable marks upon physical or radiological examination.

TABLE 32.1: Various types of physical torture and associated clinical findings

	Method	Findings
Beating *(most common method)*		
♦ Falanga/bastinado	Beating on soles by blunt objects	Hematoma of soles of feet
♦ El quirofano/operating table	Beating on abdomen while lying on a table with upper half of the body unsupported	Bruise, ruptured abdominal viscera
♦ Telefono	Repeated slapping of both the ears by open hands of torturer	Ruptured tympanic membranes
♦ Belana/ the roller	Pole pressed down with great weight on the back and then rolled up over legs and body	Crushing of soft tissue and damage to muscles of legs and body
♦ Chepuwa	Thigh placed under two wooden rods and pressed	Crushing of soft tissue and damage to muscles of legs
♦ Campana/the bell	Head is placed within a pail which is then struck repeatedly	Ruptured tympanic membranes
Forced posture		
♦ El cabellete/saw horse	Forced straddling on a bar	Perineal bruising
♦ El planton	Prolonged standing	Dependent edema and petechiae
♦ Aeroplane method	Body bent at right angle to the legs, and arms raised behind back with head bent down	Pain, nerve and muscle damage, joint injuries
♦ Tiger bench	Tied and secured to bench with his feet and legs, and heavy objects such as bricks are placed under feet	Bruising, nerve and muscle damage, joint injuries
Suspension		
♦ Palestinian hanging	Tying hands behind waist and then strung up to a ceiling beam	Bruising, nerve and muscle damage, joint injuries
♦ La bandera	Suspended by wrists	
♦ Murcielago	Suspended by ankles	
♦ Parrot's perch/pau de arara	Suspended head down from a horizontal pole placed under the knees with wrists bound to ankles	
♦ Stretching (cheera)	Forcible abduction of hips	
Asphyxial torture		
♦ Water boarding	Water is poured over mouth and nose covered with cloth which prevents it from being expelled	Sensation of drowning
♦ El submarine/wet submarine	Head repeatedly submerged underwater or in foul liquid	Fecal matter and other debris in the airways
♦ Dry submarine	Plastic bag covers the head resulting in near-suffocation	Lung petechiae
Electric torture		
♦ Buzzer/chicharra	Charged batons placed over sensitive parts of body, like nipples, genitalia or anal canal	Reddish brown lesions at points of contact, burning and scarring
♦ Electric cattle prod/picana	Current applied with a pointed object	
Burns		
♦ Black slave	Hot metal skewer inserted up the anus	Perinal or rectal burns
♦ Cigarette burns	Burning cigarette end stubbed on to skin	Circular and macular scars of 5-10 mm with a depigmented center and a hyperpigmented indistinct periphery
Irritant torture	Irritating chemicals (e.g., chillies) inserted into rectum/vagina, or applied on eyes or thrown naked onto a pile of hemp	Inflammation, extremely itchy and painful

Cause of Death

♦ Deaths usually result from severe closed blunt force head injuries with cerebral contusion and laceration, with or without skull fracture.
♦ Blunt trauma to the abdomen is the second most common cause of death due to tearing of the mesentery or laceration of internal organs.

Psychological Torture

It uses non-physical methods to induce pain in the subject's mental, emotional and psychological states. Psychological torture includes deliberate use of extreme stressors and situations, such as mock execution*, shunning, violation of deep-seated social or sexual norms or taboos, and extended solitary confinement.

---

* **Sham execution:** Victim is blindfolded and made to stand before a wall and then threatened that a vehicle is going to hit him.

It is categorized into:
i. **Deprivation technique:** Deprivation of sleep, food or water, deprivation of use of toilet, sanitary napkins, shower or change of clothes, or prohibition of eye contact and talk (social deprivation) are some of the methods.
ii. **Coercion technique:** Threats, humiliations and sexual torture are included in this category.
iii. **Communication technique:** Disinformation and conditioning of new reflexes are some of the methods.
iv. **Witness torture:** Victims are forced to witness the torture of another prisoner.

Some forms of psychological torture are:
- **Sleep deprivation:** In this, the victim could be kept awake for days at a time. It involves both physical and psychological aspects.
- **White torture:** The victim is subjected to extreme sensory deprivation and isolation in a cell where everything is white and there is no sound.
- **Force feeding:** The victim is fed against his will through a tube used to inject food into the victim's stomach.

Pharmacological Torture

- It uses psychotropic and/or other chemicals to induce pain and cause compliance with the torturer's goals.
- It includes forced ingestion or injection of psychotropic drugs (e.g., dimenhydrinate, R015-4513), or being forced to ingest (or be injected with) chemicals or other products (such as broken glass, heated water or soaps) that cause pain and internal damage.

Sexual Torture

It includes:
- Undress or paraded naked or photographed in humiliating position (usually in women).
- Sexual assault like rape/gang rape, fellatio or forced masturbation, sodomy (usually in males).
- Forced abortion.
- Pinching or biting off nipples.
- Electric baton shock of nipples and vagina.
- Inserting bottles and rods inside the vagina.
- Psychological assault, like forced nakedness, sexual humiliation or forced witness of sexual torture.

It is usual for the torturer to use more than one method to traumatize the victim.

Sequelae of Torture

i. Physical problems can be wide-ranging, e.g., STDs including AIDS, musculoskeletal pain, fractures, brain injury, post-traumatic epilepsy or chronic pain syndromes.
ii. Psychological includes post-traumatic stress disorder (PTSD), phobia, sleep disturbances, irritability, aggressiveness, sexual problems, suicide ideation, depression and anxiety disorder.
iii. Social sequele includes loss of job, stigma or rejection by society.

Management: Treatment of torture victims might require expertise and often specialized experience. Common treatments are psychotropic medication, e.g., SSRI antidepressants, counseling, cognitive behavioral therapy, family systems therapy and physiotherapy.

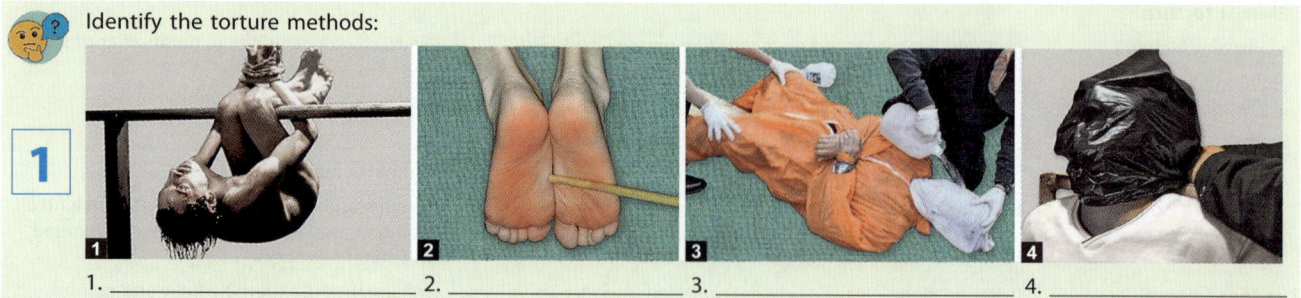

Identify the torture methods:
1. _____ 2. _____ 3. _____ 4. _____

MEDICAL PRACTITIONER AND TORTURE

At times, medicine and medical practitioners have been drawn into the ranks of torturers, either to judge what victims can endure, to apply treatments which will enhance torture, or as torturers in their own right. Medical torture may involve the use of their expert knowledge to facilitate interrogation or corporal punishment, in the conduct of unethical human experimentation, or in providing professional medical sanction and approval for the torture of prisoners.

Torture is often difficult to prove, particularly when some time has passed between the event and a medical examination. Many torturers around the world use methods designed to have a maximum psychological impact, while leaving only minimal physical traces.

Medical and Human Rights Organizations worldwide have collaborated to produce the *Istanbul Protocol*, a document designed to outline common torture methods, consequences of torture and medico-legal examination techniques. Typically, deaths due to torture are shown in an autopsy as being due to 'natural causes' like heart attack due to extreme stress.

Legal aspects: Apart from various sections relating to injury, assault and homicide, *Secs. 330 and 331 IPC* deals with voluntarily causing hurt and grievous hurt respectively for the purpose of extorting confession or any information which may lead to the detection of an offense or misconduct.

- Offenses under these sections are cognizable and non-compoundable; punishment for hurt is imprisonment for 7 years and fine, and for grievous hurt, imprisonment for 10 years and fine.

> **FM 3.31**
> Describe and discuss guidelines and Protocols of National Human Rights Commission regarding torture.

National Human Rights Commission Guidelines

The National Human Rights Commission was created by the Act of Union Parliament—the Protection of Human Rights Act, 1993.

1. Cases of death in police action are to be reported to the Commission by the SSP/SP of the district within 48 h of the incident.
2. Cases of custodial deaths/rapes are to be reported to the Commission by the DM and SPs within 24 h of their occurrence.
3. Chief Ministers and Administrators are required to send a 6 monthly statement of all cases of deaths in police action in the States/UTs to the Commission.
4. Women police officers should be associated where the arrested person is a woman. The arrest of women between sunset and sunrise should be avoided.
5. Where children or juveniles are arrested, no force or beatings should be administered.
6. The arrested person can demand that a friend/relative/person known to him be informed of the fact of his arrest and the place of his detention.
7. Whenever some person is arrested by police, there must be proper entry in Daily Dairy Report (DDR).
8. It is mandatory for the police to send the arrestee remanded to the police custody for medical examination by a doctor on the panel of approved doctors and is to be repeated every 48 h.
9. The person under arrest must be produced before the appropriate court within 24 h of the arrest (Secs. 56 and 57 CrPC).
10. The arrested person should be permitted to meet his lawyer at any time during the interrogation.
11. The interrogation should be conducted in a clearly identifiable place, which is accessible, and the relatives/friend of the person must be informed of the place of interrogation.
12. 'Lie detector test' should not be administered without the consent of the accused. Consent should be recorded before a Judicial Magistrate and the accused should be duly represented by a lawyer.

> **FM 2.15**
> Describe special protocols for conduction of medico-legal autopsies in cases of death in custody or following violation of human rights as per National Human Rights Commission (NHRC) guidelines.

CUSTODIAL DEATHS

Definition: Death in custody (Latin *custosodis*: guardian) should include the following categories:
i. The death of a person in prison/police custody.
ii. The death of a person is caused or contributed by traumatic injuries sustained, or by lack of proper care while in custody or detention.
iii. The death of a person in the process of police or prison officers attempting to detain that person.
iv. The death of a person in the process of escaping or attempting to escape from prison/police custody.

- The postmortem report is the most valuable record and considerable importance is placed on this document in drawing conclusions about the death, and hence should be carried out properly without inordinate delay in writing.
- A meticulous autopsy is needed to confirm or dispel the allegations of custodial deaths.
- Exhaustive notes must be made, including the description of how the deceased was identified.
- While dissecting, there may be many more injuries in the deeper tissues which may not be detected during external examination, particularly, the fresh deep bruises in the muscles in the back of the body or in the sole and palm. In this regard, the **Cosmetic Autopsy Incision** (developed by *Dr AJ Patowary*) is of much help where the whole circumference of the body can be visualized. For the limbs, it can be extended a little bit to expose the limbs up to the sole of foot and the palm of hands to note all the hidden injuries.

National Human Rights Commission (NHRC) Guidelines

In cases of custodial death/rapes and encounter deaths, guidelines of NHRC are:

- **Reporting:** In every case of custodial death/rape, a magisterial inquiry has to be conducted, and to report within 24 h of occurrence.
- In order to help in proper assessment of 'time since death', determination of rectal temperature and development of rigor mortis at the time of first examination at the scene is essential by a medical officer or a trained police officer.
- **Precautions to be taken:** Both the hands of the deceased should be wrapped in white paper bags and the body should be covered in 'special body bags' having zip pouches for proper transportation. Clothing should not be removed by the police or any

other person as it must be examined, preserved and sealed by the doctor conducting the autopsy. It should be sent for further examination at the FSL, a detailed note regarding examination of the clothing is to be incorporated in the postmortem examination by the concerned doctor.

- **Autopsy form:** To ensure better quality of postmortem and to plug the loopholes, a 'model autopsy form' has been prepared by the Commission with its recommendation to circulate to the States and UTs.
- **Video filming:** To prevent tampering and to supplement the postmortem report, video recording of postmortem examination is to be done. This will rule out any undue influence or suppression of material information and to facilitate an independent review of the examination at a later stage, if required. At the time of video recording, the voice of the doctor should be recorded and must narrate his prima-facie observation while conducting the postmortem examination.
- In case of alleged firearms death, the body should be subjected to radiological examination (X-ray/CT scan) prior to autopsy. While describing the injuries, the distance from heel, as well as midline must be taken in respect of each injury which will help later in reconstruction of events.
- **Photographs:** A total of 20–25 colored photographs of the whole body should be taken and some photographs should be without removing the clothes. The photographs should include profile photo—face (front, right lateral, left lateral views), back of head, front of body (up to torso—chest and abdomen) and back, upper and lower extremity—front and back, focusing on each injury/lesion—zoomed in after properly numbering the injuries, internal examination findings (two photos of soles and palms each, after making incision to show absence/evidence of any old/deep seated injury) **(Figs. 32.1A and B)**.

The photographs should be taken after incorporating postmortem number, date of examination and a scale for dimension in the frame of the photographs itself and the camera must be held at right angle to the object being photographed, and the video filming and photography of the postmortem examination should be done by a person trained in forensic photography and videography with a good quality camera having 10X optical zoom and minimum 10 MP.

- After the postmortem examination, the viscera may be sent for examination. The postmortem reports and other related documents should be sent to the Commission without waiting for the viscera report (such reports take time in being received) with the latter being sent subsequently as soon as it is available. It recommended that the facility for chemical analysis should be provided at the center so that undue delay in submitting the postmortem report could be avoided.
- All reports, viz. postmortem, videograph and magisterial inquiry reports must be sent to the Commission within 2 months of the incident.

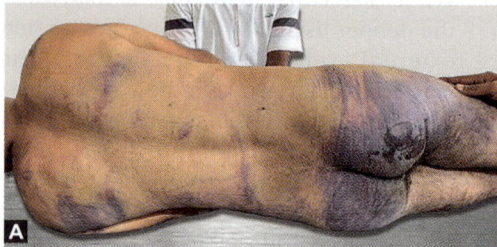 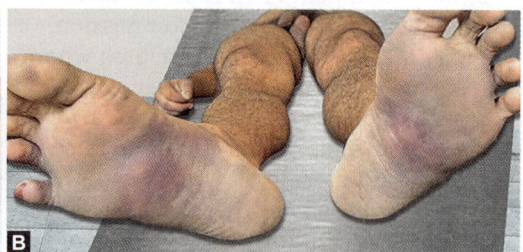

Figs. 32.1A and B: Alleged case of custodial death. Bruises over (A) Back and gluteal region; (B) Soles

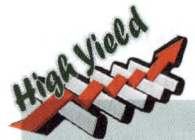

- **Torture:** Deliberate infliction of physical/mental suffering to force a person to yield information, make a confession or for any other reason *(Declaration of Tokyo)*.
- **Falanga (bastinado):** Beating the victim's soles of feet using a thin rod, cane, wooden stick or a similar object.
- **Telefono:** Repeated and simultaneous slapping of both the ears of the victim by the open palms of the perpetrator.
- **Wet submarine:** Forcing the victim's head repeatedly underwater or in foul liquid.
- **Dry submarino:** Attaching a plastic bag over the victim's head resulting in near-suffocation.
- **Strappado:** Tying the victim's hands behind his waist and then strung up to a ceiling beam by their wrists ("*Palestinian hanging*").
- **Stretching (cheera):** Forcible abduction of the hips.
- **Picana:** Electric shocks are delivered through pointed electrodes to delicate areas such as the nipples, lips or earlobes.
- **Non-invasive diagnostic method to assess torture:** Scintigraphy for bone lesion.

Interesting case

Istanbul Protocol (Case of Baki Erdogan, 1993)

Baki Erdogan, a 29-year-old university graduate in Turkey was arrested by the anti-terror department in August 1993 **(Fig. A)**. The police held him incommunicado as a dissident. He was taken to hospital after 11 days of custody and died the same day. The official autopsy stated that he died of acute pulmonary edema as a result of a 10-day hunger strike. They did not let Erdogan's father to attend the autopsy. The Turkish Medical Association investigated the death and conducted a second autopsy and submitted a report that contradicted the autopsy and official forensic report.

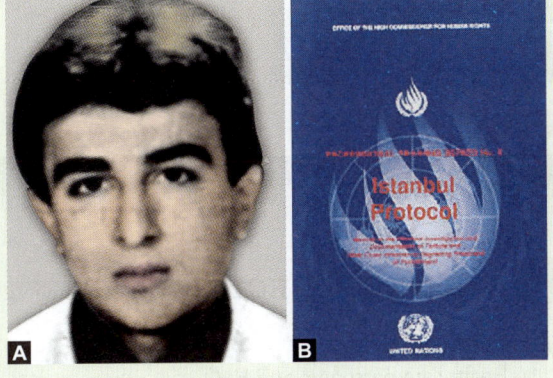

The investigation was based on the UN Manual on the Effective Prevention and Investigation of Extra-legal, Arbitrary and Summary Executions (the 'Minnesota Protocol'). It claimed there were several deficiencies and inaccuracies in the autopsy, and faults with the official medical experts' assessments of Erdogan. The conclusion was Erdogan died from blunt force trauma due to torture resulting in Acute Respiratory Distress Syndrome (ARDS). After this report, six police officers were sentenced to imprisonment on charges of torturing him to death.

After successfully challenging the case, the Turkish Medical Association hosted an international meeting and work began on a manual for the investigation and documentation of torture and other forms of ill treatment. The result was the production of the Istanbul Protocol or "The Manual on Effective Investigation and Documentation of Torture and Other Cruel, Inhuman or Degrading Treatment or Punishment"—the first set of international guidelines for documentation of torture and its consequences **(Fig. B)**. The Istanbul Protocol was finalized in 1999, reported in The Lancet and is now published in several languages in the Professional Training Series of the Office of the UN High Commissioner for Human Rights. The Istanbul Protocol is now an internationally recognized guideline for medical and legal experts.

CHAPTER 33

Medico-legal Aspects of HIV

LEARNING OBJECTIVES

Desirable to know
1. Healthcare personnel and HIV
2. Partner notification
3. Blood donation and HIV
4. HIV and AIDS Act, 2017

Describe and discuss the ethics related to HIV patients.

Hospital and healthcare workers are concerned about the transmission of acquired immunodeficiency syndrome (AIDS) from the patient's blood and body fluids. Patients are concerned that they may be exposed to AIDS from healthcare workers or other patients in the hospital-setting.

Body fluids responsible for transmitting HIV include blood, semen, vaginal secretions, breast milk, and cerebrospinal, peritoneal, amniotic, pericardial and synovial fluids. Other fluids, such as saliva, tears and urine are not implicated in the transmission of HIV, unless they contain visible blood.

HIV TESTING POLICY

Testing can be:
 i. Compulsory
 ii. Mandatory
 iii. Voluntary.

- For *compulsory testing* to be legally acceptable, there must be a strong public interest that overrides the individual's right to privacy, e.g., HIV testing of all military recruits, compulsory screening of prison inmates or applicants for immigration.
- *Mandatory testing* is recommended only for screening donors of blood, semen, organs or tissues in order to prevent transmission of HIV to the recipient of the biological products. In Andhra Pradesh, legislation was passed, making the AIDS/HIV test mandatory for all persons of marriageable age.

National AIDS Control Organization (NACO) Guidelines

The American Medical Association advises against mandatory testing, and recommends voluntary informed consent testing of patients in the high-risk groups undergoing surgery or other invasive procedures. Some States in the US allow nonconsensual antibody testing of hospital patients, when healthcare providers are immediately threatened by exposure to disease.

As per NACO policy, *HIV testing is to be carried out on a voluntary basis* with appropriate pre-test and post-test counseling. Moreover, the disclosure of HIV status of the person should not in any way affect his rights to employment, position at the workplace, right to medical care and other fundamental rights.

- HIV positive women should have the complete choice to make decisions about pregnancy and childbirth, and proper counseling should be given to them to enable them to decide whether to continue or terminate the pregnancy.
- They should be advocated to avoid pregnancy as there is a one in three chance of having an infected child.
- There should be no forcible abortion or even sterilization.
- As far as the breast-feeding is concerned, it may result in transmission of HIV from mother to child.

HIV Testing

- The result of the HIV test must be kept confidential, and even healthcare workers who are not directly involved in the care of the patient should not be told about the result.

- Surveillance of HIV positive cases in the country does not require reporting of the identification data of the patient.
- Purpose of HIV surveillance is to measure the level and trends of HIV infection in a given geographical area over a period of time.

HEALTHCARE WORKERS AND HIV INFECTION

A sensitive question is whether an employer, particularly a healthcare employer may screen employees for HIV infection and refuse to employ, terminate employment or limit employment of people who are seropositive.

The Government of India has issued a comprehensive HIV testing policy and the following issues are reiterated here:
- No individual should be made to undergo a mandatory testing for HIV.
- No mandatory HIV testing should be imposed as a precondition for employment or for providing healthcare facilities during employment.
- Equal rights to education and employment for HIV positive persons.
- HIV status to be kept confidential.

Healthcare workers who are known to have antibodies to the virus might be advised to refrain from participating in certain surgical procedures.
- When a healthcare provider is seropositive or develops AIDS, the hospital should review the staff's privileges and determine whether or not the medical condition interferes with the person's ability to perform the job, and whether the condition creates a health risk to the patients.
- The healthcare provider's performance must be continuously monitored and evaluated with the goal of protecting the patient.
- It has been recognized that certain direct patient care areas, such as surgery, may create an increased risk of transmission of HIV from the doctor to the patient. Although, NACO does not recommend that HIV-positive individuals be routinely restricted from performing surgery, it does recommend that the restrictions be determined on a case by case basis.
- There is no generally accepted medical evidence that HIV can be transmitted through normal day-to-day contact in typical private workplace settings. Since, present medical evidence indicates that the HIV infected individuals pose virtually no threat of infection to fellow workers, HIV-positive persons in most settings may be permitted to continue their employment as long as they are able to perform their job.

The Centers for Disease Control (CDC), estimates that 5.5% of all HIV positive persons are employed in the healthcare field. According to the guidelines issued by CDC, with the exception of healthcare workers and personal service workers who use instruments that pierce the skin, no testing or restriction is indicated for workers known to be infected with HIV, but otherwise able to perform their jobs.

PARTNER NOTIFICATION (CONTACT TRACING/ PARTNER COUNSELING)

It refers to activities aimed at identifying, notifying and counseling the sexual and needle sharing partners of an individual with HIV ('*index person*') about their exposure, and offering services.

There are two approaches to partner notification:
i. **Patient referral:** HIV-positive persons are encouraged to notify partners of their possible exposure to HIV, without the direct involvement of healthcare providers.
ii. **Provider referral:** HIV-positive persons give partners' names to healthcare providers or other health workers, who then confidentially notify the partners directly.

There are two approaches to informing third parties:
i. **Contact tracing:** The contact tracing approach emerged from sexually transmitted disease programmes. It is based on the patient's voluntary cooperation in providing the names of contacts, this entailed protecting the absolute confidentiality of the entire notification process, without disclosure of the identity of the index case.
ii. **Duty to warn:** This approach came out of the clinical situation where the physician knew the identity of the person deemed to be at risk, e.g., sexual partner of an HIV positive individual. It argued for disclosure to endangered persons without consent of the patient, due to his moral 'duty to warn'. It could also involve the revelation of the patient's identity.

Patient confidentiality continues to be a central issue, even in those subjects in whom the 'duty to warn' tradition has been invoked.
- Persons unknowingly placed at risk from an ethical perspective of a clinical relationship, have a moral right to information in order to protect themselves, seek testing and commence treatment, if necessary.
- Since, most public health strategies for dealing with HIV are based on individuals coming forward voluntarily for testing, counseling and treatment, failure to maintain confidentiality could threaten the continued cooperation of people with HIV.

Neither the principle of confidentiality nor the value attached to professional autonomy is absolute. Early identification of HIV infection in asymptomatic individuals has become increasingly beneficial with the availability of antiviral therapy and prophylactic antimicrobial agents.

Today, however, it is almost universally recognized that partner notification programs can make a positive contribution to a successful HIV/AIDS public health and prevention program, particularly with regard to persons who may be unaware that they are at any increased risk of HIV infection, and as a result are not informed or aware of any need to practice risk-reducing behavior. Partner notification programs can encourage these persons to seek HIV testing.

> **NOTA BENE**
>
> The Supreme Court of India has recently ruled for disclosure of the HIV positive status by the doctor to his patient's wife/spouse. Though, the decision has correctly dealt with the legal position of when confidentiality of a patient should be breached by the doctor, it has not laid down the parameters around which such disclosure should or should not be made. The judgment went on to state that persons with HIV infection who knowingly expose others to health risk are guilty of an offense punishable under law.

CLINICAL TRIALS AND HIV

The highest ethical standards must be upheld when collecting behavioral or biological data on sexually transmitted infections, including HIV/AIDS. Because of the stigma and human rights issues around HIV/AIDS, study participants may experience psychological, social, physical or economic harm, even when precautions are taken. Data collection protocols or procedures should include an explicit description of the measures that will be taken to protect the subjects.

BLOOD DONATION AND HIV

It is mandatory for every unit of blood collected at blood banks in India to undergo screening and test negative for HIV-1 and HIV-2 prior to being declared fit for transfusion and/or further processing for preparation of blood products and blood components. The result of such testing must be clearly indicated on the label.

According to guidelines laid by the Government of India, the status of HIV should not be disclosed to blood donor. The intention is to spare him of the agony of knowing the helplessness of his situation. If the blood drawn is positive, it should be discarded. Once blood sample is drawn, the register of patient identities should be kept separate and samples identified only with a code number. If the donor wants to know the result of HIV test, he should be referred to an accessible HIV testing center where supplemental tests with counseling will be offered to him.

Legal Aspects

HIV positive person has the right to marry, but only after obtaining informed consent from their prospective spouse prior to marriage. A person who knowingly communicates the disease of AIDS to other person by sexual relations or otherwise, will be guilty of an offense under **Sec. 269 IPC** (imprisonment for 6 months with/without fine) or **Sec. 270 IPC** (imprisonment for 2 years with/without fine). The conduct in order to be punishable must be malicious or negligent, so as to cause the spread of an infectious disease dangerous to life.

A civil suit may be filed to claim compensation for violation of the fundamental rights to personal liberty.

Test and Treat Policy for HIV

Ministry of Health and Family Welfare, Government of India launched this policy in 2017. According to this policy, as soon as a person is tested and found positive for HIV, he will be treated with antiretroviral therapy (ART), irrespective of the CD4 count or clinical stage. This will improve longevity, improve quality of life of those infected and will save them from many opportunistic infections, especially tuberculosis.

The Human Immunodeficiency Virus (HIV) and Acquired Immune Deficiency Syndrome (AIDS) (Prevention and Control) Act, 2017

This Act was passed in April 2017 for prohibition of discrimination, informed consent, non-disclosure of HIV status, antiretroviral therapy and opportunistic infection management, protection of property of affected children, safe working environment and appointment of ombudsman in every state. The main provisions of the act are:

1. **Prohibition of discrimination:** No person shall discriminate against the infected person on any ground, namely:
   a. the denial of, or termination from employment or occupation, unless such person poses a significant risk of transmission of HIV to other person in the workplace, or is unfit to perform the duties of the job;
   b. unfair treatment in employment or occupation;
   c. the denial/discontinuation/unfair treatment in:
      - healthcare services
      - educational establishments
      - right to reside, purchase, rent, any property
      - stand for, or hold public or private office
      - provision of insurance, etc.
   d. the denial of access to, removal from, or unfair treatment in Government or private establishment in whose care or custody a person may be;
   e. the isolation or segregation of a protected person;
   f. HIV testing as a pre-requisite for obtaining employment, or accessing healthcare services or education or for the continuation of the same.
2. **Informed consent for undertaking HIV test or treatment:** No HIV test shall be undertaken or performed upon any person; or no infected person shall be subject to medical treatment, medical interventions or research, except with the informed consent of such person or his/her representative. The informed consent for HIV test shall include pre-test and post-test counselling to the person being tested or such person's representative. The informed consent for conducting an HIV test *shall not be required*:
   a. where a court determines, by an order that the carrying out of the HIV test of any person either as part of a medical examination or otherwise, is

necessary for the determination of issues in the matter before it;
b. for procuring, processing, distribution or use of a human body or any part thereof including tissues, blood, semen or other body fluids for use in medical research or therapy, but the test report will not be shared with the donor;
c. for epidemiological or surveillance purposes where the HIV test is anonymous and is not for the purpose of determining the HIV status of a person;
d. for screening purposes in any licensed blood bank.

3. **Disclosure of HIV status:** No person shall be compelled to disclose his HIV status except by an order of the court that the disclosure of such information is necessary in the interest of justice. Also no person shall disclose or be compelled to disclose the HIV status of other person except with the informed consent of that other person or his representative. The informed consent for disclosure of HIV-related information is not required where the disclosure is made by a healthcare provider to another healthcare provider who is involved in the care, treatment or counselling of such person, when such disclosure is necessary to provide care or treatment to that person.

4. **Disclosure of HIV-positive status to partner of HIV-positive person:** A healthcare provider may disclose the HIV positive status of a person (after informing the person) under his direct care to his/her partner, if such healthcare provider reasonably believes that the partner is at the significant risk of transmission of HIV from such person who in spite of being counseled, has not informed such partner. Such disclosures should be made in person after counselling, provided that such healthcare provider shall have no obligation to identify or locate the partner of an HIV-positive person. The healthcare provider shall not be liable for any criminal or civil action for any disclosure or non-disclosure of confidential HIV-related information made to a partner.

5. **Duty to prevent transmission of HIV:** Every person, who is HIV-positive and has been counseled in accordance with the guidelines issued or is aware of the nature of HIV and its transmission, shall take all reasonable precautions to prevent the transmission of HIV to other persons.

6. **Confidentiality of data:** Every establishment keeping the records of HIV-related information shall adopt data protection measures.

7. **Women and children infected with HIV or AIDS:** The Central/State Government shall take measures to counsel and provide information regarding the outcome of pregnancy and HIV-related treatment to the HIV infected women. No HIV positive woman, who is pregnant, shall be subjected to sterilisation or abortion without obtaining her informed consent.

Interesting case

Partner Notification (The Tarasoff Case, 1969)

In 1967, Prosenjit Poddar (**Fig. A**), an Indian graduate student at the University of California met another university student named Tatiana Tarasoff (**Fig. B**) at a folk dancing class on campus. They went on several dates, but soon disagreed on the seriousness of their relationship. He became obsessed with her and began stalking her. Poddar underwent an emotional crisis and began psychological counseling at the university medical center.

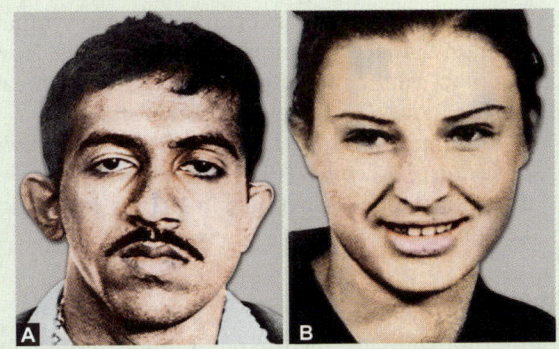

Poddar's therapist became alarmed when he confessed his intention of killing her. The psychologist believed him and notified the campus police, requesting that they have him committed. They briefly detained him, but he was soon released as he appeared to be rational and promised to stay away from her. At the order of the psychologist's superior, a psychiatrist, no further steps were taken to commit (restrict) Poddar or warn Tatiana.

In October, 1969, Poddar confronted her and she attempted to flee. He pursued her and then stabbed her to death with the kitchen knife he had been carrying. He went on trial and was found guilty of second-degree murder. He served five years in prison until a lawyer successfully appealed the conviction. Poddar was then deported to India.

Shortly after his release, Tarasoff's parents brought a civil suit against the therapists and the University of California for failure to warn them or Tatiana of her danger and for negligently failing to confine (physically restrain) Poddar. The therapists defended their actions on the grounds of their duty to their patient over a private third party and the trial court agreed with them. After the plaintiffs appealed this decision, the California Supreme Court reviewed the case and finally handed down what would become a landmark decision in 1976. In ruling the case of *Tarasoff vs. Regents of the University of California*, the court determined that the need for therapists to protect the public was more important that protecting client-therapist confidentiality. The therapists have a duty to protect potential victims if their patients made threats or otherwise behaved as if they presented a 'serious danger of violence to another'. With Tarasoff, a matter of professional discretion became a legal obligation. The Tarasoff ruling formed the basis of partner notification.

CHAPTER 34

Newer Techniques and Recent Advances

LEARNING OBJECTIVES

Desirable to know
1. Polygraph
2. Brain fingerprinting
3. Narco-analysis
4. Facial reconstruction
5. Crime search methods

Enumerate the indications and describe the principles and appropriate use of polygraph (lie detector), brain mapping and narcoanalysis.

POLYGRAPH

A **polygraph** (*'lie detector'*) is a device which makes a continuous record of several physiological variables, such as *blood pressure*, *heart rate*, *respiration* and *electrodermal reaction*,* while a series of questions are being asked, in an attempt to detect lies **(Fig. 34.1)**. The above measurements are believed to be indicators of anxiety due to sympathetic stimulation that accompanies the telling of lies. However, if the subject exhibits anxiety for other reasons, a measured response can result in unreliable conclusions.

♦ A polygraph test is also known as a *psychophysiological detection of deception* (PDD) examination.
♦ The polygraph was invented in 1921 by John Augustus Larson.

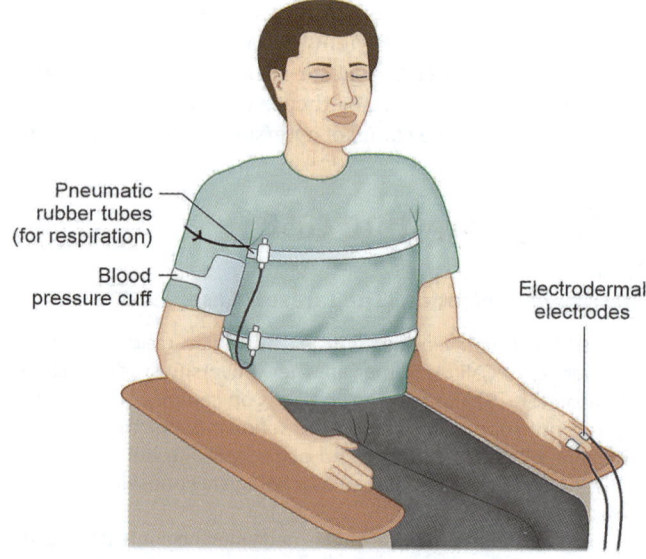

Fig. 34.1: Polygraph test

Procedure

There are two major testing techniques in use—(1) the Relevant/Irrelevant Technique (RIT), and (2) the Control Question Technique (CQT). Polygraph test starts with a pre-test interview to gain some preliminary information which will later be used for 'control questions' (CQ). Some of the questions asked are 'irrelevant' or IR, others are 'probable-lie' control questions that most people will lie about, and the remainder are the 'relevant questions', or RQ, that the tester is really interested in. The different types of questions may alternate.

Accuracy

Examiners maintain that the accuracy is 90% and the errors tend to be false negative rather than false positive, i.e., a person who actually lied is reported as 'truthful'.

Uses

1. Polygraph is useful to the police in the investigation of crime (usually sexual assaults) since it can help clear innocent persons and thus screen and eliminate suspects.

---
* It is also known as **galvanic skin response (GSR)**, **electrodermal response (EDR)** or **skin conductance response (SCR)**—a method of measuring the electrical conductance of the skin, which varies with its moisture level.

2. It can be used for security screening to identify individuals who present serious threats to national security.
3. Polygraph is used for screening of employees for government organizations.
4. It is also used for pre-employment screening in law enforcement and national security agencies.

BRAIN FINGERPRINTING (BRAIN MAPPING)

Brain mapping is a group of neuroscience techniques based on the mapping of quantities or properties (biological) onto spatial representations of the brain.

While various brain imaging techniques (e.g., CT, MRI, PET, SPECT) measure properties such as cerebral blood flow, metabolism or structural integrity, whilst QEEG (quantitative EEG) measures electrical activity of the brain which is known as *brain mapping*.

Brain fingerprinting, invented by *Lawrence Farwell*, is a computer-based test that is designed to discover, document and provide evidence of guilty knowledge regarding crimes. This test detects the presence or absence of information, and not guilt or innocence *per se*.

Procedure

- An elastic cap (headband) with 19 electronic sensors is placed on the shaven scalp of the subject and connected to the recording device that measures the EEG. The subject is shown stimuli consisting of sounds, words, phrases or pictures on a computer screen.
- It detects response to the stimuli related to the crime or other investigated situation. The theory is that the suspect's reaction to the details of an event or activity will reflect, if the suspect had prior knowledge of the event or activity. As the test is based on EEG signals, it does not require the subject to issue verbal responses to questions or stimuli.

Principle

Farwell's brain fingerprinting originally used the *P300 brain response* (emitted from an individual's brain approximately 300 milliseconds after it is confronted with a stimulus of special significance) to detect the brain's recognition of the known information. Later, he used the *MERMER* ('Memory and Encoding Related Multifaceted Electroencephalographic Response'), which includes the P300 and additional features and is reported to provide a higher level of accuracy than the P300 alone.

Uses

i. **Criminal cases:** Investigators use it to determine if a suspect is telling the truth or make him reveal facts pertaining to a case.
ii. **Medical diagnosis:** Brain functioning evaluation for early detection of Alzheimer's and other cognitive degenerative diseases.
iii. **Advertisement:** Evaluates the effectiveness of advertising by measuring brain responses.
iv. **National security:** Screening employees, especially in military and foreign intelligence and counter-terrorism.
v. **Insurance fraud**.

Drawbacks

The test may not be useful in a case in which:
- Two suspects were present at a crime—one as a witness and the other a perpetrator.
- Investigators do not have sufficient information about a crime so as to test a suspect for crime-relevant information stored in the brain.

Brain Fingerprinting vs Polygraph

Since, it depends only on information stored in the brain and cognitive brain responses, brain fingerprinting does not depend on the emotions of the subject, nor it is affected by emotional responses. Polygraph is fundamentally different from the brain fingerprinting as it measures emotion-based physiological signals. Also, unlike polygraph testing, it does not attempt to determine whether or not the subject is lying or telling the truth.

> **NOTA BENE**
> **Brain Signature Profiling (BSP) or BEOS** is another EEG procedure which was developed in 2003 by *CR Mukundan* which is similar to brain fingerprinting.

NARCO-ANALYSIS

Definition: It is a scientific procedure to obtain information from an individual in a natural sleep-like state.

Principle

The narco-analysis procedure dwells upon the effect of bio-molecules on the bioactivity of an individual.
- A person is able to lie by using his imagination. During the test, the subject's imagination is neutralized by making him semi-conscious. In this state, it becomes difficult for him to lie, and his answers would be restricted to facts he is already aware of.
- The subject is not in a position to speak up on his own, but can answer specific and simple questions.
- In such sleep-like state, efforts are made to obtain 'probative truth' about the crime.

Procedure

The individual is put to trance-like state and loses all his inhibitions by administering *sodium amytal or thiopentone sodium* (known as '**truth drug**' or '**truth serum**') 2.5–5% solution, slow IV.

Other Methods

- 0.5 mg scopolamine hydrobromide (commonly used) subcutaneously, followed by 0.25 mg every 20 minutes (average 3–6 injections), till proper stage of questioning is reached.
- 100 mg secobarbital sodium, 15 mg morphine and 0.5 mg of scopolamine hydrobromide may be given iv.

The dose is dependent on the person's sex, age, health and physical condition. A wrong dose can result in a person going into a coma or even death.

Team required: A team comprising of an anesthetist, psychiatrist, clinical/forensic psychologist, audio-videographer and supporting nursing staff does the test. The forensic psychologist will prepare the report about the revelations along with audio-video recordings.

Uses

1. The test is used by investigators to cross check their findings, determine if a suspect is telling the truth or make him reveal facts pertaining to a case.
2. It can be used for restoring speech to mute persons.
3. In case of amnesia, narco-analysis helps in reviving memory.
4. It can be used for expression of suppressed or repressed thought or conflict.

Legal Aspects

- Supreme Court has declared that deception detection tests such as narco-analysis, polygraph tests and brain-mapping cannot be done without the consent of the individual. If the person consents for such methods, then any information obtained can be used for further probe. *Results of such tests will not be admissible as evidence, even if done with consent.*
- Use of such methods are illegal and as against constitution. As per Article 20(3) of the Constitution 'No person accused of any offense shall be compelled to be a witness against himself'. Therefore, a suspect of the crime cannot be compelled to disclose facts which he can recall from his memory, and likely to implicate him in a crime in which he was involved.

FM 7.1
Enumerate the indications and describe the principles and appropriate use for facial reconstruction.

FACIAL RECONSTRUCTION

- Facial reconstruction is the process of recreating the face of an unidentified individual from their skeletal remains through a combination of both scientific methods and artistic skills.
- The goal of craniofacial reconstruction (CFR) is to recreate a likeness with the face of missing individuals which may help to identify the missing person.
- CFR is a combination of science and art.

Indications

a. Identification of an individual where the conventional/usual methods of identification (dental records examination, radiography, DNA analysis) are unsuccessful.
b. Identify the faces of the people from the ancient times, bone remains and embalmed bodies.

Prerequisites

- Before proceeding with CFR, the forensic artist need to consult many different specialists, for e.g., forensic anthropologists for estimation of age, sex and stature; forensic dentist for any racial characteristics or any unusual dental traits or anomalies.
- The police may provide information concerning items found at the recovery scene like hair, eye glasses, clothing or jewelry.

Methods for CFR can be classified into two types:

1. **Two-dimensional reconstruction:** This method used to recreate a face from the life size photographs of the skull with the use of soft tissue depth estimates. It is basically a sketch of the unidentified person.
2. **Three-dimensional manual reconstruction:** In manual methods, facial reconstruction is done by using clay, plasticine or wax directly on a replica of the victim's skull. In the computerized method, computer software produces reconstruction by using scanned and stock photographs.

3D Facial Reconstruction Methods

1. **Anthropometerical American method/Tissue depth method:** In this method, soft tissue depth data is considered. This method requires highly trained personnel and was commonly used by law enforcement agencies. It is not preferred now-a-days.
2. **Anatomical Russian method:** In this technique, soft tissue depth data was not considered but facial muscles were used in anatomical position. Reconstruction was done by shaping muscles, glands and cartilage onto the skull layer by layer. This technique is not commonly used.
3. **Manchester or combination method:** Most accepted method for facial reconstruction. In this technique, soft tissue thickness and facial muscles are taken into account.
4. **Computerized facial reconstruction:** With the development of software for computer based CFR

methods, automated creation of multiple reconstructions from the image of the skull using different modeling assumptions (like age, BMI, ancestry, sex) became possible. As a result, the computer-generated CFR process becomes accessible to a wide range of people without the need for extensive expertise.

Recent Advances

Artificial intelligence (AI) is the replication of human intellect in computers that are programmed to think, act, and imitate our behaviors—the science of computer algorithms that can learn and improve over time.
- It allows the software to anticipate outcomes accurately without having to be trained to do so.
- AI is frequently considered a subset of machine learning.
- Forensic specialist can automate their procedures with AI, allowing them to swiftly identify information and insights, saving time in the process.

Uses in Forensic Science
1. AI can be used to analyze digital evidence such as images and videos by detecting objects or faces within them. This will help investigators quickly narrow down their search and zero in on potential suspects more efficiently.
2. Deep learning algorithms analyze images from crime scenes for specific objects or patterns that may go unnoticed by the investigators.
3. **AI-enhanced virtual autopsy:** Machine learning tools will take the images of the body with the help of CT/MRI. The machine will then identify the pathological condition of an organ from the images by comparing, process the input data provided and will draw the conclusion regarding the disease condition of the organs and the cause of death.
4. Various markers in blood can be used to predict the time since death after being processed through an AI device.
5. Improves the likelihood of detecting lies (automated lie detection systems) and investigating cybercrime.

> **FM 2.18**
> Describe and discuss the objectives of crime scene visit, the duties and responsibilities of doctors on crime scene and the reconstruction of sequence of events after crime scene investigation.

CRIME SCENE INVESTIGATION

- **Crime scene:** Any location that may be associated with a committed crime.
- **Crime scene investigation** involves the use and integration of scientific methods, physical evidence, and deductive reasoning in order to determine and establish the series of events surrounding a crime.
- **Preservation:** A crime scene is preserved by setting up a blockade to control the movement in and out of a scene, as well as maintaining the scene's integrity and prevent contamination of evidence.
- **Types of crime scene:** Different types of crime scenes include outdoors, indoor and conveyance. It can be primary (area/place where the incident occurred) or secondary (area/place where physical evidence related to the incident is found).
- **Search methods:** The most commonly used search methods are geometric patterns: (a) Link, (b) Line or strip, (c) Grid, (d) Zone, (e) Wheel or ray, and (f) Spiral methods (**Table 34.1**). Each has some advantages and disadvantages and some are better suited for outside than indoor.
- **Documentation:** Photographs of all evidence are taken before anything is touched or moved. Evidence markers are placed next to each piece of evidence allowing for organization of the evidence. Sketching

TABLE 34.1: Types of search methods

Method	Procedure	Representation
Link method	*Most common method*, based upon the linkage theory; one type of evidence leads to another item; works with any scene (indoor/outdoor; small/large)	
Line/strip method	Works best in large, outdoor scenes	
Grid method	Double line search; effective method but time consuming	
Zone method	Best used on scene with defined zones or areas; effective in houses or buildings with rooms	
Wheel/ray method	Used for special situations; best used on small, circular crime scenes	
Spiral method	Inward or outward spirals; best used in crime scenes without physical barriers (e.g., open water)	

the scene is also a form of documentation at a crime scene.
- **Evidence collection:** Evidence comes in many different forms such as fingerprints, guns, bones, blood on knives, etc. It can be anything from a biological sample like blood, or everyday item like receipts or bank statements.
- **Chain of custody:** After evidence has been collected from the scene of the crime, it is placed in its appropriate container and then is labeled or tagged. The tag identifies the specific scene the evidence came from and establishes the 'chain of custody'. The chain of custody refers to the order in which evidence is handled by individuals who are involved in the case's investigation.

Objectives of crime scene visit by the doctor (forensic pathologist/autopsy surgeon):

1. It will provide the doctor with an opportunity to observe the situation and gain firsthand knowledge of circumstantial evidences needed to interpret postmortem findings.
2. It will minimize misinterpretation of facts due to introduction of artifacts due to passage of time.
3. The doctor can help in judiciously selecting biological evidences to be collected in order to achieve maximum utility. Irrational collection of evidences and overburdening the police and FSL staff can be avoided.
4. The doctors can advice regarding the best method of preserving any fragile evidence.
5. It also provides an opportunity to advise for an early analysis of evidence in a particular case, objectives of analysis, precautions in handling or transportation and place where the analysis may be undertaken.

Duties and Responsibilities of a Doctor at the Crime Scene

Prerequisites

1. Formal written requisition should be there before the visit (if not there, it should be made available afterwards on return).
2. On receipt of a request for a visit to scene of crime, a doctor should accompany the team punctually together with other members of the team.
3. He must carry a kit containing surgical gloves, hand lens, clean containers, glass slides, stethoscope, scalpel, measuring tape, chemical thermometer, disposable syringes, paper and plastic envelopes, EDTA and oxalate vials, flashlight, printed body charts and notebook.

At the Crime Scene (Fig. 34.2)

- The death scene should be secured and recorded photographically and diagrammatically.
- A doctor is not supposed to touch anything until the same has been identified, documented and photographed. He has to ask/inform the IO before moving anything. He should not lead but follow the police/detective.
- **Confirmation of death of the victim:** Check for any clinical sign (pulse, breathing and heartbeat) of life. If otherwise, the doctor should call an ambulance immediately, simultaneously doing whatever he can to save the life of the person. Dying declaration must be recorded, if death is eminent.
- **History of the case:** The doctor should try to get a brief history about incidence. An enquiry should be made about original posture and prior manipulation/handling of the body, condition of clothing and surroundings.
- The doctor should advise the photographer for any relevant photographs from medico-legal point of view.
- **Identity and age of the deceased:** Points of identification and age should be noted in unidentified bodies. Details can be recorded at the time of the autopsy.
- **General observations:** Any evidence of struggle, description of clothing and signs of struggle/assault, stains, fibers/hairs or foreign objects found should be noted. Presence of drag marks or shifting of body from some other place must be noted. Blood spatter pattern, quantity and location of blood over the body and/or weapons present at the scene must be described.
- **Evidence of sexual assault:** In case of females, any disturbance or disarray of clothing, injuries around vagina and anus, and evidence of seminal emission should be looked for.
- **Nature of injuries:** It should be noted whether the injuries are from blunt/sharp weapon or firearm, burns, vehicular, presence or absence of defense injuries, etc.
- He should make a sketch of position and condition of body in relation to surroundings and depict relevant details, e.g., injuries in assault cases, ligature material, knot, suspension point in hanging, etc., in body diagrams.

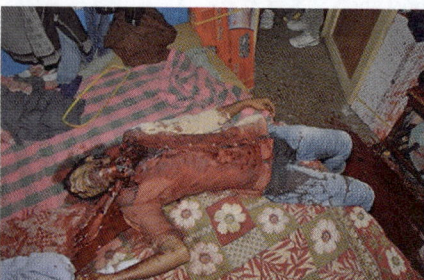 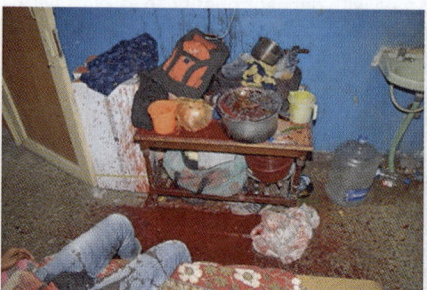 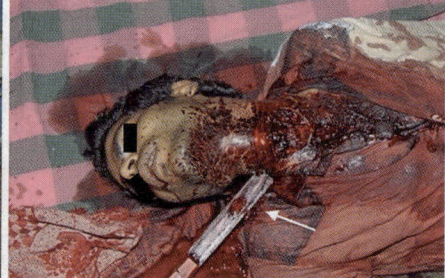

Fig. 34.2: Crime scene of cut throat injury. Note the presence of weapon at the crime scene (arrow)

- In case of poisoning, look for any peculiar odor, frothing from the mouth and nostrils, poison or drug containers lying around, etc.
- Any materials or evidences which are likely to be lost during transportation of body to the mortuary should be collected (loose fibers or hair). Perianal or vaginal swabbing in sexual assault cases, nail scrapings, swabbing of hands in firearm cases, loose ligature material, etc., can be preserved.
- Clothing of the victim should be left in situ which is removed and preserved during detailed autopsy.
- **Time of death:** Note should be made about rigor mortis, PM staining, temperature of the body (rectal temperature), signs of putrefaction to determine time since death.
- **Cause and manner of death:** The doctor should not be in a hurry to opine on the cause and manner of death. A guarded opinion based on experience should be given, and that can be later verified at autopsy. He should not voice unsubstantiated theories on non-medical matters, nor attempt to over-interpret the situation from insufficient facts.
- After complete documentation and collection of evidences, the doctor should supervise the removal and transportation of the body to the mortuary. It is best if the doctor who attends the scene is the one who conducts the autopsy.

Recent Advances
- **Artificial intelligence (AI):** AI is currently being used in digital forensics, analyze a crime scene, compare fingerprint data, and draw conclusions from photograph comparisons.
- **Nanotechnology:** Nanosensors are utilized to examine the presence of illegal drugs, explosive materials, and biological agents at the molecular level.
- **Wet-vacuum sampling device for DNA:** It is a sterile wet-vacuum (M-Vac™) which causes the DNA material to release from the substrate and to capture the cells. Collection solution is sprayed onto the surface while simultaneously being vacuumed off of the surface. It helps in collecting DNA from immovable surfaces, as well as from porous substrates, such as clothing, fabrics, cement or rocks.
- **Carbon dot powders:** Researchers have developed a fluorescent carbon dot powder that can be applied to fingerprints, making them fluorescent under UV light and hence easier to analyze.
- **Proteomes:** Proteomes are a complete set of proteins produced by an organism. Proteomes are found in blood, bones, and other biological materials which can be analyzed to find if a victim came in contact with otherwise undetectable venom or matching a severely degraded body fluid sample to a perpetrator.
- There has been an increase in the use of condoms by sexual offenders either to avoid contacting STDs or to prevent transfer of DNA evidence. However, they are less likely to consider the possibility of condom lubricant transferring onto their fingertips and then into fingerprints left at the scene. Researchers have developed a method wherein they can detect this condom lubricant. They used *MALDI-MSI* (matrix-assisted laser desorption/ionization mass spectrometry imaging), a powerful technology that can be used to map fingerprint ridge patterns.
- Forensic researchers in the UK have devised a method to detect smoking from the chemicals left behind in the fingerprints. The technique involves dusting the prints with a solution of gold nanoparticles, attached to which are antibodies that bind to *cotinine*—a metabolite of nicotine. Then the print is soaked in a fluorescent dye that binds to the antibodies.
- **Genome editing (also called gene editing)** is a group of technologies that give scientists the ability to change an organism's DNA. These technologies allow genetic material to be added, removed, or altered at particular locations in the genome. Several approaches to genome editing have been developed. A well-known one is called CRISPR-Cas9, which is short for clustered regularly interspaced short palindromic repeats and CRISPR-associated protein 9. The cutting-edge gene-editing technique CRISPR enables precise DNA changes within an organism's genome. Its development in the past few years has significantly advanced genetic engineering and biotechnology.

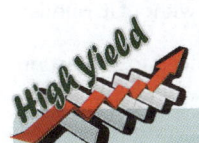

- **Polygraph/lie detector:** Device which infers deception through analysis of physiological responses to a structured but unstandardized series of questions.
- In polygraph test 'GSR' stands for Galvanic Skin Response.
- **Three indicators of polygraph assesses:** Heart rate/BP, respiration and skin conductivity.
- Brain fingerprinting was invented by Lawrence Farwell.
- Brain mapping test is based on EEG signals.
- **Narco-analysis:** Scientific procedure to obtain information from an individual in a natural sleep-like state where he loses all his inhibitions.
- **Father of truth serum:** Robert Ernest House.
- **Commonly used drug for narcoanalysis:** Scopolamine hydrobromide.
- **Truth drug/serum:** Sodium amytal or thiopentone sodium.
- Deception tests such as narco-analysis, polygraph tests and brain-mapping cannot be done without the consent of the individual.
- Results of deception tests are not be admissible as evidence, even if done with consent.
- **Best facial reconstruction method:** Combination Manchester method.
- **Types of crime scene search methods:** Link, grid, strip, wheel, zone and spiral.
- **Most common crime scene search method:** Link method.

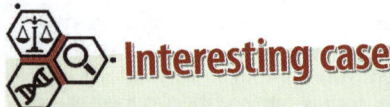

Interesting case

Crime Scene Investigation (Case of Soham Murders, 2002)

On August 4, 2002, Jessica went to a barbecue party at her best friend Holly, both 10-year-old girls living in Soham, Cambridgeshire, UK. After playing and enjoying food, the girls said to Holly's parents they were going upstairs to play. At about 6:15 pm, the girls left the house without informing anyone to buy sweets from a vending machine in a nearby sports center. By 9:55 pm, when their parents could not find the girls anywhere, the girls were reported missing to the police at that same night.

Police immediately launched a massive manhunt to locate the missing children. Next day, Ian Huntley, the caretaker at a local secondary school informed the investigators that he had spoken with the girls before their disappearance the previous afternoon. The two girls enquired about his girlfriend, who was their assistant teacher. After a brief conversation they left and saw the girls walking in the direction of a local library. But police were suspicious about Huntley. Something about his story just did not fit right.

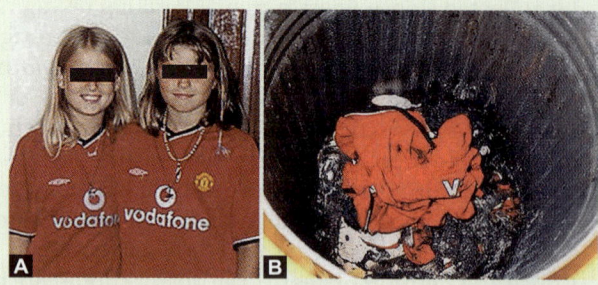

Last photograph before the girls went missing

Charred remains of jerseys which were recovered from a dustbin at Huntley's place of work with his fingerprints on dustbin

During the first week after the girls went missing, he began making media appearances and was involved in the search. He was continually contacting police to see what the status of the investigation was.

After 13 days, the bodies of two girls were found lying side-by-side in a ditch about 10 miles from where the girls went missing. In an apparent effort to destroy evidence, the murderer had attempted to burn both bodies. In addition, no clear footprints were discovered at the crime scene.

The bodies were in an advanced state of decomposition and were partially skeletonized. The pathologist was unable to determine the cause of death of either child, or whether the girls had been sexually assaulted before or after death. The bodies neither showed signs of compressive neck injuries, knife wounds, drugging or poisoning, and that both girls had most likely died of asphyxiation. The bodies of both girls were conclusively identified using DNA testing.

At the crime scene, the forensic botanist found some stinging nettles that were growing new side shoots where the bodies were found which only happens when a plant has been trampled underfoot. An analysis enabled to approximate that the actual time the bodies had been placed at this location to almost two weeks prior, which gave the investigation a timeline for the murder. It also proved that the girls had almost certainly not died at this location where discovered, and that both bodies had been placed at this location within 24 h of their deaths. Besides the nettles, pollen found in a soil sample where the bodied were found further linked to Huntley. Fiber evidence and the soil found inside his car was an exact match to the soil and fiber evidence found where the girls' bodies were dumped.

On August 20, the police arrested and charged Ian Huntley and his girlfriend (she was his alibi) after gathering sufficient physical evidence from his home, vehicle and Soham Village College **(Figs. A and B)**. The evidences from crime scene were important in his conviction. Police and prosecutors were not able to establish a motive for murders, but the case was solid enough without it. Huntley had lured the girls to his house and murdered them before dumping their bodies in a remote ditch.

Huntley was convicted in 2005 of double murder and sentenced to life imprisonment. His girlfriend was sentenced to 3½ years in prison for perverting the course of justice.

SECTION 2

Toxicology

Section Outline

35. General Toxicology   531
36. Corrosive Poisons   549
37. Inorganic Metallic Irritants—Arsenic   557
38. Inorganic Metallic Irritants—Mercury   563
39. Inorganic Metallic Irritants—Lead   568
40. Inorganic Metallic Irritants—Copper   575
41. Inorganic Metallic Irritants—Thallium   579
42. Other Inorganic Metallic Irritants   582
43. Non-metallic Irritants   587
44. Organic Irritants—Plant   592
45. Organic Irritants—Animal   599
46. Somniferous Poisons (Narcotic Poisons)   613
47. Inebriants—Alcohol   620
48. Sedative-hypnotic—Barbiturates   637
49. Deliriants—Dhatura/Datura   641
50. Deliriants—Cannabis   646
51. Deliriants—Cocaine   650
52. Spinal Poisons   654
53. Cardiac Poisons   658
54. Hydrocyanic Acid   666
55. Asphyxiants   671
56. Agricultural Poisons   677
57. Alphos (Aluminum Phosphide)   687
58. Medicinal Poisons   692
59. Drug Dependence and Date Rape Drugs   703
60. Supplement   712
61. Answer Key   737

SECTION 2

Toxicology

CHAPTER 35

General Toxicology

LEARNING OBJECTIVES

Must know
1. Toxicology, poison, xenobiotics, tolerance, idiosyncrasy
2. Classification of poisons (based on mode of action and effects)
3. Duties of a doctor in poisoning cases
4. Treatment of poisoning with unknown substance
5. Physical antidote, activated charcoal, demulcents
6. Gastric lavage, contraindications
7. Chelating agents; universal antidote
8. Dialyzable and non-dialyzable poisons
9. Antidotes in different poisoning
10. Poisons causing miosis and mydriasis
11. Ideal suicidal and homicidal poison (Diff.)
12. Diagnosis of poisoning in dead
13. Color of PM staining and odor in different poisoning
14. Poisons causing subendocardial hemorrhages
15. Hepatotoxic and nephrotoxic poisons
16. Collection and preservation of samples and viscera

Desirable to know
1. Aphrodisiac, poisons causing priapism, poisons resisting putrefaction, blister forming poisons, formication
2. NDPS Act, 1985
3. Factors modifying the action of poison
4. Analytical methods—TLC, GC, LC, AAS

Describe the history of toxicology.

History of Toxicology

- Forensic toxicology has a rich and fascinating history. The word 'toxic' is thought to be associated with the use of poisoned arrows in hunting and warfare.
- Written documents dating back to 450 BC describe the toxicity of venom in snakebite and how it can be treated.
- Socrates (470–399 BC) was sentenced to drink poisonous hemlock for supposedly corrupting the youth of Athens.
- Cleopatra (51–30 BC) is alleged to have committed suicide by a self-inflicted bite from asp (venomous snake).
- Dioscorides (40-90 AD), a Greek physician in the court of the Roman emperor Nero, authored *De Materia Medica* and made the first attempt to classify plants according to their toxic and therapeutic effect.
- Paracelsus, a 16th century physician is considered to be the '*father of toxicology*'. He determined the specific chemicals responsible for the toxicity of a plant or animal poison. He is credited with the classic toxicology maxim, '*the dose makes the poison*'.
- The origin of modern toxicology is attributed to French toxicologist and chemist Mathieu Orfila who is known as the '*father of modern toxicology*'. He wrote '*Traité des poisons*' in 1814. The book made a systemic correlation between the chemical and biological properties of the poisons.
- In 1836, English chemist James March discovered an accurate way to detect arsenic ('*inheritance powder*') in the body.
- Dr Alexander Gettler is known as father of American forensic toxicology.

Define the terms toxicology, forensic toxicology, clinical toxicology and poison.

Definitions

- **Toxicology:** Science dealing with properties, actions, toxicity, fatal dose, detection, estimation, treatment and autopsy findings (in case of death) in relation to the poisonous substances.
- **Clinical toxicology:** It deals with human diseases caused by or associated with abnormal exposure to chemical substances.

- **Forensic toxicology:** It deals with the medical and legal aspects of the harmful effects of chemicals on human beings. It involves not only the identification and quantifying of a drug, poison or substance in tissues, but also the ability to interpret the results of one's findings.
- **Xenobiotics** (Greek '*xenos*': foreign; '*bios*': life): Any foreign substances or exogenous chemicals to which an organism is exposed that are extrinsic to the normal metabolism of that organism, such as drugs, pollutants, as well as some food additives and cosmetics.
- **Poison:** It is a substance (solid, liquid or gaseous) which if introduced in the living body or brought into contact with any part thereof will produce ill-health or death by its constitutional or local effects or both. Thus, almost anything is a poison.
- **Toxin:** A poisonous substance produced by a biological organism, such as microbe, animal, plant or fungus, e.g., botulinum toxin, tetrodotoxin, aflatoxins, pyrrolizidine alkaloids, venom or amanitin.
- **Venom:** A toxic substance produced by some animals (snakes, scorpions, spiders or bees) that are injected into prey or an enemy, chiefly by biting or stinging and has an injurious or lethal effect. *All venoms are toxins and all toxins are poisons, but all poisons are not toxins and all toxins are not venoms.*
- **Toxinology:** It is the science which deals with toxins produced by plants, animals, bacteria and fungi which are harmful to human beings.
- **Acute poisoning** is caused by an excessive single dose or multiple doses of a poison taken over a short interval of time.
- **Chronic poisoning** is caused by smaller doses over a period of time, resulting in gradual worsening.
- **Subacute poisoning** shows features of both acute and chronic poisoning.
- **Fulminant poisoning** is caused by massive dose of poison where death occurs rapidly, sometimes without preceding symptoms.

Describe the laws in relations to poisons including NDPS Act, medico-legal aspects of poisons.

MEDICO-LEGAL ASPECTS OF POISONS

- In law, the real difference between a medicine and a poison is the intent with which it is given. If the substance is given with the intention to save life, it is medicine, but if it is given with intention to cause bodily harm, it is a poison. The law does not make any difference between homicide by means of poisons and homicide by any other means.
- **Sec. 284 IPC** states that whoever causes hurt/injury with rash or negligent conduct with respect to poisonous substance shall be punished with imprisonment up to 6 months with/without fine (up to ₹ 1000).
- **Sec. 328 IPC** deals with administering of any poison, stupefying or intoxicating agent with the intent to cause hurt and facilitate the commission of an offense. Punishment is imprisonment up to 10 years and also fine.

Narcotics Drugs and Psychotropic Substances Act, 1985

This Act was enacted to resolve the problems of illicit drug trafficking:
a. Cultivating or gathering any portion of coca plant.
b. Cultivating opium (poppy) or cannabis plant.*
c. Engaging in the production, manufacture, possession, sale, purchase, transportation, concealment, consumption, import, export of narcotic or psychotropic substances.
d. Dealing in any activities in narcotic drugs or psychotropics substances other than those referred to in the Act.
e. Handling or letting out any premises for carrying out any activities referred to in the Act.

- '*Narcotic drug*' means coca leaf, cannabis (hemp), opium, poppy and all drugs manufactured from them.
- '*Psychotropic substance*' means any substance, natural or synthetic, or any salt or preparation of such substance or material included in the list of psychotropic substances specified in the Schedule (76 drugs and their derivatives are listed), e.g., amphetamine, pentobarbital, psilocybin and diazepam.
- '**Small quantity**' means any quantity lesser than the quantity specified by the Central Govt. by notification if the official gazette. For e.g., cocaine: 2 g, codeine: 10 g, cannabis: 100 g, ganja: 1,000 g, heroin: 5 g; fentanyl: 0.005 g, MDMA: 0.5 g, morphine: 5 g, opium: 25 g.
- '**Commercial quantity**' means any quantity greater than the quantity specified by the Central Govt. by notification in the official gazette. For e.g., cocaine: 100 g, codeine: 1,000 g, cannabis: 1,000 g, ganja: 20,000 g, heroin: 250 g, fentanyl: 0.1 g, MDMA: 10 g, morphine: 250 g, opium: 2,500 g.

Punishment

- Under this Act, the punishment for possessing commercial quantity of the banned substance is higher than the smaller quantity.
- The Supreme Court has ruled that the quantity of neutral substances mixed with the narcotic drugs or psychotropic substances should be taken into consideration along with actual content by weight of the offending drug, while determining the "small or commercial quantity".
- If any person produces, possesses, transports, imports, sells, purchases or uses any narcotic drug/psychotropic

---

* Some states like Rajasthan, Uttar Pradesh and Madhya Pradesh have allowed cultivation of opium for medicinal use.

substance in commercial quantity, he is punished with rigorous imprisonment (RI) for 10–20 years and fine of ₹ 1–2 lakhs. Punishment for a repeat offense is RI for 15–30 years and fine of ₹ 1.5–3 lakhs.
- Punishment for more than small quantity and less than commercial quantity is RI for up to 10 years and fine up to ₹ 1 lakh.
- However, if a person is carrying 'small quantities', then the punishment is RI up to 6 months or fine up to ₹ 10,000.
- For consumption of drugs; *cocaine, morphine and heroin:* RI up to 1 year with/without fine up to ₹ 20, 000. *Other drugs:* imprisonment up to 6 months with/without fine up to ₹ 10, 000. Addicts volunteering for treatment enjoy immunity from prosecution.
- In a later enactment, the Prevention of Illicit Traffic in NDPS Act, 1988, there is a provision for preventive detention and seizure of property. The maximum punishment is death penalty, if a person is found to be trafficking ≥1 kg of pure heroin twice (despite conviction and warning on the first attempt).

NOTA BENE

Important Schedules under the Drugs and Cosmetic Rules, 1945
- Schedule C: Biological and special products
- Schedule E(1): Poisonous substances under the Ayurvedic, Siddha and Unani system of medicine
- Schedule F: Vaccines, antisera and diagnostic antigens
- Schedule G: Drugs to be taken under medical supervision (about 65 drugs)
- Schedule H: Prescription drugs
- Schedule J: Diseases for the cure of which no drug can be advertised (e.g., AIDS)

FM 8.3, 8.4
- Describe the various types of poisons, toxicokinetics and toxicodynamics, and diagnosis of poisoning in living and dead.
- Describe the general symptoms, principles of diagnosis of common poisons encountered in India.

■ CLASSIFICATION OF POISONS

According to their **mode of action**, poisons are classified as:

I. Corrosives

They produce inflammation and ulceration of the tissues; symptoms are commonly manifested immediately.

Strong acids	Strong alkalis	Metallic salts
◆ *Mineral or inorganic acids*, e.g., HCl, HNO₃, H₂SO₄	Caustic soda, caustic potash, carbonates of sodium, potassium and ammonium	Zinc chloride, ferric chloride, AgNO₃
◆ *Organic acids*, e.g., carbolic, oxalic and acetic acid		

II. Irritants

They cause inflammation of the gastrointestinal tract (GIT) and other symptoms; symptoms are usually manifested slowly.

Inorganic	Organic	Mechanical
◆ *Metallic*, e.g., arsenic, antimony, copper, lead, mercury, zinc	◆ *Plant*, e.g., abrus, castor, croton, calotropis	Powdered glass, hair, diamond dust, needles
◆ *Non-metallic*, e.g., phosphorus, chlorine, iodine, CCl₄	◆ *Animal*, e.g., snakes, cantharides, scorpions, spiders	

III. Neurotics

They act mainly on the CNS, though some have local irritant action.

Cerebral	Spinal	Peripheral
◆ *Somniferous*, e.g., opioids, barbiturates	Nux vomica, gelsemium	Curare, conium
◆ *Inebriants*, e.g., alcohol, anesthetics, ether		
◆ *Deliriants*, e.g., dhatura, cannabis, cocaine		

IV. Cardiac

Cardiac poisons have mainly action on the heart, either directly on the musculature or through its nerve supply, e.g., digitalis, oleander, aconite, nicotine, hydrocyanic acid.

V. Asphyxiants

Asphyxiants deprive the body of oxygen. They can be gases, liquids or solids, or their metabolites. For e.g., CO, CO_2, H_2S, war gases.

VI. Miscellaneous

It includes poisons having widely different pharmacological actions.

i. **Agrochemicals**

Pesticides	Fumigants	Rodenticides	Herbicides
Organophosphates, organochlorines	Aluminum phosphide, ethylene dibromide	Thallium sulfate, zinc phosphide	Paraquat, bromoxynil

ii. **Drugs of dependence:** Tranquilizers, antidepressants, hallucinogens.
iii. **Petroleum products:** Kerosene, petrol, naphtha.
iv. **Food poisoning:** Bacterial, chemical (botulism).
v. **Others:** Analgesics and antipyretics.

Classification of poisons based on their uses, effects or outcome is given in Synopsis (Summary-II).

TOXICOKINETICS AND TOXICODYNAMICS OF POISONS

- **Toxicokinetics:** Study of the time course of the absorption, distribution, elimination and uptake of potentially harmful xenobiotics leading to toxic response.
- **Toxicodynamics:** Determination and quantification of the sequence of events at cellular and molecular levels leading to toxic effects after exposure to a chemical agent.

Factors Modifying the Action of Poisons

i. **Quantity/dose:** More the quantity, more severe will be the toxic effects.
ii. **Form**
   - *Physical state:* Gases and vapors act more rapidly than liquid. Liquid poisons act more rapidly than solid ones, of which fine powders act more quickly than coarse ones.
   - *Chemical combination:* Action of poison depends upon the solubility or insolubility resulting from chemical combination, e.g., $AgNO_3$ and HCl are both strong poisons, but when combined, an insoluble salt of AgCl is formed which is harmless.
   - *Mechanical combination:* Action of poison is altered when combined mechanically with inert substances. Corrosives when sufficiently diluted with water act as irritants.
iii. **Mode of administration:** In order of rapidity of action: Inhaled in gaseous/vaporous form > Intravenous injection (IV) > Intramuscular (IM), subcutaneous and intradermal injection > Application to a wound > Application to serous surface > Ingestion > Introduction into the natural orifices, e.g., rectum, vagina, urethra and sublingual > Application to unbroken skin (e.g., nicotine patch).
   ('>' indicates more rapidly acting)
   As a rough estimate, if the active dose by mouth is considered as one unit, the rectal dose about 1½–2 times and the hypodermic dose is about ¼.
iv. **Condition of the patient**
   - *Age:* Poisons have greater effect at the two extremes of age. A child does not have fully developed drug metabolizing enzymes and effective blood-brain barrier, and as such more susceptible to the effect of most drugs.
   - *State of health:* A healthy person tolerates poisons better than a diseased person. General debility, senility, chronic or disabling disease may cause death of a person to a dose that is ordinarily safe, e.g., opium in bronchial asthma.
   - *Sleep and intoxication:* Action of poison is delayed, if a person goes to sleep soon after taking it. Action is also delayed, if one takes a poison in an intoxicated state.
   - *Tolerance and idiosyncrasy:* People have widely varying susceptibility, but tolerance can build up to a substance, so that same dose no longer has the effect that originally it had; seen with intake of alcohol, barbiturates, amphetamines, benzodiazepines, tobacco and the morphine-heroin-methadone group.
     The opposite situation is that of idiosyncrasy, where there is an inherent hypersensitivity towards drugs or food resulting in symptoms, like dyspnea, rigors, fever, diarrhea, hemorrhage from bowel and albuminuria, as seen in penicillin, aspirin, cocaine, sulfonamides, sera, certain articles of food (mushrooms, eggs, shell-fish, fruits), and heroin intake.
   - *State of stomach:* Presence of food in stomach delays the action of the poison in most cases. It also dilutes the concentration of the ingested poison.
   - *Cumulative action:* Poisons which are not excreted readily tend to accumulate in the body when given in repeated doses, and produce symptoms when their concentration reaches the threshold.

Routes of elimination: The absorbed poison is mainly excreted by the kidneys and to some extent by the skin. Other routes are bile, milk, saliva, mucus and serous secretions. Unabsorbed portion is excreted in the vomit and feces.

Action of Poison

- **Local**
  i. Chemical destruction by corrosives.
  ii. Congestion and inflammation by irritants.
  iii. Effect on motor and sensory nerves, e.g., tingling of skin and tongue by aconite or dilatation of pupils by atropine.
- **Remote:** Remote action produced are either by shock, acting reflexly through severe pain, or exerting a specific action on certain organs and tissues.
- **Combined:** Substances, like carbolic acid, oxalic acid and phosphorus have local and remote actions.

POISONING IN THE LIVING

There is no single symptom and no definite group of symptoms which are absolutely characteristic of poisoning.

Following should arouse suspicion of poisoning:
i. Symptoms appear immediately or within a short period after food or drink.
ii. Symptoms are uniform in character and increase rapidly in severity.
iii. When several persons eat or drink from the same source of food or drink at the same time, all suffer from similar symptoms at or about the same time.
iv. Discovery of poison in food taken, in the vomitus or in the excreta is strong proof of poisoning.

Symptoms Suggestive of Poisoning

i. Sudden onset of abdominal pain, nausea, vomiting, diarrhea and collapse.
ii. Sudden onset of coma with constriction of pupils.
iii. Unexplained coma, especially in children.
iv. Coma in an adult, known to have a depressive illness.
v. Rapid onset of a peripheral neuropathy, such as wrist-drop.
vi. Rapid onset of a neurological or GIT illness in persons known to be occupationally exposed to chemicals.
vii. Sudden onset of convulsions.
viii. Delirium with dilated pupils.
ix. Paralysis, especially of lower motor neuron type.
x. Jaundice and hepatocellular failure.
xi. Oliguria with proteinuria and hematuria.
xii. Persistent cyanosis.

Features Indicative of Chronic Poisoning

i. Symptoms are exaggerated after the administration of suspected food, fluid or medicine.
ii. Malaise, cachexia, depression, and gradual deterioration of general condition of the patient.
iii. Repeated attacks of diarrhea and vomiting.
iv. Removal of patient from his usual surroundings causes the symptoms to disappear.
v. Traces of poison found in the urine, blood, stool or vomit.

Systemic findings due to poisoning with various xenobiotics are given in Synopsis (Summary-II).

Pearls

Xenobiotics causing miosis (constricted pupils)
- Opioids
- Phenol
- Organophosphorus
- Carbamates
- Benzodiazepines
- Ethanol
- Barbiturates
- Muscarinic type mushrooms

Xenobiotics causing mydriasis (dilated pupils)
- Dhatura
- Cannabis
- Ergot
- Strychnine
- Atropine
- Anticholinergics
- Cocaine
- Methanol

FM 1.9, 8.9
- Describe the importance of documentation in medical practice.
- Describe the procedure of intimation of suspicious cases or actual cases of foul play to the police, maintenance of records.

DUTIES OF A DOCTOR IN A CASE OF SUSPECTED POISONING

Medical: Care and treatment to save the life of the patient is first and foremost duty.

Legal: Assist the police to determine the manner of poisoning.

1. Note preliminary particulars of the patient, viz. name, age, sex, occupation, address, date and time, brought by whom, identification marks, and history.
2. In case of *suspected homicidal poisoning*, the doctor must confirm his suspicion before expressing an opinion. For this he must:
   i. Collect vomitus and urine, and submit it for analysis.
   ii. Carefully observe and record the symptoms in relation to food, any change in color, taste or smell of food/drink, and other persons affected at the same time.
   iii. Consult in strict confidence a senior practitioner and keep him informed about the case.
   iv. Remove the patient to the hospital. If the patient refuses, the doctor should engage nurses of his confidence who should administer the medicine and food, and allow no one to be with the patient alone.
3. Once the suspicion is confirmed, he should request the removal of the patient to the hospital. If the victim is an adult, it desirable to seek his consent.
4. Any suspected articles of food, excreta and stomach wash samples should be preserved. Non-compliance is punishable under **Sec. 201 IPC**, if it is proved that the doctor did it with the intention of protecting the accused (imprisonment up to 7 years depending upon the nature of offense). In this case, the onus of proving a non-deliberate omission to collect and preserve the samples would lie on the medical practitioner.
5. A government medical officer is required to report to police *all cases of suspected poisoning*, whether accidental, suicidal or homicidal attended in the hospital.
6. If a private practitioner is convinced that the patient is suffering from homicidal poisoning, he is bound under **Sec. 39 CrPC** to inform the police or Magistrate. Non-compliance is punishable under **Sec. 176 IPC** (simple imprisonment of 1 month with/without fine of ₹ 500/-). Giving false information on such matters is punishable under **Sec. 177 IPC** (simple imprisonment for 6 months with/without fine of ₹ 1000).
7. If the private practitioner is sure that the patient is suffering from *suicidal/accidental poisoning*, he is *not bound to inform the police*, since **Sec. 309 of IPC** (attempt to commit suicide) is not included in the section of IPC for which information has to be given under **Sec. 39 CrPC**.*
   - **Sec. 43 IPC** describes the word 'illegal' and 'legally bound to do'. The word 'illegal' is applicable to everything which is an offense, prohibited by law or furnishes ground for a civil action. A person is said to be 'legally bound to do' whatever it is illegal in him to omit. *Thus, it is the duty of the medical practitioner not to do anything illegal or hide illegal acts.*

---

* Attempt to commit suicide has been decriminalized as per the Mental Healthcare Act, 2017.

- In an alleged case of attempted suicide, possibility of abetment to suicide or homicide cannot be ruled out. It is the duty of the police, not doctors, to decide whether the case was actually of attempted suicide or not, not even if the patient was successfully cured. So, it is better to inform the police. Subsequently, the patient may inform the police whether to pursue the case any further or not.
8. If the condition of the patient is serious, he must make arrangement to record the dying declaration.
9. If the patient dies, he should not issue a death certificate, but should inform the police.
10. Any opinion about the nature of poison should be given only after getting the report from the forensic science laboratory.
11. If the practitioner is summoned by the investigating officer (IO), he is bound to give all information regarding the case that has come to his notice (**Sec. 175 CrPC**). If he conceals the information, he is liable to be prosecuted under **Sec. 202 IPC** (imprisonment up to 6 months with/without fine). If he gives false information during judicial proceedings, he is liable to be charged under **Sec. 193 IPC**.

MEDICAL RECORDS

Definition: Medical records pertains to documents containing a chronological written account of the patient's medical history and complaints, physical findings, results of diagnostic tests, medications, therapeutic procedures and day-wise progress notes recorded by a medical practitioner.

- It is a part of medical training and one must make a habit of keeping records, not only in the interest of medical science, but also for his own safety and interest.
- Records are the property of the hospital, and the personal data contained in the medical record is considered confidential information and the property of the patient.
- Safe custody of the patient's confidential records, whether kept in conventional manner or in a computer, is the responsibility of the doctor.
- It serves as a documentary evidence of the patient's illness, treatment and response to the treatment. This record may be used as evidence in malpractice suits, claims of the insurances and compensations in personal injury suits. The dictum is that '*If it is not in the record—it did not occur*'.
- It is considered **professional misconduct** if a doctor does not maintain the medical records of his indoor patients for a period of 3 years and refuses to provide the same within 72 h (NMC is planning to extend it to 5 working days) when the patient requests for it.
- Original hospital record of the medico-legal case (MLC) including X-ray/CT/MRI films should not be handed over to the police. However, if the investigating officer requests, a photocopy of the record (bed-head-ticket) may be supplied and a receipt of the same must be obtained.
- Medico-legal report (MLR) and postmortem report (PMR) belongs to the requestor, i.e., the police and the same is held by the doctor in fiduciary relationship.
- If affected party is asking for a record, then attested photocopy of the MLR can be handed over to the patient or his relative and after the requisite fee has been paid by applicant.
- Request for supply of copy of MLR or PMR under the RTI Act are not maintainable under Section 8(1) (e) & Section 8(1) (h). It should not be issued to third parties (including the accused) by the hospital authorities.
- Patient's record cannot be used in clinics or conferences without the patient's consent.
- Hospitals have the right to use the records without consent for evaluating the quality of care and statistical purposes.
- X-ray films are the property of the hospital/doctor as part of the record, the patient is entitled for the skill and treatment, but copies of records and X-ray films may be given.
- As per Ministry of Health and Family Welfare guidelines (2014), hard copy of in patient's record (case sheets) should be kept for 3 years, OPD record for 3 years, and medico-legal registers and case sheets for 10 years or till the disposal of ongoing cases. Medical record of indoor patients should be stored in digitized form for at least past 10 years or as per availability. For future, all medical records of indoor patients should be kept indefinitely in digitized form.

SUICIDE/HOMICIDE/ACCIDENT

- Poisoning is one of the common methods of committing suicide among women.
- The use of poison is also a unique method of homicide and has been used for centuries. Poisoning often involve passionate and vengeful murder.
- Poisoning might result from an accidental drug overdose or taken by mistake. Accidental unintentional exposure can occur in children or in adults who are under the influence of alcohol or in psychiatric patients.

Qualities of an ideal homicidal and ideal suicidal poison is given in **Diff. 35.1**.

Parasuicide or pseudocide: Suicide attempts or gestures and self-harm where there is no actual intention to die. It is a deliberate self-harm, and acts are committed with the intention of manipulating a lover or family member. Others commit the act in hope of extricating themselves from an intolerable situation. Some of them may be psychologically disturbed persons.

DIFFERENTIATION 35.1: Ideal homicidal and ideal suicidal poison

S.No.	Feature	Ideal homicidal poison	Ideal suicidal poison
1.	Cost	Immaterial	Cheap
2.	Availability	Easily available	Easily available
3.	Physical characteristics	Colorless, odorless and tasteless	Tasteless or pleasant taste, no repulsive smell
4.	Toxicity	Highly toxic	Highly toxic
5.	Antidote	None	None
6.	Solubility in food/drink	Soluble without producing any obvious change	Should be easily taken in food or drink
7.	Signs and symptoms	Should resemble a natural disease, or delayed for the offender to escape suspicion	Capable of producing painless death
8.	Metabolism	Must be rapidly destroyed, or undetectable in urine/blood	Not particularly so
9.	Detection	Should not be detected by chemical tests or other methods	Not particularly so
10.	Postmortem changes	Should be none	Not particularly so
11.	Examples	Arsenic, aconite, thallium, oleander, insulin and other drugs	KCN, HCN, opium, barbiturates, alphos or organophosphorus

FM 8.6, 8.8

- Describe the management of common poisons encountered in India.
- Describe basic methodologies in treatment of poisoning: decontamination, supportive therapy, antidote therapy, procedures of enhanced elimination.

MANAGEMENT OF POISONING CASES

If the poison is known, specific treatment must be started. If not, treatment is given on general lines (**Flowchart 35.1**).

Main aim of treatment: Help the patient to stay alive by attention to respiration and circulation, while he is assisted in getting rid of the poison by metabolism or excretion.

Emergency Management of Symptomatic Patient

In symptomatic patients, treatment of life-threatening complications takes precedence over diagnostic evaluation.

i. **Coma:** The initial management can be remembered by the mnemonic ABCD, for airway, breathing, circulation and drugs respectively.
   - *Airway:* Establish a patent airway by positioning, suctioning or insertion of an artificial nasal or oropharyngeal airway or endotracheal intubation.
   - *Breathing:* Provide assistance, if necessary, with a bag-valve-mask device or mechanical ventilator. Provide supplemental oxygen. It is important since severe poisoning often make the patient comatose and protective airway reflexes and respiratory drive is lost.
   - *Circulation:* Measure the pulse and blood pressure, and estimate tissue perfusion (e.g., by measurement of urinary output, skin signs and arterial blood pH). Place the patient on continuous ECG monitoring.
   - *Drugs* **(Coma cocktail)**
     a. Dextrose 50%: 50–100 mL IV (unless bedside glucose is normal).
     b. Thiamine: 100 mg IM or IV.
     c. Naloxone: 0.45–2 mg IV.
     d. Consider flumazenil: 0.2–0.5 mg IV.

ii. **Hypothermia:** Gradual rewarming is preferred, unless the patient is in cardiac arrest.

iii. **Hypotension:** Most patients respond to empiric treatment (200 mL IV bolus of 0.9% saline or other isotonic crystalloid up to a total of 1–2 L). If unsuccessful, give dopamine, 5–15 µg/kg/minute (min) by infusion. Prolong hypotension is commonly seen in severe poisonings.

iv. **Hypertension:** Treat hypertension, if the patient is symptomatic or if the diastolic pressure is >105–110 mm Hg. Hypertensive patients who are agitated or anxious may benefit from a sedative, such as lorazepam 2–3 g IV. For persistent hypertension, administer phentolamine 2–5 mg IV or nitroprusside sodium 0.25–8 µg/kg/min IV.

v. **Convulsions/seizures:** Administer lorazepam 2–3 mg IV over 1–2 mins, or if IV access is not immediately available—midazolam 5–10 mg IM. If convulsions continue, administer phenobarbital 15–20 mg/kg slow IV over 30 mins, or phenytoin 15 mg/kg IV over 30 mins.

vi. **Hyperthermia:** Treat aggressively by removing all clothing, spraying with tepid water, and fanning the patient. If this is ineffective, induce neuromuscular paralysis with a nondepolarizing neuromuscular blocker (e.g., pancuronium, vecuronium). Dantrolene (2–5 mg/kg IV) may be effective for hyperthermia that does not respond to neuromuscular blockade (i.e., malignant hyperthermia).

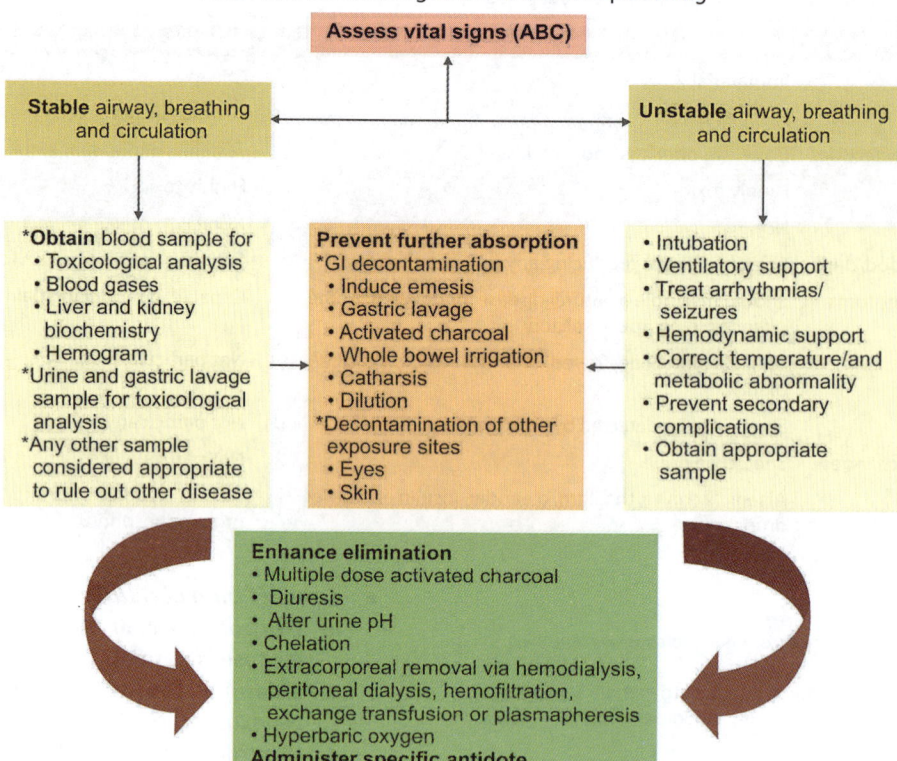

Flowchart 35.1: Management of a case of poisoning

vii. **Acidosis:** Correct acidosis. Measure arterial pH. Infuse sodium bicarbonate if <7.1.

REMOVAL OF UNABSORBED POISON

Inhaled Poisons

In case of inhalation of gaseous poisons, the patient should be removed into fresh air, artificial respiration and O_2 (6–8 l/min) should be given. Air passages should be kept free from mucus by postural drainage or by suction.

Injected Poisons

If the poison has been injected subcutaneous, a tourniquet may be applied immediately above the point of injection, which must be loosened for 1 min after every 10 mins to prevent gangrene. Immersion of the extremity in water at 10°C or below, slows capillary blood flow and limits absorption.

Contact Poisons

Immediate, copious flushing with water, saline or any other available clear liquid is the initial treatment for topical exposures (except alkali, metals, calcium oxide and phosphorus). The eyes should be irrigated with the eyelids fully retracted, for at least 20 mins. Saline is preferred for eye irrigation. A triple wash (water, soap and water) is best for dermal decontamination. The removal of liquids from body cavities, such as the vagina or rectum is done by irrigation.

Ingested Poisons (Gastric Decontamination)

1. Gastric Lavage

Gastric lavage *(stomach washing)* is most useful within 1 hour (h) after ingestion of any poison.* It is performed by sequentially administering and aspirating about 5 mL fluid/kg of body weight with a 36–40 French orogastric tube (22–28 French tube for children). It is repeated, till clear and odorless fluid comes out. If there is any bleeding, the procedure is abandoned.

♦ **Procedure:** The patient is placed in Trendelenburg (mouth is at lower level than larynx so as to aid respiratory drainage and prevent aspiration) and in left lateral decubitus position (pylorus points upward in this orientation and helps prevent the poison from passing through the pylorus during the procedure), even if an endotracheal tube is in place for ventilatory support **(Fig. 35.1)**.

♦ **Confirmation of tip in the stomach:** For confirmation, a little air in a syringe is forced down the tube, bubbling sounds are heard through the stethoscope applied over the stomach. If the tube has entered the trachea, a hissing noise is heard at the other end, and if the patient is conscious, reflex coughing takes place and bubbles

---

* Gastric lavage can be gastric irrigation/suction, stomach pumping, nasogastric lavage or orogastric lavage. It is not recommended if patient presents > 2 h after ingestion, poison/dose ingested is non-life threatening and if the patient has vomited after consumption of poison.

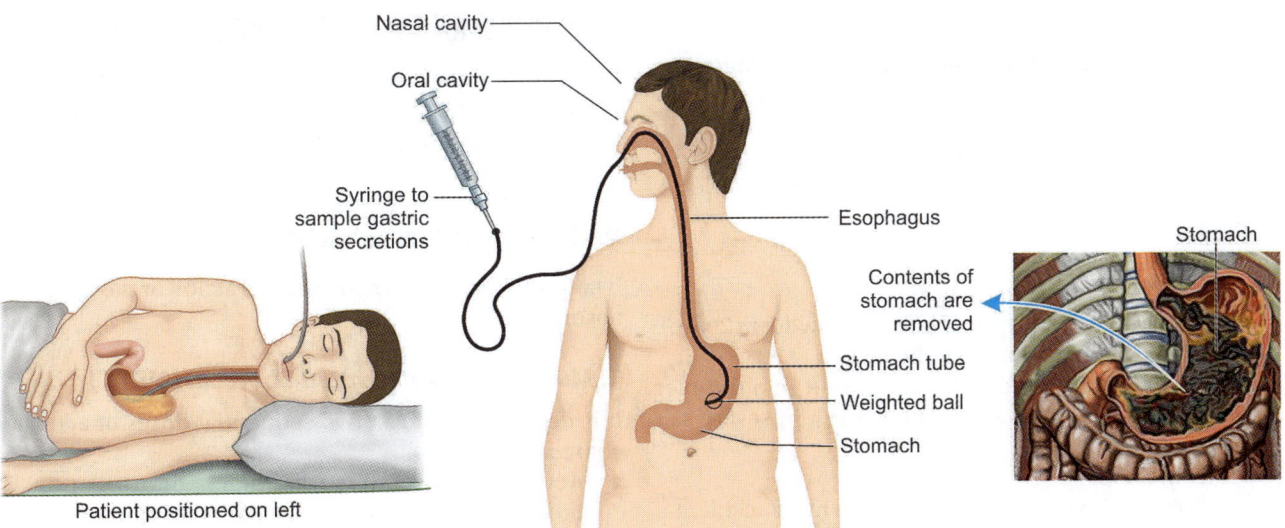

Fig. 35.1: Gastric lavage

of air will be found coming out, if outer end is dipped in water.
- After testing, about 250 mL of water is injected. Allow few minutes for fluid to act in the stomach. The fluid is then taken out and preserved for chemical analysis **(Fig. 35.1)**.
- **Fluid for gastric lavage:** Except for infants, where normal saline is recommended, tap water is acceptable. **Others agents used:** 1:5000 $KMnO_4$, 5% $NaHCO_3$, 4% tannic acid, 1% NaI/KI, 1–3% calcium lactate, saturated lime water or starch solution.
- When clear solution comes out, a small quantity of fluid is left behind to neutralize whatever small quantity of poison remains in the stomach.
- **Complications:** Aspiration is a common complication (10% of patients) and serious complications (like esophageal and gastric perforation, tube misplacement in the trachea) occur in about 1% of patients.

NOTA BENE
- Ryle's tube of appropriate size may be used for gastric lavage. In adults, it is inserted through the nose, up to the second marking wherein the tip reaches the midway of body of stomach (1st marking: at the level of cardiac end of stomach, 3rd marking: pyloric end).
- Gastric lavage is done with a stomach tube (**Ewald or Boas tube, Fig. 35.2**). It is a non-collapsible rubber tube of 1 cm diameter and 1.5 meter in length with a filter funnel attached at one end and a mark at about 50 cm from the other end which is rounded with lateral openings. At about the midway of the tube, there is a suction bulb to pump out the stomach contents. A wooden mouth gag is provided, one end of which is pointed, so that it can be forcefully inserted by the side of the mouth in non-cooperative patients.
- In the **Trendelenburg position,** the body is laid in supine position with the feet higher than the head by 15–30°.

Pearls
Contraindications for gastric lavage (starts with 'C')
- **C**orrosive poisoning (except Carbolic acid) owing to danger of perforation and further injury to esophageal mucosa*
- **C**onvulsant poison (e.g., strychnine), as it may lead to convulsions
- **C**omatose patients because of risk of aspiration into air-passages as the laryngeal reflex is impaired
- **C**ompromised unprotected airway
- Volatile poisons and hydrocarbons (petroleum distillate and kerosene oil) as there is risk of aspiration of the liquid (due to low viscosity) and chemical pneumonitis
- Risk of hemorrhage or perforation due to esophageal or gastric pathology, such as upper alimentary diseases (esophageal varices) or recent surgery
- Hypothermia or hemorrhagic diathesis
- Ingestion of a foreign body (e.g., drug packet).

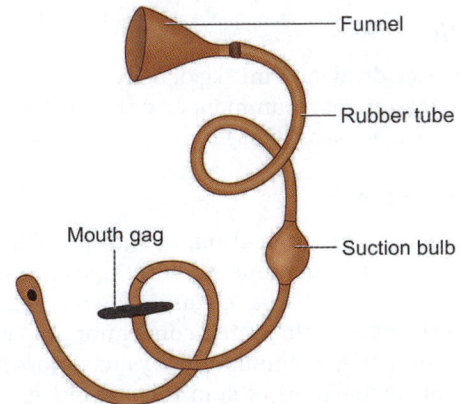

Fig. 35.2: Ewald or Boas tube for gastric lavage

---
*Corrosives are **'absolute contraindication'**; rest are relative contraindications.

2. Emetics

They should be used only if there is difficulty in obtaining gastric lavage. Vomiting can be produced if the medullary centers are still responsive. Due to danger of aspiration of gastric contents, vomiting should only be induced in a conscious patient.

Methods

a. *Household emetics*
   - Large amount of warm water.
   - A table-spoonful (15 g) of mustard powder in 200 mL of warm water—not very effective.
   - Two table-spoonful of common salt in a tumbler (200 ml) of warm water—may result in severe salt poisoning.

b. *Other methods*
   - Syrup of ipecac (home management of accidental ingestions; 30 mL for adults, 15 mL for children).
   - $ZnSO_4$, 1–2 g in 200 mL of water, repeated in 15 min, but no longer used as an emetic.
   - $(NH_4)CO_3$, 1–2 g in 200 mL of water.
   - Apomorphine, 6 mg subcutaneously followed by naloxone hydrochloride 5–10 mg IM—may cause CNS depression with an increased risk of aspiration, hence not recommended.
   - Tickling the back of throat (fauces) with a wooden tongue depressor or finger-down-the-throat technique is quick and easy method, but it is ineffective and potentially traumatic.

Side-effects include lethargy in children, and protracted vomiting. Except for aspiration, serious complications (e.g., gastric or esophageal tears and perforations) are rare.

Contraindications: Same as stomach wash, in addition to:
- Severe heart and lung diseases.
- Advanced pregnancy.
- In cases of CNS depression, seizures or rapidly acting CNS poisons (camphor, cyanide, morphine, tricyclic antidepressants, propoxyphene and strychnine).

3. Dilution

Dilution (i.e., drinking 5 mL/kg of body wt. of water or any other clear liquid) is recommended only after the ingestion of corrosives (acids or alkali).

4. Other Methods

- Endoscopic or surgical removal of poisons may be useful in rare situations, such as ingestion of a toxic foreign body that fails to transit the GIT, agents that have coalesced into gastric concentrations or *bezoars* [barbiturates, glutethimide, heavy metals (arsenic, iron, mercury or thallium), lithium, meprobamate, salicylates or sustained-release preparations].
- Patients who become toxic from cocaine due to its leakage from ingested drug packets, require immediate surgical intervention.

ADMINISTRATION OF ANTIDOTES

Definition: Antidotes are substances that act specifically to prevent, inhibit, inactivate, counteract, reverse or relieve the action or poisonous effects of a toxic agent, i.e., they are remedies used to counteract the action of poisons.

Mechanical/Physical Antidotes

It neutralizes poison by mechanical action or prevents their absorption.

1. Multiple-dose Activated Charcoal (MDAC)

It is defined as at least two sequential doses of activated charcoal.

- Activated charcoal is fine, black, odorless powder produced by destructive distillation of various organic materials, usually wood pulp and then treating at high temperature with a variety of activating agents, such as steam or CO_2, to increase its adsorptive capacity.
- **Dose:** 40–80 g (dose: 0.5–1 g/kg body wt.) is mixed with 200 mL of water to form a soup-like mixture and given orally. Palatability may be increased by adding a sweetener (sorbitol) or a flavoring agent (cherry, chocolate or cola syrup) to the suspension.
- **Action:** It acts mechanically by *adsorbing* and retaining within its pores, especially alkaloid poisons, allowing the charcoal-toxin complex to be evacuated with stool. The network of pores adsorbs 100–1000 mg of drug/g of charcoal.
- **Uses:** It is used in cases of poisoning with strychnine, morphine, atropine, nicotine, phenobarbital, *Amanita phalloides*, salicylates, KCN and phenol. Charged (ionized) chemicals, such as mineral acids, alkalis and highly dissociated salts of cyanide, fluoride, iron and lithium are not well adsorbed by charcoal. Activated charcoal does not bind metals and thus is of limited usefulness in cases of acute metal ingestion.
- **Contraindications:** Ingestion of caustic acid/alkali or aliphatic hydrocarbons like kerosene/gasoline, metallic salts, iodine, cyanide, alcohol, unprotected airway, depressed level of consciousness, functional or mechanical bowel obstruction (absent bowel sounds/ileus) and when the patient presents >2 h post-ingestion.
- **Side-effects:** Nausea, vomiting and diarrhea or constipation. Charcoal may also prevent the absorption of orally administered therapeutic agents.
- **Complications** include mechanical obstruction of the airway, aspiration, bowel obstruction and infarction caused by inspissated charcoal.

2. Demulcents

Demulcents are substances which form protective coating on the gastric mucous membrane, e.g., milk, starch, egg-white, mineral oil, aluminum hydroxide and milk of magnesia.

Contraindications: Fats and oils should not be used for oil-soluble poisons, such as kerosene, phosphorus, OPC, DDT, phenol, turpentine, aniline and CCl_4.

3. Bulky Foods

It acts as mechanical antidote to glass powder by imprisoning its particles within its meshes.

Chemical Antidotes

They counteract the action of poison by forming harmless or insoluble compounds, or by oxidizing poison when brought into contact with them.

i. **Potassium permanganate** has oxidizing properties, 1:5000 solution is used. The wash must be continued till the solution coming out of stomach is pink in color. It is effective against most of the alkaloids (opium, strychnine or atropine), barbiturates, phosphorus and cyanide.
ii. **Tannic acid** (4%) in the form of strong tea precipitates alkaloids, lead, silver, aluminum, cobalt and copper.
iii. **Dilute alkalis,** e.g., milk of magnesia, alkaline hydroxide or ammonia will neutralize acid; bicarbonates should not be given because of risk of rupture of stomach due to liberated CO_2.
iv. **Tincture iodine** or Lugol's iodine precipitates alkaloids, lead, mercury, silver and quinine.
v. **Common salt** reacts with $AgNO_3$ by direct chemical action forming insoluble AgCl.
vi. **Albumin** precipitates $HgCl_2$ and **$CuSO_4$** precipitates phosphorus.
vii. **Chemical action:** Canned fruit juice and lemon juice are other alternatives.

> **NOTA BENE**
>
> **Universal Antidote:** It was a combination of physical and chemical antidotes; used in those cases where the nature of ingested poison was unknown or when it was suspected that two or more poisons were taken.
>
> | Constituents | Quantity | Purpose/Action |
> |---|---|---|
> | ♦ Powdered charcoal (burnt toast) | 2 parts | Adsorbs alkaloids |
> | ♦ Magnesium oxide (milk of magnesia) | 1 part | Neutralizes acids |
> | ♦ Tannic acid (strong tea) | 1 part | Precipitates alkaloids, glycosides and metals |
>
> ♦ The use of universal antidote declined by the mid-1980s and is no longer available.
> ♦ Activated charcoal was found superior to the universal antidote in decreasing absorption, and that the decreased efficacy of the universal antidote was caused by tannic acid interfering with activated charcoal's adsorbance of other toxins.
> ♦ Moreover, tannic acid was found to be hepatotoxic in nature.

Physiological/Pharmacological Antidotes

These agents produce effects which are opposite to that of poison. They are used after some of the poison is absorbed into the circulation. The antagonism is usually not complete and it may itself produce undesirable side effects. For example, atropine for pilocarpine, diazepam for strychnine, naloxone for morphine, amyl nitrite for cyanide, N-acetyl cysteine for acetaminophen, atropine and oximes for OPC, and anti-snake venom for snake bite poisoning (*serological antidote*).*

Chelating Agents

Definition: Chelators are agents that form stable ligands with metal, effecting enhanced renal or biliary excretion of the drug–chelate complex.

♦ A chelator molecule binds a metal ion by two or more polar functions, such as sulfhydryl, carbonyl, amino, or hydroxyl groups.
♦ They are widely used as specific antidotes against some *heavy metal poisoning*, as they have greater affinity for the metals as compared to the endogenous enzymes. Many heavy metals have affinity for sulfhydryl (–SH) radicals, combine with them in tissues and deprive the body of the use of respiratory enzymes.

Commonly Used Chelating Agents (Table 35.1)

i. **BAL (British anti-lewisite, dimercaprol):** BAL has two unsaturated –SH groups which competes with the thiol groups of enzymes for binding with arsenic or other metals to form a stable metal-chelate complex. The formed complex is then excreted from the body through urine. It prevents the union of the metal with the –SH group of the respiratory enzyme system.
ii. **EDTA (Ethylenediaminetetraacetic acid, calcium disodium versenate):** Superior to BAL for treatment of poisoning with arsenic and mercury. Since $CaNa_2$ EDTA is ionized, it is not absorbed from GIT—must be given IV (IM is painful).
iii. **Penicillamine (cuprimine):** It is a hydrolysis product of penicillin, has got a stable –SH group. It is also useful in hepatolenticular degeneration (Wilson's disease which is due to disorder of copper metabolism), cystinuria and scleroderma. The d-isomer is used because the l-isomer and the racemate produce optic neuritis.
iv. **Deferoxamine** is also useful in hemochromatosis (characterized by excessive retention of iron in the tissues) and transfusional chronic iron overload.
   ■ Recently, *deferiprone* and *deferasirox* (20–30 mg/kg, once daily) has been developed, which are orally effective iron chelator.
v. **Succimer or DMSA (dimercaptosuccinic acid):** It is similar to dimercaprol in chelating properties, water soluble and orally effective (DMSA and DMPS are water soluble analogues of BAL). It is superior to EDTA in the treatment of lead poisoning, as it is less toxic to the kidneys and can be given in G-6-PD deficient patients.

---

* Studies have shown that the antitoxic sera do not act as chemical antidote in destroying the venom, but as physiological antidote.

TABLE 35.1: Indications and doses of chelating agents

Chelating agent	Indication	Dose	Route	Contraindications
BAL (10% sol. in oil)	As, Pb, Cu, Hg, Au, Bi poisoning	3–5 mg/kg 4 h for 2 days, 6 h on 3rd day, then 12 h for 10 days	IM (as BAL is oil based)*	Liver damage, G-6-PD deficiency, cadmium, cobalt, selenium and iron poisoning¥
EDTA	As, Hg, Pb, Cu, Cd, Fe, Ni, Co poisoning	25–35 mg/kg in 500 mL of 5% glucose or NS in 1–2 h twice daily for 5 days	IV	Renal damage
Penicillamine	Cu, Pb, Hg poisoning	30 mg/kg in 4 divided doses for 7 days	Oral	—
Desferrioxamine	Fe poisoning	2 g in 5% of laevulose repeated after 12 h (based on clinical response)	IM/IV	—
Succimer (DMSA)	Pb, Hg, As poisoning	10 mg/kg 8 h for 10 days	Oral	—

Various antidotes available for treatment of poisoning are given in Synopsis (Summary-II).

Identify the various tubes.

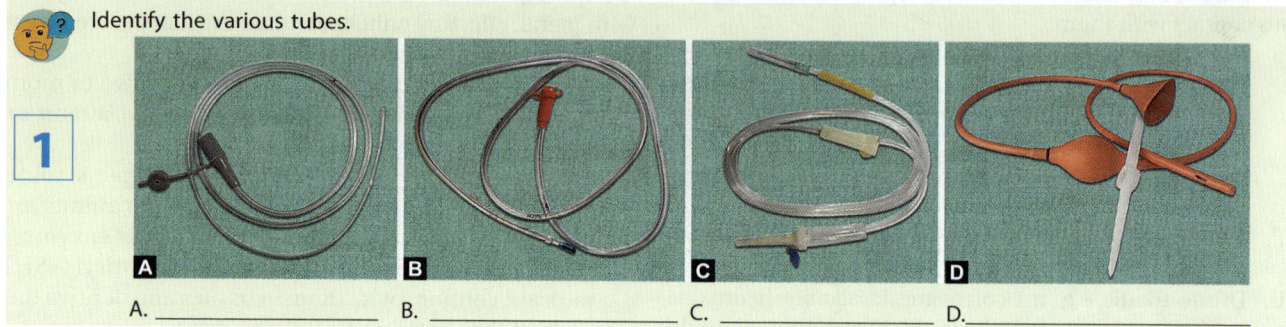

A. _____   B. _____   C. _____   D. _____

ELIMINATION OF POISON BY EXCRETION

Indications of Enhanced Elimination

- Severe poisoning and the poison is distributed predominantly in the extracellular fluid.
- Poison has low protein binding.
- Progressive deterioration, in spite of full supportive care.
- When there is high risk of morbidity and mortality.
- When normal route of excretion of poison is impaired or induced rate of elimination is faster than the normal rate.
- When poison produces delayed, but serious toxic effects.

Methods

1. Renal Excretion

Renal excretion may be improved by giving large amounts of fluid or tea orally.

2. Forced Diuresis and Alteration of Urinary pH

- *Saline diuresis* can enhance the renal excretion of alcohol, fluoride and thallium.
- *Alkaline diuresis* (producing a urine pH ≥7.5 and a urine output of 3–6 mL/kg body wt/h by adding sodium bicarbonate to an IV solution) enhances the excretion of chlorpropamide, 2,4 dichlorophenoxyacetic acid, diflunisal, fluoride, mecoprop, methotrexate, phenobarbital and salicylate.
- *Acid diuresis* can enhance the excretion of amphetamines, cocaine, local anesthetics, phencyclidine, quinidine, quinine, strychnine, sympathomimetics and tricyclic antidepressants.

However, excretion of many poisons, mainly those by hepatic metabolism, is not enhanced by forced diuresis and risk of fluid overload/electrolyte balance and renal complications (myoglobinuric renal failure) outweighs the benefits. This procedure is currently not employed.

3. Whole-bowel Irrigation

It is performed by administering a bowel-cleansing solution containing electrolytes and polyethylene glycol orally or by gastric tube at a rate of 2 L/h (0.5 L/h in children), until rectal effluent is clear.

4. Cathartics

Cathartics are salts (disodium phosphate, magnesium citrate/sulfate or sodium sulfate) or saccharides (mannitol or sorbitol) that promote the rectal evacuation of GIT contents.

- Most effective cathartic is sorbitol in a dose of 1–2 g/kg of body wt.
- *Contraindications:* Ingestion of corrosives and pre-existing diarrhea.
- Magnesium-containing cathartics should not be used in patients with renal failure.

5. Diaphoretics (Sudorifics)

Application of heat (blankets or hot water bottles) and administration of warm beverages—alcohol, ipecac,

---

* BAL is prepared in vegetable oil (peanut or arachis oil) and stabilized with benzyl benzoate. Due to its lipophilicity (ability to penetrate intracellularly), and generation of fat emboli (if given IV), it is given only deep IM.
¥ The metal complexes formed are more toxic than the free metal ions.

pilocarpine, opium, sweet spirits of nitre and salicylates will cause increased perspiration and speeds up the excretion of toxic agents, but its usefulness is doubtful.

6. Extracorporeal Removal

Peritoneal dialysis, hemodialysis, charcoal or resin hemoperfusion, hemofiltration, plasmapheresis and exchange transfusion are capable of removing any toxin from the bloodstream.

Pearls

Dialysis is useful in poisoning with:
- Acetone
- Bromide
- Cocaine
- Ethanol
- Ethylene glycol
- Salicylates
- Barbiturates
- Chloral hydrate
- Cannabis
- Methanol
- Isopropyl alcohol
- Heavy metals (possibly)

Dialysis is NOT useful in poisoning with:
- Kerosene oil
- Organophosphorus
- Benzodiazepines
- Amphetamine
- Copper sulfate
- Digitalis
- Digoxin

Hemoperfusion should be considered in cases of severe poisoning due to caffeine, CCl_4, hypnotic sedatives (barbiturates, meprobamate or methaqualone), mushrooms (amatoxin-containing) and paraquat.

Symptomatic Treatment

It should be applied as indications arise. Morphine is given to relieve pain, O_2 or artificial respiration for respiratory failure, and anesthetic, barbiturates or diazepam for convulsions, sodium bicarbonate to treat acidosis, glucose infusion for hypoglycemia, and restoration of electrolyte imbalance.

Maintenance of Patient's General Condition

Patient should be kept warm and comfortable, prevent development of urinary tract infection, particularly those unconscious, prophylactic antibiotics, and physiotherapy to prevent bed sores are indicated.

Describe the diagnosis of poisoning in dead.

DIAGNOSIS OF POISONING IN DEAD

Evidence of poisoning will depend on postmortem examination, chemical analysis, experiments on suitable animals and circumstantial evidence.

Postmortem Examination

External Findings

i. The **color changes** in the corroded skin and mucous membrane due to some common poisons is given in **Table 35.2**.

TABLE 35.2: Color changes in skin and mucous membrane due to poisoning

S.No.	Poison	Color observed
1.	Sulfuric, oxalic and hydrochloric acid	Gray, becoming black from blood
2.	Nitric acid	Brown or yellow
3.	Hydrofluoric acid	Reddish-brown
4.	Carbolic acid, caustic alkali	Grayish-white
5.	Mercuric chloride	Bluish white
6.	Zinc chloride	Whitish
7.	Chromic acid, potassium chromate	Orange and leathery

ii. **Color of PM staining** in poisoning **(Table 35.3)**.
iii. **Smell** present about the mouth and nose is given in **Table 35.4**.
- The natural orifices, e.g., mouth, nostrils, rectum and vagina may show presence of poisonous material or the signs of it.
- *Injection marks* should be looked for with care.

TABLE 35.3: Color of PM staining in some poisons

S.No.	Poison	Color of PM staining
1.	Carbon monoxide (CO)	Cherry red
2.	Carbon dioxide (CO_2)	Deep blue (reduced hemoglobin)
3.	Cyanide	Bright red/pink
4.	Phosphorus or copper	Dark brown/yellow
5.	Hydrogen sulfide	Bluish-green
6.	Opiates	Bluish-black
7.	Nitrites, aniline, nitrobenzene, chlorates (methemoglobin formation)	Chocolate or coffee-brown

TABLE 35.4: Smell due to various poisons

S.No.	Poison	Odor
1.	Phosphorus, heavy metal poisoning (arsenic, selenium, thallium), parathion, malathion, alphos	Garlic-like
2.	Ethanol, methyl or propyl alcohol, chloroform, nitrites, acetone, chloral hydrate	Sweet fruity
3.	Paraldehyde	Acrid
4.	H_2S, mercaptans, disulfiram	Rotten eggs
5.	HCN	Bitter almond
6.	Carbolic acid	Phenolic
7.	Organophosphates	Kerosene-like
8.	Zinc phosphide	Fishy (musty)
9.	Methyl salicylates	Oil of wintergreen
10.	Marijuana, opium	Burnt rope
11.	Camphor, naphthalene	Mothballs
12.	Nitrobenzene	Shoe polish
13.	Nicotine	Tobacco

- Skin should be examined for lesions, like hyperkeratosis and pigmentation seen in chronic arsenic poisoning.
- Jaundice may occur in poisoning with phosphorus and potassium chlorate.

Internal Findings

i. **Smell:** The skull should be opened first to detect unusual odors in the brain, since the opening of the body masks such odors.
ii. **Mouth and throat:** Examine for any evidence of inflammation, erosion or staining. Areas of necrosis of the pharynx may be seen in death associated with agranulocytosis caused by amidopyrine, thiouracil, dinitrophenol, sulfonamide and barbiturates.
iii. **Respiratory system:** Corrosives may cause edema of glottis, and congestion and desquamation of mucous membrane of trachea and bronchi due to trickling of acid or alkali into the respiratory tract.
iv. **Esophagus:** Corrosive alkalis produce marked softening and desquamation of the mucous membrane.
v. **Heart:** *Subendocardial hemorrhages* in left ventricle are seen in poisoning with arsenic, antimony, barium, mercury, phosphorus and viper bite, and in certain conditions, such as heat stroke, acute infectious disease, e.g., influenza, and traumatic asphyxia.
vi. **Stomach:** Hyperemia of mucous membrane (ridges are more involved) is caused by irritant poison, usually at the cardiac end and greater curvature of stomach (empty stomach).
   - Redness of mucosa is also found during digestion, in asphyxial deaths, venous congestion and when exposed to the atmosphere.
   - Hyperemia due to disease is spread uniformly over the whole surface and not in patches.
   - Color changes of mucous membrane of stomach seen in different poisoning are given in **Table 35.5**.
   - *Softening:* Softening of mucous membrane of the stomach, especially at cardiac end and greater curvature is usually caused by corrosives, especially alkaline corrosives.
   - *Ulcers:* Ulceration due to corrosives or irritants is usually found at greater curvature, ulcer from disease is usually seen on the lesser curvature—margins are well-defined, thickened and indurated.
   - *Perforation:* Usually observed when strong mineral acids, especially H_2SO_4 has been taken. The stomach in such cases is blackened and extensively destroyed. Acid escapes into the abdomen and causes peritonitis.
vii. **Duodenum and intestines:** A strong acid reaction from its constituents is of greater significance than that of stomach contents. Normal GIT rules out poisoning by corrosives (acids, alkalis and phenol), mercury and arsenic.
viii. **Liver (hepatotoxic poisons) and kidneys (nephrotoxic poisons) (Table 35.6).**

Chemical Analysis

The most important proof of poisoning is the analytical detection of poison in the parenchyma of the organs of the body. The finding of poison in the food, medicine or fluid alleged to have been taken is corroborative.

Experiments on Animals

The suspected food, medicine or fluid or poison extracted from viscera can be fed to domestic animals, such as dogs or cats. The poison affects these animals in the same way as human beings.

Circumstantial Evidence

Clues regarding recent purchase of poison by the victim or accused, his behavior, the conduct of those living with the victim, suicide note and history of quarrel or financial problems may provide valuable information.

TABLE 35.5: Color of mucous membrane of stomach due to poisoning

S.No.	Poison	Color
1.	Copper sulfate, amytal capsule	Blue
2.	Ferrous sulfate	Green
3.	Sulfuric, hydrochloric or acetic acid	Black/charred
4.	Nitric acid	Yellow
5.	Carbolic acid	Buff/white
6.	Arsenic	White particles
7.	Mercury	Slate
8.	Cresols	Brown

TABLE 35.6: Hepatotoxic and nephrotoxic poisons

Hepatotoxic poisons	Nephrotoxic poisons
Acute liver necrosis: As, Fe, Tl, phosphorus, CCl_4, chloroform, trinitrotoluene, paracetamol, aluminum phosphide and zinc phosphide	*Acute tubular necrosis:* As, Hg, Cr, oxalic acid, carbolic acid, CCl_4, cantharides, turpentine, paraquat, mushrooms, aluminum phosphide and zinc phosphide
Fatty liver: As, CCl_4, amanita phalloides, $FeSO_4$.	*Parenchymatous degenerative changes:* Metal and cantharidin poisoning
Jaundice: Phosphorus and potassium chlorate	
Granulomatous hepatitis: Cu, salicylates	
Fibrosis and cirrhosis: Ethanol	

> **FM 8.5, 8.9**
> - Describe medico-legal autopsy in cases of poisoning including preservation and dispatch of viscera for chemical analysis.
> - Describe the procedure of preservation and dispatch of relevant samples for laboratory analysis.

SAMPLES PRESERVED FOR TOXICOLOGICAL ANALYSIS

Usually, toxicological procedures require the collection of blood, urine, stomach contents, liver and 'scene residues'—material found at the scene of incident, like tablets or empty containers **(Table 35.7)**. However, other specimens such as hair, sweat, saliva, spleen, kidneys, brain and exhaled air have also been used to determine poisoning and/or drug use (details in Chapter 7). The samples must be sealed and meticulously labeled with the patient's name, address, hospital number and the date of collection. The doctor's signature should also be placed on the label. The sample should be handed to a specific person, often a police officer, whose name is noted, and who will take the sample to the laboratory—maintaining the chain of evidence.

Collection of Specimens

i. **Blood:** It is important to obtain blood samples from the correct site, when postmortem analysis is to be carried out. During life, any venous sample is usually satisfactory, except in unusual circumstances where arterial blood is required. However, at autopsy, the results of analysis can be distorted by an incorrect sample.
   It should not be taken from the heart or great vessels in the chest, as postmortem contamination can occur from the stomach or even from aspirated vomit in the air passages. *The best place to obtain blood is from the femoral or iliac veins, or from the axillary veins.*

ii. **Vomit and stomach contents:** Vomit is placed either in a clean glass jar or a plastic tub with a tight-fitting lid.

iii. **Feces:** The contents of the rectum are not required for analysis, except in suspected heavy metal poisoning, such as arsenic, mercury or lead. A sample of 20–30 g should be taken in a plain screw-topped jar or in a plastic container with a snap-on-lid.

iv. **Liver and other organs:** Liver concentrates many drugs, making them identifiable when the blood and urine concentrations may have declined to very low levels. After examination, 300 g of liver along with gallbladder should be placed in a clean container. Sometimes, bile may be required for analysis, it is particularly useful for seeking presence of chlorpromazine and morphine.

v. **Hair and nail clippings:** If a heavy metal poison is suspected, such as antimony, arsenic or thallium, some hair, cut or pulled at the roots, together with nail clippings, should be submitted for analysis. These metals are laid down in keratin in a sequence depending on the time of administration, and their detection may be possible by *neutron-activation analysis*.

Toxicological analysis of urine and blood (and occasionally of gastric contents and chemical samples) can confirm or rule out suspected poisoning. A negative result means that substance is not detectable by the test used or that its concentration is too low for detection at the time of sampling. In the latter case, repeating the test at a later time may yield a positive result.

> **FM 8.7**
> Describe simple bedside clinic tests to detect poison/drug in a patient's body fluids.

Quantitative analysis is useful for poisoning with acetaminophen, alcohol, barbiturates, heavy metals, paraquat, salicylate, carboxyhemoglobin and methemoglobin.

Some of the bedside chemical tests that are used to screen biological specimens for toxic substances are given in **Table 35.8**. Other bedside tests are discussed along with the respective poisons.

> **NOTA BENE**
> - **'Screening tests'** are said to be *'qualitative'*, where a test is either positive (indicating that the drug/toxin is present) or negative (indicating that the drug/toxin is not present).
> - When specific levels of drugs or toxins are determined, the tests are said to be *'quantitative'*.

FAILURE TO DETECT POISON

In some cases, no trace of poison is found on analysis, although from other circumstances, it is almost or quite certain that poison was the cause of illness or death.

Possible explanations for negative findings:
i. Poison may have been eliminated by vomiting and diarrhea, e.g., irritant poison.
ii. Poison has disappeared from the lungs by evaporation or oxidation.

TABLE 35.7: Sample preservation

Sample	Quantity	Preservative
Whole blood	10 mL	Lithium heparin or EDTA tube; fluoride/oxalate, if alcohol is suspected
Urine	20–50 mL	No preservative, sodium fluoride is added, if alcohol is suspected
Gastric contents	25–50 mL	No preservative
Scalp hair	About 100–200	No preservative
Exhaled air	As required	No preservative
Scene residues	As appropriate	No preservative

TABLE 35.8: Bedside tests applied to detect some xenobiotic

S.No.	Tests	Xenobiotic
1.	Marquis test	Opiates and amphetamines
2.	Mandelin's test	Cocaine, heroin, morphine
3.	Scott test	Cocaine
4.	Dille-Koppanyi test	Barbiturates
5.	Duquenois-Levine test	Marijuana
6.	Ehrlich's test (Van Urk reagent)	LSD
7.	Bratton-Marshall test	Benzodiazepines
8.	Fujiwara test	Halogenated hydrocarbons
9.	Forrest test	Phenothiazines
10.	Reinsch test	Arsenic, mercury
11.	Folin-Ciocalteu test	Phenols
12.	Sodium dithionite test	Paraquat and diquat
13.	Furfuraldehyde test	Carbamates
14.	Test for cholinesterase inhibitors	OPCs
15.	Trinder's test, ferric chloride test	Salicylates

iii. Poison after absorption may be detoxified, conjugated and eliminated from the system.
iv. Some alkaloidal poisons cannot be definitely detected by chemical methods.
v. Some drugs are rapidly metabolized, making extraction difficult.
vi. Biological toxins and venoms which may be protein in nature, cannot be separated from body tissues.
vii. Some organic poisons, especially alkaloids and glucosides may detoxify by oxidation during life or due to faulty preservation or from decomposition of the body, and cannot be detected chemically.
viii. In a slow acting poison, death may be delayed and by then the poison may have been completely excreted following production of irreversible changes.
ix. Many drugs may be present in small amount and these may require considerable amount of viscera for their identification.
x. Wrong or insufficient material may have been sent for analysis.

Describe the general principles of analytical toxicology and give a brief description of analytical methods available for toxicological analysis.

- **Analytical toxicology:** Detection, identification, and measurement of xenobiotics in biological and other specimens.
- **Analytical methods:** Set of techniques that qualitatively (identify and isolate) and/or quantitatively detect the composition of any material and chemical state in which it is located.

CHROMATOGRAPHY

Definition: A physical method of separation in which the components are separated based on their differential interactions distributed between two phases: a mobile phase and a stationary phase.

- The mixture is dissolved in a fluid (*mobile phase*), which carries it through a structure holding another material (*stationary phase*). The various constituents of the mixture travel at different speeds, causing them to separate. The separation is based on differential partitioning between the mobile and stationary phases.
- The instrument that is used to perform a separation in chromatography is known as a chromatograph. For instance, in GC the instrument is a gas chromatograph.

Techniques Based on Chromatographic Bed Shape

- **Column chromatography:** Separation technique in which the stationary bed is within a tube.
- **Planar chromatography:** Separation technique in which the stationary phase is present as or on a plane. The plane can be a paper (*paper chromatography*) or a layer of solid particles spread on a support such as a glass plate (*thin-layer chromatography*).

Techniques Based on Physical State of Mobile Phase

- Gas chromatography
- Liquid chromatography

1. **Thin-layer chromatography (TLC)** is a widely used laboratory technique to separate different biochemicals on the basis of their relative attractions to the stationary and mobile phases. The stationary phase involves the use of a thin layer of adsorbent like silica gel, alumina or cellulose on a metal, plastic or glass plate. It is routinely used to identify and compare samples of drugs, explosives, inks and biological samples such as saliva, urine, blood for the presence of drugs. Various hypnotics, sedatives, anticonvulsants, tranquilizers, antihistamines steroids can be tested qualitatively.
2. **Gas chromatography (GC)/gas-liquid chromatography (GLC)** is a separation technique in which the mobile phase is a gas. Gas chromatographic separation is always carried out in a column. GLC is widely used for analysis of body fluids for the presence of illegal substances, testing of fiber and blood from a crime scene and to detect residue from explosives.
3. **Liquid chromatography (LC)** is a separation technique in which the mobile phase is a liquid. It can be carried out either in a column or a plane. Present-day liquid chromatography that generally utilizes very small packing particles and a relatively high pressure is referred to as high-performance liquid chromatography

(HPLC). In HPLC, the sample is forced by a liquid at high pressure (the mobile phase) through a column that is packed with a stationary phase composed of irregularly or spherically shaped particles or a porous membrane. HPLC is used in identification and quantification of illegal and therapeutic drugs, urine testing for performance enhancing drugs, pesticides and other organic poisons from body fluids, explosive and ink analysis, and fibers.

Atomic Absorption Spectroscopy

Atomic absorption spectroscopy (AAS) is a spectroanalytical procedure for the quantitative determination of elements using the absorption of radiation (light) by free atoms in the gaseous state. In AAS, the total amount of absorption depends on the number of free atoms present and the degree to which the free atoms absorb the radiation. At the high temperature of the AA flame, which may be either oxyacetylene or nitrous oxide/acetylene, the sample is broken down into atoms and it is the concentration of these atoms that is measured. AAS is used for gunshot powder residue analysis and toxicological examinations in suspected heavy metal poisoning cases.

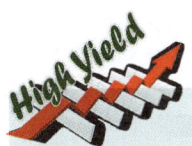

- **Forensic toxicology** deals with medico-legal aspects of the harmful effects of chemicals on human beings.
- **Poison:** Any substance which if introduced or brought in contact with the body will produce ill-health or death by its constitutional or/and local effects.
- All venoms are toxins and all toxins are poisons, but all poisons are not toxins and all toxins are not venoms.
- **Tolerance:** Same dose no longer has the effect that originally it had; seen with alcohol, barbiturates, amphetamines, benzodiazepines and morphine-heroin-methadone group.
- **Idiosyncrasy:** Inherent hypersensitivity towards drugs or food; seen with penicillin, aspirin, cocaine, heroin, sulfonamides, sera, food (mushrooms, eggs, shell-fish, fruits).
- **Antidotes:** Remedies used to counteract the action of poisons.
- **Narcotic drug:** Coca leaf, cannabis (hemp), opium, poppy and all drugs from them.
- **Psychotropic substance:** Any substance included in the list of psychotropic substances specified in the schedule of NDPS Act, e.g. amphetamine, pentobarbital, psilocybin and diazepam.
- **Schedule H:** Prescription drugs.
- Action of poison is delayed, if a person goes to sleep soon after taking it. Action is also delayed, if one takes a poison in an intoxicated state.
- Presence of food in stomach delays the action of the poison in most cases.
- Government or private doctor should report to police all cases of suspected poisoning, whether accidental, suicidal or homicidal. Non-compliance is punishable under Sec. 176 IPC.
- **Sec. under which doctor needs to inform police in homicidal poisoning:** Sec. 39 CrPC.
- Any suspected food articles and stomach wash samples should be preserved. Non-compliance is punishable under Sec. 201 IPC (if the doctor did it with the intention of protecting the accused).
- If the doctor summoned by investigating officer conceals information regarding the case, he is liable under Sec. 202 IPC.
- Embalming without issuing death certificate is punishable under Sec. 201 IPC.
- Homicide by means of poisons is punishable under Sec. 302 IPC.
- **Coma cocktail** consists of dextrose, thiamine, naloxone and flumazenil.
- Gastric lavage is most useful within 1 h after ingestion of poison.
- **Contraindications of gastric lavage:** Corrosives *(except carbolic acid)*, convulsants, comatose patients, compromised unprotected airway, kerosene oil ingestion.
- **Activated charcoal is useful for:** Alkaloids—strychnine, morphine, atropine, nicotine poisoning *(adsorbs poisons)*.
- **Activated charcoal is *not* useful for:** Metals, mineral acids, alkalis, cyanide, fluoride, iron poisoning.
- **Universal antidote:** Combination of physical and chemical antidotes comprising of charcoal, magnesium oxide and tannic acid.
- Anti-snake venom is a *serological antidote* (physiological antidote).
- Chelating agents are specific antidotes against *heavy metal poisoning*.

- **BAL is contraindicated in:** Cadmium and iron poisoning.
- **Alkaline diuresis:** Useful in poisoning with phenobarbital and salicylates.
- **Acid diuresis:** *Not recommended* because of potential CVS and renal complications.
- **Dialysis is useful** for poisoning with barbiturates, cocaine, cannabis, ethanol, methanol and salicylates.
- **Dialysis not indicated** in toxicity with benzodiazepines, kerosene oil, OPC and $CuSO_4$.
- PM staining in CO poisoning is cherry red in color, nitrites: chocolate brown, H_2S: bluish-green and opiates: bluish black.
- Smell in poisoning with phosphorus, arsenic, parathion, malathion and alphos is garlic-like, marijuana: burnt rope, nitrobenzene: shoe polish, OPC: kerosene-like and HCN: bitter almond.
- **Bluish discoloration of gastric mucosa is seen in:** Copper sulphate and amytal sodium poisoning.
- **Constricted pupil (miosis):** Opioids (morphine), phenol, OPC, carbamates, muscarinic type mushrooms, ethanol poisoning.
- **Dilated pupil (mydriasis):** Dhatura, atropine, cannabis, cocaine, strychnine, HCN, methanol poisoning.
- **Test to determine heavy metal poisoning in hair and nails:** Neutron-activation analysis.

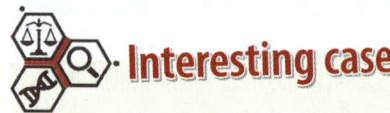

Interesting case

Activated Charcoal (Case of Pierre-Fleurus Touéry, 1852)

Pierre-Fleurus Touéry, a 19th century French scientist whose research focused on two distinct fields: pure chemistry and practical pharmacy **(Fig. A)**. The first of these works was of extracting the active principle from plants, while the second which was the masterful work of Touéry on the virtues of animal charcoal is a reference in the history of modern pharmacy **(Fig. B)**.

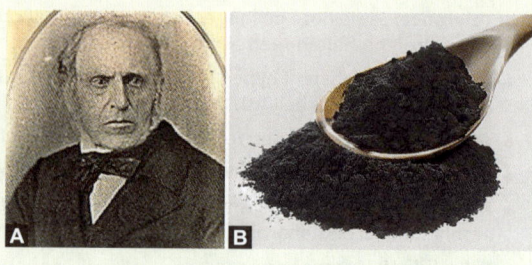

In 1831, through a letter to the *Academie de Medicine*, Paris he explained how activated charcoal could act as an antidote to strychnine, which he claimed to have verified by first poisoning a dog and then himself with a toxic decoction of *Strychnos nux-vomica* nut. However, the result did not convince the audience at the Academy. Around 1851, Touéry intensified his work and carried out no less than 56 experiments, based on the neutralization of cantharidine and strychnine, which he communicated to the Academy. Bouchardat and Deschamps only made a summary report, and Orfila, who is considered as a pioneer of toxicology, turned down his research. In 1852, to prove his point, Touéry, in front of a large sceptical audience on the floor of the Academy ingested ten times the lethal dose of strychnine mixed with charcoal—he survived the stunt unharmed without any ill-effects.

However, it took almost another decade for charcoal to be accepted widely by the medical practitioners as a 'universal antidote'. It was not until 1984 that the American Medical Association attested to the value of the experiments of Touéry and chemist Bertrand, who also achieved similar results in 1813*. Today, charcoal has become one of the most widely used decontamination agents in industry and hospitals, to the great memory of Pierre-Fleurus Touéry.

---

* The first use of charcoal as an antidote occurred in 1813, when French chemist Michel Bertrand reportedly ingested charcoal with 5 g of arsenic trioxide, and survived.

CHAPTER 36

Corrosive Poisons

LEARNING OBJECTIVES

Must know
1. Signs and symptoms, treatment and PM findings in corrosive acid poisoning
2. Vitriolage
3. Carbolism
4. Carboluria

Desirable to know
1. Chemical colitis
2. Oxalic acid poisoning
3. Ochronosis
4. Alkali poisoning

Introduction

- A caustic is a xenobiotic that causes both functional and histologic damage on contact with tissue surfaces.
- They are most commonly categorized into *acids and alkalis*. An acid is a proton donator and causes significant injury at a pH <3, and an alkali is a proton acceptor, which causes significant injury at a pH >11.
- **Table 36.1** list common caustics and commercial products that contain them.
- The ingestion of caustic agents frequently produces adverse effect on the esophagus and the stomach or on both.

TABLE 36.1: Common caustic and its sources

Caustic	Uses
Sulphuric acid	Bleaches, cleansers
Nitric acid	Dishwashing gel, woodworking, metal cleaners
Hydrochloric acid	Toilet bowl cleaners
Boric acid	Roach powder, water softeners, germicide
Oxalic acid	Disinfectants, household bleach, antirust products, furniture refinisher
Carbolic acid	Antiseptics, preservatives
Ammonia	Toilet bowl cleaners, hair dyes, glass cleaners, wax removers
Sodium hydroxide	Detergents, paint removers, drain cleaners and openers, oven cleaners
Sodium carbonates	Detergents, dishwasher gel, water softeners

 FM 9.1

Describe general principles and basic methodologies in treatment of poisoning with regard to caustic inorganic—sulphuric, nitric and hydrochloric acids.

MINERAL/INORGANIC ACIDS

- Mineral acids produce coagulative necrosis, precipitate proteins with resultant hard eschar or scab (which may protect the underlying tissue from further damage), have no remote action and act as irritants when slightly diluted, but as stimulants when well diluted.
- Acids usually cause second degree, deep partial thickness burns, tend to be clearly demarcated and are dry, hard and mildly edematous.
- The stomach is the most commonly involved organ following acid ingestion. This may due to some natural protection of the esophageal squamous epithelium.

Common acids are:
- Sulphuric acid (oil of vitriol, H_2SO_4)
- Nitric acid (*aqua fortis*, HNO_3)
- Hydrochloric acid (HCl)

The signs and symptoms, fatal dose, fatal period, post-mortem appearances and medico-legal aspects of these acids are given in **Table 36.2**.

TABLE 36.2: Salient features of sulphuric acid, nitric acid and hydrochloric acid poisoning (Figs. 36.1A to C)

Feature	H$_2$SO$_4$	HNO$_3$	HCl
Physical properties	Colorless, odorless, burning taste, oily, non-fuming	Colorless, pungent, choking, burning taste, fuming	Colorless, pungent, sour, burning taste, fuming
Action			
Local	Corrosive	Corrosive Respiratory distress (inhalation)	Corrosive Respiratory tract inflammation
Indirect	• Shock, asphyxia • Perforation of stomach • Chemical peritonitis • Esophageal stricture	Pain → circulatory failure	Pain → circulatory failure
Fatal dose (concentrated)	5–10 mL	10–15 mL	15–20 mL
Fatal period	12–18 hours (h)	12–24 h	18–30 h
Signs and symptoms			
• Oropharyngeal burns and burning pain in throat, epigastrium	Present	Present	Present
• Dysphagia, dysphonia and dyspnea	Present	Present	Present
• Eructation, vomiting	Present	Present	Present
• Thirst	Present, drinking causes more vomiting	Same	Same
• Vomitus	Strongly acidic, with altered blood and mucous shreds	Same	Same
• Teeth	Chalky white, brittle	Yellowish coating (due to xantho-proteic reaction), not brittle	No change
• Constipation	Usually present	Same	Same
• Urination	Suppressed	Same	Same
• Tenesmus	Present	Present	May be present
• Nature of stool	Mucus, altered blood	Same	Same
• Tenderness over abdomen	Present	Present	Present
• Stiffness of abdomen	Present, due to peritonitis	Present, due to distension	Present, due to distension
• Abdominal distension	Not usual	Present, due to gas in stomach	Present, due to gas in stomach
• Erosion of skin, mucous membrane of mouth and tongue	Over angles of mouth, lips, fingers with blackening, excoriation	Over angles of mouth, lips, fingers with yellow discoloration	Usually no erosion, epidermis may fall off after few days
• Perforation of stomach	Common	Less common	Less common
Cause of death	• Shock • Perforation of stomach • Peritonitis • Laryngeal spasm • Malnutrition (due to esophageal stricture)	• Shock • Perforation of stomach • Peritonitis • Laryngeal spasm • Respiratory distress	• Shock • Laryngeal spasm • Pulmonary edema (due to inhalation of vapor)
Postmortem findings (Fig. 36.1)	• Erosion of skin, angles of mouth, lips • Corrosion of the trachea and larynx • Blackish charring of the stomach, peppery feel • Perforation of the stomach • Toxic swelling of the liver and kidneys	• Yellow discoloration of skin • Corrosion of skin • Larynx and trachea: congested • Stomach wall is soft, friable and ulcerated	• Not much corrosion of skin • Brownish parchmentization • Inflammation of respiratory passages • Stomach contains brownish fluid
Medico-legal aspects	• Accidental, mistaking it for glycerin • Suicidal: common • Homicide is rare • Abortifacient • Vitriolage	• Accidental or suicidal • Homicide is rare	• Mostly suicidal • Accidental: few • Homicide and abortifacient: rare

CHAPTER 36 : Corrosive Poisons

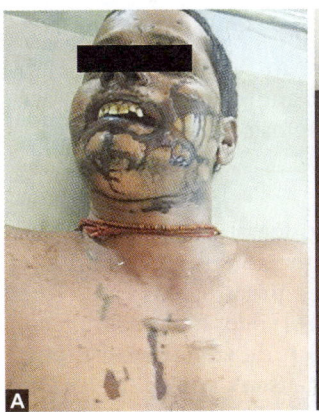
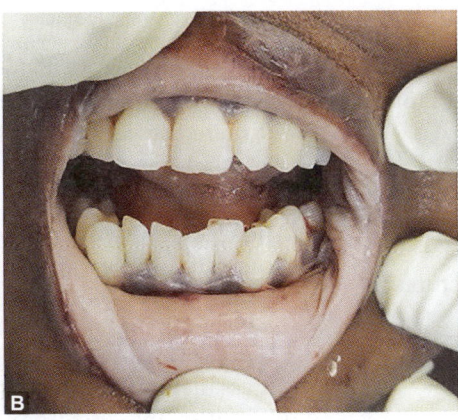
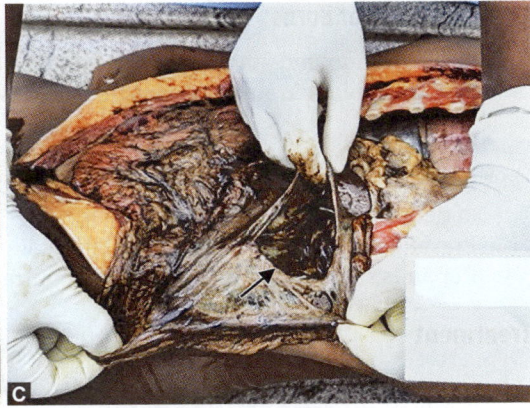

Figs. 36.1A to C: Corrosive poisoning: (A) Erosion of skin, angles of mouth, lips, blackening and trickle marks over cheeks, chin and chest; (B) Chalky white teeth; (C) Blackish viscera and perforation of stomach (arrow)

Treatment

i. Avoid gastric lavage or emetics.
ii. Acid should be immediately diluted by giving a glass of milk or water to drink, and 4 tablespoonfuls of aluminum hydroxide gel.
iii. Give a demulcent, like olive oil, milk, egg white, starch water or butter.
iv. Do not give bicarbonate or other neutralizing agents.
v. Prednisolone 60 mg/day may be given in divided doses.
vi. Correct circulatory shock, IV fluids and blood products are administered in the event of significant bleeding or vomiting. Antibiotics should be given, if evidence of perforation exists.
vii. Tracheostomy, if there is edema of glottis.
viii. Give nothing by mouth. Nutrient substances are given by IV route for about a week. Then, try liquids, soft food and finally a regular diet.
ix. Morphine to relieve pain.
x. Symptomatic treatment.

Skin burns are washed with large amounts of water for 20 minutes (min). No chemical antidotes are used as the heat of the reaction may cause additional injury.

Complications: Delayed perforation may occur as many as 4 days after an acid exposure. Delayed upper GI bleeding may occur in acid burns 3–4 days after exposure as the eschar sloughs. Gastric outlet obstruction may develop 3–4 weeks after an acid exposure.

Preservative: Viscera and skin are preserved in absolute alcohol or rectified spirit and the clothes are sent without any preservatives.

> **NOTA BENE**
> ◆ **Abandonment of neutralizing agents for caustic ingestion:** Earlier, recommendations for the treatment of acid ingestion included the use of magnesium hydroxide, lime water or calcium carbonate, and for alkali ingestions included vinegar (acetic acid), lemon juice or dilute HCl. However, due to the rapid onset of action of corrosive agents, it may be too late to reverse the caustic process. Furthermore, the addition of neutralizing agents could increase the potential for a consequential exothermic reaction and/or gas production. Such reaction in an already weakened hollow viscus may lead to extension of the tissue injury or perforation. Hence, the use of neutralizing agents is no longer recommended.
> ◆ **Magenstrasse** (street of the stomach): In stomach, the injuries are common in the antrum due to "magenstrasse" flow of liquid acids along the lesser curvature of the stomach with resultant pooling in the pylorus secondary to acid-induced pylorospasm **(Fig. 36.2)**. The relative sparing of the duodenum may be due to the pylorospasm and the alkaline pH of the duodenum, but injury does occur. To preserve the pathology, the stomach must be opened along the greater curvature.

VITRIOLAGE (VITRIOL THROWING)

Definition: It is the throwing of any corrosive, not necessarily sulphuric acid, on a person with malicious intent **(Fig. 36.3)**. Sulphuric acid is most commonly used for this purpose, hence it is called vitriolage.

Other substances used: Nitric acid, carbolic acid, caustic soda, caustic potash, iodine, marking nut juice or calotropis.

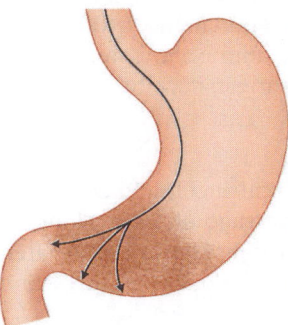
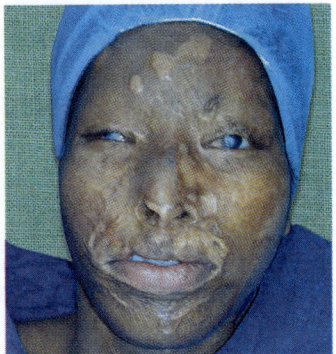

Fig. 36.2: Pathway of corrosive agent in stomach

Fig. 36.3: A case of vitriolage (*Courtesy:* Dr Ish Kumar Garg, SPS Apollo Hospital, Ludhiana)

Characteristics of Burns

i. Discoloration and staining of the skin and clothings (brown or black in sulphuric acid, and yellow in nitric acid).
ii. Trickle marks.
iii. Painless burns with absence of vesication and red line of demarcation.
iv. Presence of chemical substance in the stains.
v. Repair is slow, and scar tissue causes contractures.

Treatment

i. Wash the parts with plenty of water and soap.
ii. Apply thick paste of MgO or carbonate.
iii. Cover raw surface with antibiotic ointment.
iv. For *eye burns,* the conjunctiva and corneal surfaces are anesthetized with topical anesthetic drops (e.g., proparacaine) and irrigated with water* for 15 min holding the eyelids open. Repeat irrigation using 0.9% saline, till pH is near 7.0. Eye drops containing antibiotics and steroids are helpful.

Medico-legal Aspects

- These fluids are usually thrown on the face with the objective of destroying vision or causing facial disfigurement, and this results in *grievous hurt* (**Sec. 320 IPC**).
- It is punishable under **Sec. 326-A IPC** (voluntarily causing grievous hurt by use of acids)$ for 10 years to life imprisonment and fine paid to the victim, and under **Sec 326-B IPC** (voluntarily throwing or attempting to throw acid) with imprisonment for 5–7 years and fine.

CHEMICAL COLITIS

Definition: Chemical colitis is characterized by an inflammation of the colon due to the exposure of colonic mucosa to various toxic chemicals.

Agents Involved

Sulphuric/hydrochloric acid, acetic acid, sodium hydroxide, hydrogen peroxide, alcohol, radiocontrast agents, glutaraldehyde, formalin, ergotamine, hydrofluoric acid, household disinfectants, ammonia, soap, herbal medicines and potassium permanganate.

Signs and Symptoms

Intermittent abdominal pain, fecal incontinence, severe diarrhea, and *hematochezia* (passage of fresh blood in stools). However, severe mucosal injury may be associated with peritonitis, ischemic colitis, colonic strictures and rectovaginal fistulas.

Treatment

Discontinuation of exposure to the toxic agent, fluid resuscitation, broad-spectrum antibiotics, steroids, bowel rest, if there is evidence of necrosis—resection.

Medico-legal Aspects

- Chemical colitis may be accidental, deliberate (suicidal, homicidal or sexual—intentional use of corrosive enemas as sexual practice), or iatrogenic (prescribed medication, contamination of endoscopic instruments).
- High-risk individual include those with mental illness, depression, Munchausen's syndrome, learning difficulties, and certain groups who use enemas regularly.

> **FM 9.1**
> Describe general principles and basic methodologies in treatment of poisoning with regard to caustic organic—oxalic and carbolic acid (phenol).

OXALIC ACID (ACID OF SUGAR)

Physical properties: Colorless, transparent, prismatic crystals and resembles $MgSO_4$ and $ZnSO_4$. Oxalic acid is a naturally occurring component of plants and is found in relatively high levels in dark-green leafy foods, e.g., beet leaves, purslane, spinach, rhubarb and parsley.

Uses: Oxalic acid forms soluble chelates with iron. This property makes it useful for removing blood and rust stains, cleaning metals other than iron and flushing car radiators. It is used in many chemical processes like bleaching and dyeing. It may be used to remove signatures/writings from documents in cases of forgery.

Action: It acts locally as a corrosive on both skin and mucosa, and remotely affects several systems after being absorbed.
- CVS → shock → death
- Electrolyte system → extracts tissue calcium → hypocalcemia
- Renal system → tubular necrosis → uremia → death

Signs and Symptoms

Poisoning presents in three forms:

i. **Fulminating poisoning:** Intake of large dose (>15 g) produces immediate symptoms and death within minutes. There is a burning, sour or bitter taste in the mouth with a sense of constriction around the throat and burning pain from the mouth to stomach, radiating all over the abdomen. Nausea and eructation are immediately followed by vomiting which contains altered blood, mucus and has a **coffee-ground appearance** (black in color). Severe thirst, diarrhea, electrolyte imbalance, and ultimately death occurs.
ii. **Acute poisoning:** All findings are due to hypocalcemia—tingling and numbness of fingers and

---

*Other solution that can be used—0.9% NaCl, Ringer lactate, balanced salt solution.
$ The Delhi High Court has defined the word 'acid' as any substance with an acid/burning/corrosive nature capable to cause bodily injury leading to scars or disfigurement, or temporary or permanent disability.

limbs, weakness, parasthesia, carpopedal spasm,* hyperirritability of peripheral nerves (**Chvostek/Weiss sign**), tetany, convulsions, coma and death. There may be dilated pupils, metabolic acidosis, ventricular fibrillation, and renal failure.

iii. **Delayed poisoning:** It is characterized by nephritis—uremia, scanty urine, hematuria, albuminuria, *oxaluria* (envelope-shaped calcium oxalate crystals in the urine is seen under microscope).

Fatal Dose

15–20 g of oxalic acid.

Fatal period: 1–2 h. In case of renal failure, death may occur between 2 days to 2 weeks.

Treatment

i. Gastric lavage with calcium lactate (2 teaspoons/lavage).
ii. **Antidotes:** Limewater, calcium lactate, calcium gluconate or calcium chloride when given orally (150 mg/kg) act as specific antidotes and form insoluble calcium oxalate, and are excreted.
iii. **Calcium gluconate:** 10 mL of 10% solution IV frequently.
iv. Parathyroid extracts: 100 units IM.
v. Demulcent drink, bowel washes by enema and purgatives.
vi. Hemodialysis and exchange transfusion can be helpful.
vii. Symptomatic treatment.

Postmortem Findings

External: No specific findings. Burns may be present on face and skin.

Internal

i. Mucosa of the mouth, tongue, pharynx and esophagus are bleached and corroded. There are desquamation and hemorrhages.
ii. **Stomach:** Mucosa is reddened and punctate due to erosions, giving velvety red or blackish appearance. Wall of the stomach is softened, but no perforation and contains gelatinous brown material (due to acid hematin formation).
iii. **Kidneys:** Swollen and congested. Tubules on histopathology show oxalate crystals. Renal tubules are necrosed, primarily the PCT.
iv. All other viscera are congested.

Medico-legal Aspects

- Usually consumed accidentally, mistaken for $MgSO_4$ or sodium bicarbonate.
- Suicidal or homicidal cases are rare due to it sour/bitter taste.
- Abortifacient to induce criminal abortion.

CARBOLIC ACID (PHENOL)

Physical properties: Pure phenol is colorless, prismatic needle-shaped and crystalline in form. On exposure to air, it turns pink and liquefies.

Uses: It is used as an antiseptic or disinfectant. *Lysol* is a 50% solution of cresol in saponified vegetable oil. *Dettol* is a chlorinated phenol with turpineol.

Absorption: It is ingested, inhaled and absorbed through skin, per rectum/per vaginum.

Metabolism and Excretion

- Phenol is metabolized in the liver, wherein it gets converted into *hydroquinone and pyrocatechol* and excreted in the urine, partly free and partly in an unstable combination with glucoronic acid. Further oxidation of hydroquinone and pyrocatechol cause a dark smoky *green coloration* of the urine known as **carboluria**.
- It may also cause pigmentation in the cornea and various cartilages, a condition called **ochronosis**.

> **NOTA BENE**
>
> **Ochronosis** is the bluish black discoloration of tissues, such as the ear cartilage and the ocular tissue (sclera, between the margin of the cornea and the outer or inner canthus), seen with alkaptonuria (autosomal recessive metabolic disorder caused by deficiency of homogentisic acid oxidase). It can also occur from exposure to various substances, such as phenol, trinitrophenol, resorcinol, mercury, picric acid, benzene, hydroquinone and antimalarials.

Signs and Symptoms

Poisoning by carbolic acid is known as **carbolism.**

System	Signs and symptoms
Local	Damage to nerve endings with initial tingling sensation *(pins and needles sensation)*. Later, there is numbness, coagulation necrosis and gangrene of tissues that becomes a grayish white slough. Painless, white, opaque eschar is formed and falls off in few days and leaves a brown stain.
GIT	Initially, there is burning and tingling sensation, and later on anesthesia. Diarrhea, pain in abdomen, but vomiting is rarely seen.
RS	Odor of phenol in breath. Inhalation of phenolic vapors causes laryngeal and pulmonary edema. Stertorous breathing and cyanosis are seen.
MS	Muscular spasms, convulsions.
CNS	Headache, giddiness, tinnitus, pupils are constricted.
CVS	Pulse is rapid, feeble and irregular. Skin is cold, clammy and sweating. Collapse, unconsciousness and coma.

(GIT: Gastrointestinal tract; RS: Respiratory system; MS: Muscular system; CNS: Central nervous system; CVS: Cardiovascular system)

Cause of death: Phenol being fat-soluble, attacks the nervous system and causes paralysis of respiratory and CVS centers leading to death.

---

* The hands are flexed at the wrist, fingers are flexed at the metacarpophalangeal joints and the thumb adducted to the palm—so called **Accoucher's hand (Trousseau's sign)**.

SECTION 2: Toxicology

Fatal Dose
1–2 g of phenol, or 25–50 mL of household phenol.

Fatal period: 3–4 h.

Diagnosis: Add 1 mL of 10% ferric chloride to 10 mL of urine; a purple or blue color is formed which persists even on heating. Cresol gives green color.

Treatment
i. Stomach is washed carefully with plenty of lukewarm water containing charcoal, olive oil, $MgSO_4$ or Na_2SO_4. Medicinal liquid paraffin or 30 g of $MgSO_4$ may be left in the stomach after the lavage.
ii. Demulcents may be given.
iii. Saline containing 7 g of $NaHCO_3$/l is given IV to combat circulatory depression, dilute carbolic acid in blood and encourage diuresis.
iv. If phenol falls on the body, contaminated clothing should be removed at once, skin cleaned, and the area washed with soap and water. To prevent further absorption, apply olive oil/methylated spirit.

There is not much of a role for emetics.

Postmortem Findings (Figs. 36.4A and B)

External: Grayish or brownish corrosions at the angle of the mouth, chin, front of the body, arms and hands with phenolic odor. Putrefaction is retarded.

Internal
i. Corrosion of the GIT mucosa, and laryngeal and pulmonary edema.
ii. **Stomach:** Marked corrosion of gastric mucosa and swelling of mucosal folds with coagulated grayish or brownish slimy mucus on it.

- Intervening normal mucosal folds appear dark red in color.
- Hardening of the stomach wall—**leathery stomach**.
- Vomitus and gastric lavage collection show partially detached gastric mucosa.

iii. **Kidneys:** Hemorrhagic nephritis.

Medico-legal Aspects
- It is used for suicidal purposes.
- Accidental poisoning may occur.
- Phenol is rarely used for homicidal poisoning because of its odor and taste.
- Sometimes, it is used as an abortifacient.

Chronic Poisoning (Phenol/Carbol Marasmus)

It is characterized by anorexia, progressive weight loss, excess production of saliva, headache, vertigo, dark urine, and pigmentation of skin and sclera (ochronosis). It was a common occupational disorder of physicians and their assistants during the mid 19th century when carbolic acid sprays were commonly used for antisepsis in operating rooms.

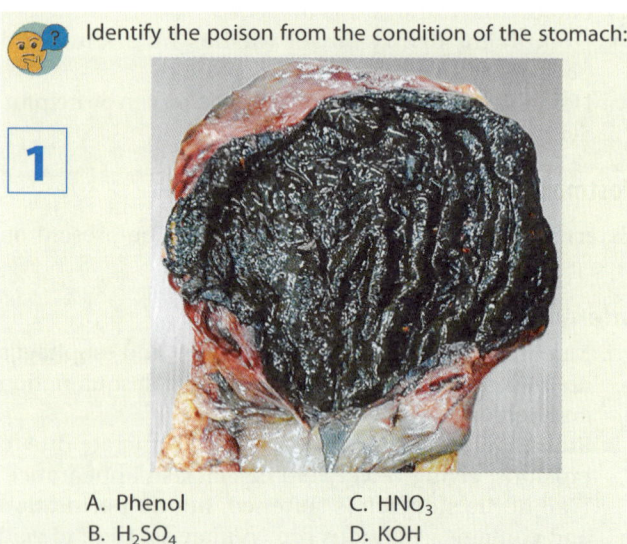

Identify the poison from the condition of the stomach:

A. Phenol
B. H_2SO_4
C. HNO_3
D. KOH

FM 9.6 Describe general principles and basic methodologies in treatment of poisoning with regard to ammonia.

STRONG ALKALIS (CAUSTIC ALKALIS)

Common poisons are ammonia, potassium hydroxide, sodium hydroxide, and carbonates of ammonia, potassium and sodium.

Action: Caustic alkalis produce more severe injury than acids, because they absorb water from tissues, precipitate protein and produce liquefaction necrosis resulting in

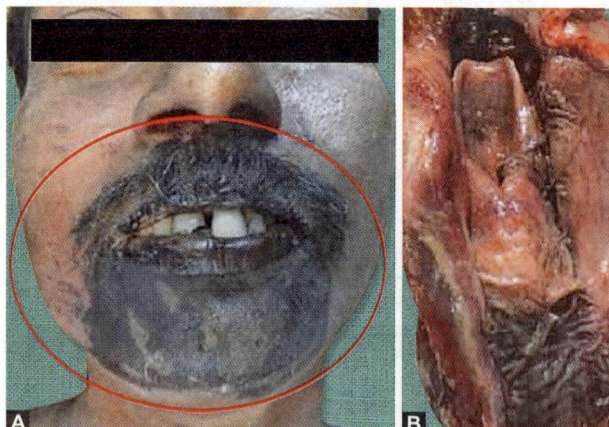

Figs. 36.4A and B: Carbolic acid poisoning: (A) Grayish discoloration of skin over lips and chin; (B) Grayish corrosion of esophageal mucosa.
(*Courtesy:* Dr Jamshid P, Assistant Professor, Department of Forensic Medicine, MES Medical College, Kerala)

deeper penetration and saponification of fats with marked edema.
♦ Agents of alkaline pH usually result in esophageal injury; squamous epithelium lining the esophagus is sensitive to alkaline agents.

Signs and Symptoms

Lesions caused by caustic alkalis are of same extent and distribution as those of acids.
i. There is caustic taste and sensation of burning heat from the throat to the stomach. The vomited matter is alkaline and does not effervesce on contact with the ground. It is at first thick and slimy, but later contains dark altered blood and shreds of mucosa.
ii. Purging is a frequent symptom accompanied by severe pain and straining.
iii. Motions consist of mucus and blood.
iv. Blisters and brownish discoloration is seen on the lips and the skin around the mouth.
v. Mucosa of the digestive tract is soft, swollen with gray slough which readily detaches.
vi. Esophageal stricture formation is a major long-term complication.

Ammoniacal vapor when inhaled causes congestion and watering of eyes, violent sneezing, coughing and choking. Sudden collapse and death may occur from suffocation.

Fatal Dose

♦ KOH and NaOH: 5 g.
♦ Ammonia: 30 g.
♦ Sodium and potassium carbonate: 15–30 g.

Fatal period: 24 h.

Treatment

i. Gastric lavage or emetics are contraindicated.
ii. Dilute immediately with water.
iii. Demulcents, like egg white and milk may be given.
iv. In case of inhalation of ammonia vapor, O_2 inhalation should be given.
v. Keep airway patent, tracheostomy if necessary.
vi. Give adequate parenteral analgesics and antibiotics.
vii. Steroid is of no benefit and is contraindicated in case of esophageal perforation.

Complications: Airway edema or obstruction may occur immediately or upto 48 h following alkali ingestion.

Postmortem Findings

i. Characteristic odor in case of ammonia.
ii. The marks about the mouth become dark in color and parchment-like after death.
iii. Inflammatory edema with corrosion and sliminess of the tissues of the esophagus and stomach are prominent features. Most severely affected is the *squamous epithelium of the esophagus* with the stomach much less frequently involved after alkaline ingestions.
iv. Mucosa may be brownish due to formation of alkali hematin.
v. Perforation of the esophagus or stomach is rare.
vi. Kidneys are inflamed and congested.

Medico-legal Aspects

♦ Accidental poisoning is common in children.
♦ Homicidal cases are rare, and few suicidal cases are seen.
♦ Poisoning by ammonia is more common than with other alkalis.

A 41-year-old male presented with vomiting, altered sensorium, with GCS E2V2M4. BP 80/60 mm Hg, tachypenic with bilateral contricted pupils. There was grayish discoloration of lips and gums. On catheterization, greenish colored urine was seen. What is your provisional diagnosis?

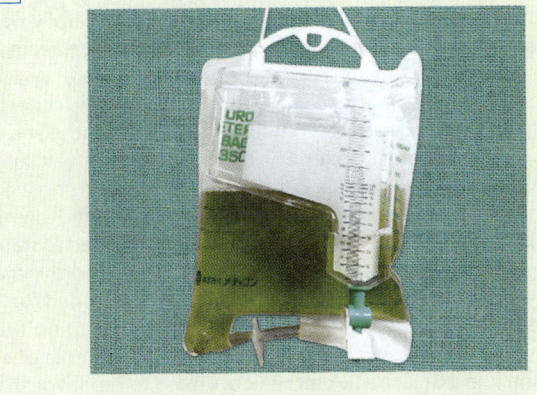

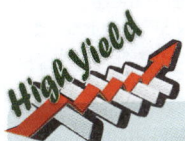

♦ **Most common organ involved in acid ingestion:** Stomach.
♦ **Most common organ involved in alkali poisoning:** Squamous epithelium of esophagus.
♦ Perforation of stomach is seen in ingestion of sulphuric acid.

- **Most common substance used in vitriolage:** Sulphuric acid.
- **Vitriolage causing grievous hurt is punishable under:** Sec. 326-A IPC.
- Gastric lavage and emetics are contraindicated in acid poisoning.
- In stomach, the injuries are common in antrum due to 'magenstrasse' flow of acids along the lesser curvature of stomach.
- In deaths due to acid poisoning, viscera and skin are preserved in absolute alcohol or rectified spirit.
- Burns in vitriolage are painless with absence of vesication and red line of demarcation.
- Oxalic acid is naturally occurring component of plants and is found in dark-green leafy foods, e.g., beet leaves, purslane, spinach, rhubarb and parsley.
- In oxalic acid poisoning, envelope-shaped calcium oxalate crystals in the urine (*oxaluria*) are seen under microscope.
- Tetany is caused by poisoning with oxalic acid.
- Trousseau sign is positive in oxalic acid poisoning.
- Coffee-ground appearance of vomit is seen in oxalic acid poisoning.
- In deaths due to oxalic acid poisoning, kidney tubules show oxalate crystals.
- Green-colored urine is seen in carbolic acid (phenol) poisoning (carboluria—oxidation of *hydroquinone and pyrocatechol*).
- Ochronosis is seen in poisoning with carbolic acid poisoning.
- In phenol poisoning, pupils are constricted.
- Gastric lavage can be done in carbolic acid poisoning.
- **Ferric chloride test is done to diagnose:** Carbolic acid poisoning.
- Leathery stomach is seen in carbolic acid poisoning.

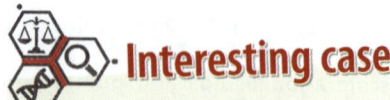

Interesting case

Vitriolage (Case of Laxmi Agarwal, 2005)

Laxmi Agarwal, a girl belonging to a middle-class family was attacked with acid at age of 15 in Delhi's Khan Market in 2005 by her acquaintances, Naeem Khan alias Guddu and Rakhi, when she rejected the romantic advances of the former.

She survived the vitriolage attack, but her face and other body parts were disfigured, and she suffered severe mental and physical strain. For months, she was unable to wear any clothes and would stay under a blanket. She had to undergo seven surgeries and was so traumatized that she contemplated suicide. But thinking of the pain she would cause her parents, she decided to end such thoughts. Instead, Laxmi chose to confide in her parents, who encouraged her to seek counselling. She gained confidence and decided to start her diploma in vocational training. She also decided to take her case to the court, and the trial went on for 4 years. Naeem was sentenced to 10 years in jail, and Rakhi was imprisoned for 7 years.

Simultaneously, she filed public interest litigation (PIL) in 2006, seeking a ban on the sale of acid, citing an increasing number of incidents of such attacks on women across the country. In 2013, the Supreme Court ruled in her favor that led to the regulation of the sale of acid, compensation for the victims, after-care and rehabilitation of the survivors, limited compensation from the government, reservation in educational institutions and easier access to jobs. Under the new regulations, acid could not be sold to any individual <18 years and he has to furnish a photo identity card before buying. The IPC was amended to introduce a section that exclusively dealt with acid attacks. In 2015, the SC also issued a directive that made it mandatory for private and public hospitals to treat acid attack victims free of charge. Acid attack survivors are now given rights under the Rights of Persons with Disabilities Act, 2016.

Laxmi received the Women Courage Award by Michelle Obama in the year 2014. In 2020, the film '*Chhapaak*' was released which was based on her life story with Deepika Padukone playing the role of Laxmi **(Fig. A)**. She is a now motivational speaker on an international level.

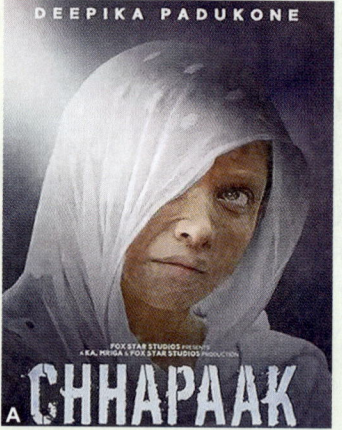

37 CHAPTER

Inorganic Metallic Irritants—Arsenic

LEARNING OBJECTIVES

Must know
1. Signs and symptoms of chronic arsenic poisoning
2. Postmortem findings in arsenic poisoning
3. Raindrop pigmentation
4. Mees lines
5. Arsenic poisoning and cholera (Diff.)
6. Advantages and disadvantages of arsenic as an ideal homicidal poison

Desirable to know
1. Signs and symptoms and treatment of acute arsenic poisoning
2. Blackfoot disease
3. Laboratory investigations in arsenic poisoning

FM 9.3
Describe general principles and basic methodologies in treatment of poisoning with regard to arsenic.

Introduction

Physical properties: Metallic arsenic (black in color) is not poisonous, as it is not absorbed from the GIT. It is a normal constituent of all animal tissues, in minute amounts.

Toxic Compounds and its Uses

i. **Arsenious oxide or arsenic trioxide (Fig. 37.1A)** (*sankhya, somalkhar*, white arsenic or arsenic): Most toxic form of arsenic. It has no taste or smell and is sparingly soluble in water. It is used in fruit sprays, sheep-dips, weed-killers, insecticides, rat poisons, flypapers, calico-printing, wallpapers, artificial flowers and as mordant in dyeing.

ii. **Copper arsenite** (*Scheele's green*) and **copper acetoarsenite** (*Paris green or emerald green*) **(Fig. 37.1B):** It is used as coloring agent for substances including confectionary.
iii. **Sodium and potassium arsenate**.
iv. **Arsenic sulfide:** Yellow orpiment (*hartal*) or arsenic trisulfide, and red realgar or arsenic disulfide are used as depilatory, coloring pigment and in flypaper.
v. Arseniuretted hydrogen or arsine is a colorless gas with garlic-like odor.
vi. The **natural sources** of arsenic are soil, water and some sea fish (mussels, prawns). High arsenic content of soil and subsoil water of some places is the cause of endemic toxicity (from shallow tube-wells inserted for drinking water).
vii. Tobacco smoke, particularly cigars also contain arsenic, and in some beers as impurities.

Action

♦ Arsenic interferes with cellular respiration by uncoupling mitochondrial oxidative phosphorylation and combining with the sulfhydryl groups of mitochondrial enzymes, especially pyruvate dehydrogenase and certain phosphatases. Consequently, conversion of pyruvate to acetyl CoA is decreased, citric acid cycle activity is decreased and production of cellular ATP is decreased.
♦ It inhibits cellular glucose uptake, gluconeogenesis, fatty acid oxidation and further production of acetyl CoA.

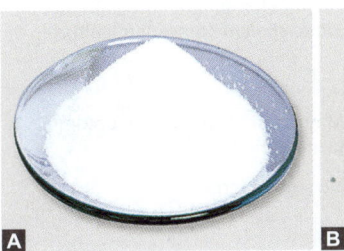 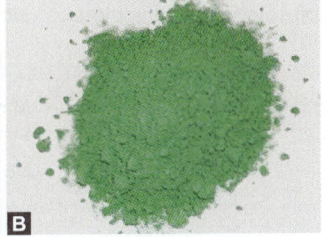

Figs. 37.1A and B: (A) Arsenious oxide; (B) Copper acetoarsenite

- Locally, it causes irritation of the mucous membranes, and remotely, depression of the nervous system.
- Arsenic is a carcinogenic substance since lung, skin and bladder (transitional cell) carcinoma has been observed in populations with multiple exposures.

Absorption and Excretion

It is absorbed orally through the GIT, skin and lungs (arsine) or parenterally.
- It is present in almost all tissues, and found in the greatest quantity in the liver, followed by kidneys and spleen.
- In cases, where the patient survives, it is found in the muscles (for months), bones, hair, nails and skin (sulfhydryl groups in keratin) for years. Normally, the hair contains <2 parts/million arsenic.
  It is excreted mainly by the kidneys (urine), but some part through feces, bile, sweat, milk, nails and hair.
- The arsenic is excreted in the hair and nails within few hours of ingestion, and in cases of intermittent chronic poisoning there will be successive deposits of arsenic in the hair and nails.
- Arsenic is secreted into the stomach and intestines after absorption, even when given by routes other than mouth.

SIGNS AND SYMPTOMS (ACUTE POISONING)

Clinical features manifest in virtually all body systems. Symptoms usually appear by 10 minutes (min) to 1 hour (h) after ingestion, but may be delayed, if arsenic is taken with food.

System	Signs and symptoms
GIT	Sweetish metallic taste, nausea, persistent vomiting, burning in mouth and throat, and difficulty in swallowing, garlic odor in breath, intense thirst, pain in esophagus and abdomen, purging accompanied by tenesmus, pain and irritation about the anus. Initially, defecation is frequent and involuntary, dark-colored, but later, it become colorless, odorless and watery resembling *rice-water*.
Renal	Oliguria, uremia, albuminuria, red cells and casts, pain during micturition.
CVS	Hypotension, pulmonary edema, ARDS, circulatory collapse, ventricular tachycardia and fibrillation.
Hepatic	Fatty infiltration.
MS	Pain in limbs, weakness.
CNS	Headache, vertigo, hyperthermia, tremors, convulsions, coma, general paralysis.
Skin	Delayed loss of hair, skin rash and eruptions.

- *Acute exposures* generally manifest with the cholera-like gastrointestinal symptoms of nausea, vomiting, abdominal pain and severe diarrhea **(Diff. 37.1)**. Respiratory failure and pulmonary edema are common features of acute poisoning.
- In *fulminant type*, when large dose (>3 g) is taken, the GIT symptoms are absent and death occurs in 1–3 h from shock and peripheral vascular failure.

DIFFERENTIATION 37.1: Arsenic poisoning and cholera

S.No.	Feature	Arsenic poisoning	Cholera
1.	GIT symptoms (in order of appearance)	Pain in throat ↓ Vomiting ↓ Purging*	Purging ↓ Vomiting ↓ Pain in throat
2.	Vomitus	Contains mucus, bile and blood	Watery, without mucus, bile or blood
3.	Stools	Rice-watery, may contain blood	Rice-watery, no blood, and passed in a continuous involuntary jet
4.	Tenesmus** and pain around anus	Present	Absent
5.	Voice	Not affected	Rough and whistling
6.	Conjunctiva	Inflamed	Not inflamed
7.	Laboratory investigation	• Radiopaque shadow (X-ray abdomen) seen in arsenic trioxide • Level of urinary coproporphyrin III may be increased • Arsenic in chemical analysis	*Vibrio cholerae* present in culture
8.	Circumstantial evidence	Poisoning may be present in an individual or a family or a group	May occur in sporadic or epidemic form in the locality
9.	Motive	Homicidal, rarely accidental	No such thing

* Evacuate/empty his/her bowels
** Persistent and painful desire to evacuate the bowel, despite having an empty colon.

- In *narcotic type*, the GIT symptoms are less. There is giddiness, formication, tenderness of the muscles, delirium, coma and death. Rarely, there is complete paralysis of the extremities.
- *Arsine gas exposure* causes hemolysis, damages the liver and kidneys (hemoglobinuria and renal failure) and depresses the CNS. There is nausea, vomiting, shaking chills, backache and anemia. The urine appears black due to hemoglobinuria. Death may be preceded by anuria and convulsions.

Fatal Dose

- Inorganic arsenic: 0.6 mg/kg/day
- Arsenic trioxide: 120–200 mg (adults) and 2 mg/kg (children).

Fatal period: 1–2 days.

Laboratory Investigations

Urine, stool, blood, vomit, hair and nails from patients, and in addition, stomach and intestinal contents, bone, liver, bile and kidneys from dead bodies are tested.

- *Urine:* Excretion of arsenic >50 µg/L in 24 h urine is indicative of recent poisoning. Metabolites of arsenic including methylarsonic acid and dimethylarsenic acid may be recovered in a urine specimen.
- *Blood* (serum arsenic >0.9 µg/dL), stool, liver, kidneys and bones show presence of arsenic. As with all heavy metals, microcytic hypochromic anemia is common.
- *Hair:* Arsenic >75 µg% is suggestive of poisoning. Levels between 1.0–3.0 mg/kg indicate acute poisoning, while 0.1–0.5 mg/kg indicates chronic poisoning.
- *Nails:* Presence of >100 µg% of arsenic is suggestive of poisoning.
- Radiopaque sign on abdominal *X-ray*.
- *ECG:* QRS broadening, QT prolongation, ST depression and T-wave flattening.
- *Marsh, Reinsch and Gutzeit tests* are obsolete.

Neutron activation analysis and atomic absorption spectroscopy helps in estimating concentration of arsenic in hair, nails and bone.

TREATMENT

Hemodynamic stabilization is of primary importance, and large amounts of crystalloid solutions may be required because of significant GI losses (i.e., vomiting and diarrhea).

i. Gastric lavage is done repeatedly with large amount of warm water and milk; activated charcoal does not adsorb arsenic appreciably and is not recommended in patients whom co-ingestants are not suspected.
ii. Demulcents (butter or greasy substances) prevent absorption.
iii. Whole bowel irrigation with polyethylene glycol may be effective to prevent GIT absorption of arsenic.
iv. **Antidote** is *BAL* or *dimercaprol*, given in a dose of 3–5 mg/kg IM 4 hourly for 2 days, 6 hourly for 1 day and then 12 hourly for 10 days. Oral *succimer* (DMSA), 10 mg/kg every 8 hourly for 10 days or *dimerval* (DMPS, *drug of choice for treating most heavy metal poisonings*), 200 mg IV 4 hourly until oral product can be given in a dose of 100 mg TDS or QID may be used instead of BAL.
v. Alkalis should not be given by mouth as they increase the solubility of arsenic.
vi. Purgatives (castor oil/magnesium sulfate) are given to remove unabsorbed poison from intestine.
vii. Glucose-saline with sodium bicarbonate is helpful to combat shock and improve alkali reserve.
viii. Hemodialysis or exchange transfusion may be done.

> **NOTA BENE**
> Earlier, *freshly precipitated ferric hydroxide* (**antidotum arsenici**) was used for stomach wash in the treatment of arsenic poisoning which formed ferric arsenite, is no longer recommended.

POSTMORTEM FINDINGS

External

i. The body looks emaciated due to dehydration.
ii. Rigor mortis appears early.
iii. Putrefaction is delayed due to anti-bacterial action of arsenic and partly due to dehydration.
iv. The eyeballs are sunken and the skin is cyanosed.
v. Blood tinged vomitus and fecal matter may be present on the body and clothes.

Internal

i. The mucous membrane of the mouth, pharynx and esophagus may show inflammation or ulceration.
ii. Hemorrhages may be found in the abdominal organs and mesentery, and occasionally in the larynx, trachea and lungs.
iii. **Lungs:** Congested, pulmonary edema with subpleural ecchymoses.
iv. **Heart:** Subendocardial petechial hemorrhages of the ventricle may be found, even when the stomach shows little signs of irritation.
v. **Stomach:** Mucosa is swollen, edematous, desquamated and red, either generally or in patches, especially in the pyloric region. Usually, groups of petechiae are seen scattered over the mucosa, but sometimes large submucosal and subperitoneal hemorrhages may be seen—**red velvety appearance**. A mass of sticky mucus covers the mucosa in which

particles of arsenic may be seen. Congestion is most marked along the crest of the rugae. Inflammation is more marked at the greater curvature, posterior part and the cardiac end of the stomach.

vi. **Small intestine:** It contains large flakes of mucus with very little fecal matter. The mucosa is pale-violet and shows signs of inflammation with submucous hemorrhages along its whole length.

vii. **Cecum and rectum** show slight inflammation.

viii. **Liver, spleen and kidneys:** Congested, enlarged and show cloudy swelling, and occasionally fatty degeneration. Nephritis and scarring of renal cortices are seen.

ix. **Brain:** Edema with patchy necrosis or hemorrhagic encephalitis. The meninges are congested.

CHRONIC ARSENIC POISONING

Chronic arsenic poisoning may occur due to:
- Recovery from an acute poisoning.
- Accidental ingestion of small doses repeatedly by those working with the metal.
- Intake of food/drink in which there are traces of arsenic (may be homicidal in nature).

Tolerance: Some people take arsenic daily as a tonic or as an aphrodisiac and they acquire tolerance to 250–300 mg or more in one dose. Such people are known as *arsenophagists*.

Signs and Symptoms

It is divided into four stages **(Table 37.1)**:
i. GIT disturbances
ii. Catarrhal changes
iii. Skin rashes
iv. Nervous disturbances

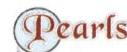

Conditions in which Mees' lines can be seen:
1. Poisoning (arsenic, thallium, fluorosis)
2. Severe infection
3. Renal disease
4. Cardiac failure
5. Malignant disease

- A metallic taste, excessive salivation, and garlic odor of breath and sweat may indicate chronic arsenic poisoning.
- Melanosis and leucomelanosis with or without keratosis are the earliest symptoms of arsenicosis.

TABLE 37.1: Signs and symptoms in chronic arsenic poisoning

System	Signs and symptoms
GIT	Nausea, vomiting, abdominal cramps, loss of appetite, constipation or diarrhea, salivation.
Ocular	Congestion, watering of the eyes, photophobia.
RS	Cough, hoarseness of voice, bronchial catarrh, hemoptysis, dyspnea.
Skin and nails (Figs. 37.2A to C)	There may be a rash resembling fading measles rash. Speckled brown pigmentation, mostly on the skin flexures, temples, shoulders, eyelids and neck (**raindrop pigmentation**). Macular areas of depigmentation may appear on normal/hyperpigmented skin—**leucomelanosis**. Hyperkeratosis of the palms and soles with irregular thickening of the nails and development of white bands of opacity in the nails of fingers and toes (called **Aldrich-Mees lines**). Brittle nails and alopecia are also seen.
CNS	Peripheral neuropathy with tingling, numbness of hands and feet, polyneuritis, anesthesia, paresthesia with painful swelling (*erythromelalgia*), encephalopathy. Neuritis resembles chronic alcoholism.
CVS	Hypertension, ischemic heart disease, cardiac failure, dependent edema.
Renal	Chronic nephritis, urine may be red or green in color, dysuria and anuria may develop from renal tubular necrosis.
Hepatic	Hepatomegaly, jaundice, cirrhosis of the liver.
Hematologic	Bone marrow suppression, hypoplasia, anemia, thrombocytopenia and leukemia.

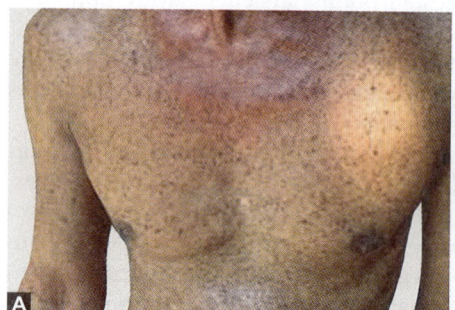
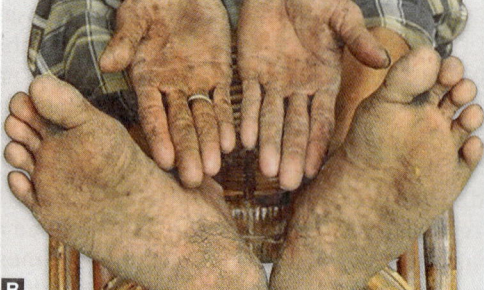
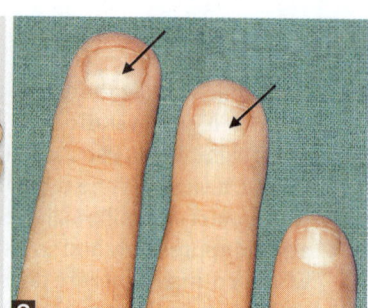

Figs. 37.2A to C: Chronic arsenic poisoning: (A) Raindrop pigmentation; (B) Hyperkeratosis of palms and soles; (C) Aldrich-Mees' lines in nails (arrows)

- Chronic exposure also causes diabetes, vasospasm and peripheral vascular insufficiency (**blackfoot disease**—peripheral vascular disease characterized by systemic arteriosclerosis resulting in dry gangrene and spontaneous amputations of lower extremities).
- Squamous and basal cell carcinomas, and Bowen disease may occur.

> **Mnemonic for chronic arsenic poisoning: ARSENIC**
> A: **A**ldrich-Mees' lines; R: **R**aindrop pigmentation; S: **S**oles hyperkeratosis; E: **E**rythromelalgia; N: **N**europathy (peripheral); I: **I**cterus (jaundice); C: **C**irrhosis

Treatment

i. Remove the patient from the source of exposure and gastric decontamination should be done, if there is evidence of arsenic in GIT. Vigorous scrubbing with soap and water will remove arsenic from skin.
ii. Administer BAL in usual doses.
iii. Vitamin B complex and IV sodium thiosulfate are useful; hemodialysis is not indicated.
iv. Mineral supplements and antioxidant therapy are beneficial.
v. Symptomatic treatment.
vi. When homicidal intent is suspected, all hospital visitors should be closely monitored and outside food should be forbidden.

POSTMORTEM FINDINGS

External

Emaciation, pigmentation, keratosis, alopecia, white streaks on nails, jaundice, wasting of muscles, and ulceration of nasal septum.

Internal

i. **Stomach:** It may be normal or may show a chronic gastritis. Some rugae may show patchy inflammatory redness or focal ulceration.
ii. **Small intestine:** Reddish with thickened mucosa.
iii. **Liver:** Hepatomegaly, fatty degeneration or even necrosis with non-cirrhotic portal fibrosis.
iv. **Kidneys:** Tubular necrosis.
v. **Heart:** Myocardial necrosis may be seen.
- Bone marrow histopathology will show hypoplasia.
- If arsenic poisoning is suspected, hair or tissue samples should be obtained for confirmation.

Medico-legal Aspects

Arsenic poisoning can be homicidal, suicidal, accidental, occupational, environmental, iatrogenic or unintentional.

i. **Homicide**

> Arsenic was a popular homicidal poison because:*
> - Onset of symptoms is gradual
> - Symptoms simulate those of cholera
> - Small quantity is required to cause death
> - Can be administered easily with food, drink or betel leaf (paan)
> - Chronic cases causing debility resemble certain diseases
> - Cheap
> - Colorless
> - Tasteless
> - Odorless
> - Easily obtainable

Disadvantages of arsenic as homicidal poison:
- It retards putrefaction.
- It can be detected in decomposed/buried bodies.
- Arsenic can be found in bones, hair and nails for several years.
- It can be detected in charred bones or ashes.

ii. **Suicide** is rare, because it causes too much of pain.
iii. **Accidental** death may be due to admixture with articles of food or from its improper medicinal use.
iv. Arsenic exposure can be **occupational** in those working in metal foundry, mining, glass production or in the semiconductor industry.
v. **Environmental contamination** of water sources has become a major problem in many countries, including India. Chronic poisoning results from drinking well water containing arsenic.
vi. It is sometimes ingested or applied locally in the form of a paste or ointment on abortion sticks to procure abortion.
vii. It may be used as cattle poison.

POSTMORTEM IMBIBITION OF ARSENIC

- Arsenic is the 12th most abundant element on earth. This makes it obvious that in postmortems after exhumations, the possibility of imbibition from the surrounding earth should be considered. Adequate controls should be taken from surrounding and distant soil and ground water, as any arsenic found in the body may found its way by percolation from natural sources.
- Keratin tissues absorb arsenic by contamination from outside. The concentration in hair and nails thus contaminated is likely to be much greater than the concentration of arsenic in the contaminating fluid.
- In poisoning cases, the concentration of arsenic should be more than in the soil/ground water.

---

* Arsenic became notorious as '*inheritance powder*' because people would use it to kill their family members to gain the inheritance.

SECTION 2 : Toxicology

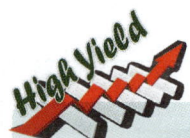

- Metallic arsenic is not poisonous, as it is not absorbed from the GIT.
- **Most toxic form of arsenic:** Arsenic trioxide.
- Natural sources of arsenic are soil, water and some sea fish (mussels, prawns).
- High arsenic content of soil and subsoil water—cause of endemic toxicity.
- Heavy metals like arsenic, mercury, copper, cadmium combine with the sulfhydryl groups of mitochondrial enzymes → interferes with cellular respiration.
- Acute arsenic poisoning manifests with *cholera-like GIT symptoms*.
- In acute arsenic poisoning, stools are dark-colored initially, but later it becomes *rice-water like*.
- **Tests to detect arsenic:** Marsh test, Reinsch test and Gutzeit test.
- **Technique to detect arsenic in hair, nails, bone:** Neutron activation analysis and AAS.
- **Preferred specimen for acute arsenic poisoning:** Urine.
- **Preferred specimen for chronic arsenic poisoning:** Hair.
- **Antidote for acute arsenic poisoning:** BAL or dimerval (DMPS—*drug of choice for heavy metal poisoning*).
- **Red velvety stomach mucosa is seen in:** Arsenic poisoning.
- *Raindrop pigmentation, leucomelanosis and Aldrich-Mees lines* are characteristic of chronic arsenic poisoning.
- *Blackfoot disease* is caused due to chronic arsenic poisoning.
- Chromic arsenic poisoning mimics Guillain-Barre syndrome.
- Arsenic was a popular homicidal poison since symptoms simulate cholera.
- **Disadvantages of arsenic as homicidal poison:** Retards putrefaction and can be detected in decomposed/buried bodies.

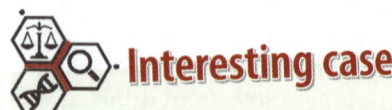

Arsenic Poisoning (Case of Cynthia Sommer, 2008)

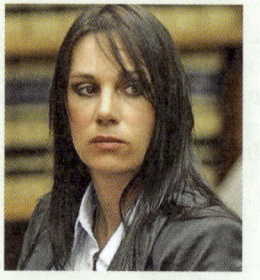

Todd Sommer, a healthy young Marine collapsed and died in February 2002 at his home in San Diego. He was having GIT distress for the last 10 days—vomiting, diarrhea, nausea, stomach cramping, which he thought was due to food poisoning. On that day, he felt well enough to go on a family outing to an amusement park. But when he returned home, he collapsed and died unexpectedly. The doctor ruled death as a result of cardiac arrhythmia and cause of death as a heart attack. His wife donated his tissues and organs to research and his body was cremated. But more than a year later, military forensic investigators reported finding extremely high levels of arsenic in his liver and kidneys—although not in other body tissues. The medical examiner opined that it was a case of acute arsenic poisoning and he died of the direct effect of arsenic on the heart. Cynthia, his wife was arrested and charged with his murder in November 2005.

The prosecutor built the case largely on the lab tests and her promiscuous behavior after Todd's death. She collected $250,000 in life insurance. The prosecution introduced dubious witnesses who testified that Cynthia had obtained breast augmentation, entered a wet T-shirt contest and engaged in sex with several men after Todd's death. She had opportunity and the motive and arsenic was present in Todd's body. But expert witnesses on both sides testified that there were some inconsistencies in the test results. The significantly high levels in his liver and kidney should have resulted in elevated levels in his blood, urine, brain and other organs. Moreover, the prosecutors had no evidence, no purchasing records, electronic paper trail or any direct link to prove that she had access to the arsenic that killed her husband.

In January 2007, a jury convicted Cynthia of first-degree murder with the special circumstances of murder by poison and murder for financial gain. But the trial judge vacated her conviction and granted her a new trial based on ineffective assistance of her counsel. She got a new attorney for the new trial and he pursued the issue of the unreliability of the laboratory results. He gathered all the tissue samples that had been taken from Todd's body, including some that were not tested before during the first trial. He then sent the samples to an internationally-renowned lab for testing. Testing on the newly found materials, including samples from liver and kidneys were negative for arsenic. An expert also suggested that earlier samples in which arsenic was found must have been contaminated. In April 2008, based on these new tests, the court dismissed the charges against Cynthia and she was released.

She was wrongfully convicted of murdering her husband with arsenic based on false toxicological and gender-biased evidence. However, Todd Sommer's death is still officially listed as a homicide.

38 CHAPTER

Inorganic Metallic Irritants— Mercury

LEARNING OBJECTIVES

Must know
1. Toxic compounds of mercury
2. Danbury tremors/hatter's shakes
3. Mercurial erethism
4. Mercurialentis
5. Acrodynia (Pink disease)
6. Minamata disease

Desirable to know
1. Signs and symptoms and fatal dose of acute mercury poisoning
2. Treatment of acute mercury poisoning
3. Diagnosis of mercury poisoning
4. Medico-legal aspects of mercury poisoning

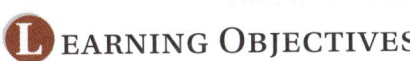

Describe general principles and basic methodologies in treatment of poisoning with regard to mercury.

Introduction

Mercury (*quicksilver/para*) has three forms:
  i. **Elemental mercury** is a heavy, silvery liquid and volatile at room temperature **(Fig. 38.1A)**. It is non-poisonous, if swallowed, since it is poorly absorbed from the GIT. But mercury vapor can give rise to acute toxicity.
 ii. **Inorganic salts** toxicity occurs in several forms: metallic mercury (Hg), mercurous mercury (Hg$^+$), or mercuric mercury (Hg^{2+}).
iii. **Organic compounds** are found in three forms: aryl and short- and long-chain alkyl compounds. Organic salts are better absorbed from the GIT than the inorganic salts because of its intrinsic properties, such as lipid solubility. It can cross the blood-brain barrier to accumulate in the brain, hence CNS effects are more predominant. In contrast, the kidney is the main storage organ for inorganic compounds.
  ♦ Mercury exposures occur chiefly through inhalation of elemental mercury vapor via occupational or dental amalgam* exposure or through ingestion of mercury bonded to organic moieties, primarily from seafood.

Toxic Compounds

A. *Inorganic salts*
  i. **Mercuric chloride** (*corrosive sublimate*): Colorless, odorless, prismatic crystals or white crystalline powder, but has a nauseous metallic taste. It is the most toxic inorganic salt, and *common cause* of acute poisoning.
 ii. **Mercurous chloride** (calomel): Heavy, amorphous, white and tasteless powder.
iii. **Mercuric sulfide** (*cinnabar* or *vermilion*): It is not absorbed through skin, and is as such non-poisonous (red crystalline powder) **(Fig. 38.1B)**.
iv. **Mercuric cyanide, oxide** and **iodide** (scarlet red powder).

B. *Organic salts* include methyl mercury (most toxic), dimethyl mercury, ethyl mercury and phenyl mercury.

Uses

  ♦ **Medicine:** Disinfectant, dental amalgam, purgative and diuretic, and earlier used in the treatment of syphilis. A controversial source of organic mercury exposure is *thimerosal*, a preservative used in vaccines (DTP and hepatitis B) to prevent bacterial contamination.
  ♦ **Industry:** Manufacture of thermometer, barometer, calibration instruments, fluorescent and mercury

---
* **Amalgam** is also known as '*silver fillings*' because of its color. It contains 45–52% of mercury and rest is copper, tin, silver and zinc.

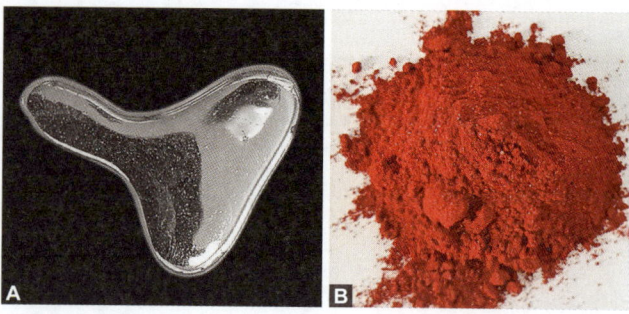

Figs. 38.1A and B: (A) Elemental mercury; (B) Mercuric sulfide

vapor lamp*, electrical equipment, explosives and fireworks.
- **Miscellaneous:** Electroplating, photography, insecticide, germicide, fingerprint powder, paints and embalming fluid.

Action

- Mercury binds with sulfhydryl groups resulting in enzyme inhibition and pathological alteration of cellular membranes.
- Elemental mercury and methyl mercury are toxic to the CNS. Metallic mercury vapor is also a pulmonary irritant. Inorganic mercury salts are corrosive to the skin, eyes and GIT, and nephrotoxic. Inorganic and organic forms may cause contact dermatitis.

Absorption and Excretion

- It is absorbed through the GIT and respiratory tract.
- After absorption, mercury gets deposited in all tissues, particularly in the liver, kidneys, spleen and bones. When inhaled, the maximum concentration occurs in the brain.
- Mainly excreted through the kidneys (urine), liver (bile) and colonic mucous membrane (feces). It passes rapidly to the fetus through placental circulation.

■ SIGNS AND SYMPTOMS (ACUTE POISONING)

- **Mercurialism** is poisoning resulting from the ingestion or inhalation of mercury or its compound. It can be acute or chronic.
- The three types of mercury have different manifestations.
- The target organ for inhaled mercury vapor is mainly the brain, mercurous and mercuric salts damage the gut lining and kidneys, while methyl mercury is widely distributed throughout the body.

Elemental (Metallic) Mercury

As a vapor, it is rapidly absorbed through the lungs, reaching the blood and entering the brain. The clinical picture can be divided into three phases—*initial phase* manifests itself as metal fume fever, *intermediate phase* in which severe multiorgan symptoms are seen, and *late phase* when only CNS symptoms persist.
- *Inhalation* causes headache, nausea, cough, chest pain, bronchitis, chemical pneumonitis, pulmonary edema, gingivostomatitis, fine tremor punctuated by coarse shaking, and CNS symptoms like insomnia, ataxia, restriction of visual field, paresis, delirium and polyneuropathy.
- Subcutaneous nodules or granulomas are seen, if injected.

Ingestion of Inorganic Mercuric Salts

It produces extensive precipitation of intestinal mucosal proteins and mucosal necrosis causing hemorrhagic gastroenteritis and massive fluid loss resulting in shock. If the patient survives, acute renal failure may follow.

System	Signs and symptoms
GIT	◆ Metallic taste, feeling of constriction in the throat, hoarse voice. ◆ Mouth, tongue and fauces become corroded, swollen, and mucous membrane appears grayish white. ◆ Hot burning pain from the mouth to the stomach, and pain radiating over the abdomen followed by nausea, retching and vomiting. Vomitus contains grayish, slimy, mucoid material with blood and shreds of mucous membrane. ◆ This is followed by diarrhea, often bloody with tenesmus (*gastroenteritis*).
Renal	Oliguria, albuminuria and hematuria ending in renal failure or nephrotic syndrome.
CVS	Hypertension, tachycardia, difficulty in breathing and circulatory collapse.

Organic Mercury

Acute exposures tend to have a latency period of one or more weeks. Symptoms typically involves the CNS, such as visual field constriction, ataxia, paresthesias, hearing loss, dysarthria, tremors, neurobehavioral impairment, paralysis and death.

Fatal Dose

- 1–4 g of mercuric chloride (30–50 mg/kg)
- 10–60 mg/kg of methyl mercury
- 10 mg/m³ of mercury vapor.

Fatal period: 3–5 days.

Diagnosis

Acute mercury poisoning can be detected by measuring blood levels, whereas urine and hair analysis help confirming chronic exposure.

---

* Fluorescent and compact fluorescents lamps (CFL) contain mercury; incandescent bulbs contain lead and mercury, while LED bulbs contain lead and nickel. In the US, the symbol 'Hg' is now required on all fluorescent lamps that contain mercury.

- The DMPS provoked urine challenge test is sometimes performed for chronic exposure.
- Blood mercury level >10 µg/dL, and 24 hours (h) urinary excretion of mercury >20 µg/L (50 µg/L as per US federal biological exposure index) indicates toxicity. A hair mercury level >5 ppm indicates chronic toxicity.
- Urine and blood mercury levels are assessed by atomic absorption spectrophotometer. Mercury concentration of hair is best assessed by neutron activation analysis.

NOTA BENE

- Urine is useful for assaying elemental and inorganic mercury. Value >100 µg/L produce neurological signs, while concentration >800 µg/L results in death.
- In general, mercury concentrations in the hair is <10 mg/kg. In moderate intoxications, it is about 200–800 mg/kg, in severe case it is >2400 mg/kg.

TREATMENT

i. In case of *inhalation*, the victim is immediately removed from source of exposure and supplemental oxygen is given, and observed for the development of acute pneumonitis and pulmonary edema.
ii. Egg whites, milk or activated charcoal to precipitate mercury. Efficacy of activated charcoal is controversial. Emesis is not induced because of the risk of serious corrosive injury.
iii. Gastric lavage with 250 mL of 5% *sodium formaldehyde sulfoxylate*. About 100 mL of this solution is left in the stomach. Lavage can be done with egg-white solution or 2–5% solution of sodium bicarbonate.
iv. Polythiol resins helps in binding mercury in the GIT.
v. High colonic lavage with 1:1000 solution of sulfoxylate twice daily. Whole bowel irrigation may be done.
vi. BAL is the traditional chelator of choice (10% solution in oil, 3–5 mg/kg IM every 4 h for 2 days, tapered to 6 hourly for 1 day and then 12 hourly for 7 days), but oral agents are preferable.
vii. **DMSA or succimer** (10 mg/kg orally every 8 h for 5 days and then 12 hourly for 2 weeks) is a good oral chelator with increased mercury excretion.
viii. **D-penicillamine** is an alternative oral treatment, but it may be associated with more side-effects and less efficient Hg excretion.
ix. There is no role of dialysis, hemoperfusion or repeat dose charcoal in removing metallic mercury or inorganic salts. However, hemodialysis/peritoneal dialysis may be required in case of renal failure.
x. Maintain electrolyte and fluid balance.
xi. Symptomatic treatment.

Recent Advances
- **Application of nano-medicine in the diagnosis of mercury poisoning:** The use of gold nanoparticles (AuNPs) is a sensitive detection method. Hg^{2+} binds thymine (thymine-mercury-thymine) and form base pairs in DNA. These bases are absorbed onto AuPNs surfaces. This combination develops Hg^{2+} sensors, based on the function of DNA and lysozyme gold. After the combinations of DNA with AuNPs, Hg^{2+} is detected by colorimetric sensors. Silver nanoparticles (AgNPs) have been used as a sensitive detector of low concentration Hg^{2+} ions in homogeneous aqueous solutions. On the other hand, ultrasensitive surface-enhanced Raman scattering (SERS) nanosensor has been developed for Hg^{2+} detection based on 4-mercaptopyridine (4-MPY) functionalized AgNPs (4-MPY-AgNPs) in the presence of spermine. This reagent determines mercury up to 0.34 nmol.
- **New DMSA analogues and combination therapy with chelating agents:** Recently, esters of DMSA have been found to be more effective antidotes for heavy metal poisoning. *Mono isoamyl ester of DMSA (MiADMSA)* is more effective chelating agent for reducing mercury, lead and cadmium burden. However, co-administration of DMSA with MiADMSA has been found more effective than mono-therapy with MiADMSA.

POSTMORTEM FINDINGS

i. Body looks emaciated.
ii. **GIT:** Mucosa shows inflammation, congestion and grayish corrosion. Ulceration or even gangrene of large intestine may be seen.
iii. **Kidneys:** Acute proximal tubular damage and glomerular degeneration or glomerular nephritis (membranous glomerulopathy) may be seen.
iv. **Liver:** Congested and shows cloudy swelling or fatty change.
v. **Heart:** Fatty degeneration and subendocardial hemorrhage.

CHRONIC MERCURY POISONING (HYDRARGYRISM)

Chronic poisoning results from:
- Continuous accidental absorption by workers.
- Excessive therapeutic use.
- Recovery from a large dose.
- If an ointment is used as an external application for a long time.

In the US, exposure to organic mercury is primarily through ingestion of contaminated fish (seafood).

Signs and Symptoms

- Chronic intoxication from *inhalation of mercury vapor* produces a triad of tremors, neuropsychiatric disturbances and gingivostomatitis.
- Chronic poisoning with *inorganic mercury compounds* is characterized by non-specific early symptoms, such as anorexia, insomnia, abnormal sweating, headache, lassitude, increased excitability, tremors, gingivitis, hypersalivation, loosening of teeth with blue line in the gum, jaundice, increased urination, personality changes, and memory and intellectual deterioration. Glomerular and tubular damage may occur in chronic exposure.

- Exposure to *organic mercuric compounds* is characterized by paresthesia of lips, hands and feet, ataxia, tremors, dysarthria, constriction of visual fields, deafness, and impairment of motor speed, memory and coordination.

SPECIFIC FEATURES/DISEASES

Intention Tremors (Danbury Tremors/Shaking Palsy)
- It occurs first in the hands, then progresses to the lips and tongue, and finally involves the arms and legs.
- Tremor is moderately coarse and is interspersed by jerky movements every few minutes. The patient may not display much tremor during an accustomed job, but if he is being observed, he may begin to shake violently.
- In the advanced stage, the person is unable to dress himself, write legibly or walk properly. They are also called **hatter's shakes or glass blower's shakes**, as they are common in persons working with mercury in hat and glass-blowing industries. The most severe form of tremors is known as **concussion mercurilis**.

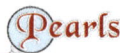

Xenobiotics causing tremors
- Mercury
- Phosphorus
- Carbon monoxide
- Caffeine and theophylline
- Alcohol
- Phenothiazines
- Antidepressants (tricyclic)

Mercurial Erethism

Erethism is seen in chronic *inorganic mercury toxicity*. This cluster of symptoms was first described by *Kussmaul* in persons working with mercury in mirror manufacturing firms, and the term is used to refer to the *neuropsychiatric effects* of mercury toxicity. These include:

Insomnia	Loss of confidence
Depression	Feeling of embarrassment
Anxiety	Suicidal melancholia
Timidity and shyness	Emotional instability, e.g., sudden attacks of anger
Amnesia	Delusions
Frequent blushing	Hallucinations
Explosive irritability	

Mercurialentis

It is a peculiar eye change due to exposure to mercury vapor.
- It is due to brownish deposit of mercury through the cornea on the anterior lens capsule.
- Slit-lamp examination gives a malt-brown reflex from the anterior lens capsule.
- It is bilateral and has no effect on visual acuity.

Acrodynia or Pink Disease

It is seen mostly in children due to idiosyncratic hypersensitivity reaction to repeated ingestion or contact with mercury (*allergic reaction to inorganic mercury*).

Signs and symptoms: There is pinkish morbilliform/acral rashes, desquamation of palms and soles, pain in the extremities, flushing, itching, swelling, tachycardia, hypertension, excessive salivation or perspiration, weakness, irritability, photophobia, anorexia, insomnia, and constipation or diarrhea.

Minamata Disease

It is due to *chronic organic mercury intoxication* caused by eating contaminated fish and shellfish.

Symptoms include disturbances in hand coordination, gait and speech, chewing and swallowing difficulties, visual blurring, tremors, rigidity, seizures and clouding of consciousness.

> **Mnemonic for chronic mercury poisoning: HG-MERCURI** (Hg is the chemical symbol of mercury)
> H: **H**atter's shakes; G: **G**ingivostomatitis;
> M: **M**ercurialentis/Minamata disease; E: **E**rethism;
> R: **R**enal changes; C: **C**erebral palsy; U: **U**rticaria;
> R: **R**ashes (in Pink disease); I: **I**ntention tremors

NOTA BENE
- **Hatter's shake:** In the UK and US (Danbury, CT), during 18–19th century, *mad hatter syndrome* was seen due to occupational exposure of mercury among people making felt hats. Mercuric nitrate was used to mat animal furs to make felt. The workers developed neurotoxic effects including tremors, shyness and irritability characteristic of erethism.
- **Minamata disease:** In Minamata Bay (Japan), a factory discharged inorganic mercury into the water. The mercury was methylated by bacteria and subsequently ingested by fish. Local villagers ate the fish and began to exhibit signs of chronic mercury poisoning.

Treatment

i. Remove the patient from the source of exposure.
ii. N-acetyl penicillamine is the chelator of choice. However, DMPS may improve the neurological features.
iii. Oral hygiene.
iv. Demulcent drinks.
v. Saline purgatives.

Postmortem Findings

External

Emaciated body with pale skin. Erosions of oral mucosa, gum of lower jaw may show bluish gray lines of pigment deposition, along with loosening of teeth.

Internal

- **Brain:** In organic mercury poisoning, the brain is predominantly affected. The gyri of both hemispheres are usually atrophic and the sulci widened. This is more prominent in the calcarine cortex and pre- and

post-central gyri which probably reflect the three characteristic manifestations seen: constriction of visual fields, ataxia and sensory disturbance.
♦ Inorganic mercury poisoning may cause cerebral infarctions, pneumonia, renal cortical necrosis and disseminated intravascular coagulopathy.

Medico-legal Aspects

a. Suicidal and homicidal poisoning is rare. However, cases of deliberate intravenous or subcutaneous metallic mercury injection have been reported.

b. Accidental poisoning may occur from:
- Ingestion of broken thermometers.
- Ingestion of antiseptic solutions containing mercuric chloride/cyanide.
- Soluble salts employed as vaginal douches.
- Absorption of mercurial preparations applied to the skin.
- Intravenous administration of organic mercurials, such as diuretics.
- In children, swallowing the sulfocyanide of mercury tablet, the constituent of *Pharaoh's serpents,* or elemental mercury because of its bright gray appearance.

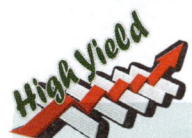

- ♦ **Mercurialism:** Poisoning resulting from the ingestion/inhalation of mercury or its compound.
- ♦ LED bulbs are not associated with mercury pollution.
- ♦ Elemental mercury is non-poisonous, if swallowed, since it is poorly absorbed from the GIT.
- ♦ **Most toxic inorganic salt of mercury:** Mercuric chloride (common cause of acute poisoning).
- ♦ Vermilion is mercuric sulfide.
- ♦ Acute mercury poisoning presents as *gastroenteritis*.
- ♦ Chronic mercury poisoning affects both peripheral and central nervous system.
- ♦ Danbury tremors/hatter's shakes/glass blower's shakes are seen in chronic mercury poisoning *(classical feature)*.
- ♦ Intention tremor starts from hands → lips and tongue → arms and legs.
- ✗ **Xenobiotics causing tremors:** Mercury, alcohol, phosphorus, phenothiazines, CO, antidepressants, caffeine and theophylline
- ♦ Mercurial erethism are psychiatric effects seen in chronic inorganic mercury toxicity.
- ♦ Mercurialentis is brownish deposit of mercury on the anterior lens capsule due to exposure to mercury vapor.
- ♦ Acrodynia/Pink disease is due to allergic reaction (pinkish rashes) to inorganic mercury.
- ♦ Minamata disease seen in chronic organic mercury intoxication is due to eating contaminated fish and shellfish.
- ♦ **Chelator of choice for mercury poisoning:** BAL (acute poisoning) and N-acetyl penicillamine (chronic poisoning).

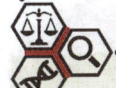 **Interesting case**

Mercury Poisoning (Case of Karen Wetterhahn, 1997)

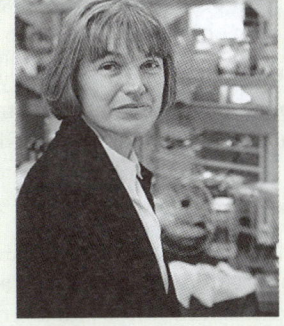

Karen Wetterhahn was a Professor of Chemistry at Dartmouth College, New Hampshire, US. In August 1996, she was pipetting a small amount of dimethylmercury under a fume hood in her lab when she accidentally spilled 1–2 drops of the colorless liquid onto the dorsum of her latex gloved hand. Dimethylmercury was the common calibration standard for ^{199}Hg NMR spectroscopy. She proceeded to clean up the area prior to removing her protective clothing.

About three months later, Karen began experiencing brief episodes of nausea, vomiting, abdominal discomfort and noted significant weight loss. In January 1997, there was tingling in her lower extremities, slurred speech, brief flashes of light in both eyes and her sight and hearing were impaired (distinctive neurological symptoms of mercury poisoning). There was progressive deterioration in balance, gait, field of vision and speech and she was admitted in the hospital in January. Physical examination showed upper-extremity dysmetria, dystaxic handwriting and slurred speech. Her urinary mercury content was 234 µg/L; its normal range is 1–5 µg/L and the toxic level is >50 µg/L. She was diagnosed with mercury poisoning. She told doctors about the dimethylmercury spill in her office. This was an incident she had to actively recall as it was so minor and incidental. Despite aggressive chelation therapy, her condition rapidly deteriorated. In early February 1997, she went into a coma. She remained in a vegetative state until she died in June 1997.

Tests later revealed that dimethylmercury can rapidly permeate different kinds of latex gloves and enter the skin within about 15 secs and offered no protection. As a result, it is now recommended to wear Silver Shield laminate gloves beneath abrasion-resistant outer gloves for those working with dimethylmercury.

CHAPTER 39

Inorganic Metallic Irritants— Lead

LEARNING OBJECTIVES

Must know
1. Plumbism
2. Treatment of chronic lead poisoning

Desirable to know
1. Signs and symptoms of acute lead poisoning
2. Diagnosis of chronic lead poisoning

Describe general principles and basic methodologies in treatment of poisoning with regard to lead.

Introduction

♦ Lead (*shisha*) is ubiquitous in our environment but has no physiologic role in biological systems.
♦ Acute toxicity is related to occupational exposure and is quite uncommon, while chronic toxicity is much more common (*commonest heavy metal causing toxicity*).
♦ Central nervous system (CNS) and neuromuscular manifestations result from intense exposure, while gastrointestinal tract (GIT) features result from exposure over longer periods.
♦ The nervous system appears to be the most sensitive and chief target for lead induced toxicity. The effects on the peripheral nervous system are more pronounced in adults while the CNS is more prominently affected in children.

Physical properties: Heavy, steel-gray metal. Salts are variously colored. Contrary to many other pure metals, metallic lead is absorbed through GIT, being soluble in gastric juice.

Toxic Compounds

It can be inorganic (lead oxides, metallic lead and lead salts) or organic (tetraethyl lead and tetramethyl lead). Common toxic compounds and their uses are given in **Table 39.1**.
♦ Features of poisoning differ depending on whether the agent is an organic or an inorganic one.
♦ Organic lead is usually more toxic than inorganic lead; symptoms appear rapidly (due to its lipid solubility), and primarily affects the CNS.

TABLE 39.1: Toxic compounds and its uses

Compounds	Uses
i. Lead acetate (sugar of lead) **(Fig. 39.1A)**	Earlier used as an astringent and local sedative for sprains
ii. Lead tetraoxide (red lead or vermilion) **(Fig. 39.1B)**	Used as *sindoor*
iii. Tetraethyl lead	Antiknock for petrol
iv. Lead sulfide (*surma*; least toxic)	Applied on the eyes
v. Lead carbonate (white lead)	Manufacture of paints

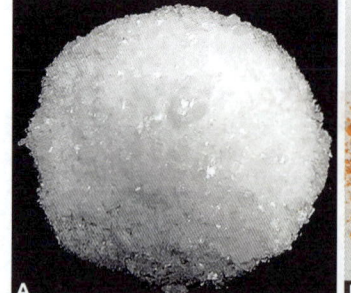 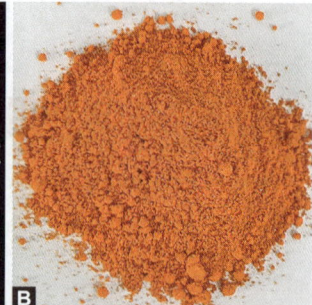

Figs. 39.1A and B: (A) Lead acetate; (B) Lead tetraoxide

Action

i. Lead combines with sulfhydryl groups and interferes with mitochondrial oxidative phosphorylation, ATPases, calcium-dependent messengers, and enhances oxidation and cell apoptosis. This causes defective heme synthesis, proximal renal tubular and osteoblast dysfunction.
ii. In the CNS, it has deleterious effects on the nerve cells and myelin sheaths, and also causes cerebral edema. Since developing, immature brain is more

susceptible to toxic effects, neuropsychiatric effects are predominantly seen in children.

Absorption and Excretion

- Lead is absorbed through the GIT, respiratory tract (dust and fumes) and skin (lead tetraoxide). In blood, 95–99% of lead is sequestered in RBCs.
- Absorption of lead compounds is directly proportional to solubility and inversely proportional to particle size. GIT lead absorption is increased by iron deficiency and low dietary calcium, and decreased by coingestion with food.
- It is a cumulative poison. In chronic exposure, it deposits in tissues, mostly in the bones (90%), liver and kidneys.
- It is mainly excreted through the urine (70%), but rate of excretion is low; smaller amounts are eliminated via feces, and scant amounts via the hair, nails and sweat.

Signs and Symptoms (Acute Poisoning)

It manifests as GIT and CNS disturbances.
- **GIT:** Metallic taste, dry throat, thirst, vomiting, nausea, burning abdominal pain (colic) and blood-stained diarrhea leading to circulatory collapse.
- **CNS:** Headache, lethargy, arthralgia, myalgia, anorexia, insomnia, paresthesia, depression, coma and death.

Fatal Dose

- Lead carbonate: 40 g.
- Lead acetate: 20 g.

Fatal period: 1–2 days.

Laboratory diagnosis
i. Porphyrinuria due to coproporphyrin III.
ii. Blood lead level >70–100 µg/dL. Protoporphyrin >35 µg/dL.
iii. Urine lead level >0.15–0.3 mg/L.

Treatment

i. Gastric lavage with 1% solution of sodium or magnesium sulfate (forms insoluble lead sulfate), above salts are also given in purgative dose.
ii. Whole-bowel irrigation with a polyethylene glycol electrolyte solution at 1–2 L/hour (h) for adults (25–40 mL/kg/h for children), if lead chips are visible on abdominal X-ray.
iii. Demulcents and repeated cathartics, as indicated.
iv. Calcium chloride 5 mg as 10% solution IV or calcium gluconate 10 mL of 10% solution IV causes deposition of lead in bones from blood (to combat acute crisis).
v. Calcium disodium ethylenediaminetetraacetic acid (CaNa$_2$EDTA) 50 mg/kg/day in 4–6 divided doses or as a continuous infusion for 5 days. Some add BAL, 4–5 mg/kg IM every 4 h for 5 days.
vi. Vitamin C (weak, but natural chelating agent) may be given.
vii. Peritoneal or hemodialysis in patients with renal failure.
viii. Symptomatic treatment.

Postmortem Findings

i. Body appears emaciated, rigor mortis appears early.
ii. Stomach wall is swollen, mucous membrane is congested, grayish in color and softened with eroded patches. Characteristic reddish color of mucosa is seen in acute lead tetraoxide ingestion (**Figs. 39.2A and B**).

CHRONIC LEAD POISONING (PLUMBISM/SATURNISM)

- It was also called *colica pictorum* (the colic of painters), **painter's colic** or **Devonshire colic**.
- Lead is a cumulative poison, remains accumulated in bones as phosphate and carbonate.
- High calcium level favors storage, while calcium deficiency causes lead to be released into the blood stream.
- Other factors promoting release of stored lead: acidosis, fever, sweating, consumption of alcohol and exposure to sunlight.

Causes

- Lead is ingested or inhaled. The most common source is ingestion of lead-containing dust.
- Lead paint dust is the most common source of lead exposure for children. Children <3 years are at the greatest risk for lead poisoning as they are more likely to put things containing lead into their mouths (*pica*—persistent eating of non-nutritive material for 1 month or more) and their brains are rapidly developing.
- Inhalation of lead dust and fumes by makers of white lead, lead paints, plumbers, glass polishers, printers and glass blowers.
- Absorption from drinking water stored in lead cisterns, from tinned food contaminated with lead from solder, and use of hair dyes and cosmetics containing lead.
- Percutaneous absorption of tetraethyl lead in persons who handle petrol and gasoline.
- Absorption of *vermilion* applied to scalp.

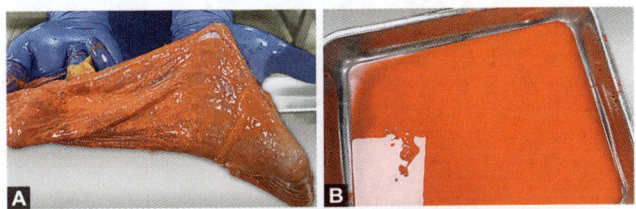

Figs. 39.2A and B: Lead tetraoxide poisoning: (A) Reddish mucosa; (B) Contents in a tray

Chronic lead poisoning results from daily intake of 1–2 mg of lead.

SIGNS AND SYMPTOMS

Chronic poisoning is insidious with fatigue, sleep disturbance, headache, irritability, slurred speech, stupor, ataxia, convulsions, anemia and renal failure. CNS symptoms, such as delirium, insomnia, cognitive deficits, tremors, hallucinations and convulsions are seen commonly with organic lead compounds.

Characteristic features are **(Fig. 39.3)**:
1. **Anemia:** In early stages, there may be polycythemia with polychromatophilia, but later, there is anemia with karyorrhexis and dyserythropoiesis [*punctate basophilia* **(Fig. 39.4)**, *Cabot's rings, reticulocytosis, poikilocytosis, anisocytosis*], nucleated red cells and increase in mononuclear cells in peripheral blood and ringed sideroblasts in bone marrow. However, polymorphonuclear cells and platelets are decreased. RBC count comes down to 3.5 million/dL and hemoglobin level to 6.5 g%.
   Cause of anemia:
   - Impairment in heme synthesis from protoporphyrin and of porphobilinogen from δ-aminolevulinic acid.
   - Increased fragility of RBCs due to loss of intracellular potassium (there is an increased permeability of cell membrane to K$^+$).

> **NOTA BENE**
> ◆ Lead inhibits heme synthesis through inhibition of delta ALA-dehydratase, ferrochelatase, porphobilinogen synthase, coproporphyrinogen oxidase and other enzymes, resulting in the buildup of aminolevulinic acid, coproporphyrins and free erythrocyte protoporphyrin. It also inhibits enzyme pyrimidine 5′-nucleotidase, thus increasing erythrocyte fragility.
> ◆ *Karyorrhexis*: Rupture of the RBC cell nucleus with chromatin disintegration into granules that are extruded from the cell.
> ◆ *Punctate basophilia/basophilic stippling*: Presence of dark blue colored pinhead sized spots in the cytoplasm of the RBCs representing aggregated ribosomes, due to the toxic action of lead on porphyrin metabolism (seen in 25% of patients) **(Fig. 39.4)**.
> ◆ *Cabot's rings*: RBCs containing mitotic spindle remnants appearing as fine, thread-like filaments of bluish purple color in the shape of a single ring or a double ring **(in the form of figure 8)** on Wright-stained smears. They have been observed in lead poisoning, megaloblastic anemia, leukemia, myelodysplastic syndromes and other cases of dyserythropoiesis.
> ◆ *Ringed sideroblasts*: Erythroblasts with large iron granules (iron-laden mitochondria) forming a partial or complete ring around the nucleus.
> ◆ *Anisocytosis*: Presence of abnormal size erythrocytes.
> ◆ *Poikilocytosis*: Presence of abnormal-shaped erythrocytes.

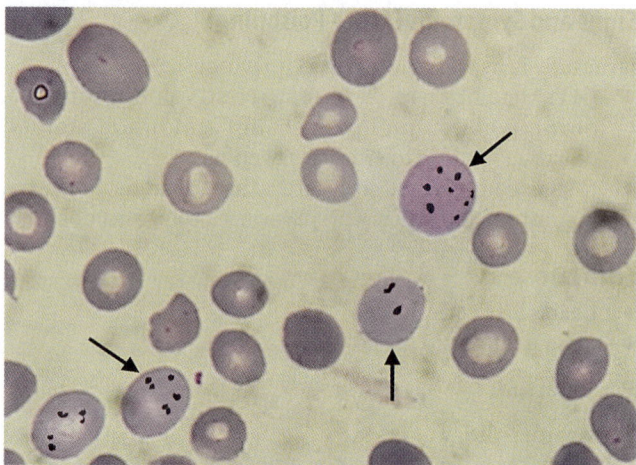

Fig. 39.4: Basophilic stippling of RBCs (arrows)

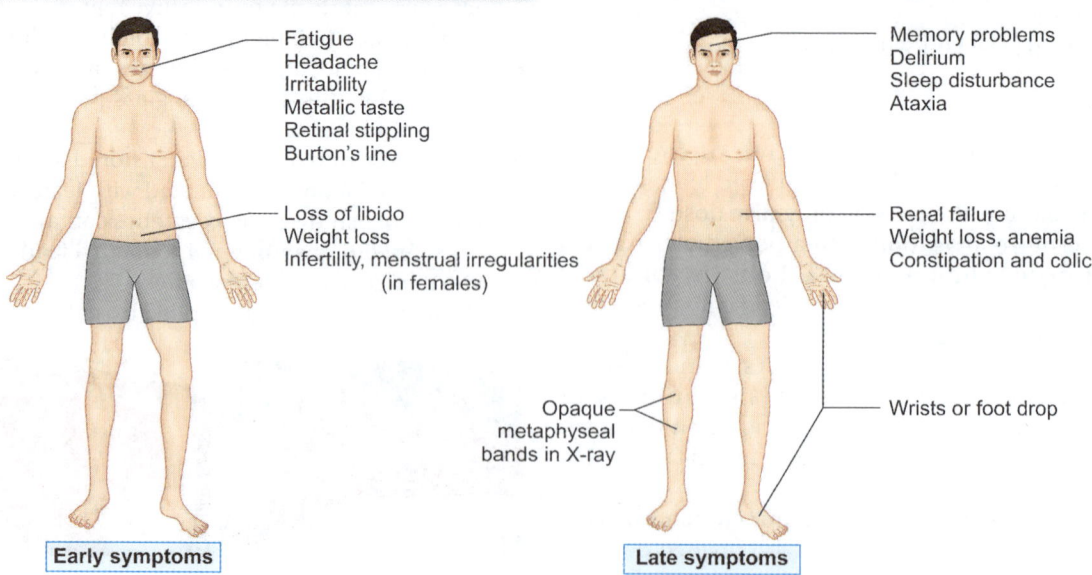

Fig. 39.3: Signs and symptoms of chronic lead poisoning

2. **Burton's/Burtonian line:** A stippled *blue line* is seen on the gingival surface in 50–70% cases.
   - It is due to subepithelial deposit of granules at the junction of teeth, especially near dirty or carious teeth of the upper jaw, within a week of exposure.
   - It is due to formation of lead sulfide by the H_2S formed from decomposed protein in the mouth.

Pearls

Xenobiotics causing blue line on the gums
1. Lead
2. Mercury
3. Copper
4. Silver
5. Bismuth
6. Iron

3. **Colic:** It is usually a late symptom, involving both large and small intestines, ureters and blood vessels.
   - Seen in 85% of cases.
   - The pain is spasmodic, paroxysmal, occurs at night and may be very severe (**saturnine colic**). During pain, the abdomen is tense.
   - Individual attacks last only for few minutes, but may recur after several days and weeks.
   - Pain is slightly relieved by application of pressure over the abdomen.
4. **Constipation:** Common feature and usually precedes colic. During pain, there is a desire for defecation. Diarrhea and vomiting may occur.
5. **Lead palsy (drops):** It is a late and uncommon phenomenon, seen in <10% of cases.
   - It is common in adults than in children, and males are particularly affected.
   - It occurs due to degeneration of nerves and atrophy of muscles as a result of interference with phosphocreatine metabolism.
   - The muscle groups affected are those most prone to fatigue.
   - Sensory nerves are not clinically affected.
   - There may be tremors, numbness, hyperesthesia and cramps before the actual muscle weakness.
   - Later, the extensor muscles of wrist *(wrist drop)* are affected **(Fig. 39.5)**, but the deltoid, biceps, anterior tibial *(foot drop)*, and rarely muscles of eye or intrinsic muscles of hand and foot are also affected.

Pearls
- Heavy metals causing peripheral neuropathy: Lead, arsenic, thallium and mercury.
- Lead damages more to motor nerves than sensory, and thallium causes sensorimotor pain.
- Mercury affects both PNS and CNS.

6. **Lead encephalopathy:** Minor degree of involvement of brain function, commonly in children is present in almost every case.
   - This may be due to inactivation of MAO as a result of combination of lead with –SH radical of the enzyme.
   - *Symptoms* include changes in personality, restlessness, hyperkinetic and aggressive behavior, fatigability, mental dullness, learning disorders, refusal to play, headache, insomnia, vomiting, raised intracranial pressure, papilledema, visual disturbances and irritability. In others, there may be acute conditions, such as persistent vomiting, hallucinations, delirium, convulsions, ataxia, coma and death (due to cerebral edema).
7. **Facial pallor:** *Earliest sign;* seen around the mouth. It is due to vasospasm and produced by contraction of the capillaries at the arterial side.
8. **Effects on reproductive system:** Lead may cause sterility in both male and female patients. In males, there may be loss of libido and erectile dysfunction. In females, there may be infertility, menstrual irregularities, such as amenorrhea, dysmenorrhea and menorrhagia. It may result in abortion in pregnant females due to atrophy or spasmodic contraction of uterus.
9. **Optic atrophy:** Few patients may develop blindness due to optic atrophy.
10. **Retinal stippling** is noticed by ophthalmoscope as grayish glistening lead particles in the early phase of chronic lead poisoning.
11. **Lead osteopathy:** In children and young adults, lead is deposited beyond the epiphysis of growing long bones. The deposition is promoted by calcium and vitamin D, and is detectable by radiological examination. Deposition of lead at the growing ends may lead to their abnormal development.
12. **Effects on circulatory system:** Lead causes vascular constriction leading to hypertension and arteriolar degeneration.
13. **Effect on kidneys:** Renal functional abnormality can be of two types: acute and chronic nephropathy. *Acute nephropathy* is characterized by abnormal excretion of glucose, phosphates and amino acids without any proteins in urine (*Fanconi's syndrome*).

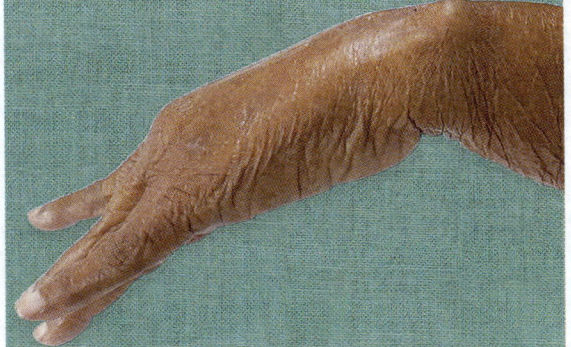

Fig. 39.5: Wrist drop
(*Courtesy:* Dr Ajay Kumar, DMCH, Ludhiana)

Chronic nephropathy is characterized by glomerular and tubulointerstitial changes, resulting in renal breakdown, hypertension and hyperuricemia.

14. **Effects on liver:** Acute or chronic degeneration leading to dyspepsia, anorexia, emaciation, general weakness and foul breath.
15. **Effect on peripheral nerves:** In addition to meningoencephalitis, it may cause degeneration of anterior horn cells and demyelination leading to peripheral neuritis.
16. **Hair:** There may be alopecia.

> **Mnemonic for chronic lead poisoning: ABCDEFGHI**
> i. **A**nemia/Anorexia/Arthralgia/Abortion/Atrophy of optic nerve
> ii. **B**asophilic stippling/Burton's line
> iii. **C**olic/Constipation/Cerebral edema
> iv. **D**rop (wrist, foot)
> v. **E**ncephalopathy/Emaciation/Erectile dysfunction
> vi. **F**acial pallor/Foul smell of breath/Fanconi syndrome
> vii. **G**onadal dysfunction/Gout-like picture (*Saturnine gout*)
> viii. **H**ypertension/Headache/Hallucination
> ix. **I**nfertility/Insomnia/Irritability

Diagnosis

- **History:** History should be thorough to assess the risk of lead exposure—occurs after occupational or home exposure.
- **Clinical features:** Abdominal pain, irritability, lethargy, anorexia, anemia, Fanconi's syndrome, peripheral neuropathy, pyuria and azotemia in children. Neurodevelopmental delays, convulsions and coma may be seen.
  - In adults, additionally, there are headaches, arthralgias, myalgias, depression, impaired short-term memory, and loss of libido. The blue line on the gums is a valuable but variable clue to diagnosis.

Laboratory Diagnosis

i. Normocytic and normochromic, a microcytic, hypochromic anemia may be seen with mixed etiology.
ii. Punctate basophilia: >200 cells/cu mm.
iii. Elevated free erythrocyte protoporphyrin or zinc protoporphyrin (>35 µg/dL) level and azotemia.
iv. Urine lead level >80 µg/dL (in 24 h sample).
v. Blood lead levels are an indicator of recent lead exposure, not of the total body burden. The CDC (US) have set the standard elevated blood lead level for adults as 10 µg/dL and for children 5 µg/dL of the whole blood. Blood lead >70 µg/dL (severe toxicity) and >50–70 µg/dL (moderate toxicity).
vi. Coproporphyrin in urine >15 µg/dL.
vii. δ-aminolevulinic acid in urine >5 mg/L.
viii. Plasma lead >0.1 mg/mL.
ix. *X-ray:* Radio-opaque bands or **'lead lines'** (*metaphyseal sclerosis*)* at the metaphyseal plate of long bones are seen in children. These growth arrest lines are not pathognomonic, but are associated with lead levels >40 µg/dL over long period of time. With recovery, the lead line becomes broader and less dense and may eventually disappear.
  - Whole body lead can be measured in bones noninvasively by X-ray fluorescence—*best measure* of cumulative exposure and total body burden.
  - X-rays may also reveal lead-containing foreign materials, such as paint chips in the GIT.

TREATMENT

i. Remove the patient from the source of exposure.
ii. Potassium or sodium iodide 1–2 g TDS orally.
iii. Sodium bicarbonate 20–30 g in 4 or 5 divided doses orally.
iv. $MgSO_4$ or sodium sulfate 8–12 g orally.
v. **$CaNa_2EDTA$** IV in usual doses. Chelation therapy is indicated for adults with blood lead >70 µg/dL and for children with encephalopathy or blood lead >45 µg/dL.
vi. **BAL:** Chelator of choice in case of renal impairment. DMSA is given in mild to moderate toxicity in a dose of 10 mg/kg orally every 8 h for 5 days, then every 12 h for 2 weeks.
vii. N-acetylcysteine (NAC) has shown a significant reduction in the blood lead levels.
viii. **Dietary management:** Correction of dietary deficiencies of iron, calcium, magnesium and zinc lowers lead absorption. Natural antioxidants [vitamins (particularly B6, B1, C and E), flavonoids, quercetin] have been found useful. These vitamins may chelate lead from the tissues along with restoring the pro/antioxidant balance. Iron supplementation is withheld during chelation therapy.
ix. Ammonium chloride 1 g, 3–4 times given daily. By this, lead deposited in the bones is mobilized into the blood and excreted.
x. Mannitol for cerebral edema, and diazepam IV for seizures associated with lead encephalopathy; hemodialysis in cases of renal failure.
xi. Symptomatic treatment.

> **Recent Advances**
> The major drawback in the usefulness of antioxidants is their poor bioavailability due to low solubility and rapid clearance. *Lipid-based nanoencapsulation* of antioxidants provides improved biodistribution and bioavailability.

---

* This is due to increased density along transverse lines in the metaphyses of growing long bones, representing increased mineralization owing to interference with metabolism of the bony matrix—implies chronic lead exposure.

POSTMORTEM FINDINGS

i. A blue line may be seen on the gums in patients with poor oral hygiene, but it is not a constant feature.
ii. Paralyzed muscles show fatty degeneration.
iii. **Heart:** It may be hypertrophied and there may be atherosclerosis of aorta.
iv. **Stomach and intestines:** It may show ulcerative or hemorrhagic changes with contraction and thickening.
v. **Liver and kidneys:** Contracted and hard.
vi. **Brain:** Pale (almost white), and swollen with flattening of gyri.

> **NOTA BENE**
>
> **Histopathology**
> - *RBC:* Basophilic stippling of erythrocytes.
> - *Liver and kidneys:* Characteristic eosinophilic intra-nuclear inclusions may be seen in hepatocytes and cells of the proximal tubules of kidneys. Chronic nephritis with tubular degeneration.
> - *Brain:* PAS-positive pink homogenous material in the perivascular spaces along with cell necrosis.
> - *Bone marrow* shows hyperplasia of leucoblasts and erythroblasts ('immature' white and red blood cells).

Medico-legal Aspects

- Acute and homicidal poisoning is rare.
- Chronic poisoning is common. There is a risk of failure to recognize the possibility of lead poisoning as the symptoms and signs are subtle and easily overlooked.
- Accidental chronic poisoning occurs in people working with lead.
- Lead oleate or red lead is used as a local application for abortion. It is also used alone or mixed with arsenic as cattle poison.
- A person can develop lead poisoning from retained lead bullets or projectiles. It is a well-known clinical problem that is frequently encountered since the bullet (or shots) is often not removed by the surgeons if not lodged near a major vessel or plexus.*
- Spinal tap performed on the patients with lead encephalopathy and increased intracranial pressure can precipitate cerebral herniation and death.

> **NOTA BENE**
>
> - The 1st, 2nd, 3rd and 6th hazards on the list in Toxic Substances and Diseases Registry of the US are heavy metals: lead, mercury, arsenic and cadmium.
> - Methods for measuring lead in biological media were developed in the late 1960s. First, the dithizone method and later atomic absorption spectrophotometry.
> - **L-line-X-ray fluorescence** (LXRF) is being used to make in vivo measurements of lead levels in cortical bone which reflect cumulative exposure over many years in contrast to blood levels, which reflect recent exposure.

---

* Curtis '50 Cent' Jackson, who had speech-altering shrapnel lodged in his tongue, was advised by his doctors to leave it in because it might do more damage to his nerves and taste buds.

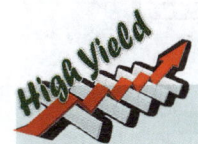

- **Commonest heavy metal causing toxicity:** Lead.
- PICA is associated with lead poisoning.
- **Heavy metal poisoning affecting the motor nerves:** Lead.
- **Most sensitive and chief target organ:** Nervous system.
- Effects on peripheral nervous system are more in adults while CNS is affected more in children.
- *Sindoor* is lead tetraoxide (red lead or *vermilion*).
- Sideroblasts are seen in lead poisoning.
- Plumbism/saturnism is chronic lead poisoning.
- **Earliest sign of plumbism:** Facial pallor.
- Anemia seen in chronic lead poisoning is normocytic and normochromic.
- Punctate basophilia, Cabot's rings, reticulocytosis, poikilocytosis, anisocytosis are seen in peripheral blood smear in plumbism.

- **Cause of anemia in plumbism:** Impairment in heme synthesis from protoporphyrin and of porphobilinogen from δ-aminolevulinic acid.
- Lead inhibits heme synthesis through inhibition of delta ALA-dehydratase, ferrochelatase, porphobilinogen synthase and coproporphyrinogen oxidase.
- Punctate basophilia/basophilic stippling are due to aggregated ribosomes in the cytoplasm of RBCs.
- **Burton's/Burtonian line:** In chronic lead poisoning, blue line on the gingival surface is seen due to the formation of lead sulphide.
- **Blue line on the gums seen in poisoning due to:** Lead, mercury, iron, copper, silver and bismuth.
- Colic is a late symptom in plumbism, involving both large and small intestines, ureters and blood vessels which is relieved by application of pressure.
- Lead palsy is a late and uncommon phenomenon seen in plumbism where there is wrist drop or foot drop.
- **Heavy metals causing peripheral neuropathy:** Lead, arsenic, thallium and mercury.
- Lead encephalopathy with minor degree of involvement of brain function is present in plumbism, more commonly in children.
- Retinal stippling is seen in chronic lead poisoning.
- A diagnostic blood lead level in adults is >10 µg/dL (recent lead exposure).
- **Punctate basophilia:** >200 cells/cu mm (*biological marker*) is diagnostic of plumbism.
- In chronic lead poisoning, δ-aminolevulinic acid levels increases in urine.
- In plumbism, 'lead lines' (radio-opaque bands) at the metaphyseal plate of long bones in children are seen in X-ray.
- **Chelator of choice in case of renal impairment:** BAL.

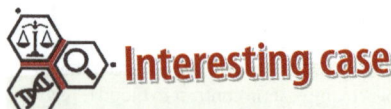

Interesting case

Lead Poisoning (Case of Louisa Taylor, 1883)

Louisa Taylor was a 37-year-old widow and had no savings to survive on **(Fig. A)**. In 1882, to help make ends meet, she took a live-in job as a nurse to the wife of a friend of her former husband, William Tregellis at Plumstead in Kent (now part of Greater London). His wife, Mary Ann who was 82-year-old agreed, and Louisa shared her room while William moved to the front room. She stayed with them for 3 months till William reported Louisa to the police for stealing items from the house which she took to pawn shops.

A day or two later after her arrest, Mary was found in a state of collapse and near to death. The frail old woman was in a terrible state and her gums showed a dark blue line at their edge. She

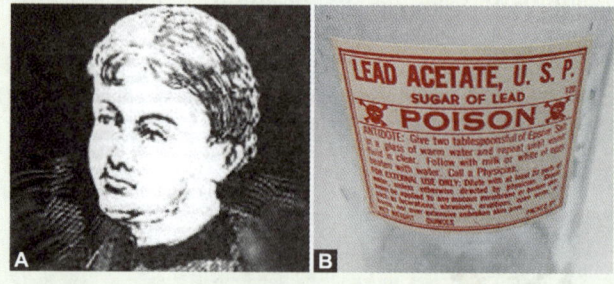

recovered enough to give a deposition. In her statement, she mentioned that until Louisa had come to stay, she had been in good health. During her stay, Mary began to have fits and attacks of vomiting. She pointed to Louisa and stated she had seen her pour a white powder into her medicine. Her vomit became black and it hurt her throat. The family doctor Dr John Smith reportedly tried to get Louisa to retain a sample of the vomit for analysis but she had always conveniently forgotten to do so.

After few days, she began to lose her voice again and gradually became paralysed. Three days later, she died in October 1882. During autopsy, the blue lead line on her gums was visible. However, her brain, lungs, liver, heart, and spleen were all apparently healthy although there were dark patches on parts of her stomach and intestines. Samples of tissue were sent to Guy's Hospital in London for analysis. The analyst found significant amounts of lead in each kidney and traces in the lungs, intestines and spleen and concluded that Mary had been given a dose of lead acetate very recently **(Fig. B)**.

Louisa, already in custody, was charged with the murder. The Coroner's inquest was held in November 1882 and the jury convicted her of wilful murder. Mrs Smith (who was runing the pharmacy of Dr Smith) also testified that she had sold 'sugar of lead' (lead acetate) multiple times to Louisa for a fictitious skin complaint.

However, the Lancet in an article after her conviction said that the primary cause of death of Mrs Tregillis was due to a heart attack few days before she died. The lead given to her by Louisa may have hastened her end but could not with certainty be said to have caused it. But the Lancet's opinion carried little weight. Louisa was hanged in January 1883.

CHAPTER 40

Inorganic Metallic Irritants— Copper

Learning Objectives

Must know
1. Signs and symptoms, treatment and PM findings in acute copper poisoning
2. Toxic compounds of copper
3. Medico-legal aspects of copper poisoning

Desirable to know
1. Chronic copper poisoning
2. Chalcosis oculi
3. Vineyard sprayer's lung

FM 9.3 Describe general principles and basic methodologies in treatment of poisoning with regard to copper.

Introduction

Copper *(tamba)* as a metal is not poisonous. In human body, the copper content is about 100–150 mg which is present as an integral and functional moiety of proteins and enzyme systems including catalase, cytochrome C oxidase, dopamine β-hydroxylase and serum ceruloplasmin. However, as the body cannot synthesize copper, the human diet must supply regular amounts for absorption.

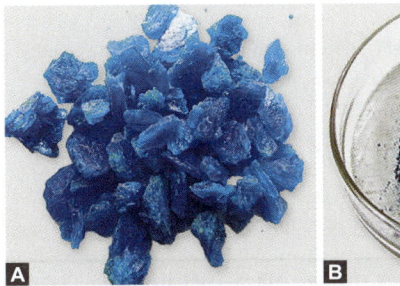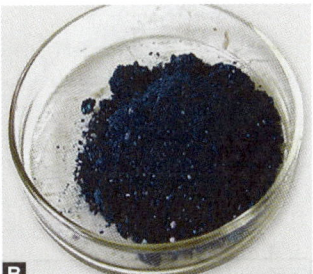

Figs. 40.1A and B: (A) Copper sulfate; (B) Copper subacetate

Toxic Compounds and its Uses

i. **Copper sulfate** (blue vitriol, bluestone, *nila tutia*, $CuSO_4$): It occurs as large blue crystals, freely soluble in water and having a styptic/astringent taste (**Fig. 40.1A**). It is used as algicide, molluscicide and plant fungicide, as mordant in electroplating, as an agent for leather tanning and hide preservation and can be used as an emetic. It was being used as a precipitator in heavy metal poisoning, and treat gastric and topical exposure to phosphorous.

ii. **Copper subacetate** *(verdigris)*: It occurs as a powder or as bluish-green masses, and is frequently used in the field of arts and external medicine (**Fig. 40.1B**).

iii. **Copper carbonate** is a blue-green compound forming part of the verdigris patina that is found on weathered brass, bronze and copper. It is used as fungicide.

Action

Toxicity of copper is exerted on enzymes whose activities depend on sulfhydryl and amino groups, because it has high affinity for ligands containing nitrogen and sulfur donors (as in other heavy metals). Besides, nucleic acid may also be targets of copper toxicity.

♦ Copper ions can oxidize heme iron to form methemoglobin which may cause cyanosis (clinically) and chocolate brown color blood.

Absorption and Excretion

♦ The principal route of exposure is through ingestion, but inhalation of copper dust and fumes occurs in industrial settings and in miners.

- After ingestion, maximum absorption of copper occurs in the stomach and jejunum. Absorbed copper is initially bound to albumin and is transported from the GIT to the liver where it is transferred to ceruloplasmin.
- Copper is eliminated mostly through the feces after excretion into the bile. Urinary excretion of copper is low in humans. Adults have urinary excretion of 25 µg/24 hours (h).
- Copper toxicity affects the following in the order of severity—erythrocytes, liver and kidneys.

SIGNS AND SYMPTOMS

Acute Ingestion

Symptoms of hypercuprosis appear in 15–30 minutes (min) after swallowing.

System	Signs and symptoms
GIT	Metallic taste, ptyalism (increased salivation), burning pain in stomach, thirst, colicky abdominal pain, nausea, eructation and repeated vomiting. Vomitus is greenish-blue. Diarrhea with much straining, hemorrhagic gastroenteritis.
Renal	Oliguria, hematuria, hemoglobinuria, albuminuria and uremia.
Hepatic	Jaundice, tender hepatomegaly, hepatic encephalopathy.
MS	Cramps or spasms of legs, paralysis of limbs, rhabdomyolysis.
CVS	Breathing difficulty, cold perspiration, methemoglobinemia, hypotension, tachycardia, circulatory collapse and shock.
CNS	Frontal headache, lethargy, drowsiness, insensibility, irreversible coma and death occurs.

> **Mnemonic for copper poisoning: COPPER**
> C: **C**olicky abdominal pain, cramps, circulatory shock, coma;
> O: **O**liguria; P: **P**aralysis of limbs; P: **P**erspiration (cold);
> E: **E**mesis (greenish blue), eructation; R: **R**habdomyolysis

- Hemolysis and hemoglobinuria are present in severe cases. Individuals with G-6-PD deficiency may be at increased risk of hematologic effects of copper.
- Multiorgan dysfunction syndrome may occur.
- Early death is attributed to hypotension and shock, late death to hepatic and/or renal failure.

Inhalation

Acute inhalation of large doses of copper dusts or fumes can cause metal fume fever, nausea, gastric pain and diarrhea.
- Upper respiratory tract irritation may result in sore throat and cough.
- Conjunctivitis, palpebral edema and sinus irritation may occur.
- Nasal mucous membrane may show atrophy with perforation.

Contact

Exposure of skin to copper compounds may cause irritant contact dermatitis, and severe exposure may cause a greenish-blue discoloration of skin.

Fatal Dose

- Copper subacetate: 15 g
- Copper sulfate: 10–20 g (0.15–0.3 g/kg)

Fatal period: 18–24 h, but it may extend to 1–3 days

Diagnosis: In acute poisoning, whole blood copper levels correlate better with the severity of poisoning than do serum copper. Normal serum copper level range is 12–20 µmol/L.
- Neutron activation analysis and atomic absorption spectroscopy can detect copper. Merocyanine dye allows copper to be detected using fluorescence spectroscopy.

TREATMENT

i. No need to use emetics as vomiting occurs in 5–10 min after ingestion. Moreover, emetics should be avoided to prevent re-exposure of the esophagus to the corrosive agent.
ii. Gastric lavage with 1% *potassium ferrocyanide*, which acts as antidote by forming cupric ferrocyanide (insoluble). If not available, plain water can be used.
iii. **Demulcents:** Egg white or milk (form insoluble albuminate of copper). Sucralfate may help to relieve the symptoms of mucosal injury.
iv. Castor oil is given to remove poison from the intestines.
v. Patients with methemoglobinemia should be given methylene blue (dose is 1–2 mg/kg of 1% solution IV over 5 min).
vi. **Chelating agents:** *D-penicillamine* given in usual doses is very effective. The hydrophilic dithiol chelators DMSA and DMPS are more efficient and suitable alternatives. EDTA or BAL in usual doses are other alternatives.
vii. Allay pain by injecting morphine, and use diuretics, if urine is suppressed.
viii. Hypotension is treated with fluids, dopamine and noradrenaline.
ix. Symptomatic treatment to maintain electrolyte and fluid balance.
x. For severe cases associated with anorexia and hematuria, hydrocortisone 50–100 mg IM thrice daily is recommended. However, routine use of steroids is doubtful.
xi. Hemodialysis is ineffective, but may be indicated in patients with renal failure secondary to copper poisoning.

POSTMORTEM FINDINGS

i. Skin may be yellow due to jaundice.
ii. Greenish-blue froth from the mouth and nostrils.
iii. Mucous membrane of the mouth and tongue may have bluish or greenish-blue tinge.
iv. Internally, bluish or greenish-blue discoloration is present in the mucous membrane of the esophagus, stomach and intestines (Fig. 40.2A). Caustic burns of esophagus, superficial and deep ulcers in the stomach and small intestine may be seen.
v. **Stomach:** Gastric mucosa is congested with desquamation and hemorrhages at places (Figs. 40.2B and C).
vi. **Small intestine:** Mucosa (upper part) may show necrosis.
vii. **Liver:** Soft and fatty. It shows centrilobular necrosis and biliary stasis.
viii. **Kidneys:** It may show acute proximal tubular necrosis. Hemoglobin casts may be seen in the tubules.

CHRONIC COPPER POISONING

Cause

- Chronic copper toxicity may occur from eating acidic foods cooked in uncoated copper cookware, or from exposure to excess copper in drinking water or food contaminated with verdigris, or other environmental sources.
- It may also occur among workers using copper and its salts due to inhalation of copper dust or fumes—welders may develop *metal fume fever*.

Signs and Symptoms

i. Green or purple line on the gums, a constant metallic taste, nausea, dyspepsia, vomiting and diarrhea with colicky pain.
ii. Giddiness and headache.
iii. Laryngitis and bronchitis.
iv. Renal damage.
v. General signs of progressive emaciation, viz. anemia, malaise and debility.
vi. Peripheral neuritis with wrist drop or foot drop and atrophy of muscles.
vii. Copper dust may cause inflammation of the conjunctiva and ulceration of the cornea.
viii. Skin becomes jaundiced. Urine and perspiration become green.
ix. Bronze diabetes may be present.

Treatment

i. After removing the cause, patient should be given a massage and a warm bath. Patient should be exposed to fresh air.
ii. Attention should be paid to his diet and dyspepsia.
iii. Symptomatic treatment.

Postmortem Findings

- *Liver:* Fatty degeneration
- *Kidneys:* Degeneration of the epithelial cells.

Medico-legal Aspects (Acute and Chronic)

- Suicidal cases are common.
- Accidental poisoning results from eating food contaminated with verdigris (formed from action of vegetable acids on copper cooking vessels).
- Toxicity may develop from the copper absorbed systemically from the wire used in certain intrauterine contraceptive devices, or from the tubing used in hemodialysis equipment.
- Rarely, it is used for homicide because of its color and metallic taste.
- Poisoning may be caused by ingestion of food to which copper has been added to keep the color of vegetables green.
- Children may swallow copper sulfate crystals attracted by its color.
- Rarely, it is used as cattle poison.

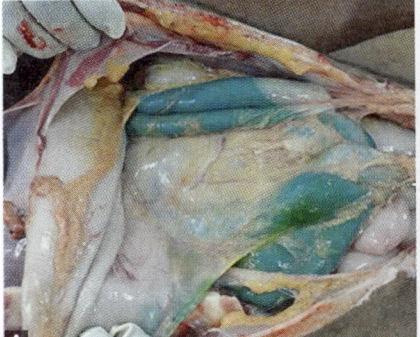 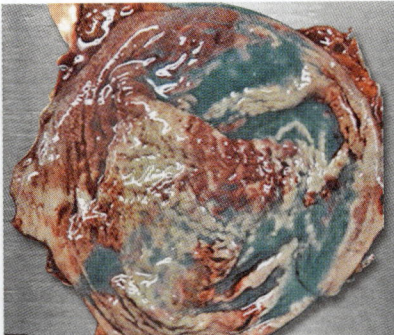 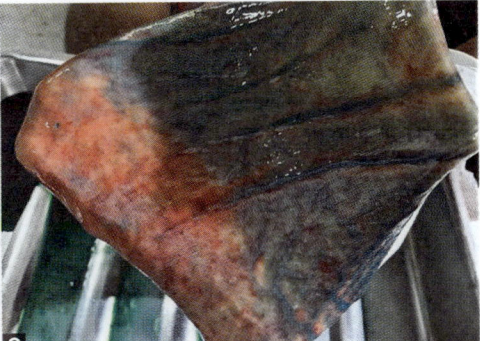

Figs. 40.2A to C: (A and B) Acute copper sulfate poisoning. Bluish color GIT and desquamation and hemorrhages in stomach; (C) Acute copper subacetate poisoning: Bluish-green color and submucosal hemorrhages in stomach

- Copper occurs in small medicinal doses in tablets with sulfate of iron and manganese.
- Copper sulfate was used as an antidote in phosphorus poisoning and in wound debridement.

NOTA BENE

- **Tetrathiomolybdate** is suggested to be useful as chelating agent in case of acute copper poisoning, since urinary excretion is enhanced by increased molybdenum intake.
- **Chalcosis oculi** (Greek *chalkos*: *copper*): Chronic ophthalmic exposure to particulate elemental copper or one of its alloys may result in its deposition in the cornea, lens, vitreous and retina. Copper deposits in the cornea (*chalcosis corneae*) appear as golden brown, ruby red or green pigment ring in the peripheral Descemet's membrane (**Kayser-Fleischer ring**). Lens opacities (*chalcosis lentis*) occur in the form of anterior **subcapsular cataract** ('*sunflower' cataract*, and typically greenish in color).
- **Vineyard sprayer's lung**: It is an occupational disease seen in Portuguese vineyard workers due to chronic exposure to Bordeaux solution (1–2% copper sulfate solution neutralized with lime). The patients develop interstitial pulmonary fibrosis and histiocytic granulomas containing copper. The radiographic picture resembles that of silicosis with micronodular disease in the early stages and progressive massive fibrosis in later stages. Besides Bordeaux mixture, paraquat and organophosphates can cause significant pulmonary fibrosis.

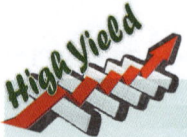

- Copper is not poisonous.
- Copper content in our body: 100–150 mg.
- Copper ions oxidize heme iron to form met-Hb which causes cyanosis and *chocolate brown color blood*.
- **Compound acting both as poison and antidote:** Copper sulfate.
- Acute copper sulfate poisoning presents with acute hemolysis.
- Color of vomitus in acute copper sulfate poisoning is greenish-blue.
- **Chelator of choice in acute copper poisoning:** D-penicillamine.
- In copper poisoning, greenish-blue froth from the mouth and nostrils can be seen during PM examination.
- In copper poisoning, mucous membrane of the mouth, tongue, esophagus and stomach may have bluish or greenish-blue tinge.

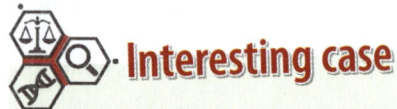

Copper Poisoning

Aurore Moussiegt *et. al.*, reported an unusual case of a 40-year-old female patient who presented to the emergency department with diarrhea, abdominal pain and anuria. She had a rectal enema using a blue powder sent from Cameroon 48 h back in the belief that this would help her get pregnant.

At the time of admission, she was conscious and hemodynamically stable, urinary output was only a few mL of 'port-colored' urine (**Fig. A**). After 6 h, O_2 saturation on pulse oximetry dropped to 74% without breathlessness. Arterial blood gas analysis at that time showed: pH 7.18, pO_2 70 mm Hg, pCO_2 30 mm Hg, HCO_3^- 11.2 mmol/L and SpO_2 99%. Methemoglobinemia level was 13% and explained the saturation gap.

The patient was admitted in the ICU. High-flow nasal oxygen was given and intermittent hemodialysis was done. MetHb rose to 23% and one dose of methylene blue was given. The laboratory could not test the blood for potassium levels, hepatic enzymes or bilirubin as it was black and viscous. After 48 h, she developed severe anemia (4.2 g/dL) due to massive hemolysis. The troponin level also continued to rise, without any ECG changes. She was treated with 8 packed red blood cell transfusions, and received 80 mg of methylprednisolone. After 72 h post admission, the patient suffered a cardiac arrest, recovering after cardiac massage, adrenaline and mechanical ventilation. The diagnosis of toxic myocarditis was made. Dobutamine infusion and nitric oxide therapy were necessary for 24 h. Toxicology report about a week later of the powder she had taken came positive for copper sulfate. She was extubated on day 15 of hospitalization. She recovered with urine output of about 250 cc/day but developed chronic renal failure.

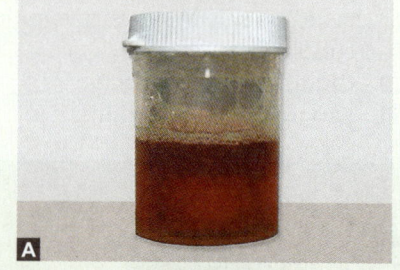

Source: Moussiegt A, Ferreira L, Aboab J, Silva D. She has the blues: an unusual case of copper sulfate intoxication. Eur J Case Rep Intern Med. 2020;7: doi:10.12890/2020_001394

41 CHAPTER

Inorganic Metallic Irritants—Thallium

LEARNING OBJECTIVES

Desirable to know
1. Signs and symptoms and fatal dose of acute thallium poisoning
2. Treatment of thallium poisoning
3. Medico-legal aspects of thallium poisoning

FM 9.3

Describe general principles and basic methodologies in treatment of poisoning with regard to thallium.

Introduction

Physical properties: Thallium is a soft, heavy metal having a tin-white lustrous color, which tarnishes on exposure to air due to formation of thallous oxide.
- Currently, the toxicity is through occupational exposure, environmental contamination and accumulation in food, mainly vegetables grown on contaminated soil.

Toxic Compounds and its Uses

i. **Thallium acetate:** Colorless and almost tasteless. It was used as a depilatory in the treatment of ringworm of scalp, for removing the superfluous hair, as constituent of some proprietary depilatory creams, in fireworks and as a rodenticide and insecticide.

ii. **Thallium sulfate** is used for killing rats and ants.

Action

- Thallium and its salts are corrosive to the GIT.
- After absorption, it replaces potassium in numerous potassium-dependent enzyme systems (similar atomic radius to thallium). In addition, thallium damages the ribosomes, resulting in impaired protein synthesis. This results in failure of aerobic respiration and cellular energy production.
- In the peripheral nervous system (PNS), thallium causes a 'dying-back' or Wallerian degenerative sensory neuropathy due to acute myelin fragmentation and axonal degeneration. Motor neuropathy may occur, since it impairs depolarization of muscle fibers.
- Hair loss is caused by stunted mitosis of hair follicle epithelial cells and by destruction of hair shaft cells.

Absorption and Excretion

- Thallium is absorbed through the skin and mucous membrane of the GIT and respiratory tract. It is a cumulative poison, and is deposited in the epididymis, liver, kidneys, muscles, hairs and bones.
- Excretion is through the kidneys, and it is also excreted through the milk.

SIGNS AND SYMPTOMS

In **acute poisoning**, signs and symptoms start between 12–36 hours (h) to 12 days **(Table 41.1)**.
- The effects are the most severe in the nervous system.
- Unlike exposure to most metal salts, GIT symptoms are relatively minor, and constipation is more characteristic than diarrhea.
- In *mild cases*, the symptoms are joint pains in the legs and feet, loss of appetite, stomatitis, drowsiness, and hypochlorhydria. These generally pass off in few days.
- In *sub-acute cases*, there is encephalopathy with white stripes across the nails (*Mees lines*).
- In *chronic exposure*, these symptoms appear in milder forms. The diagnosis may be difficult because it is often unsuspected. The cardinal features (triad) are *gastroenteritis, peripheral neuropathy and alopecia*.
  - A symmetrical mixed peripheral neuropathy is characteristic with distal nerves more strongly affected than proximal nerves.
  - There may be extreme sensitivity of the legs, followed by 'burning feet' syndrome and paresthesia.
- In *fatal cases*, death is preceded by delirium, convulsions and coma.

TABLE 41.1: Signs and symptoms of thallium poisoning

System	Signs and symptoms
GIT	Irritation, metallic taste in mouth, nausea, vomiting, hematemesis, abdominal pain, anorexia, dryness of mouth, colic, diarrhea or constipation.
RS	Distress, running nose, respiratory depression.
Ocular	Conjunctivitis, scotoma, blindness.
MS	Polyneuritis, tingling and pain sensation in hands and feet ('pins and needles'), 'glove-stocking' numbness, muscular weakness with paralysis of some muscles (peripheral neuropathy), tremors.
CNS	Confusion, nystagmus, insomnia, psychosis, ataxia, organic brain syndrome, coma. Dysfunction of cranial nerves II, III, IV and VI, which govern oculomotor and visual function are most common.
Others	Loss of scalp hair, lateral eyebrows*, body and axillary hair (10–14 days after exposure), and deafness.

Causes of death usually are related to the CNS, cardiac and renal system effects.

Fatal Dose

- *Adults*: 200 mg–1 g (10–15 mg/kg).
- *Children*: 8 mg/kg body wt.

Fatal period: Variable, usually 24–36 h.

Diagnosis

- GIT and polyneuritic symptoms (pain and dysesthesias occurring in the feet) together with the falling of hair from head, eyebrows and axilla should lead to suspicion of thallium poisoning.
- A brownish black pigmentation close to the hair root is characteristic of thallium exposure and may appear as early as 3rd–4th day (seen in blonde hair).
- Opacity in the liver on X-rays has been reported.

Laboratory Diagnosis

Thallium toxicity can be monitored in blood, urine and hair.
- Eosinophilia is a common phenomenon.
- Thallium >40 µg% in blood, and >150 µg/L in urine (levels up to 20 µg/L is considered normal) is significant. Hair levels <15 ng/g are considered normal.
- Urine may be green, with proteinuria, diminished creatinine clearance, elevated blood urea nitrogen.

TREATMENT

i. Patient should be kept warm.
ii. Emesis is indicated within 4–6 h of ingestion.
iii. Multiple-dose of activated charcoal may be given, followed by saline purgative. Whole bowel irrigation with polyethylene glycol electrolyte lavage solution may be useful.
iv. Stomach wash is performed with 1% sodium or potassium iodide solution. It forms insoluble iodide salts of thallium. Iodide also acts as a *systemic antidote*.
v. **Prussian blue or Berlin blue** (potassium ferric hexacyanoferrate)¥ which acts to sequester the ions in the intestine and preventing their absorption is given in a dose of 250 mg/kg/day in 2–4 divided doses orally.
vi. Although chelating agents including BAL and EDTA are contraindicated in the treatment, sodium-diethyl-dithio-carbamate 25 mg/kg body wt in 500 mL of 5% glucose IV once daily may be given.
vii. Pilocarpine in usual doses is also a *physiological antidote*.
viii. Potassium chloride promotes renal excretion of thallium. Administration of *sodium polystyrene sulfonate* as sodium-thallium exchange resin may be helpful.
ix. Hemodialysis/peritoneal dialysis may be useful within 48 h of ingestion.
x. Stimulants, dextrose and calcium salts are used according to necessity.

POSTMORTEM FINDINGS

i. There is anemia and loss of hair.
ii. **Stomach:** Mucous membrane may be inflamed and there may be submucous petechial hemorrhages.
iii. **Spleen:** Congested.
iv. **Liver:** Congested, and shows centrilobular necrosis and fatty degeneration.
v. **Kidneys:** Congested, glomeruli are swollen, convoluted tubules show cloudy swelling and necrosis of the cells.
vi. **Trachea and bronchi:** Congested.
vii. **Lungs:** Congested with subpleural hemorrhages.
viii. **Heart:** Fatty degeneration.
ix. **Brain:** Meningeal vessels may be congested.
x. Cells of adrenal cortex, thyroid and hair follicles show vacuolization and degenerative changes.

Medico-legal Aspects

- Poisoning by thallium is rare in contrast to poisoning by lead or mercury, probably due to its infrequent use.
- Thallium was used as an ideal homicidal poisoning in some European countries and Australia, where it was used as rodenticide.
- It is tasteless and odorless, dissolves completely in liquid, rapidly and completely absorbed, and they defy detection on routine toxicological screens.

---

* Medial part of eyebrow are in a resting phase, and not affected by thallium poisoning.
¥ Potassium is exchanged preferentially for thallium entering the enterohepatic circulation. As Prussian blue sequesters thallium, a concentration gradient is established for the continued movement of thallium into the gut.

CHAPTER 41 : Inorganic Metallic Irritants—Thallium

- Accidental intoxication may result from its therapeutic use as a depilatory cream or abortifacient, or from its accidental ingestion when used as a rodenticide.
- Chronic poisoning occurs from occupational exposure.
- Suicidal cases are also seen sometimes.

NOTA BENE

- *Thallium stress test*: In clinical practice, thallium 201 is used as a radioactive tracer in heart scintigraphy to detect myocardial ischemia.
- Accidental poisoning has become rare in the domestic setting since the 1970s, when thallium-based rodenticides were banned in many countries. The majority of reported cases of thallium poisoning in the last two decades have been caused by deliberate poisoning.
- Thallium may be detected in the urine 1 h after ingestion (normal level <0.003 µmol/L; a level of >0.98 µmol/L is toxic), but most clinical laboratories may not have the facilities to quantitatively analyze the thallium content.
- A rapid quantitative urine test can be done by mixing urine with 0.4% sodium bismuth in 20% nitric acid and 10% sodium iodide. A red precipitate indicates that thallium is present.
- Microscopic examination of hair after application of 10% sodium hydroxide may reveal dark bands of pigmented material characteristic of presence of thallium.

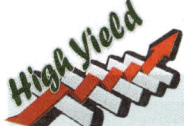

- Thallium toxicity is through occupational exposure, environmental contamination and accumulation in food.
- Thallium causes sensorimotor pain.
- **Cardinal features of thallium toxicity are:** Gastroenteritis, peripheral neuropathy and alopecia.
- In thallium toxicity, a symmetrical mixed peripheral neuropathy is characteristic with distal nerves more commonly affected.
- Prussian blue (potassium ferric hexacyanoferrate) is used in the treatment of thallium toxicity.
- BAL and EDTA are contraindicated in the treatment of thallium poisoning.
- Thallium was used as an ideal homicidal poisoning in some European countries and Australia, where it was used as rodenticide.

Interesting case

Thallium Poisoning (Case of Tianle Li, 2011)

In mid January 2011, Xiaoye Wang, a 39-year-old computer engineer admitted himself in a hospital in Princeton, New Jersey with flu-like symptoms. He complained of nausea, abdominal pain, severe joint pains and trembling of legs. Doctors at the hospital tried one treatment after another but Wang only became weaker. During his hospital stay, he developed alopecia, thickened skin and loss of sensation of his hands and feet. Suspecting thallium poisoning, they sent his blood and urine samples for testing out of State. The lab reported a very high level of thallium in Wang's body. Since, thallium is a dangerous and carefully regulated poison in US, the doctors considered it as either attempted suicide or homicide*.

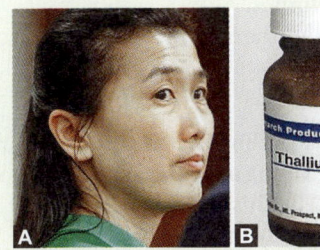

By the time, the doctors were able to secure the antidote Prussian blue, it was too late. Wang's condition worsened and he went into a coma. He died in late January 2011 and his wife Tianle 'Heidi' Li, a research chemist at Bristol-Myers Squibb was arrested 2 days later **(Fig. A)**. She was charged with murder and hindering her own apprehension for telling authorities at first that she never ordered or used thallium at work. The murder charge was lodged after an autopsy confirmed Wang was poisoned with thallium.

Prosecutors proved that Tianle had specialized knowledge and access to thallium. Testimonies were given during the trial that she had obtained four bottles of thallium through her work at the pharmaceutical company in the two months before her husband's hospitalization **(Fig. B)**. Tianle began poisoning her husband as early as November 2010, and continued to do so even when he was admitted in the hospital. She intentionally chose a rare poison for which doctors would not immediately test when admitted to the hospital. Wang had filed for divorce in 2010 and the couple was supposed to finalize their divorce in the court on the day of his hospitalization. She tried to flee unsuccessfully back to China, with her son and an aunt, just before her husband's death, but was unable to pay for the tickets. She also visited websites for criminal attorneys and the State judiciary system, the day before his death. She was found guilty by the Jury and convicted of murder and of hindering the prosecution by lying, and has to spend the life in prison.

---

* Murder mystery writers like Agatha Christie's knew long before that thallium appears to be a near perfect homicidal poison which she exploited in the 1961 murder mystery story 'The Pale Horse'.

Other Inorganic Metallic Irritants

Learning Objectives

Must know
1. Cadmium, barium and zinc toxicity
2. Metal fume fever

Desirable to know
1. Itai-itai disease
2. Polymer fume fever

Describe general principles and basic methodologies in treatment of poisoning with regard to cadmium.

CADMIUM

Cadmium is a soft, white metal, used in welding, metal-plating, battery and plastic industries.
- Cadmium exposure occurs from cigarette smoking (significant source), ingestion of contaminated food or water, drugs and dietary supplements.
- Poisoning may occur from the inhalation of cadmium dust or fumes.
- Kidneys are the main organ affected in long-term exposure.

Action

- It binds to sulfhydryl groups, denaturing proteins and/or inactivating enzymes. The mitochondria are severely affected by this process, which may result in increase susceptibility to oxidative stress.
- It also interferes with calcium transport mechanisms leading to intracellular hypercalcemia, and ultimately apoptosis.

Absorption and Metabolism

- Cadmium (2–7%) is absorbed through the GIT and its absorption is enhanced when the diet is deficient in calcium, iron or protein. Absorption through the respiratory tract is more efficient, ranging from 15–50% of an inhaled dose.
- It binds to RBCs, plasma albumin and metallothionein, which is synthesized in the liver. Cadmium is initially detoxified in the liver through the formation of a metallothionein-cadmium complex, which is slowly released from that organ.

Signs and Symptoms

Toxicity by inhalation is far greater than by ingestion.
- **On inhalation:** Symptoms develop usually after 4–8 hours (h). They are influenza-like and similar to those seen in *metal fume fever*. It is characterized by sneezing, sore throat, irritant cough, nausea, excessive salivation, metallic taste, headache and cyanosis ('**cadmium blues**'). After a latent period of 24–36 h, *chemical pneumonitis* develops which is characterized by fever, dyspnea, bronchospasm and pleuritic chest pain, along with tachycardia, oliguria and noncardiogenic pulmonary edema.
- **On ingestion:** Symptoms occur in 1 h. These are increased salivation, nausea, vomiting, cramps in the abdomen, diarrhea, myalgia, collapse, and rarely death.
- **Chronic exposure** causes anosmia, yellowing of teeth *(cadmium ring formation)*, emphysema, bone pain, fractures with osteomalacia (*itai-itai disease* is the most severe form) and chronic renal failure (hypercalciuria, proteinuria, azotemia). In males, it decreases libido, fertility and serum testosterone level, and in females, the function of ovary and development of oocytes may be inhibited. Hypertension and hypochromic anemia may be seen.
- Cadmium is said to be carcinogenic, and increased incidence of lung, prostate, pancreas and bladder carcinoma has been reported.

Fatal Dose

Serum cadmium >100 mg. Symptoms are seen with serum cadmium >5 mg/dL (normal range 0.2–6.0 ng/mL) and urinary cadmium >100 nmol/L.

Fatal period: 5–7 days.

Diagnosis: Blood cadmium levels are a reflection of acute cadmium exposure; urine levels appear to provide a better measure of chronic exposure. Urinary beta-2 microglobulin test is an indirect method of measuring cadmium exposure.
- Blood cadmium is measured by atomic absorption spectrophotometry or plasma mass spectrometry.
- Cadmium levels in hair and nails samples are often determined in chronic toxicity. Saliva analysis can be an excellent method for diagnosis (mean tolerable level of cadmium is <0.55 μg/L).

Treatment

i. Avoid further exposure, O_2 and steroids may be given in case of inhalation of fumes.
ii. Stomach is washed with tannin or egg albumin, and activated charcoal may be given.
iii. Sodium sulfate as a purgative is given.
iv. Succimer (10 mg/kg/dose 8 h) may be given (decreases the GIT absorption and improves survival without increasing cadmium burden in target organs) in case of acute poisoning, and dithiocarbamates in chronic poisoning.
v. Vitamin D is given for osteomalacia.
vi. Hemoperfusion and hemodialysis are not useful.

> **Recent Advances**
> - **Dithiocarbamates:** N-tetramethylene dithiocarbamate enhances the urinary and biliary excretion of cadmium.
> - **New DMSA analogues:** *Monoisoamyl* DMSA *(MiADMSA)* has been found effective for lead, cadmium, mercury and gallium arsenide overdose.
> - **Combination therapy:** Combination therapy of DMSA and MiADMSA is administered and more effective than single agent. A combination of DMSA and calcium trisodium diethylene triaminepen taacetate (CaDTPA) has been effectively used in acute toxicity.
> - **Antioxidants**, such as vitamins C and E have protective effect against cadmium toxicity.
> - **Nanoparticle:** Cadmium can be adsorbed by Al_2O_3 nanoparticles.

Postmortem Findings

i. **GIT:** Mucous membranes of the esophagus, stomach and intestines are congested and inflamed.
ii. **Lungs:** Pulmonary edema and emphysema. There may be degeneration and/or loss of bronchial and bronchiolar epithelial cells.
iii. **Heart and liver:** Fatty degeneration.
iv. **Kidneys:** Proximal tubular necrosis (interstitial nephritis in chronic cases).
v. **Brain:** Congested.

Medico-legal aspects: Poisoning with cadmium is rare, but may occur as an industrial disease.

> **NOTA BENE**
> - Cadmium poisoning occurred in 1946 from the contamination of food and water by mining effluents in Japan resulting in outbreak of *'itai-itai' ('ouch-ouch')* disease, so named as cadmium-induced bone toxicity led to painful bone fractures.
> - In chronic exposure, cadmium is bound to intracellular metallothionein, which greatly reduces its toxicity. Any attempt to remove cadmium from these deposits risks redistributing cadmium to other organs, thus exacerbating toxicity, as is known to occur with BAL therapy (exacerbate nephrotoxicity).

> **FM 9.2**
> Describe general principles and basic methodologies in treatment of poisoning with regard to barium.

BARIUM

Physical properties: It is a heavy, white, tasteless, odorless powder and insoluble in water. Barium sulfate is used for the X-ray examination of the GIT ('barium-meal').

Toxic compounds: Soluble salts are most toxic. These are barium chloride, barium nitrate, barium carbonate (rodenticide) and barium sulphide (used as a depilatory cream). In Kiating, China, a subacute form of barium poisoning (*pa-ping*) was endemic because of use of contaminated table salt.

Action: It acts locally as an irritant poison. After absorption it acts both on voluntary and involuntary muscles. Barium seems to act as potassium antagonist and calcium agonist.

Absorption

Toxicity of barium compounds depends on their solubility. The free ion is absorbed from the lungs and GIT, but barium sulfate remains unabsorbed. After absorption, it accumulates in the skeleton and in pigmented parts of the eye.

Signs and Symptoms

Ingestion

The most characteristic features are areflexia and paralysis (Ba^{2+} ion is a muscle poison).

System	Signs and symptoms
GIT	Nausea, vomiting, salivation, abdominal pain and diarrhea.
MS	Tingling sensation, tremors, cramps, stiffness of the muscles, paralysis of the tongue and larynx, myoclonus, myalgia, flaccid quadriplegia.
CVS	Hypertension, arrhythmia, ectopic beats, ventricular fibrillation, irregular pulse, shock, cardiac arrest.
RS	Pulmonary edema, respiratory failure.
CNS	Mydriasis, vertigo, headache, confusion, convulsions.

Inhalation

Inhalation of barium sulfate dust causes a benign pneumoconiosis ('baritosis') with conspicuous radiographic manifestation, but no impairment of pulmonary functions.

Differential diagnosis: Gastroenteritis with hypokalemic paralysis and botulism.

Diagnosis

- Hypokalemia: Serum level of potassium is usually 1.1–2.8 mmol/L (most important manifestation).
- Characteristic changes of ECG: Prolongation of PR interval, ST segment depression with U waves and T wave inversion.

Fatal Dose

About 0.8–1 g of barium chloride/sulfide/nitrate.

Fatal period: Usually within 12 h.

Treatment

i. **Decontamination:** Gastric lavage with sodium or magnesium sulfate (5–10 g) solution to precipitate the barium as insoluble sulfate.
ii. **Saline diuresis:** Administer 0.45% of NaCl in D5W and a diuretic (furosemide 1 mg/kg) to obtain a urine flow of 3–6 mL/kg/h to flush out barium by diuresis.
iii. **Intravenous potassium supplementation:** Administration of large amounts of potassium parenterally (KCl 20–40 mEq/L) is indicated (potassium infusion is an effective antidote).
iv. 10 mL of 10% sodium sulfate IV every 15 min to convert barium into insoluble sulfate.
v. Purgation with magnesium sulfate and repeated bowel washes.
vi. Aggressive respiratory assistance and bicarbonate administration are essential to manage the life threatening respiratory paralysis and acidosis.
vii. Sodium nitrite 30–60 mg for hypertension.
viii. Procainamide 500 mg slow IV for ventricular fibrillation.
ix. Hemodialysis is effective in patients with severe poisoning.
x. Symptomatic treatment.

Postmortem findings: Non-specific. Subendocardial hemorrhage in the ventricles, submucosal hemorrhages in the GIT and fatty changes in the liver may be seen. **Histopathology** may show degenerative changes and amorphous, flocculent foamy materials in the renal tubules.

Medico-legal Aspects

- Suicidal cases may be seen.
- Homicidal cases are rare.
- Accidental poisoning with barium sulfide may occur, if taken by mistake as barium sulfate for X-ray examination.

Unintentional mixing of barium carbonate with food resulting in accidental poisoning has been reported.

Describe general principles and basic methodologies in treatment of poisoning with regard to zinc phosphide.

ZINC

Zinc is normally present in our body. Poisonous salts are compounds of chloride, phosphide, sulfate (*white vitriol*), oxide and stearate.

Uses: Zinc chloride is used to clean metals before soldering. Zinc phosphide is used as rodenticide. Zinc stearate is used as a cosmetic (baby powder).

Action: Salts of zinc are locally irritating, and after absorption cause metabolic acidosis, hypocalcemia, damage to the liver and kidneys, and affects the CNS.

Signs and Symptoms

Ingestion

On ingestion, there is a metallic taste, nausea, vomiting, pain in the abdomen and diarrhea. The vomitus and the stool may contain blood. There is ulceration of the mucous membrane of mouth, esophagus and stomach wall with occasional perforation. Collapse due to shock may occur.

- *Zinc phosphide* releases phosphine gas under acidic conditions in the stomach (similar to aluminum phosphide). In addition to the above features, the vomitus gives the smell of garlic. Dyspnea, lethargy, hypotension, cardiac arrhythmias, pulmonary edema, metabolic acidosis, convulsions, circulatory collapse, coma and death may occur.

Inhalation

Inhalation of *zinc oxide* vapor in industries causes chill and fever, a condition known as 'metal fume fever' or 'zinc shakes' (when exposed daily to concentrations of >8–12 mg/m^3).

- Inhalation of *zinc stearate* used in baby powder may cause pneumonitis.

Fatal Dose

- Zinc chloride: 40–70 mg/kg.
- Zinc phosphide: 20–40 mg/kg.
- Zinc sulfate: 15 g (10–30 g).
- Zinc oxide fumes: 500 mg/m^3 (recommended exposure limit: 5 mg/m^3).

Fatal period: 3–5 h to few days.

Treatment

i. Gastric lavage is done with alkaline solution. Demulcents and castor oil may be given.

ii. Sodium bicarbonate with water is given orally.
iii. Purgatives are given for elimination.
iv. Symptomatic treatment.

Postmortem Findings

i. Non-specific external signs may be seen. Garlicky odor from the mouth and on opening the stomach may be observed in case of zinc phosphide poisoning.
ii. Signs of irritation of the GIT with degenerative changes in the stomach wall and occasional perforation may be there.
iii. Degenerative changes in the liver, kidneys and heart may occur.
iv. Visceral organs are congested.

Medico-legal Aspects

- Suicidal poisoning is seen with the phosphide.
- Accidental cases occur with chronic exposure in industries, acute poisoning may occur with consumption of food stored and cooked in zinc galvanized metal containers.
- Homicidal cases are rare.
- It may be used as an abortifacient.

METAL FUME FEVER

- Metal fume fever (MFF) is a self-limiting acute febrile illness associated with inhalation of metal oxide fumes. It is also called *smelter's shakes, brass chills or Monday morning fever* (symptoms become more severe after weekend).
- **Signs and symptoms:** This influenza-like syndrome starts 4–8 h after exposure of fumes, which is characterized by headache, fever, chills, cough, dyspnea, cyanosis, myalgia, metallic taste, salivation, sweating and tachycardia. Symptoms subside within 24–36 h, only to return on repeated exposure.
- **Metals involved:** It is caused by acute exposure to fumes/smoke of oxides of zinc (*commonest cause*), copper, magnesium, nickel, mercury, lead, iron, chromium, cadmium, cobalt, antimony, tungsten, titanium, manganese and silver.
- **Pathophysiology:** The inhalation of ZnO particles causes changes in composition of bronchoalveolar lavage fluid, including early increase in pro-inflammatory cytokines, inflammatory marker and recruitment of inflammatory cells in the lungs.
- A proper occupational history (those involved in welding, melting or flame cutting galvanized metal or in brass foundry operations) should make the diagnosis evident. WBC count may be elevated, chest X-ray is usually normal.
- **Treatment:** Supplemental oxygen, bronchodilators (if there is wheezing) and symptomatic treatment.

NOTA BENE

Polymer fume fever is a separate and distinct occupational disease that has been associated with inhalational exposure to specific fluorinated polymer products, such as polytetrafluoroethylene or Teflon. Overheating of Teflon-coated cookware is one of the more common mechanisms for exposure. The clinical presentation is indistinguishable from MFF, with an exposure history being necessary to distinguish the two entities.

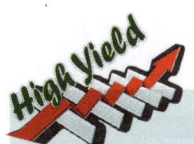

- **Target organ in cadmium poisoning:** Kidneys (proximal tubular necrosis).
- Chemical pneumonitis is seen in cadmium poisoning; characterized by fever, dyspnea, bronchospasm and pleuritic chest pain.
- **Itai-itai disease:** Cadmium-induced bone toxicity leading to painful bone fractures.
- Succimer is given in case of acute cadmium poisoning, and dithiocarbamates in chronic poisoning.
- **Characteristic features of barium poisoning:** Areflexia and paralysis (muscular weakness).
- Zinc phosphide releases phosphine gas in stomach (similar to Alphos). Vomitus gives garlicky smell.
- **Metal fume fever (smelter's shakes):** Inhalation of zinc oxide vapor in industries causes chill and fever.
- **Commonest metal indicated in metal fume fever:** Zinc.

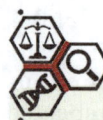 **Interesting case**

Barium Poisoning (Case of Damian Skipper, 2015)

In March 2016, police found a charred body from a truck that had been set on fire at night. His body was found on the floor between the front and back seats. The Coroner's office later identified the body as Arthur Noflin, a 42-year-old man from New Orleans, Louisiana. An autopsy showed no signs of trauma and he did not inhale any smoke indicating that he was dead before his body was burnt. The cause and manner of his death remained unclassified. Police investigated the death as a homicide.

A few days after his body was found, Meshell Hale, a 50-year-old female **(Fig. A)** lodged a missing person report of her husband who turned out to be Noflin. The police started investigating Meshell after the suspicious death of her husband and the resulting investigation revealed startling evidence. They found that Noflin had become sick several months before his death. He was recently 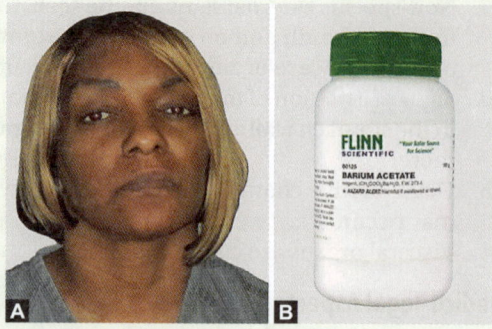 hospitalized with symptoms, such as abdominal pain, diarrhea, vomiting, weakness and low potassium. Investigators at some point discovered, Skipper, Meshell's 41 year live-in boyfriend died in June 2015 after being hospitalized several times with abdominal pain and related symptoms. It was believed he died of a heart attack, and he was buried without an autopsy. Noflin became sick with the same symptoms 6 months after Skipper died.

In May 2016, a search of Meshell's home turned up several phones and computers with search-engine histories around barium acetate and its poisoning effects **(Fig. B)**. In the months before Skipper died, Meshell made two purchases of barium acetate. Her financial records revealed these purchases. Hale repeated the barium purchases in January 2016 using her credit card and was researching on poison-related queries in the months leading up to the death of Noflin. In June 2015, search queries included 'Transamerica Employee Benefits Damian Skipper health claim form'. After Skipper's death, Meshell claimed to be his wife and received $10,000 from his life insurance policy. She also was trying to collect $750,000 in life insurance proceeds as the sole beneficiary on Noflin's policy.

Noting that Meshell had bought barium acetate prior to Skipper's death, investigators contacted the Coroner. His body was exhumed and toxicologists found lethal levels of barium acetate and reclassified his death as a homicide by barium poisoning. The police arrested Meshell and charged her with first-degree murder in the June 2015 death of Skipper, but not charged in the suspicious death of Noflin. Coroner's office does not know what caused his death, so they have not classified it as a homicide. Evidence relating to Noflin's death would be offered to prove motive because in both murders Meshell financially benefited from the victim's deaths.

43 CHAPTER

Non-metallic Irritants

LEARNING OBJECTIVES

Must know
1. Signs and symptoms, fatal dose, treatment and PM findings in acute phosphorus poisoning
2. Phossy jaw
3. White and red phosphorus (Diff.)

Desirable to know
1. Medico-legal aspects of phosphorus poisoning
2. Iodine poisoning

> **FM 9.2**
> Describe general principles and basic methodologies in treatment of poisoning with regard to phosphorus.

PHOSPHORUS

Introduction

The most common allotropes of phosphorous (Greek '*phos*': light, '*phorus*': bringing) are* **(Diff. 43.1)**:
  i. **White or crystalline:** Samples of white phosphorus always contain some red phosphorus and therefore appear yellow (also called '*yellow phosphorus*').
  ii. **Red or amorphous:** White phosphorus gradually changes to red phosphorus. This transformation is accelerated by heat and light.

Action: It is a protoplasmic poison and affects cellular oxidation. The metabolism of cells reduces, leading to necrobiosis which is predominantly seen in the liver (periportal injury).

SIGNS AND SYMPTOMS

Contact Injury

White phosphorus exposure results in painful penetrating second and third degree burn injuries. The burn typically appears as a necrotic area with a yellowish color and characteristic garlic-like odor. White phosphorus is lipid soluble, and hence results in rapid dermal penetration and delayed wound healing.

DIFFERENTIATION 43.1: White and red phosphorous (Figs. 43.1A and B)

S.No.	Feature	White phosphorus	Red phosphorus
1.	Color	White or yellow	Reddish-brown
2.	Appearance	Crystalline, waxy, translucent	Amorphous or crystalline, opaque
3.	Solubility ♦ Organic solvents ♦ Water	Yes Very low (~3 mg/l)	No Insoluble
4.	Odor	Characteristic garlicky odor	Odorless
5.	Taste	Garlicky	Tasteless
6.	Chemiluminescence	Luminous in dark	Non-luminous
7.	Ignitability	Inflammable, spontaneous ignition in air at room temperature (emits white fumes) and in chlorine	Non-inflammable, ignites only at >260°C; heat is necessary for ignition in chlorine
8.	Reaction with aqueous alkali	Produces phosphine	None
9.	Toxicity	Highly toxic	Low toxicity
10.	Uses	Fertilizers, insecticides, rodenticide, incendiary bombs, smoke screens and fireworks	On sides of match box**

---
* There are more than 10 allotropes of phosphorous; black phosphorous is the most stable form.
** Red phosphorous is mixed with abrasives like tiny fragments of glass to create heat through friction.

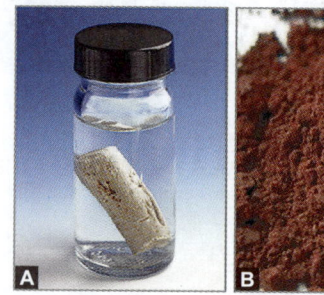
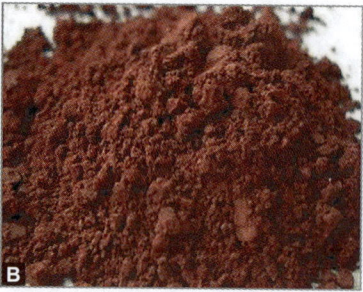

Figs. 43.1A and B: (A) White phosphorous; (B) Red phosphorous

Acute Ingestion

The clinical effects can be divided into three stages:

First Stage

Within ½–6 hours (h), yellow phosphorus produces burning pain in the throat and abdomen with intense thirst, nausea, vomiting, diarrhea and abdominal pain. Breath, vomitus and feces have garlic-like odor. Luminescent 'smoking' vomit and feces are diagnostic.

Second Stage

This stage (1–4 days), which may last for several days, is essentially a symptom-free period, but liver enzyme levels become elevated, and toxic hepatitis begins to spread.

Third Stage

The third stage may progress to multiorgan failure—acute liver and renal failure with metabolic derangements, encephalopathy, coagulopathy, arrhythmia and cardiogenic shock.

System	Signs and symptoms (Third stage)
GIT	Nausea, vomiting, hematemesis, diarrhea.
Hepatic	Tender hepatomegaly, jaundice, pruritus.
Renal	Oliguria, hematuria, casts, albuminuria, sometimes anuria.
CNS	Restlessness, anxiety, insomnia, headache, confusion, hallucinations, convulsions, delirium, coma.
PNS	Paresthesia, carpopedal spasm, tetany, laryngeal stridor, opisthotonus (because of hypocalcemia).
Hematologic	Purpura, epistaxis, hemorrhage in mucous membrane and viscera.

Fulminating poisoning (death within 12 h) may be seen when the patient takes a large dose.

Cause of death
- Early death is due to cardiac dysrhythmias, secondary to electrolyte abnormalities, such as hypocalcemia and hyperkalemia.
- Death after the first 24 h is due to hepatic failure.

Fatal Dose

White phosphorous: 60–120 mg (1 mg/kg).

Fatal period: Within 24 h, but may be delayed by 5–7 days.

Diagnosis: Oral and skin burns, luminescent 'smoking' vomitus and stools with a garlic odor, and GIT and biliary damage characterize white phosphorus poisoning.

Treatment

Management is usually supportive as there is no antidote. Liver transplantation may be lifesaving in patients with acute hepatic failure.

i. Life support measures—airway support and fluid maintenance should be provided.
ii. External burns should be washed and cleaned with mild disinfectant soap and water, and covered with antibiotic ointment.
iii. Activated charcoal is given.
iv. Demulcents (oily or fatty substances) are contra-indicated, as phosphorus gets dissolved and gets absorbed.
v. Purgatives (magnesium sulfate) may be given.
vi. Vitamin K 20 mg IV in repeated doses, or blood transfusion (fresh frozen plasma).
vii. Transfusion of glucose-saline and plasma with vitamins is useful to protect the liver and to correct shock and dehydration.
viii. Peritoneal or hemodialysis may be required (for correction of hyperphosphatemia, hyperkalemia and hypocalcemia).
ix. N-acetylcysteine, ubiquinone and sulfate have been tried to prevent liver damage.
x. Anti-cholestatic modalities, such as cholestyramine, ursodeoxycholic acid and sertraline are also used.

NOTA BENE

- Identifiable phosphorous particles from the skin are removed by thorough debridement and the area covered with saline-soaked gauze to prevent further combustion. Copper sulfate solution is sometimes recommended for conversion of phosphorous particles to blue-black cupric phosphide.
- Alternatively, application of silver nitrate may prevent ignition of phosphorus by depositing a film of silver over the phosphorous.
- In the past, acute poisoning management involved removal of the toxin with gastric lavage using $KMnO_4$ (as chemical antidote), which oxidizes phosphorus into less toxic phosphoric acid and phosphates. The administration of $KMnO_4$ is not safe and is no longer recommended in the treatment of phosphorus poisoning.
- Stomach can also be washed with 0.2% copper sulfate solution. Since, copper sulfate itself can cause acute copper poisoning and inhibit G-6-PD leading to lethal hemolysis, it is not recommended.
- There is a danger of explosion and fire because of entry of oxygen into the stomach or exit of phosphorous through the nasogastric tube. This is minimized by connecting the external end of the tube to a syringe filled with water; confirmation of placement is done by instilling water rather than air or by withdrawing gastric contents.

POSTMORTEM FINDINGS

External

i. Emaciation, purpuric hemorrhages in the skin, jaundice and smell of garlic may be present.
ii. Mucous membrane of the mouth is corroded.
iii. PM staining is dark brown in color.

Internal

i. Multiple hemorrhages are seen in the muscles, serosal and mucosal membranes of the GIT and respiratory tract, liver, kidneys, endocardium, pericardium, epicardium, peritoneum, lungs and brain **(Figs. 43.2A and B)**.
ii. **Stomach and intestines:** Mucous membranes are yellowish or grayish-white in color, softened, thickened, inflamed and corroded in patches; luminous material may be found in the stomach. Contents may smell of garlic.
iii. **Liver:** Swollen, yellow, soft, fatty and easily ruptured **(Fig. 43.3A)**.
iv. **Kidneys:** Enlarged, greasy, yellow **(Fig. 43.3B)**.
v. **Heart:** Flabby, pale and shows fatty degeneration.
vi. **Lungs:** Fat emboli may be found in the pulmonary arterioles and capillaries.

Histopathology: Toxic hepatitis with extensive necrosis, ballooning degeneration, and steatosis.

Medico-legal Aspects

- Accidental poisoning in children due to chewing of fireworks or by eating rat paste* may occur.
- It is not preferred for suicide because of painful symptoms and prolonged suffering.

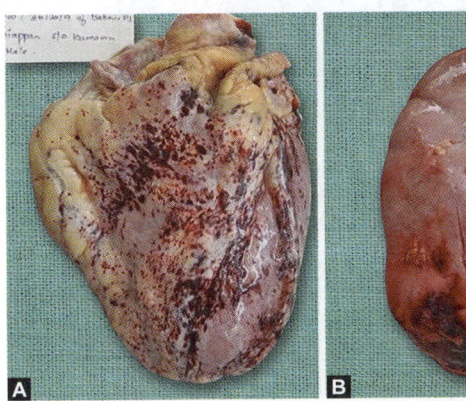

Figs. 43.2A and B: Yellow phosphorous poisoning (Ratol paste). Hemorrhages in heart and kidney

- It may be used for homicide purpose by mixing with alcohol or coffee to mask the taste and smell, and administered, since:
  a. Symptoms resemble acute liver disease.
  b. There is delay in the appearance of symptoms.
  c. The poison is oxidized in the body, hence cannot be detected.
  d. Death occurs after few days.
- Sometimes, it is taken by mouth or introduced into the vagina to procure abortion.
- Poisoning may result from industrial accidents in developed countries.
- Cases of poisoning may occur during war when phosphorus enters the body with fragments of hand grenades, smoke screens, bombs or bullets.
- For arson, white phosphorus covered with dung or wet cloth is thrown on huts. When the covering becomes dry, the roof catches fire.

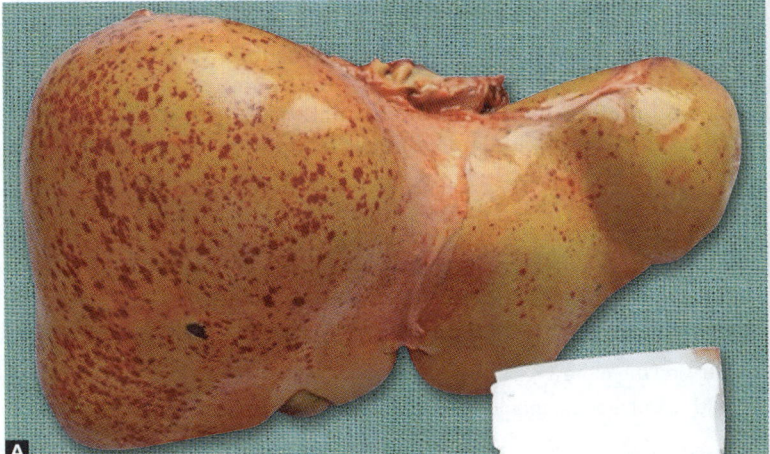
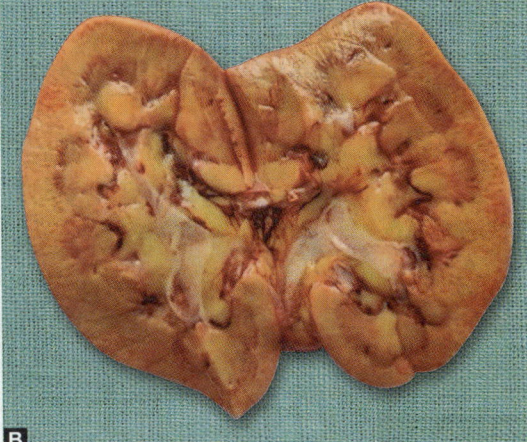

Figs. 43.3A and B: Yellow phosphorous poisoning: (A) Liver showing hemorrhages and yellowish discoloration; (B) Kidney showing yellowish discoloration of the renal parenchyma
(*Courtesy:* Dr K Chavali, Professor of Forensic Medicine, AIIMS, Raipur, Chattisgarh)

---

* Yellow phosphorus pose a problem as the product directions suggest that the paste be applied to bread to enable ingestion by rodents, thus making it appealing to children as well. Sometimes, it may be mistaken for toothpaste.

CHRONIC PHOSPHORUS POISONING

- The frequent inhalation of fumes over a period of years causes necrosis of the lower jaw in the region of a decayed tooth.
- Initially, there is toothache which is followed by swelling of the jaw, loosening of the teeth, necrosis of the gums and sequestration of bone in the mandible with multiple sinuses discharging foul-smelling pus. This is known as **'phossy jaw'** *(glass jaw or Lucifer's jaw)* in which osteomyelitis and necrosis of jaw occurs.
- *Constitutional symptoms* include nausea, vomiting, anorexia, pain in the abdomen, indigestion, purging, pain in the joints, weakness, loss of weight, bronchitis, cirrhosis, jaundice, ascites and anemia.

> **FM 9.2**
> Describe general principles and basic methodologies in treatment of poisoning with regard to iodine.

IODINE POISONING

Introduction: Iodine occurs as blackish crystals with a metallic taste, characteristic odor and acrid taste.

Uses: It is commonly used as a disinfectant (tincture povidone iodine), antiseptic, emetic and for treatment of thyroid cancer (radioactive iodine). It is also used in chemical industry, photography and dye manufacturing.

Lugol solution is 5% iodine and 10% iodide in water. Iodophors such as povidone-iodine (Betadine) consist of iodine linked to a large molecular weight molecule.

Action: Toxicity is due absorption, ingestion or inhalation. Iodine is both a corrosive and irritant poison. It directly damages the cell by precipitating proteins.

Signs and Symptoms

- **On ingestion:** Brownish discoloration of lips and oral mucosa, pain in mouth and unpleasant taste, intense thirst and abdominal pain with vomiting and diarrhea (corrosive gastroenteritis). Vomitus and stool may be dark colored (blue colored, if starchy food are present in the stomach) with peculiar odor of iodine. Micturition is painful and there may be oliguria or anuria. Marked depression, feeble pulse, delirium and collapse may occur.
- **Inhalation of iodine vapors** may cause edema of glottis, pulmonary edema and death from asphyxia.
- **Skin contact** causes erythema, desquamation and sometimes vesication.

Fatal Dose

- Iodine vapor: 2 ppm (immediately dangerous to life)
- Ingestion: 2–4 g of free iodine (30–60 mL of tincture).

Fatal period: 24 h.

Treatment

i. Gastric lavage should be done immediately with 1% starch solution or 5% solution of sodium thiosulfate.
ii. Demulcents, such as starchy foods, eggs, milk, oils, etc., should be left in the stomach.
iii. IV hydrocortisone (reduces edema of glottis) and antihistamines should be given.
iv. Tracheostomy, if respiratory distress occurs.
v. Symptomatic treatment.

Postmortem Findings

i. Characteristic iodine odor.
ii. Brownish or yellowish stains of skin and mucosa. The mucosa of GIT will appear bluish if starch solution had been administered during treatment of the patient.
iii. Congestion of viscera, particularly kidneys.

Medico-legal Aspects

- Poisoning in children is usually due to accidental ingestion of iodine solution at home.
- Poisoning may be suicidal.
- Homicidal poisoning is rare due to its bad taste.

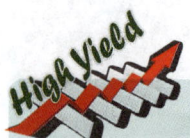

- White/crystalline phosphorus contains some red phosphorus and therefore appears yellow ('*yellow phosphorus*').
- White phosphorous has a garlicky odor, luminous in dark with spontaneous ignition in air (kept under water to prevent its contact with oxygen).
- Contact with white phosphorus results 2° and 3° burns. Burn typically appears as a necrotic area with a yellowish color and characteristic garlic-like odor.
- **Diagnostic of phosphorous poisoning:** Luminescent 'smoking' vomit and feces.
- Acute phosphorous poisoning may progress to multiorgan failure—acute liver and renal failure with metabolic derangements.
- Early death is due to cardiac dysrhythmias, secondary to electrolyte abnormalities, such as hypocalcemia and hyperkalemia.

- Death after the first 24 h is due to hepatic failure.
- There is no antidote to phosphorus poisoning.
- Copper sulfate was used as an antidote for phosphorous poising.
- Liver transplantation is life saving in patients with acute hepatic failure.
- Liver is soft, yellow, fatty and easily ruptured in deaths due to phosphorous poisoning.
- Phossy jaw (glass jaw/Lucifer jaw) is seen in chronic phosphorous poisoning.
- Brownish discoloration of oral mucosa is seen in iodine poisoning.
- Gastric lavage with starch or sodium thiosulphate is indicated in iodine poisoning.

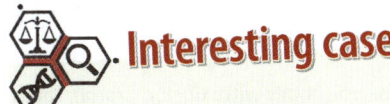

Interesting case

Phosphorous Poisoning

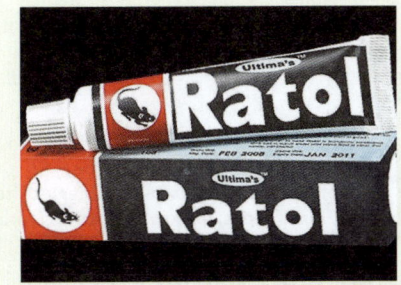

Soni JP et al. reported a case of suicidal poisoning of yellow phosphorus. A 30-year-old female patient was admitted to the hospital complaining of burning sensation in mouth, nausea, and vomiting. There was garlicky odor from the vomitus. Her husband gave history of 10–12 g Ratol paste (3% yellow phosphorous) ingestion about 2 h before. She was conscious with stable vitals. Gastric lavage was done with 1:5000 $KMnO_4$ and activated charcoal given. Symptomatic management was done along with N-acetylcysteine (NAC).

On the 2nd day, her clinical status improved, and she was asymptomatic. The patient and their relative took discharge despite medical advice to contrary. On the 4th day, the patient returned to the hospital with generalized weakness, bodily pain, drowsiness, and breathing difficulty. She was drowsy with hypotension, tachycardia and tachypnea. On examination, icterus was present. USG showed hepatomegaly and fatty changes. A provisional diagnosis of yellow phosphorus poisoning with hepatic encephalopathy and multiorgan failure was made. On the 5th day, the patient developed sudden onset of bradycardia, hypotension and rapidly led to the patient's death, with no possibilities to perform liver transplantation.

An autopsy was conducted. Scleral icterus was present. Both pleural cavities were filled with hemorrhagic fluid. Pinpoint to pinhead size petechial hemorrhages were present over the mesenteries, liver, and kidneys. Yellowish discoloration of the liver, kidneys, and brain surfaces was present.

Source: Soni JP, Ghormade PS, Akhade S, Chavali K, Sarma B. A fatal case of multi-organ failure in acute yellow phosphorus poisoning. Autopsy Case Rep (Internet). 2020;10(1):e2020146.
(*Courtesy:* Dr K Chavali, Professor of Forensic Medicine, AIIMS, Raipur, Chattisgarh)

44 CHAPTER

Organic Irritants—Plant

LEARNING OBJECTIVES

Must know
1. Active principles and identification of: *Ricinus, Croton, Abrus, Semecarpus, Capsicum, Calotropis*
2. Suis
3. Medico-legal aspects of marking nut
4. Artificial and true bruise (Diff.)

Desirable to know
1. Signs and symptoms of poisoning with: *Castor, Croton*, rati, marking nut, *Capsicum*, and *Calotropis*
2. Toxalbumin
3. Hunan hand

 FM 14.17

To identify and draw medico-legal inference from common poisons, e.g., *Castor*, *Abrus* seeds, marking nut, *Capsicum*, and *Calotropis*.

◼ RICINUS COMMUNIS (CASTOR)

Distribution: It grows all over India, especially in wastelands.

Identification of Seeds (Fig. 44.1)

- Seeds are variable, smooth, flattened-oval, mottled with light and dark brown markings, bright and polished.
- They are of 2 sizes, small and big.
- Small seeds are about 1.2 × 0.8 cm in dimensions and resemble croton seeds.

Active Principle

- The entire plant is poisonous, containing toxalbumin *ricin*, a water-soluble glycoprotein and a powerful allergen. Seeds contain the highest level.
- It is easily and inexpensively produced, highly toxic, and can be in the form of a powder, mist or pellet, or it can be dissolved in water or weak acid.
- Ricin makes up 3–5% of the waste material ('white mash') left over from processing castor beans into castor oil (used as purgative oil), which can be separated by chromatography.
- Castor oil is nonpoisonous as it does not contain ricin.

Unbroken seeds are not poisonous when swallowed or cooked. Toxicity is caused when castor beans are thoroughly chewed or blenderized, even though the quantity of ricin so produced is small and is poorly absorbed from the GIT.

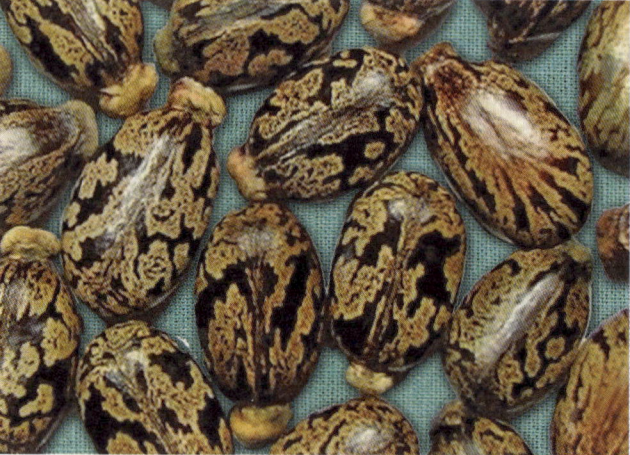

Fig. 44.1: *Ricinus communis* (seeds)

NOTA BENE

Toxalbumin or phytotoxin is a toxic protein that disable ribosomes and thereby inhibit protein synthesis, and present in the plants like in castor, croton or rati.
- It is antigenic in nature, agglutinates red cells, causes hemolysis and cell destruction.
- Toxalbumins are similar in structure to the toxins found in cholera, tetanus, diphtheria, pseudomonas and botulinum; and their physiological and toxic properties are similar to those of viperine snake venom.

Action

- Ricin blocks protein synthesis through inhibition of RNA polymerase. It belongs to a group of poisons known as A-B toxins (protein virulence factors secreted by many bacterial pathogens).
- Ricin has a special binding protein that gains access to the endoplasmic reticulum in the GIT mucosal cells causing diarrhea.

Signs and Symptoms

Inhalation is more potent than oral ingestion.

Dust of seeds may cause:
- Watering of eyes and conjunctivitis
- Headache, pharyngitis
- Gastric upset
- Acute nasal inflammation and sneezing
- Asthmatic bronchitis
- Dermatitis

Inhalation causes non-cardiogenic pulmonary edema, diffuse necrotizing pneumonia, interstitial and alveolar inflammation, and edema.

On ingestion [seen within 10 hours (h) of ingestion]
- **GIT:** Burning pain in throat, colicky abdominal pain/cramping, nausea, thirst, vomiting and diarrhea (often bloody) leading to volume depletion, hypovolemic shock and renal failure.
- **CNS:** Vertigo, drowsiness, delirium, convulsions and coma.
- Uremia, jaundice, rapid feeble pulse, cold clammy skin and dehydration.

Local injection induces erythema, induration, blisters and localized necrosis at the injection site, and swelling of regional lymph nodes.

These symptoms may progress to seizures, hypotension, shock, organ failure, pulmonary edema and respiratory failure. Consciousness is retained till death in some cases.

Laboratory Diagnosis

- Liquid chromatography-mass spectrometry and immunoassays.
- Ricinine, an alkaloid can be detected in serum and urine. Comprehensive untargeted urine drug screening testing is highly valuable.
- Ricin-antibody conjugates can be detected in surviving patients after 2 weeks.

Fatal dose: 3–10 µg/kg body wt (by inhalation or injection). Oral exposure to ricin is far less toxic, and lethal dose is about 20 µg/kg (10–20 seeds).

Fatal period: 3–5 days.

Treatment

No known antidote or other specific treatment, although a vaccine has been developed by the US military.

- After suspected ricin inhalation or exposure to powdered ricin, remove clothings and wash skin with water.
- In case of ingestion:
  i. Gastric lavage.
  ii. Emetics and demulcents.
  iii. Administration of glucose and saline for dehydration.
  iv. 2–5 g of sodium bicarbonate is given 8 hourly by mouth to alkalinize the urine.
  v. Blood transfusion may be needed in some patients.

Postmortem Findings

Deaths caused by ingestion of castor plant seeds are rare, because of its indigestible capsule.

i. Mucosa of the GIT is congested, softened and inflamed with occasional erosions and submucous hemorrhages.
ii. Fragments of seeds may be found in the stomach and intestines.
iii. Dilation of heart, hemorrhages in the pleura, edema and congestion of the liver, kidneys, spleen and lungs may be seen.

Medico-legal Aspects

- Accidental poisoning may occur in children through the ingestion of castor beans.
- Rarely, powdered seeds are given for homicide.
- Ricin can be used an agent of biological warfare or a weapon of mass destruction (WMD).
- The powdered seeds causes conjunctivitis when applied to the eye.

NOTA BENE

- **Chemical warfare:** The toxin has been linked with terrorist activity among anti-government militia in the US and the Al Qaeda.
- In 2003, ricin was detected in a facility that handled mail for the White House. In 2013, envelopes addressed to the then US President Barack Obama tested positive for ricin.
- Ricin is commonly used as part of immunotoxins for clinical tumor research and application in cancer therapy.

CROTON TIGLIUM (JAMALGOTA)

Distribution: It grows all over India, and belongs to Euphorbiaceae family. The processed seeds are used in Indian medicine for treating flatulence, dyspepsia, colic, edema, dyspnea and persistent cough.

Identification of Seeds (Fig. 44.2)

- Seeds are 1.2 × 0.8 cm in dimensions.
- Oval or oval-oblong and odorless.
- Dark brown or brownish-gray shell.

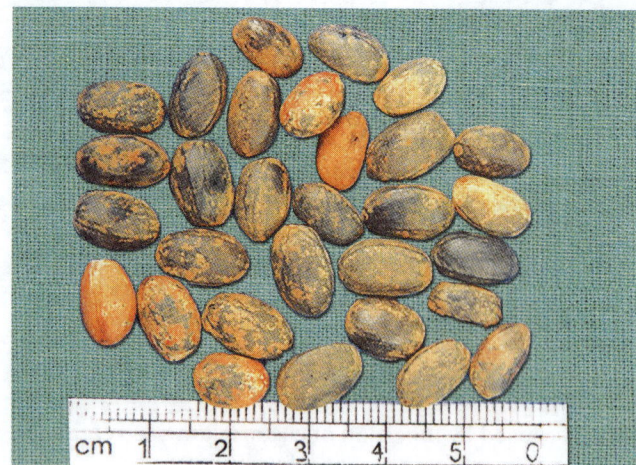

Fig. 44.2: *Croton tiglium* (seeds)

- Resemble castor seeds, but they are not shiny and not mottled.

Active Principles

All parts are poisonous, but seeds contain the maximum concentration of the active principles. *Crotin,* a toxalbumin and *crotonoside,* a glycoside are the active principles.

Signs and Symptoms

- **On ingestion**, there is hot burning pain from the mouth to stomach, salivation, nausea, vomiting, purging, vertigo and bloody stools with severe griping pain, followed by prostration, circulatory and respiratory collapse and death.
- **Applied to the skin**, the oil produces burning, redness and vesication.

Fatal dose: 4 crushed seeds or 3 drops of oil (1.5 mL).
Fatal period: 6 h to 3 days.

Treatment

i. Stomach wash.
ii. Administration of demulcent drinks, such as milk or egg white.
iii. Morphine with atropine to allay pain and reduce intestinal secretions.
iv. Glucose and saline are given IV to combat collapse and dehydration.

Postmortem findings: Same as castor.

Medico-legal Aspects

- Accidental poisoning results from swallowing croton oil by mistake or from traditional Chinese herbal medicines.
- Suicide and homicide is rare.
- Root and oil are taken internally as an abortifacient.
- Oil is used as an arrow poison.

ABRUS PRECATORIUS (RATI/ROSARY PEA/GUNCHI/JEQUIRITY)

Distribution: It is found all over India, and belongs to Leguminosae family. All parts of the plant are poisonous.

Identification of Seeds (Fig. 44.3)

- Seeds are egg shaped and scarlet in color with a black spot at one end. White seeds are also found.
- Seeds are tasteless and odorless.
- 0.83 × 0.62 cm in dimensions; having a weight of 105 mg.
- It was used by Indian goldsmiths for weighing silver and gold.

Active Principles

Seeds contain active principles, *abrin*, a thermolabile toxalbumin; *abrine*, an amino acid; *hemagglutinin*, a lipolytic enzyme; and *abralin*, a glycoside.

Signs and Symptoms

- **On ingestion**, there is abdominal pain, nausea, vomiting, hematemesis, bloody diarrhea (*classical features*), weakness, cold perspiration, trembling of hands, weak pulse, bleeding, tachycardia, headache, dilated pupils, raised intracranial pressure, papilledema, hallucinations, drowsiness, tetany and circulatory collapse, seen in 6 h but may be delayed to 1–3 days.
- When extract of seeds is **injected** under the skin, symptoms resemble *viperine snakebite,* and as such poisoning is not suspected. There is inflammation, edema, oozing of hemorrhagic fluid from site of puncture and necrosis may occur.
- If injected into an animal, it drops down and does not take feed, and dies in 3–4 days. Tetanic convulsions occur or the animal becomes cold, drowsy or comatose and dies.

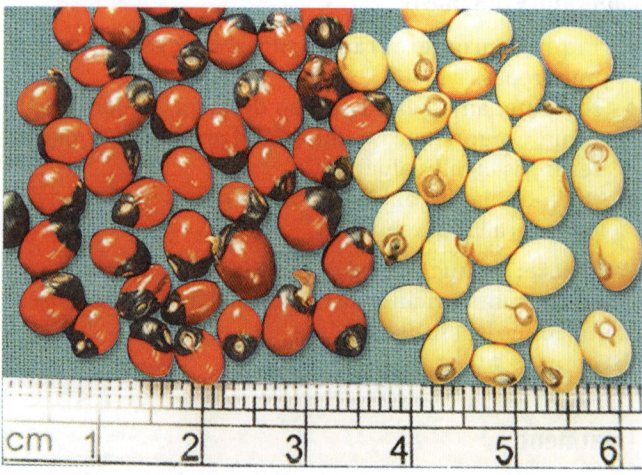

Fig. 44.3: *Abrus precatorius* (red and white seeds)

Fatal dose: 90–120 mg of abrin injected or 1–2 crushed seeds orally (0.1–1 µg/kg body wt.).

Fatal period: 3–5 days.

Treatment

There is no antidote. Treatment is supportive with intravenous fluids.
  i. Gastric lavage and emetics may be used with caution due to necrotizing action of abrin.
  ii. Needle should be dissected out.
  iii. Alkaline diuresis with sodium bicarbonate—urine is maintained at an alkaline pH.

Postmortem Findings

- Fragments of needle may be found. Edema at the site of injection.
- Petechial hemorrhages may be seen under the skin, pleura, pericardium and peritoneum.
- *GIT*: Hemorrhages, edema and congestion (commonly affected on ingestion).
- Internal organs are congested and show focal hemorrhages in the intestines, brain, myocardium and pleura (on parenteral exposure).
- Necrosis, hemorrhages and edema are also seen in lymph nodes and kidneys.

Medico-legal Aspects

- Suicidal cases—the seeds are crushed and taken orally.
- Accidental cases—on account of the attractive color of seeds, children may ingest them. Poisoning may result from traditional herbal remedy in the treatment of urinary schistosomiasis (reported from Zimbabwe).
- Commonly used as cattle poison in Indian villages to get the hide or for taking revenge. The toxic principle is injected into the animal in the form of fine needle-shaped structures called *'suis'*.
- Powdered seeds are used by malingerers to produce conjunctivitis.
- Seeds are also used as abortifacient and as arrow poison.

SUIS

The seeds of *Abrus precatorius* are decocted (boiling down to extract an essence; resulting liquid) and mixed with dhatura, opium and onion, and made into paste with spirit and water. From this paste, small sharp pointed spikes or needles or *'suis'* are made, which are dried in the sun.

- The needles are 15 mm long and weigh 90–120 mg. Two needles are inserted by their base into holes in a wooden handle and a blow is struck to the animal with great force which drives the needle into the flesh (so as to resemble snakebite) **(Fig. 44.4)**.
- For homicide, two needles are kept between the fingers and the person is slapped which drives the needle into the body.

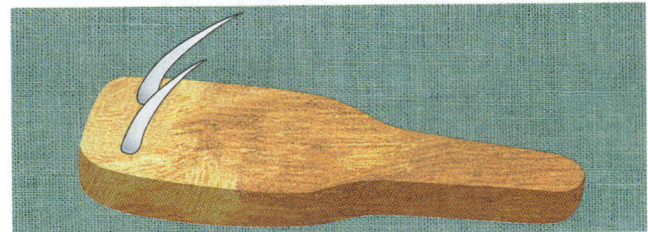

Fig. 44.4: Suis inserted on a wooden handle

- **Signs and symptoms:** At the site of injection, painful swelling and ecchymosis develops with inflammation and necrosis of muscle and regional lymph nodes. Faintness, vertigo, vomiting, anorexia, fever, headache, dyspnea and prostration are seen. Convulsions may occur before death. Weakness may develop within 5 h after injection, but onset of symptoms may be delayed by 10–12 h.

SEMECARPUS ANACARDIUM

The fruit of this plant is known as '*ballataka*', '*bhilawa*', or 'oriental cashew nut'.
- It is also called 'marking nut' as the nut leaves an indelible ink and used by washerman/laundries to inscribe number on the clothes.
- Marking nut is recognized to have caused washerman's dermatitis among British soldiers in the 1940s.

Identification of Seeds (Fig. 44.5)

Seeds are black, cone or heart-shaped with a rough projection at the base. They have a thick, pericarp containing the irritant juice which is brownish, oily and acrid, but turns black on exposure to air.

Active Principles

Anacardic acid, bhilawanol (a mixture of phenolic compounds, including isomers of urushiol), semecarpol, cardol, catechol, anacardoside, etc.

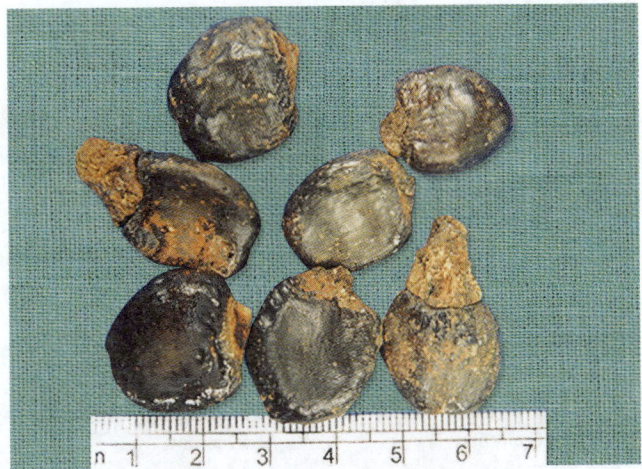

Fig. 44.5: *Semecarpus anacardium* (seeds)

Signs and Symptoms

- When the juice is **applied to the skin**, it causes irritation, itching, redness, burning sensation, painful blisters containing acrid serum and eczematous contact dermatitis. The lesion resembles a bruise. The rash takes 1–2 weeks to heal and normally does not leave scars. Severe cases have small (1–2 mm) clear fluid-filled blisters on the skin. Sometimes, an ulcer may be produced with sloughing. Constitutional symptoms such as fever, painful micturition with brown color urine may be seen.
- **Orally**, if a large dose of juice is taken, blisters in mouth and throat, severe GIT irritation, dyspnea, tachycardia, hypotension, cyanosis, loss of reflexes, delirium, coma and death may result.

Fatal dose: 5–10 g/5–8 seeds.

Fatal period: 12–24 h.

Treatment: Wash the contaminated part of the skin with soap and water. Bland liniments are applied. Demulcents drinks and symptomatic treatment are given.

Postmortem Findings

- Bruise-like lesion with small blisters may be seen near the angle of the mouth or lips. Blisters are also seen in the mouth and throat.
- **Stomach:** Congested and inflamed.
- **Liver:** It may show degenerative changes.
- **Other organs:** Congested.

Medico-legal Aspects

- Accidental poisoning may result from the administration of juice by quacks for treatment of rheumatic pain and worm infestation.
- Cases of contact dermatitis (due to urushiol) related to its use as hair dye, voodoo treatment, remedy for eczema or tattoo removal have been reported. Anaphylaxis due unintentional oral ingestion related to marking nut has also been reported.
- Juice may be introduced into the vagina, as a punishment for infidelity.
- For criminal abortion, juice is applied to the cervical os by means of abortion stick.
- It may be used by malingerers to produce conjunctivitis or to support a false charge of assault; lesions produced *simulate bruises* (**Diff. 44.1**).
- The juice may be thrown on the face to cause injury (*vitriolage*).
- Homicidal and suicidal poisoning is rare.

CAPSICUM ANNUUM

Capsicum or chilli fruits are universally employed as a condiment, the powdered form being known as red pepper or *lal mirch*. It has a pungent smell and a burning irritating taste. The seeds, about 0.3 cm long and wide, *resemble dhatura seeds* (**Fig. 44.6**).

Active Principles

The fruits contain two main capsaicinoids, capsaicin and dihydrocapsaicin which are exceedingly acrid, volatile, non-alkaloidal and non-fatal substances.

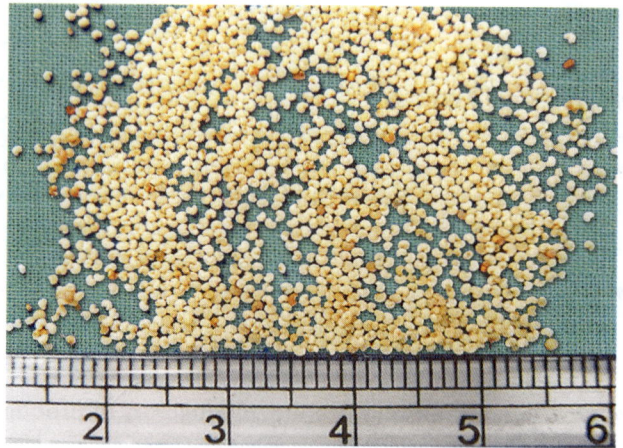

Fig. 44.6: *Capsicum annuum* (seeds)

DIFFERENTIATION 44.1: Artificial and true bruise

S.No.	Feature	Artificial bruise	True bruise
1.	Cause	Juice of marking nut, *Calotropis* or *Plumbago rosea*	Trauma
2.	Color	Dark brown	Typical color changes
3.	Shape	Irregular	Round
4.	Site	Exposed accessible parts	Anywhere
5.	Margins	Well-defined and regular, covered with small vesicles/blisters	Not well-defined, diffuse and irregular, no vesicles/blisters
6.	Redness and inflammation	Seen in surrounding skin	Seen at the site
7.	Itching	Present	Absent
8.	Vesicles/blisters	May be found on fingertips due to scratching	Absent
9.	Contents	Acrid serum	Extravasated blood
10.	Chemical tests	Positive for the chemical	Negative

Signs and Symptoms

- When it is *applied to the skin*, it causes irritation and vesication.
- When *thrown into the eyes*, it causes lacrimation, burning pain and redness.
- On *ingestion* in large quantity, it acts as an irritant poison and causes burning sensation in the mouth, throat, esophagus and stomach.

Treatment

i. When applied to the skin, it should be washed out with water and treated symptomatically.
ii. When ingested, the tongue should be scraped by a blunt edged instrument and ice given to suck.
iii. When thrown into the eyes, they should be washed in saline and antibiotics applied. Corticosteroid drops may be helpful.

Medico-legal Aspects

- It may be thrown into the eyes to facilitate robbery.
- The powder is used as a means of torture to extort money or a confession of some guilt by introducing it into the eyes, urethra, vagina or rectum, burning it under the nose or rubbing it on the female breasts.
- Superstitious people use the fumes from burning chillis to scare away devils and ghosts.

> **NOTA BENE**
>
> 'Hunan hand' ('*Chilli Willy*') is a painful contact dermatitis seen in people with continuous and prolonged exposure to chilli peppers containing capsaicin. This is paradoxical to the use of capsaicin as local application for relief of pain in various conditions, such as diabetic neuropathy and postherpetic neuralgia.

■ CALOTROPIS (RUBBER BUSH)

Distribution: *Calotropis* plant grows wild almost everywhere in India. There are two varieties—*Calotropis gigantea* (*akdo, akand*) with purple flowers and *Calotropis procera* (*madar*) with white flowers **(Fig. 44.7)**.

Active Principles

Uscharin, calotoxin, calactin, gigantin and calotropin.

Signs and Symptoms

- When the juice is **applied on the skin**, it becomes red with formation of blisters which excoriate later.
- When **instilled into the eyes**, it produces keratoconjunctivitis, corneal edema and gross dimness of vision over a period of 2–4 h, but without any pain (after initial burning sensation).

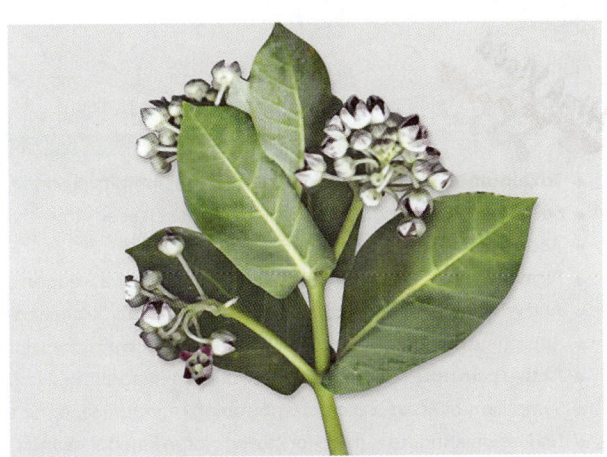

Fig. 44.7: *Calotropis*

- When **ingested**, it acts as a GIT and cerebrospinal poison. There is an acrid bitter taste, burning pain in the mouth, throat and abdomen along with nausea, vomiting and diarrhea. Pupils are dilated, and there may be tetanic convulsions. Circulatory collapse and death may occur.

Fatal dose: Uncertain.

Fatal period: About 12 h.

Treatment: The patient is treated symptomatically; gastric lavage is done with warm water, demulcents and morphine to relieve pain.

Postmortem Findings

Findings are non-specific.
i. Dilated pupils and froth from the nostrils may be seen.
ii. Stomatitis, acute inflammation of the GIT with ulcerated patches/perforation in the stomach may be present.
iii. Viscera and the brain are congested.

Medico-legal Aspects

- All the parts of the plant are used in Indian medicine, the flowers as digestive stimulants, the powdered root as emetic, and the milky juice as a vesicant, depilatory and for treatment of chronic skin conditions—all may lead to poisoning.
- Juice may be taken orally or applied on an abortion stick to procure abortion.
- It may be mixed with milk for infanticide, rarely for suicide or homicide.
- It may be used as cattle poison by mixing with fodder or inserting a cloth smeared with the juice inside the rectum of the animal.
- Sometimes, it is used to produce an artificial bruise.
- It may be used as an arrow poison.
- The dried latex and dried root are used as an antidote for snake poisoning in some parts of Andhra Pradesh.
- The roots of *Calotropis procera* are highly poisonous to cobras and other poisonous snakes, and hence used by snake charmers to control them.

SECTION 2 : Toxicology

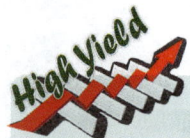

- **Toxalbumin/phytotoxin:** Toxic protein that inhibits protein synthesis; present in plants, such as castor, croton or rati.
- Seeds are most poisonous, although unbroken seeds (mostly) are not poisonous when swallowed or cooked.
- **Active principle in *Ricinus communis* (castor):** Ricin.
- Ricin can be used an agent of chemical warfare or a weapon of mass destruction.
- **Active principles in *Croton tiglium* (jamalgota):** Crotin and crotonoside.
- *Abrus precatorius* (rati) was used by Indian goldsmiths for weighing silver and gold.
- **Active principles of *Abrus*:** Abrin, abrine, hemagglutinin and abralin.
- Symptoms of *Abrus precatorius* poisoning resemble viperine snakebite.
- No known antidote is there for castor/croton/rati poisoning.
- The toxic principle of *Abrus* is injected into the animal in the form of fine needle-shaped structures called *'suis'*.
- *'Suis'* are small sharp pointed needles made from decocted seeds of *Abrus precatorius,* datura, opium and onion.
- The nut of *Semecarpus anacardium* (*bhilawa*, marking nut) leaves an indelible ink and used by washerman to inscribe number on the clothes.
- **Active principles in *Semecarpus anacardium*:** Bhilawanol, semecarpol.
- Marking nut may be used by malingerers to produced artificial bruises.
- The juice may be thrown on the face to cause vitriolage.
- Artificial bruises can be made by juice of marking nut, *Calotropis, Plumbago rosea*.
- Capsicum or chilli seeds resemble dhatura seeds.
- **Active principles in capsicum:** Capsaicin and dihydrocapsaicin.
- Hunan hand is seen due to prolonged exposure to capsicum.
- **Active principles in *Calotropis*:** Uscharin, calotoxin, calactin, gigantin and calotropin.

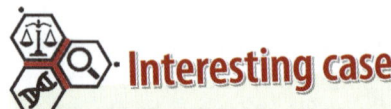

Ricin Poisoning (Case of Georgi Markov, 1978)

Georgi Markov was a well-known novelist and playwright in Bulgaria prior to his defection in 1969 **(Fig. A)**. He settled in UK and became a broadcast journalist for the BBC World Service, London. In September 1978, while waiting for a bus on Waterloo Bridge, Markov felt a sharp pain, such as a bug bite or sting on the back of his thigh. He looked behind and saw a man picking up an umbrella off the ground. The man was facing away from Markov. He apologized, and then hailed a taxi and left. Markov later remembered that the apology was made in a foreign accent.

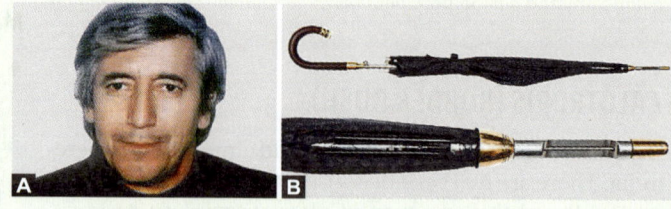

When he arrived at his work, Markov noticed a blood spot on his jeans and a small red pimple at the site of the sting he had felt earlier. The pain had not lessened or stopped. He told his colleagues at the BBC about this incident. That evening he developed a high grade fever and was admitted to a London hospital. The next day he went into shock, his condition worsened and was not responding to any medications. After four days of hospitalization, he died. The preliminary diagnosis of his cause of death was kept as 'septicemia, possibly a result of kidney failure'.

Due to the circumstances and statements Markov made to doctors expressing the suspicion that he had been poisoned, the police ordered a thorough autopsy. The forensic pathologist discovered a spherical metal pellet the size of a pin-head embedded in his leg. Further examination of the pellet showed that it contained traces of toxic ricin. The Coroner ruled that Markov had been unlawfully killed and cause of death was poisoning from a ricin-filled pellet.

The event was recognized as the '*Umbrella Murder*' case. An umbrella with a hidden pneumatic mechanism which injects a small poisonous pellet containing ricin must have been used to assassinate Markov **(Fig. B)**. British scientists later estimated that only about 450 μg was used to kill him. The Markov murder case remains officially unsolved since no one was ever arrested in connection with his death, though the KGB and Bulgarian spies are widely suspected to have been behind the killing.

CHAPTER 45

Organic Irritants—Animal

Learning Objectives

Must know
1. Signs and symptoms and PM findings in ophitoxemia
2. Management of snakebite poisoning
3. Fatal dose and fatal period of common venomous snakes
4. Identification of common snakes
5. Venomous and non-venomous snakes (Diff.)
6. Neurotoxic and vasculotoxic venom (Diff.)

Desirable to know
1. Cobra and viper (Diff.)
2. Components of snake venom
3. Cantharides toxicity
4. Scorpion bite toxicity
5. Bees and wasps bite toxicity
6. Spider bite toxicity

FM 11.1
Describe features and management of snake bite, scorpion sting, bee and wasp sting and spider bite.

SNAKES

Nomenclature (Flowchart 45.1)

Phylum	Chordata
Class	Reptilia
Order	Squamota
Suborder	Serpentes

Flowchart 45.1: Nomenclature

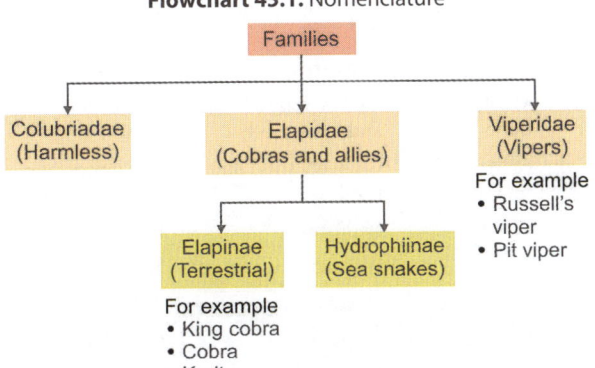

Classification of Snakes

Snakes are classified into two types:
  i. **Venomous (poisonous) snakes (Table 45.1)**
  ii. **Non-venomous (non-poisonous) snakes**, e.g., rat snake, common watersnake, Indian python, sand boa and mud snake.

The differences between venomous and non-venomous snakes, and between cobra and viper are given in **Differentiations 45.1** and **45.2** respectively.
- In tropical regions of the world including India, most of the snakebite cases are caused by four venomous snakes often referred to as '**big four**' snakes—common cobra, common krait, Russell's viper* and saw scaled viper.

TABLE 45.1: Classification of venomous snakes

S.No.	Type	Examples
1.	Elapidae (neurotoxic)	◆ Common cobra *(Naja naja)* ◆ King cobra *(Ophiophagus hannah)* ◆ Krait: Subgrouped into common krait *(Bungarus caeruleus)*, banded krait *(Bangarus fasciatus)*, coral snake, tiger snake, mambas and death adder
2.	Viperidae (vasculotoxic)	◆ Pitiless vipers: Russell's viper *(Daboia rusellii)*, saw-scaled viper *(Echis carinatae)* ◆ Pit vipers: Pit viper-crotalidae, common green pit viper
3.	Hydrophidae (myotoxic)	◆ 20 types of sea snakes are found in India—all venomous

---

*The Russell's viper is considered one of the most deadly land dwelling snakes.

SECTION 2 : Toxicology

DIFFERENTIATION 45.1: Venomous and non-venomous snakes

S.No.	Feature	Venomous snakes	Non-venomous snakes
1.	Head scales (Figs. 45.1A and B)	Small (vipers). Large scales are seen with: ◆ Heat-sensing pit anteroinferior to the eye (pit viper) (Fig. 45.2) ◆ 3rd labial touches eye and nasal shields (cobra) (Fig. 45.3) ◆ Central row of scales on back enlarged; under surface of mouth has only four infralabials, 4th being largest (kraits) (Figs. 45.4A and B)	Large, with exception as mentioned under the poisonous snakes
2.	Belly scales (Figs. 45.5A and B)	Large and cover the entire breadth of belly	Small, such as those on back and do not cover the entire breadth
3.	Fangs	Long and canalized, such as hypodermic needle	Short and solid
4.	Scales distal to anal plate (Figs. 45.6A and B)	Single row	Double row
5.	Tail	Compressed	Not markedly compressed
6.	Habits	Nocturnal	Not so
7.	Bite marks	Two fang marks, with or without small marks of other teeth	Number of small teeth marks in a row

DIFFERENTIATION 45.2: Cobra and viper (Figs. 45.2 and 45.3)

S.No.	Feature	Cobra	Viper
1.	Head	Small, covered by large scales or shields	Large, broader than the body, triangular, covered by small scales
2.	Body	Long and cylindrical	Short with narrow neck
3.	Pupils	Circular/round	Vertical, slit like
4.	Maxillary bone	Carries poison fangs and other teeth	Carries only poison fangs
5.	Fangs	Grooved, short and fixed	Canalized, long and movable
6.	Venom	Neurotoxic	Hemotoxic
7.	Tail	Less tapering (round)	Tapering
8.	Other teeth	Present in upper jaw	Absent
9.	Reproduction	Oviparous	Ovo-viviparous

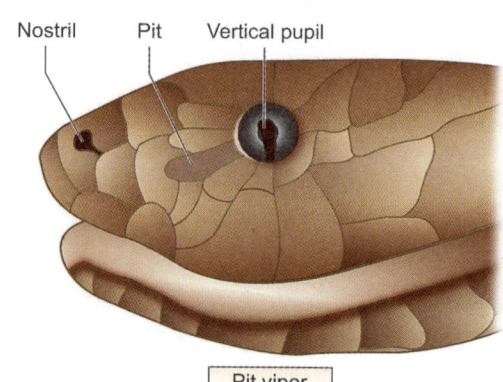

Fig. 45.2: Large head scales with a pit between the eye and nostril

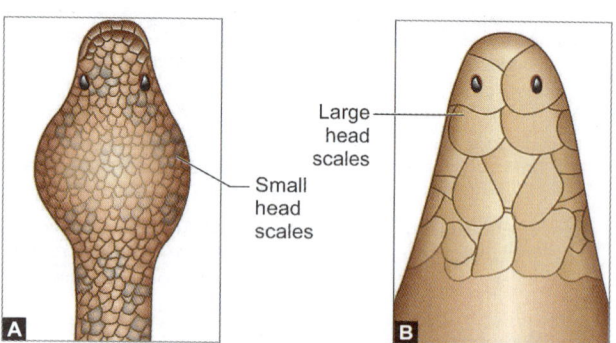

Figs. 45.1A and B: Head scales of: (A) Venomous; (B) Non-venomous snakes

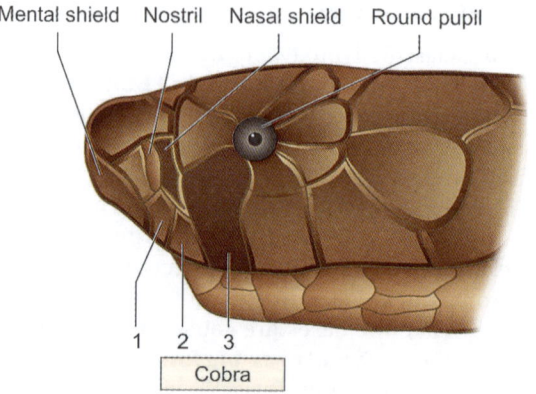

Fig. 45.3: Large head scales and third labial touches the eye and nasal shields

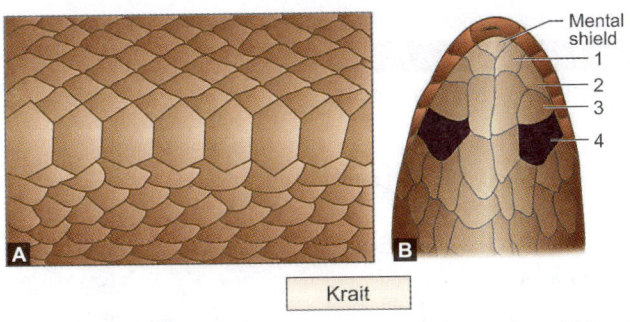

Figs. 45.4A and B: (A) Central hexagonal scales on the middle of back; (B) Fourth infralabial is the largest

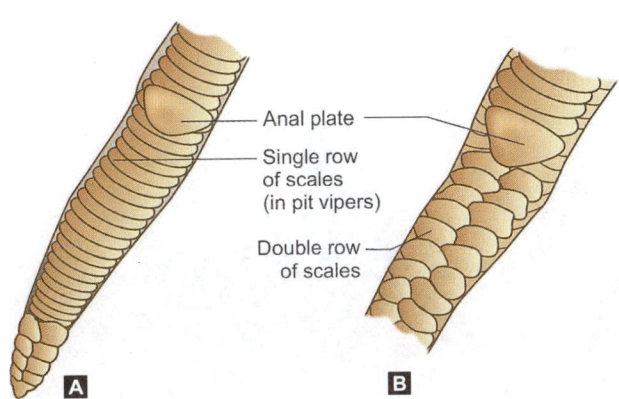

Figs. 45.6A and B: (A) Venomous; (B) Non-venomous snakes

Features of Common Venomous Snakes

Some features of common venomous snakes are given in **Table 45.2**.

Poison apparatus: It is a *modified salivary gland* consisting of:
- *Gland*: Lies just below and behind the eyes, one on each side of the head, above the upper jaw.
- *Duct*: Arises from the gland to carry the poisonous venom from gland to the fangs.
- *Fangs*: Two in number. These are curved teeth situated on the maxillary bones and lie along the jaws **(Figs. 45.7A and B)**. They are like hollow hypodermic needles (solid in non-venomous snakes).

Snake venom: Venom is the saliva of snake, ejected from the poison apparatus (modified parotid gland) during the act of biting. It can be neurotoxic, vasculotoxic or myotoxic in its action **(Diff. 45.3)**.
- *Physical appearance*: Faint transparent yellow and viscous, when fresh.

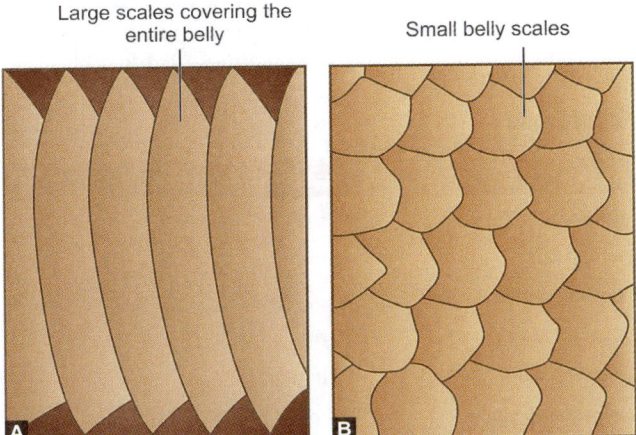

Figs. 45.5A and B: Belly scales of: (A) Venomous; (B) Non-venomous snakes

- In Indian setting, almost 2/3rd of bites are attributed to saw-scaled vipers, about 1/4th to Russell's viper, and only a small proportion to cobras and kraits.

TABLE 45.2: Features of common venomous snakes

Feature	Common cobra	King cobra	Common krait	Banded krait	Russell's viper
Head and neck	Hood present, bears a double/single spectacle mark	Hooded without spectacle mark	Head covered with large shields	Head covered with large shields	Flat, triangular with distinct 'V' mark and small scales
Belly	Smooth scales	Scales looks shiny, but is dry to touch	Creamy white	Triangular in cross-section	White with broad plates
Back	Spectacled white or yellow pattern, which sometimes forms ragged bands	Yellow or black bands or broad chevron like markings	Single/double white bands with central row of hexagonal scales	Alternate black and yellowish bands	Three rows of diamond-shaped black/brown spots
Color	Brown/black/green	Yellow/green/brown/black with white cross-bands	Steel-blue/black	Resembles common krait	Brown/buff
Length	1.5–2 meters	3–4 meters	1.25–1.5 meters	2 meters	1.5 meters
Habitat	Throughout India	Thick jungles/forests	Close to human dwelling	Assam, Bengal, South India	Throughout India

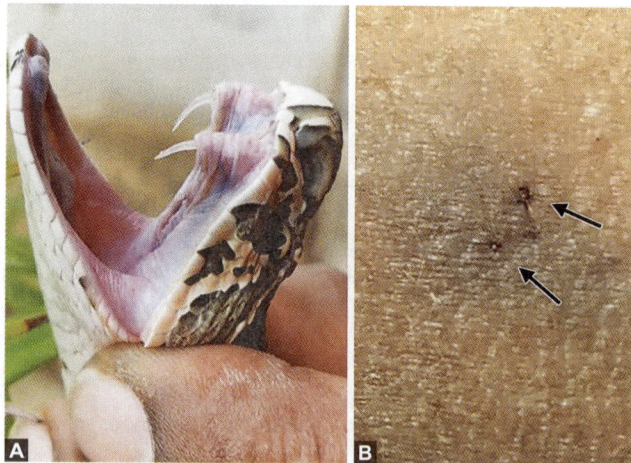

Figs. 45.7A and B: Fangs and fang marks (arrows)

TABLE 45.3: Components of snake venom and their actions

Venom components	General clinical effect
Phospholipase A$_2$ (lecithinase)	Myotoxic, cardiotoxic, neurotoxic, increases vascular permeability
Serine proteases and other proteases	Hemolysis
Hyaluronidase	Local tissue destruction
Acetylcholinesterase (elapids)	Neurotoxic, relaxe muscles
Neurotoxins	
◆ α-bungarotoxin and cobrotoxin	Postsynaptic inhibition
◆ β-bungarotoxin, crotoxin	Presynaptic inhibition

♦ *Toxic principles*: Proteinous in nature, most of which are glycopolypeptides and are enzymatic in action. About 80–90% of viperidae and 25–70% of elapidae venom consists of enzymes **(Table 45.3).**

DIFFERENTIATION 45.3: Neurotoxic and vasculotoxic venom

S.No.	Feature	Neurotoxic venom	Vasculotoxic venom
1.	Action	It causes muscular weakness of legs and paralysis of muscles of face, throat and respiration	It causes enzymatic destruction of cell walls and coagulation disorders
2.	Site	Acts on motor nerve cells and resemble curare	Acts on endothelial cells of blood vessels, and red cells are lysed—hemolysis
3.	Local symptoms	Minimum	Severe—swelling, oozing of blood and spreading cellulitis
4.	Symptoms	Cobra venom produces both convulsions and paralysis, while krait causes only paralysis	Hemorrhage from external orifices is common
5.	Examples	Elapids, such as cobra or kraits	Vipers

Note: **Myotoxic venom** produces generalized muscular pain ending in respiratory failure in fatal cases, e.g., sea snakes.

Fatal Dose

Snake	Fatal dose *(dried form)*
Cobra	15 mg
King cobra	12 mg
Common krait	2.5–6 mg
Banded krait	10 mg
Russell's viper	40 mg
Saw-scaled viper	8 mg

Russell's viper injects 63 mg of venom on an average. The range of venom injected is 5–147 mg.

Fatal period: Death may occur immediately from shock due to fright.

♦ *Cobra*: ½–24 hours (h)
♦ *Viper*: 1–4 days
♦ *Krait*: 12–24 h

SIGNS AND SYMPTOMS OF OPHITOXEMIA

Ophitoxemia characterizes the clinical spectrum of snakebite envenomation.
♦ *Epidemiology*: Snakebite is more prevalent in rural than urban areas, commonly seen in summers, in males,

Identify the common venomous snakes:

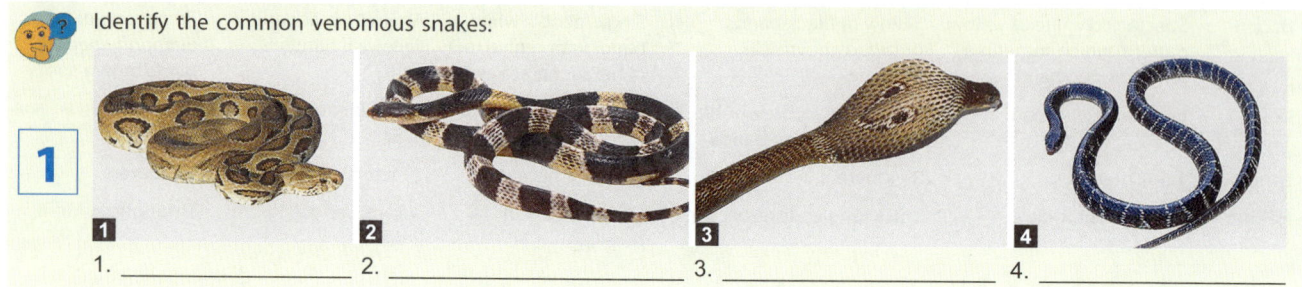

1. _____ 2. _____ 3. _____ 4. _____

farmers and mostly at night. Most of the bites in tropical countries are on lower extremities since the victims are bitten by treading on or near the snake, while in non-tropical countries most bites are on fingers and hands because of deliberate handling of the snake.
- *History:* The time elapsed since the bite is important to determine if the process is confined locally or if systemic signs have developed. Obtain a description of the snake to determine its species.
- Onset of symptoms and sudden progression are more common with elapidae bite rather than viperidae. Most cobra, krait and sea snakebites would show symptoms within the first 6 h, the shortest time is for the sea snakes.
- Many bites by the venomous snakes are dry bites implying that the snakes fail to inject the venom. In general, about 70% of bites are due to non-venomous snakes, and of the rest, 15% are dry bites and only 15% bites cause envenomation.
- The likelihood of a 'dry bite' is most common with a cobra.
- Early and intense pain implies significant envenomation.
- *Local signs and symptoms:* Fang marks, pain, bleeding, bruising, lymphangitis, lymph node enlargement, inflammation, blistering, local infection, abscess formation and necrosis.

Cobra (Diff. 45.4 and Fig. 45.8A)

Local symptoms start within 6–8 minutes (min).
- A small reddish wheal develops at the site of the bite. Bitten area is tender with a burning pain. Local necrosis

DIFFERENTIATION 45.4: Signs and symptoms of elapinae and viperine bite

S.No.	Feature	Elapinae bite	Viperine bite
1.	Local reaction	Minimal	Extensive
2.	Skip lesions*	Typically seen	Not so
3.	Speech and deglutition	Affected	Not so
4.	Tongue	Paralyzed	Not affected
5.	Saliva	Hypersalivation	Not so
6.	Pupils	Normal	Dilated
7.	Gait	Staggering	Not so
8.	Gangrene	Wet type, early onset	Dry type, late onset
9.	Blood pressure	Normal	Hypotension
10.	Pulse	Initially normal, later irregular	Weak, irregular
11.	Respiration	Slow, weak and labored	Quick and labored
12.	Coagulation	Not affected	Greatly affected
13.	Hemorrhagic manifestations	Absent	Prominent feature
14.	Cause of death	Respiratory paralysis	Circulatory failure

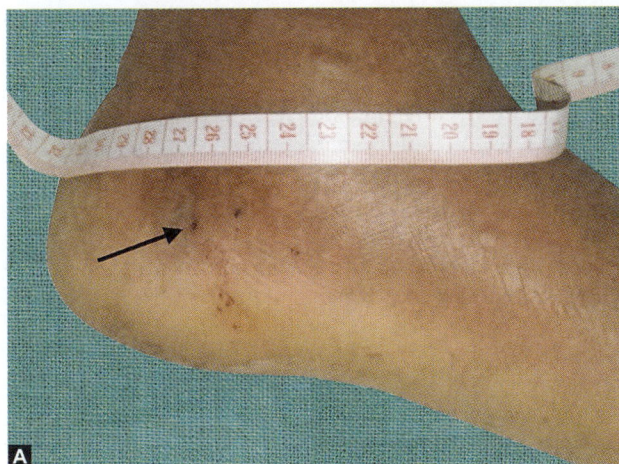
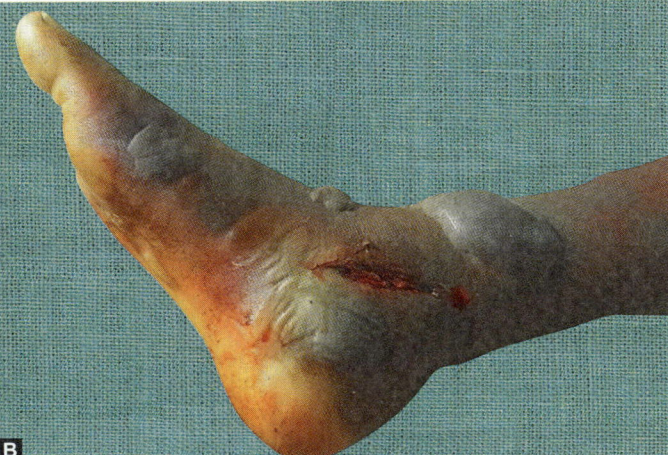

Figs. 45.8A and B: Local signs: (A) Cobra (arrow); (B) Viper bite

* Areas of necrosis separated by strips of unaffected skin caused by proximal spread of venom in lymphatic vessels—characteristic of spitting cobra bites.

causes 'wet gangrene' with a characteristic putrid smell due to the direct cytolytic action of the venom in 1-2 days.
- *Early symptoms* include vomiting, heaviness of eyelids, blurred vision, paresthesia around mouth, hyperacusis, headache, dizziness, vertigo, hypersalivation, congested conjunctiva and gooseflesh.
- Muscles of the extremities become weak. Paralysis starts in the lower limbs, which ascends gradually affecting the respiratory muscles, including the diaphragm. Respiratory muscle paralysis is indicated by poor neck lift, falling single breath count, falling SpO_2, hypoxic symptoms, such as cyanosis, altered sensorium and coma.
- Drooping of the head, lower lip and eyelids with blurring of vision and external ophthalmoplegia. Ptosis is one of the *commonest and earliest manifestations* of neuroparalytic snakebite.

Krait

Signs and symptoms are similar to cobra poisoning, but less rapid.
- Abdominal pain, ptosis, dysarthria, dysphagia, chest pain, quadriparesis, respiratory paralysis and death may occur.
- There is no nausea and froth, but drowsiness is more.
- Common krait hunt nocturnally and are quick to bite people sleeping on the floor, often without waking their victims, since the venom is painless. Victims wake up early morning, paralyzed—mistaken for STROKE.

Viper (Diff. 45.4 and Fig. 45.8B)

- More local reaction is seen along with pain and oozing.
- Local necrosis is extensive which may lead to gangrene.
- Serous and serosanginous blisters sometimes appear.
- Bilateral parotid swelling ('*viper head*'), conjunctival edema and subconjunctival hemorrhage.
- Petechial hemorrhages, epistaxis, gum bleeding, hemoptysis, hemetemesis, hematuria, fundal hemorrhage, and bleeding from the bite site and rectum are common.
- Acute renal failure evidenced by oliguria, anuria and rising serum creatinine due to DIC or circulatory collapse and shock may be seen (common with Russell viper, hump nosed pit viper).

Death is due to circulatory failure in early phase, and hemorrhagic complications later.

Sea Snake

- The bite is usually painless with minimal or no local swelling or involvement of local lymph nodes.
- Early symptoms include headache, a thick feeling of the tongue, thirst, sweating and vomiting.

- *Generalized rhabdomyolysis*: Muscles, especially of the neck, trunk and proximal part of the limbs may become tender and painful on active or passive movement (segmental myopathic lesions), and later may become paralyzed with ptosis as in elapid envenoming. Trismus (spasm of jaw muscles causing 'lockjaw') is common.
- Myoglobinuria may be seen within 3 h after the bite.
- Myoglobin and potassium released from damaged skeletal muscle can cause renal failure, while the hyperkalemia may lead to cardiac arrest.

Snake Venom Ophthalmia

If the 'spat' venom enters the eyes, there is immediate and intense burning, stinging pain, followed by profuse watering of the eyes with production of whitish discharge, congested conjunctiva, spasm and swelling of the eyelids, photophobia and blurring of vision.

> **NOTA BENE**
>
> Signs and symptoms of ophitoxemia depend upon:
> **i. Patient characteristics**
> - *Age, size, sex and health of the patient*: Men have more resistance than women. Children are more vulnerable as they have lesser body mass and fat, and more rapid circulation.
> - *Location of bite*: Bites on the extremities, bony part, through clothing or foot wear or in adipose tissue are less dangerous (absorption delayed due to poor blood supply and loculation) than those on the head (richly vascular and proximity to systemic circulation), trunk or directly into blood vessel. Nearly 98% of snakebites occur over extremities.
>
> **ii. Snake characteristics**
> - The length of time the snake holds on.
> - The extent of anger or fear that motivates the snake, and nature of bite.
> - The condition of its fangs and venom glands.
> - Species and size of the snake.
> - The amount of venom injected. It is poisonous when injected subcutaneously, IV or IM, and has no ill effects when taken by mouth as it is not absorbed from gastric mucosa.

Diagnosis

20 min whole blood clotting test (20 WBCT): This is very useful and informative bedside test.
- Place a few mL of freshly sampled venous blood in a clean, dry, glass tube/bottle.
- Leave it undisturbed for 20 min at room temperature.
- Gently invert the tube.
- If the blood is still unclotted and runs out, the patient has hypofibrinogenemia ('incoagulable blood') as a result of venom-induced consumption coagulopathy.

A normal 20 WBCT and clot lysis would exclude viperidae species.

Simultaneously, a *single breath counting test** is done in suspected elapidae bites, and the same is repeated at 15 min interval over the first 2 h.

---
* Single breath counting is how far an individual can count in normal speaking voice after a maximal inspiration.

> **NOTA BENE**
>
> *Clinical examination*
> - To exclude early neurotoxic envenoming, the patient is asked to look up, and observe whether the upper lids retract fully.
> - Eye movements are tested for evidence of early external ophthalmoplegia.
> - The patient is asked to open his mouth and protrude his tongue; early restriction in mouth opening may indicate *trismus* (sea snake envenoming) or more often paralysis of pterygoid muscles.
> - Other muscles innervated by the cranial nerves (facial muscles, tongue and gag reflex) are checked. The muscles flexing the neck may be paralyzed, giving the '*broken neck sign*.'

MANAGEMENT

- All patients with a history of snakebite should be observed for 8–12 h after the bite, if the skin is broken and the offending snake cannot be positively identified as non-venomous.
- The Latin maxim '*primum non nocere*' (first, do no harm) has significant meaning here because many traditional and popular, but poorly substantiate treatments may cause more harm than good. These methods include making an incision over the bite, mouth suctioning, tourniquet around the limb, use of snake stones, ice packs or electric shock.

Prevention of Spread of Venom

Spread of venom through the body is mostly by diffusion through lymph circulation.
- **Reassurance:** The victim is reassured since most bites are non-venomous.
- **Immobilization:** The bitten limb should be immobilized with a splint or sling (any movement or muscular contraction hastens systemic absorption of venom), and should be kept below the level of the heart.
- **Pressure-immobilization** for elapid bites is recommended, as it may delay systemic absorption of venom (indicated if the patient is >1 h from medical care).
- **Avoid manipulation:** Any interference with the bite wound may introduce infection, increase absorption of venom and increase local bleeding. Any constriction bands, pressure bandages, jewelry, watches and rings adjacent to the bite site should be removed.

> **NOTA BENE**
>
> - The first aid can be remembered by the mnemonic 'Do it RIGHT': R—Reassurance, I—Immobilize, GH—Get to hospital immediately, T—Tell doctor about any systemic symptoms that developed on the way to hospital.
> - **Pressure immobilization technique** is recommended for elapid bites, including sea snakes but should not be used for viper bites (may cause local necrosis). A compression bandage (e.g., elastic/crepe bandage or torn clothing, and not a tourniquet) should be wrapped firmly (maintaining a pressure of 50–70 mm Hg) from the bite site upwards **(Figs. 45.9A and B)**. This procedure (*Sutherland wrap*) is to occlude the lymphatic circulation without impeding the arterial or deep venous flow (if occluded, it could result in gangrene or necrosis). The bandage should allow for the insinuation of one finger, and peripheral pulse (radial, posterior tibial, dorsalis pedis) is palpable.
> - **Pressure pad or 'Monash technique':** In this method a hard pad of rubber or cloth is applied directly to the wound in an attempt to reduce venom entering the system.
> - *Tourniquets*: Tight rope, belt, string, cloth has been traditionally used to stop venom flow into the body following snakebite.
> - Washing increases the flow of venom into the system by stimulating the lymphatic system.
> - If there is an ulcer or wound in the mouth, sucking may allow the venom to get into bloodstream.

The issue which confronts the doctor when attending to a patient with snakebite is assessment of the degree of systemic envenomation and decision on dose of ASV.

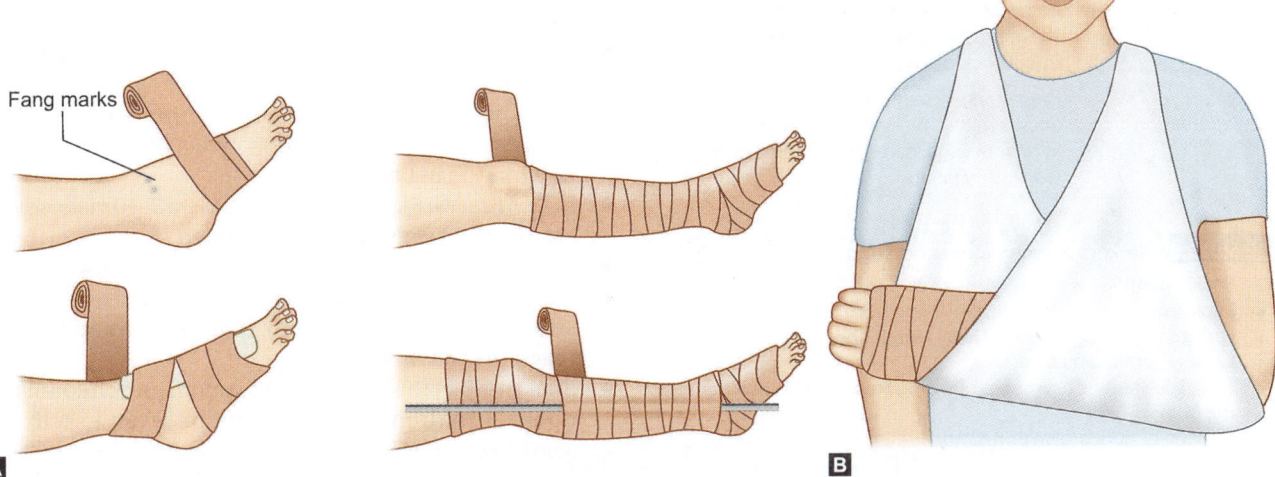

Figs. 45.9A and B: (A) Pressure immobilization technique for lower limbs; (B) Forearm

Using the **snakebite envenomation severity scale (SESS)**, the severity of envenomation should be graded (**Table 45.4**). Clues for severe snake envenomation should be sought (**Box 45.1**). Antivenom is indicated for patients with clinical manifestations attributable to snake venom who are graded as moderate and severe according to the SESS (**Flowchart 45.2**).

Antivenom Treatment

- The **polyvalent antisnake venom (ASV)** serum available in India is effective against common venomous snakes (cobra, common krait, saw scaled viper and Russell's viper).
- *Dose:* Freeze-dried (lyophilized)* antivenom serum is dissolved in water (10 mL vial). About 80–100 mL serum should be diluted in 200–500 mL of isotonic saline and given slow IV.
- The recommended initial dose of ASV is 8–10 vials administered slowly via IV route over a period of 1 h. Repeat doses for *vasculotoxic species* is based on the 6 h rule (depending on the coagulation profile); maximum recommended dose is 30 vials. Repeat doses for *neurotoxic* is based on the 1–2 h rule (depending on whether patients have not improved, or worsened); maximum dose is 20 vials. However, evidence-based medicine found no difference in the outcome in low-dose ASV regimen to standard recommended dose.

TABLE 45.4: Assessment of severity of envenomation

Category	Findings
No envenomation	Absence of local or systemic reactions, fang marks +/–
Mild envenomation	Fang marks, moderate pain, minimal local edema (0–15 cm), erythema +, ecchymosis +/–, no systemic reactions
Moderate envenomation	Fang marks +, severe pain, moderate local edema (15–30 cm), erythema +, ecchymosis +, systemic weakness, sweating, syncope, nausea, vomiting, or thrombocytopenia and anemia
Severe envenomation	Fang marks +, severe pain, severe local edema (> 30 cm), erythema +, ecchymosis +, hypotension, paresthesia, coma and respiratory failure

Box 45.1 Markers of severe envenomation

- Snake identified is a venomous one.
- Rapid early extension of local swelling from the site of the bite.
- Early tender enlargement of local lymph nodes.
- Early systemic symptoms.
- Early spontaneous systemic bleeding (especially bleeding from the gums).
- Passage of dark brown urine.

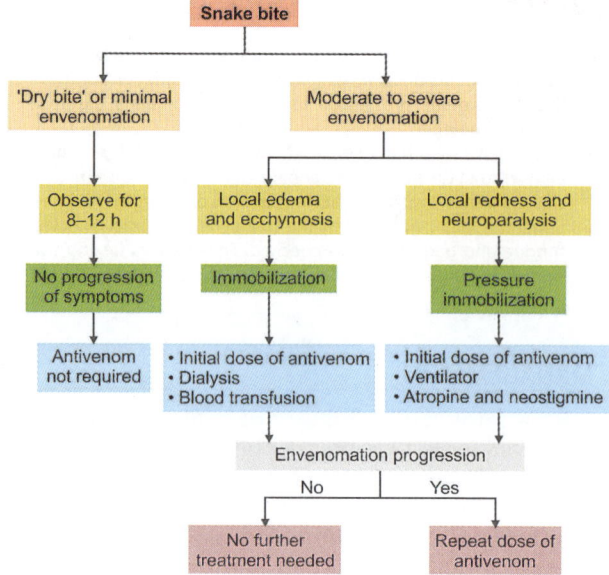

Flowchart 45.2: Management of snake bite poisoning

NOTA BENE

Indications for antivenom administration

Systemic envenoming
- *Hemostatic abnormalities*: Spontaneous systemic bleeding, coagulopathy or thrombocytopenia
- *CNS*: Ptosis, external ophthalmoplegia, paralysis
- *CVS*: Hypotension, shock, cardiac arrhythmia, abnormal ECG
- *Acute renal failure:* Oliguria/anuria, elevated creatinine/urea
- *Hemoglobin/myoglobinuria*, other evidence of intravascular hemolysis or generalized rhabdomyolysis

Local envenoming
- Local swelling involving more than half of the bitten limb (in the absence of a tourniquet)
- Swelling after bites on the digits (toes, and especially fingers)
- Rapid extension of swelling
- Enlarged tender lymph node draining the bitten limb

- Antivenom treatment should be given, as soon as it is indicated. Ideally, ASV should be administered within 4 h, but effective even if given within 24 h.
- *Contraindications:* There is no absolute contraindication to ASV treatment.
- ASV should not be used indiscriminately because it carries a risk of severe adverse reactions, and is costly and may be in limited supply.
- In mild cases: 5 vials; moderate cases: 5–10 vials; severe cases: 10–20 vials are recommended.
- ASV should not be given locally at the site of snakebite.
- Patients must be closely observed for at least 1 h after starting IV antivenom, so that early anaphylactic reactions can be detected.
- Snakes inject the same dose of venom into children and adults. Children must therefore be given exactly the same dose of ASV as adults.

---

* Low temperature dehydration process that involves freezing the products, lowering the pressure and then removing the ice by sublimation.

> **NOTA BENE**
>
> **Antivenom reactions**
> - *Anaphylactic or type I (immediate) hypersensitivity reactions* may develop (itching, urticaria, glottis edema, wheezing, cough, nausea, vomiting, fever and tachycardia). Adrenaline, 0.5–1.0 mL of 0.1% solution (1 in 1000, 1 mg/mL) is given subcutaneously in adults; in children the dose is 0.01 mL/kg.
> - *Serum sickness* is a *type III (delayed) hypersensitivity reaction* which is characterized by fever, urticaria, lymphadenopathy and arthritis, and may develop in 3 days to 3 weeks. Serum sickness is dose-related, as it occurs when > 8 vials of polyvalent ASV are administered.

Supportive Treatment

Ventilatory Care for Bulbar Paralysis and Respiratory Failure

- Patient should be nursed in lateral position, and salivation should be cleaned timely to prevent aspiration.
- Endotracheal intubation, O_2 supplementation and tracheostomy may be needed in neuroparalytic bite.

Care of Bitten Part

- Broad spectrum antibiotics should be given, if there is wound infection.
- Tetanus toxoid or tetanus immunoglobulin of human origin is given.

Surgical Excision

Early surgical intervention is needed to prevent extension of infection and development of gangrene. Surgical debridement of necrotic tissue is helpful, but the use of fasciotomy is highly questionable. Fasciotomy does not remove or reduce any envenomation. It is indicated only for compartment syndrome **(Fig. 45.10)**.

Anticholinesterase (ACE)

- ACE is effective and safe in elapid bite.
- Atropine (0.6 mg in adults and 50 μg/kg in children) is given IV (to prevent undesirable muscarinic effects of acetylcholine, such as increased secretions, sweating, bradycardia and colic) followed by an IV injection of neostigamine (0.01–0.04 mg/kg every 1–3 h).
- Patient can be then maintained on neostigmine and atropine (4 hourly continuous infusions).

Hypotension and Shock

- Fluid resuscitation with normal saline or Ringer's lactate should be initiated.
- Plasma expander, 5% albumin (10–20 mL/kg), fresh whole blood or fresh frozen plasma should be infused, if CVP is low.
- Dopamine (starting dose 2.5–5 μg/kg/min IV) can be given.

Oliguria and Renal Failure

- Cautious rehydration, diuretics (furosemide) or dopamine should be tried in case urine output drops to < 400 mL/24 h.
- Hemofiltration or peritoneal or hemodialysis, as indicated (acute renal failure seen in vasculotoxic bite).

Hemostatic Disturbances

- **For coagulopathy:** Fresh blood, fresh frozen plasma, cryoprecipitate or platelet concentrates, as needed in viperine snakebites.
- **For clotting abnormalities:** Heparin 1000–5000 IV may be given, (e.g., DIC). Use of heparin should be weighed against risk of bleeding, and hence caution is advocated.

Corticosteroid therapy: No beneficial effects.

Snake venom ophthalmia: The eye or mucous membrane should be washed immediately using large volumes of water or other bland fluid.

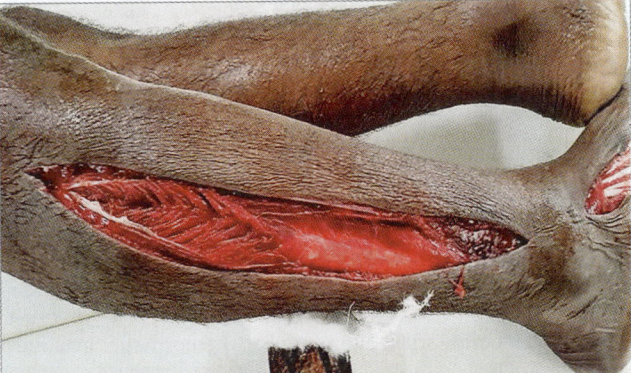

Fig. 45.10: Surgical fasciotomy wound in right leg following viperine snake bite

> **NOTA BENE**
>
> **Antivenom** is immunoglobulin [usually the enzyme refined F(ab)2 fragment of IgG] purified from the serum/plasma of a horse or sheep that has been immunized with the venoms of one or more species of snake. It is of two types:
> i. **Monovalent (specific) antivenom:** ASV has been raised against the venom of the snake that has bitten the patient and it contains specific antibody that will neutralize that particular venom.
> ii. **Polyvalent (polyspecific) antivenom:** It neutralizes the venoms of several different species of snakes, usually the most prevalent in a particular geographical area. It is less potent, less immunogenic and less effective than movovalent, and has more adverse effects (caused particularly by non-neutralized part of the polyvalent ASV).
>   - In India, polyvalent ASV is raised in horses using the venoms of the four most important venomous species (cobra, krait, Russell's viper and saw-scaled viper).
>   - The most commonly used ASV in the US for pit viper (rattlesnake, copperhead and water moccasin) is *CroFab*, which has a much lower incidence of acute or delayed allergic reactions compared to the older ASV.

SECTION 2: Toxicology

> **Recent Advances**
> - **Neostigmine** appears to have no useful role in confirmed presynaptic envenoming (kraits and Russell's viper). It is effective in postsynaptic neurotoxins (cobra). Their use helps reduce the consumption of ASV, which is generally limited.
> - **Oral ASV:** Alginate coated polyvalent ASV administered by oral route has been found to be effective in entrapping all the structural components of ASV, which on release and intestinal absorption effectively reconstituted the function of antivenom in neutralizing viper and cobra venom.
> - **Species identification:** DNA swab taken from fang marks on people bitten by snakes can correctly identify the species of the biting snake. Most of the time, the snake is not brought to the hospital, and hence, the species cannot be identified. Positive identification of the species of snake is critical for effective treatment.
> - **Species identification:** DNA swab taken from fang marks on people bitten by snakes can correctly identify the species of the biting snake. Most of the time, the snake is not brought to the hospital, and hence, the species cannot be identified. Positive identification of the species of snake is critical for effective treatment.
> - Radio-immunoassay (RIA) and enzyme-linked immunosorbent assay (ELISA) can identify the nature of venom from the bite site, based on antigens in the venom.
> - Recent studies have reported the beneficial effects of IV immunoglobulin (IVIg) which may improve coagulopathy, though its effect on neurotoxicity is doubtful.
> - *Snake venom metalloproteases (SVMPs)* are responsible for hemorrhage and tissue degradation at viperine bitten site. Antivenom's inability to offset viper venom-induced local toxicity has been a basis for an insistent search for SVMP inhibitors. In this context, N-acetyl cysteine (NAC), compound 5d and *Cassia auriculata* leaf methanol extracts are potent agents and its results are encouraging.
> - A compound extracted from the plant *Hemidesmus indicus* (2-hydroxy-4-methoxybenzoic acid) has been found to have potent anti-inflammatory, antipyretic and antioxidant properties, particularly against Russell's viper venom.
> - An aqueous extract of *Mimosa pudica* root possesses compounds which can neutralize the toxic effects of the cobra and krait venoms.

Complications: Compartment syndrome, tissue necrosis and bleeding diathesis. CVS and hematologic complications and pulmonary collapse may occur.

POSTMORTEM FINDINGS

- Venomous snakes leave two fang marks (occasionally one) slightly separated from each other and also small marks of other teeth **(Fig. 45.11A)**.*
- Non-venomous snakes leave a semicircular set of teeth-marks **(Fig. 45.11B)**.
- The bite marks are 1–1.5 cm deep in colubrine and 2.5 cm deep in viperine bites. These should be searched for with a magnifying lens, if not visible to the naked eye.
- **In viperine bite,** there is discoloration, swelling and cellulitis about the mark, and hemorrhages occur from the puncture site and mucous membranes. Petechiae are also found in mucosa of the urinary bladder, stomach and intestines. The regional lymph nodes are swollen and hemorrhagic. Hemorrhages into the bowel and lungs, and endocardial hemorrhages may be seen. Kidneys are inflamed, and may show medullary hemorrhages, tubular necrosis, cortical necrosis and interstitial nephritis **(Fig. 45.12)**. Internal organs are congested.
- **In elapidae bite,** the site of bite contains fluid and hemolyzed blood causing staining of vessels, and there are no definite appearances indicating the cause of death, except the signs of asphyxia.

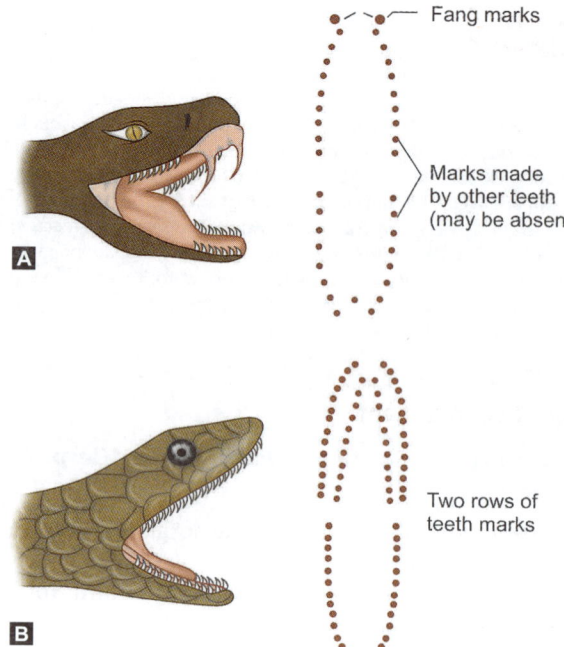

Figs. 45.11A and B: External features of snakebite: (A) Venomous snake; (B) Non-venomous snake

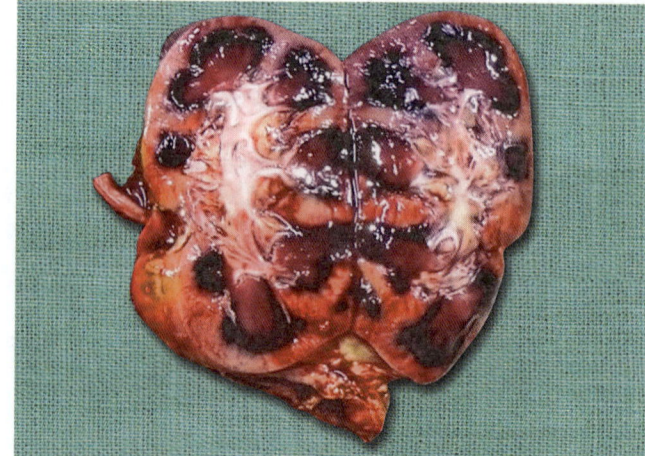

Fig. 45.12: Viperine snakebite: Medullary hemorrhages in kidneys

---
* The bite may not show the characteristic arched row of teeth, and sometimes, it is hard to demonstrate even a single fang bite mark in the skin, especially in kraits.

Medico-legal Aspects

- Whether or not antivenom is given, any patient with signs of envenomation should be observed in hospital for at least 24 h.
- Allegation of negligence may be leveled against the doctor in failure to authenticate and identify the snake (when killed snake is brought along with the patient) with subsequent development of envenomation and death, especially when the snake was initially claimed to be a non-venomous snake.
- Poisoning is usually accidental.
- Snakebite is a well-known occupational hazard amongst farmers, plantation workers and other outdoor workers.
- Recently, addicts are getting deliberately bitten by a venomous snake on the tongue or lips to experience the euphoric effects of recreational drugs.* Drugs made from snake venom (K-72 or K-76) are also popular in rave parties.
- Occasionally, a murder is committed by throwing a venomous snake on the bed of sleeping person.
- It is very rarely used for suicide. Queen Cleopatra is said to have committed suicide after her forces were defeated in battle. She chose to submit to the bite of an *asp* (venomous snake), rather than humiliation by her enemies.
- The bodies of animals killed by snake poisoning may be eaten without ill-effects, but their blood is poisonous and is fatal, if injected into the human body.
- Cattle are sometimes poisoned by snake venom.

Describe features and management of scorpion sting.

SCORPIONS

Introduction: About 100 species of scorpions are found in India. These are eight-legged arthropods and the end part of tail has two poisonous glands and a sting. Fatal cases have been reported from Maharashtra and Bihar due to acute pulmonary edema caused by Indian red scorpion (*Mesobuthus tamulus*).

Physical properties: The venom is a clear, colorless, proteinous toxalbumen, having hemolytic and neurotoxic effect. Its toxicity is more than that of snakes, but only a small quantity is injected.

Action: The venom is a potent autonomic stimulator, resulting in the release of massive amounts of catecholamines from the adrenals. It has also some direct effect on the myocardium.

Signs and Symptoms

- In case of hemolytic venom, reaction is mainly local and simulates viperine bite, but the scorpion sting bite shows only one hole in the center of the reddened area at the site of bite.
- Neurotoxic bite simulates cobra bite.
- Dysfunction of cranial nerve and hyperexcitability of skeletal muscles develop within hours.

Local: Little swelling, but prominent radiating pain, reddening, paresthesia, and hyperesthesia which is accentuated by tapping on the affected area (*tap test*).

Systemic effects are nausea, vomiting, restlessness, fever, headache, giddiness, blurred vision, abnormal eye movement, profuse sweating and salivation, lacrimation, rhinorrhea, slurred speech, muscular fasciculations, jerking and shaking (may be mistaken for a seizure), slow pulse, cyanosis, convulsions, coma and respiratory depression, and death may occur from pulmonary edema or cardiac failure in children.

Complications: Tachycardia, hypertension, arrhythmias, hyperthermia, rhabdomyolysis and acidosis.

Treatment

i. The limb is immobilized and a pressure bandage is applied proximal to the site of sting.
ii. The site may be incised and washed with water or weak solution of ammonia, borax or $KMnO_4$.
iii. **Prazosin therapy:** Prazosin 30 μg/kg/dose (1 mg for adult, 500 μg for children) is given orally and then after every 3 h till extremities are warm, dry and peripheral veins are visible.
iv. **Scorpion antivenom** (SAV) is specific antidote to scorpion venom. SAV against Indian red scorpion is available. Recovery is better by simultaneous administration of SAV and prazosin compared with prazosin alone.
v. Calcium gluconate 10 mL of 10% solution slow IV is given for pains, cramps and edema.
vi. Barbiturates/chlorpromazine is given to sedate and control convulsion.
vii. Atropine to prevent pulmonary edema.
viii. Symptomatic treatment.

Postmortem Findings

Affected site is swollen. Sting may be found at the site. The area may show ecchymosis. Pulmonary edema and myocardial infarction may be seen.

Medico-legal aspects: Poisoning is usually accidental.

---

* The neurotoxins in snake venom seems to have psychoactive properties—they induce symptoms like sleepiness, sense of grandiosity, pain- and stress-relief, sexual arousal, and sense of well-being in the addicts. The most commonly used snakes are cobra, common krait and green snake.

BEES AND WASPS

Introduction
- A bee sting is strictly a sting from a bee (honey bee, bumblebee or sweat bee). In common parlance, it can mean a sting of a bee, wasp, hornet or yellow jacket.
- When a honey bee stings a person, it cannot pull the barbed stinger back out. It leaves behind not only the stinger, but also part of its abdomen and digestive tract, muscles and nerves. This massive abdominal rupture kills the honey bee. Honey bees are the only species of bees to die after stinging.
- Painful and sometime, fatal reactions occur in humans.

Active Principles
- Bee venom contains dopamine, histamine, neurotoxin enzymes and toxic peptides.
- Wasp venom, in addition, contains serotonin and kinins.
- Ant venom mainly contains alkaloids, solenopsin-A and proteins.

Signs and Symptoms (Fig. 45.13)

Locally, there is pain, itching, redness and slight swelling at the site of the sting. Stings of the mouth, throat, and sometimes of the face, neck or upper limbs may cause edema of the larynx or pharynx and obstruction.

Systemic reactions occur due to multiple stinging with signs of GIT disturbance (nausea, vomiting and diarrhea), sweating, bronchospasm, hypotension, shock and unconsciousness.

Immediate **anaphylactic reactions** may be seen in some cases. Nausea, vomiting, diarrhea, urticaria, swelling, tachycardia, hypotension, respiratory distress, faintness and unconsciousness may be seen. Death may occur in 2–15 min.

Treatment
i. Tourniquet is applied proximal to the site of the sting and incision is given. The sting is located and removed by scraping or using tweezers. Ice or cold packs are applied.
ii. The area is then cleaned with soap and water, and tincture of iodine or local application of antihistamine or hydrocortisone cream is useful.
iii. Adrenaline is given to combat systemic reactions.
iv. Calcium gluconate 1–2 g IV.
v. Glucocorticoids are useful for urticaria.
vi. Artificial respiration and O_2 inhalation is given.
vii. Tetanus immunization is recommended.

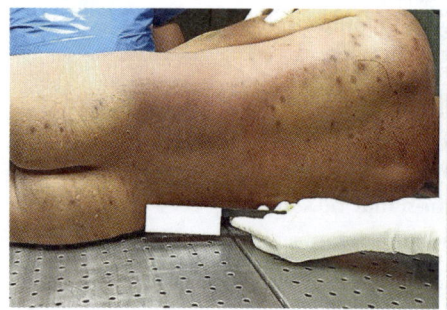
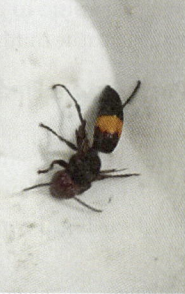

Fig. 45.13: Case of multiple stinging by wasps. The child had sudden onset of stridor, hematuria and went into coma and died within 4 h

SPIDERS

Introduction: Spider bites are common in some parts of the world. In India, it is not so common and fatalities are rare.
- Most spider bites are harmless and causes only local irritation, but some spider bites can cause significant morbidity and rarely, mortality.
- Some of the bites occur while people are asleep or dressing.

Signs and Symptoms
- Bites by **brown recluse spiders** (*Loxosceles* species) cause skin ulcer and necrotic eschars, intravascular hemolysis and acute renal failure. Initially, bites are painless and unnoticed, but a burning sensation develops after few hours with swelling and characteristic macular wheal showing surrounding rings of red vasodilatation, white vasoconstriction and blue prenecrotic cyanosis (*red-white-blue sign*).
- Bites by *Poecilotheria* species ('Mysore Ornamental'/Indian Tarantula) may cause headache, nausea and mild blurring of vision along with pain, redness and swelling. It causes immediate intense pain and swelling at the bite site with severe generalized muscle cramps, tremors, lymphadenopathy, fever, tachycardia, hypertension, restlessness.

Complications: Muscle cramps, intravascular hemolysis, acute renal failure and neurotoxicity.

Treatment
i. **Symptomatic and supportive treatment is sufficient:** Gentle cleansing, tetanus prophylaxis, analgesia, antipruritic medications and immobilization, if needed.
ii. **Contraindicated:** Early wound excision, corticosteroids, cyproheptadine and electric shocks at the bite site.

CHAPTER 45 : Organic Irritants—Animal

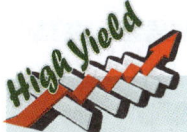

- **Snakes are classified into two types:** Venomous snakes and non-venomous snakes.
- Poison apparatus is a *modified salivary gland*.
- Snake venom is proteinous in nature; can be neurotoxic, vasculotoxic or myotoxic in its action.
- Venomous snakes are small head scales, compressed tail, large belly scales, fangs are long and canalized (leave two fang marks on the skin).
- **Neurotoxic venom** causes muscular weakness of legs and paralysis of muscles of face, throat and respiration (e.g., cobra or kraits).
- **Vasculotoxic venom** causes enzymatic destruction of cell walls and coagulation disorders causing hemorrhage from external orifices, e.g., vipers.
- **Myotoxic venom** produces generalized muscular pain ending in respiratory failure in fatal cases, e.g., sea snakes.
- **Fatal dose:** Cobra 15 mg; common krait 2.5–6 mg, Russell's viper 40 mg; saw-scaled viper 8 mg.
- Bites on the extremities, bony part, through clothing or foot wear or in adipose tissue are less dangerous than those on the head, trunk or directly into blood vessel.
- Venom is *not* poisonous when taken by mouth as it is not absorbed from gastric mucosa.
- Ophitoxemia characterizes the clinical spectrum of snakebite envenomation.
- Cobra belongs to elapidae family.
- Cobra bite produces both convulsions and paralysis, while krait causes only paralysis.
- 'Dry bite' is most common with a cobra.
- **Commonest and earliest manifestation of cobra bite**: Ptosis.
- At the cobra bite site, local necrosis causes '*wet gangrene*' with a characteristic putrid smell.
- **5Ds and 2Ps of elapid bites:** Dyspnea, dysphonia, dysarthria, diplopia, dysphagia; Ptosis, paralysis.
- Common kraits venom is painless, bite nocturnally and bite people sleeping on the floor. Victims wake up early morning, paralyzed—mistaken for STROKE.
- In viper bites, there is more local reaction with pain and oozing from the bite site, petechial hemorrhages, epistaxis, hemoptysis, hemetemesis, hematuria etc.
- In viper bite, there is bilateral parotid swelling ('*viper head*').
- Sea snake bite is usually painless with minimal local swelling but with *generalized rhabdomyolysis and myoglobinuria*.
- **Poison causing rhabdomyolysis:** Alcohol, CO, drugs of abuse (heroin, cocaine, amphetamine, LSD, phencyclidine), sea snake and insect venom.
- **Cause of death in cobra bite:** Respiratory paralysis.
- **Cause of death in viper bite:** Circulatory failure in early phase, and hemorrhagic complications later.
- **Diagnosis of snakebite:** 20 min whole blood clotting test for viperidae; and single breath counting test for elapids.
- **Broken neck sign:** Muscles flexing the neck gets paralyzed; seen in neurotoxic envenoming (cobra).
- In sea snake envenoming, *trismus* is observed.
- **Most important first aid measure in snake bite:** Reassurance since most bites is non-venomous.
- **Contraindicated in snakebite treatment:** Incision over the bite, mouth suctioning, tourniquet around the limb, use of snake stones, ice packs or electric shock.
- **Not recommended in treatment of snakebite:** Washing with soap and water (avoid manipulation).
- To prevent spread, pressure-immobilization (ligature pressure should be 50–70 mm Hg) for elapid bites (not be used for viper bites) is indicated.
- Antivenom is immunoglobulin purified from serum/plasma of a horse or sheep that has been immunized with the venoms of one or more species of snake.
- Monovalent antivenom contains specific antibody that will neutralize that particular venom.
- Polyvalent antisnake venom (ASV) serum is effective against cobra, common krait, saw scaled viper and Russell's viper.

- Polyvalent ASV is *not* effective against pit viper bite.
- In snake envenomation, effective ASV treatment is started by giving a dose of 10 vials.
- Polyvalent ASV may cause Type III hypersensitivity reactions *(serum sickness)*.
- **Drug to treat muscarinic symptoms in cobra bite:** Neostigmine.
- Atropine premedication should be used before administering neostigmine in cobra bite.
- Priaprism is seen in cantharide poisoning.
- Scorpion venom resembles snakebite (having hemolytic and neurotoxic effect) envenomation.
- **Drug to treat scorpion bite:** Prazosin.
- Red-white-blue sign is seen in bites by brown recluse spiders.

Interesting case

Snakebite Poisoning (Case of Uthra, 2020)

In 2018, Uthra **(Fig. A)**, a homemaker got married to Sooraj **(Fig. B)**, who worked in a private finance company. He was not so well off, but she was from an affluent family in Kerala. Soon after tying the knot, the couple had marital issues and Uthra was allegedly harassed for dowry, although nearly 100 gold coins, a car and cash were given at the time of marriage.

In March 2020, she was bitten by a venomous viper snake at her husband's house. She was taken to a hospital unconscious where doctors were able to save her. She was discharged in April and went to her parents' home to recover. In May 2020, her mother found Uthra unconscious when she went to wake her up in the morning. She was rushed to a hospital, where doctors declared her dead and informed that she had been bitten by a snake again. The autopsy revealed that she was bitten twice by the snake. Later, a cobra

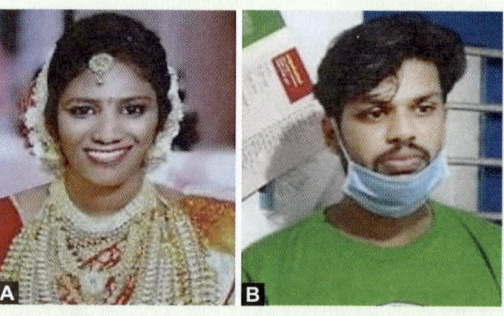

was found under a cupboard in her bedroom and killed. Sooraj was with Uthra at her parents' home on the eve of her death. Her parents became suspicious when he tried to secure ownership of his wife's property just after her death. They approached the police saying there was something suspicious about her death as she was bitten by a snake earlier as well.

The initial investigation pointed that although the cause of death was snakebite, but it was homicide plotted by her husband who had bought the snake. Police found digital evidence on his mobile phone. He had been watching snake-related videos on YouTube since the last three months, apparently to get trained in handling them. His phone records showed that he had been in contact with serpent handlers too. Sooraj bought a viper from a snake handler and attempted to kill his wife at their house using the snake. After the first attempt failed, he bought a cobra from his friend in April. He allegedly starved the snake for 11 days (to make the snake aggressive and dangerous) and brought the snake hidden in a glass bottle. He sedated Uthra on that night before dropping the snake while she was asleep. He sat in the bed and hit the snake with a stick to force it to bite. Sooraj reportedly tried to bag the snake again but it slithered away. He remained awake all night to ensure that he could escape unscathed. He left the room in the morning and started reading a newspaper in the verandah as if nothing happened.

The police arrested Sooraj in connection with the death of his wife due to snakebite. They also arrested three family members and recovered the victim's gold ornaments buried in two packets on the premises of their house. They were booked for domestic violence, anti-dowry provisions, abetment to crime and destroying evidences.

To gather more evidence, the police conducted postmortem of the snake carcass from the premises of Uthra's house where it was buried. The postmortem confirmed that it was a cobra. The fangs of the snake remains were collected to compare with the wound on Uthra's left hand. The bottle used to store the snake was also found which will be examined for fingerprints, any secretions or scales of the snake.

CHAPTER 46

Somniferous Poisons (Narcotic Poisons)

LEARNING OBJECTIVES

Must know
1. Signs and symptoms, treatment and PM findings in morphine poisoning
2. Active principles in opium
3. Medico-legal aspects of morphine poisoning
4. Body packers
5. Toxidromes

Desirable to know
1. Alkaloids
2. Clinical toxidrome
3. Marquis test
4. Chronic morphine poisoning
5. Chasing the dragon

FM 10.1 Describe general principles and basic methodologies in treatment of poisoning with regard to narcotic analgesics.

Definitions

- **Narcotic:** It refers to a sleep inducing xenobiotic, and initially used to mean the opioids. Currently, the term is used by law enforcement agencies to indicate any illicit psychoactive substance.
- **Opiate:** It refers to natural alkaloids derived directly from the poppy plant.
- **Opioids:** They are broader class of xenobiotics that are capable of producing opium-like effects on binding to opioid receptors. Endogenous neural polypeptides such as endorphins and enkephalins are natural opioids.
- **Toxidrome:** A constellation of clinical examination findings that assists in the diagnosis and treatment of the patient who presents with an exposure to an unknown agent.

OPIUM

Introduction

Opium is derived from *Papaver somniferum*, an annual plant with white or red flowers growing on a central bulbous pod (**Fig. 46.1**). Crude opium has a characteristic odor and bitter taste.

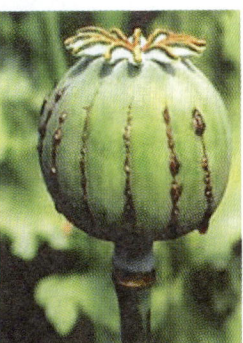

Fig. 46.1: *Papaver somniferum*

Distribution: Worldwide.

Common names: Poppy, *afim*, *kasoomba* or *madak chandu*.

Toxic Part

Unripe fruit capsule, latex juice.
- Latex is obtained by lacerating ('scoring') the immature seed pods; the latex leaks out and dries to a sticky brown residue (**Fig. 46.1**). This is scraped off the fruit.

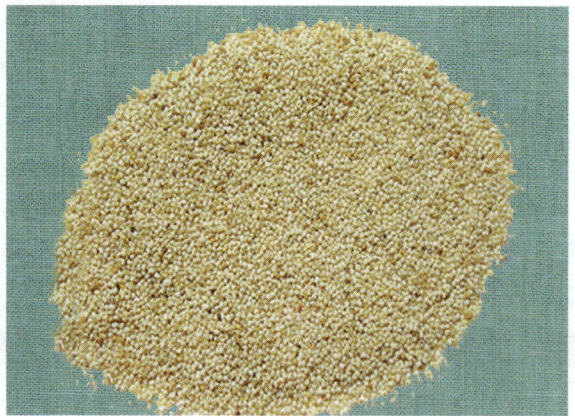

Fig. 46.2: Poppy seeds (non-poisonous)

- Seeds are non-poisonous and are called *'khaskhas'* which constitutes a condiment in cooking **(Fig. 46.2)**.*

Active Principles

The latex juice of opium has about 25 alkaloids, divided into two groups:

a. **Phenanthrene derivatives** (main narcotic constituents)
   i. *Natural alkaloids*
      - Morphine (10%): White powder/crystals, bitter taste and alkaline in reaction.
      - Codeine (0.5%).
      - Thebaine (0.3%).
   ii. *Semi-synthetic opioids:* They are produced by chemical modification of an opiate and include hydromorphone, diacetylmorphine *(heroin, brown sugar or smack)*, oxymorphone and oxycodone.
   iii. *Synthetic opioids:* These compounds are not derived from an opiate, but binds to an opioid receptor and produce opioid effects clinically. It includes methadone, fentanyl, pentazocine, tramadol and meperidine (pethidine).

b. **Benzyl-isoquinoline derivatives** (no significant CNS effects)
   i. Papaverine (1%)
   ii. Noscapine (6%).

> **NOTA BENE**
> - **Alkaloids** are complex substance having nitrogenous base, and is found in various plants. Chemically, it behaves like an alkali as it unites with acids to form salts. Its basic quality depends on the pyridine nucleus. In nature, they are usually combined with certain acids to from salts. They act mainly on the CNS, each compound having its own individual action.
> - **Important alkaloids:** Atropine, hyoscine, morphine, quinine, strychnine, cocaine and codeine. Some synthetic substances, such as amphetamine, heroin, pethidine and methadone also behave chemically like alkaloids.

Action

- Opioids act by binding to opioid receptors on neurons distributed throughout the nervous system and immune system.
- Four major types of opioid receptors have been identified: mu, kappa, delta and the recently recognized OFQ/N. These receptors are the binding sites for endogenous peptides.
- Activation of opioid receptors results in inhibition of synaptic neurotransmission in the CNS and PNS.

Routes of intake: It can be taken by snorting, smoking or heating and inhaling the vapor (*chasing the dragon*), intravenously (*mainlining*) and subcutaneously (*skin popping*).** It can be mixed with cocaine (known as **speed balling**) and then taken by addicts.

Metabolism

- Most opioids are metabolized by hepatic conjugation to inactive compounds that are excreted readily in the urine.
- Certain opioids (e.g., propoxyphene, fentanyl and buprenorphine) are more soluble in lipids and can be stored in the fatty tissues of the body.

> **Clinical toxidrome**
> Some poisons may produce a collection of symptoms (toxidromes) that can assist in making diagnosis and are also useful for anticipating other symptoms that may occur **(Table 46.1)**.

SIGNS AND SYMPTOMS

- The symptoms of an opiate/narcotic toxidrome include the *classic triad* of respiratory depression, pin-point pupils and impairment of sensorium.
- Peak effects are seen in 10 minutes (min) with IV route, 10–15 min after nasal insufflations, 30–45 min with IM, 90 min after taking orally and 2–4 hours (h) after dermal application.

I. Stage of Excitement

It is of short duration. There is euphoria, increased sense of well-being, freedom from anxiety, talkativeness and laughter. Hallucinations, flushing of face, conjunctival injection and rapid heart rate are seen.

II. Stage of Stupor

Headache, nausea, vomiting, weakness, heaviness in limbs, giddiness, drowsiness, diminished sensibility and strong tendency to sleep from which the patient can be aroused by painful stimuli.

- Pupils are constricted, and face and lips are cyanosed.
- Pulse and respiration: Almost normal.

---

* All parts of the opium poppy, including the seeds, contain morphine and codeine. Consumption of poppy seeds may give a positive drug test. The seeds contain between 0.5–10 µg of morphine/g of seeds.
** Method of injecting illicit drugs, especially opiates, cocaine and barbiturates, into the skin with the goal of achieving slower absorption, decreased risk of overdose, and easier administration than with IV drug use.

CHAPTER 46 : Somniferous Poisons (Narcotic Poisons)

TABLE 46.1: Clinical toxidromes

Toxidrome	Clinical features	Common poisons	Treatment	Site of action
Opiate	Respiratory depression and oxygen desaturations, miosis, decreased GI motility, bradycardia, hypothermia and coma	Morphine, codeine, oxycodone, fentanyl	Naloxone	Opioid receptor
Anticholinergic	Tachycardia, hyperthermia (mild to severe), agitation, delirium, seizures, mydriasis, dry, flushed skin, urinary retention, decreased intestinal motility	Dhatura, atropine, scopolamine, antihistamines	Physostigmine	Muscarinic acetylcholine receptors
Cholinergic (Organophosphate and carbamates)	Bradycardia, respiratory depression, miosis, SLUDGE (salivation, lacrimation, urination, defecation, GIT distress, emesis) CNS: Seizures, coma Muscle: Fasiculations, paralysis	DDT, parathion, malathion, diazinon	Atropine Pralidoxime (for OP insecticides)	Nicotinic and muscarinic acetylcholine receptors
Sympathomimetic	Hypertension, tachycardia, pyrexia, pupillary dilatation, diaphoresis, altered mental status	Cocaine, amphetamines	Benzodiazepines	α and β adrenergic receptors
Sedative hypnotic (Benzodiazepines)	Sedation or coma, normal vital signs, diplopia, ataxia, impaired motor function, slurred speech, anterograde amnesia, anxiety, hallucinations, delirium	Alprazolam, flunitrazepam, oxazepam	Flumazenil	ϒ-aminobutyric acid receptors

III. Stage of Narcosis/Coma

Patient passes into deep coma from which he cannot be aroused. In this stage:

- Muscles: Flaccid and relaxed; muscular rigidity with rapid IV injection may be seen
- Face: Pale
- Reflexes: Absent
- Conjunctiva: Congested
- Skin: Cold with profuse perspiration, all other secretions are suspended
- Pupils: Constricted to *pin-point* (Fig. 46.3), non-reacting
- Blood pressure: Hypotension
- Temperature: Hypothermia
- Pulse: Weak, feeble
- Respiration: Slow, stertorous (4–6 breaths/min)
- Sphincter tone: Increased (can lead to urinary retention).
- CNS: Seizures due to hypoxia.

Cause of death: During the terminal stages, ARDS develops and pink froth comes from the mouth (*'foam cone'*), pulse is slow, irregular and imperceptible, respiration becomes Cheyne-Stokes, and ultimately deep coma and death due to respiratory depression and cardiorespiratory arrest.

> **Mnemonic for morphine poisoning: MORPHINES**
> M: **M**uscle relaxation; O: **O**rthostatic hypotension;
> R: **R**espiratory depression, reflexes absent; P: **P**in-point pupil;
> H: **H**allucinations; I: **I**rregular, feeble pulse;
> N: **N**ausea; E: **E**uphoria; S: **S**edation

Fatal Dose

- Opium: 2 g.
- Morphine: 200 mg.
- Codeine: 50 mg.

Fatal period: 6–12 h.

Differential Diagnosis

- **Intracranial hemorrhage:** Cerebrovascular accidents or brain trauma.
- **Poisoning:** Alcohol, barbiturates, benzodiazepine, carbolic acid, carbon monoxide or organophosphorus.
- **Metabolic conditions:** Diabetic and uremic coma.
- **CNS infections:** Meningitis, encephalitis, encephalopathy or cerebral malaria.
- **Others:** Epileptic or hysterical coma, or heat hyperpyrexia.

■ TREATMENT

Support vitals through ventilator and other emergency procedures.

I. Decontamination and Elimination

i. Stomach wash frequently with 1:5000 KMnO$_4$ leaving some solution in stomach to oxidize the alkaloid that might be secreted in stomach after absorption. Lavage should be carried out even after IV/IM injection of drug, as it is secreted in the stomach.

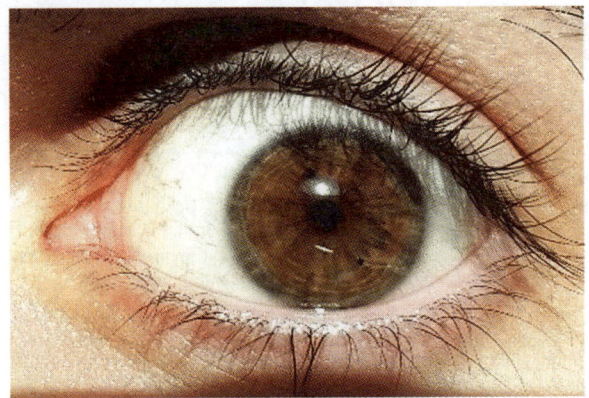

Fig. 46.3: Pinpoint pupil

ii. Administer activated charcoal—method of choice for decontamination following ingestion.
iii. Enema with 30 g of sodium sulfate twice daily.
iv. Whole-bowel irrigation in body packers.

II. Antidote

Narcotic antagonist **naloxone** in an initial dose of 0.4–2 mg IV/IM repeated every 2–3 min up to 10 mg, if no response occurs.

If there is little response to naloxone alone, possibility of an overdose with a benzodiazepine should be considered, and a challenge with flumazenil, 0.2 mg/min IV up to maximum of 3 mg in an hour might be used.

Detection

- **Marquis test:** It is a simple spot-test to presumptively identify opiates and amphetamines. Three milliliters of concentrated H_2SO_4 +3 drops of formalin are added to the suspected sample. Purple-red color is observed which gradually changes to violet if opiates are present.
- **Mandelin test:** This test can be used to test for a variety of alkaloids. The reagent consists of ammonium vandanate in concentrated sulfuric acid. The alkaloids produce characteristic color changes: morphine: blue-gray, codeine: olive, heroin: brown, and methadone: green to blue.

> **NOTA BENE**
>
> **Microcrystalline tests:** A more precise test for such drugs is based on their crystalline structure. When a particular drug is treated with a few drops of a specific reagent, small crystals with characteristic shapes, color or dichroism may result, which can be examined under a polarizing microscope and compared with recorded images. For example, morphine with K_2HgI_4 forms brownish brushes, fans or rosettes; and heroin with $HgCl_2$ forms fine dendritic crystals.

POSTMORTEM FINDINGS

External

i. Smell of opium.
ii. Face/body is bluish, deeply cyanosed or blackish.
iii. Postmortem staining is purple or blackish.
iv. Froth at the nostrils.
v. Pupils are constricted, can be dilated also.
vi. Allergic reactions to IV heroin may be seen.
vii. Needle tracks are found occasionally, depending on the route of intake.

Internal

i. Diffuse cerebral edema.
ii. All organs are congested, trachea contains frothy secretions.
iii. Blood is dark and fluid.
iv. Stomach may show presence of small, soft brownish lumps of opium, and smell of drug may be perceived.

Medico-legal Aspects

- Negligence may be alleged in cases of prehospital discharge-on-scene after naloxone treatment followed in most Western countries, since this practice is sometimes associated with risk of death due to rebound toxicity after such episodes.
- Opioid poisoning nowadays is from street drugs which not only have brown sugar, but also therapeutic opioids like hydrocodone or oxycodone, codeine taken with glutethemide, and abuse of Subutex (buprenorphine hydrochloride).
- It is a poison of choice to commit suicide (*ideal suicidal poison*), since death is painless.
- Homicide is rare, because of bitter taste and characteristic odor.
- Morphine is one of the favored drugs for euthanasia.
- Infanticide by breastfeeding an infant by a woman who had smeared her nipple with tincture opium.
- Accidental opium poisoning is also common among addicts. Drugging of children by opium to keep them quiet, and overdose of medicines may result in accidental poisoning.*
- Various nonproprietary formulations, folk remedies, and herbs may contain opium, and administration of these results in unintentional poisoning.
- Heroin and oxycodone have been reportedly smuggled by body packers.
- Sometimes opium is used for doping racehorses.
- It is said to increase libido, hence used as an aphrodisiac.
- Some criminals take opium to build courage before committing a crime.
- Opium disappears with putrefaction, so it may not be detected in putrefied bodies.

> **NOTA BENE**
>
> - It should be noted that opioid exposure does not always result in pupillary constriction, and respiratory depression is the most specific sign. Other important presenting signs are ventricular arrhythmias, acute mental status changes and seizures.
> - *Acute lung injury* is known sequelae of heroin, propoxyphene and methadone overdose, and present in fatal cases of opioid overdose. The findings are cyanosis, dyspnea, pink frothy sputum, rales (crepitations), tachypnea and tachycardia.

---

* In the early 18th century in the UK, with industrial revolution, 18 h workdays, extra cost in feeding and loss of sleep due to infant's cries, various concoctions of opium were specifically designed for the purpose of quieting unruly children.

CHAPTER 46 : Somniferous Poisons (Narcotic Poisons)

- Earlier opioid overdose was treated with analeptics. In 1950s, specific antidotes were introduced: *nalorphine and levallorphan* which were capable of reversing the respiratory effects by blocking the opioid receptors. However, they have a mixed agonist-antagonist properties that significantly limited their usefulness. *Naloxone* with its pure opioid antagonistic properties completely replaced nalorphine and levallorphan in the treatment of opioid overdose.
- *Nalmefene and naltrexone* are newer opioid antagonists that have longer half-lives than naloxone (4–8 h and 8–12 h vs 1 h). The routine use of a long-acting antagonist in the patient who is unconscious for unknown reasons is not recommended.

Body Packers/Body Stuffers

- Multiple-wrapped packets of illicit drugs (cocaine or heroin—*most common*) may be ingested or inserted into body cavities by '*swallowers*', '*internal carriers*', '*couriers*', or '*mules*' to intentionally transport drugs from one country to another. After they arrive at their destination, cathartics are administered so that the packets can be passed and delivered.
- Body packers often swallow 50–100 packages containing 0.5–1 g of xenobiotic.
- Packages are often made of latex, plastic bags/wraps, condoms, balloons, cellophane, tape, rubber gloves, surgical ligature, paraffin and fiberglass.
- When the authorities discover such individuals or when individuals in custody become ill, they may be brought to a nearby hospital for evaluation and management. Although, these patients generally are asymptomatic on arrival, they are at risk for delayed, prolonged or lethal poisoning as a consequence of packet rupture (**Figs. 46.4A to C**).
- If there is a suspicion of body packing or body stuffing, careful cavity searches of the rectum and vagina are done.

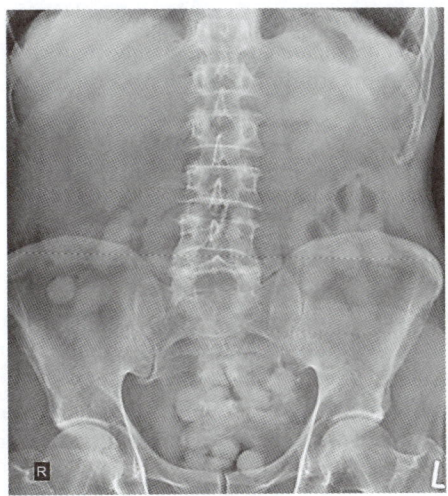

Fig. 46.5: Body packers: 'Double-condom' sign (radiolucent rim of air trapped between the multiple layers of packing surrounding each drug packet)
(*Courtesy:* Dr Íomhar O' Sullivan, Emergency Medicine Consultant, Cork, Ireland)

- An abdominal X-ray can confirm the diagnosis (**Fig. 46.5**). Ultrasonography and CT are other recommended diagnostic modalities.
- Polyethylene glycol electrolyte lavage solution is used to flush out the packets. Intestinal perforation or obstruction by the packets may require surgical intervention.

Chasing the Dragon

- Intravenous injection and nasal insufflation are the preferred means of heroin self-administration in the US. In the other countries, including the Netherlands, UK and Spain, the prevalent method is '*chasing the dragon*'.*
- In this, users inhale a thick, white pyrolysate that is generated by heating heroin base on aluminum

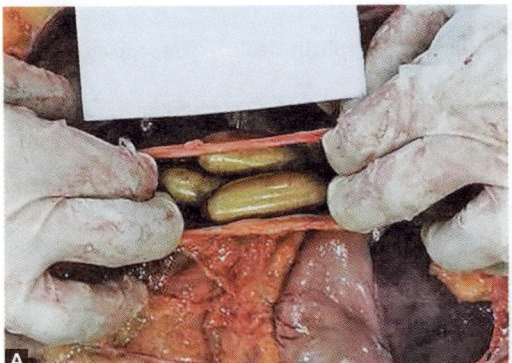 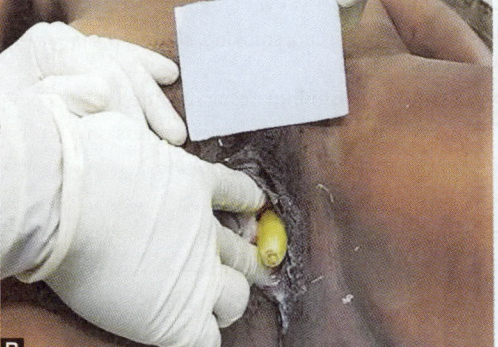 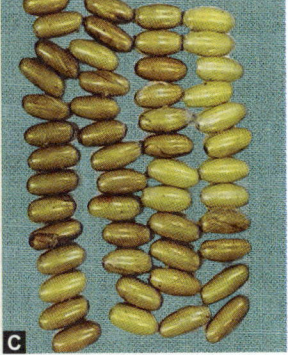

Figs. 46.4A to C: 'Body packer' syndrome: The female arrested at the airport suddenly collapsed and died due to effects of heroin concealed within: (A) GIT; (B) Vagina; (C) Recovered pellets (3 pellets were found damaged)

---

* This method is also quite prevalent in Punjab among drug abusers where it is referred to as '*chitta*' (diacetylmorphine, traditionally referred to just heroin, but include other synthetic drugs like LSD and methamphetamines).

foil using a hand-hold flame (the smoke looks like a 'dragon'). This means of administration produces heroin concentration similar to those observed following IV administration.
- Chasing the dragon is not a new phenomenon, but it has gained acceptance recently among both IV heroin users and non-addict individuals.

CHRONIC MORPHINE POISONING (MORPHINISM)

- Opioid dependence is seen among patients with chronic pain syndromes, and the physicians, nurses and pharmacists because of its easy access.
- The most important dependence-producing derivatives are *morphine and heroin.* Heroin is more addicting than morphine and can cause dependence after a short period of exposure. Tolerance to heroin occurs rapidly and can be increased to more than 100 times the first dose needed.
- The important complications of chronic opioid use may include one or more of the following:
   i. *Due to illicit drug (contaminants)*: Peripheral neuropathy, amblyopia, degeneration of globus pallidus, Parkinsonism and transverse myelitis.
   ii. *Due to intravenous use:* Skin infections, thrombophlebitis, AIDS, hepatitis, pulmonary embolism, endocarditis, osteomyelitis, pneumonia, septicemia and tetanus.

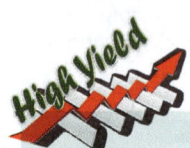

- **Opiate:** Natural alkaloids derived directly from the poppy plant.
- **Opioids:** Xenobiotics capable of producing opium-like effects on binding to opioid receptors.
- **Toxidrome:** Constellation of clinical examination findings that assists in the diagnosis and treatment of the patient who presents with an exposure to an unknown agent.
- **Alkaloids:** Substances having nitrogenous base, and found in various plants. Act mainly on the CNS.
- **Important alkaloids:** Atropine, hyoscine, morphine, quinine, strychnine, cocaine and codeine.
- Opium (poppy, *afim*) is derived from *Papaver somniferum*.
- Crude opium has a characteristic odor and bitter taste.
- **Toxic part of plant:** Unripe fruit capsule, latex juice.
- Latex is obtained by lacerating the immature seed pods; the latex leaks out and dries to a sticky brown residue.
- Seeds are non-poisonous *(khaskhas)* which constitutes a condiment in cooking.
- Active principles in opium are classified into phenanthrene and benzyl-isoquinoline derivatives.
- **Natural alkaloids:** Morphine, codeine, thebaine.
- **Semi-synthetic opioids:** Hydromorphone, diacetylmorphine (heroin/brown sugar/smack), oxymorphone and oxycodone.
- **Synthetic opioids:** Methadone, fentanyl, pentazocine, tramadol, meperidine (pethidine).
- Most important dependence-producing derivatives are morphine and heroin.
- **Routes of administration of opium:** Snorting, smoking, *chasing the dragon*, IV (*mainlining*) and subcutaneously (*skin popping*). It can be mixed with cocaine *(speed balling)*.
- **Classic triad of symptoms in opium poisoning:** Respiratory depression, pin-point pupils and impairment of sensorium.
- **Most common feature of opiate poisoning:** Respiratory depression.
- Pin-point pupil (miosis) is seen in opium/morphine poisoning.
- **Fatal dose:** Opium: 2 g; morphine: 200 mg.
- **Antidote for opium/morphine poisoning:** Naloxone.
- **Detection of opiate:** Marquis test (for opiates and amphetamines) and Mandelin test (detects variety alkaloids).
- **PM findings in opium poisoning:** Smell of opium; PM staining is purple or blackish.
- Morphine is an ideal suicidal poison since death is painless.
- Morphine is one of the favored drugs for *euthanasia*.
- *Infanticide* may result from by breastfeeding an infant by a woman with nipple smeared in opium.
- **Body packers:** Multiple-wrapped packets of illicit drugs (cocaine and heroin—*most common*) may be ingested or inserted into body cavities to transport drugs from one country to another.

Interesting case

Morphine Poisoning

In December 2019, five babies, aged between one day and five weeks, some of them prematurely born, suddenly developed life-threatening breathing difficulties at roughly the same time and in the same hospital room at the Ulm University Hospital, Germany **(Fig. A)**. It was only due to the immediate medical attention by the staff that the babies' were saved and were not expected to suffer any further health problems. The neonatologists initially suspected the infants had caught an infection, but this was ruled out by the urine tests whose results came back positive for morphine— although none of the infants were receiving the drug at that particular time. Morphine is sometimes used to treat withdrawal symptoms in babies born to drug-addicted mothers. A morphine overdose can lead to life-threatening respiratory failure. The hospital notified the police the following day after the reports came.

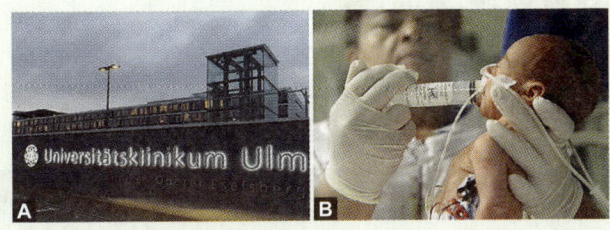

The authorities searched the lockers of hospital staff who were on duty at the time of the incident and found a syringe containing breast milk among the nurse's possessions. Initial testing showed the syringe had been laced with morphine. The nurse was arrested of attempted manslaughter on suspicion of poisoning the babies with morphine. It is common for premature and newborn babies who are too weak to drink from a bottle to be fed orally through a syringe **(Fig. B)**. But the breast milk or formula, they are given is never combined with medication. The nurse rejected the accusations against her.

Ulm prosecutor told afterwards that the initial test was found to be wrong, after further analysis showed the syringe did not contain morphine after all. The woman was released from custody after four days with an apology from the prosecutor. The decision to act based on the preliminary test result was a mistake, which had not been checked against a control sample. The error came to light after the mother whose breast milk was in the syringe volunteered to give a control sample, which also tested positive for morphine. The lab which carried out the analysis then discovered that the solvent used in the tests had been contaminated with morphine, for unknown reasons. Follow-up tests by another lab confirmed that neither the syringe nor the control sample contained any morphine.

However, the nurse remains a suspect in the case, along with two doctors and three other nurses who were on duty that night because of their close proximity to the infants at the time of the incident. The six employees are currently barred from working at the hospital in southern Germany. Use of morphine is strictly regulated in German hospitals and is stored in a locked cupboard and a log is kept of when it is administered and to which patients. The hospital in Ulm has admitted finding 'some inconsistencies' in the logs.

CHAPTER 47

Inebriants—Alcohol

LEARNING OBJECTIVES

Must know
1. Signs and symptoms, fatal dose and treatment of acute alcohol intoxication
2. Signs and symptoms, fatal dose, treatment and PM findings in methanol poisoning
3. Medico-legal aspects of alcohol intoxication
4. Drunkenness
5. Percentage of alcohol in different beverages
6. McEwan's sign, blackout, hangover
7. Treatment of alcoholism
8. Delirium tremens
9. Korsakoff's psychosis
10. Wernicke's encephalopathy
11. Widmark's formula

Desirable to know
1. Proof of spirit
2. Zieve syndrome
3. Mellanby effect, pathological intoxication
4. Holiday heart syndrome
5. Field impairment tests
6. Laboratory investigations for alcohol estimation
7. Ethylene glycol poisoning

Describe general principles and basic methodologies in treatment of poisoning with regard to ethanol.

Introduction

- Ethanol (ethyl alcohol) is a transparent, colorless, volatile liquid having a characteristic odor (odorless in pure state; odor in primarily due to congeners formed during fermentation and aging) and a burning taste with a specific gravity of 0.79.
- Ethanol is produced by the enzymatic action of yeasts on vegetable substrate containing sugars. Direct fermentation cannot raise the concentration to ≥12–15% as the yeast is killed, but distillation of primary fermentation can concentrate the alcohol to 40–60% strength. Different types of beverages with percentage of alcohol are given in **Table 47.1**.
- At low doses, alcohol is said to have beneficial effects, such as decreased rates of myocardial infarction, diabetes, stroke, gallstones and possibly Alzheimer's dementia, but consumption of two standard drinks per day increases the risk of health problems in many organ systems. Regular consumption of 20–32 g/day for men and 14–27.2 g/day for women are considered as safe limits for drinking, if liver damage is to be avoided

TABLE 47.1: Approximate percentage of alcohol by volume in beverages

Beverage	Alcohol by volume
Spirits (whisky, brandy, rum, gin, vodka)	35–50%
Port (fortified with brandy), sherry	17–21%
Wine	10–15%
Champagne	10–13%
Beers, stout, cider	4–8%

(difference between the sexes is due to the lower weight and water-to-body-mass ratio of women).

NOTA BENE

- Earlier, weekly safe limit was recommended [168–210 g/week (≤21 units) of alcohol for men and 98–140 g for women (≤14 units)]. This is not advised, since a study showed that many people were in effect 'saving up' their units and using them at the end of the week for *binge drinking* where the primary intention is to become intoxicated by heavy consumption of alcohol over a short period of time.
- Units of alcohol are a measure of the volume of pure alcohol in alcoholic beverages used as a guideline in some countries. One unit of alcohol is defined as 10 mL in the UK and as 10 g (12.7 mL) in Australia. A standard drink is 30 mL of spirits; 330 mL can of beer or 100 mL glass of wine.
- To calculate standard drinks, the following formula is used: Volume of container (liters) × % alcohol by volume (mL/100 mL) × 0.789 = Number of standard drinks.

Commercial Preparations of Alcohol

- *Absolute alcohol* contains 99–100% ethanol (not more than 1% water).
- *Mineralized methylated spirit* (denatured alcohol) consists of 90% ethanol, 9.5% wood naphtha (methanol) and 0.5% pyridine, and is colored pink for easy identification.
- *Industrial methylated spirit* contains 95% ethanol and 5% methanol, with no coloring agent.
- *Surgical spirit* (rubbing alcohol) consists of 95% of ethanol or isopropyl alcohol, and 5% methanol with oil of wintergreen to give it a sweetish flavor.

Proof of spirit indicates a mixture containing 57.1% by volume or 49.28% by weight of absolute alcohol. In the US, the term proof refers to twice the percentage of alcohol by volume. So, the common 80-proof whisky sold in the US contains 40% alcohol by volume. In India, the spirit (whisky, rum or brandy) is usually 42.8% by volume and 75-proof.

The concentration written on the labels of most bottles is v/v, i.e., volume of alcohol per volume of drink.

Action

Ethanol acts mainly on the CNS. It acts as a depressant of specialized and sensitive cells of cerebral cortex (centers regulating conduct, judgment and self-criticism) with release of inhibitory tone, leading to unrestrained behavior. This is followed by depression of vital centers of medulla producing coma and death.

Alcohol also acts a hypnotic, diaphoretic, and in small doses as an appetizer.

Metabolism

Absorption occurs mainly in the stomach (70%), and in the duodenum (25%), while only a small percentage occurs in the remaining intestinal tracts. Following absorption, the concentration of alcohol in the blood reaches a maximum in about 45–90 minutes (min) after ingestion. The **blood alcohol concentration (BAC)** is often represented by a graph. The major determinants of the timing and peak of the BAC include body size, sex, amount and type of beverage ingested, duration of drinking, and the presence and type of food (**Table 47.2**).

- With an empty stomach, there is a rapid rise and slow decline (**Fig. 47.1**).
- With diluted drinks or a full stomach, the rise is slower and the maximum peak is lower with a flatter BAC curve. If subsequent drinks are taken, the new alcohol is superadded to the existing curve.

Factors that interfere with absorption are (**Table 47.2**):
- Presence of food (especially fats and proteins) in stomach retards absorption.

TABLE 47.2: Factors affecting rate of absorption of alcohol

Factors enhancing absorption	Factors decreasing absorption
Femaleness	Maleness
Empty stomach	Full stomach
Drugs: Cholinergic agents, parasympathomimetic agents, aspirin, erythromycin, metoclopramide, H_2-receptor antagonists	Drugs: Anticholinergic agents, sympathomimetic agents, nicotine or caffeine, tricyclic antidepressants, amphetamines, opiates
Gastric resection, gastric ulcers, gastritis	Malignant gastric neoplasm, pyloric stenosis
Carbonated drinks	Fatty foods

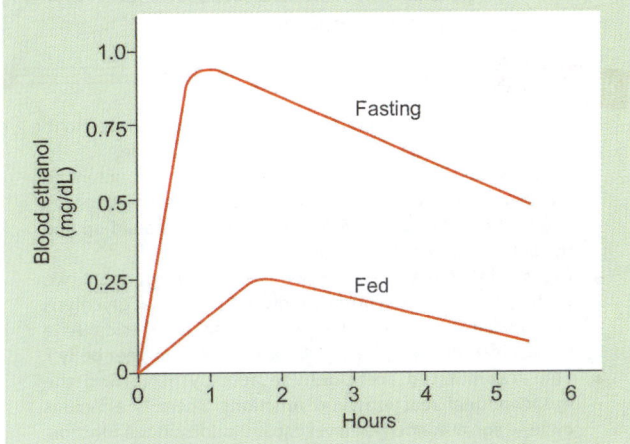

Fig. 47.1: Blood alcohol concentration in relation to presence of food

- Strength of alcoholic beverages taken—higher the strength more rapid will be the rate of absorption.
- Diluted drinks, such as beer may take double the time to absorb, compared to stronger drinks.
- Carbonated drinks hasten absorption as the bubbles greatly increase the surface area carrying alcohol.
- Warm alcoholic drinks which dilate gastric mucosal capillaries are more quickly absorbed than iced drinks of same strength.

Distribution

Ethanol is distributed evenly throughout the body, passing the blood-brain barrier easily to affect cerebral function. However, it is poorly soluble in body fat; females of same body size as males will produce a higher BAC for the same amount of drink, as their aqueous compartment is smaller.

It attains equilibrium with a constant blood alcohol concentration and concentration of alcohol in other body fluids, the ratio being:
- Blood: Urine = 1:1.33
- Blood: Exhaled air (breath) = 1:2300

- Blood: Saliva = 1:12
- Blood: CSF = 1:1.17

Detoxification

Ninety percent of ethanol is metabolized in the liver, while the kidneys and lungs help to excrete about 10% only. In the liver, alcohol is oxidized by alcohol dehydrogenase **(Flowchart 47.1)**.

- Non-habituated persons metabolize ethanol at 13–25 mg/dL/h. In alcoholics, this rate increases to 30–50 mg/dL/h. Because of tolerance, BACs must be interpreted in conjunction with history and clinical presentation.
- Excretion of alcohol is mainly by the kidneys, lungs and skin through urine, breath and sweat respectively. If is also secreted in saliva and milk.

> **NOTA BENE**
>
> A number of metabolic effects from alcohol are directly linked to the production of an excess of both NADH and acetaldehyde.
> - NADH is utilized in the conversion of pyruvic acid (intended for conversion into glucose by gluconeogenesis) to lactic acid. The final result may be acidosis from lactic acid build-up and hypoglycemia from lack of glucose synthesis.
> - Excess NADH may be used as a reducing agent in two pathways—one to synthesize glycerol (from a glycolysis intermediate) and the other to synthesis fatty acids. As a result, heavy drinkers may initially be overweight ('**beer belly**').
> - The accumulated acetaldehyde acts by inhibiting the mitochondrial reactions and functions. There is a vicious cycle—high acetaldehyde level impairs mitochondria function, metabolism of acetaldehyde to acetic acid decreases, more acetaldehyde accumulates and causes further liver damage—hepatitis and cirrhosis.
> - Acetaldehyde may be responsible for the development of alcohol addiction.

SIGNS AND SYMPTOMS (ACUTE POISONING)

I. Stage of Excitement
(Blood level: 50–150 mg%)

- Person will be euphoric (sense of well-being). Actions, speech and emotions are less restrained due to lowering of the inhibition normally exercised by the higher centers of the brain. It alters time and space perception.
- He may perform dancing, thrilling shows, carelessly and fearlessly.
- He might disclose secrets (*'in vino veritas'*—in wine there is truth).
- Person might show increase in confidence, but lack of self-control.
- There is lowering of visual acuity. Nystagmus present.
- Mental concentration is poor and judgment impaired.
- Faculty of attention deteriorates.
- Recall memory is disturbed, person cannot accurately recall certain situations or names of individuals.
- It increases the desire for sex, but markedly impairs performance resulting in prolonged intercourse without ejaculation.

II. Stage of Incoordination
(Blood level: 150–250 mg%)

- Due to further depression of higher centers, the person may be morose/cheerful/irritable/ill-tempered/excitable/sleepy—depending on the dominant impulses released.
- Centers of perception and skilled movements are involved—there is clumsiness, incoordination of fine and skilled movements, and alterations in speech and fine finger movements.
- Nausea and vomiting.
- Face: Flushed.
- Pulse: Rapid.
- Sense of touch, taste, smell and hearing are diminished.
- Prolonged reaction time.
- Hypothermia.
- Breath smells of alcohol.
- Pupils are dilated and react sluggishly to light.

III. Stage of Coma
(Blood level >250 mg%)

- Dysarthria; speech is thick and slurred.
- Coordination is markedly affected—becomes giddy, stagger and fall.

Flowchart 47.1: Metabolism of ethanol in liver [(A) causes increased blood acetaldehyde levels and (B) causes increased dopamine levels]

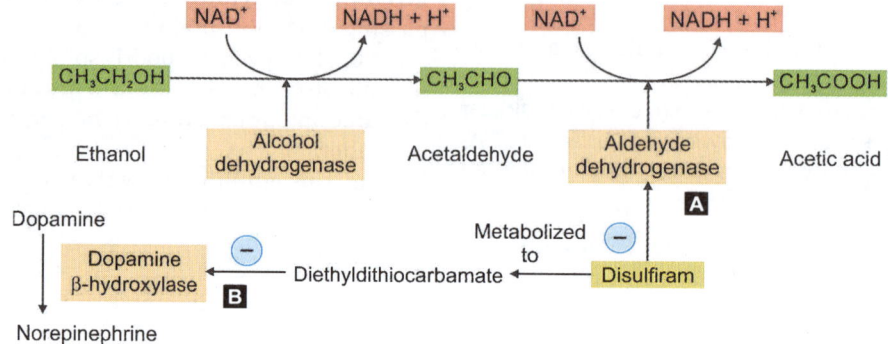

- Pulse is rapid.
- Hypothermia.
- Amnesia.
- Diplopia: Pupils are constricted, but on stimulation of the person, e.g., by pinching or slapping causes them to dilate with slow return **(McEwan's sign)**.
- Patient passes into coma with steatorous breathing.

The physiologic effects of alcohol are more pronounced when the blood level is rising, as compared to levels attained at peak or plateau, or when the level is falling. This is known as the **Mellanby effect** and is believed to result from an acute tolerance to alcohol that develops during intoxication.

Recovery

Unless a large quantity of alcohol is consumed in a short time, recovery is the rule.

- About 35% of drinkers may experience a **blackout**, an episode of temporary anterograde amnesia in which the person forgets all or part of what occurred during a drinking session.
- At times, a small dose of alcohol may produce acute intoxication in some persons which is known as **pathological intoxication**.

With recovery, coma gradually lightens into deep sleep. Person will wake up in 8–10 hours (h) with acute depression of mood, nausea and headache—**alcohol hangover**.

Cause of death: If the victim does not recover from coma within 5 h, prognosis is bad and may result in death due to shock, depression of respiratory center or aspiration of vomit.

Fatal Dose (Non-addict)

- 150–250 mL of absolute alcohol consumed in 1 h.
- Risk of death is increased if BAC >300 mg/dL, and death is typical if the BAC is between 400–500 mg/dL.*

Fatal period: 12–24 h.

Diagnosis of Intoxication

- Ethanol concentrations are not predictive of intoxication, despite the legal limit of 30 mg/dL for driving. Intoxication is a clinical diagnosis. The terms alcohol intoxication and drunkenness are often used interchangeably.
- The distinctive aroma of alcohol may assist in diagnosis. Attributing an altered mental status (AMS) because of its odor on a patient's breath is potentially dangerous and misleading. Small amounts of alcohol and its congeners generally produce the same breath odor as do intoxicating amounts. Conversely, when an extremely high level of BAC is confirmed by laboratory, it is dangerous to ignore other possible causes of AMS.
- The diagnostic features of alcoholic intoxication developed by the American Psychiatric Association include a requirement that there must have been recent ingestion of alcohol. The diagnostic criterion for alcohol intoxication as per ICD-11 is given in **Box 47.1**.
- Confirmation is done by analysis of blood (serum glucose level should be done along with it).
- Possibility of intoxication with other drugs should be considered and a blood or urine sample is indicated to screen for opioid and other CNS depressants, particularly benzodiazepines and barbiturates.

> **Box 47.1** Diagnostic criteria for alcohol intoxication (ICD-11)
>
> - Transient and clinically significant disturbances in consciousness, cognition, perception, affect, behavior or coordination that develop during or shortly after the consumption or administration of alcohol.
> - Symptoms must be compatible with the known pharmacological effects of alcohol, and their intensity is closely related to the amount of alcohol consumed.
> - Presenting features may include impaired attention, inappropriate or aggressive behavior, lability of mood and emotions, impaired judgment, poor coordination, unsteady gait, and slurred speech. At more severe levels of intoxication, stupor or coma may occur.
> - Symptoms of intoxication are time-limited and abate as alcohol is cleared from the body.
> - Symptoms are not better accounted for by another medical condition or another mental disorder, including another disorder due to substance use (e.g., withdrawal from a different substance).

TREATMENT

Outline of management is given in **Flowchart 47.2**.

I. Patient Stabilization

i. Patient must be kept warm and placed in a quiet environment, and made to lie on the side to minimize risk of aspiration.
ii. In comatose and extremely intoxicated patient with severe respiratory depression, endotracheal intubation and ventilator is useful.
iii. Gastric lavage with alkaline solution within 2 h of ingestion.
iv. One liter of normal saline with 10% glucose and 15 units of insulin or 50% dextrose (50 in 100 mL) is given IV.

---

*Amy Winehouse, Grammy-winning British singer and songwriter died of accidental alcohol poisoning in 2011. Her BAC was 416 mg% at the time of her death.

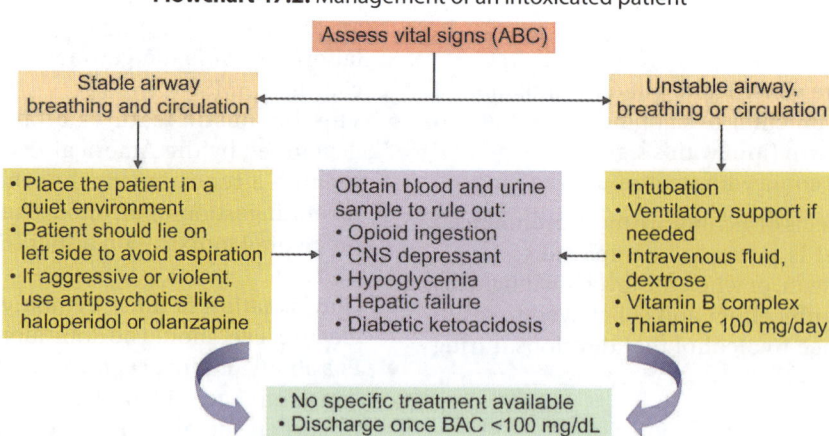

Flowchart 47.2: Management of an intoxicated patient

v. Thiamine 100 mg in 500 mL glucose solution IV. Multivitamins with folate and magnesium may be added to it.
vi. Respiratory support and O_2 therapy for hypoxia.
vii. Hemodialysis and peritoneal dialysis may be used.

II. Patient Sedation

In case of aggressive behavior, non-threatening force by intervention team (physical restraint should be avoided) or sedation (using midazolam or droperidol) may be adopted.

III. Acceleration of Ethanol Elimination

Single dose metadoxine (300–900 mg IV) has been found useful to accelerate ethanol elimination from blood.

Complications

- **Holiday heart syndrome:** Patient may exhibit cardiac dysrhythmias (especially atrial fibrillation and ventricular arrhythmias) after a heavy drinking episode.
- Hypoglycemia, gastritis, pancreatitis and toxic psychosis may also occur.
- In teenagers, it may lead to anemia, macrocytosis, and elevation of enzymes, bilirubin and uric acid.

NOTA BENE

Zieve syndrome: It is an acute alcohol hepatitis seen in patients following alcohol binge and consists of *triad of symptoms:* transient hemolytic anemia, cholestatic jaundice and hyperlipidemia. Patient presents with right upper quadrant pain and fever. Treatment consists of alcohol abstinence, blood transfusion, and administration of glutathione, diuretics, ursodeoxycholic acid and vitamin supplements. Most patients recover in 4–6 weeks.

Postmortem Findings

i. Odor of alcohol around the mouth and nose.
ii. Congestion of conjunctiva.
iii. Rigor mortis is prolonged and decomposition is retarded.
iv. Acute inflammation of the stomach with coating of mucus.
v. All viscera are congested and smells of alcohol.
vi. Blood is fluid and dark.

Medico-legal Aspects

- The ICD-11 criteria require that any medical or drug-related (non-alcohol) conditions must be excluded before the diagnosis of alcohol intoxication is made. This is important, since allegation of negligence can be brought against the doctor in assessing an intoxicated individual in police custody when death may occur because of failure to exclude any pathological conditions.
- Patients with alcohol intoxication should be evaluated for coexisting injuries and metabolic disorders. A presumably 'inebriated' comatose patient who is still unarousable 3–4 h after initial assessment should be considered to have head injury, a cerebrovascular accident, CNS infection or another toxic etiology for the AMS, until proven otherwise. Hypoglycemia should always be sought in such cases.
- There is a strong association between binge drinking and violent crimes, such as homicide, assault, robbery and sexual offenses.
- An increased risk of injury and traffic accident has been found in individuals with alcohol intoxication.
- In an embalmed body, determination of ethanol or methanol carries no legal value, since embalming fluid itself contains both.
- Routine use of BAC is controversial because it is unlikely to affect management in a patient who is awake and

alert. It is safe to discharge the patient once he is clinically (not numerically) no longer intoxicated.
- There should not be any delay in waiting for laboratory tests (to confirm the presence of alcohol) before starting the treatment.
- **Sec. 85 IPC:** Nothing is an offense which is done by a person who at the time of doing it, by reason of intoxication, is incapable of knowing the nature of the act, or what he is doing is either wrong or contrary to law; provided that thing which intoxicated him was administered to him without his knowledge or against his will.
- Voluntary drunkenness is not an excuse for commission of crime.
- **Sec. 510 IPC:** Misconduct by a drunken person in public is punishable with imprisonment up to 24 h.

FM 1.9, 14.16
- Describe the importance of documentation in medical practice (issuance of drunkenness certificate).
- To examine and prepare medico-legal report of drunk person in a simulated/supervised environment.

DRUNKENNESS

Definition: Drunkenness is a condition which results from excessive intake of alcohol to a degree that mental and physical faculties are noticeably impaired.

The person under its influence shows the following:
 i. Loss of control over his mental faculties.
 ii. Inability to perform the duties in which he is engaged.
 iii. Dangerous to himself or/and to the community.

Consent for Examination

- The detained person should not be examined and blood, urine or breath should not be collected without his written consent.
- If the person becomes unconscious or incapable of giving consent, examination and treatment can be carried out, but the doctor should not disclose any information obtained during examination and wait for his consent, till he regains consciousness.
- Under **Sec. 53 (1) CrPC**, examination of an accused can be carried out by a doctor at the request of the police, even without his consent and by use of force, if necessary. Such examination may include taking of body fluids in cases of suspected intoxication.

Diagnosing a Case of Drunkenness

Preliminary data, such as name, age, sex, address, time of examination, two identification marks and person escorting the patient should be noted.

History: The history of relevant events should be obtained from the person while observing him. Enquire about past illnesses and drug treatment. Note, if he admits having taken alcoholic drinks. If so, the nature, quantity and time of consumption should be recorded.

> **NOTA BENE**
> **Exclusion of Injuries and Pathological Conditions**
> Before diagnosing the case as drunkenness, it is better to rule out the following conditions, which simulate alcoholic intoxication:
> - Head injury.
> - *Metabolic disorders:* Hypoglycemia, diabetic precoma, uremia and hyperthyroidism.
> - *Neurological conditions:* Intracranial tumors, epilepsy, Parkinsonism and disseminated sclerosis.
> - *Drug overdose:* Insulin, barbiturates, antihistamines, cocaine, morphine, atropine, hyoscine and tranquilizers.
> - *Psychological disorders:* Hypomania and general paresis.
> - Febrile illnesses.
> - Exposure to carbon monoxide.

Clinical Examination

General Appearance

- Manner of dressing—properly dressed or not, and soiling of clothes.
- Posture—whether over-erect and over smart, can stand steady or not, leans to a side or stoops forward, and can stand without support or not.

General Examination

The scalp should be inspected and palpated for evidence of any head injury. Any other injury present is noted. Injuries could have been sustained in a motor vehicle accident or as a result of resistance to arrest. Careful documentation of these injuries needs to be done.

Specific Physical Examination

 i. **Gait** is observed for any unsteadiness, staggering, bumping into people or furniture. The best way is to watch him approaching the examination facility, or to ask the person to go to the weighing machine, and while doing so, watch the gait. Gait on turning (normal, unsteady, stumbling) is also noted.
 ii. **Orientation and memory:** Ask him about incidents which have occurred few hours prior to examination to check his memory (clear, vague or confused) and mental alertness. Ask him about the date, time and place where he is at present (good, moderate, bad or indefinite).
 iii. **Behavior:** Whether noisy, jovial, boastful, rude, emotional, talkative, excited, nervous or uncontrollable. If the subject is cooperative, state it.
 iv. **Face:** Note his face, whether normal, flushed or pale. Alcohol is vasodilatatory, and redness of the face is indicative of this.

v. **Speech:** Record whether the patient can understand, and whether his speech is normal, thick and slurred, stuttering or confused. Speech is also observed for incoherence, unintelligible, aggressive, offensive or over precise.
vi. **Tongue:** Examine the tongue, whether dry, moist and clean or furred. Dry tongue is seen in thirst, and waning phase of BAC. Moist tongue may be indicative of having taken any drink including water.
vii. **Signs of vomiting and salivation:** As soon as the alcohol reaches a concentration of about 20% in the intestines, an ileus follows which is responsible for vomiting. Nausea is responsible for abnormal salivation. Salivation and drooling may also be the result of suppression of swallowing reflex. It is, therefore, only found in the severely intoxicated.
viii. **Smell of alcohol:** Strong, moderate, faint or none. The smell is dependent on the capabilities of the examiner, and smell acuity differs from person to person. The smell of the breath may confirm that alcohol has been taken and the type of drink, but is no guide whatsoever to the amount, e.g., certain liquors, such as vodka have a lesser odor than that of beer.
ix. **Ears:** Examine the ears for any discharge and any chronic disease. Any middle ear condition may have an impact on the balance and the maintaining thereof in the subject (vertigo, ataxia) or inability to hear questions or commands.
x. **Handwriting:** The person is asked to copy a few lines from a book or newspaper, and handwriting should be assessed. Note the time taken, ability to write in line and any repetition or omission of words. The individual can be asked to sign his name and compared with his driving license. Drawing simple patterns, such as triangle and diamond may be preferable, if the person is illiterate.
xi. **Eyes:** Examine the eyes, noting the state of the conjunctiva (normal or congested), pupillary size (normal, equal, unequal, mydriasis or miosis), response to light, visual fields and acuity (reading the time on a clock across a room), and the presence of nystagmus (coarse, fine, continuous or absent). Note should be made of use of spectacles or contact lens and any other abnormal eye findings. In drunkenness, drooping and swollen eyelids, congestion of conjunctiva and horizontal nystagmus may be seen, and convergence test is negative (difficulty in convergence).

- *Conjunctiva*: Alcohol is known for its vasodilation and hence suffusion.
- *Response to light*: The person is asked to look at an object in the room while a light is shone into the eye. This will eliminate the possibility of pupil size change as a result of accommodation. The reaction may be normal, delayed (intoxication), or non-reacting (severe intoxication).
- *Nystagmus*: The head is held in the neutral position. The subject is asked to follow with the eyes of an object held about 30–40 cm in front of him/her. The object is moved from side to side to a maximum angle of about 45° **(Fig. 47.2)**. If the object is moved to a more acute angle, the muscles of eye movement will be stressed and nystagmus can be elicited in a sober person.

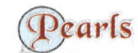

Conditions showing nystagmus
Alcohol intoxication, fatigue, emotion, postural hypotension, and ingestion of sedatives and tranquilizers.

xii. **Tests to determine incoordination:** Watch the patient unbutton his shirt, dressing, undressing or handling objects like picking up a pen. Carry out a series of *standardized field impairment tests (FITs)* to check muscle coordination. These consist of Romberg test, Walk and Turn test, One Leg Stand test and Finger Nose test **(Box 47.2)**.
xiii. **Knee reflexes** are elicited to check whether normal, exaggerated or depressed. Reflexes are equally depressed in intoxication. Sometimes, the subject may exaggerate to impress the examiner, but they are usually not equal in magnitude.

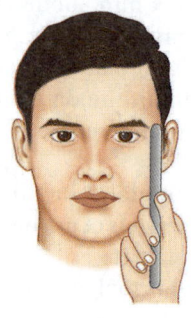 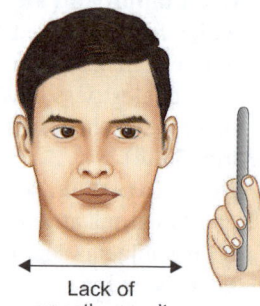 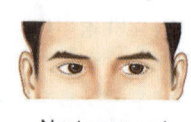 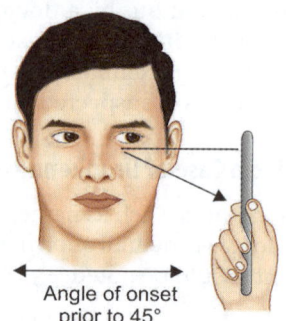

Fig. 47.2: Horizontal gaze nystagmus test.

Box 47.2 Standardized field impairment tests (Fig. 47.3)

- **Romberg test:** The person is asked to stand up straight with feet together and arms down by the sides. When told to start, he should tilt his head back slightly and close his eyes. Tell him to keep the head tilted backwards with eyes closed for about 30 secs, and then bring his head forward. Assessment is based on ability to stand still during instructions, whether he sways excessively or unable to complete the test (*positive sign*). The essential feature is that the patient is unsteadier than with open eyes. With severe intoxication, a positive Romberg is seen even with open eyes or in the sitting position.
- **Walk and turn test:** Identify a real or imaginary line. The person with his arms by the sides is asked to put his left foot on the line, then his right foot on the line in front of the left touching heel to toe. When told to start, the person should take nine heel-to-toe steps along the line. On each step, the heel of the foot must be placed against the toe of the other foot. When the ninth step has been taken, he then leaves the front foot on the line and turns around using a series of small steps with the other foot. After turning, he then takes another nine heel-to-toe steps along the line. The person is assessed as whether he is able to stand during instructions, start too soon or late, stops walking, incorrect turn, misses heel to toe, steps off line, raises arms and incorrect step count.
- **One leg stand test:** The person is asked to stand with his feet together and arms by the sides. When told to start, he should raise his foot 6–8 inches off the ground, keeping his leg straight and toes pointing forward, with the foot parallel to the ground. He should keep looking at his elevated foot while counting out loud in the following manner, 'one…two…three…four…' and so on until the examiner tells him to stop. The person is assessed as to whether he sways, hops, puts his foot down or raises arms.
- **Finger nose test:** The person is asked to stand with her feet together. The arms extended with both hands closed and out in front or on sides, with the index finger of both hands extended. When the examiner instructs, she should close her eyes and touch the tip of her nose with the tip of her finger and lower her hand once done. The examiner calls out the hands in the following order: left, right, left, right. The person is assessed whether she sways her body, use incorrect hand, and any other comments.

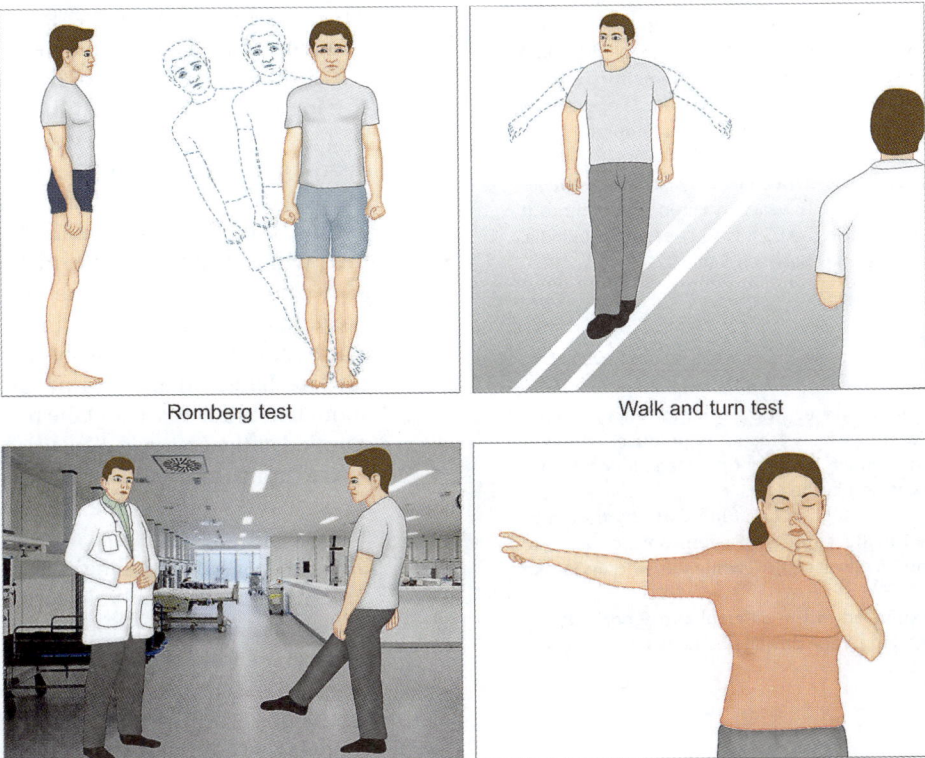

Fig. 47.3: Field impairment tests

xiv. **Examine for drug abuse:** Look for needle marks, shivering, yawning, rhinorrhea, gooseflesh and lacrimation.

xv. Examine the **cardiovascular system** noting pulse, blood pressure (slight rise in BP may occur, often the systolic pressure), temperature and heart sounds.

xvi. **Respiratory** (hurried, slow, shallow, deep, stertorous, sighing or gasping, any added sounds) and **gastrointestinal system** (soft, tender, bowel sounds, enlarged liver or spleen, ascites) examinations are done both to exclude other diagnosis and to find out complications related to acute or chronic alcohol consumption.

Opinion

The report should be written at that time, and at the end the police informed about the doctor's opinion (based on examination and laboratory findings). The opinion can be drafted with any one of the following statements:
i. He/she has not consumed alcohol.
ii. He/she has consumed alcohol, but is not under the influence of it.
iii. He/she has consumed alcohol and is under its influence.

> **NOTA BENE**
> - **Driving under the influence of alcohol or drunk driving:** Operating a motor vehicle after having consumed alcohol or other drugs to the degree that mental and motor skills are impaired.
> - Authorities around the world have laid down their own standards for permissible maximum BAC **(Table 47.3)**.
> - According to the **Motor Vehicles (Amendment) Act, 2019,** in case of drunken driving, imprisonment up to 6 months with/without fine of up to ₹ 10,000 in case of first time offense. For the second offense, the punishment is 2 years imprisonment with/without fine of ₹ 15,000. There can be arrest without warrant, a breath test and a laboratory test can also be carried out.
> - The *age for possession and consumption of alcoholic beverages* in Australia and Canada is 18 years, in European countries it is between 16–18 years, in the US it is >21 years, and in India, it is between 18–25 (varies between States).

> **NOTA BENE**
> - **Auto-brewery syndrome or gut fermentation syndrome** is a rare condition in which ethanol is produced through endogenous fermentation by fungi or bacteria (*Candida* and *Saccharomyces* families) in the GIT.
> - Patients usually have high-sugar, high-carbohydrate diet and present with the signs and symptoms of alcohol intoxication and an elevated BAC while denying an intake of alcohol.
> - It should be considered in the differential diagnosis of any individual arrested for drunk driving and denying any alcohol consumption.

TABLE 47.3: Permissible BAC in different countries

Permissible BAC (mg/dL)	Countries
0	Hungary, Pakistan, Saudi Arabia, UAE
20	Norway, Poland, Sweden
30	India, China, Japan
50	Australia, France, Germany, Italy, Spain, Netherlands, Russia, Denmark
80	Canada, UK, US (100 mg/dL in some States)

LABORATORY DIAGNOSIS

The common laboratory tests include estimation of alcohol from:
i. Blood
ii. Urine
iii. Breath
iv. Vitreous fluid, bile and other tissues (during autopsy).

Measurement of Alcohol

- The *BAC* is *the most useful measure,* as there is rapid equilibration across the blood-brain barrier, therefore BAC reflects the concentration of alcohol currently affecting the brain.
- *Urine alcohol*: BAC is a direct method for the determination of a blood alcohol level whereas urine analysis is an indirect method. The pool of urine in the bladder at any given time is an accumulation of secreted urine since the last emptying of the bladder.
    - At any given point in time, urine alcohol concentration (UAC) will be different from the BAC. After the cessation of drinking, the BAC may rise for a period of time. At this point, the UAC will be less than the BAC because of absorption and distribution throughout the body fluids. Thereafter, the BAC and UAC curves will cross. For some period of time, the UAC will continue to rise, whereas the BAC will remain constant or begin to decrease. In the post-absorptive state, the UAC will always exceed the BAC. Hence, a urine level in bladder is a combination of continuously changing BAC.
    - UAC is reliable when two urine samples are collected about half to 1 h apart, and the bladder is completely emptied at the first void. The urine sample collected second time is formed within the period of the first and second void samples. The difference in UAC values also provides information concerning the state of the UAC curve (rising or falling). In addition, the alcohol content of the second void represents the average alcohol concentration of the urine formed between the first and second void. An average 1.33:1 ratio of urine alcohol to blood alcohol is generally used.
- *Breath alcohol*, unlike urine, is in equilibrium with blood, even though in a very small concentration of about 1: 2300. At 37°C, a level of 1 mg/dL in blood will be equivalent to about 0.43 µg/dL in breath. The exact ratio of blood/breath alcohol is temperature dependent and varies slightly with other factors, such as the depth of respiration and concentration of alcohol.

Widmark's formula is used to estimate *blood* **alcohol level.**

$$a = cpr$$

where, a – the total amount of alcohol (in grams) absorbed in the body

- c – the concentration of alcohol in blood (in g/kg)
- p – the weight of the person (in kg)
- r – constant (0.68 in men and 0.5 in women)

Alcohol level from *urine* is estimated with the formula:

$$a = 3/4\ qpr$$

where, q – concentration of alcohol in urine (in g/L) and 'a', 'p' and 'r' are same as above.

Kozelka and Hine method or Cavett method: It involves aeration/distillation or diffusion of alcohol under low pressure. It utilizes the principle that alcohol is easily oxidized to acetic acid by oxidizing agents, such as potassium dichromate and sulphuric acid.

Other Methods

i. *Gas liquid chromatography (GLC)*: Most reliable method. It is extremely sensitive and produces accurate quantitative results. In high performance liquid chromatography (HPLC), the sample is in liquid state at the time of analysis, rather than in volatile state as in GLC.*

ii. *Alcohol dehydrogenase (ADH) method*: It is highly specific and accurate.

> **NOTA BENE**
>
> Any method to determine ethanol in blood and urine can be classified into:
> - Macro (requiring 1–2 mL of specimen)
> - Micro (requiring 0.1–0.2 mL of specimen or less)
>
> The methods are:
> i. **Chemical**: Widmark method, Cavett method, etc.
> ii. **Biochemical**: ADH method
> iii. **Physical**: GLC
>
> - **Chemical methods**: It depends on reduction of a dichromate/sulfuric acid by alcohol vapor.
> - **Biochemical method**: *ADH method*: Micro-method, alcohol is oxidized by the ADH enzyme in the presence of a coenzyme; the reduced coenzyme is then determined calorimetrically by a separate method, from the result of which the alcohol content of the original sample is calculated.
> - **Breathalyzer (or breath analyzer)** is a device for estimating BAC from a breath sample. In 1954, *Dr Robert Borkenstein* invented the breathalyzer which used chemical oxidation and photometry to determine alcohol concentration (breath passes through a solution of potassium dichromate, which oxidizes ethanol to acetic acid, changing color in the process). Subsequent breathalyzers have converted primarily to *infrared spectroscopy*.
> - **Ethanol saliva testing** (*saliva dipstick*) is an alternative to breath ethanol analysis in patients regardless of their mental status. Fatty acid ethyl esters may be a highly sensitive test for recent ethanol use as they remain in the body for at least 24 h. Ethyl glucuronide and ethyl sulfate are nonoxidative direct metabolites in urine which can be detected for recent ethanol intake.

COLLECTION OF SAMPLES IN THE LIVING

- **Blood:** Soap and water is used to clean the site to be venipunctured. The blood is collected from antecubital or femoral vein using a disposable syringe. Blood container should be tightly stoppered to prevent loss of alcohol by evaporation, and labeled with name, date, time of taking the specimen and signature of the medical officer.
- **Urine:** Full quantity of urine passed must be collected. The patient is asked to pass urine in a toilet where there is no water source (preventing him to dilute alcohol concentration by adding water). It is collected in a large clean, sterilized, screw capped bottle. The urine is preserved, and labeled with name, date, time of taking the specimen and signature of the medical officer.
- **Breath:** The patient is asked to blow into a rubber balloon with a glass tube filled with yellow crystals. The bands of crystals in the tube change color from yellow to green depending on concentration of alcohol in the blood (manual test).

Postmortem Samples

Details are given in Chapter 7.

In temperate climates, postmortem blood alcohol determination is completely valid for 36 h after death.

> **Erroneous BAC results can be obtained due to:**
> - Postmortem diffusion from other body fluids and tissues
> - Improperly preserved sample
> - Putrefaction
> - Samples stored at room temperature for >1 week
> - Hemolysis
> - Clot formation

ALCOHOLISM

Alcoholism: A chronic, progressive disease characterized by tolerance and physical dependence to ethanol and pathological organ changes.

These is a gradual physical, mental and moral deterioration.

1. **Physical:** There is lack of personal hygiene, loss of appetite, chronic gastroenteritis, wasting, peripheral neuropathies, erectile dysfunction, sterility, fatty changes in liver and heart, cirrhosis, tremors, insomnia, red eyes and intermittent infections.
2. **Mental:** There is loss of memory, impaired power of judgment and dementia.

> **Clinical syndromes associated with chronic alcoholism:**
> - Delirium tremens
> - Alcoholic hallucinosis
> - Korsakoff's psychosis
> - Wernicke's encephalopathy
> - Marchiafava-Bignami syndrome
> - Alcoholic paranoia
> - Alcoholic seizures

3. **Moral:** It manifests as crimes which the addict commits to get his drink. He becomes morbidly jealous and suspicious of his wife's fidelity, and may assault her.

---

* Gas chromatography-Mass spectrometry (GC-MS) is the only method of analysis that is 100% specific.

Treatment

i. Sudden withdrawal of alcoholic drinks.
ii. **Antabuse** *(disulfiram)* is given as an aversion technique. Disulfiram (tetraethyl thiuram disulfide) blocks metabolism of alcohol at the acetaldehyde stage (*see* **Flowchart 47.1**). Acetaldehyde accumulates in blood causing disulfiram-ethanol reaction (*aldehyde syndrome*).
   - **Symptoms**: Flushing, palpitation, nausea, vomiting, anxiety, tightness of chest, hypotension, sweating, throbbing headache, giddiness, sense of impending doom and abdominal cramps appear due to which patient dislikes alcohol. Duration of the syndrome (1–4 h) depends on the amount of alcohol consumed.
   - **Dose**: The initial dose is 250–500 mg for 1–2 weeks (taken before bedtime) followed by a maintenance dose of 250 mg/day (range 125–500 mg). The total daily dosage should not exceed 500 mg.
   - **Contraindications**: Coronary artery disease, liver failure, chronic renal failure, peripheral neuropathy, muscular disease, history of psychosis and pregnancy (1st trimester).
iii. Citrated calcium carbimide (*Temposil*): 100 mg/day in 2 divided doses instead of antabuse may be given.
iv. Metronidazole, nitrafezole and methyltetrazolethiol are other alternatives.
v. Nutrients, vitamins and gradual return to a normal balanced diet.
vi. Symptomatic treatment.

Withdrawal Symptoms

Tremulousness or shakes or jitters (*most common sign*), weakness, pain in muscle, cold sweat, insomnia, loss of appetite, vomiting, diarrhea, restlessness, exaggerated reflexes, raised temperature, fluctuating BP, hallucinations, loss of memory and delirium tremens.

Many alcoholics experience '*the shakes*' approximately 12–24 h after their last drink. The shakes are tremors caused by over excitation of the CNS. Tremors may be accompanied by tachycardia, diaphoresis, anorexia, and insomnia. After 24–72 h, the alcoholic may have '*rum fits*' (i.e., generalized seizures).

NOTA BENE

- **Disulfiram** action was discovered accidentally, as the substance was intended to provide a remedy for parasitic infestations. However, workers testing the substance on themselves reported severe symptoms after alcohol consumption.

   It is also being studied as a treatment for *cocaine dependence*, as it prevents the breakdown of dopamine (neurotransmitter whose release is stimulated by cocaine), the excess dopamine results in increased anxiety, higher blood pressure, restlessness and other unpleasant symptoms (*see* **Flowchart 47.1**).

- Animal charcoal, fungus (*Coprinus atramentarius*), sulfonylureas and certain cephalosporins also cause a disulfirum-like action.
- **CAGE questionnaire:** Developed by *Dr John Ewing*, CAGE is an internationally used assessment instrument for identifying alcoholics.
   i. Have you ever felt you should **C**ut down on your drinking?
   ii. Have people **A**nnoyed you, by criticizing your drinking?
   iii. Have you ever felt bad or **G**uilty about your drinking?
   iv. Have you ever had a drink, first thing in the morning, to steady your nerves or to get rid of a hangover (**E**ye opener)?

   Scoring: Item responses on the CAGE are scored 0 or 1, with a higher score an indication of alcohol problems. A total score of 2 or greater is considered clinically significant.

FM 5.5

Describe and discuss delirium tremens.

DELIRIUM TREMENS

This is an acute organic brain syndrome, usually seen within 2–4 days of complete absence from heavy alcohol drinking in chronic alcoholics, and most severe alcohol withdrawal syndrome.

Causes

- Sudden excess or sudden withdrawal of alcohol.
- Long continual ingestion of alcohol.
- Shock due to severe trauma, e.g., fracture in a chronic alcoholic.
- Acute infections, such as pneumonia or influenza in a chronic alcoholic.

Signs and Symptoms

There is an **acute attack of insanity** in which there is:
i. Clouding of consciousness with disorientation in time and space.
ii. Coarse muscular tremors of face, tongue and hands.
iii. Insomnia with reversal of sleep-wake cycle, and loss of memory.
iv. Psychomotor agitation, ataxia, uncontrollable fear, and tendency to commit suicide/homicide/violent assault or cause damage to property.
v. Marked autonomic disturbances with tachycardia, fever, sweating, hypertension and pupillary dilatation.
vi. Peculiar type of *delirium of horrors* due to hallucinations of sight and hearing. *Tactile hallucinations* of insects and ants crawling under the skin or on the beds may occur.

Treatment

(For both withdrawal symptoms and delirium tremens)
i. Diazepam (40–80 mg/day in divided doses) is used.
ii. Oral multi-B vitamins, including thiamine 50–100 mg is given daily for a week or more.

iii. Chlordiazepoxide (80–200 mg/day in divided doses) or haloperidol 20 mg or more/day may be used.
iv. Intravenous fluids are avoided, unless there is evidence of bleeding, vomiting or diarrhea.
v. In some withdrawal symptom cases, only restoration of alcoholic drinks helps.
vi. In cases of urgent sedation as in delirium tremens—phenobarbitone or chlorpromazine injection can be given, and then detoxification and maintenance of nutrition is carried on with 5% dextrose solution IV and thiamine.
vii. Symptomatic treatment.

Medico-legal Aspects

- It is a medical emergency and should be treated on an inpatient basis.
- When a person in delirium tremens commits any illegal act, he is not held responsible by the reason that he is considered to be mentally unsound during this state **(Sec. 84 IPC)**.

Alcoholic Hallucinosis

- It is a state of hallucination, mainly auditory with systematized *delusions of persecution* lasting from weeks to months.
- Occurs during abstinence in 2% of patients who have been on regular alcohol till then.
- It is a psychiatric emergency, requiring hospitalization, sedation and close monitoring. Usually, recovery occurs in a month.
- Patient may become homicidal or suicidal in response to his hallucination.
- **Treatment:** Same as delirium tremens.

WERNICKE'S ENCEPHALOPATHY

This is an acute reaction due to severe thiamine deficiency (vitamin B-1), the commonest cause being chronic alcohol abuse. Characteristically, the onset occurs after a period of persistent vomiting.

Signs and Symptoms

i. **Ocular**: Coarse nystagmus and ophthalmoparesis (usually the VIth cranial nerve is involved). Pupillary irregularity, retinal hemorrhages, papilledema and impairment of vision.
ii. **CNS**: Disorientation, confusion, recent memory disturbances, poor attention span and distractibility. Apathy and ataxia are early symptoms.
iii. Peripheral neuropathy and serious malnutrition are often coexistent.

Pathologically, neuronal degeneration and hemorrhage is seen in the thalamus, hypothalamus (mammillary bodies) and midbrain.

KORSAKOFF'S PSYCHOSIS

Korsakoff first identified this condition in 1887. Korsakoff's psychosis often follows Wernicke's encephalopathy, so they are referred to as *Wernicke-Korsakoff syndrome*.

Cause: Severe, untreated thiamine deficiency, secondary to chronic alcohol abuse.

Signs and Symptoms

It presents as an *organic amnestic syndrome*, characterized by inability to learn new information, impairment of short-term memory and compensatory confabulation. Insight is often impaired.

The *pathological lesion* is usually widespread, but changes are seen in bilateral dorsomedial nuclei of thalamus and mammillary bodies. The changes are also seen in periventricular and periaqueductal gray matter, cerebellum and parts of brainstem.

Sometimes, **alcohol dementia** may be associated with Wernicke-Korsakoff syndrome, which is caused by long-term or excessive drinking resulting in neurological damage and impairment of memory.

Treatment

i. Intravenous thiamine (in the form of *Pabrinex,* two vials 8 hourly for 48 h) initially, followed by oral (100 mg 8 hourly).
ii. Supplementation of electrolytes, particularly magnesium and potassium, may be required in addition to thiamine.

- **Alcoholic peripheral neuropathy:** Symptoms of alcoholic polyneuritis are weakness, pain in extremities, wrist and foot drop, unsteady gait, loss of deep reflexes and tenderness of muscles of arms and legs.
- **Alcoholic paranoia:** In this, there is a fixed delusion, but no hallucinations. Patient becomes suspicious of the motives and actions of those he meets and of his family members.
- **Marchiafava-Bignami syndrome:** This is a rare disorder characterized by disorientation, epilepsy, ataxia, dysarthria, hallucinations, spastic limb paralysis, and personality and intellectual deterioration. There is a widespread demyelination of corpus callosum, optic tracts and cerebellar peduncles. The cause is probably some alcohol-related nutritional deficiency.
- **Alcoholic seizures ('rum fits'):** In alcohol dependence persons, generalized tonic clonic seizure may occur after 12–48 h of heavy bout of drinking alcohol. Multiple seizures are more common than single seizure. Sometimes, status epilepticus and delirium tremens may be precipitated.

NOTA BENE

- Thiamine is absorbed from the duodenum; alcohol interferes with its active transport, and chronic liver disease causes decreased capacity of the liver to store thiamine.
- Thiamine is converted to its active form *thiamine pyrophosphate* in neuronal and glial cells which serves as a cofactor for several enzymes (transketolase, pyruvate dehydrogenase and alpha ketoglutarate). The main function of these enzymes in the brain is lipid (myelin sheath) and carbohydrate metabolism, production of amino acids and production of glucose-derived neurotransmitters.

FM 9.4 Describe general principles and basic methodologies in treatment of poisoning with regard to methanol.

METHYL ALCOHOL (METHANOL)

Introduction

Methanol (carbinol, wood alcohol, wood naphtha or wood spirits) is found in cleaning materials, solvents, paints, varnishes, formaldehyde solutions, antifreeze, windshield washer fluid (30–40% methanol) and duplicating fluids.

Physical properties: Colorless, volatile liquid with odor similar to ethyl alcohol and a burning taste.

Uses: In industries as solvent, in laboratories with ethanol as an antiseptic spirit.

Routes of intake: Ingestion, dermal absorption and inhalation.

Absorption and Excretion

It is rapidly absorbed from the stomach, intestines, lungs and skin, and achieves a maximal concentration 30–90 min after ingestion.
- Oxidation is slow, 15% of that of ethyl alcohol, and acts as a cumulative poison.
- During metabolism, it is converted into formaldehyde and formic acid which is metabolized to folic acid, folinic acid, carbon dioxide and water **(Flowchart 47.3)**. Eighty percent is excreted unchanged from lungs and 3–5% in urine.
- Without competition for alcohol dehydrogenase, methanol undergoes zero-order metabolism and is excreted at a rate of 8.5–20 mg/dL/h. Once methanol experiences competitive inhibition from ethanol or fomepizole, the metabolism changes to first order.

Action

- It causes ethanol-like CNS depression and increased serum osmolality.
- Formic acid causes an high anion-gap metabolic acidosis and retinal toxicity.
- Mechanism of cellular toxicity is similar to that of cyanide or CO poisoning.

Signs and Symptoms

- Symptoms occur 12–24 h after ingestion. Unlike ethanol or isopropanol, methanol does not cause much of an inebriated state.
- Initially, the symptoms from methanol intoxication are similar to those of ethanol, often with disinhibition and ataxia.
- Methanol causes severe metabolic acidosis, visual disturbances and permanent neurological deficit.

System	Signs and symptoms
GIT	Nausea, vomiting, cramps in abdomen, spirit-like odor in the nostrils and mouth, dehydration.
RS	Dyspnea, cyanosis, respiratory depression.
CNS	Headache, dizziness, vertigo, restlessness, muscular weakness, hypothermia, delirium, amnesia, convulsion (terminal event), coma.
Renal	Acidosis, strongly acidic urine, scant urine.
Ocular	Pupils: Fixed and dilated. Visual disturbances, such as photophobia, '**halo vision**'*, blurred or misty vision (**snowfield vision**), central or peripheral scotoma, decreased light perception, concentric diminution of visual fields (**tunnel vision**) causing temporary or complete *blindness due to optic neuritis and atrophy* from accumulation of formic acid within the optic nerve. Retinal edema and hyperemia may be seen.
Pancreas	Pancreatitis may occur.

*Bright circles that surround the light source.

Levels >20 mg/dL are considered toxic, and treatment should be initiated based on blood levels alone.

Cause of death: Respiratory failure due to pulmonary edema, circulatory failure due to shock or coma due to cerebral and cerebellar hemorrhage.

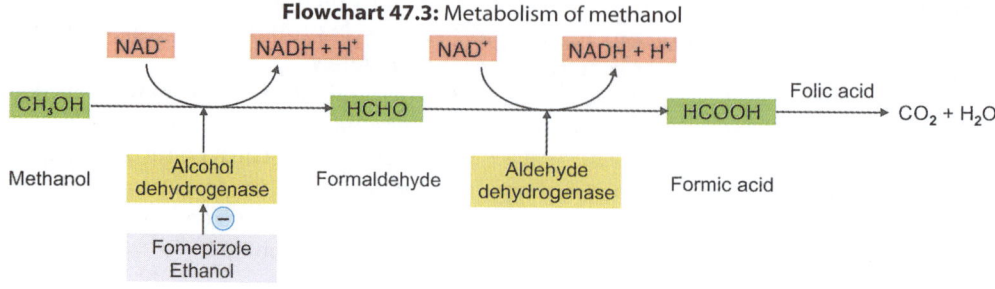

Flowchart 47.3: Metabolism of methanol

Fatal Dose

Range is 30–240 mL, but 60–140 mL of methanol is usually fatal (>150 mg/dL in blood).

Fatal period: 24–36 h.

Diagnosis: Color test involves the oxidation of methanol to formaldehyde using $KMnO_4$. Sodium bisulfate and chromotropic acid are then added, followed by layering of concentrated H_2SO_4. A purple color at the acid/filtrate interface indicates positive test.

Treatment

i. **Preventing absorption by gastric lavage**: Five percent sodium bicarbonate solution is used and 500 mL is left in the stomach.
ii. **Use of bicarbonate to combat acidosis**: Oral administration of sodium bicarbonate, 2 g in 250 mL of water, 4 hourly.
iii. **Folate therapy**: Calcium folinate/leucovorin (calcium salt of folinic acid) IV tends to reduce blood formate levels by enhancing its metabolism. High dose of folinic acid (50–75 mg every 6 hourly) is indicated. Thiamine and pyridoxine may be given. Vitamin B_{12} is not used.
iv. **Administration of ethanol as competitive antagonist**: Ethanol has a much higher affinity for alcohol dehydrogenase than methanol and ethylene glycol. Presence of ethanol will therefore inhibit formation of toxic metabolites from methanol and ethylene glycol.
Dose: Loading dose of 0.8–1 mL/kg orally of 95% ethanol (v/v) in 200 mL of orange juice or 7.6–10 mL/kg IV of 10% ethanol (v/v) in D5W over 30 min, and then maintenance dose of 0.15 mL/kg/h orally or 1.4 mL/kg/h IV. Desired serum ethanol concentration is 100–150 mg/dL.
v. **Antidote**: 4-methylpyrazole (**fomepizole**) is a competitive inhibitor of alcohol dehydrogenase. It blocks the formation of formaldehyde and formic acid, and can be used instead of ethanol.
Dose: Loading dose of 15 mg/kg over 30 min, followed by 10 mg/kg every 12 h for 4 doses, then 15 mg/kg every 12 h.
vi. **Other measures**
   - Eyes should be kept covered to protect them from light.
   - *Hemodialysis,* as soon as possible in case of severe poisoning.
   - Symptomatic treatment.

Postmortem Findings

External

Signs of asphyxia with cyanosis and prominent postmortem staining are observed. Froth from the mouth may be seen. Pyridine may give the skin a purple color.

Internal

i. **GIT:** Mucous membrane of stomach and duodenum are congested and inflamed with small hemorrhages.
ii. **Lungs**: Congested and edematous.
iii. **Liver**: Necrobiosis and fatty change.
iv. **Kidneys**: Tubular degeneration.
v. **Brain**: Edematous and cerebral infarction—ischemic, as well as hemorrhagic, selectively affecting the putamen and sub-cortical white matter.
vi. **Urinary bladder**: Mucosa congested.
vii. **Blood**: Dark and fluid.

Medico-legal Aspects

- Mostly accidental, due to consumption of adulterated liquor containing methyl alcohol (which is often a component of *'bootlegged alcohol'*) by lower socio-economic classes that results in mass poisoning (**'hooch tragedy'***).
- Sometimes, it is used as intoxicating beverage when ethanol is not available.
- Suicides and homicides may occur, but not common.
- Accidental poisoning may be seen in children as methanol is a constituent of commonly available liquids.

NOTA BENE

- **Metabolic acidosis** is reduction in HCO_3^- with compensatory reduction in pCO_2; pH may be low or slightly subnormal. It is categorized as *high or normal anion gap* based on the presence or absence of un-measured anions in serum. Causes include accumulation of ketones and lactic acid, renal failure and drug or toxin ingestion (high anion gap); and GI or renal HCO_3^- loss (normal anion gap).
  Signs and symptoms include nausea and vomiting, lethargy, and hyperpnea. *Diagnosis* is clinical and with ABG and serum electrolyte measurement. The cause is treated; IV $NaHCO_3$ may be indicated when pH is very low.
  - Toxins causing high-anion gap acidosis: Alcohol, methanol, ethylene glycol, paraldehyde and salicylates. Lactic acidosis may be caused by carbon monoxide, cyanide and iron.
  - Most common cause of normal anion gap acidosis is diarrhea followed by renal tubular acidosis.
- Any alcoholic beverage made under unlicensed conditions is called **illicit liquor**. Usually substandard raw material is used; often this is spiked with other chemicals. Under unregulated conditions, methanol may be produced along with ethanol. Sometimes, industrial methyl alcohol or denatured spirit is added by illicit brewers to save costs and in mistaken belief that it will increase potency. There have been incidents where chemicals, such as OPCs have been added to illicit liquor. Gujarat is the only State in India that has death penalty for those found guilty of making and selling spurious liquor.
- Although the eye is the primary site of organ toxicity, in the later stages specific changes may be seen in the basal ganglia.
- If vision is impaired, ocular examination may reveal dilated pupils that are unreactive to light with hyperemia of the optic disc. After several days, the red disc becomes pale and the patient may become blind. Typically, subjective complaints precede physical findings in the eye.

---

* The term '*hooch*' for liquor comes from the Hoochinoo Indians, known for their ability to make liquor so strong, it could knock someone out.

Describe general principles and basic methodologies in treatment of poisoning with regard to ethylene glycol.

ETHYLENE GLYCOL

Ethylene glycol is the major constituent of antifreeze solutions. It is a clear, colorless, odorless, non-volatile liquid with a bitter-sweet taste. It is not absorbed through the skin.

Action: Ethylene glycol itself is not toxic, but the toxicity is due to metabolites glycolic and oxalic acids, which inhibits oxidative phosphorylation.
- Oxalic acid combines with calcium to form calcium oxalate crystals which accumulates in the proximal convoluted tubules causing renal failure.
- Metabolic acidosis occurs from glycolic acid.

Signs and Symptoms

It can be divided into neurological, cardiorespiratory and renal.
- **CNS symptoms** usually develop within half hour to 12 h after ingestion. The individual develops nausea, vomiting, slurred speech, tipsy sensation, severe headache, delusions, dizziness, feeling of breathlessness, convulsions and coma.
- **Cardiorespiratory symptoms** usually appear 12–24 h after ingestion. Tachycardia, tachypnea and congestive heart failure are present.
- **Renal:** Acute tubular necrosis. This usually is seen 24–72 h after ingestion. Oxalate crystals are seen in the urine.

Cause of death: Death occurs from renal failure or heart attack.
- **Fatal dose:** 100–200 mL.
- **Fatal period:** Few hours to 3 days.

Treatment: Gastric lavage is done. Charcoal is not very effective. Treatment is similar as for methanol.

Postmortem Findings

Non-specific findings.
i. Organs are congested.
ii. Mucous membrane of the GIT is congested and inflamed.
iii. Cerebral edema, chemical meningoencephalitis, liver and kidney damage may be seen.
iv. Oxalate crystals are seen in the brain, spinal cord and kidneys.

Medico-legal aspects: Poisoning is accidental or suicidal in nature.

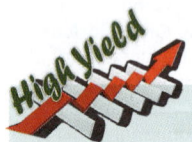

- Absolute alcohol is 99–100% ethanol (<1% water).
- Empty stomach, female sex, carbonated drinks, gastritis enhances absorption.
- Fatty foods, male sex, opiate delays absorption of alcohol.
- Blood alcohol: Exhaled air (breath) alcohol = 1:2300
- *McEwan's sign* is seen in acute alcohol intoxication.
- **Mellanby effect:** Behavioral impairment is more pronounced when BAC is rising or falling.
- **Alcohol hangover:** Acute depression of mood, nausea and headache seen during recovery after alcohol intoxication.
- **Fatal blood alcohol level:** 300–400 mg/dL.
- In *holiday heart syndrome*, patient may have atrial fibrillation and ventricular arrhythmias after a heavy drinking episode.
- **Permissible legal limit of ethanol:** 30 mg/dL for driving.
- Criminal responsibility of an intoxicated person is dealt under **Sec. 85 IPC**.
- Detained person should not be examined, and blood, urine or breath alcohol should not be collected without his written consent.
- Under **Sec. 53 (1) CrPC**, an accused can be examined at the request of the police, even without his consent and by use of force.
- **Tests to determine incoordination:** Romberg test, Walk and Turn test, One Leg Stand test, and Finger Nose test.
- Most useful level to determine concentration of alcohol affecting the brain is BAC.
- Soap and water is used to clean the site to be venipunctured for BAC and not alcohol swabs.
- **Methods to estimate BAC:** Widmark method, Cavett method, Nickolls method, Southgate and Carter method, Kozelka and Hine method.
- *Widmark's formula* is used to estimate blood alcohol concentration.
- Chemical tests for BAC depend on reduction of a dichromate/sulfuric acid by alcohol vapor.

- *Dr Robert Borkenstein* invented breathalyzer/breath analyzer.
- Breathalyzers currently use *infrared spectroscopy* to determine alcohol level.
- **Most reliable, sensitive method for blood alcohol:** Gas liquid chromatography.
- **Specific for alcohol level:** Gas chromatography-Mass spectrometry (GC-MS).
- **Treatment of alcoholism:** Antabuse *(disulfiram)*.
- **Most common sign of alcohol withdrawal syndrome:** Shakes or jitters.
- CAGE questionnaire was developed by *Dr John Ewing* and used for identifying alcoholics.
- **Delirium tremens:** Acute attack of insanity, seen 2–4 days of complete absence from alcohol in chronic alcoholics, and *most severe alcohol withdrawal syndrome*.
- **Features of delirium tremens:** Delirium of horror, tactile hallucination and coarse muscular tremors.
- **Treatment for withdrawal symptoms and delirium tremens:** Diazepam.
- **Wernicke's encephalopathy** seen in chronic alcohol abuse due to thiamine deficiency. There is coarse nystagmus and opthalmoparesis.
- **Korsakoff's psychosis** seen in chronic alcohol abuse due to thiamine deficiency. There is inability to learn new information, impairment of short-term memory and confabulation.
- Thiamine is converted to its active form *thiamine pyrophosphate* in neuronal and glial cells which serves as a cofactor for several enzymes.
- Methanol causes metabolic acidosis, visual disturbances and permanent neurological deficit.
- *Snowfield vision or misty vision* is seen in methanol poisoning.
- In methanol poisoning, blindness due to optic neuritis and atrophy occur due to accumulation of formic acid within the optic nerve.
- **Fatal dose of methanol:** 60–140 mL (>150 mg/dL in blood).
- **Antidote for methanol and ethylene glycol poisoning:** 4-methylpyrazole (fomepizole).
- Ethanol as competitive antagonist in the treatment of methanol and ethylene glycol poisoning.
- 'Hooch tragedy' is due to consumption of adulterated liquor containing methanol.
- Ethylene glycol itself is not toxic, but toxicity is due to metabolites glycolic and oxalic acids.
- In ethylene glycol poisoning, there is acute tubular necrosis, and oxalate crystals are seen in urine.

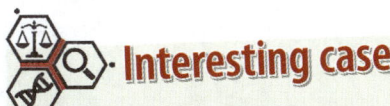

Ethylene Glycol Poisoning (Case of James Keown, 2004)

James Keown and Julie met in college and dated for a few years before marrying in 1996 and settling in Kansas City, Missouri **(Figs. A and B)**. Julie worked as an ICU nurse before joining a company that provides healthcare information technology. James worked in a local radio station and then a job doing marketing for a nonprofit educational consulting group. In 2004, he announced that he had been accepted in Harvard Business School on a scholarship, and they relocated to Waltham, Massachusetts. They had each worked out deals to work remotely for their employers while James attend Harvard.

But eight months after they moved, Julie started developing flu-like symptoms that quickly worsened. Her symptoms included slurred speech and dizziness. She was admitted in the hospital. After a 3-day stay, her condition improved. But she was informed that she has chronic kidney disease and would require dialysis in future. She was discharged from the hospital. After two weeks, Julie had another attack of GIT ailments, slurred speech and confusion. This time her symptoms were even more serious. Once again her motor skills were severely impaired, and within a short time, she slipped into a coma. She was put onto life support. The doctors tested her blood and found ethylene glycol (EG). She died in September 2004. An autopsy revealed she had ingested EG. After her death, James left Waltham and headed back to his hometown and got a new job as a radio talk show host. He informed his new friends and colleagues that his wife was either the victim of a 'tragic illness' or that she had committed suicide.

After more than a year of investigation, Waltham police arrested him on first degree murder charges for slowly and methodically poisoning his wife to death. During the trial, prosecutors claimed Keown killed his wife to collect her $250,000 life insurance policy. He was involved in embezzlement and forged an admission letter to Harvard Business School and then relocated to Waltham after being fired by his employer. He tried to escape from dire financial situation. The prosecution presented a computer forensics analysis of Keown's laptop, which revealed he surfed the internet for ways to buy or make various poisons prior to Julie's death. He searched terms like 'antifreeze death human' and 'poison recipe'; evidence that the taste of ethylene glycol can be masked by putting it in 'Gatorade' and the defendant had been insistent that the victim drink Gatorade in the days and weeks before her death; and testimony by the medical examiner that the victim's symptoms suggested that she had been given small doses of EG over a length of time and then a lethal dose prior to her final admission to the hospital. Although police never found antifreeze or Gatorade at his home, Julie's friend testified that she had heard James calling out reminding his wife to drink Gatorade while she was ill **(Fig. C)**.

The medical examiner further testified that the victim's manner of death was inconsistent with suicide. When defense lawyers tried to force the medical examiner to accept that poisoning is not always a homicide, she replied that a registered nurse would never kill herself in such a horrific way. The defense also claimed during the trial that Julie had ingested the EG to commit suicide because she was depressed about an underlying kidney disease, and there was no direct evidence that Keown was involved in his wife's death, including the absence of any antifreeze.

In 2008, the Jury convicted James Keown guilty of first-degree murder for slowly poisoning his wife by spiking her drink with antifreeze. He was sentenced to life in prison without the possibility of parole.

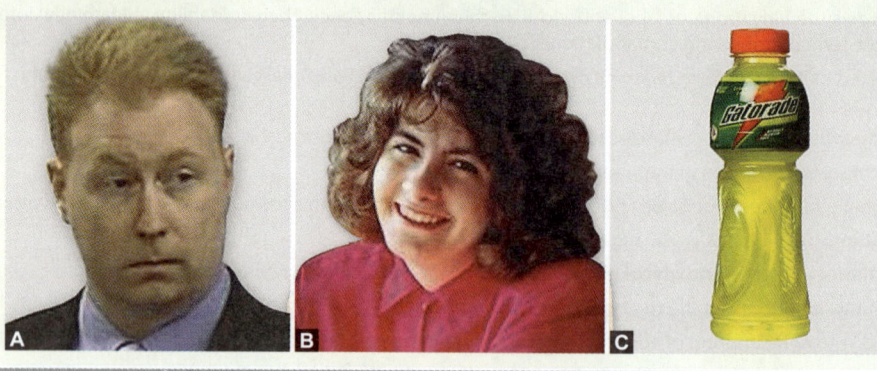

CHAPTER 48: Sedative-hypnotic—Barbiturates

LEARNING OBJECTIVES

Must know
1. Signs and symptoms, fatal dose, treatment, and PM findings in barbiturate poisoning
2. Medico-legal aspects of barbiturate toxicity
3. Barbiturate automatism

Desirable to know
1. Forced alkaline diuresis
2. Scandinavian method of treatment of barbiturate toxicity

 FM 10.1
Describe general principles and basic methodologies in treatment of poisoning with regard to barbiturates.

Introduction

Barbiturates are the earliest class of sedative-hypnotic agents to be developed and were first used in medicine in the early 1900s. They are also used as anticonvulsants, anesthetics and tranquilizers. Commonly abused barbiturates are secobarbital, pentobarbital and amobarbital. In recent years, their use has decreased markedly, as less toxic hypnosedative benzodiazepines have replaced barbiturates for a majority of clinical indications.

Physical properties: It is a white, crystalline, odorless powder and bitter in taste.

Common names: Sleeping pills, goof balls, yellow jackets, red devils, bluebirds and downers.

Classification

Barbiturates are chemical derivatives of barbituric acid and depending on their duration of action, they can be classified as:

Long acting (8–24 hours)	Short acting (3–6 hours)	Ultra-short acting (0.5–2 hours)
Phenobarbital	Butobarbital	Thiopental
Mephobarbital	Secobarbital	Methohexital
Pentobarbital	Hexobarbital	Thiamylal

Action

- Barbiturates act at the GABA: BZD receptor—Cl^- channel complex and potentiate GABAergic inhibition by increasing the lifetime of Cl^- channel opening induced by GABA.
- At very high concentration, it directly increases Cl^- conductance and inhibit Ca^{2+} dependent release of neurotransmitters.
- It also depresses the Na^+ and K^+ channels.

Absorption and Metabolism

- After oral/rectal administration, absorption is usually rapid and complete. The rate of absorption is increased when the barbiturate is formulated as a liquid, when the stomach is empty and when alcohol is ingested concurrently. After IV administration, the onset of action is immediate for amobarbital and pentobarbital, and within 5 minutes for phenobarbital.
- Once absorbed, the barbiturates are rapidly distributed to all tissues and fluids. High concentrations are seen in the brain, liver and kidneys.
- Barbiturates are slowly metabolized in the liver, and these metabolites are mostly inactive, water-soluble and excreted in the urine. Only small amounts of barbiturates are excreted unchanged by the kidney.

SIGNS AND SYMPTOMS

The poisoning is characterized by stupor or coma and areflexia; and in late cases, severe respiratory depression, hypotension and hypothermia.

System	Signs and symptoms
CNS	Drowsiness, dysarthria, clumsy movement, trembling, unsteady gait, nystagmus, disorientation, stupor, delirium, hallucinations, ataxia, coma with loss of superficial and deep reflexes and gradual loss of response to painful stimuli. Corneal reflexes are lost. Conjugate doll's eye movements are absent. Pupils are usually constricted (may dilate in terminal phases), pupillary light response is minimal. Babinsky toe sign may be positive.
RS	Rapid and shallow or slow and labored breathing with reduced minute volume. Respiration may be irregular, sometimes Cheyne-Stokes in character.
CVS	Hypotension, cyanosis, bradycardia, fall in cardiac output, cold clammy skin.
MS	Flaccid, tonicity of muscles is lost.
Renal	Urine scanty or suppressed, dark in color and may contain sugar, albumin and hematoporphyrin. Incontinence may occur.
Skin	Blisters (**barbiturate/'barb' blisters**) are found on the skin (friction areas, such as axilla, inner aspects of knee, calf and interdigital clefts). Blisters contain serous fluid and on rupture, leave a red, raw surface which dries to a brown parchment-like area.
Others	Absent bowel sounds, hypothermia (as low as 31°C), fever indicates bronchopneumonia.

Cause of death: Death may be due to respiratory failure or ventricular fibrillation in early stages, and bronchopneumonia, ARDS, cerebral edema, renal failure or multiorgan failure in later stages.

Fatal Dose and Blood Level

Category	Fatal dose	Blood level
Ultra-short acting	1–2 g	3 mg/dL
Short acting	2–3 g	7 mg/dL
Long acting	3–5 g	10 mg/dL

Fatal period: 1–2 days.

Diagnosis

- Acute barbiturate intoxication should be clinically evaluated to differentiate it from other forms of coma or CNS injury.
- History of possible trauma, associated ingestion of alcohol, previous psychiatric illnesses and attempts at suicide and drug usage should be obtained.
- The effect of barbiturates is potentiated by alcohol, narcotics, tranquilizers and antidepressants.
- Urine, gastric lavage and blood are specimens of choice. Quantify serum alcohol and barbiturate concentrations (particularly phenobarbital). A urine drug screen may help establish co-ingestants.
- Some capsules may be suggestive by color—pentobarbital: yellow or brown, seconal: red, amytal: blue, tuinal: blue and red.

NOTA BENE

Dille-Koppanyi test: This is commonly used as a presumptive test for barbiturates. If a barbiturate is present in the sample, the mixture turns violet blue.

TREATMENT

The management of barbiturate poisoning is supportive. Maintenance of ABC is vital for patient survival. Once the patient is stabilized, gut decontamination and elimination enhancement is done.

I. Airway Support

Mechanical ventilation with O_2 (artificial respiration) is given. If the patient is comatose, prompt intubation is recommended because of the fear of impending, worsening respiratory failure.

II. Cardiovascular Support

Hypotension responds to crystalloid bolus, and vasopressors (dopamine or norepinephrine) are rarely required.

III. Decontamination and Elimination

- Gastric lavage with $KMnO_4$ and activated charcoal is administered 2–4 hours (h) apart as barbiturates re-enter the GIT through enterohepatic circulation.
- Bowels are evacuated by enema.
- *Forced alkaline diuresis* by sodium bicarbonate (2–3 ampoules) in 1 liter of 5% dextrose with rate of infusion at 30 mL/kg/h is useful for *phenobarbital toxicity*. The goal is to maintain a urine output of 150–250 mL/h.
- *Extracorporeal drug removal:* Hemodialysis or hemoperfusion is indicated in phenobarbital poisoning. In hemodynamically unstable patient, sustained low efficiency dialysis may be used instead of conventional dialysis. Newer technique of *lipid dialysis* (which removes lipid-soluble substances from the blood) can extract long-acting drugs in greater quantity.

IV. Supportive Care

The most important aspect of management is close observation and quality nursing care.
- Patient is kept warm (passive rewarming) and mucus removed from the throat.
- Endotracheal intubation for first 3 days, but after this tracheostomy should be done.
- Good oral hygiene, temperature maintenance, posture change at regular intervals, antibiotics and symptomatic treatment.

> **NOTA BENE**
> - Multiple doses of activated charcoal may be effective for substances that undergo enterohepatic recirculation (e.g., phenobarbital, theophylline) and for sustained-release preparations.
> - Urinary alkalinization enhances the elimination of phenobarbital and other long acting barbiturates by ion trapping in renal tubular cells, but it is not recommended as first line treatment (as multiple-dose activated charcoal is superior) or for short acting barbiturate toxicity.
> - **Analeptic drugs:** Earlier analeptics were used in the treatment of barbiturate overdose. They are nonspecific arousal agents such as strychnine, camphor, caffeine, picrotoxin, pentylenetetrazol, nikethamide, amphetamine, megride and methylphenidate. The principal goal of analeptic therapy was to awaken the patient. Adverse effects such as hyperthermia, dysrhythmias, seizures and psychoses were associated with its use.
> - **Scandinavian method:** *Clemmensen and Nilsson* proposed this conservative procedure which abandoned the use of analeptics in the treatment of barbiturate poisoning. It consists of gastric lavage, oxygen, prophylactic antibiotics, determining fluid balance, administration of vitamins, administration of heat or cold for hypo- or hyperthermia respectively, and prevention of bed or eye sores and mouth lesions.

POSTMORTEM FINDINGS

External

i. Mainly those of asphyxia.
ii. Cyanosis is present.
iii. Froth is seen from the mouth and nostrils.
iv. Congested face, and prominent postmortem staining.
v. Barbiturate blisters may be seen.

Internal

i. **Esophagus:** Thickened, dark red-brown, sometimes filled with colored jelly.
ii. **Stomach:** White particles may be seen (rarely). Gastric mucosa may be eroded. Fundus may be thickened, granular and hemorrhagic.
iii. **Lungs:** Congested and edematous. Bronchopneumonia, and/or petechial hemorrhages may be present.
iv. **Heart:** Subendocardial hemorrhages may be seen.
v. **Kidneys:** Degeneration of convoluted tubules.
vi. **Brain:** Edematous. In delayed deaths, there is symmetrical necrosis of globus pallidus and corpus callosum, and focal necrosis in cerebrum and cerebellum.
vii. **Other organs:** Congested.

Medico-legal Aspects

- Mostly suicidal, rarely homicidal.
- It is a popular drug of abuse and used for recreational purpose (e.g., amytal, seconal, tuinal)
- Barbiturates are used as '*date rape*' drugs, since they can be easily placed into drinks and produce a state of relaxation and disinhibition.
- Accidental poisoning occurs due to an overdose **(automatism)**.
- Addiction due to excessive use of barbiturates.
- Barbiturates are used for euthanasia. They are also used for narco-analysis as '*truth serum*'.
- It is used in some states of the US for judicial execution (sodium thiopental).
- *Occupational hazards*: Barbiturates may impair the mental and/or physical abilities required for the performance of tasks, such as driving a vehicle or operating machinery. Patients should be warned accordingly.
- Following the use of barbiturates in OPD procedures, patients should be warned against driving vehicles for the rest of the day.

BARBITURATE AUTOMATISM (SELF-POISONING)

Definition: It is taking of barbiturate tablets repeatedly, because of mental confusion.

Cause: The patient develops a state of toxic delirium after ingestion of one or several doses of drug, and in the delirium or automatism state, takes additional doses of drug in order to get to sleep without any intention to commit suicide and without realizing it.

Medico-legal aspects: Barbiturate automatism may be more pronounced with alcohol consumption. Such deaths are considered 'accidental' and not suicidal.

> **NOTA BENE**
> - Barbiturate in high doses is used for physician-assisted suicide, and in combination with a muscle relaxant for euthanasia and for capital punishment by lethal injection.
> - Thiopental is used IV for the purposes of euthanasia. The Belgians and the Dutch have created a protocol that recommends sodium thiopental as the ideal agent to induce coma, followed by pancuronium bromide.
> - Barbiturates including thiopental (sodium pentothal) and sodium amytal (amobarbital) are used as a '*truth serum*'.

SECTION 2 : Toxicology

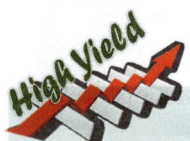

- Commonly abused barbiturates are secobarbital, pentobarbital and amobarbital.
- Barbiturates are used as *'date rape'* drugs, for recreational purpose, for euthanasia and judicial execution (sodium thiopental) and as *'truth serum'* (thiopental and sodium amytal).
- **Slangs used:** Sleeping pills, goof balls, yellow jackets, red devils, bluebirds and downers.
- **Features of barbiturate poisoning:** Stupor or coma, areflexia, respiratory depression (rapid and shallow breathing), hypotension, bradycardia, and hypothermia.
- Pupils are constricted in barbiturate poisoning.
- **Barbiturate blisters:** In barbiturate poisoning, blisters are seen on friction areas of skin such as axilla, interdigital clefts.
- **Fatal dose of barbiturates:** Short acting: 2–3 g; Long acting: 3–5 g.
- **Dille-Koppanyi test:** Presumptive test for barbiturates.
- Forced alkaline diuresis is useful for treatment of *phenobarbital* toxicity.
- *Scandinavian method* is a conservative method of treatment for barbiturate toxicity.
- **Barbiturate automatism:** Taking of barbiturate tablets repeatedly, because of mental confusion and amnesia.

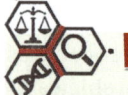

Interesting case

Barbiturates Poisoning (Case of Marilyn Monroe, 1962)

Marilyn Monroe **(Fig. A)** was an American actress, model and singer. Although she was a very successful actor, her troubled private life received much attention. She struggled with addiction, depression and anxiety. Her marriages to retired baseball star DiMaggio and to playwright Miller were highly publicized, and both ended in divorce.

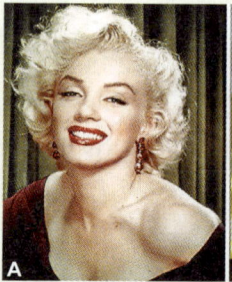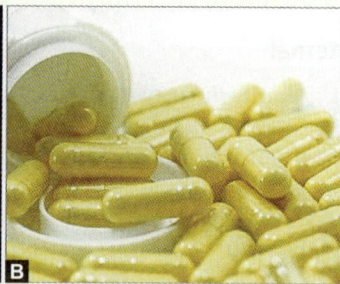

In June 1962, she was fired publicly by the film production company as she often failed to show up on set because of sickness caused by mixing sedatives with alcohol. She had developed insomnia and was prescribed different psychoactive drugs, mostly barbiturates, but also other hypnotic drugs. During the last few months of her life, she suffered from several mental health problems, including substance abuse, depression, bipolar disorder, along with physical ailments, such as endometriosis and gallbladder disease.

On August 4th 1962, she was facing problems with sleep and was acting annoyed and moody. She went to her bedroom at 8 pm. Early morning, at about 3.25 am, Eunice Murray, her housekeeper could see the lights in her bedroom, but the door was locked and she did not respond to shouts to open it up. She appeared unresponsive when she looked into the bedroom through a window. Eunice alerted her doctor, who arrived and entered the room by breaking a window and found Marilyn unresponsive and was declared dead.

During autopsy, there were no signs of needle marks, external wounds or bruises on the body to suspect foul play. Based on the advanced state of rigor mortis at the time her body was discovered, it was estimated that she had died between 8.30 to 10.30 pm. There were no tablets or yellow discoloration of stomach as was expected in Nembutal ('yellow jackets') overdose **(Fig. B)**. The toxicologist reported that she took a lethal dose of barbiturate and a large dose of chloral hydrate ('knockout drops/Mickey Finn'). She had 4.5 mg% of pentobarbital and 8 mg% of chloral hydrate in her blood, and 13 mg% of pentobarbital in her liver. The police found empty bottles of these medicines next to her bed. The medical examiner listed her cause of death as 'acute barbiturate poisoning—ingestion of overdose' and classified her death a 'probable suicide'. However, no suicide note was found. Accidental overdose was ruled out since barbiturates found in her body were several times over the lethal limit.

Despite the coroner's findings, several conspiracy theories suggesting murder or accidental overdose have been proposed since the mid-1960s. It was alleged that the overdose that killed Marilyn was neither swallowed nor injected, but instead administered via an enema, based on the congestion and discoloration of her colon and complete lack of injection marks on her body. The high dose of choral hydrate prevented Marilyn's body from metabolizing the remaining barbiturates in her system, a drug interaction that eventually proved fatal.

Due to the prevalence of these theories in the media, her case was reviewed in 1982, but found no credible evidence to support them and did not disagree with the findings of the original investigation. In 1983, the medical examiner in his memoirs explained that hemorrhages of the stomach lining indicated that the medication had been administered orally, and since Marilyn had been an addict for several years, the pills would have been absorbed more rapidly than in the case of non-addicts. He also denied that Nembutal leaves yellow residue. He said that based on his observations, the most probable conclusion is that Marilyn committed suicide.

49 CHAPTER

Deliriants—Dhatura/Datura

LEARNING OBJECTIVES

Must know
1. Signs and symptoms (11 Ds) and treatment of dhatura poisoning
2. Fatal dose of dhatura
3. Medico-legal aspects of dhatura poisoning
4. Dhatura and capsicum seeds (Diff.)

Desirable to know
1. *Atropa belladonna* poisoning
2. *Hyoscyamus niger* poisoning

FM 14.17
To identify and draw medico-legal inference from common poisons, e.g., dhatura.

Plants that contain the tropane alkaloids include the following:
♦ *Datura stramonium*
♦ *Atropa belladonna* (deadly nightshade)
♦ *Hyoscyamus niger* (henbane)
♦ *Mandragora officinarum* (mandrake).

NOTA BENE
A subgroup of the alkaloids is the alkaloid amines. The three major groups of alkaloid amines are:
  i. Hallucinogenic alkaloid amines
  ii. Stimulant alkaloid amines
  iii. Anticholinergic tropane alkaloids (belladonna alkaloids or bicyclic alkaloids).

DHATURA/DATURA

Introduction

Dhatura, a member of the Solanaceae family and belongs to the genus *Datura*, which consists of nine species, such as *Datura ferox*, *Datura alba*, *Datura fastuosa*, etc.

Common names: Thorn apple (fruits are spherical and have sharp spines), Jimson weed,* Hell's bell and devil's trumpet (for their large trumpet-shaped flowers) **(Fig. 49.1A)**.

Toxic Part

♦ All parts of these plants are poisonous—fruit, flowers and seeds (highest concentrations of alkaloids are found in roots and seeds).
♦ The seeds resemble chilli seeds **(Fig. 49.1B and Diff. 49.1)**. Poisoning occurs only if seeds are masticated and swallowed.

Routes of intake: The usual route is ingesting seeds or other plant parts as tea, although smoking dried leaves also are common.

Active Principles

The plant contains belladonna alkaloids whose primary actions are anticholinergic. Most important are:
1. Hyoscine (scopolamine)
2. Hyoscyamine
3. Atropine.

Action

♦ Atropine and hyoscine block the acetylcholine receptor and produces sympathomimetic or parasympatholytic actions.
♦ CNS stimulant in early phase, but later CNS depression occurs, especially of the respiratory center.
♦ Vagolytic action resulting in stimulation of the heart.

---
* A shortened version of 'Jamestown weed', named after the first recorded accidental ingestion occurred in Jamestown, Virginia, US in 1676.

SECTION 2: Toxicology

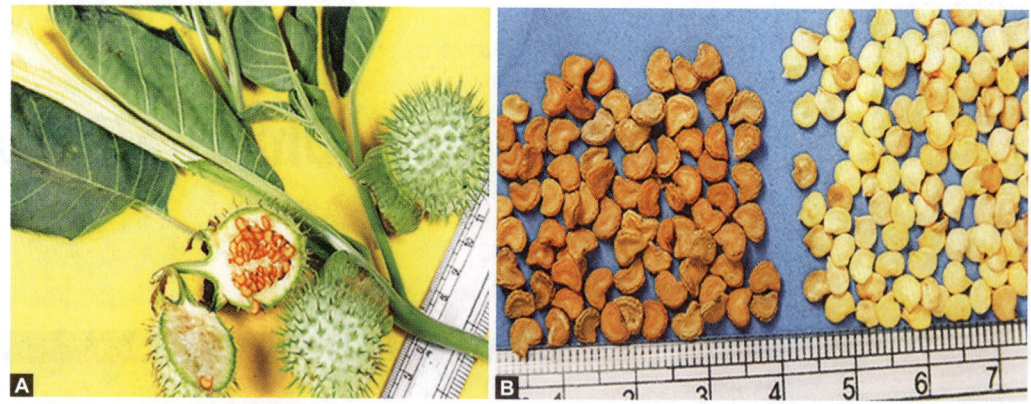

Figs. 49.1A and B: (A) Dhatura fruit (thorn apple), flower and leaves; (B) Dhatura and capsicum seeds

DIFFERENTIATION 49.1: Dhatura and capsicum seeds

S.No.	Feature	Dhatura seeds	Capsicum seeds
1.	Size	Large and thick	Small and thin
2.	Shape	Kidney-shaped	Rounded
3.	Color	Dark brown	Pale yellow
4.	Convex border	Double edge	Single edge
5.	Smell	Odorless	Pungent
6.	Surface	Small depression	Smooth
7.	Taste	Bitter	Pungent
8.	On cut section (LS) **(Fig. 49.2)**	Embryo curved outwards	Curved inwards like figure '6'

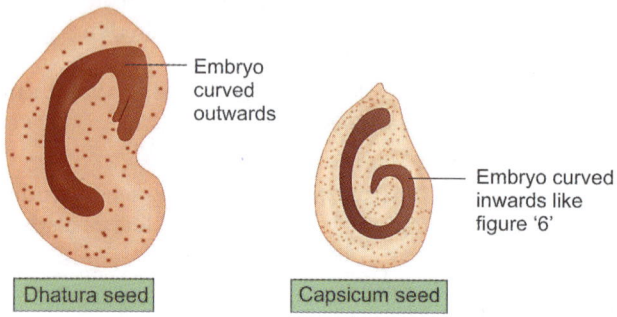

Fig. 49.2: Longitudinal section of dhatura and capsicum seed

Absorption and Excretion

- The alkaloids are absorbed through the mucous membrane of the GIT and respiratory tract, and through the skin and conjunctiva.
- It is destroyed in the liver by enzyme atropinase.
- Part of it is excreted through the urine.

SIGNS AND SYMPTOMS

Anticholinergic syndrome may follow the ingestion of any part of the above mentioned plants, and a wide variety of prescription and over-the-counter medications including illicit street drugs (e.g., heroin "cut" with scopolamine).

There is considerable heterogeneity in the clinical expression of the 'toxidrome' including the peripheral and central manifestations.

- Symptoms are seen 30–60 minutes (min) after ingestion and may continue for 24–48 hours (h) because tropane alkaloids delay gastric emptying and absorption.
- The simile '*red as a beet, dry as a bone, blind, as a bat, mad as a hatter, hot as a hare and full as a flask*' is useful to remember the anticholinergic toxidrome.

Signs and symptoms of dhatura poisoning can be summarized as 11 Ds:

1. **Dryness of the mouth** (*dry as a bone*), bitter taste, burning pain in stomach and vomiting.
2. **Dysphagia** (difficulty in swallowing).
3. **Dysarthria** (difficulty in talking) due to inhibition of salivation—mumbling in quality and is often incomprehensible.
4. **Dilatation of cutaneous blood vessels** (*red as a beet*). Face is flushed and conjunctiva congested.
5. **Diplopia** due to dilated pupil (mydriasis) with loss of accommodation for near vision, developing into temporary blindness (*blind as a bat*) and photophobia **(Fig. 49.3)**. Light reflex is sluggish, and later absent.
6. **Dry hot skin** (*hot as a hare*): Fever is seen due to inhibition of sweat and stimulation of heat regulating center. There is dry mucous membrane with dry axillae. Temperature is raised by 1–2°C.
7. **Distention of urinary bladder** (*full as a flask*) due to urinary retention.
8. **Drunken gait:** There is giddiness, confusion, restlessness, agitation and unsteady gait, the patient staggering like a drunken individual.
9. **Delirium** (*mad as a wet hen*): There is altered mental status; mutters indistinct words, exhibits typical **pill-rolling movements (Fig. 49.4)** or pulls imaginary thread from fingertips or clothes (**carphologia**) and tries to run away from his bed. Visual and auditory hallucinations may be present. Patient

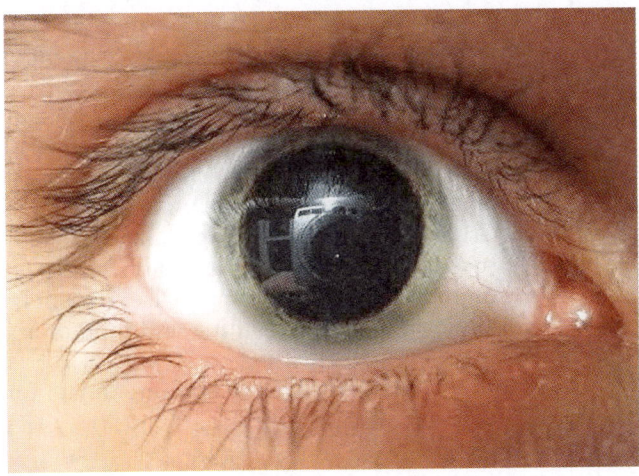

Fig. 49.3: Dilated pupil

cannot recognize relatives and friends. Undressing behavior is common. The changes in mental status are characteristic of delirium.

10. **Diminished bowel sounds**, patients may present with a paralytic ileus (pseudo-obstruction).
11. **Drowsiness:** Delirium passes off and patient becomes drowsy, may progress to stupor, coma, or rarely to death from respiratory paralysis.

Additionally, there may be:
- Rapid pulse (120–140/min), full and bounding, but later becomes weak and irregular.
- Increased respiration.
- Scarlatiniform rash over the body.
- Amnesia regarding events following ingestion is common.

Fatal Dose

- Seeds: 75–125 (stupefying dose: 40–50 seeds).
- Hyoscine: 15–30 mg.

Fatal period: 24 h.

Differential diagnosis: Drunkenness and heat stroke.

Diagnosis: Atropine can be detected by radioimmunoassay, GS-MS, thin layer chromatography and liquid chromatography. Scopolamine can be analyzed in plasma and urine by radio-receptor assay and GC-MS.

> **NOTA BENE**
> - **Pill-rolling movement:** The index finger of the hand tends to get into contact with the thumb, and they perform a circular movement together (commonly seen in Parkinson's disease) (Fig. 49.4).
> - **Carphologia (floccillation):** It is an aimless lint-picking behavior that is often a symptom of a delirious state, such as picking or grasping at imaginary objects, as well as the patient's own clothes or bed linens.

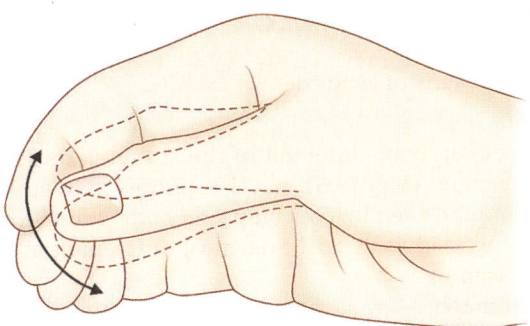

Fig. 49.4: Dhatura poisoning: Pill-rolling movement

TREATMENT

Treatment in a low stimulus environment and control of anticholinergic toxicity usually by supportive measures. Agitation can be controlled with intravenous benzodiazepines.

i. Emetics.
ii. Gastric lavage with tannic acid, $KMnO_4$ or activated charcoal. First dose of activated charcoal may be given with cathartic (e.g., sorbitol). One or two additional doses may be given at 1–2 h intervals to ensure adequate gut decontamination.
iii. **Physiological antidote:** *Physostigmine salicylate* (reversible acetylcholinesterase inhibitor capable of directly antagonizing CNS manifestations of anticholinergic toxicity) 0.5–1 mg slow IV over 5 min with ECG monitoring (0.02 mg/kg/dose).
iv. Purgatives and colonic lavage is recommended.
v. Tepid sponge baths to control high temperature, and diazepam IV for sedation and seizures. Morphine is avoided.
vi. Delirium is controlled by short acting barbiturates.
vii. Hallucinations often respond to reassurance and do not require specific treatment, unless they also have significant psychomotor agitation.
viii. O_2 inhalation and artificial respiration.
ix. Hemodialysis and hemoperfusion are generally ineffective (tropane alkaloids are lipophilic and cross the blood-brain barrier).
x. Catheterization in case of urinary retention.

Moistening of the tongue and change in the size of pupils point towards normalization and are useful as guidelines for adequate management.

> **NOTA BENE**
> - Physostigmine can induce a life-threatening cholinergic crisis such as seizures, respiratory depression and asystole. Since most patients can be safely treated without this antidote, physostigmine preferably should be used in consultation with a poison control center. As such, it is generally not recommended.
> - Physostigmine is contraindicated in patients receiving tricyclic antidepressants, disopyramide, quinidine, procainamide and cocaine.

POSTMORTEM FINDINGS

External: Signs of asphyxia.

Internal

i. Seeds may be detected in the stomach and small intestines **(Fig. 49.5)**. It resists putrefaction and may be found even in a decomposed body. Identification of ingested seeds can be diagnostic of tropane alkaloid poisoning.
ii. **Stomach:** Mucosa may show inflammation.
iii. **Lungs:** Edematous and congested.
iv. **Heart:** Petechial hemorrhages in endocardium.

Medico-legal Aspects

- In India, dhatura is employed mainly as a *stupefying poison* prior to robbery, kidnapping and rape. It is sometimes known as *rail-road poison,* as it is commonly encountered during a journey. Many a time, robbers disguised as saints offer '*prasad*' mixed with dhatura seeds and rob the passengers.
- Teenagers, especially those with history of substance abuse, voluntary ingest the seeds, drink tea or smoke cigarettes for its hallucinogenic and euphoric effects which may result in unintentional poisoning.
- Occasionally, it is used for suicidal purpose and for criminal abortion. In Mexico, dhatura is taken by *Yaqui* women to lessen pain of childbirth.
- Accidental poisoning is common in children who may chew the fruit. Sometimes, it may be due to intake of seeds mistaking them for chilli seeds.
- Unintentional overdose from therapeutic use may occur. Chinese herbal medicines containing tropane alkaloids have been used to treat asthma, chronic bronchitis, pain and flu symptoms. In Africa, a common use is to smoke leaves of dhatura to relieve asthma and pulmonary problems.
- Scopolamine is an alternative to sodium amytal for narco-analysis in interrogations.
- Homicide is rare.
- It is used as an adulterant in country liquor for enhancing the 'kick' effect.
- Sometime, it is used as an aphrodisiac.

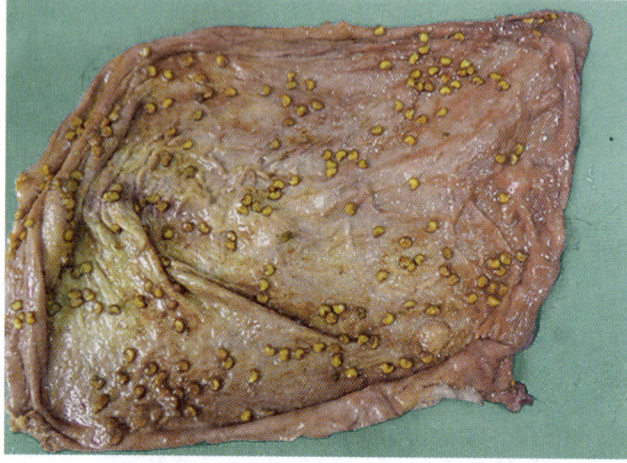

Fig. 49.5: Dhatura seeds in the stomach
(*Courtesy:* Raghvendra Kumar Vidua, AIIMS, Bhopal)

NOTA BENE

Atropa belladonna
- *Atropa belladonna* belongs to Solanaceae family, and grows abundantly in India in the Himalayan ranges. All parts of this plant are poisonous.
- **Active principles:** It contains three alkaloids—atropine, hyoscine and belladonine, but the most important of them is atropine.
- **Action:** It acts by inhibiting the muscarine effects of acetylcholine.
- **Absorption and metabolism:** They are absorbed from the skin and parenteral sites, and detoxicated in the liver.
- **Signs and symptoms** resemble those of poisoning by dhatura.
- **Fatal dose:** Atropine: 100–130 mg.
- **Fatal period:** Within 24 h.
- **Treatment:** Same as for dhatura poisoning.
- **Postmortem findings:** Similar to those found in poisoning by dhatura.
- **Medico-legal aspects:** Poisoning by belladonna occurs accidentally from an overdose of its pharmacopoeial preparations or from swallowing 'eye drops' by mistake. Accidental poisoning is also seen in children and adults from the plant being grown in the garden, either willfully or accidentally.

Hyoscyamus niger
- It yields the active principles hyoscyamine, hyoscine and atropine. It also produce signs and symptoms similar to dhatura.
- **Fatal dose:** Hyoscyamine: 200 mg.
- **Fatal period:** Within 24 h.
- **Treatment:** Similar to that for dhatura.

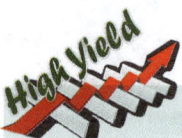

- **Common name:** Thorn apple, Jimson weed, Hell's bell and devil's trumpet.
- Seeds of dhatura resemble chilli seeds.
- Poisoning with dhatura occurs only if seeds are masticated and swallowed.

- All parts of dhatura plant are poisonous—fruit, flowers and seeds.
- **Active principles in dhatura:** Hyoscine (scopolamine), hyoscyamine and atropine.
- Poisoning due to dhatura gives rise to anticholinergic toxidrome.
- **Signs and symptoms of dhatura (11 Ds):** Dry mouth, dysphagia, dysarthria, dilatation of cutaneous blood vessels, diplopia, dry hot skin, distention of urinary bladder, drunken gait, delirium, diminished bowel sounds and drowsiness.
- Pupils are dilated in dhatura poisoning.
- Pill-rolling movements or pulling imaginary threads *(carphologia)* is characteristic of dhatura poisoning.
- **Fatal dose:** Seeds: 75–125 (stupefying dose: 40–50 seeds).
- **Antidote for dhatura poisoning:** Physostigmine salicylate (physiological antidote).
- Dhatura is used as a *stupefying poison* prior to robbery, kidnapping and rape.
- Dhatura is also known as *rail-road poison*.
- Active principles in *Atropa belladonna* are three alkaloids—atropine, hyoscine and belladonine.
- **Fatal dose:** Atropine: 100–130 mg.
- Active principles in *Hyoscyamus niger*—hyoscyamine, hyoscine and atropine.

Interesting case

Atropine Poisoning (Case of Maxime Masseron, 1977)

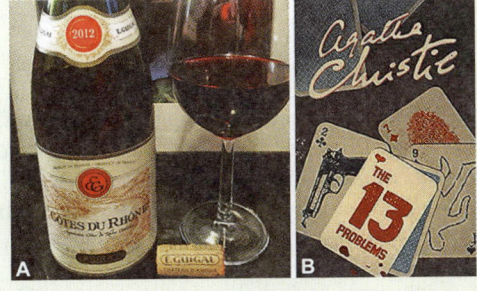

In December 1977 in Créances, France, Maxime Masseron, an 80-year-old man and his wife sat down for their Christmas Eve meal. They had decided to open a bottle of Côtes du Rhône (a type of red wine) given to them by Roland Roussel, their nephew, in the summer **(Fig. A)**. The elderly couple normally abstained from drinking alcohol and they had saved the bottle for a special occasion. A few minutes later Masseron lay dead and his wife became unconscious.

Ms Masseron was rushed to a hospital by neighbors and was in coma for 11 days. Doctors thought it was a case of accidental food poisoning and the police was not alerted. However, the diagnosis came into question a few days later when the couple's son-in-law and the local carpenter went to the house to place Masseron's body in a coffin. Finding wine on the table, both men decided to drink a glass, and they immediately feel ill and collapsed on the floor unconscious. But timely medical treatment saved their lives and both recovered. Now it was clear that it was not food poisoning that had affected the Masserons and the police were called to investigate the incident. Analysis of the remaining wine revealed it was not just red wine in the bottle, but there was atropine mixed with it.

Suspicion fell on to Roussel, who had presented the wine to the Masserons. A police search of his apartment yielded some incriminating evidence. There were bottles of medicine and poisons, magazine and newspaper articles on poisons, and several Agatha Christie novels. Roussel had focused his attention and underlined several key passages on a short story collection—*The Thirteen Problems*, and in particular *The Thumb Mark of St* Peter which features atropine **(Fig. B)**. Christie's story is about an elderly man plotting against his son who he believes is planning to put him in an asylum.

Rousell confessed that he poured an eye drop into the bottle of red wine, but the poisoning had all been a terrible accident. He never intended to murder his uncle. Knowing that his uncle and aunt did not drink, he had expected them to offer the wine to a friend of theirs; a woman he believed had killed his mother. She was a frequent visitor and known to drink wine at their house.

Source: A is for Arsenic: The Poisons of Agatha Christie By Kathryn Harkup

CHAPTER 50

Deliriants—Cannabis

LEARNING OBJECTIVES

Must know
1. Signs and symptoms and treatment of cannabis toxicity
2. Various preparations, active principle and fatal dose of cannabis
3. Medico-legal aspects of cannabis toxicity
4. Run-amok

Desirable to know
1. Cannabinoid hyperemesis syndrome
2. Intravenous marijuana syndrome

Describe features and management of abuse/poisoning with cannabis.

Introduction

Cannabis sativa (marijuana/marihuana/hashish), a deliriant cerebral neurotic hemp plant which has several varieties: *Cannabis indica* (India), *Cannabis mexicana* (Mexico) and *Cannabis americana* (US). It is the *most commonly abused illegal substance* in India and the US, particularly among adolescents, and the most commonly abused substance in the world after nicotine, alcohol and caffeine.

Distribution: Grows all over India. Whole plant is poisonous.

Common names: Pot, grass, weed, ya(r)ndi, rope, mull, dope, joint, Mary Jane, skunk, hash, chronic, reefer, cone or shit.

Active Principle

It is not an alkaloid, but a fat-soluble oleoresin, cannabinol, the active form being δ-9-tetrahydrocannabinol (*THC*). It also contains benzopyrene, a known carcinogen which is also found in tobacco.

Preparations of Cannabis (Table 50.1 and Fig. 50.1)

- **Bhang** is the mildest of cannabis concoctions. It consists of dried cannabis leaves that are ground to a fine paste, mixed with a combination of sugar, spices and fruit.
- **Hashish** is a highly potent, concentrated cannabis resin which is dried and pressed into bricks.
- **Charas** is the handmade form of hashish.
- **Marijuana** refers to tobacco-like preparations of dried leaves and flowers, and is the most common form of drug in the US. It is usually smoked, although it is occasionally baked into foods such as brownies or brewed as tea for drinking.
- **Majum:** Sweetmeat made with bhang.
- **Hash oil:** A lipid soluble plant extract which is mixed with tobacco and smoked. It may contain THC up to 25–50%, and may be added to hashish and marijuana to enhance its THC concentration.

TABLE 50.1: Preparations of cannabis

Features	Bhang (siddhi, patti)	Ganja	Charas (hashish)
Source	Dried leaves and shoots	Flowering tops of female plant	Resinous exudates from leaves, flowers and stems
Color	Brownish	Rusty green color	Dark green or brown
Active principle	2–5% *(least potent)*	5–8%	10–20% *(most potent)*
Uses	Beverage	Mixed with tobacco and smoked in pipe/*hukka*	Mixed with tobacco and smoked in pipe/*hukka*

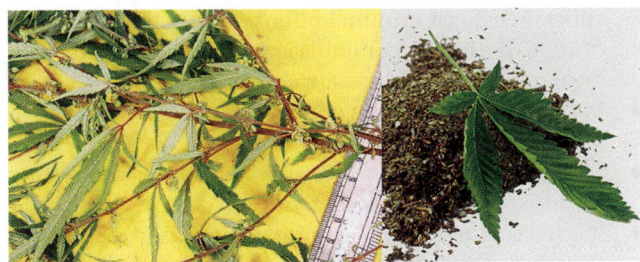

Fig. 50.1: Cannabis (fresh and dried leaves)

- **Sinsemilla** (means 'without seeds') is unpollinated/unfertilized flowering tops from the female plant (similar to ganja). THC content is 6–11%.

THC is also available in synthetic forms (dronabinol and nabilone) which are used as an appetite stimulant for AIDS-related anorexia and as treatment for vomiting associated with cancer chemotherapy.

Routes of intake: Cannabis is usually smoked in cigarettes (joints or reefers)* or pipes, added to food (usually cookies, brownies or sweetmeat) or mixed with milk (*bhang*) (Fig. 50.2).

Drug combinations: Cannabis is frequently combined with other drugs, including heroin, cocaine, LSD and ecstasy.

Action

- THC which binds to anandamide receptors in the brain may have stimulant, sedative or hallucinogenic actions, depending on the dose and time after consumption.
- Both catecholamine release (resulting in tachycardia) and inhibition of sympathetic reflexes (resulting in orthostatic hypotension) may be seen.

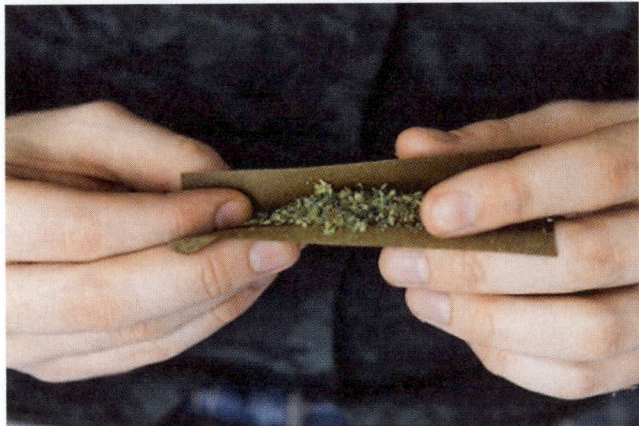

Fig. 50.2: Joints or reefers

SIGNS AND SYMPTOMS

Onset of symptoms occurs within a few minutes of smoking and within half hour of oral ingestion. The duration of action is usually 6–12 hours (h); symptoms are most marked in the first 1–2 h.

I. Stage of Excitement

i. Feeling of euphoria, detachment, well-being/grandiosity, dreaminess, subjective sense of slowing of the passage of time, increased self-confidence, rapidly changing emotions, talkativeness and laughing. Some may experience unpleasant psychological reactions, such as panic, fear or depression.
ii. Impairment of thinking and short-term memory, decreased concentration, disorientation, illusions, visual hallucinations, altered sexual feelings, impaired judgment, slow reaction time, and perceptual and psychomotor dysfunctions resulting in impaired driving and motor vehicle accidents.
iii. Increased appetite (the '*munchies*'), thirst, nausea, headache, conjunctival injection (bloodshot eyes), dizziness, dry mouth, slurred speech, postural hypotension, tachycardia and increased urinary frequency.

II. Stage of Narcosis

i. Giddiness, incoordination, confusion, ataxia and paresthesias.
ii. The person passes into deep sleep and wakes up without depression/nausea/hangover.
iii. Rarely, drowsiness may be followed by respiratory failure, coma, collapse and death (due to cardiac arrest or apnea).

> **Intravenous marijuana syndrome:** Intravenous injection of marijuana broth produces a distinct clinical syndrome wherein emesis, myalgia and hypotension are seen. There may be fatal anaphylaxis following injection.

Fatal Dose

There is no authentic reported case of death attributable to cannabis in the medical literature. Most deaths are attributed to multiple drug intoxication. However, researchers have estimated the fatal dose as follows:
- Bhang: 10 g/kg body wt.
- Charas: 2 g.
- Ganja: 8 g.

Fatal period: About 12 h.

Diagnosis is based on the history and typical findings. Serum and urine concentrations of THC metabolites

---

*It is a type of cigarette used for intoxication, containing 0.3–0.6 g of marijuana which is dipped in tincture of cannabis and dried.

are useful for confirmatory testing. Enzyme-multiplied immunoassay technique (EMIT) and radioimmunoassay (RIA) are useful; gas-chromatography-mass spectrometry (GC-MS) is the most specific (can detect up to 7 days post-exposure in urine).

> **NOTA BENE**
>
> **Duquenois-Levine test:** A presumptive test for cannabis/marijuana. Two reagents and chloroform comprise this reaction. The three solutions are added to the sample being tested, which forms multiple layers. If the chloroform layer develops a purple color, marijuana may be present in the sample.

TREATMENT

Immediate management is supportive, including cardiovascular and neurological monitoring, and placement in a quiet room.
  i. Gastric lavage with warm water.
  ii. Strong tea/coffee.
  iii. Artificial respiration.
  iv. Saline purgatives.
  v. 100 mL of 50% glucose or dextrose, 2 mg naloxone and 100 mg thiamine IV.
  vi. Diazepam, 5–10 mg IV, if patient is violent and aggressive.
  vii. Haloperidol to control psychotic manifestations.

Postmortem findings: Non-specific. Mostly features of asphyxia are seen.

Medico-legal Aspects

- Most cases of poisoning are accidental, particularly in young children, or due to overindulgence during recreational use. It is the most commonly abused drug among pregnant women and women of childbearing age in most Western societies. Unintentional ingestion by children has also been reported.
- *Driving under the influence of cannabis*: Driving is impaired if cannabis is ingested along with alcohol.
- *Concomitant poisoning*: Lead and mercury poisoning have been reported in marijuana abusers.
- Medical practitioners face ethical challenges which go beyond indications for use with patients requesting medical cannabis.
- Medical use is legal in about a dozen countries, including Canada and parts of Australia.
- Passive smoke inhalation does not produce concentrations high enough to be detected in most urine drug screens.
- In India, possession, trade, transport and consumption of marijuana (among other narcotic and psychotropic substances) is a criminal offense under the NDPS Act of 1985. In the US, cannabis is subject to contradictory legal regulation under state and federal law.
- Majum and charas are sometimes used by thieves to stupefy persons to facilitate robbery.
- Sometimes, it is taken by criminals before committing a criminal act to strengthen nerves.
- It is used as an aphrodisiac and is supposed to increase duration of coitus.
- Its use in chocolates causes intense craving among children for its euphoric effects.

RUN-AMOK

An addict often suffers from mental disorders, such as hallucination and delusion of persecution, presenting with a desire to destroy life and property willfully; or commit homicide out of jealousy; however, there is no recollection afterwards.

- Run-amok is a psychic disturbance resulting from continued use or sudden consumption of cannabis, and is characterized by a peculiar homicidal mania.
- After intake, there is a period of depression, followed by excitation, confusion and a violent attempt to kill people (*impulse to murder*).
- The addict first kills a person against whom he may have real or imaginary enmity and then kills anyone who comes in his way, until the homicidal tendency lasts. The person may then commit suicide or surrender himself to the law enforcement authority.
- **Criminal responsibility:** The person is not held responsible for his acts since 'run amok' is considered a disorder of mind and not intoxication, unless he had taken it purposefully to strengthen himself before commission of the offense.

> **NOTA BENE**
>
> **Cannabinoid hyperemesis syndrome**
> - Cannabinoid hyperemesis syndrome (CHS) is due to the paradoxical effects of marijuana on the GIT and CNS (although anti-emetic properties are well known). The mechanism is unknown.
> - CHS is characterized by chronic cannabis use, cyclic episodes of nausea and vomiting, and frequent compulsive hot bathing.
> - There are three distinct phases: prodromal, hyperemetic and recovery. During the prodromal phase, the patient develops early morning nausea, a fear of vomiting, and abdominal discomfort. Afterward, the hyperemetic phase consists of incapacitating nausea and profuse vomiting. In most patients, there is dehydration, mild abdominal pain and weight loss. Patients are relieved by taking hot showers/baths.
> - Haloperidol is useful for acute CHS management, and long-term treatment is abstinence from cannabis.

CHAPTER 50 : Deliriants—Cannabis

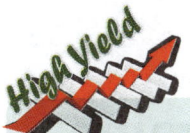

- *Cannabis sativa* is a deliriant cerebral neurotic hemp plant.
- Most commonly abused illegal substance in India.
- Most commonly abused substance in the world after nicotine, alcohol and caffeine.
- **Common names:** Pot, grass, weed, rope, mull, dope, joint, Mary Jane, hash, reefer, cone or shit.
- **Active principle:** δ-9-tetrahydrocannabinol (THC).
- *Bhang* is obtained from dried leaves and shoots (*least potent*).
- *Ganja* is obtained from flowering tops of female plant.
- *Charas (hashish)* is resinous exudates from leaves, flowers and stems (*most potent*).
- *Marijuana* is tobacco-like preparations of dried leaves and flowers.
- Cannabis can be smoked in cigarettes known as *joints/reefers*.
- **Signs and symptoms:** Euphoria, laughing, hallucinations, conjunctival injection, dry mouth, slurred speech, increased appetite, nystagmus, incoordination, ataxia, deep sleep and wakes up without hangover.
- **Fatal dose:** Bhang: 10 g/kg body wt; charas: 2 g, ganja: 8 g.
- **Duquenois-Levine test:** Presumptive test for cannabis.
- Management of cannabis toxicity is supportive.
- **Run-amok:** Psychic disturbance resulting from continued use or sudden consumption of cannabis, and is characterized by *homicidal mania* (impulse to murder).

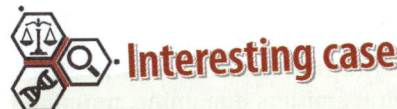

Medical Cannabis

Kevin O'Brien reported a case of a 7-year-old boy JJ who lived with his mother in California. He had severe behavioral disorder—he was hyperactive and aggressive and diagnosed with PTSD, bipolar disorder and impulse control disorder. He told therapists that he hears voices telling him to kill his mother. His mother pursued all forms of medical help from medications to behavior therapy. During the last four years, she consulted 16 physicians who prescribed multiple medications. Most of the time JJ was overmedicated; he had slurred speech and was unable to walk. She questioned the wisdom of all the medications and believed that most of his symptoms may have resulted from the side-effects of the medicines and not the underlying behavior.

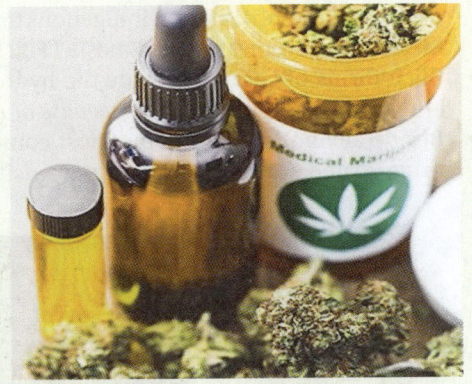

In May 2001, she discovered in the course of her research that medical marijuana might help him. When all other medical treatments failed, she discussed the intake of small amount of marijuana with case workers, team members and several physicians. After consulting them, she decided to give it a try.* She notified the medical team that JJ is no longer on any psychotropic medications and begun treatment with medical marijuana. He started taking it in a muffin—half in the morning and half in the evening monitored by pediatrician who adjusted the dosage.

The treatment resulted in significant improvement and his behavior took a remarkable turn. His demeanor became polite and he interacted with zeal with students and staff. He was able to use words and expressed his feelings—his likings and disliking. When the officials heard of medical marijuana being used to treat a child, they tried to remove JJ from his mother's care, but she was able to keep custody with legal help.

---

* The medical use of cannabis is legalized (with a doctor's recommendation) in many states of US. Since cannabis is banned in India, there is no medical marijuana program.
Source: O'Brien K, S Clark PA. Case study: Mother and son: The case of medical marijuana. The Hastings Center Report 2002;32(5):11-13.

51 CHAPTER

Deliriants—Cocaine

LEARNING OBJECTIVES

Must know
1. Signs and symptoms and treatment of cocaine toxicity
2. Medico-legal aspects of cocaine toxicity
3. Magnan's syndrome

Desirable to know
1. Cocaine washed-out syndrome
2. Cocainomania
3. Crack lung

Describe features and management of abuse/poisoning with cocaine.

Introduction

Cocaine is a colorless, odorless, crystalline substance with bitter taste and slightly soluble in water, but freely soluble in alcohol.

- It is an alkaloid deliriant, obtained from dried leaves of *Erythroxylum coca*, a shrub indigenous to Peru, Bolivia, Mexico, West Indies and Indonesia **(Fig. 51.1)**.
- Illicit forms of cocaine include the hydrochloride salt and its alkalization products, *freebase or crack*.
- Beside alcohol, cocaine is the most common cause of drug-related emergency department visits in the US.

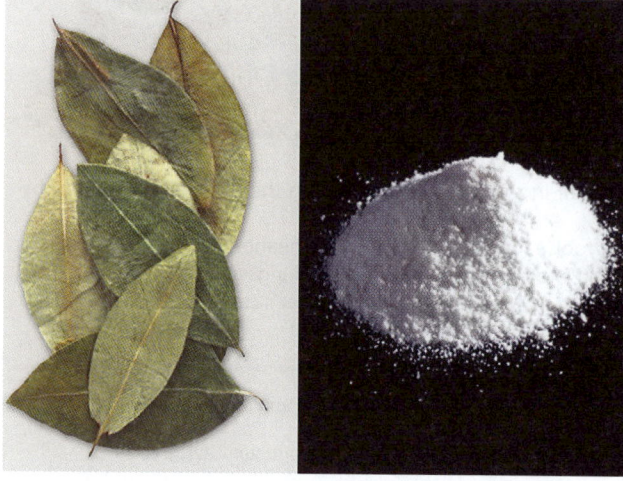

Fig. 51.1: Erythroxylum coca leaves and cocaine

Common names: Crack, pasta, bazooka, snuff, coke, snow or white lady.

Action

- Cocaine produces a hyperadrenergic state.
- It increases the synaptic concentrations of the monoamine neurotransmitters dopamine, norepinephrine and serotonin by binding to transporter proteins in presynaptic neurons and blocking uptake.
- It is also a local anesthetic, as it blocks initiation and conduction of nerve impulse by decreasing axonal membrane permeability to sodium ions.
- It stimulates the cortex for a short time, followed by depression.

Absorption and Excretion

- Cocaine is rapidly absorbed from the mucous membranes and subcutaneous tissues.
- About 30–50% of cocaine is metabolized by hepatic esterases and plasma pseudocholinesterase, resulting in the formation of *ecgonine methyl ester*. Spontaneous nonenzymatic hydrolysis of another 30–40% results in *benzoylecgonine*.
- Only 1–5% of cocaine is excreted unaltered through the kidneys within 6 hours (h) of use.
- A metabolite of cocaine, *cocaethylene* has been found in blood and urine of patients who abuse both alcohol and cocaine.

Routes of intake: Chewing, application to nasal mucous membrane (snorting), smoking *(free basing)* and IV.

Cocaine may be inhaled through a straw or rolled-up paper currency, or a spoon containing 5–20 mg of the drug **(Fig. 51.2)**.

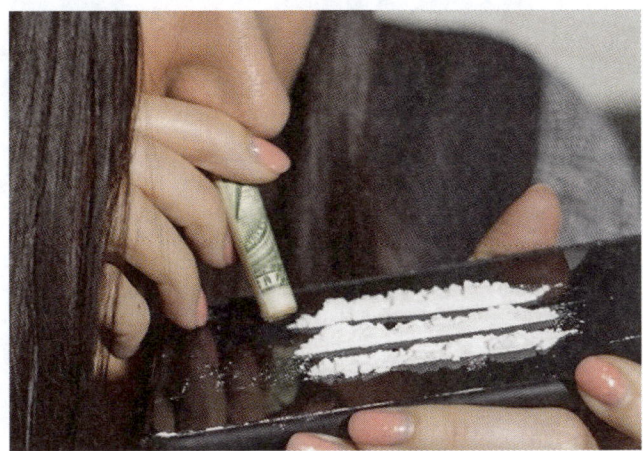

Fig. 51.2: Snorting cocaine

SIGNS AND SYMPTOMS

Signs and symptoms of acute poisoning include elevated pulse, blood pressure, respiration and temperature. Onset occurs within 7 seconds after inhalation, 15 seconds after taking IV, 3 minutes (min) after nasal insufflations and 10 min after oral ingestion. The initial stimulatory effects *(rush)* are followed by depression *(crush)*.

I. Stage of Excitement

System	Signs and symptoms
Local	Feeling of numbness or tingling at the place of application
Face	Flushed
Skin	Pale
GIT	Bitter taste, dryness of mouth, vomiting, diarrhea, hyperactive bowel sounds
CNS	Headache, bruxism, feeling of well-being, euphoria, restlessness, excitement, talkativeness, delirium, maniacal, hallucinations, nonintentional tremors (e.g., twitching of small muscles, especially facial and finger) and tonic-clonic seizures. Reflexes are exaggerated
RS	Tachypnea, dyspnea, cyanosis
CVS	Tachycardia, hypertension, ventricular arrhythmias
Temperature	Hyperthermia
Ocular	Mydriasis, resulting in blurred vision

II. Stage of Depression

After an hour, respiration becomes slow, there is profuse sweating, and patient becomes calm and dull.

System	Signs and symptoms
CNS	Coma, areflexia, pupils fixed and dilated, flaccid paralysis and loss of vital support functions
CVS	Ventricular dysrhythmias result in weak, rapid, irregular pulse and hypotension, circulatory failure and cardiac arrest
RS	Cheyne-Stokes respirations, apnea, pulmonary edema, cyanosis, respiratory failure

Tea colored urine may indicate rhabdomyolysis and potential renal failure.

Cause of death: In fatal cases, the onset and progression are accelerated, with convulsions and death from respiratory failure, cerebral hemorrhage or cardiac failure, frequently occurring in 2–3 min.

Fatal Dose

Cocaine: 20 mg IV; 500 mg to 1.2 g orally.

Fatal period: Few minutes to 1–2 h.

Differential diagnosis: Lithium toxicity, cyclic antidepressants toxicity, neuroleptic malignant syndrome, acute withdrawal from sedatives or ethanol, thyroid storm and other hyperadrenergic states.

Diagnosis: Qualitative toxicological analysis of blood and urine.

- Finding cocaine and metabolites in the urine supports the diagnosis. However, urinalysis can detect cocaine metabolites 2–4 days post-exposure, a positive screen does not equate with clinical toxicity.
- Urine, blood, gastric contents and unknown substances found on patients, such as on a moustache, may be sent for toxicological evaluation.

> **NOTA BENE**
> - **Mandelin test:** The reagent consists of ammonium vandanate in concentrated sulfuric acid. Cocaine gives an orange color with the reagent.
> - **Scott test:** Cobalt thiocyanate is used for this test. If cocaine is present in the sample, a blue precipitate will form.

TREATMENT

There is no specific antidote; therapy consists of treatment of symptoms until the acute effects (which are generally short lived since half-life of cocaine is about 1 h) are gone.

i. If injected, apply tourniquet above the part; if applied to nose or throat, wash-out with warm water or saline. If swallowed, gastric lavage should be done with $KMnO_4$ and/or activated charcoal.
ii. *Control seizures:* Diazepam in doses up to 0.5 mg/kg IV may be given over an 8 h period. Physical restraint should be avoided due to risks of rhabdomyolysis and hyperthermia.
iii. Dysrhythmias should be treated according to standard advanced cardiac life support (ACLS) protocols. Ventricular arrhythmia is managed by giving 0.5–1 mg of propranolol IV.
iv. Short acting, direct vasodilator (esmolol) and short acting beta-blockers are indicated for tachycardia and hypertension.
v. Thiamine 100 mg IV.
vi. Airways are kept clean, artificial respiration and O_2 inhalation as required.

Complications

- *CNS:* Cerebrovascular accidents (frequent cause of stroke in <45 years), subarachnoid or intracerebral hemorrhage and cerebral vasculitis.
- *CVS:* Myocardial, bowel and kidney ischemia, myocardial infarction, skin necrosis and aortic dissection.
- Pulmonary infarcts, eosinophilia with granuloma formation.
- *Inhalational exposure* can result in cough, hemoptysis, reactive airway disease, pneumonitis (*'crack lung'*) and barotrauma due to forceful Valsalva maneuver that are performed during smoking (e.g., pneumothorax).

Postmortem Findings

Non-specific findings.
  i. Patients may have linear excoriations, 'crack pipe' burns of the fingers or thumbs, thermal burns of the face and upper airway.
  ii. Track marks in the usual sites, such as the antecubital fossae, and at unusual sites, such as under the tongue and on top of the feet may be seen.
  iii. Intense asphyxial signs and cardiac dilatation may be seen.

Blood should be preserved by adding fluoride.

Medico-legal Aspects

- Accidental cases occur from urethral, vesical and rectal injection. Oral overdose can occur in body packers and body stuffers.
- Cocaine is rarely used for homicide or suicide.
- Intentional criminal poisoning wherein prenatal (known ingestion of cocaine by pregnant female), infant and child deaths determined to be homicide has been reported.
- It is believed to increase the libidinal drive and increase the duration of sexual act by paralyzing sensory nerves of glans penis.
- It causes lowering of moral values, loss of decency and self-respect.
- It is rapidly destroyed in the body and is difficult to detect by chemical analysis.

> **NOTA BENE**
>
> **Cocaine washed-out syndrome**
> There is depressed mental status, ranging from lethargy to deep coma, following binge use of cocaine.
> - The mechanism is due to depletion of dopamine.
> - On examination, patients are difficult to arouse for upto 24 h and unable to speak or follow simple commands.
> - They assume normal sleep postures and can be aroused to full orientation—contrast to patients with intracranial hemorrhages, like SAH.
> - All reflexes, pupillary size, cranial nerve examination are usually normal with mild hypotension and mild bradycardia.

> **NOTA BENE**
>
> - 'Crack' is produced when the hydrochloride molecule is removed by ether extraction, which frees the basic cocaine molecule (*'freebase'*). The term 'crack' describes the crackling sound heard when cocaine freebase is smoked.
> - Illicit drugs are frequently admixed with additional chemicals either to increase the apparent quantity of the street drug or to enhance its effect. For example, 8–20% of stimulants available on the street contain cocaine and methamphetamine hydrochloride. Other adulterants may include quinine, talc, ascorbic acid, boric acid, chalk, laundry detergent, laxatives and lactose.
> - **'Crack baby':** The term *'crack baby'* was used to describe children who were exposed to crack as fetuses in the US during 1980–90 in the midst of a crack epidemic.
> - **'Crack lung'** may occur 1–48 h after cocaine smoking. It is a hypersensitivity pneumonitis wherein there is chest pain, cough, hemoptysis, dyspnea, bronchospasm, pruritus, fever, diffuse alveolar infiltrates without effusions, and pulmonary and systemic eosinophilia.
> - **'Crack dancing'** refers to the extrapyramidal phenomena and other movement disorders that are sometimes associated with cocaine abuse.

Cocainism (Cocainomania/Cocainophagia)

- Cocainomania is an irresistible craze, crave or impulse to intoxication by cocaine, or any of its salts or combinations, at all risks. It is addiction and morbid craving for cocaine.
- Many users take repeated doses to keep the high going and avoid the 'crash' or try to modify the effects with other drugs like alcohol, tranquilizers or heroin. This rush-and-crash pattern leads to toxic levels of cocaine in the bloodstream and reinforces the highly addictive nature of cocaine.
- Abusers can tolerate up to 10 g/day.

Signs and Symptoms

- Emaciation, anorexia, digestive disturbances, significant loss of libido, erectile dysfunction, gynecomastia, galactorrhea and major derangements in menstrual cycle in women—amenorrhea and infertility.
- Face is pale, shifty gaze, sunken eyes, dilated pupils, tongue and teeth are black, and ulceration of nasal septum.
- Degeneration of CNS with hallucinations, convulsions and delirium may occur.

Magnan's Syndrome/Cocaine Bugs

- Magnan's syndrome is seen in cocaine addicts, usually with IV users.
- It is a type of *tactile hallucination*.
- There is a feeling as if grains of sand are lying under the skin or small insects ('bugs') are creeping on the skin giving rise to itching sensation (*formication*).

- The patients may cause self-inflicted cuts and scratches in an attempt to remove the imagined parasites.
- This syndrome is now called *'delusional parasitosis'* and not confined to cocaine abusers only. It may be seen with psychotic disorders, such as schizophrenia and organic mental disorders, or even in dementia.

NOTA BENE

- **Ekbom syndrome (delusional parasitosis)** is a psychiatric disorder in which individuals incorrectly believe they are infested with parasites, insects or bugs, whereas in reality no such infestation is present.
- **Formication** (Latin *formica*: ant): Tactile hallucination involving the sensation that tiny insects are crawling over the skin. Causes of formication can be actual physical conditions, including diabetic neuropathy, menopause, skin cancer or herpes zoster, and may also be physical or psychological side effect of substance abuse (cocaine, amphetamines and alcohol withdrawal along with delirium tremens).

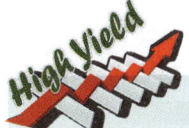

- Cocaine is an alkaloid deliriant, obtained from dried leaves of *Erythroxylum coca*.
- **Common names:** Crack, pasta, bazooka, snuff, coke, snow or white lady.
- Taking cocaine through smoking route (in a purified/concentrated form) is called *free basing*.
- **Characteristic features of cocaine poisoning:** Elevated pulse, BP, respiration and temperature.
- **Signs and symptoms of cocaine poisoning:** Initial stimulatory effects (*rush*—euphoria, talkativeness, delirium, maniacal, hallucinations, tachypnea, tachycardia, hypertension) are followed by depression (*crush*—coma, areflexia, flaccid paralysis, weak and irregular pulse, hypotension, apnea).
- Tea colored urine may indicate rhabdomyolysis and potential renal failure.
- **Fatal dose of cocaine:** 20 mg IV; 500 mg to 1.2 g orally.
- *Mandelin* and *Scott tests* are presumptive test for cocaine.
- Oral overdose can occur in body packers and body stuffers.
- Management of toxicity is supportive with diazepam, propranolol and esmolol.
- **Magnan's syndrome/cocaine bugs:** Seen in cocaine addicts; type of *tactile hallucination (formication)*.
- **Ekbom syndrome (delusional parasitosis):** Psychiatric disorder in which patients falsely believe they are infested with parasites, insects or bugs.

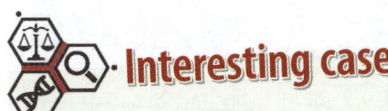

Cocaine Poisoning

Nolte KB *et al.* reported a case wherein they determined cocaine poisoning as the cause of death by analyzing insect larvae specimens. The maggot infested remains of a 29-year-old male intravenous drug abuser was found prone, lightly covered with snow, and partially embedded in frozen earth in a densely wooded area less than a mile from where he was last seen. He was reported missing 5 months back.

During autopsy, the clothing had no unusual cuts, tears, or holes. Skeletal muscle from the legs, Calliphoridae (blow fly) larvae and pupa **(Fig. A)** were collected at autopsy and frozen. Initial screening for cocaine and benzoylecgonine was performed using radioimmunoassay. Confirmation of the presence of cocaine in muscle was accomplished by full spectrum gas chromatography/mass spectrometry (GC/MS). Quantitative evaluation of cocaine in muscle and larval specimens was performed with gas chromatography using a nitrogen-phosphorus detector. Benzoylecgonine was determined using an automated quantitative program. Findings indicated that no ethanol or other volatile hydrocarbons were present in muscle screened by GC. Further, no opiates, benzodiazepines or barbiturates were detected in muscle screened by radioimmunoassay. Cocaine, lidocaine, and caffeine were qualitatively identified in muscle analyzed by GC/MS.

The cause of death was given as cocaine poisoning based on toxicological report from insect larvae, combined with autopsy findings and circumstances of the case.

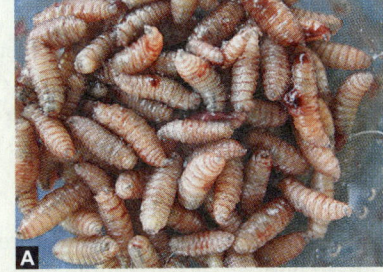

Source: Nolte KB; Pinder RD; Lord WD. Insect larvae used to detect cocaine poisoning in a decomposed body. J Forensic Sci. 1992;37(4):1179-85.

52 CHAPTER

Spinal Poisons

LEARNING OBJECTIVES

Must know
1. Signs and symptoms and treatment of strychnine poisoning
2. Fatal dose of strychnine
3. Risus sardonicus
4. Strychnine poisoning and tetanus (Diff.)

Desirable to know
1. Medico-legal aspects of strychnine poisoning

 FM 14.17
To identify and draw medico-legal inference from common poisons, e.g., Nux-vomica.

STRYCHNOS NUX-VOMICA

Introduction

Strychnos nux-vomica (family Loganiaceae) is an evergreen tree native to Southeast Asia, especially India and Myanmar from which strychnine is obtained, one of the oldest poisons known to man.

Common names: Nux vomica, poison nut, Quaker buttons, strychnine tree, *kuchila, yetti, maqianzi*.

Identification of Seeds (Fig. 52.1)

- The ripe fruit contains seeds which are poisonous. They are flat, circular discs, 10–30 mm diameter and 4–6 mm thick, slightly concave on one side and convex on the other, ash gray in color, have a shiny surface and are covered with silky hairs.
- They look like enlarged RBCs.
- Unbroken seeds when ingested are not poisonous, as the hard pericarp is not soluble in digestive juices.

Active Principles

i. Strychnine—alkaloid
ii. Brucine—alkaloid
iii. Loganin—glucoside.

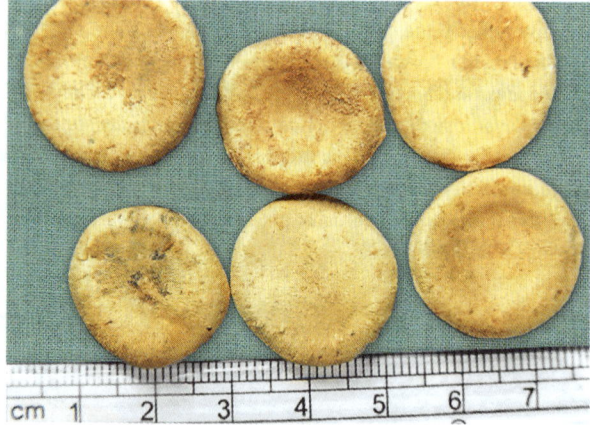

Fig. 52.1: Strychnos nux-vomica (seeds)

- Minor alkaloids present in the seeds are protostrychnine, vomicine, n-oxystrychnine, pseudostrychnine, isostrychnine and chlorogenic acid.
- Alkaloids are mostly found in the seeds, but it can be isolated from all parts of the plants including bark, leaves and roots.

Properties of strychnine: Colorless, bitter, odorless, rhombic prism-shaped crystals. Dissolves sparingly in water or ether, but dissolves well in alcohol and benzene.

Uses: It is used as a respiratory stimulant, rodenticide, and for killing stray dogs. Strychnine is still available as herbal and homeopathic remedies, as a purgative, appetite suppressant and as a constituent of nerve tonics. It can be found as an adulterant in some street drugs (cocaine, heroin and amphetamines).

Action

Strychnine competitively antagonizes the inhibitory neurotransmitter *glycine* by blocking its post-synaptic uptake by brainstem and spinal cord receptors.

- The inhibiting effect of glycine is reduced and nerve impulses are triggered with lower levels of neurotransmitters.
- When there is no inhibitory effect, the motor neurons do not stop their stimulus, and the victim will have constant muscle contractions (*release excitation*).
- Its action is particularly in the anterior horn cells (especially in Renshaw cells of the spinal cord).

GABA, the neurotransmitter for presynaptic inhibitory neurons is *not affected* by strychnine.

Metabolism: Up to 80% of ingested strychnine is eliminated through hepatic metabolism and the remaining 20% is excreted in urine.

SIGNS AND SYMPTOMS

Signs and symptoms are seen within 15–30 minutes (min) of ingestion. A '*conscious*' seizure is the characteristic presentation of strychnine poisoning. Findings associated with poisoning are:

i. Bitter taste.
ii. Choking sensation in throat, and stiffness of the neck and face.
iii. *Prodromal symptoms:* Restlessness, increased acuity of perception, increased rigidity of muscles and muscular twitchings.
iv. *Face:* Cyanosed, look is anxious, eyes are staring, eyeballs are prominent and the pupils are dilated. Mouth is filled with bloodstained froth.
v. *Convulsions:* The threshold for CNS stimulation is lowered with the result that any sensory stimulus (light, pain, touch or noise) may produce violent muscular spasm. Initially, clonic but eventually become tonic, and affect all the muscles at the same time.
   - **Risus sardonicus** (Latin, scornful laughter or devilish grin) or **risus caninus** (Latin, dog's laughter or grinning) results from raising of patient's eyebrows, bulging of eyes and contraction of the jaw and facial muscles in which the corners of the mouth are drawn back leading to an evil looking grin (**Fig. 52.2**). This expression can be seen in tetanus too.
   - Convulsions are most marked in anti-gravity muscles resulting in hyperextension (**opisthotonus**) (**Fig. 52.3**).
   - Sometimes, the spasm of the abdominal muscles may bend the body forward (**emprosthotonus**) or sideways (**pleurosthotonus**).
   - Duration of convulsions is about half to 2 min and may recur for 12–24 hours (h). During convulsions, the patient remains awake and aware of everything around him, since strychnine does not cross the blood-brain barrier.
   - In between convulsions, muscles are completely relaxed and breathing is resumed. Patient is usually in pain, exhausted, anxious and anticipating the next series of convulsions.
   - After 5–15 min, on the slightest impulse, such as sudden noise, current of air or on gently touching the patient, another convulsion occurs with increased intensity.

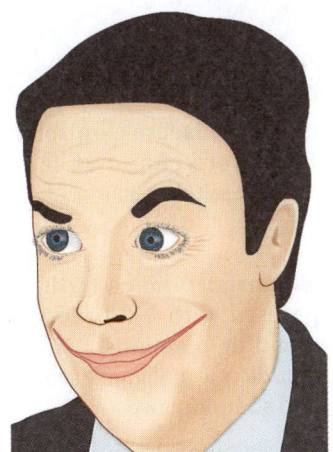

Fig. 52.2: Risus sardonicus

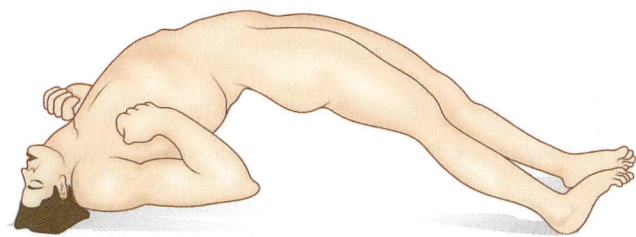

Fig. 52.3: Opisthotonus

- Increased muscle tone, hyperreflexia, agitation, restlessness and convulsions lead to profound lactic acidosis, rhabdomyolysis and hyperthermia.
- Death occurs within 4–5 convulsions as the patient cannot breathe. Consciousness is not lost and the mind remains clear till death. At the time of death, the body 'freezes' even in the middle of convulsions resulting in '*cadaveric spasm*'.

Cause of death: Death is due to medullary paralysis or asphyxia due to spasm of respiratory muscles or due to exhaustion from convulsions.

> **NOTA BENE**
> - **Clonic contractions:** Alternate involuntary muscular contraction and relaxation in rapid succession.
> - **Tonic contractions** is characterized by continuous tension or contraction of the muscles.

Fatal Dose

- Strychnine: 15–50 mg (1–2 mg/kg body wt).
- 1 crushed seed.

The US Centers for Disease Control and Prevention quantify the dose of strychnine that is 'immediately dangerous to life and health' as 30 mg.

Fatal period: 1–2 h.

Differential diagnosis: Tetanus **(Diff. 52.1)**, epilepsy (patient is depressed with obtunded mental status), hysteria, dystonic drug reactions, picrotoxin exposure, hypocalcemia, neuroleptic malignant syndrome, malignant hyperthermia, and stimulant use.

Diagnosis: Confirmation of strychnine poisoning is done by urine or gastric aspirate analysis utilizing a qualitative test such as thin layer chromatography (TLC). GC-MS and high-performance liquid chromatography are also sensitive methods to detect strychnine.

> **NOTA BENE**
> - **Mandelin test:** When the reagent is added to the extract, a violet-blue color forms, which soon changes to yellow on standing.
> - **Wenzell test:** The suspected material is treated with a solution of $KMnO_4$ in sulfuric acid; even a small amount of strychnine will cause color reactions.

TREATMENT

There is no specific antidote for strychnine poisoning. Treatment involves supportive care with minimization of external stimulus and prevention of convulsions.

i. Maintain clear airway and adequate ventilation including endotracheal intubation.
ii. **Control of convulsions:** Dark room, free from noise and disturbance. Diazepam 0.1–0.5 mg/kg IV slowly. If ineffective, general anesthetics and/or muscle relaxants, such as gallamine should be given.
iii. Barbiturates, such as pentobarbital sodium or sodium amytal are antidotes. *Dose:* 300–600 mg IV.
iv. Gastric lavage with $KMnO_4$ *may be done cautiously* after securing the airway with an endotracheal tube, if there are no convulsions. Activated charcoal is recommended as it adsorbs strychnine and may reduce its absorption if given 1 h of ingestion.
v. Hyperthermia is treated by active cooling with ice water immersion, cooling blanket or mist and fan.
vi. Intravenous fluid is given to maintain a urine output > 1 mL/kg/h, since metabolic acidosis and renal failure may occur.
vii. Hemodialysis is not effective, as strychnine is rapidly distributed to the tissues.
viii. Symptomatic treatment.

Postmortem Findings

i. Not characteristic.
ii. Rigor mortis appears early.
iii. Signs of asphyxia.
iv. Extravasated blood may be found in the muscles.
v. Viscera are congested.

Strychnine can be easily detected in blood, urine, gastric fluid, bile and fixed liver and kidney samples in autopsy.

Medico-legal Aspects

- Death is usually accidental due to overdose, exposure to rodenticide, quack remedies and poison mistaken for some other harmless drug, or in children eating the seeds.
- Intentional self-harm has also been reported. However, homicide is rare because of its bitter taste and strychnine is detectable in food in very low concentrations, hence, it is impossible to disguise in food and beverages.
- It is used as an aphrodisiac, as cattle and arrow poison, and to kill dogs and rats.
- It is used as an adulterant in street drugs, such as cocaine, heroin and amphetamines.
- Tolerance develops on repeated consumption.
- It can be detected easily even in a decomposed body (detectable as low as 0.01 ppm in tissue).

DIFFERENTIATION 52.1: Strychnine poisoning and tetanus

S.No.	Feature	Strychnine poisoning	Tetanus
1.	History of injury	None	Present
2.	Onset	Sudden (in hours)	Gradual (several days)
3.	Site of action	Postsynaptic membrane	Presynaptic membrane
4.	Muscles affected	All muscles affected at the same time	Not affected at the same time
5.	Trismus or lock jaw	Does not start in, nor especially affect the jaw	Starts in and affects the lower jaw
6.	Muscular condition	Relaxed in between convulsions	Rigid throughout
7.	Fatal period	1–2 h	>24 h
8.	Chemical analysis	Strychnine found	No poison
9.	Culture	No growth	*Clostridium tetani* found
10.	Progression	Steadily worse/steadily better	Progress rarely steady. Variations and longer remission not uncommon

CHAPTER 52 : Spinal Poisons

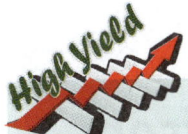

- Ripe fruit with seeds are poisonous.
- Seeds are flat, circular discs, slightly concave on one side and convex on the other, ash gray in color and look like enlarged RBCs.
- Unbroken seeds when ingested are not poisonous.
- **Active principles of *Strychnos nux-vomica*:** Strychnine, brucine and loganin.
- Strychnine antagonizes *glycine* by blocking its post-synaptic uptake by brainstem and spinal cord receptors.
- GABA, the presynaptic neurotransmitter is not affected by strychnine.
- **Characteristic feature of strychnine poisoning:** 'Conscious' seizure (convulsion).
- **Signs seen in strychnine poisoning:** Risus sardonicus (can be seen in tetanus too) and opisthotonus.
- Pupils are dilated in strychnine poisoning.
- During convulsions, the patient remains awake and aware of everything around him.
- **Differential diagnosis of strychnine poisoning:** Tetanus, epilepsy, hysteria.
- **Cause of death due to strychnine poisoning:** Medullary paralysis or asphyxia due to spasm of respiratory muscles.
- **Fatal dose:** Strychnine: 15–50 mg or 1 crushed seed.
- Mandelin and Wenzell tests are presumptive tests for strychnine poisoning.
- **Antidote for strychnine poisoning:** Barbiturates (pentobarbital sodium/sodium amytal).
- Rigor mortis appears early in deaths due to strychnine poisoning.

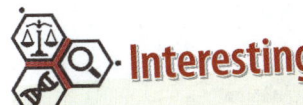

Strychnine Poisoning (Case of Jane Stanford, 1905)

Jane Stanford, co-founder of Stanford University **(Fig. A)**, funded and operated the University almost single-handedly after her husband's death in 1893. Since the death of her husband, Jane had lived alone in their Nob Hill Mansion in San Francisco, with just a few trusted servants. In January 1905, Jane, then 76-year-old drank a glass of mineral water placed in her room before going to bed. Detecting a bitter taste, she immediately vomited it out and called her staff to taste it. Both the maid and her secretary agreed that the bottled water tasted strange, and sent it to a laboratory to be analyzed. The analysis showed that the water had been poisoned with toxic dose of strychnine. Deeply shaken, Jane quickly planned a trip to Hawaii to leave the city and the assassination attempt behind her.

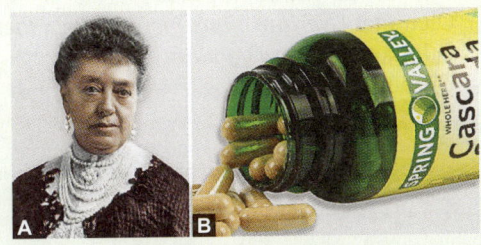

In February 1905, at the Moana Hotel, Honolulu, she asked her secretary Bertha Berner (a trusted employee and the only other person who was present during the previous incident) to bring her a laxative and bicarbonate of soda at 8:15 pm, as she was not feeling well after a heavy lunch. Bertha prepared the solution which she drank and retired to bed soon after. At around 11 pm, Jane cried out for her servants and hotel staff to call for a doctor, as she supposed of being poisoned again. This time, attempts to induce vomiting were unsuccessful. Within few minutes, the hotel doctor arrived. He had a stomach pump fetched, but it was too late. He tried to administer a solution of bromine and chloral hydrate. But she was unable to take it as her jaws were stiff. Thereafter, she had a tetanic spasm that progressed to a state of severe rigidity and her body twisted with opisthotonus convulsions. Finally, her respiration stopped and she was declared dead.

An inquest was held. In her room, police found the glass of bicarbonate of soda, little amount of vomit and the cascara capsules (a laxative) on the nightstand which they preserved for analysis **(Fig. B)**. Chemical analysis revealed the presence of strychnine in samples from the bicarbonate and laxative pills she had taken, as well as traces of the poison in her tissues. The forensic pathologist testified that the symptoms found at the autopsy were typical of strychnine: extreme rigidity of the limbs, a locked jaw and purple discoloration of the body. The cause of death was strychnine poisoning. At the end of the inquest, the Jury concluded that Jane Stanford was murdered.

The testimony revealed that the bottle in question was purchased in California and accessible to anyone in her residence, and had not been used until the night of her death. Bertha admitted the prescription for the cascara capsules was hers; she had filled it in San Francisco for years, often for her own use as well as Jane's. The source of the strychnine was never identified.

53 CHAPTER

Cardiac Poisons

LEARNING OBJECTIVES

Must know
1. Signs and symptoms of aconite poisoning
2. Identification of aconite (root)
3. Hippus
4. Medico-legal aspects of aconite poisoning

Desirable to know
1. Signs and symptoms and treatment of poisoning with tobacco, digitalis, oleander, odollam

These are poisonous plants having an action mainly on the heart, either directly or through the nerves. Important poisonous plants and compounds in this group are:
- Aconite (*Aconitum napellus, Aconitum ferox*)
- Nicotine (*Nicotiana tabacum*)
- Digitalis (*Digitalis purpurea*)
- Oleander (*Nerium odorum, Cascabela thevetia*)
- Odollam (*Cerbera odollam*)
- Quinine.

Describe general principles and basic methodologies in treatment of poisoning with regard to aconite.

ACONITE

Introduction

All parts of the plant are poisonous, however, the root and root tubers are the most potent.

Dry root is conical or tapering, shows bases of the broken rootlets and shriveled with longitudinal wrinkles (**Fig. 53.1A**). It is 5–10 cm long, 1.5–2 cm thick at the upper end and dark brown in color. Roots are mistaken for horseradish root (**Fig. 53.1B**).

Common names: Monk's hood, mitha zaher, bish, wolf's bane, women's bane, devil's helmet or blue rocket.

Active Principles

Aconitine, mesaconitine, hypaconitine, pseudoaconitine, indaconitine, picraconitine and aconine.

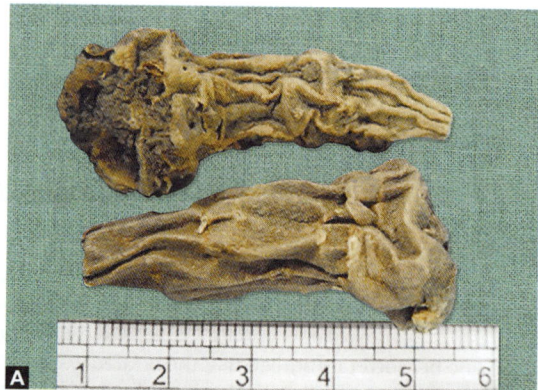

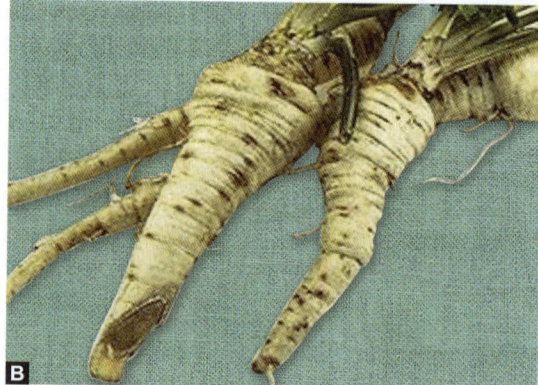

Figs. 53.1A and B: (A) Aconite (root); (B) Horseradish root

Properties of aconitine: Colorless, transparent, rhombic crystals. Insoluble in water, but readily soluble in benzene and chloroform.

Action

- Toxicity of aconitine and related alkaloids are due to their actions on the voltage-sensitive sodium channels of the cell membranes of excitable tissues. Aconitine first stimulates and then paralyzes the peripheral terminations of sensory and secretory nerves, CNS, and nerves of the myocardium, skeletal and smooth muscles.
- It does not affect the higher centers of the brain as consciousness remains intact till the end.

Signs and Symptoms

Patients present mainly with a combination of gastrointestinal, cardiovascular and neurological (sensory and motor) features.

System	Signs and symptoms
GIT	Bitter-sweet taste, severe burning and tingling of tongue, mouth, perioral area and throat, followed by numbness. Nausea, vomiting, salivation, pain in the abdomen and diarrhea
CVS	Hypotension, chest pain, palpitations, bradycardia, sinus tachycardia, ventricular ectopics and ventricular tachycardia/fibrillation. Pulse is slow, feeble and irregular
CNS	Paresthesia and numbness of face and all the four limbs; vertigo, restlessness, headache, giddiness
MS	Weakness of the muscles of the limbs with twitchings and spasms
RS	Respiration is slow, labored and shallow
Ocular	Pupils alternately contract and dilate (**hippus** or **pupillary athetosis**). Diplopia and impaired vision occurs
Others	Temperature is subnormal and skin is cold

- Terminal stages are marked by severe pain and paralysis of facial muscles.
- Many victims remain conscious until near death; some complain of yellow-green vision and tinnitus.

Cause of death: Death is due to respiratory failure or ventricular fibrillation.

Fatal Dose

- Root: 1–2 g.
- Aconitine: 2–5 mg.

Fatal period: 2–6 hours (h).

Treatment

There is no specific antidote for aconite and treatment is supportive.
  i. Gastric lavage with tannic acid/activated charcoal.
  ii. Inotropic therapy is required if hypotension persists, and atropine (0.5–1 mg IV) should be used to treat bradycardia.
  iii. Ventricular arrhythmia is treated with amiodarone and flecainide (first-line treatment). In refractory cases and cardiogenic shock, early use of cardiopulmonary bypass is recommended.
  iv. Symptomatic treatment.

Postmortem Findings

  i. Not specific, those of asphyxia.
  ii. Organs are congested.
  iii. **Stomach:** Fragments of root may be found in the stomach.
  iv. **Lungs:** Hemorrhagic pulmonary edema.
  v. **Heart:** Diffuse contraction-band necrosis in myocardium.

Medico-legal Aspects

- It is often regarded as **an ideal homicidal poison**. *Advantages are*:
  a. It is cheap and easily available.
  b. Lethal dose is small and the fatal period is short.
  c. Color can be disguised by mixing it with pink colored drinks.
  d. Taste can be masked by mixing it with sweets or by giving it with betel (*paan*) leaves.
  e. Extremely unstable and destroyed by putrefaction, hence cannot be detected by chemical analysis.
- Accidental poisoning occurs due to:
  a. Eating the roots mistaking it for horseradish.
  b. Use of quack remedies.
  c. Taking of liquor mixed with aconitine to increase intoxication.
  d. Consumption of herbal decoction made from aconite roots.
- It is also used as an abortifacient, cattle and arrow poison.
- Suicide is not common.

NOTA BENE

- **Horseradish** is a perennial plant with long, rough, tapering pungent root (belong to same family as mustard and wasabi) (**Fig. 53.1B**). It is grated and mixed with vinegar for a condiment.
- **Hippus** (Greek *hippos*: horse) is spasmodic, rhythmic, but irregular dilating and contracting pupillary movement of the sphincter and dilator muscles, independent of changes in illumination or in fixation of the eyes. The rhythm of the contractions represents galloping horse. The occurrence of hippus is normal. However, pathologic hippus (increased oscillation or amplitude) is associated with aconite poisoning, altered mental status, trauma, cirrhosis, multiple sclerosis, neurosyphilis, myasthenia gravis, cerebral tumors and renal disease.
- The term '*wolf's bane*' comes from its use to poison meat laid out for wolves.
- In ancient Rome, aconite was widely used by professional poisoners, and cultivating the plant was considered capital offense. On the Greek island of Chios, it was used for euthanasia of the old and infirm.

FM 12.1 Describe features and management of abuse/poisoning with tobacco.

NICOTIANA TABACUM (TOBACCO)

Introduction

- All parts of the plant are poisonous, except the ripe seeds.
- Leaves contain toxic alkaloids, like nicotine, anabasine, nornicotine and lobeline (in Indian tobacco).
- Dried leaves contain 1–8% nicotine **(Fig. 53.2)**.
- An average cigarette delivers 1–3 mg of nicotine.

Properties of nicotine: Colorless, hygroscopic oily liquid. Burning acrid taste and disagreeable odor.

Action

- It acts on the autonomic ganglia, which are stimulated initially, but are depressed and blocked at the later stages.
- It also acts on the somatic neuromuscular junction and afferent fibers from sensory receptors.

Signs and Symptoms

Acute Poisoning

i. **CVS:** Tachycardia followed by bradycardia, hypotension, arrhythmia, tachypnea followed by respiratory depression and collapse.
ii. **GIT:** Burning acid sensation, nausea, vomiting, abdominal pain, salivation and odor of tobacco.
iii. **CNS:** Headache, restlessness, confusion, vertigo, sweating, convulsions and coma.

Chronic Poisoning

i. **RS:** Cough, wheeze, dyspnea, chronic bronchitis, and lung cancer may develop.

ii. **CVS:** Anemia, palpitations, irregularity of heart, angina pectoris and Buerger's disease.
iii. **GIT:** Anorexia, vomiting and diarrhea.
iv. **CNS and others:** Impaired memory, blindness, tremors, insomnia, anxiety and headache.

Fatal Dose

- Nicotine: 60–100 mg.
- Tobacco: 15–30 g.

Fatal period: 5–15 minutes.

Treatment

i. Gastric lavage with charcoal, $KMnO_4$.
ii. Purgatives.
iii. Cardiac monitoring.
iv. Atropine to correct hypotension, and diazepam for convulsions.
v. Symptomatic treatment.

In chronic poisoning, clonidine has shown encouraging result.

Postmortem Findings

i. Brownish froth at mouth and nostrils.
ii. Stomach may contain fragments of leaves or smell of tobacco.
iii. Features of asphyxia are seen.

Medico-legal Aspects

- Accidental poisoning results from ingestion, excessive smoking and application of leaves or juice to wound or skin.
- Common drug of addiction.
- For the purpose of malingering, leaves are soaked in water for some hours and placed in axilla at bed time, poisonous symptoms are seen by next morning.
- Suicidal/homicidal cases are rare.

NOTA BENE

Green tobacco sickness commonly occurs in tobacco growing States. Workers handling leaves may absorb alkaloids through skin. Symptoms include nausea, vomiting, diarrhea, diaphoresis and weakness that usually resolve with symptomatic treatment.

FM 10.1 Describe general principles and basic methodologies in treatment of poisoning with regard to digitalis.

DIGITALIS PURPUREA (FOXGLOVE)

Introduction

Digitalis purpurea is a biennial plant, often grown as an ornamental plant due to its colorful flowers which range

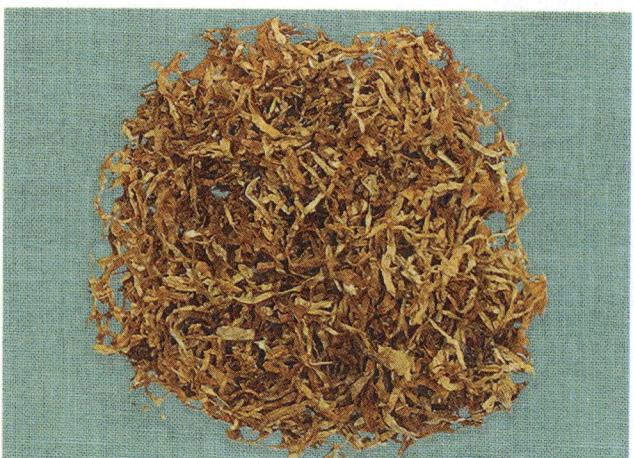

Fig. 53.2: Dried tobacco leaves

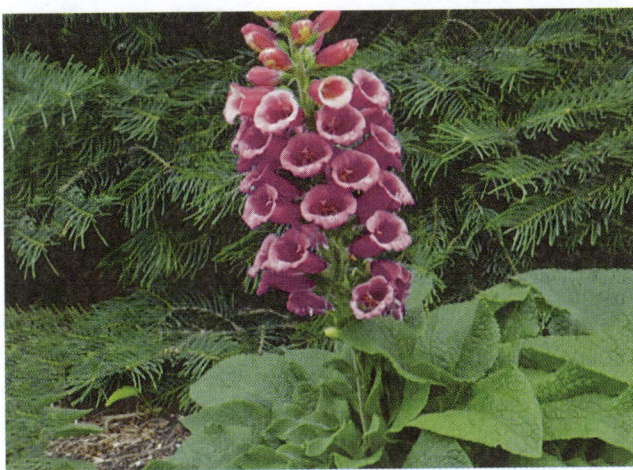

Fig. 53.3: *Digitalis purpurea*

from various purple tints through pink, and purely white (Fig. 53.3). It is cultivated commercially as source of cardiac stimulant drug digitalis (digoxin). The drug is obtained from the dried leaves.

Active Principles

Its roots, leaves and seeds contain several glycosides—digitoxin, digitalin, digitalein and digitonin, and are most poisonous.

Action

The glycosides act directly on the heart muscle (prolong diastolic period) and improve the function of the failing heart. In toxic doses, excitability is increased with extrasystoles.

> **NOTA BENE**
>
> **Glycosides** are substances found in plants, and are composed of a sugar and a non-sugar compound, the latter having toxicological action.

Signs and Symptoms

Toxic symptoms are due to overdose or by a cumulative action.

System	Signs and symptoms
GIT	Nausea, vomiting, pain in abdomen, burning sensation, diarrhea
CVS	Bradycardia, extrasystoles, ventricular tachycardia and fibrillation, atrial fibrillation, faintness, precordial oppression, heart block
CNS	Headache, fatigue, confusion, anxiety, depression, disorientation, drowsiness, hallucinations, delirium
RS	Labored and sighing respiration
Ocular	Transient amblyopia, blurring, photophobia, scotoma, diplopia, color aberration
Skin	Urticaria

The patient becomes drowsy and the condition may deepen into coma. Convulsions may precede death.

Cause of death: Death occurs from cardiovascular collapse.

Fatal Dose

- Digitalis: 2–3 g.
- Digoxin: 5 mg.
- Digitalin: 15–20 mg.
- Powdered leaves: 2.5 g.

Fatal period: 1–24 h.

Treatment

ECG monitoring is necessary as a guide to treatment.
 i. Gastric lavage is done with a solution of tannic acid.
 ii. Activated charcoal is given.
 iii. Purgatives may be given.
 iv. Atropine is given in a dose of 0.6 mg IV to treat bradycardia.
 v. Potassium chloride may be given to reduce extrasystoles.
 vi. **Digoxin-specific antibody fragments** (Digoxin-Fab) is indicated in all patients with life-threatening arrhythmias and an elevated digoxin concentration. In acute poisoning, a small bolus of 80 mg, titrated against clinical effect is beneficial (*repeat if necessary*).
 vii. Specific antidote for cardiac arrhythmias is lignocaine 100 mg IV or novocaine or propranolol.
 viii. Trisodium EDTA may help to lower serum calcium.
 ix. Symptomatic treatment.

Postmortem Findings

Non-specific changes are seen. There may be irritation of the gastric mucosa, and digitalis leaves or seeds may be found in the stomach.

Medico-legal Aspects

- Accidental poisoning due to overdose of a medicinal preparation or from eating leaves by mistake.
- It is a cumulative poison, and persons taking it for a long time may suddenly develop symptoms of poisoning.
- Homicidal poisoning cases may be seen, and no suspicion of poisoning may arise in such cases as it will simulate heart disease.

> **FM 10.1**
>
> Describe general principles and basic methodologies in treatment of poisoning with regard to oleander.

OLEANDER (KANER)

The oleander plant grows wild in India. There are two varieties:
- *Nerium odorum:* Bears white, dark red or pink flowers.
- *Cascabela thevetia:* Bears yellow bell-shaped flowers, globular fruits, light green in color, about 5 cm in

diameter containing a single nut, triangular in shape and light brown in color. The nut contains five pale yellow seeds.

NERIUM ODORUM

Common names: White Oleander/Kaner (**Fig. 53.4A**)
All parts of the plant are poisonous.

Active Principles

Nerin consisting of three glycosides—neriodorin, neriodorein and karabin.

Action

It is similar to that of digitalis causing death from cardiac failure. Neriodorein causes muscular twitching and tetanic spasm which is more powerful than strychnine. Karabin acts on the heart like digitalis and on the spinal cord like strychnine.

Signs and Symptoms

- **Locally**, contact dermatitis.
- **Inhalation** of flowers may cause headache, dizziness, respiratory difficulty and nausea.
- **Ingestion** causes vomiting, pain in the abdomen, frothy salivation, difficulty in swallowing and articulation. Later on, there is restlessness, muscular twitchings, tetanic spasms and lock jaw. The pulse is slow and weak, respiration is rapid, blood pressure falls, and there is fibrillation and AV block. This is followed by exhaustion, drowsiness, coma, respiratory paralysis and death from heart failure.

Fatal Dose

Root: 15–20 g; leaves: 5–15.
Fatal period: 24 h.

Treatment

i. Gastric lavage.
ii. Administration of an anesthetic is usually necessary.
iii. Morphine injection seems to be beneficial.
iv. Symptomatic treatment.

Postmortem Findings

Non-specific findings. Petechial hemorrhages on the heart are characteristic feature. Organs are congested.

Medico-legal Aspects

- Suicide is common among village girls, using it as a paste or decoction.
- It is used as an abortifacient, applied both locally and internally.
- Homicide is rare.
- Accidental poisoning is sometimes met with when decoction is used:
  a. Externally to reduce swelling.
  b. As a remedy for venereal diseases.
  c. As a *love-philter* (increases attraction between the giver and taker).
  d. For treatment of cancer and ulcers.
- It is used as cattle poison.
- *Nerium odorum* resists heat and can therefore be detected even from the burnt remains of the dead body.

CASCABELA THEVETIA

All parts of the plant are poisonous. Milky juice exudes from all parts of the plant (**Fig. 53.4B**).
Common names: Yellow Oleander/Pila Kaner.

Active Principles

Glycosides—thevetin, thevotoxin, cerberin and peruvoside. Thevetin is a powerful cardiac poison. Thevotoxin is less

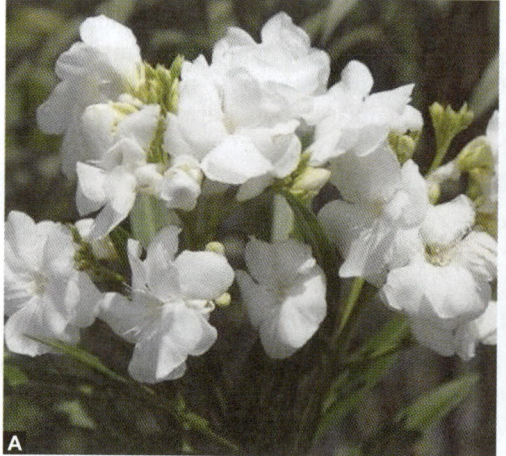
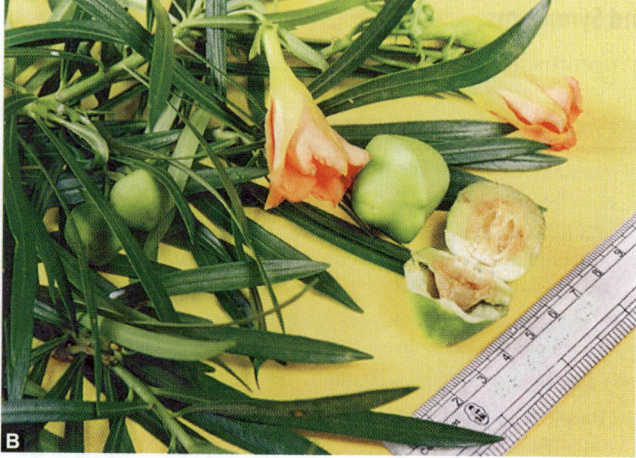

Figs. 53.4A and B: (A) *Nerium odorum*; (B) *Cascabela thevetia* (oleander)

toxic than thevetin and resembles the glycosides of digitalis in action. Cerberin acts like strychnine.

Signs and Symptoms

Locally, the sap of the plant may cause inflammation.

On ingestion, there is burning sensation in the mouth with tingling of the tongue, dryness of throat, vomiting, diarrhea, headache, dizziness, dilated pupils, drowsiness and loss of muscular power. Pulse is rapid, weak and irregular, blood pressure falls. Heart block, collapse and death is due to peripheral circulatory failure.

Fatal Dose

Seeds: 8–10; root: 15–20 g.
Fatal period: 2–3 h.

Treatment

i. Gastric lavage. Single-dose activated charcoal is beneficial and safe.
ii. Molar solution of sodium lactate IV and 5% glucose to combat acidosis.
iii. Atropine 1 mg, 2 mL of adrenaline 1:1000 and 2 mg of noradrenaline (if blood pressure is low) to counteract heart block.
iv. Digoxin-specific antibody fragments is effective in reverting life-threatening cardiac arrhythmias.
v. Symptomatic treatment.

Postmortem Findings

Non-specific:
i. Signs of GIT irritation may be seen.
ii. Stomach and duodenum may be congested and may show fragments of seeds.
iii. Congestion of visceral organs is seen.

Medico-legal aspects: Same as *Nerium odorum*.

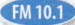
Describe general principles and basic methodologies in treatment of poisoning with regard to odollam.

CERBERA ODOLLAM

Introduction

Cerbera odollam is a tree belonging to the poisonous Apocynaceae family, which includes the yellow and common oleanders. The plant grows in wet areas in South India, Madagascar, and Southeast Asia. The fruit resembles mango and its kernel (core of the fruit) contains various toxic principles **(Fig. 53.5)**.

Common names: Suicide tree, Buddha tree, sea mango, *pong-pong, othalanga*.

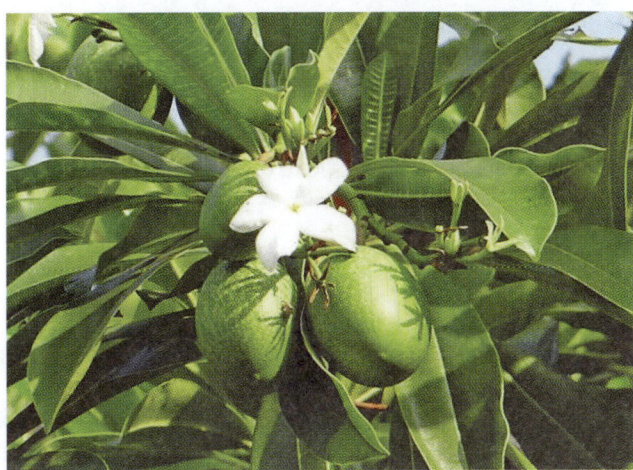
Fig. 53.5: *Cerbera odollam*

Active Principles

The seeds contain cardiac glycosides cerberin, cerberoside neriifolin and diacetlytanghinin.

Action: Cerberin has a mechanism of action similar to digoxin (binds and inhibit Na^+, K^+ ATPase in cardiac myocytes); hence, *its* toxicity is similar to acute digoxin poisoning.

Signs and Symptoms

Toxic effects resemble those produced by digitalis.
♦ **On ingestion,** there is bitter taste, nausea, vomiting, chest pain, palpitations, bradycardia, syncope, hyperkalemia, thrombocytopenia and ECG abnormalities.
♦ Death is due to 'heart attack' produced by the poison.

Fatal Dose

Kernel of one fruit.
Fatal period: 12–24 h.

Treatment

Supportive therapy for bradycardia and hyperkalemia (similar to digoxin toxicity).
i. Atropine followed by temporary cardiac pacing.
ii. Administration of digoxin immune Fab.
iii. Extracorporeal membrane oxygenation.

Postmortem Findings

Non-specific changes.
i. Signs of GIT irritation may be seen.
ii. Stomach and duodenum may be congested and may show fragments of seeds.
iii. Congestion of visceral organs is seen.

Medico-legal Aspects

- It is used both for suicide and homicide.
  - Common suicidal agent in Kerala (more in females).
  - It can be used for homicide as kernel may be added to toddy, liquor or food to disguise its bitter taste.
- Accidental poisoning can occur from eating the fruit by mistake.
- The identification is difficult unless sophisticated tests are employed (TLC or LC-MS).

- Aconite is also called Monk's hood, mitha zaher (bitter-sweet taste), bish.
- **Active principles in aconite:** Aconitine, pseudo-aconitine, mesaconitine.
- Aconitine does not affect the higher centers of brain as consciousness remains intact till death.
- Acute poisoning shows hypotension, palpitations, bradycardia, VT and VF, slow, feeble and irregular pulse.
- *Hippus* (alternate contraction and dilatation of pupil) is seen in aconite poisoning, altered mental status, trauma, cirrhosis, multiple sclerosis, neurosyphilis, myasthenia gravis, cerebral tumors and renal disease.
- **Fatal dose of aconite:** Root: 1–2 g, aconitine: 2–5 mg.
- In deaths due to aconite poisoning, heart shows diffuse contraction-band necrosis in myocardium.
- Aconite is considered as *an ideal homicidal poison*.
- **Tobacco:** Whole plant is poisonous, except ripe seeds.
- **Active principles in tobacco:** Nicotine, anabasine, nornicotine and lobeline.
- Acute tobacco poisoning shows tachycardia followed by bradycardia, hypotension, arrhythmia, tachypnea followed by respiratory depression and collapse.
- **Fatal dose:** Nicotine: 60–100 mg; tobacco: 15–30 g.
- **Active principle in *Digitalis purpurea* (foxglove):** Digitoxin.
- Acute digitalis poisoning shows bradycardia, extrasystoles, VT and VF, AF, faintness, heart block.
- **Fatal dose:** Digitalis: 2–3 g, digoxin: 5 mg.
- Digoxin-specific antibody fragments (Digoxin-Fab) is use to treat digitalis toxicity.
- **Active principle in *Nerium odorum*:** Nerin.
- **Common names:** Common oleander, *kaner*.
- Acute oleander poisoning shows restlessness, muscular twitchings, tetanic spasms, lock jaw, slow and weak pulse, rapid respiration, hypotension, fibrillation and AV block.
- **Fatal dose *N. odorum*:** Root: 15–20 g; leaves: 5–15.
- *Nerium odorum* resists heat and can be detected even from remains of burnt dead body.
- **Active principles in *C. thevetia*:** Thevetin, thevotoxin, cerberin.
- **Common names:** Yellow oleander, *pila kaner*, lucky nut.
- Acute oleander poisoning presents with tingling of tongue, drowsiness, dilated pupils, loss of muscular power, rapid, weak and irregular pulse, hypotension, heart block, collapse and death.
- **Fatal dose *C. thevetia*:** Seeds: 8–10; root: 15–20 g.
- **Active principle in *Cerbera odollam*:** Cerberin.
- **Common names:** Suicide tree, *Pong-pong*, *othalanga*.
- Acute odollam poisoning shows hyperkalemia, thrombocytopenia, ECG abnormalities.
- **Fatal dose of *C. odollam*:** Kernel of one fruit.
- Odollam is used both for suicide and homicide.

Interesting case

Nicotine Poisoning (Case of Paul Curry, 1994)

In 1989, Paul Curry and Linda met each other at the San Onofre nuclear plant where they worked. They started dating and 3 years later, in 1992 they decided to marry. Paul Curry was in his mid-thirties and Linda was approaching her fifties **(Figs. A and B)**.

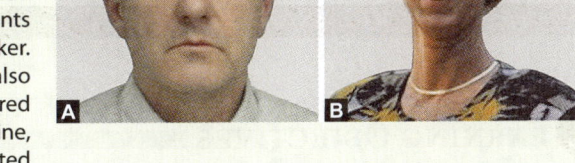

In June 1994 near midnight, Curry called 911 and said that his wife was not breathing. Paramedics arrived but were unable to revive Linda. Linda was pronounced dead in the hospital. An autopsy revealed fatal amounts of nicotine in Linda's body, despite the fact that she was a non-smoker. A needle puncture was discovered behind her right ear. There was also evidence of toxic levels of sedative in her system. Her death was declared a homicide, but there was no evidence to connect Curry to the nicotine, sleeping pills or syringe so that he could be charged. Paul Curry collected $419,000 from two of Linda's life insurance policies and her retirement plan. He also began collecting her retirement benefit of $564 every month.

The case was reopened in 2007, and investigators discovered new evidence that revealed a shorter time frame for the nicotine injection. According to prosecutors, Linda started falling ill nine months into the marriage. She was suffering unusual bouts of stomach pains, diarrhea and vomiting. Her GIT problems led to hospitalization twice in 1993. On both occasions, her IV bag was found to have been tampered with, right after her husband's visits. On the first occasion, nurses discovered that the IV bag had been punctured and laced with Lidocaine, a local anesthetic and cardiac depressant that Linda had not been prescribed with. On the second occasion at a different hospital, something similar happened again. In a police interview recorded before her death (after her first admission), she was asked if anyone had reason to hurt her and she mentioned that 'the only person I could think of that would have a motive to do it would be Paul'.

Police also questioned Leslie, the former wife of Curry. She also relayed similar incidents during her final year of marriage. She began to suffer from a 'debilitating' sickness that left her bedridden and doctors were unable to diagnose the cause of her illness. Leslie said her health problems disappeared after her divorce.

A toxicology expert reviewed the evidence and testified that the nicotine injection would have killed Linda within a few hours of her being exposed to it. Curry's story had always been that on the night Linda died, the two of them were at home alone for about 6 hours. He was the only person who could have sedated Linda, before injecting her with nicotine.

Sixteen years after his wife's death, Curry was arrested in 2010 and charged with murder and insurance fraud. During the trial, prosecutors argued that Curry had poisoned his wife with nicotine for insurance money and benefits that amounted to half a million dollars. The defense argued that the high level of nicotine in her blood was due to a self-administered nicotine enema which she used as a holistic treatment for her GIT symptoms, but could not explain the sedative in her blood. The Jury found Paul Curry guilty of first-degree murder with special circumstances for poisoning and murder for financial gain. In November 2014, he was sentenced to life in prison without possibility of parole.

54 CHAPTER

Hydrocyanic Acid

LEARNING OBJECTIVES

Must know
1. Signs and symptoms and treatment of hydrogen cyanide poisoning
2. Postmortem findings in cyanide poisoning
3. Medico-legal aspects of cyanide toxicity

Desirable to know
1. Judicial execution using hydrogen cyanide

Describe general principles and basic methodologies in treatment of poisoning with regard to hydrogen cyanide and derivatives.

Introduction

Hydrogen cyanide (HCN) is a highly toxic chemical. Hydrocyanic acid (Prussic acid, cyanogens) is a bluish-white solution of HCN in water, either 2% or 4%, the latter being called *Scheele's acid*.

Physical properties: Pure acid is a colorless gas with **bitter almond odor**. All persons cannot smell the gas, and the ability to detect it is a *sex-linked recessive trait*. Cyanides of sodium/potassium are white powders. HCN is liberated from these by reacting with acids (e.g., HCl in stomach).

Sources and Uses

- *Natural:* It is found in many fruits, seeds, bean and leaves, such as bitter almond (slightly broader and shorter than the sweet almond) **(Figs. 54.1A and B)**, apricot, peach, apple, cherry and plum, and in certain oilseeds and beans where it exists in the form of glucoside *amygdalin* which is harmless, but usually co-exists with a group of enzymes, the emulsion complex which hydrolyzes it and liberates HCN in the GIT leading to poisoning.
- *HCN gas:* It is used for fumigation of ships.
- HCN is often used in laboratory and industries connected with photography, electroplating, silver coating and tanning.
- It is normal constituent of the body (15–30 µg).

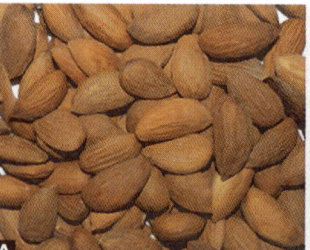 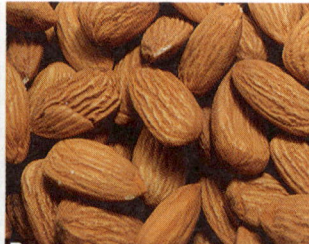

Figs. 54.1A and B: (A) Bitter almonds; (B) Sweet almonds

> **NOTA BENE**
> *Linseed oil* (flax seed oil), is a yellowish drying oil derived from the dried ripe seeds of the flax plant *(Linum usitatissimum)*. Linseed meal (after extraction of oil) can have cyanide, if made from immature seeds. The meal is safe, if boiled.

Action

- HCN is a protoplasmic cytotoxic poison.
- Cyanide ions (CN^-) bind to, and inhibit the ferric (Fe^{3+}) heme moiety form of mitochondrial cytochrome oxidase, carbonic anhydrase and other enzyme systems of cellular respiration.
- It blocks the final step of oxidative phosphorylation and prevents the formation of ATP, resulting in the arrest of aerobic metabolism and death from *histotoxic anoxia*. The inhibition of oxidative metabolism puts increased demands on anaerobic glycolysis, which results in lactic acid production and may produce severe acid-base imbalance.
- It also acts as a corrosive on mucosa.

Cyanides may become less effective, if they are kept too long (they tend to change into carbonates) and if the person suffers from *achlorhydria* (since HCl acts on cyanides to liberate hydrocyanic acid).

Absorption and Excretion

- Hydrocyanic acid is rapidly absorbed by all routes—ingestion, inhalation, dermal and parenteral.
- Cyanide gas is absorbed from the respiratory tract, and the acid and cyanide salts from the stomach.
- Absorption is delayed when cyanide is taken on a full stomach or with a large quantity of wine.

■ SIGNS AND SYMPTOMS

This is *most rapid of all poisons.* The dose of cyanide required to produce toxicity is dependent on form (gas or salt), duration of exposure, dose and route of exposure.
- When inhaled as gas, its action is instantaneous.
- If a large dose is ingested, symptoms appear at once, but in some cases symptoms appear after few minutes, during which the victim may perform certain voluntary acts, such as throwing away the bottle or walking a little distance.
- In case of dermal application, latent interval can be several hours.

System	Signs and symptoms
Local	Corrosive effect on the mouth, throat and stomach
CNS	Headache, vertigo, faintness, anxiety, excitement, confusion, drowsiness, prostration, opisthotonus, lockjaw, hyperthermia, epileptiform or tonic convulsions, paralysis, stupor and coma
CVS	Initially hypertension with tachycardia, sinus arrhythmia, later on bradycardia with hypotension and cardiovascular collapse
GIT	Bitter acid burning taste, constriction or numbness of throat, clenched jaw, salivation, froth, nausea, rarely vomiting
RS	Odor of bitter almonds in breath, initially tachypnea and dyspnea, followed by rapid slowing of respiratory rate with severe respiratory depression and absence of cyanosis
Skin	Perspiration, bullae, pinkish or brick-red color*
Ocular	Glassy, prominent eyes, pupils dilated and unreactive, bright retinal veins
Renal	Acidosis

- Additionally, after inhalation, there is nasal and laryngeal irritation, dyspnea, feeling of suffocation and chest tightness and air hunger. Cyanosis is usually absent, unless respiratory depression supervenes.

Cause of death: Death occurs from respiratory failure.

Fatal Dose

(Blood levels >2.5 mg/L is fatal)
- Pure acid: 50–60 mg.
- NaCN and KCN: 200–300 mg.
- Pharmacological preparation: 30 drops.
- Crude oil of bitter almonds: 60 drops or 50–60 beans.
- Airborne concentration: 270 ppm (μg/mL) of HCN for few minutes.

Fatal period
- HCN: 2–10 minutes (min), sometimes immediate.
- KCN or NaCN: 30 min.

Differential diagnosis: Neurotoxic organophosphates.

Diagnosis: The triad of laboratory findings is suggestive of cyanide poisoning:
  i. A narrow arterial-venous oxygen difference
  ii. An anion gap metabolic acidosis
  iii. An elevated lactate concentration.
- Measurement of whole blood cyanide in an anticoagulant tube (not done with plasma or serum, since cyanide is sequestered in RBCs) can confirm toxicity.
- HCN is also measured by gas chromatography or spectrophotometry (shows characteristic bands).

> **NOTA BENE**
>
> **Lee Jones test:** A few small crystals of ferrous sulfate are added to 5 mL of gastric aspirate, and 4–5 drops of 20% NaOH solution are added to precipitate the iron. The mixture is boiled, cooled and acidified with few drops of 10% HCl. A greenish-blue precipitate (ferricyanide) which intensifies on standing indicates the presence of cyanide. Similar color change may occur with salicylate too.

■ TREATMENT

If the patient is symptomatic, emergency life support measures are started; oxygen (100%) should be given immediately followed by specific antidote.

I. Stabilization

Assisted ventilation, 100% oxygen and cardiac monitoring. In cases of respiratory compromise, shock or seizures, patient is treated according to advanced life support (ALS) protocols.

II. Decontamination

Remove the person from the source of poisoning.
- Healthcare provider should always be protected from potential dermal contamination by using protective devices such as water-impervious gowns, gloves and eyewear.

---

* Pink color results from increased venous hemoglobin saturation due to decreased utilization of O_2 at tissue level. On fundoscopic examination, veins and arteries may appear similar in color.

- For patients with dermal exposure, remove clothing, brush off any powder from the skin and flush the skin with water.
- In case of ingestion, gastric lavage is done with 5–10% solution of sodium thiosulfate, followed by potassium carbonate to form Prussian blue which is inert. Activated charcoal is ineffective (because of low binding of cyanide), but can be given in patient with patent airway. Emetics should not be used.

III. Antidotal therapy

The 3-step *cyanide antidote kit* is used. It contains amyl nitrite, sodium nitrite and sodium thiosulfate.

i. 0.3 mL ampoule of amyl nitrite pearl is broken in a gauze and the victim is made to inhale for 30 seconds, every minute *(1st step)*, and use a new pearl every 3 min. Stop amyl nitrite, if systolic BP is <80 mmHg.

ii. 10 mL of 3% solution (300 mg) of sodium nitrite (weak vasodilator; large doses sufficient to generate enough metHb, can be injected IV without producing hypotension) is injected IV slowly over 5 min *(2nd step)*, followed by 50 mL of 25% solution (12.5 g) of sodium thiosulfate over 10–20 min, by the same needle *(3rd step)*.

Alternative Therapy

- Two 20 mL ampoules of 1.5% dicobalt tetracemate (*Kelocyanor*) are given IV followed by 20 mL of 50% glucose.
- 50 mL of 1% sterile aqueous solution of methylene blue may also be used as an antidote.

In case of KCN/NaCN poisoning: Hydroxocobalamin (vitamin B_{12}) 4–5 g IV is given as infusion over 15 min.

In case of mercury cyanide poisoning: Inject BAL also.

IV. Supportive Measures

- Administer crystalloids and vasopressors for hypotension, and $NaHCO_3$ for acidosis (1 mEq/kg IV).
- Control seizures with anticonvulsants, and cardiac monitoring to evaluate and treat dysrhythmias.

Survival for 4 hours after poisoning is usually followed by recovery.

> **NOTA BENE**
> - The principle of treatment is to reverse the cyanide-cytochrome combination. This is done by converting hemoglobin to methemoglobin by giving nitrites. Methemoglobin has a higher binding affinity for cyanide than cytochrome oxidase complex and removes cyanide from cytochrome oxidase.

- Cyanides combine with methemoglobin and form non-toxic *cyanmethemoglobin** which in the presence of rhodanese and sulfate donors, such as thiosulfate, converts cyanide to thiocyanate which is excreted in urine.
- Cyanide is directly converted to thiocyanate by complexing of cyanide with thiosulfate under the influence of enzyme rhodanese.
- Cyanide is also converted to cyanocobalamin by complexing with hydroxocobalamin.

> Cytochrome oxidase + NaCN → Cytochrome oxidase cyanide
> Sodium nitrite + Hemoglobin → Methemoglobin
> Methemoglobin + NaCN → Cyanmethemoglobin
> Cyanmet Hb + sod. thiosulfate → MetHb + sod. thiocyante
> (excreted in urine)

- *Cyanide kit* is proposed by WHO as contingency antidotes and the mainstay of antidotal therapy in the US.
- In Europe, 4-dimethylaminophenol (3 mg/kg) is the methemoglobin-inducing agent of choice in place of sodium nitrite, which is coadministered with thiosulfate. PAPP (p-aminopropiophenone) can also form methemoglobin, but its action is slow.
- Methemoglobin-inducing agents are no longer utilized in France, and dicobalt EDTA is prescribed.
- *Stroma-free methemoglobin* (oxidized hemoglobin from which cell membrane has been removed) is an investigational tool—provides exogenous methemoglobin to bind cyanide without compromising the oxygen-carrying capacity of hemoglobin, and removal of cell membrane eliminates antigenicity.

POSTMORTEM FINDINGS

Usually, those of asphyxia.

External

i. Smell of bitter almonds near the body.
ii. Face, lips and body surfaces show irregular pink patches, or rarely, cyanotic tinge.
iii. Fine froth at the mouth.
iv. *Eyes*: Bright, glistening, prominent with dilated pupils.
v. Rigor mortis appears early.
vi. Jaws are firmly closed.

Internal

i. In case of suspected cyanide poisoning, cranial cavity should be opened first as the odor of bitter almonds is well marked in the brain tissue.
ii. *Brain and meninges*: Hyperemic, diffuse cerebral edema with loss of gray-white differentiation.
iii. Potassium or sodium cyanide produces slight corrosion of the mouth. Mucosa of the stomach may be eroded and blackened due to formation of alkaline hematin.
iv. Bloodstained froth in the trachea/bronchi.
v. Pleura and pericardium may show petechial hemorrhages.

---

* Cyanmethemoglobin formed may again disassociate to release cyanide. Therefore, sodium thiosulfate is given to form sodium. thiocyante which is poorly dissociable and is excreted in the urine. Cytochrome and other oxidative enzymes are thus protected from cyanide; even when the enzyme which is complexed with CN is reactivated.

- Cyanide concentration can be measured in whole blood, gastric contents, tissues and urine.
- Extremely volatile substance—viscera for chemical examination must be sent in air tight bottles. Lungs should be preserved and sealed in nylon bag.
- Spleen is said to be the *best specimen* for cyanide analysis, since it has the highest concentration of the poison owing to its presence of RBCs.

NOTA BENE

Exposure to cyanide vapors has been associated with toxic symptoms of cyanide in autopsy personnel (stomach contents containing ingested cyanide salts present the highest risk because the gastric acid converts cyanide salts to volatile HCN gas). Autopsies on victims of cyanide poisoning should be performed in a negative-pressure isolation room and using adequate protective devices.

Medico-legal Aspects

- It is commonly used for suicidal purposes—*ideal suicidal agent*. A fruit-flavored drink laced with KCN was the causative agent in the mass suicide of the members of the People's Temple in Jonestown, Guyana, in 1978. Suicides by ingestion of KCN used by goldsmiths or textile industry workers are common.
- Accidental incidences may be seen occasionally—eating bitter almonds, workplace exposure (chemists or technicians handling cyanides in laboratories), smoke inhalation in fire in enclosed spaces (from combustion of materials such as wool, silk, synthetic rubber and polyurethane).
- Homicide is rare—quick action and peculiar smell and taste. In ancient Rome, Emperor Nero reportedly used cyanide in the form of cherry laurel water to poison enemies and family members.
  - In case of homicidal poisoning, the defense frequently insists upon the poison developing internally through fruit previously eaten. It is advisable for the analyst to make quantitative analysis of fruits the deceased supposedly or known to have eaten.
- Iatrogenic poisoning may occur during use of nitroprusside for management of hypertension.
- Cyanide has been used as an agent of genocide in gas chambers in Nazi concentration camps in World War II.
- Embalming can remove/destroy cyanide.
- Small amount of cyanides may be formed in the tissues due to putrefaction.
- Normal cyanide levels are higher in cigarette smokers than in nonsmokers, and in whole blood as compared to plasma. Smokers may have whole blood cyanide levels of 0.4 mg/L, >2.5 times the mean of non-smokers.

Chronic cyanide poisoning occurs from repeated exposure among photographers or gilders. Such people suffer from headache, vomiting, diarrhea, cachexia and mental disturbances. Hydrogen cyanide has not been associated with any carcinogenic effects or developmental defects.

JUDICIAL EXECUTION

In some countries, hydrocyanic gas is used for legal execution.

Procedure

The condemned person is strapped in a metal chair with perforated seat, and the straps applied across his upper and lower legs, arms, thighs and chest. A long stethoscope is also affixed to the person's chest so that a doctor sitting outside can monitor the heart beat and pronounce death.

Beneath the chair is a bowl filled with sulfuric acid mixed with distilled water, with sodium cyanide pellets suspended in a gauze bag just above it. After the door is sealed, the executioner in a separate room operates a lever that releases the cyanide into the liquid. This causes a chemical reaction that releases hydrogen cyanide gas which rises through the holes in the chair.

$$2NaCN + H_2SO_4 = 2HCN\uparrow + Na_2SO_4$$

Prisoners are advised to take deep breaths after the gas is released as this will considerably shorten their suffering. Unconsciousness takes place very rapidly, although the heart continues to beat for 10–20 min.

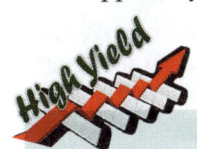

- Most rapid of all poisons; instantaneous death on inhalation.
- HCN has *bitter almond odor*—ability to detect it is a *sex-linked recessive trait*.
- HCN is liberated by reacting with acids (e.g., HCl in stomach).
- If the person suffers from *achlorhydria*, cyanides may not cause poisoning.
- Cyanide inhibits cytochrome oxidase causing *histotoxic anoxia*.
- **Fatal dose:** NaCN and KCN: 200–300 mg.
- **Fatal period** HCN: Immediate to 2–10 min; KCN or NaCN: 30 min.
- **Presumptive test for cyanide:** Lee Jones test.
- **Antidotal for cyanide poisoning:** Cyanide antidote kit which contains *amyl nitrite (given by inhalation), sodium nitrite and sodium thiosulfate*.

- **Principle of treatment:** Reverse the cyanide-cytochrome combination by converting hemoglobin to methemoglobin. Cyanides combine with methemoglobin and form non-toxic *cyanmethemoglobin*.
- **Alternative therapy:** Dicobalt tetracemate (*Kelocyanor*), methylene blue, hydroxocobalamin (vitamin B_{12}).
- **PM findings in cyanide poisoning:** Smell of bitter almonds, bright red/pink PM staining, fine froth at mouth, rigor mortis appears early.
- **Best specimen for cyanide analysis:** Spleen.
- HCN is commonly used for suicidal purposes—*ideal suicidal agent*.
- Embalming can remove/destroy cyanide.
- Small amount of cyanides may be formed in the tissues due to putrefaction.
- **Judicial execution:** In some countries, hydrocyanic gas is used for legal execution.

Interesting case

Cyanide Poisoning (Case of Robert Ferrante, 2013)

Dr Robert Ferrante, 64-year-old was the Co-Director of the Center of ALS Research and Visiting Professor of Neurology at the University of Pittsburgh Medical School (UPMC) and his wife, Dr Autumn Klein, 41-year-old was a neurologist at UPMC **(Figs. A and B)**. They lived with their 6-year-old daughter in Pittsburgh, Pennsylvania. Autumn was having difficulty getting pregnant with her second child. Her husband had been encouraging her to take creatine, a nutritional supplement to help her conceive. On April 17, 2013, Ferrante sent a text message in which he inquired if she had taken the supplement. She returned home from the hospital at about 11:30 pm and collapsed suddenly while complaining of a headache. Ferrante called 911 and the paramedics found her on the kitchen floor. Next to her body, they noticed a bag of white powder, later identified as creatine.

In the emergency, the patient was crashing; her BP and pulse were dropping fast; eyes were open and glassy and her breaths were shallow. There was a vacant look on her face. Pupils were reactive to light, but patient was unresponsive. After some time, the pupils were non-reacting to light. Her arms were contorted and her face twisted up and over her left shoulder. Doctors suspected a brain hemorrhage (as she had been complaining of headaches) and ordered a CT scan which turned out to be normal. They asked additional CT scans and ECG which showed no abnormalities. The emergency team was in a dilemma as to what else could cause such a dramatic decline so fast.

Shortly after the patient was admitted into the hospital, doctors ordered a broad panel of blood tests, gases, and chemistries to check her organ function. When a preliminary serological analysis revealed a high level of metabolic acidosis, the doctor ordered toxicological tests for cyanide poisoning, which came out to be positive.* Autumn died on April 20, 2013. Three days later, at Ferrante's insistence, her body was cremated, and as a result, there was no autopsy. The medical examiner, based on the toxicology reports, determined that Autumn had died of cyanide poisoning and ruled her death a homicide.

In July 2013, the prosecutor charged Ferrante with first-degree murder. Prosecutors got the purchase order form for cyanide which Ferrante got two days before his wife collapsed **(Fig. C)**. He had used the UPMC credit card to buy it and asked the vendor to ship it to his laboratory overnight. Investigators searched his lab and found that 8.3 g of cyanide was missing from the bottle. Detectives believed that the suspect mixed the cyanide into the dietary supplement. According to friends of the victim, Robert suspected that Autumn was having an affair and she was planning to leave him.

During the trial, medical toxicologist also testified that the victim's symptoms ruled in favor of cyanide poisoning. Ferrante's defense attorney pointed out the circumstantial nature of the prosecution's case, inconsistent crime toxicology reports and absence of an autopsy. However, in November 2014, the Jury found Dr Robert Ferrante guilty of first-degree murder and sentenced him to life imprisonment without parole.

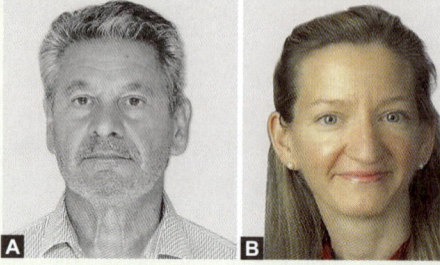
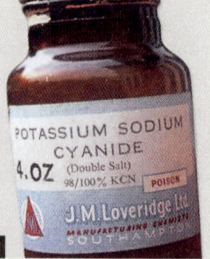

A B C

* Cyanide can become undetectable from 1 min to 3 h after ingestion. Had samples of Autumn's blood not been taken immediately after her admission, there would have been no physical evidence of poisoning beyond the contents of the bag of white powder found lying on her kitchen floor.

CHAPTER 55

Asphyxiants

LEARNING OBJECTIVES

Must know
1. Signs and symptoms, treatment and postmortem findings in CO poisoning
2. Medico-legal aspects of CO poisoning

Desirable to know
1. Asphyxiant gas, tear gas, methyl isocyanate
2. Delayed neuropsychological sequelae in CO poisoning

Introduction

Asphyxiant gas is a non-toxic or toxic gas which causes respiratory embarrassment leading to unconsciousness or death by asphyxiation. The brain is commonly affected.

There are two broad categories of asphyxiants: simple and chemical.

i. **Simple asphyxiants:** They are physiologically inert gases that displace O_2 from ambient air resulting in fall in partial pressure of O_2 in the alveoli, e.g., acetylene, CO_2, argon, helium, ethane, nitrogen and methane.

ii. **Chemical asphyxiants:** They interfere with the transportation or absorption of O_2 in the body and interfere with cellular metabolism causing cells to become O_2 starved. It can be:
   a. *Irritant gases:* They produce toxic effect by destruction of the integrity of the mucosal barrier of the respiratory tract (damage to both type I and type II pneumocytes), e.g., ammonia, H_2S, formaldehyde, phosgene and SO_2.
   b. *Systemic asphyxiants:* They produce significant systemic toxicity by various mechanisms, e.g., CO, cyanide and smoke.

 FM 9.6
Describe general principles and basic methodologies in treatment of poisoning with regard to carbon monoxide.

CARBON MONOXIDE (CO)

Properties

- CO is a colorless, tasteless, non-irritative and odorless gas, and lighter than air.
- It is produced by incomplete combustion of carbonaceous material.
- It combines with chlorine and forms carbonyl chloride—commonly called *phosgene*.

Sources

- Common sources of CO include tobacco smoke, house fires, automobile exhaust (1–7% CO), industrial processes, unvented or faulty heating units (stove gas, water heater, burning fossil fuel or furnace) and fires.
- Coal gas (mixture of CO, methane and hydrogen).
- Endogenous CO.

Action

- CO combines reversibly with hemoglobin to form carboxyhemoglobin (COHb) producing *anemic hypoxia* (blood O_2-carrying capacity is reduced). It has a high affinity for Hb (about 250 times more than O_2).
- It inhibits the electron transport by blocking cytochrome A_3 oxidase and cytochrome P450 and hence *intracellular respiration*.
- About 15% of CO present in extracellular tissues combines with myoglobin (affinity constant—40). A '*rebound effect*' with delayed return of symptoms may be due to late release of CO from myoglobin with subsequent binding to hemoglobin.

Signs and Symptoms

Presenting symptoms are mostly nonspecific and depend on the duration of exposure and levels of COHb.

Most frequent acute symptoms are headache (dull, frontal and continuous), dizziness, weakness, nausea and confusion.

COHb (%)	Signs and symptoms
0–10	No symptoms
10–20	Breathlessness, mild headache, abdominal pain
20–30	Throbbing headache, irritability, emotional instability, buzzing in the ears
30–40	Severe headache, nausea, vomiting, dizziness, dimness of vision, confusion, ataxia
40–50	Increasing confusion, hallucinations, rapid respiration, staggering and incoordination—**mistaken for drunkenness**
50–70	Weak thready pulse, hypotension, irregular respiration, convulsions, coma and death
>80	Rapid death from respiratory arrest

- On examination, there may be tachycardia, hypertension or hypotension, hyperthermia, flame-shaped retinal hemorrhages and bright red retinal veins. Classic cherry red skin is rare; pallor is present more often.
- CNS is most sensitive followed by heart (MI, dysrhythmias) due to their high oxygen demand. Patients display memory disturbance (most common) including retrograde and anterograde amnesia with amnestic confabulatory state.

NOTA BENE

Two features of CO poisoning may create confusion:
i. Bullous lesions on the body which simulate 2nd-degree thermal burn, deep coma, early putrefaction, antemortem and postmortem gasoline exposure.
ii. Tendency of the dying victim to wild, flailing movements inside the room, disturbing clothing and furniture which gives an impression of a violent tussle, thus creating a suspicion of homicide.

Severity of CO Poisoning

Normal COHb level is <5%, up to 9% in cigarette smokers. Serious toxicity is associated with levels >25%, and risk of fatality at 70%.

COHb (%)	Severity of poisoning
10–30	Mild
30–40	Moderate-severe
>40	Very severe

Fatal Dose and Fatal Period

The normal atmospheric concentration of CO is usually <0.001% (10 ppm). The atmospheric concentration can exceed 0.01% (100 ppm) in heavy urban traffic and during periods of atmospheric stagnation.

CO concentration (%)	Fatality (hours)
0.2	4
0.4	1
10	½

Diagnosis: Misdiagnosis is common because of the vagueness and broad spectrum of complaints; symptoms often are attributed to viral illness (influenza).

- *History:* Following should alert suspicion: winter months, exposed to the previously named sources and when more than one patient in a group or household in a particular enclosed site presents with similar complaints.
- *Laboratory diagnosis:* COHb analysis can be done by direct spectrophotometric measurement in specific blood gas analyzers. Bedside pulse CO-oximetry is available. Breath CO monitoring is an alternative to pulse CO-oximetry.

NOTA BENE

- **CT:** Symmetric low density areas in the region of globus pallidus, putamen and caudate nuclei are frequently seen within 12 h of CO exposure that resulted in unconsciousness.
- **Laboratory diagnosis**
  i. *Spectroscopic test:* Shows two absorption bands similar to oxyhemoglobin, but placed nearer the violet end.
  ii. *Hoppe-Seyler's test:* Few drops of blood + 10% NaOH → Greenish brown (normal blood), pink/red (COHb).
  iii. *Kunkel's test:* Diluted blood (1: 10) + few drops of 3% tannic acid (shake) → Deep brown (normal), Crimson-red coagulum (COHb).
  iv. *Potassium ferrocyanide test:* 15 mL of blood + 15 mL of 20% potassium ferrocyanide + 2 mL diluted acetic acid → Dark brown coagulum (normal), bright-red coagulum (COHb).
  v. *Katayama's test* using ammonium sulfide and acetic acid is less sensitive.

Differential Diagnosis

- Alcoholic intoxication
- Diabetic/Insulin coma
- Cerebral hemorrhage
- Head injury
- Uremia
- Barbiturates/Narcotic poisoning

Delayed neuropsychological sequelae in CO poisoning: Delayed neuropsychological sequelae (DNS) commonly occur after recovery from acute CO poisoning. Most frequently include a broad spectrum of neurological deficits, cognitive impairments and affective disorders (Table 55.1).

TREATMENT

Treatment consists of removal from the source of exposure, immediate administration of high-flow or 100% O_2 and aggressive supportive measures.

TABLE 55.1: Features of DNS due to CO toxicity

Neurological sequelae	Cognitive and psychological sequelae
• Gait and motor disturbances	• Cognitive impairment
• Bradykinesia	• Concentration deficit
• Intention tremors	• Memory loss
• Postural instability	• Personality changes
• Cortical blindness	• Insomnia
• Hearing loss, tinnitus, vertigo	• Anxiety
• Recurrent headache	• Depression
• Fecal/urinary incontinence	• Extreme emotional lability
• Dysphasia, dyspraxia	• Psychosis

Recent Advances
- Early administration of erythropoietin (EPO) in patients with CO poisoning may improve neurological outcomes and reduce the incidence of DNS.
- Anti-oxidant such as N-acetylcysteine can be used as a treatment in CO poisoning. N-acetyl cysteine is effective for traumatic brain injury, cerebral ischemia and other neurological disorders.
- Anti-inflammatory and immunosuppressant steroids such as dexamethasone or methylprednisolone could be used for severe inflammations in CO poisoning.
- Hydrogen-rich saline is an antioxidant and is currently used in Japan for human metabolic disorders. It has been found to decrease neuronal necrosis and apoptosis and improve neurobehavioral function, following CO poisoning.

i. Remove the victim from source of exposure.
ii. Maintain patent airway, fresh air and orthobaric oxygen (100% oxygen at atmospheric pressure) by tight-fitting high-flow reservoir face mask or endotracheal tube. Oxygen therapy is started if COHb >10% and should be given for 4–6 hours (h). The immediate effect of oxygen is enhancement of the dissociation of COHb.
iii. The use of hyperbaric oxygen (HBO) is controversial. HBO has been postulated to reduce the incidence of neurological sequelae. It is indicated in cases of unconsciousness, cardiovascular instability or ischemia, and persistent mental and/or neurologic deficits. HBO at PO_2 of 2–3 atmospheric pressure mixed with 5% CO_2 may be given through mask or intratracheal tube.
iv. Blood transfusion, if required.
v. Gastric lavage to prevent aspiration pneumonia.
vi. Cerebral edema is treated by mannitol 500 mL IV as 20% solution over 15 minutes (min), followed by 500 mL of 5% dextrose over next 4 h.
vii. Hypotension is initially treated with IV fluids followed by inotropic agents. Standard ACLS protocols are followed to treat dysrhythmias.
viii. Antibiotics and symptomatic treatment.

POSTMORTEM FINDINGS

External

i. **Cherry red coloration** of the skin, mucous membranes, PM staining, blood, tissues and internal organs **(Fig. 55.1)**. The cherry-red PM staining is usually associated with a COHb level >30%. In dark-skinned individuals, fingernail beds can be examined.
ii. Fine froth at the nostrils/mouth.
iii. Blisters of skin over dependent areas or bony pressure points such as buttocks, calves, wrists and knees due to cutaneous edema.

Internal

i. **Lungs:** Edema and congestion.
ii. **Heart:** Lesions vary from petechial hemorrhages to myocardial necrosis.
iii. Rhabdomyolysis from the direct toxic effects of CO, and prolonged immobility lead to renal failure.
iv. **CNS:** Neuronal hypoxic injury is most pronounced in the deep gray matter, particularly in basal ganglia. Punctiform hemorrhages and softening of cerebral cortex and corpus striatum—particularly bilateral globus pallidus.

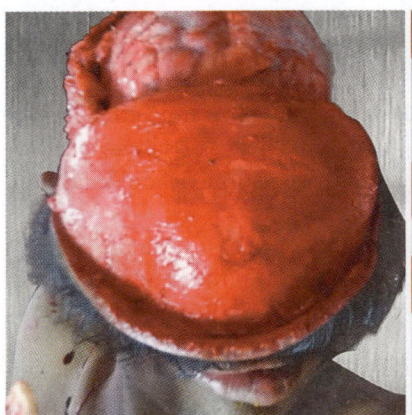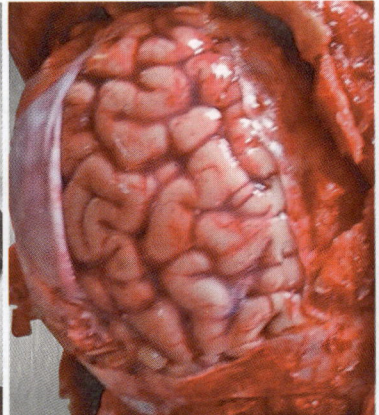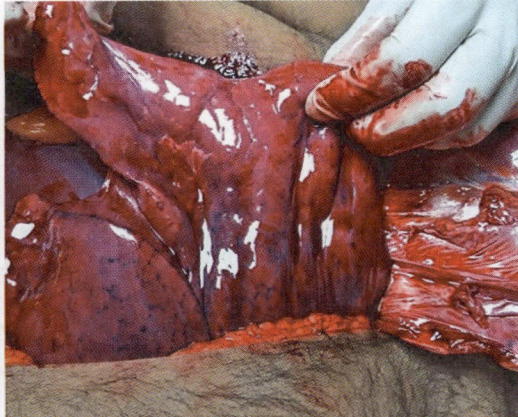

Fig. 55.1: CO poisoning: Cherry-red coloration of blood

In addition to routine viscera, lungs and brain are preserved for analysis. If blood is not available for CO determination, spleen, liver or skeletal muscle can be utilized.

Medico-legal Aspects

- It is a *common mode of suicidal poisoning* in the West (by inhaling motor vehicle exhaust), but rare in India. Suicide is also committed by sealing off door and windows and burning charcoal and papers—common in Hong Kong, Southern China and Singapore.
- *Accidental cases:* Common in India from cooking gas leakage, and incomplete combustion of wood, charcoal or coal in ill-ventilated rooms.
    - Unintentional fatalities occur in stationary vehicles from malfunctioning exhaust systems or operation in an enclosed space.
    - CO presents greater risk to firefighters and victims than thermal injury or oxygen deprivation.
    - Malfunctioning heating systems (e.g., blocked chimney) using combustible fuels can cause fatal CO poisoning.
- Homicide is uncommon (e.g., exhaust fumes used to poison an immobilized person). A victim of CO poisoning can be placed in a bed to simulate a natural death.
- Masochistic sexual asphyxia may be due to CO.
- COHb can be detected even in a putrefied or embalmed body, and it is not a product of putrefaction.

Chronic CO Poisoning

The symptoms of low level chronic CO intoxication are non-specific and unlikely to arouse suspicion of CO as the cause. Patients present with bizarre behavioral abnormalities, declining intellect, memory disturbances, chronic cough or diarrhea. The condition is often misdiagnosed as chronic fatigue syndrome, viral, bacterial, pulmonary, gastrointestinal infection or immune deficiency. COHb is usually not excessively elevated.

Describe general principles and basic methodologies in treatment of poisoning with regard to tear (riot control) gases and methyl isocyanate.

War Gases

Definition: War gases are chemicals (gas, liquid or solid) which are used for producing destruction or damage, mostly at times of war. These also include chemicals being used for dispersing unruly mobs.

Chemical warfare (CW) involves using the toxic properties of chemical substances as weapons.

Types of Chemical Warfare Agents (CWAs)
i. Asphyxiants or lung irritants
ii. Vesicants or blister gases
iii. Lacrimators or tear gases or riot control agents
iv. Sternutators or nasal irritants
v. Nerve gases
vi. Paralysants
vii. Miscellaneous, e.g., methyl isocyanate

TEAR GASES

Introduction

Tear gas (riot control agents) are chemical compounds that make people temporarily incapacitate to function by causing irritation to the eyes, mouth, throat, lungs and skin.

Common Agents

CN (chloroacetophenone) and CS (chlorobenzylidene malononitrile) and OC (oleoresin capsicum), or pepper spray or its synthetic form known as *PAVA spray*.

- These agents' cause significant lacrimation and rhinorrhea due to irritation and hence called 'tear gases'.
- The designation of tear gases is inappropriate since most of these agents are solids dispersed as aerosols.

Signs and Symptoms

System	Signs and symptoms
Ocular	Sensation of conjunctival and corneal burning leading to lacrimation, blepharospasm, conjunctival injection, photophobia, temporary blindness
RS	Nasal irritation, rhinorrhea, congestion, bronchorrhea, sore throat, cough, sneezing, tightness of chest, feeling of suffocation
GIT	Metallic taste, burning of mouth, excess salivation, nausea, vomiting, abdominal pain
Skin	Burning and erythema

Toxic dose: Very low concentration (.003 mg/m^3) can lead to ocular irritation.

Treatment

Symptoms diminish within 30 min after exposure. Redness and edema persists for 1–2 days postexposure. No antidote is available.

i. Contaminated clothing should be removed.
ii. Copious flushing with tepid water or saline; washing with soap and water may speed the decontamination process.
iii. Patient's eyes are flushed for atleast 15 mins.
iv. In case of 'pepper spray', magnesium-aluminum hydroxide suspension is applied over affected area of skin for 30 mins.
v. Topical antibiotics, humidified oxygen, assisted ventilation, bronchodilators are helpful.

Medico-legal aspects: These agents are used for riot control and crowd suppression.

METHYL ISOCYANATE (MIC)

Introduction

Methyl isocyanate is a colorless, highly flammable liquid with a pungent odor that evaporates quickly when exposed to the air.

The mass fatalities at Bhopal in 1984 make MIC an important toxin for historical reasons.

- **Uses:** It is used in the production of pesticides, polyurethane foam and plastics.
- **Routes of exposure:** Inhalation (major route), direct contact and ingestion.

Signs and Symptoms

Toxicity develops 1-4 h after exposure.

System	Signs and symptoms
RS	Dyspnea, chest pain, severe cough, pulmonary edema, distress, pneumonitis, pneumonia
Ocular	Lacrimation, burning, photophobia, blurred vision, blepharospasm, corneal ulcer, conjunctival congestion
GIT	Nausea, vomiting, persistent diarrhea, anorexia, abdominal pain
Dermal	Chemical burns

Cause of death: Death is due to respiratory failure from acute lung injury or acute respiratory distress syndrome (ARDS).

Fatal dose: 3 ppm.

Treatment

There is no antidote for methyl isocyanate.

i. Treatment consists of removal of the victim from the contaminated area and support of respiratory (supplemental oxygen, bronchodilators and/or steroids) and cardiovascular functions.
ii. In case of ocular injury, continue irrigation for at least 15 minutes. Immediately consult an ophthalmologist in case of severe corneal injuries.
iii. In case of ingestion, do not induce emesis. Gastric lavage is useful to remove caustic material and prepare for endoscopic examination.

PM findings: Severe necrotizing lesions in the lining of the upper respiratory tract, as well as in the bronchioles, alveoli, and lung capillaries.

Medico-legal aspects: It can cause accidental and occupational poisoning.

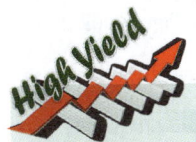

- CO is non-irritative and odorless gas.
- **Sources of CO:** Tobacco smoke, fires, automobile exhaust, industries, faulty heating units (stove gas, water heater, burning fossil fuel or furnace).
- CO combines reversibly with hemoglobin to form carboxyhemoglobin (COHb) producing *anemic hypoxia*.
- It inhibits cytochrome oxidase and cytochrome P450 and hence *intracellular respiration*.
- No symptoms are seen when COHb level is 0–10%.
- There is confusion, hallucinations, tachypnea, staggering, incoordination *(mistaken for drunkenness)* when COHb level is 40–50%.
- Death is common when COHb level is >70%.
- Bullous lesions seen in CO poisoning simulate 2nd-degree thermal burn, deep coma, early putrefaction, antemortem and postmortem gasoline exposure.
- **Presumptive tests for CO:** Spectroscopic test, Hoppe-Seyler's test, Kunkel's test, potassium ferrocyanide test, Katayama's test.
- Bedside pulse CO-oximetry is available COHb analysis.
- **Differential diagnosis:** Alcoholic intoxication, head injury, diabetic/insulin coma, uremia, cerebral hemorrhage, barbiturates/narcotic poisoning.
- Treatment of CO poisoning is fresh air and orthobaric oxygen. Use of hyperbaric oxygen is controversial.
- In CO poisoning, PM staining is **cherry red** in color.
- CO inhalation is common mode of suicidal poisoning in West, Hong Kong, Singapore.
- Accidental cases common in India from cooking gas leakage, and incomplete combustion of wood or coal in ill-ventilated rooms.
- COHb can be detected even in a putrefied or embalmed body, and it is not a product of putrefaction.
- **Most common riot control agents:** CN (chloroacetophenone) and CS (chlorobenzylidene malononitrile).
- Accidental release of methyl isocyanate was implicated in the Bhopal disaster.

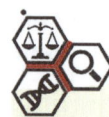

Interesting case

Vx Poisoning (Case of Kim Jong-nam, 2017)

In February 2017, Kim Jong-nam, the estranged half-brother of North Korea's reclusive ruler Kim Jong-un was scheduled to catch a flight from Kuala Lumpur to Macau **(Fig. A)**. Kim was approached by two women near the airport self check-in kiosk and one of them came from behind and splashed a liquid on his face and the other woman covered his face with a handkerchief laced with a liquid. Feeling giddy, he then went to an airport assistance counter to seek medical help and was taken to a clinic on the premises. He was sweating, in pain and unresponsive. At the clinic, Kim was given atropine and adrenaline. He required tracheal intubation, and the saliva, vomit and blood in his mouth needed to be suctioned out. They decided to call an ambulance and send him to the hospital. He died en route within 20 mins of the incident.

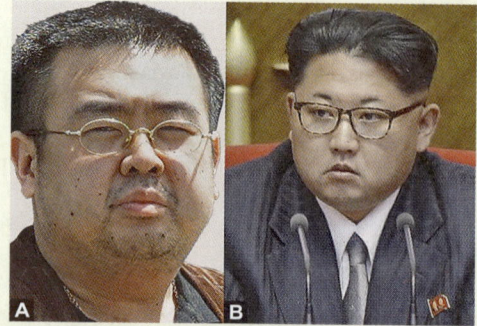

He was traveling under the pseudonym 'Kim Chol', and officials did not immediately confirm that Kim Jong-nam was the man killed. Police initially described the incident as a 'sudden death' pending the results of an autopsy. The autopsy was conducted in the presence of several North Korean officials. His lungs, brain, liver and spleen were congested. Kim did not suffer a heart attack and had no puncture wounds, such as those a needle would have left. The autopsy also verified his identity as 'Kim Jong-nam' after his son provided DNA samples for testing. Tests conducted found traces of toxin VX and its precursor on swabs of the eye mucosa, face and blood, and traces of VX were also found on the deceased's T-shirt and blazer and his bag. The final autopsy report concluded that Kim died of VX nerve agent poisoning.

On 15–16 February, the Malaysian police arrested two women, one Vietnamese, the other Indonesian through security footage at the airport. The prosecution charged the duo with murder. The women told the police that they were instructed by four men who were travelling with them to smear Kim Jong-nam's face with the liquid. The police also charged the four North Korean suspects who took separate flights out of Malaysia shortly after the assassination without being arrested. South Korea's National Intelligence Service (NIS) believed that he may have been poisoned by intelligence agents acting on behalf of Kim Jong Un **(Fig. B)**. North Korea vehemently denied any involvement in Kim's death and rejected that version of the events. It argued that the women would have died had a lethal chemical been on their hands.

A chemical pathologist testified during trial that blood tests done on the two female suspects showed that their cholinesterase levels were normal while that for the victim was low. The normal readings could indicate that the two suspects were never in contact with any VX nerve agent, but she said it could also mean they were exposed to only low amount or that it was washed off quickly. The defense claimed that the two women were duped into believing they were participating in a television show prank and had no idea who the victim was. In 2019, the murder charges were dropped against them.

CHAPTER 56

Agricultural Poisons

Learning Objectives

Must know
1. Signs and symptoms and treatment of OPC poisoning
2. Classification of OPCs
3. Mechanism of action of OPCs
4. Medico-legal aspects of OPC poisoning

Desirable to know
1. Delayed complications in OPC poisoning
2. Endrin poisoning
3. Paraquat poisoning
4. Pyrethroids poisoning

Introduction

Pesticides are varied group of agents used to control livings organisms that pose health or economic threats. Often the term is misunderstood to refer only to 'insecticides', but it also applies to herbicides, fungicides and various other substances used to control pests.

- They can be manmade (synthetic) or naturally occurring (biological) and may be active against a narrow (selective) or wide (broad-spectrum) range of pests.
- *Classification*: Pesticides are often grouped by the pest they control (e.g., insecticides, rodenticides, fungicides, etc.) or categorized by chemical structure (e.g., insecticides are categorized as organophosphate, carbamate, organochlorine, synthetic-pyrethroid, and microbial and insect growth regulators). WHO classifies pesticides by hazards they pose based on Globally Harmonized System (GHS) from Category 1 (LD_{50} <5 mg/kg body wt) to Category 5 (LD_{50} 2000–5000 mg/kg body wt) as given in **Table 56.1**.

TABLE 56.1: Classification of pesticides based on hazard

WHO Class		Oral LD_{50}* (mg/kg body weight)
Ia	Extremely hazardous	<5
Ib	Highly hazardous	5–50
II	Moderately hazardous	50–2000
III	Slightly hazardous	>2000
U	Unlikely to present acute hazard	>5000

* LD50 value is a statistical estimate of the number of mg of toxicant per kg of body weight required to kill 50% of a large population of test animals: the rat is used unless otherwise stated.

- *Commonest types* of insecticide/pesticide substance causing poisoning are organophosphates, chlorinated hydrocarbons, aluminum phosphide, and paraquat.

> **NOTA BENE**
>
> Another method of classification of insecticides is based on their *mode of penetration*, i.e., whether they cause effect upon ingestion (stomach poisons), penetration of the body covering (contact poisons) or inhalation (fumigants).
> - **Stomach poisons** are toxic only if ingested through the mouth and are useful against those insects that have biting or chewing mouth parts, such as caterpillars and grasshoppers, e.g., arsenicals like copper acetoarsenite (Paris green), calcium arsenate and lead arsenate; and fluorine compounds like NaF and cryolite.
> - **Contact poisons** penetrate the skin of the pest and are used against those arthropods that pierce the surface of a plant and suck out the juices. These can be divided into two groups: naturally occurring (nicotine, pyrethrum, rotenone and oils) and synthetic organic insecticides. The main synthetic groups are the organic phosphates (organophosphates), carbamates and chlorinated hydrocarbons.
> - **Fumigants** are toxic compounds that enter the respiratory system of the insect through its spiracles or breathing openings, e.g., HCN, naphthalene, methyl bromide and nicotine.

Describe general principles and basic methodologies in treatment of poisoning with regard to organophosphates and carbamates.

ORGANOPHOSPHORUS COMPOUNDS (OPCs)

Organophosphorus compounds and carbamates are one of the most common causes of self-poisoning seen in India.

They are used as insecticides, herbicides, antihelminthics, ophthalmic agents, in chemical industry, and as nerve gas in chemical warfare.

Classification

Based on Chemical Composition

- *Alkyl phosphates:* Tichlorfos, dimefox, HETP, TEPP and malathion.
- *Aryl phosphates:* Parathion (Follidol), paraoxon, chlorthion and diazinon (Tik-20).

Based on Toxicity

- Agriculture insecticide (highly toxic): TEPP, parathion.
- Animal insecticide (moderately toxic): Trichlorfon, ronnel.
- Household insecticide (low toxicity): Malathion, Tik-20.

Common OPCs: Chlorpyriphos (Chlorofos 20), temephos, diazinon (Tik-20), malathion (Finit), dimethoate, parathion, trichlorphon (Diptrenex) and glyphosate (Weed off) **(Fig. 56.1)**.

Common carbamates: Aldicarb (Temik), carbaryl (Sevin 50), propoxur (Baygon), carbaryl + gamma BHC (Sevidol), physostigmine, neostigmine, pyridostigmine, edrophonium and ambenonium **(Fig. 56.1)**.

Action

- The primary mechanism of action of OPCs and carbamates is inhibition of acetylcholinesterase (AChE) and plasma or butyrylcholinesterase (pseudo-cholinesterase or BuChE) by phosphorylating the serine hydroxyl residue on AChE or BuChE. Hence, these compounds are called *cholinesterase inhibitors*. It blocks the conversion of acetylcholine to its degradation products—acetic acid and choline **(Fig. 56.2)**.
- There is a covalent phophorous-enzyme bond formation that is extremely stable, and its hydrolysis in water occurs

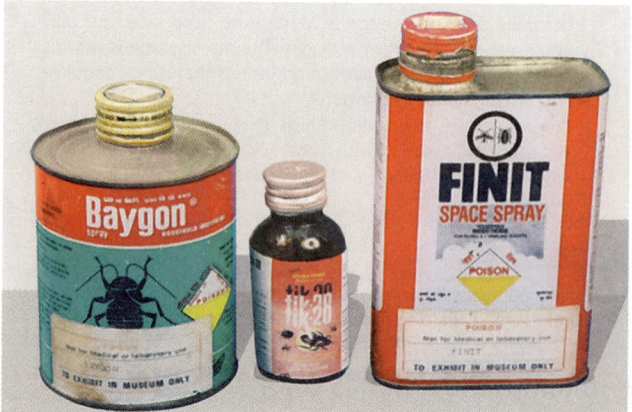

Fig. 56.1: OPC and carbamate

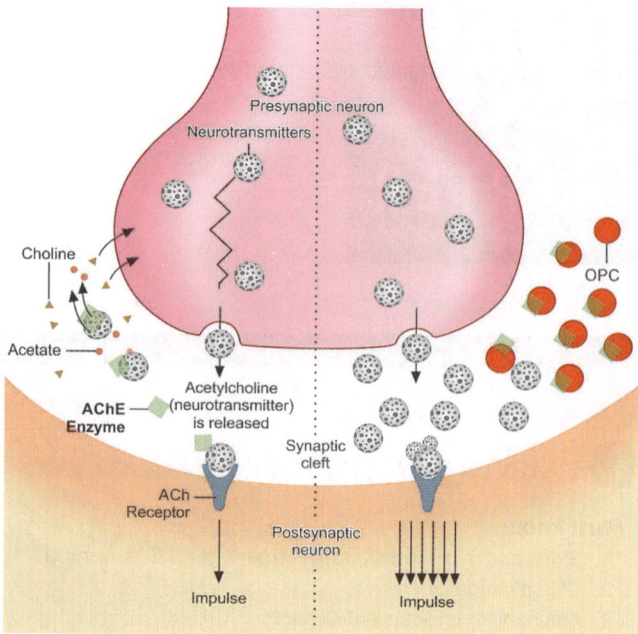

Fig. 56.2: OPCs 'lock' the AChE enzyme which prevents it to break acetylcholine

at a slow rate. This phosphorylated enzyme complex may undergo a process called as *'aging'* which further strengthens the phosphorous-enzyme bond, leading to inactivation of AChE. Once AChE has been inactivated, acetylcholine accumulates in the autonomic nervous system, somatic nervous system and brain, resulting in overstimulation of muscarinic and nicotinic receptors.
- Organophosphorus insecticides irreversibly inhibit AChE, but carbamates are eliminated rapidly by serum and liver enzymes.
- Carbamates do not penetrate the CNS to the same extent, resulting in limited CNS toxicity.

Absorption: OPCs and carbamates are absorbed by many routes including transdermal, transconjunctival, inhalational, across the GIT and through direct injection.

Metabolism: Most OPCs are hydrolyzed by the enzymes A esterases or paroxonases which are not inhibited by it. These enzymes are found in the plasma and in the hepatic endoplasmic reticulum. The metabolic products are then excreted in the urine.

SIGNS AND SYMPTOMS

- The acute effects of OPCs depend on the site of exposure, which can be inhalation, skin or eye contact, or ingestion. However, all exposure routes cause similar effects with large doses.
- Time of exposure to onset of toxicity varies from half hour to 2 hours (h).

Signs and symptoms can be divided into three broad categories **(Fig. 56.3)**.

CHAPTER 56: Agricultural Poisons

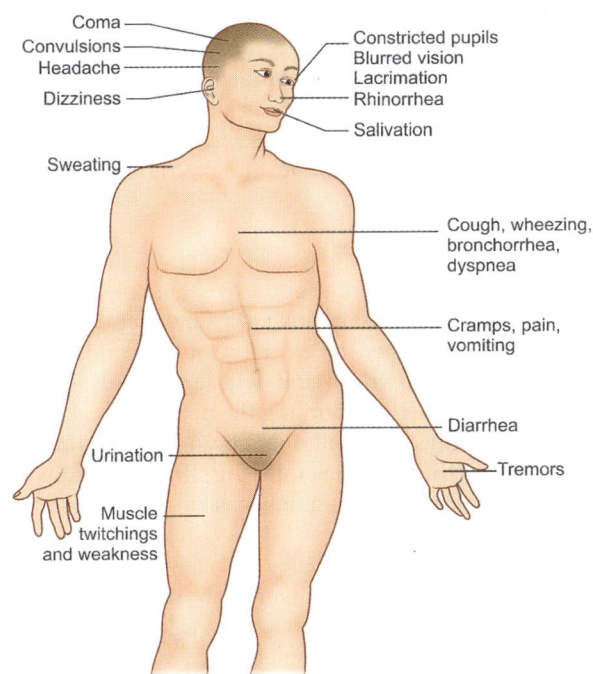

Fig. 56.3: Signs and symptoms of OPC poisoning

I. Muscarinic or Parasympathetic Effects (Figs. 56.4A and B)

System	Signs and symptoms
GIT	Increased salivation, nausea, vomiting, retrosternal pain, abdominal cramps, diarrhea, fecal incontinence
CVS	Bradycardia, hypotension
RS	Rhinorrhea, bronchospasm, bronchorrhea, cough, wheezing, dyspnea
Ocular	Blurred vision, miosis
Glands	Increased lacrimation, **chromodacryorrhea** (shedding of red tears due to accumulation of porphyrin in lacrimal glands), sweating

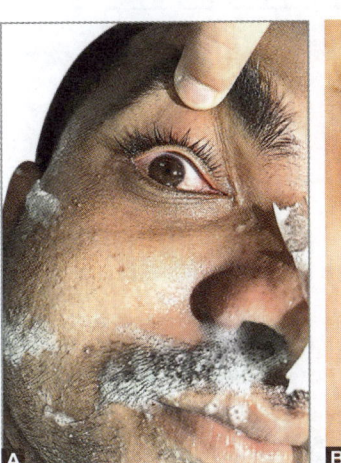
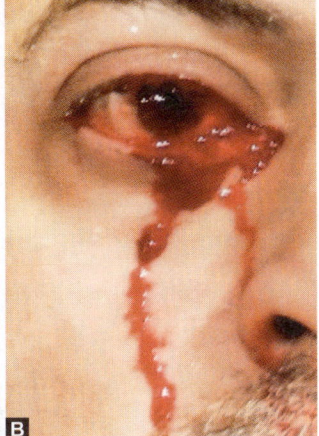

Figs. 56.4A and B: OPC poisoning: (A) Constricted pupils, rhinorrhea, and bronchorrhea; (B) Chromodacryorrhea

OPCs are usually mixed with a solvent aromax, which is responsible for kerosene-like smell in the breath and body secretions.

> **Mnemonics for OPC poisoning**
> - **SLUDGE: S**alivation; **L**acrimation; **U**rination; **D**iarrhea; **G**astrointestinal distress; **E**mesis.
> - **DUMBELS: D**iaphoresis, diarrhea; **U**rination; **M**iosis; **B**radycardia, bronchospasm, bronchorrhea; **E**mesis; **L**acrimation; **S**alivation.

II. Nicotinic or Autonomic Ganglionic and Somatic Motor Effects

It includes muscle fasciculations, cramps and weakness, twitchings and diaphragmatic failure, and can progress to paralysis, areflexia and respiratory failure. Autonomic effects include hypertension, tachycardia, mydriasis and pallor.

III. CNS Effects

It includes restlessness, emotional lability, headache, tremors, drowsiness, confusion, slurred speech, ataxia, generalized weakness, Cheyne-Stokes respiration, delirium, coma, absent reflexes, seizures, psychosis and death.

Signs and symptoms also depends on the degree of exposure

Mild exposure	Moderate exposure	Severe exposure
GIT: Nausea, anorexia, cramping	SLUDGE	SLUDGE
CNS: Fatigue, headache, dizziness, tremors of tongue and eyelids, anxiety	*CNS:* Anxiety, confusion, lethargy, incoordination	*CNS:* Convulsions, coma, loss of sphincter tone, paralysis, autonomic dysfunction
MS: Minimal muscle weakness	*RS:* Respiratory muscle weakness	*RS:* Insufficiency, pulmonary edema
Ocular: Miosis, decreased visual acuity	*MS:* Tremors, muscle fasciculations, followed by flaccid paralysis	*CVS:* Bradycardia, heart block

Most patients recover within 24–48 h, but fat-soluble OPC may cause effects for weeks to months.

Cause of death: Death is usually due to respiratory failure (due to bronchoconstriction and increased bronchial secretion).

> **NOTA BENE**
> - For most OPCs, dermal absorption through the skin is the most common way of poisoning in occupational exposure. Initial local effects include muscular fasciculation's and sweating at the site, malaise and weakness.
> - Exposure to low-vapor levels can cause visual disturbances, rhinorrhea, and/or dyspnea. Eye contact causes miosis that may be accompanied by deep eye pain, conjunctival irritation and visual disturbances. Inhalation of high-vapor concentration can induce unconsciousness within 1–2 min and then cause seizures, flaccid paralysis and apnea and the victims may die within 30 min in the absence of immediate medical care.

Fatal Dose

- Malathion and diazinon 1 g.
- Parathion: 175 mg.
- TEPP: 100 mg.
- HETP: 350 mg.

Fatal period: Usually within 24 h in untreated cases and within 10 days in treated cases, if unsuccessful.

Laboratory Diagnosis

The diagnosis of OPC poisoning is made primarily based on the history and a combination of clinical features, including the typical odor of the insecticide.

The essential finding in laboratory diagnosis is *depression of cholinesterase activity* **(Table 56.2)**. In acute poisoning, signs and symptoms generally occur when >50% of cholinesterase is inhibited.

- *RBC (true) cholinesterase:* It is found in the CNS gray matter, RBCs and motor endplate.
- *Plasma (pseudo or butyryl) cholinesterase:* It is found in the CNS white matter, plasma, liver, pancreas and heart.

Red blood cell (RBC) cholinesterase is considered more accurate of the two; however, plasma cholinesterase activity is easier to assay and generally more readily available, but declines rapidly. Blood cholinesterase level should be estimated *for 3 weeks in non-fatal parathion poisoning*.

NOTA BENE

- **P-nitrophenol test**: P-nitrophenol is a metabolite of some OPCs (e.g., parathion, ethion) and is excreted in the urine. Its presence in the urine can be used as a confirmation test of OPC poisoning. This test can also be done on vomitus or gastric lavage contents.
- Quantitative analysis of OPCs and their degradation products in plasma and urine by *mass spectrometric method* is more specific, but is expensive and limited to specialized laboratories.
- Electrophysiological tests may be required for the diagnosis of delayed neuropathy of OPC poisoning.

Differential Diagnosis

Gastroenteritis, asthma, heat prostration, influenza, exhaustion, hypoglycemia, pneumonia, carbon monoxide poisoning, narcotic overdose, ketoacidosis, sepsis, meningitis, encephalitis, Reye's syndrome, neurologic disorders and subdural or epidural hematoma.

TABLE 56.2: Severity grading based on cholinesterase levels

Grade	BuChE activity (%)	AChE activity (%)
Mild	40–50	50–90
Moderate	10–40	10–50
Severe	<10	<10

TREATMENT

The patient is treated according to the severity of the symptoms as shown in **Flowchart 56.1**. Among all approaches, external decontamination and early atropinization are only likely to be beneficial in OPC poisoning, and oxime use is unlikely to be effective.

I. Decontamination

- Patient is removed from source of exposure, stripped of his clothes and the skin flushed with water.
- Doctor and nurses should be protected with water-impermeable gowns, masks with eyeshields, and use double gloves while handling the patient.
- *Gastric lavage:* It should only be undertaken once the patient is stable. Gastric emptying should be done with continuous suction via a nasogastric tube with 1:5000 $KMnO_4$. Activated charcoal should be administered in doses of 1 g/kg body wt.
- Patients with ocular exposures should have copious eye irrigation with normal saline or lactated Ringer's solution. If these are not available, tap water can be used.

II. Atropinization

Atropine blocks the muscarinic manifestations and has no effect on nicotinic receptors (on muscle weakness or paralysis) and does not affect the rate of regeneration of inhibited AChE.

Dose: 2–4 mg IV repeated after every 5–15 min till atropinization, the dose should be adjusted to maintain

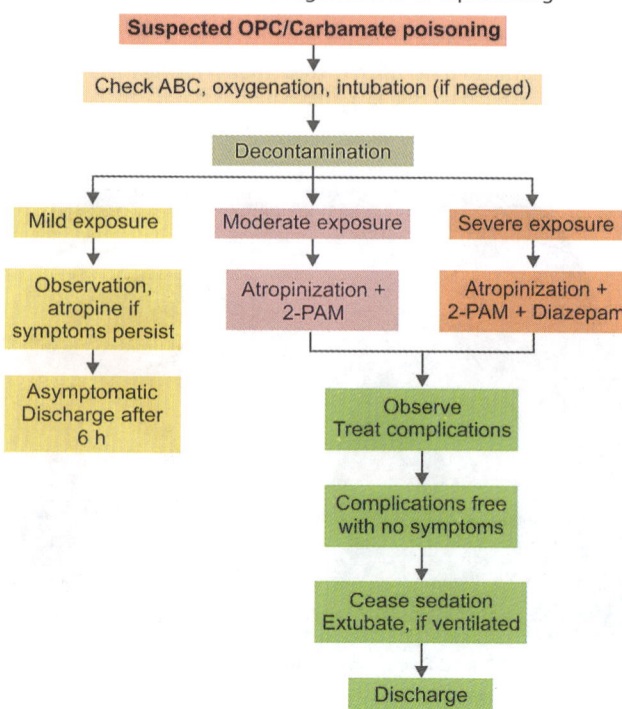

Flowchart 56.1: Management of OPC poisoning

this effect for at least 24 h (maintenance dose: 0.02–0.05 mg/kg).
- Atropine therapy should be monitored to maintain systolic BP >80 mm Hg, pulse >80 beats/min and clear chest on auscultation.
- Mild to moderate atropinization includes dryness of tongue, reduced secretion of oropharyngeal and bronchial tree, tachycardia (>100 beats/min) and flushing. *Mydriaris is an early response to atropine and is not a therapeutic endpoint.* A common failure of therapy is not maintaining adequate atropinization.
- *Glycopyrrolate* may be substituted, if there is no evidence of central toxicity.

III. Oximes

Pralidoxime (2-PAM), a nucleophilic oxime, most effective when treatment is started early and if used within 48 h, and helps in regenerating AChE associated with skeletal muscle neuromuscular junctions (overcome the nicotinic effects of OPCs).

Dose: 1–2 g IV (20–40 mg/kg) over 5–20 min dissolved in 0.9% normal saline solution, may be repeated at 1–2 h if muscle weakness is not relieved, and again after 8–10 h. Transient dizziness, blurred vision, diplopia and elevations in diastolic BP may occur depending on the administration rate.

Alternatively, continuous infusion (200–400 mg/h) of 2-PAM is more effective because of shorter duration of action of single dose.

NOTA BENE

- Atropine and 2-PAM given together are synergistic against the signs and symptoms of cholinesterase inhibition, thus decreasing atropine requirements.
- PAM is ineffective in reversing the CNS effects of organophosphate because its positive charge prevents entry into the CNS. *Diacetyl monoxime (DAM)* crosses the blood-brain barrier and can regenerate some of the CNS cholinesterase.
- The use of oximes in acute OPC poisoning remains conflicting and controversial. Some randomized controlled trials showed no benefit in moderate and severe poisoning, and concluded that PAM has no role in the routine management of patients with OPC poisoning.
- PAM is *not recommended* for the reversal of inhibition of acetylcholinesterase by carbamate poisoning.* But its use is safe, particularly if administered in conjunction with atropine in case of unknown pesticide or in mixed poisoning.

IV. Diazepam

Addition of diazepam for treatment of seizures and neuropathy improves survival (must not be used with other CNS depressants). It decreases the cardiac and brain morphologic damage resulting from OPC seizures.

Dose: 0.5–2 mg IV every 15 min.

V. Supportive Care

- Foot-end of the bed is raised to ensure drainage of respiratory secretions.
- Suction as required, to remove respiratory secretions.
- Treat bronchospasm with atropine and not bronchodilators.
- Intubate in case of respiratory distress.
- The use of other medication, including opioids for sedation may worsen CNS manifestations and the degree of respiratory depression.
- Dextrose: 2–4 mL/kg of 50% dextrose IV.
- Antibiotics to prevent pulmonary infection.
- Vitamin K may also be given.

Recent Advances

Newer therapies: Several new therapies have been studied, but there is insufficient evidence to recommend their use:

- **Magnesium sulfate** blocks ligand-gated calcium channels, resulting in reduced acetylcholine release from presynaptic terminals, thus reduce CNS overstimulation. Administration on the first day decreases hospitalization period and improve outcomes.
- **Clonidine** also reduces acetylcholine synthesis and release from presynaptic terminals.
- **Sodium bicarbonate IV** infusion in place of oximes has been found beneficial in nerve gas poisoning.
- Removing OPCs from the blood by hemodialysis and hemofiltration could allow optimum action of other therapies. Fresh frozen plasma or albumin is also a useful therapy through clearing of free OPC.
- **Enzyme bioscavengers** are being developed as a pretreatment to sequester highly toxic OPCs. BuChE purified from human plasma (HuBChE) scavenges OPCs in plasma, reducing the amount available to inhibit AChE in synapses.
- **Neuroprotective drugs**: Delayed management of convulsion and neuroprotection in OPC poisoning can be done with anticholinergic and antiglutamatergic agents. The CNS toxic affects results from increased release of glutamate (an excitatory amino acid) which causes over-activation of the N-methyl-D-aspartate (NMDA). *Gacyclidine, tezampanel, ketamine and huperzine A* are useful in treatment of nerve gas induced seizures when administered 1 h after ex posure.
- **Recombinant bacterial phosphotriesterases or hydrolases** that are able to transfer organophosphorous-degrading enzymes are very promising in delayed treatment of OPC poisoning.
- **Antioxidants**: Vitamin E treatment may be beneficial in OPCs induced oxidative stress.
- Encapsulation of drugs or enzymes in *nanocarriers* has been proposed to enhance the blood–brain barrier crossing.
- **Inhalable submicronic atropine respiratory fluid or nasal drops** may be a safe and efficacious emergency treatment of OPC poisoning. Its advantages include early blood bioavailability and atropinization, and capability of mass treatment.

Complications

Immediate	Delayed
Pulmonary edema	Paralysis
Aspiration pneumonia	Neurotoxicity
Chemical peritonitis	Guillain-Barre syndrome
Hyper-/hypoglycemia	
Coagulation abnormalities	

---

* The site on which oximes bind and reactivate the enzyme—the anionic site, is occupied by carbamates.

POSTMORTEM FINDINGS

External (Figs. 56.5A to D)
i. Kerosene-like smell from nostrils and mouth.
ii. Cyanosis of lips, fingers and nose.
iii. Deep postmortem staining.
iv. Congested face.
v. Frothy discharge, often bloodstained from the nose and mouth.

Internal
i. Mucosa of the stomach and intestine is congested.
ii. Stomach content may give kerosene-like smell.
iii. Respiratory passages are congested, contain frothy hemorrhagic exudates.
iv. Petechial hemorrhage may be present subpleurally.
v. Edema and congestion of the lungs and other visceral organs.
vi. Edema of brain.

Medico-legal Aspects
- Hospitalizing all symptomatic patients for at least 4–6 days following resolution of symptoms is recommended, because of the risk of development of respiratory depression or intermediate syndrome after resolution of an acute crisis.
- The symptoms of OPC poisoning can mimic other toxidromes and diseases. The clinician must keep in mind that misdiagnosis is a potential medico-legal pitfall.
- Accidental and occupational poisoning occurs in manufacturers, packers, sprayers and in children. OPC residue in fruits and vegetables may not induce toxic features, but could affect the health.
- Suicidal poisoning is common in our country, both in rural and urban areas. OPCs are also common suicidal agents in Pakistan, Sri Lanka and the other Asian and South East Asian countries.
- Homicidal poisoning does not occur due to detectable smell of the diluents, and signs and symptoms appear rather early.
- It is used for chemical warfare, e.g., nerve gases.

> **NOTA BENE**
>
> **Neurological manifestations**
> Neurological manifestations are the most important sequelae of OPC poisoning. Three types of paralyses are recognized based on the time of occurrence, and differ in their pathophysiology (Table 56.3).
>
> **Other neurological manifestations**
> Various other neuropsychiatric manifestations have been described:
> i. *Chronic organophosphate-induced neuropsychiatric disorder (COPIND):* It occurs without cholinergic symptoms and is not dependent on AChE inhibition. COPIND appears with a delay and is long-lasting.
> *Symptoms* include mood change, cognitive deficit, memory loss, lethargy, autonomic dysfunction, peripheral neuropathy and extrapyramidal symptoms.
> ii. *Extrapyramidal manifestations* include dystonias, resting tremor, cog-wheel rigidity and choreoathetosis. It develops in 4–40 days following poisoning and lasts for about 1–4 weeks.
> iii. *Neuro-ophthalmological sequelae* including optic atrophy, degeneration of retina, myopia owing to spasm or paresis of accommodation.

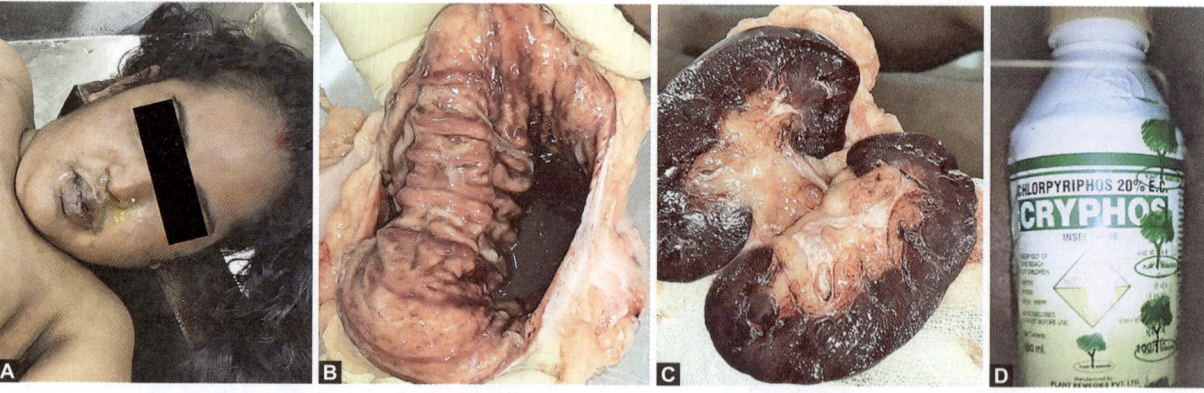

Figs. 56.5A to D: OPC poisoning: (A) Cyanosed face with frothy discharge; (B) Congested stomach mucosa and hemorrhagic fluid; (C) Congested kidney; (D) Bottle of the poison ingested

TABLE 56.3: Types of paralyses in OPC poisoning

Type	Acute paralysis (Type I)	Intermediate syndrome (Type II)	Delayed neurotoxicity/polyneuropathy (Type III)
Occurrence	Within 24–48 h	24–96 h	1–3 weeks
S/s	Muscle cramps, fasciculations, weakness (upper motor neuron)	Cranial nerve palsies, weakness of neck flexors and proximal limb muscles, respiratory distress	Symmetric weakness of legs, cramps, pain, and glove and stocking paresthesias, foot drop, ataxia, steppage gait
Treatment	Atropine	Does not respond to oximes or atropine	Does not respond to oximes or atropine

> **FM 9.5**
> Describe general principles and basic methodologies in treatment of poisoning with regard to organochlorines.

Chlorinated Hydrocarbons

The chlorinated hydrocarbons can be divided into four categories:
  i. *DDT and analogues:* DDT and methoxychlor.
  ii. *Benzene hexachloride:* Gamma hexachlorobenzene (Lindane).
  iii. *Cyclodienes and related compounds:* Endrin, aldrin, chlordane, chlordecone, dieldrin, endosulfan, hepatachlor, isobenan and mirex.
  iv. *Toxaphene* and related compounds.

All these pesticides are absorbed through skin, orally and via inhalation.

The *agents that are commonly used are:* DDT, endrin, gammexane and dieldrin.* The chemical prototype for the group is chlorophenothane which is commonly known as DDT. However, since endrin poisoning is quite common, it is described here.

ENDRIN

Introduction
- Endrin, a crystalline organochloride with mild odor and bitter taste, is the most toxic of all the chlorinated insecticides.
- The preparations available in market contain endrin in 20–50% concentration mixed with 50–80% of solvent, such as aromax, a petroleum hydrocarbon smelling like kerosene.
- It is also called *'plant penicillin'* because of its broad spectrum of activity against various insect pests.
- It is extensively used in India, and in Andhra Pradesh the poisoning is occurring at an alarming rate, both in urban and rural populations.

Action
Endrin interferes with nerve impulse transmission. It produces a noncompetitive inhibition of GABA-regulated chloride transport, blocking the stimulation of chloride influx into the neuron, causing hyperexcitability of the CNS initially, followed by depression.

Metabolism: Endrin is partially metabolized in the liver, and directly excreted in the urine, feces and milk; it is rapidly metabolized and eliminated, and does not persist in body tissues.

Signs and Symptoms
Toxic effects rapidly follow ingestion, inhalation or skin contamination. These begin between 1–6 h.

System	Signs and symptoms
GIT	Salivation, nausea, vomiting, abdominal pain, rarely diarrhea, oozing of fine froth, occasionally bloodstained from mouth and nostrils
CNS	Headache, giddiness, restlessness, irritability, dilated pupils, incoordination, ataxia, mental confusion, tremors, tonic and clonic convulsions, coma
RS	Hoarseness of voice, cough, dyspnea

In some cases, convulsions herald the onset of symptoms. Recovery is within 24 h in non-fatal cases.

Cause of death: Death is due to respiratory failure.

Fatal Dose
- **Endrin:** 5–6 g.
- **DDT:** 10–20 g.

Fatal period: 1–2 h, may be more.

Treatment
Mainly symptomatic treatment is given. There is no specific antidote.
  i. Maintain adequate airway, breathing and circulation.
  ii. Decontamination of the body should be carried out and the airway cared for, similar to OPCs.
  iii. Gastric lavage is done and emetics, activated charcoal and cathartics are given. Castor oil, fats and milk are not given as they enhance the absorption.
  iv. **Cholestyramine** (non-absorbable bile acid binding anion exchange resin) increases the fecal excretion of organochlorines, is given in a dose of 16 g/day in divided doses for few days.
  v. Calcium gluconate is given in a dose of 10 mL of 10% solution IV every 4–6 h.
  vi. Diazepam is given IV to control convulsions.

Recovery is likely, if onset of convulsions is delayed by more than an hour or if convulsions can be controlled readily.

Postmortem Findings
These are suggestive of asphyxia.

External
  i. Kerosene-like smell from the mouth and nostrils, may be found even in decomposed bodies.
  ii. Fine white froth, occasionally bloodstained from the mouth and nostrils.
  iii. The face and fingernails are cyanosed.
  iv. Conjunctiva is congested and the pupils are dilated.

Internal
  i. Mucosa of the esophagus, stomach and intestine is congested, and emits a kerosene-like smell.
  ii. Blood is dark and fluid.

---

* Organochlorine pesticides aldrin, DDT, dieldrin and endrin (persistent organic pollutant) have been banned from use as a pesticide in the UK.

iii. Respiratory passages contain frothy mucus and the mucosa is congested.
iv. Petechial hemorrhages over the lungs and heart.
v. Lungs are congested and edematous.
vi. Liver, kidneys and brain are also congested with fatty degeneration of liver.

Medico-legal Aspects

- Endrin is mostly used for suicidal purposes as it is freely available and cheap, despite its unpleasant taste and painful death.
- It may be used for homicidal purposes by mixing it with alcohol, sweets or other food to mask its smell.
- Accidental deaths may occur.
- It resists putrefaction and can be detected in exhumed bodies.
- Since alcohol is generally used to mask the smell of endrin, the viscera for chemical examination should be preserved in saturated saline in suspected cases of poisoning.

Chronic poisoning: Long-term exposure to some of these compounds results in cumulative toxicity characterized by weakness, loss of weight, ataxia, tremors, mental changes, oligospermia, increased tendency to leukemia, purpura, aplastic anemia and liver carcinoma.

> **NOTA BENE**
>
> **Endosulfan** (an organochlorine) toxicity manifestations are mostly neurological (low sensorium, generalized seizures including *status epilepticus*), although other organ dysfunction like hepatic transaminase elevation, azotemia, metabolic acidosis and leukocytosis also occurs. There is no effective antidote; prompt treatment of toxicity, mechanical ventilation and anticonvulsant therapy are recommended.

FM 9.5
Describe general principles and basic methodologies in treatment of poisoning with regard to paraquat.

PARAQUAT

Introduction: It is used as herbicide and weed-killer, available under the trade name, 'Gramoxone' and 'Weedol'.

Action

Paraquat undergoes a NADPH dependent reduction to form a free radical which acts with molecular oxygen to reform the cation to produce superoxide (O_2^-) and hydroxyl radical (OH^-) which disrupt cellular function leading to cell death.

Absorption and Excretion

Absorption through inhalation, skin or eye contact is minimal. About 5–10% of the ingested dose is absorbed and the rest is excreted in feces. It is distributed in all the organs, but highest concentrations are found in kidneys and lungs, followed by muscles. More than 90% of the absorbed paraquat is excreted unchanged in the urine within the first 24 h, but can be detected in urine up to 3 weeks after ingestion.

Signs and Symptoms

System	Signs and symptoms
Local	Irritation and inflammation of skin, cornea, conjunctiva and nasal mucosa
GIT	Ulceration and corrosion of mouth and tongue ('*paraquat tongue*')* **(Fig. 56.6A)**, oropharynx, and esophagus; nausea, vomiting, hematemesis, diarrhea, dysphagia
RS	Cough, hemoptysis, dyspnea due to pulmonary edema, aphonia, aspiration
Renal	Oliguria, renal failure
CVS	Hypovolemia, shock, arrhythmias
Hepatic	Cholestasis
CNS	Coma, convulsions, cerebral edema

Cause of death: Death occurs from multiorgan failure, corrosive effects in the GIT or progressive pulmonary fibrosis leading to ARDS.

Fatal Dose

Paraquat: 4 mg/kg; 5 mL of 'Gramoxone' or 1–2 g of 'Weedol' or 10 mL of 200 g/L concentrate.

Fatal period: 2–7 days.

> **NOTA BENE**
>
> **Diagnosis:** A semi-quantitative test using bicarbonate and sodium dithionite can be used. In an alkaline medium, sodium dithionite reduces paraquat to a bluish purple color (if the urine paraquat concentration is >1 mg/L), and indicates a very poor prognosis. Diquat will produce green color.

Treatment

i. Remove all clothings, and wash the patient thoroughly with soap and water.
ii. Gastric lavage is done with water; emetics are contraindicated.
iii. One liter of aqueous suspension of clay (Fuller's earth or 7% bentonite) is given to adsorb paraquat, followed by 200 mL of 20% mannitol. Dose may be repeated. Otherwise, administer repeated doses of activated charcoal every 2 h for 3–4 doses.
iv. Charcoal hemoperfusion, 8 h/day for 2–3 weeks.
v. Supplemental oxygen is withheld, as it may contribute to the pulmonary damage.
vi. Analgesics are given to allay pain.

Postmortem Findings

External: There may be ulceration around the lips and mouth due to dribbling and ulceration of the tongue.

---

* Initially, tongue becomes erythematous and swollen but later (about 3–5 days) develops erosion and ulcerations which is covered with yellowish necrotic debris.

Internal (Figs. 56.6B and C)

i. **Esophagus**: Reddened and desquamated.
ii. **Stomach**: Erosions and patchy hemorrhages.
iii. **Lungs**: Pulmonary edema, effusions and hemorrhages. In delayed deaths—large, rigid and stiff lungs are seen.
iv. **Liver**: Fatty degeneration and centrilobular necrosis.
v. **Kidneys**: Cortical pallor and diffuse tubular damage.

Medico-legal aspects: Poisoning is mostly accidental and suicidal (which is increasing significantly). Rarely, homicide is possible, and the poisoning may be mistaken for viral pneumonia.

> **FM 9.5**
> Describe general principles and basic methodologies in treatment of poisoning with regard to pyrethroids.

PYRETHRINS AND PYRETHROIDS

Introduction: Pyrethrins are extracted from *Crysanthemum cinerariaefolium* plant. Pyrethroids are synthetic analogues. Toxicity is very low due to their rapid metabolism.

Uses: As insect repellents, insecticides and pesticides. They are available as sprays, dusts, powders, mats and coils. For example, d-allethrin, pyrethrum, allethrin, deltamethrin, decamethrin, cypermethrin and fenvalerate.

Action: They prolong the inactivation of the sodium channel by binding it in the open state.

Signs and Symptoms

Skin contact causes dermatitis and blisters.

On ingestion, there is nausea, vomiting, headache, vertigo, restlessness, paresthesias, fasciculations, muscular weakness, hyperthermia, altered mental state, convulsions, pulmonary edema and coma. Respiratory failure may occur.

Inhalation causes rhinorrhea, sore throat, wheezing and dyspnea.

Fatal Dose

Pyrethroids: 1 g/kg body wt.

Treatment

i. Gastric lavage is done.
ii. Activated charcoal is given.
iii. Oils and fats should be avoided.
iv. Atropine and oximes are contraindicated.
v. Skin should be washed with soap and water.

Medico-legal aspects: Exposure is usually accidental. Suicide/homicide is rare.

In **chronic cases**, the patient gets sensitized with allergic manifestations. It may increase the risk for cardiovascular disease and early deaths.

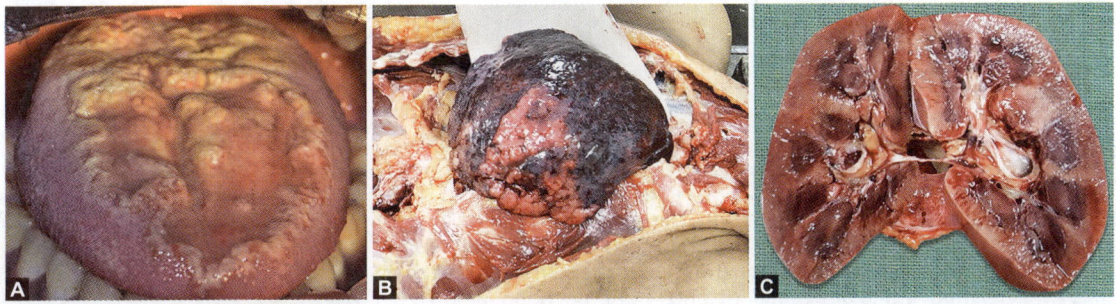

Figs. 56.6A to C: Paraquat poisoning: (A) Paraquat tongue*; (B) Congested, stiff lungs; (C) Cortical pallor in kidneys
[*Courtesy:* (A) Dr Balasubramanian Madhan, Professor of Dentistry, JIPMER, Puducherry]

* Case published in BMJ Case Reports: Madhan B, Arunprasad G, Krishnan B. Paraquat tongue. Case Reports 2014; 2014: bcr2014206581.

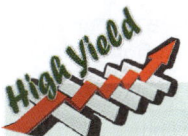

- **Commonest types of insecticide/pesticide:** Organophosphates, carbamates, chlorinated hydrocarbons, aluminum phosphide and pyrethroids.
- **Commonest pesticide poisoning:** OPCs and carbamates.
- **Classification of insecticides**
- *Based on mode of penetration*, i.e., whether they cause effect upon ingestion (stomach poisons), penetration of the body covering (contact poisons) or inhalation (fumigants).
- *Based on chemical composition:* Alkyl phosphates and aryl phosphates.
- **Common OPCs:** Chlorpyriphos, temephos, diazinon (Tik-20), malathion (Finit), parathion, trichlorphon, glyphosate (Weed off).
- **Common carbamates:** Aldicarb, carbaryl (Sevin 50), propoxur (Baygon), physostigmine, neostigmine, pyridostigmine, edrophonium.
- OPCs inhibits acetylcholinesterase (AChE) and plasma or butyrylcholinesterase (pseudocholinesterase)—*cholinesterase inhibitors.*

SECTION 2: Toxicology

- **Signs and symptoms of OPC poisoning:** Salivation; Lacrimation; Urination; Diarrhea; Gastrointestinal distress; Emesis (SLUDGE).
- Pupils are constricted (miosis) in OPC poisoning.
- Chromodacryorrhea (shedding of red tears) is seen in OPC poisoning.
- OPCs are usually mixed with a solvent aromax, which is responsible for kerosene-like smell in the breath and body secretions.
- **Fatal dose:** Malathion and diazinon 1 g; parathion: 175 mg.
- **Confirmatory test of OPC poisoning:** P-nitrophenol test.
- **Treatment of OPC poisoning:** Atropine *(antidote)* and pralidoxime (PAM).
- Atropinization includes mydriasis, dryness of tongue, reduced oropharyngeal secretion *(most specific sign)*, tachycardia, flushing.
- PAM helps in regenerating AChE associated with skeletal muscle NM junctions, and ineffective in reversing CNS effects of OPCs.
- PAM is *not recommended* for carbamate poisoning.
- Kerosene-like smell from nostrils, mouth and stomach contents is seen in deaths due to OPC poisoning.
- **Most important sequelae of OPC poisoning:** Neurological manifestations.
- **Commonly used chlorinated hydrocarbons:** DDT, endrin, gammexane and dieldrin.
- **Most toxic chlorinated insecticides:** Endrin.
- Endrin is called *'plant penicillin'* because of its broad spectrum of activity against various pests.
- Pupils are dilated in endrin poisoning.
- **Fatal dose of endrin:** 5–6 g (DDT: 10–20 g).
- **Treatment of endrin poisoning:** Gastric lavage, activated charcoal, cathartics, cholestyramine, calcium gluconate.
- Kerosene-like smell from the mouth, nostrils and stomach is seen in deaths due to endrin poisoning.
- Endrin resists putrefaction and can be detected in exhumed bodies.
- Paraquat is herbicide and weed-killer ('Gramoxone' and 'Weedol').
- There is ulceration and corrosion of mouth and tongue in paraquat poisoning *('paraquat tongue')*.
- **Fatal dose of paraquat:** 4 mg/kg; 5 mL of 'Gramoxone' or 1–2 g of 'Weedol'.

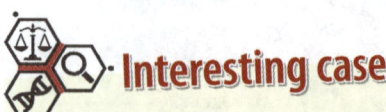

OPC Poisoning

Chheda *et al.* reported a rare case of OPC poisoning in neonates. A 15-day-old healthy breastfed girl baby presented in the emergency department with complaints of excessive secretions from mouth, roving eye movements (slow, conjugate, lateral, to-an-fro excursions) and poor feeding for the past 3 h. The baby was referred with a differential diagnosis of bronchopneumonia or late onset sepsis. There was no history of fever, convulsions or trauma. Her vital signs were: heart rate was 126/min, respiratory rate 34/min irregular, and peripheral pulses well felt. There were excessive secretions from mouth, irregular jerky respiration and nystagmus. However cry, activity and tone were good. Oxygen was given by continuous positive airway pressure, patient was kept nil by mouth on maintenance IV fluids and antibiotics were started. Arterial blood gas revealed pH of 7.43, PaO_2 of 108 mm Hg, and oxygen saturation of 97%. Complete blood count revealed polymorphonuclear leucocytosis. Serum creatinine, blood urea, bilirubin, liver enzyme levels and ionic calcium were within normal limits. CRP was negative, blood culture showed no growth and the chest X-ray was normal.

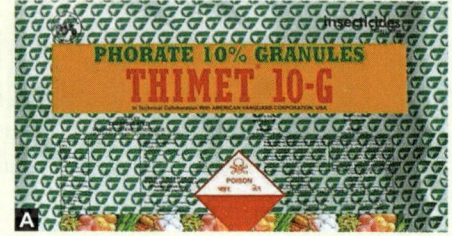

Within 3 h of admission, her condition deteriorated and she developed shallow irregular respiration. Heart rate decreased to 100/min, activity was depressed and hypotonia appeared. Pupillary examination revealed pinpoint pupils not reactive to light. Patient was intubated and ventilated in view of shallow respiration and poor sensorium.

In view of cholinergic signs, OPC poisoning was suspected and on questioning, history of homicidal ingestion of Thimet (10% phorate–OPC) granules was elicited **(Fig. A)**. The toxic substance was fed 3 h before reaching the hospital. Atropine was given as 0.05 mg/kg bolus over 10 mins and repeated every 10 mins till complete atropinization occurred and then an infusion of 0.02 mg/kg/hour was given for first 36 h. Serum acetyl cholinesterase level was 466 units (normal: 2710–11510 units), confirming the diagnosis of OPC poisoning. Pralidoxime was given at 25 mg/kg over 1 h, repeated every 12 h for 5 times. Repeat cholinesterase levels on second day showed minimal improvement (566 units). Patient showed initial clinical improvement with the disappearance of cholinergic signs and heart rate was 130/min after 48 h, however patient started having hypotension requiring inotrope support and increased oxygen requirement and developed pneumonia resulting in multiorgan failure. Patient died on the fourth day of hospitalization. Gastric lavage analysis was inconclusive. A postmortem examination was done which confirmed OPC poisoning.

Source: Chheda AH, Hiremath A, Khadse S, Kulkarni R, Valvi C, Shobi A. Organophosphorus poisoning in a neonate. Pediatr Oncall J. 2014;11:48-49. (*Courtesy:* Dr Akash Chheda, Assistant Professor, Department of Neurology, Seth GS Medical College and KEM Hospital, Mumbai)

Alphos (Aluminum Phosphide)

LEARNING OBJECTIVES

Must know
1. Signs and symptoms, treatment and PM findings in Alphos poisoning
2. Fatal dose of Alphos

Desirable to know
1. Laboratory diagnosis of Alphos poisoning

Describe general principles and basic methodologies in treatment of poisoning with regard to aluminum phosphide.

Introduction

- Alphos or AlP (*quickphos, celphos, phosfume, phostoxin, talunex*), a solid fumigant pesticide, and widely used as a grain preservative in Northern India. Although, the *commonest pesticide poisoning* is organophosphates, AlP poisoning has reached to epidemic proportions in Punjab, Haryana, Chandigarh, Uttar Pradesh, Delhi and Rajasthan.
- AlP's toxic effect in humans is due to liberation of phosphine gas (PH_3) and a small amount of diphosphine when it comes in contact with the moisture of grains and HCl of the stomach.
- AlP is available as tablets (3 g, release 1 g PH_3) or as pellets (0.6 g, releases 0.2 g of PH_3). The tablets are green, brown or gray, and each tablet contains 56% AlP and 44% ammonium carbonate (it is added to prevent self-ignition of PH_3) **(Fig. 57.1)**.
- Phosphine is a colorless and odorless gas, but on exposure to air it gives characteristic *garlic/decaying fish-like odor*. It is spontaneously inflammable and violently combines with oxygen and halogen.
- Phosphine may induce an exothermic reaction at higher temperatures, especially above 30°C. When phosphine burns, it produces a dense white cloud of 'phosphorus pentoxide', a severe respiratory tract irritant.
- Phosphine in air reacts with hydroxyl radical and is removed by it. The non-toxic residues left in grains are *phosphite and hypophosphite of aluminum* which is harmless.

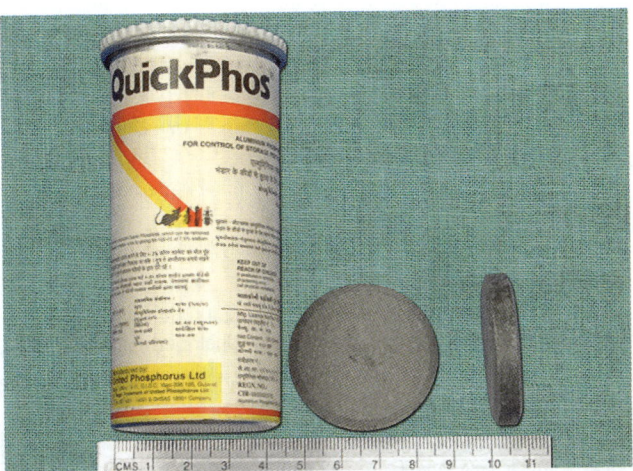
Fig. 57.1: Aluminum phosphide

Action

- AlP is a protoplasmic poison which inhibits protein and enzyme synthesis.
- Phosphine interrupts the stages of mitochondrial electron transport by inhibiting cytochrome C oxidase and oxidative phosphorylation, which eventually results in ATP depletion and cell death.
- It is also thought that superoxide anions and free radicals are in excess, and their decreased destruction leads to lipid peroxidation and change in fluidity of cell membrane and ultimately cell drops out.
- In addition, phosphine and phosphides have corrosive actions.

This process is *fully reversible* and full recovery occurs in patients who survive without any residual effect.

Absorption and Excretion

- Phosphine is rapidly absorbed from the GIT by simple diffusion and cause damage to internal organs. It is also absorbed rapidly from lungs after inhalation.
- After ingestion, some AlP is absorbed and metabolized in the liver and phosphine is slowly released, accounting for the prolongation of symptoms.
- Phosphine is oxidized slowly to hypophosphite and excreted in the urine. It is also excreted through the lungs in unchanged form.

SIGNS AND SYMPTOMS

It depends on the dose and severity of poisoning.

On Ingestion

Mild intoxication produces:
- Nausea and vomiting
- Headache
- Abdominal pain.

Recovery is usual.

Moderate to severe poisoning produces:

System	Signs and symptoms
GIT	Nausea, vomiting, diarrhea, abdominal pain
CVS	Refractory hypotension, arrhythmias, myocarditis, pericarditis, acute CHF, shock
RS	Cough, dyspnea, cyanosis, pulmonary edema, respiratory failure
Hepatic	Jaundice, hepatitis, hepatomegaly
Renal	Oliguria, renal failure
CNS	Headache, dizziness, altered mental state, restlessness, convulsions, acute hypoxic encephalopathy, coma
Others	Rarely, muscle wasting, tenderness, bleeding diathesis due to capillary damage

Mnemonic for Alphos poisoning: ALPHOS
A: **A**bdominal pain, arrhythmia, altered mental state, acidosis;
L: **L**ung failure; P: **P**ulmonary edema;
H: **H**ypotension; O: **O**liguria; S: **S**eizures

On Inhalation

Mild exposure	Moderate exposure	Severe exposure
Mucous membrane irritation	In-coordination and paralysis	Pulmonary edema
Respiratory distress	Numbness	Arrhythmias
Tightness of chest	Tremors	CHF
Headache	Diplopia	ARDS
Dizziness	Paresthesia	Convulsions
Fatigue	Jaundice	Coma
GIT disturbances	Muscular weakness	
	Ataxia	
	Multiple organ failure	

Cause of death: Metabolic acidosis or mixed metabolic acidosis and respiratory alkalosis, and acute renal failure are frequent.
- Within the first 24 hours (h) after ingestion: Cardiac arrhythmia.
- After 24 h: Refractory shock, acidosis and ARDS.

Fatal Dose
- Ingestion: 150–500 mg (1 tablet is fatal).
- Inhalation: Level >50 ppm in air is dangerous; 400–600 ppm is fatal within ½ hour.

Fatal period: 1–4 days (initial 24 h is critical).

Laboratory Findings

- Chemical analysis for PH_3 in blood or urine is not recommended as PH_3 is rapidly oxidized.
- There is leukopenia, increased serum glutamic oxaloacetic transaminase (SGOT) and serum glutamic pyruvic transaminase (SGPT), metabolic acidosis, decreased plasma magnesium and serum cortisol and raised plasma renin levels.

Laboratory Diagnosis

i. Five mL of gastric aspirate is added to 15 mL of H_2O in a flask and its mouth is covered with a filter paper impregnated with silver nitrate ($AgNO_3$). The flask is heated at 50°C for 15–20 minutes (min). If phosphine is present, the filter paper turns black due to silver phosphate.
ii. **Silver nitrate impregnated paper test**
   - It may be carried out on vomitus, lavage fluid and breath.
   - It is carried for bedside confirmation of AlP poisoning.
   - The test depends on property of phosphine to react with $AgNO_3$ and turning it into black.
   - Sensitivity is <100% with gastric juice, 50% with breath (positive in breath, if >6 g is ingested).
   - Specificity is high, but it sometimes gets blackened due to presence of H_2S in air as impurity. Its presence can be differentiated by using lead acetate paper, i.e., both papers will turn black in the presence of H_2S. Confirmation of PH_3 can be done by putting a drop of ammonium molybdate solution on the black-turned filter paper, the color of the paper will change to blue.
iii. The most specific and sensitive method for detecting phosphine is gas chromatography with a nitrogen-phosphorous detector (gastric contents and viscera during autopsy are collected in air tight jars).
iv. For spot sampling of phosphine in air, detector tubes and bulbs are available.

TREATMENT (FLOWCHART 57.1)

Since, there is no specific antidote, the only effective approach is intensive care to maintain blood pH, electrolytes

Flowchart 57.1: Management of AlP poisoning

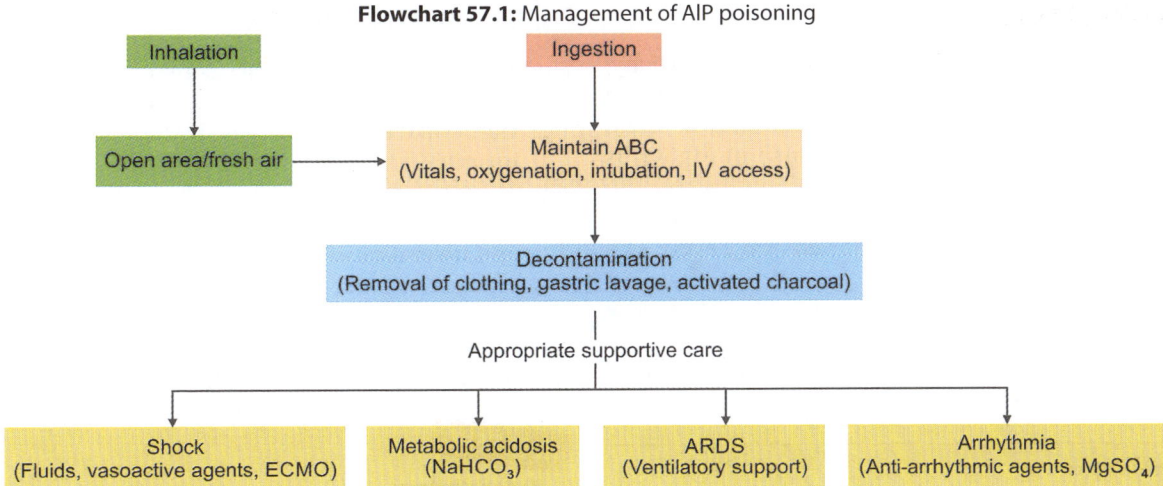

and blood pressure. The most important factor for survival is resuscitation of shock and correction of metabolic acidosis.
- The doctor must take personal protection measures, including face mask and rubber gloves during decontamination.
- In case of inhalation, remove the patient to fresh air and give supplemental oxygen.
- Patient's clothes should be removed, and the skin and eyes decontaminated with water.

I. Stabilization
- Confirm airway patency and protect the airways with endotracheal tube, if required. Requirement of endotracheal intubation and mechanical ventilation usually depends on the severity of the lung injury and poor mental status (prevent aspiration pneumonitis).
- O_2 is given for hypoxia.

II. Decontamination
a. *Reduction of absorption from GIT*
   i. Gastric lavage with $KMnO_4$ (1:10,000) in first 30–45 min after ingestion (oxidizes phosphine to phosphate). Repeated 2–3 times.
   ii. Activated charcoal 100 g orally.

> **NOTA BENE**
> **4-step-gastric lavage:** Suction of gastric contents, 3 vials of sodium bicarbonate (7.5%) orally, potassium permanganate (1:10,000) lavage and again 3 vials of sodium bicarbonate orally is said to be more effective washing method.

   iii. Antacids reduce absorption of phosphine. Liquid paraffin may also be given.
   iv. Antiemetic and H_2 receptor antagonist—gives symptomatic relief, reduces the gastric acidity and prevent further liberation of PH_3 gas.

b. *Enhancement of excretion*
   i. Phosphine is excreted through the lungs and kidneys. So, adequate hydration and renal perfusion must be maintained by IV fluids.
   ii. Diuretics like furosemide can be given, if systolic BP is >90 mm Hg.
   iii. Sorbitol solution (dose 1–2 mL/kg) may be used as cathartic.

III. Combating Shock
   i. Fluids (3–4 liters are given in the first 3–6 h, 50% of which is NS) guided by central venous pressure (CVP) and pulmonary capillary wedge pressure (PCWP) monitoring.
   ii. Hydrocortisone (dose 200–400 mg 4–6 h).
   iii. Low dose dopamine is given for hypotension and shock (dose 4–6 μg/kg/min)—should be used cautiously, as it can induce arrhythmias.
   iv. For refractory hypotension, norepinephrine or phenylephrine can be used. Digoxin is also useful for cardiogenic shock.
   v. All types of dysrhythmias should be treated with standard antidysrhythmics.
   vi. Advanced measures, such as *extracorporeal membrane oxygenation (ECMO) or extracorporeal life support (ECLS)*[*] can be employed in toxic myocarditis with refractory shock. Intra-aortic balloon pump (IABP) has been used successfully to treat cardiogenic shock.

IV. Correction of Acidosis
   i. Sodium bicarbonate IV (dose 50–100 mEq every 8 h) till the bicarbonate level rises to 18–20 mEq/L.
   ii. Hemodialysis (not very effective in removing PH_3) is helpful in severe metabolic acidosis or fluid overload and acute renal failure.

---

[*] It is an extracorporeal (outside the body) technique of maintaining the circulation in the body by providing both cardiac and respiratory support. While outside the body, hemoglobin becomes fully saturated with O_2 and CO_2 is removed.

V. Reduction of Toxicity

Magnesium sulfate is supposed to reduce organ toxicity, correct hypomagnesemia and arrhythmias. It has an antiperoxident effect and it combats free radical stress due to PH_3. At present, the routine use of $MgSO_4$ is questionable.

Dose: 3 g bolus followed by 6 g as infusion over 12 h for 5–7 days; or 3 g as infusion over 3 h followed by 6 g every 24 h for 3–5 days.

- Hyperglycemia is seen in many cases. Plasma glucose level should be corrected.
- DC cardioversion and temporary pacemaker should be available at the bedside.

Recent Advances
Apart from supportive treatment, novel therapies have been suggested but not recommended for routine use:
- **Oral administration of coconut oil:** Coconut oil has been reported to inhibit the release of phosphine gas from AlP due to physicochemical properties of AlP and non-miscibility with fat.
- **Antioxidant agents:** N-acetylcysteine, glutathione, melatonin, vitamin C and beta carotene may be used.
- **Trimetazidine** (anti-ischemic drug) reduces oxygen consumption and may have a potential role to check CVS manifestation.
- Other agents that have been used reportedly are infusion of GIK (glucose-insulin-potassium), oral liothyronine, vitamin E, digoxin, hyperbaric oxygen, Mg^{2+} carrying nanoparticles, N-omega-nitro-L-arginine methyl ester (L-NAME), atropine + pralidoxime, vitamin C + methylene blue.
- PH_3 is trapped and neutralized by boric acid $[B(OH)_3]$ which can be used as an antidote.

Complications

Pericarditis	Acute GIT bleed
Acute CHF	Acute respiratory failure
DIC	Hepatitis
Ascites	Acute tubular necrosis
Rhabdomyolysis	Pancreatitis

NOTA BENE
Good prognostic factors
- Freshness and dose of compound—fully exposed compound and lesser dose have low morbidity and mortality.
- Immediate and more frequent vomiting and early availability of supportive care.

Poor prognostic factors
- Ingestion of 'unexposed tablets'.
- Requirement of mechanical ventilation, lack of vomiting after ingestion and delay in seeking treatment after exposure.
- Shock, altered mental status, high APACHE II score, acute renal failure, low prothrombin time, and hyperglycemia.
- Abnormalities of arterial pH, serum bicarbonate level and ECG, and serum PH_3 >1.6 mg/dL.

POSTMORTEM FINDINGS

Findings of vital organs are suggestive of cellular hypoxia.
i. Blood tinged froth from mouth and nostrils.
ii. Garlic-like odor in the gastric contents, mouth and nostrils.
iii. Mucosa of the lower part of esophagus, stomach and duodenum are congested. Hemorrhages and ulcerations in stomach and duodenum may be seen.
iv. Decreasing congestion of the GIT is seen in small intestine from cephalic to caudal end.
v. Congested and edematous viscera.

NOTA BENE
Histopathology
- **Stomach:** Congested, edematous, leukocytic infiltration and sloughing of gastric mucosa.
- **Lungs:** Congested, edematous, desquamation of respiratory epithelium, atelectasis, round cell infiltration around bronchioles, thickened alveolar wall and lymphocytic infiltration.
- **Heart:** Congested, edematous, focal necrosis, myocyte vacuolation and leukocytic infiltration.
- **Liver:** Microvesicular and macrovesicular steatosis, centrilobular necrosis, dilatation and engorgement of hepatic central veins, sinusoids, and areas showing nuclear fragmentation, mononuclear infiltration and fatty changes.
- **Kidneys:** Congested, necrosis and tubular degeneration.
- **Adrenals:** Congested, hemorrhagic necrosis and areas of lipid depletion in cortex.
- **Brain:** Congested and edematous. There may be capillary dilation, paucity of glial cells, degenerated Nissl granule in the cytoplasm and deeply stained eccentric nucleus, degeneration of neurons and appearance of necrotic patches.

Medico-legal Aspects

- Poisoning is mostly suicidal, but homicidal cases may be seen in children. AlP is considered as '*ideal suicidal*' *poison* since it is cheap, easily available, highly toxic, can be taken with food or drink, and has no effective antidote.
- Accidental and occupational poisoning may occur.
- Its gaseous form and toxicity makes it a potential agent for chemical terrorism.

NOTA BENE
Each tablet of AlP has the capacity to liberate 1 g of phosphine (PH_3) gas.

$$AlP + 3HCl \rightarrow AlCl_3 + PH_3\uparrow$$
$$AlP + 3H_2O \rightarrow Al(OH)_3 + PH_3\uparrow$$
$$(NH_4)_2CO_3 + H_2O \rightarrow 2NH_4OH + CO_2\uparrow \rightarrow 2NH_3\uparrow + 2H_2O + CO_2\uparrow$$

Therefore, gases liberated during fumigation or after ingestion are CO_2, NH_3 and phosphine (PH_3) and a non-toxic residue aluminum hydroxide. The former two gases provide inert media for phosphine to act.

CHAPTER 57 : Alphos (Aluminum Phosphide)

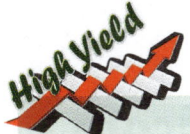

- Toxic effect of Alphos is due to liberation of phosphine gas when it comes in contact with HCl of the stomach.
- Phosphine acts by inhibiting cytochrome oxidase and oxidative phosphorylation.
- Phosphine gives characteristic *garlic/decaying fish-like odor*.
- **Signs and symptoms of Alphos poisoning:** Abdominal pain, arrhythmia, altered mental state, metabolic acidosis, lung failure, pulmonary edema, hypotension, oliguria, seizures.
- **Cause of death in Alphos poisoning:** Metabolic acidosis and acute renal failure.
- **Fatal dose:** 150–500 mg (1 tablet is fatal).
- **Test for Alphos poisoning:** Silver nitrate test.
- There is no antidote for Alphos poisoning.
- Treatment is conservative—treatment for shock, ARDS, metabolic acidosis and arrhythmia.
- Alphos is considered as '*ideal suicidal*' poison.

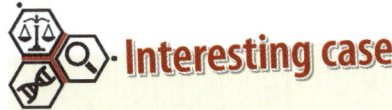

Alphos Poisoning

Mirakbari reported an interesting case of ignition with the release of phosphine from AIP poisoned patient that can affect not just the patient but also pose a health hazard to emergency physicians and medical staff.

A 34-year-old woman was brought to the emergency department with alleged history of taking AIP tablets. Her relatives brought the can and alleged she had taken two tablets 30 minutes before. On arrival, she was drowsy and was not responding to verbal commands. Her body was cold and hypotonic, and her skin was pale with mottling. Her vital signs were: pulse 110/min regular, BP 70/52 mm Hg, respiratory rate 20/min shallow, and body temperature 36.1°C. The ECG showed sinus tachycardia, pulse oximetry showed O_2 saturation of 91% on room air and arterial blood gas analysis showed metabolic acidosis with pH of 7.1. The history, symptoms and presentation of ALP tablets favored a diagnosis of AIP poisoning.

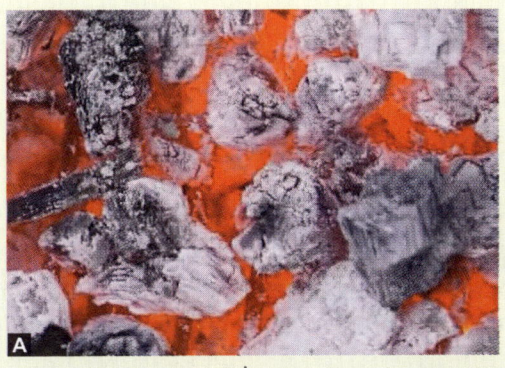

The patient was intubated and a nasogastric tube was inserted. Normal saline was administered by IV. After gastric lavage with sodium bicarbonate, potassium permanganate (1:10,000) was used and then activated charcoal (100 g) was administered **(Fig. A)**. Shortly afterwards, she vomited 'hot charcoal' filled with small bubbles covered with white smoke that led to thermal burning of the left side of the her face. A simultaneous cough splashed some vomit on the emergency personnel's clothes. She was immediately transferred to an isolated room and underwent infusion of calcium gluconate and magnesium sulfate. The patient's situation progressively deteriorated. There was decreased sensorium and apnea necessitating resuscitation and mechanical ventilation. After 3 h of admission, the patient died from cardiac arrest.

Source: Mirakbari SM. Hot charcoal vomitus in aluminum phosphide poisoning—A case report of internal thermal reaction in aluminum phosphide poisoning and review of literature. Indian J Anaesth. 2015;59:433-36.
(*Courtesy:* Dr SM Mirakbari, Associate Professor, Department of Clinical Toxicology, Bu Ali Hospital, Qazvin University of Medical Sciences, Iran)

CHAPTER 58: Medicinal Poisons

LEARNING OBJECTIVES

Must know
1. Paracetamol toxicity
2. Benzodiazepine toxicity
3. Aspirin toxicity
4. Iron toxicity
5. Antipsychotic drugs toxicity
6. Muscle relaxants toxicity
7. Anesthetics toxicity
8. Insulin toxicity

Desirable to know
1. Antidepressants toxicity
2. Lithium toxicity
3. Phenytoin toxicity
4. Antibiotics toxicity

Describe general principles and basic methodologies in treatment of poisoning with regard to paracetamol.

PARACETAMOL (ACETAMINOPHEN)

Introduction: Paracetamol (PCM) or acetaminophen (N-acetyl-para-aminophenol, APAP) is a common analgesic in many nonprescription and prescription products.

Action

- PCM inhibits prostaglandin synthesis.
- It produces liver damage through accumulation of a toxic intermediate metabolite: *N-acetyl-p-benzoquinone imine* (NAPQI). Hepatic glutathione normally inactivates the metabolite, but in PCM poisoning, the glutathione becomes depleted.
- It also causes renal tubular necrosis.

Metabolism: After absorption, it is metabolized by glucuronidation and sulfation, and by cytochrome P450 oxidase system.

Signs and Symptoms

- Usually four stages of presentation are seen **(Table 58.1)**.
- Paracetamol toxicity is manifested primarily in the liver. Risk factors associated with fatal outcome include long-term alcohol ingestion, fasting, and treatment with drugs that induce the cytochrome P450 2E1 enzyme system.

TABLE 58.1: Signs and symptoms of PCM poisoning

Stage/Phase	Time of ingestion	Signs and symptoms
I (Initial)	0–24 hours (h)	Nausea, vomiting, diaphoresis, malaise, pallor
II (Middle)	24–72 h	Discomfort disappears, giving a false sense of relief. Upper abdominal pain may be present
III (Hepatic)*	72–96 h	Vomiting, jaundice, hepatic pain, bleeding, confusion, coma, asterixis (*flapping tremor*), hepatic encephalopathy, cardiac arrhythmia, hemorrhagic pancreatitis, DIC
IV (Recovery)	4 days–2 weeks	Resolution of liver function occurs in about 2–3 months

* Death usually occurs in stage III. If not, then patient passes into stage IV.

Diagnosis

- PCM levels are assessed in the blood by enzyme immunoassay and high performance liquid chromatography (HPLC).
- Emergency measurement of blood levels is essential in assessment of poisoning.
- There is a marked elevation of liver enzymes (peak alanine transaminase >1000 IU/L) and an increased PT may be seen.
- *Rumack-Matthew nomogram* can help in planning treatment.

Fatal Dose

- *Adults:* 10–15 g (20–30 tablets).
- *Children:* 150 mg/kg body wt.

Fatal period: 2–4 days.

> **NOTA BENE**
>
> **Test for acetaminophen:** HCl is added to urine or a protein-free filtrate of blood and heated to 100°C. A blue color on adding o-cresol in water and NH_4OH constitutes positive test.

Treatment

i. Activated charcoal and gastric lavage within 1–2 h of ingestion.
ii. **Antidote:** *N-acetyl cysteine* (NAC)* 150 mg/kg in 200 mL of 5% glucose over 15 minutes (min), followed by serial infusion of 50 mg/kg in 500 mL of 5% glucose in 4, 8 and 8 h (total 300 mg/kg in 20 h). Administration of NAC within 8 h of ingestion is nearly 100% hepatoprotective. Oral *methionine* is an alternative, but is unreliable in patients who are vomiting.
iii. Liver transplantation is life saving for fulminant hepatic necrosis.
iv. **Supportive measures:** Intravenous electrolytes, rehydration, vitamin K for bleeding, and mannitol for cerebral edema.

Postmortem Findings

- **External:** Jaundice, petechiae in skin.
- **Internal:** Congestion of the GIT, centrilobular hepatic necrosis, acute tubular necrosis, cerebral edema and myocardial necrosis.

Medico-legal aspects: Most cases of poisoning are suicidal. Accidental overdose may occur.

> **NOTA BENE**
>
> In January 2014, the FDA recommended that combination prescription pain relievers containing more than 325 mg of PCM per tablet, capsule or other dosage unit should not be prescribed because of a risk of liver damage.

FM 9.3
Describe general principles and basic methodologies in treatment of poisoning with regard to iron.

IRON

Introduction: Commonly available preparations are ferrous sulfate (20% elemental iron), ferrous gluconate (12% elemental iron) and ferrous fumarate (33% elemental iron) which are used for supplemental therapy in case of iron deficiency anemia. Rarely, the source of poisoning may be from tanning, dyeing and from inks.

Action

Increased capillary permeability, release of hydrogen ions, inhibition of mitochondrial enzymes and corrosive action on gastric mucosa.

Signs and Symptoms

They are divided into four stages. Symptoms begin with acute gastroenteritis, followed by a quiescent period, then shock and liver failure.

i. **Stage I:** Nausea, vomiting, abdominal pain, gastrointestinal hemorrhage, hypotension, pallor and lethargy. These symptoms occur half an hour to 6 h post-ingestion.
ii. **Stage II:** Mild acidosis, hyperventilation, oliguria and hypotension; occur 6–24 h post-ingestion. Overall, the patient seems to show apparent improvement.
iii. **Stage III:** Multiorgan dysfunction involving GIT, CVS, CNS, hepatorenal systems with anion-gap metabolic acidosis, depression, hepatitis, coagulopathy, convulsions, disorientation, shock, coma and death. It occurs 24–48 h to few days post-ingestion.
iv. **Stage IV:** It is seen 2–6 weeks post-ingestion and includes complications, like gastric stricture and pyloric obstruction.

Fatal Dose

Elemental iron: 20–30 g (200–250 mg/kg).
Fatal period: 24–48 h.

Diagnosis

- *Abdominal X-ray:* Radiopaque tablets may be seen.
- *Serum iron level* >350 µg/dL indicate toxicity. It is measured 2–6 h post-ingestion.
- *Desferrioxamine challenge test:* It is given in a dose of 25 mg/kg which imparts a reddish 'vin rose' color to the urine (iron-desferrioxamine complex).

Treatment

Treatment is usually whole-bowel irrigation and chelation therapy.

i. **Fluid resuscitation:** If patient is in shock, normal saline drip or lactated Ringer's solution, dopamine and whole blood transfusion may be given depending upon the cause. Dextrose for hypoglycemia, and sodium bicarbonate for acidosis is given.
ii. **Decontamination:** Gastric lavage or whole bowel irrigation with normal saline or polyethylene glycol-

---

* NAC stimulates glutathione biosynthesis, promotes detoxification and acts directly as a scavenger of free radicals.

electrolyte solution. After this, 1% sodium bicarbonate/magnesium hydroxide solution is added to precipitate the residual iron as insoluble ferrous carbonate/hydroxide.
iii. **Chelation therapy:** *Desferrioxamine* (antidote) in a dose of 10–15 mg/kg/h as continuous infusion to a maximum of 6 g, till there is significant reduction of systemic toxicity.
iv. **Supportive therapy**
- Hemodialysis or exchange transfusion in severe cases.
- Endoscopy or gastrostomy, if there is clinical toxicity and a large amount of tablets are visible on the X-ray.

Postmortem Findings

Usually, internal findings are seen.
i. **GIT:** Hemorrhagic necrosis and perforation of the gastric or jejunal wall.
ii. **Lungs:** Pulmonary hemorrhage.
iii. **Liver:** Centrilobular necrosis may be seen.
iv. **Kidneys:** It may show necrosis of tubules.

Medico-legal Aspects

- Usually, accidental poisoning from overdose (children are attracted by its color and pleasant flavor), prolonged therapy or IV administration.
- Suicidal cases may occur in older children and adults.

Describe general principles and basic methodologies in treatment of poisoning with regard to: phenytoin, lithium, haloperidol, neuroleptics, tricyclic antidepressants.

PHENYTOIN

Introduction: Phenytoin (e.g., Dilantin) is most widely used anticonvulsants for seizure disorders.

Action

Phenytoin is a sodium channel blocker and acts on both neuronal and cardiac tissue.

Signs and Symptoms

Acute oral ingestion results in CNS (more common) and CVS toxicity.

System	Signs and symptoms
CNS	Confusion, nystagmus, slurred speech, tremor, irritability, ataxia, depressed conscious state, seizures, coma
CVS	Arrhythmias, bradycardia, hypotension, asystole
GIT	Nausea, vomiting

Cause of death: Death is rare but may occur due to neurologic depression and respiratory failure.

Fatal Dose

Serum level >125 mg/L.

Treatment

The mainstay of therapy is supportive care. There is no specific antidote for phenytoin poisoning.
i. Activated charcoal is given, if the patient presents early.
ii. Bradycardia is managed according to standard ACLS protocols.
iii. Hypotension is treated with an initial bolus of isotonic solution. If unresponsive, vasopressors can be given.
iv. Antiemetics for nausea and vomiting. Seizures can be controlled by benzodiazepines and phenobarbital.

Medico-legal Aspects

- Acute ingestion leading to overdose can be intentional or accidental.
- There have also been reports of crack cocaine being adulterated with phenytoin, which can lead to an unintentional overdose.

> **NOTA BENE**
>
> **Purple glove syndrome:** Rare side effect that can occur with IV administration of phenytoin; characterized by worsening distal limb edema and discoloration which can lead to extensive skin necrosis and limb ischemia.

LITHIUM

Introduction: Lithium is used for the treatment of major depressive and bipolar (manic-depressive) disorders.

Action

The mechanism of action of lithium is not well understood but is believed to involve a decrease in neuronal responsiveness to neurotransmitters.

Signs and Symptoms

Acute lithium poisoning is most often associated with GIT symptoms (within 1 h of ingestion), cardiotoxic effects and late developing neurological signs.

System	Signs and symptoms
GIT	Nausea, vomiting, abdominal pain, diarrhea
CVS	Arrhythmias, bradycardia, hypotension
CNS	Restlessness, confusion, coarse tremors, muscle fasciculations, hyperreflexia, nystagmus, ataxia, hyperthermia, delirium, convulsions, coma

Cause of death: Death is uncommon, but can be secondary to CNS effects with subsequent cardiovascular collapse.

Fatal Dose

Serum level >2–3 mEq/L (>2 mmol/L).

Treatment

Management is supportive care, and there is no antidote for lithium poisoning.
 i. Gastric lavage should be done; activated charcoal is contraindicated.
 ii. Whole bowel irrigation with polyethylene glycol solution 2–4 h after ingestion. Sodium polystyrene sulfonate may be useful.
 iii. Hemodialysis.
 iv. Seizures can be controlled with benzodiazepines, phenobarbital or propofol.

Medico-legal Aspects

Suicidal or accidental ingestion of excessive amount of lithium tablets result in acute or acute-on-chronic overdose settings.

ANTIPSYCHOTIC DRUGS (TRANQUILIZERS)

Introduction: These drugs relieve anxiety and mental tension without producing sedation, and are used in various neurotic conditions, anxiety states, relief of tension, and as anesthetics because of their muscle relaxant properties.

Classification

Phenothiazines	**Examples**
♦ Aliphatic	Chlorpromazine, Triflupromazine
♦ Piperazine	Trifluoperazine, Prochlorperazine
♦ Piperidine	Thioridazine, Mesoridazine
Butyrophenones	Haloperidol, Droperidol
Thioxanthenes	Thiothixene, Flupenthixol
Others	Pimozide, Reserpine, Loxapine
Atypical neuroleptics	Clozapine, Risperidone

Action

They have an inhibitory effect on a variety of receptors including dopaminergic (mainly D_2 receptor), cholinergic, alpha1 and alpha$_2$-adrenergic, histaminic and serotonergic receptors ($5HT_2$).

Absorption and excretion: They are completely absorbed from the GIT. Excretion is mainly via feces (50%), and the kidneys (30%) as metabolites; less than 4% is excreted in the unchanged form.

Signs and Symptoms

Toxic manifestations can be divided into CNS and non-CNS effects.

CNS Effects

♦ Depression, agitation, seizures, somnolence and coma.
♦ *Behavioral reactions:* Oversedation, impaired psychomotor function and paradoxical effects, such as agitation, excitement, insomnia and toxic confusional states.
♦ *Extrapyramidal signs:* Dystonia (acute), akathisia, Parkinsonism (akinesia), neuroleptic malignant syndrome and tardive dyskinesia.

Non-CNS Effects

System	Signs and symptoms
CVS	Orthostatic hypotension, ventricular tachycardia, torsades de pointes, ventricular fibrillation, atrioventricular block
GIT	Dry mouth, decreased colonic motility resulting in constipation, pseudo-obstruction
Ocular	Mydriasis; visual acuity, visual fields and color vision perception may be altered
Genitourinary	Urinary retention, priapism.
Hematologic	Agranulocytosis, aplastic anemia, leukopenia, eosinophilia, thrombocytopenia, anemia, pancytopenia
Hepatic	Cholestatic jaundice

Fatal Dose

Antipsychotics: 2–5 g (25–30 times of therapeutic dose).

Diagnostic trial: For a suspected case of poisoning, administration of diphenhydramine (dose: 1–2 mg/kg, maximum—25 mg) results not only in resolution of dystonia or oculogyria, but also assists in the diagnosis.

> **NOTA BENE**
>
> **Forrest test:** 1 mL of Forrest reagent is added to 0.5 mL of urine and the mixture is stirred for 5 sec. A dark green color is a positive result. Phenothiazines will also produce a color with this reagent.

Treatment

There is no specific antidote for acute phenothiazine poisoning.

Initial Stabilization

 i. *ABCs:* Oxygen is given. Intubation may be necessary.
 ii. *Emesis:* Contraindicated due to the risk of development of seizures and sedation.

iii. *Gastric lavage* must be done followed by administration of activated charcoal; beneficial even up to 6 h following ingestion.
iv. *Catharsis*: Following gastric lavage, a saline cathartic (sodium or magnesium sulfate) may be introduced and left in the stomach.
v. *Diuresis*: Mannitol solution is given slow IV in a dose of 5 mL/kg initially, followed by 2 mL/kg every 6 hourly for 2 days.
vi. *Correction of hypotension*: Elevate the foot end of the bed. Give adequate IV fluids (0.9% NS). Treatment of resistant hypotension is done with norepinephrine, 1–2 µg/kg/min (titrated to blood pressure).

Management of Specific Condition

i. *Ventricular dysrhythmia:* Administer sodium bicarbonate. Ventricular dysrhythmias are treated with lidocaine (loading dose: 1 mg/kg IV repeated after 5–10 min, maintenance dose: 2–4 mg/min IV) or phenytoin (15–20 mg/kg IV).
ii. *Dystonic reactions:* Administer diphenhydramine, 0.5–1 mg/kg IV (maximum 50 mg) or benztropine mesylate, 1–2 mg IV or IM (0.01–0.02 mg/kg).
iii. *Malignant hyperthermia:* Administer dantrolene (2–5 mg/kg IV) or bromocriptine (2.5–7.5 mg orally daily).
iv. *Seizures:* Treat seizures initially with diazepam, 0.2–0.5 mg/kg IV, repeat after 10–15 min. Phenobarbital or phenytoin can be used for persistent seizures.
v. *Other measures:* Hypothermia may occur, maintain normal body temperature and avoid overheating.

Medico-legal Aspects

- These drugs are the most frequent cause of acute accidental poisoning in children and mostly involve children <6 years of age.
- Unintentional overdose and suicidal ingestion are also common.

TRICYCLIC ANTIDEPRESSANTS

Introduction: Tricyclic antidepressants (TCAs) are one of the oldest classes of antidepressants and are still used extensively. Before the introduction of selective serotonin reuptake inhibitors (SSRIs), TCAs were the standard treatment for depression.

TCAs include:
- Imipramine
- Amitriptyline
- Trimipramine
- Doxepin
- Clomipramine
- Desipramine
- Nortriptyline
- Dothiepin

Action

- TCAs have complex actions. It inhibits monoamine uptake and interact with variety of receptors, viz. muscarinic, α-adrenergic, dopaminergic, GABA-ergic, histaminergic and serotonergic.
- They have potent anticholinergic and antiarrhythmic activity.

Signs and Symptoms

Features of poisoning appear in 1 h, and maximum intensity is seen in 4–12 h.
- **Anticholinergic effects:** Dry skin and mouth, flushing, decreased bowel sounds, constipation, epigastric distress, urinary retention, dilated pupils, blurred vision and palpitations.
- **CNS:** Drowsiness, sleepiness, unresponsive to pain, depressed brainstem reflexes, seizures and coma.
- **CVS:** Tachycardia and hypotension.
- **MS:** Myoclonus, later on flaccid paralysis.
- Respiration is depressed, and temperature is decreased.

Cause of death: Metabolic acidosis and cardiorespiratory depression.

Treatment

i. Gastric lavage, respiratory support, fluid infusion, maintenance of BP and body temperature. Acidosis is corrected by sodium bicarbonate infusion.
ii. Diazepam may be given IV to control convulsions and delirium.
iii. Propranolol or lidocaine may be used for ventricular arrhythmias.
iv. Physostigmine 0.5–2 mg IV reverses the central, peripheral and cardiac effects, but seldom used, since arrhythmias and hypotension are sometimes worsened by this treatment.

Medico-legal Aspects

Poisoning is frequent with suicidal attempts by the depressed individuals.

> **NOTA BENE**
> Tricyclic antidepressants are the leading cause of death by drug overdose in the US.

> **FM 10.1**
> Describe general principles and basic methodologies in treatment of poisoning with regard to benzodiazepines.

BENZODIAZEPINES (BZDS)

Introduction: They are used mainly as anti-anxiety and muscle relaxant agents. The commonly used preparations are: diazepam, flurazepam, chlordiazepoxide, nitrazepam, oxazepam, flunitrazepam, alprazolam and lorazepam.

Addiction may occur with these drugs. They can be ultra-short acting (e.g., midazolam), short acting (e.g., alprazolam) and long acting (e.g., diazepam).

Action

They enhance the inhibitory actions of the neurotransmitter GABA located in the brain.

Signs and Symptoms

The classic presentation of isolated BZD overdose is CNS depression with normal vital signs (no irregularity in respiration or BP).

- Confusion, dizziness, anxiety, vertigo, slurred speech, nystagmus, diplopia, dysarthria, ataxia, hallucinations, weakness, impairment of cognition, amnesia, sedation, somnolence, respiratory depression and coma.
- If taken alone, they are not fatal, but mixing with alcohol or drugs like opioids can lead to death, with advanced age as additional risk factor.

Cause of death: Death after admission is rare, and is due to respiratory depression with aspiration of gastric contents.

Fatal Dose

Benzodiazepines: 100–300 mg/kg body wt.

Diagnosis: Immunoassay screening techniques are performed most commonly. These tests typically detect BZDs that are metabolized to desmethyldiazepam or oxazepam; thus, a negative screening result does not rule out the presence of a BZD.

> **NOTA BENE**
>
> **Bratton-Marshall test:** A screening test for BZDs wherein it is converted to benzophenones by acid hydrolysis and heating. Following extraction, color reagent is added. A purple color indicates positive result.

Treatment

i. **Decontamination:** GIT decontamination with activated charcoal (not beneficial in isolated BZD ingestion).
ii. **Antidote:** *Flumazenil* selectively blocks the central effects of BZDs by competitive inhibition, 0.2 mg over 30–60 seconds given slow IV, repeated in 0.5 mg increments up to a total of 3–5 mg. However, it may itself induce seizures. A long-acting drug, such as chlordiazepoxide or diazepam is useful to prevent complications (may not be effective in seizures).

Medico-legal aspects

- BZDs are commonly used for suicidal poisoning. Usually, diazepam is safer in overdose or intentional attempts to suicide, but the newer agents, such as temazepam, flurazepam, zopiclone and triazolam have relatively low toxic doses and fatal levels, and are more often found as the cause of death in suicides.
- Flunitrazepam is frequently used as '*date rape*' drug.
- It may be mixed with food or drinks to facilitate robbery during travel.

Signs and Symptoms of Chronic Poisoning

- **CNS:** Headache, anxiety, insomnia, muscle spasms, tremors, rarely convulsions and psychiatric disturbances.
- **GIT:** Anorexia and vomiting.
- **RS:** Respiratory depression is rare.

High dose, long-term therapy may produce withdrawal symptoms when stopped suddenly.

The *withdrawal syndrome with BZDs* include fits and psychosis. In addition, anxiety symptoms, such as sweating, insomnia, headache, tremors, nausea and disordered perception, such as feelings of unreality, abnormal bodily sensations and hypersensitivity to stimuli may be seen.

> **FM 9.1, 10.1**
>
> Describe general principles and basic methodologies in treatment of poisoning with regard to acetylsalicylic acids (salicylates).

ACETYLSALICYLIC ACID (ASPIRIN)

Introduction: Salicylate can be found in hundreds of over-the-counter medications. It is popular as an antipyretic and analgesic. Toddlers are most vulnerable to acute salicylate poisoning.

Physical properties: It is a white, odorless, crystalline powder, having a slight acid taste.

Action

Initially, there is direct stimulation of respiratory center leading to hyperventilation and respiratory alkalosis. Later on, due to inhibition of Krebs cycle, uncoupling of oxidative phosphorylation, gluconeogenesis, increase lipid metabolism and inhibition of amino acid metabolism, patient develops metabolic acidosis. It is also neurotoxic.

Absorption and excretion

- It is rapidly absorbed from the stomach and to a slightly lesser extent from the small intestine.
- Metabolism occurs chiefly in the liver. Excretion is mainly through urine.

Signs and Symptoms

System	Signs and symptoms
GIT	Burning pain in the throat and abdomen, nausea, vomiting, thirst, hematemesis and melena
CNS	Ataxia, vertigo, tinnitus, slurred speech, delirium, hallucination, headache, confusion, convulsion, stupor, coma—known as **salicylate jag** secondary to hyperthermia and altered glucose metabolism
CVS	Tachycardia
Hepatic	Reye's syndrome
RS	Initially, tachypnea and hyperpnea, followed by Kussmaul's breathing secondary to metabolic acidosis, pulmonary edema
Electrolyte	Dehydration, hypokalemia, hypo-/hypernatremia, hypo-/hyperglycemia
Hematologic	Hemorrhagic tendency
MS	Rhabdomyolysis, tetany
Others	Hyperpyrexia, dilated pupils, diaphoresis rapid and irregular pulse

Fatal Dose

Blood level >100 mg/dL is fatal.
Sodium salicylate and aspirin: 15–20 g (200 mg/kg body wt.).

Fatal period: Few hours.

Mnemonic for aspirin toxicity: ASPIRIN: **A:** Altered mental status (coma); **S: S**weating; **P: P**ulmonary edema; **I: I**ncreased vital signs (hypertension, tachycardia, tachypnea), **R: R**inging in ears; **I: I**rritable; **N: N**ausea and vomiting.

NOTA BENE

Reye's syndrome may develop in children <15 years on intake of aspirin. The main features are acute onset of hepatic failure and encephalopathy with residual neurological manifestations.

Investigations

- **Bedside diagnosis:** Presence of salicylic acid in the urine can be detected by *ferric chloride test* which involves combining 1 mL of patient's urine to few drops of ferric chloride solution. If salicylate is present, solution will turn to brown-purple color.
- **Blood salicylate level:** Best indicator of the severity of intoxication. It should be done 6 h after ingestion and then repeated every 4–6 hourly for serial estimation and response to therapy.

Differential Diagnosis

- Diabetic ketoacidosis
- Methanol toxicity
- Ethylene glycol toxicity
- Lactic acidosis
- Renal failure

Treatment

i. Decontamination

- Gastric lavage is done. At the end of the lavage, activated charcoal should be left in the stomach which will bind the unabsorbed salicylate.
- Elimination can be enhanced by whole bowel irrigation with polyethylene glycol.

ii. Fluid and Electrolyte Management

- Correction of dehydration is done by crystalloids to replace the fluid loss.
- *Alkalization of urine (enhances renal salicylate excretion)* and treatment of acidosis: Add 100 mEq (2 ampoules) of sodium bicarbonate to 1 liter of 5% dextrose in 0.2% saline and infuse this solution IV at a rate of about 150–200 mL/h. Add 20–30 mEq of potassium chloride to each liter of IV fluid.
- Hypocalcemic tetany is treated with 10% calcium gluconate.
- Seizures are controlled with diazepam or phenobarbitone.
- Vitamin K should be injected, if PT is prolonged.
- If patient develops respiratory failure, positive pressure ventilation should be started.

iii. Hemodialysis

Hemodialysis is preferred over hemoperfusion and peritoneal dialysis as it helps in removal of salicylate, and maintenance of fluid and electrolyte balance.

Postmortem Findings

External: Pupils are dilated. Skin rashes may be present.

Internal

i. **Stomach:** Gastric mucosa is congested and petechial hemorrhages are seen in the mucous and serous membranes.
ii. **Lungs:** Subpleural petechial hemorrhages, congested, edematous and collapsed.
iii. All organs are congested.
iv. If the patient survives for few days, the myocardium, liver and kidneys are usually soft, dirty in appearance and greasy to touch. Hepatitis may be present. Petechial hemorrhages are seen in various organs.

Medico-legal Aspects

Aspirin is the most common salicylate in regular use, so both accidental and suicidal ingestion is common.

Describe general principles and basic methodologies in treatment of poisoning with regard to anti-Infectives (common antibiotics—an overview).

◼ ANTIBIOTICS

Introduction: Antibiotics are among the most frequently used pharmaceuticals in both the inpatient and outpatient setting. While diarrhea is a commonly associated adverse effect of many antibiotics, toxic effects on the CNS are also quite common.

CNS symptoms range from ototoxicity, neuropathy and neuromuscular blockade to confusion, non-specific encephalopathy, seizures and non-convulsive status epilepticus (NCSE), coma.

It may be difficult to make a proper diagnosis of antibiotic toxicity since the overall clinical picture, such as changes in mental status may be considered as part of the infectious process for which the antibiotic treatment was started.

Treatment

i. Discontinuation of the offending antibiotic and replacing with a non-neurotoxic agent.
ii. In cases of seizures or NCSE, anticonvulsants can be given.
iii. Hemodialysis or hemofiltration is useful.

Describe general principles and basic methodologies in treatment of poisoning with regard to muscle relaxants and anesthetics.

◼ MUSCLE RELAXANTS

Introduction: Muscle relaxants reduce skeletal muscle tension without abolishing voluntary motor control. Most compounds in this group act as simple sedative-hypnotic agents that provide skeletal muscle relaxation indirectly.

Uses: Adjuvant in general anesthesia, intubation and endoscopies, acute muscle spasm, anxiety and tension, manage spasticity and malignant hyperthermia.

Classification: Most of their effects occur at various levels of the CNS, but some also act directly within the muscle.
a. Peripherally acting, e.g., succinylcholine
b. Centrally acting skeletal muscle relaxants, e.g., baclofen, diazepam
c. Direct acting skeletal muscle relaxants, e.g., dantrolene

Signs and Symptoms

Onset of symptoms is seen within 0.5–1.5 h of ingestion.

System	Signs and symptoms
CNS	Lethargy, agitation, slurred speech, ataxia, hyporeflexia, hypotonia, hypothermia, convulsion, coma
CVS	Hypotension, bradycardia or tachycardia, respiratory depression

Toxic dose: Ingestion of more than 3–5 times the therapeutic dose may cause stupor or coma.

Treatment

There is no antidote for muscle relaxant overdose; aggressive supportive care and intensive monitoring are needed.
i. Gastric lavage, activated charcoal, and whole bowel irrigation.
ii. Hemodialysis.
iii. For hypotension—intravenous crystalloid boluses, bradycardia—atropine, and for psychomotor agitation or seizures—benzodiazepines are indicated.

Medico-legal Aspects

Carisoprodol and baclofen have been abused as recreational drugs.

◼ LOCAL ANESTHETICS

Introduction: Local anesthetics (LAs) are commonly used medicines in clinical settings. They are used for pain management during minor interventional treatments and for postoperative care after major surgeries. Allergic reactions are seen in few cases, especially with the use of ester structure drugs.

Signs and Symptoms

Manifestations of LAs toxicity appear 1–5 mins after the injection (range from 30 sec to 60 mins). Toxicity can be local or systemic (CVS and CNS).

System	Signs and symptoms
Local effects	Neurovascular manifestations, such as prolonged anesthesia and paresthesias
CVS	Palpitations, arrhythmias, sinus bradycardia, hypotension, collapse
CNS	Circumoral tingling, metallic taste, tinnitus, slurred speech, irritability, drowsiness, disorientation, sudden alteration in mental state, agitation or loss of consciousness, convulsions
Hematologic	Methemoglobinemia, cyanosis

Cause of death: Death may be due to cardiac arrest in cases of large overdose, especially those involving inadvertent IV injection.

Treatment

i. Airway management.
ii. Seizure is treated with benzodiazepines.
iii. Management of cardiac dysrhythmias as per standard protocol.
iv. Lipid emulsion therapy (lipid emulsion reverse the cardiac and neurologic effects of LAs toxicity).

Medico-legal Aspects

Acute toxicity may be due to inadvertent IV administration or cumulative large dose.

PROPOFOL

Introduction: Propofol is an intravenous short-acting general anesthetic (GA) widely used to induce and maintain general anesthesia and to provide procedural sedation. It is a phenol derivative.

Propofol is currently the most frequently administered GA drug that largely replaced barbiturates as an induction agent due to its favorable side effects profile.

Action

It depresses all excitable tissues and produces a reversible state of unconsciousness, with absence of pain sensation over the entire body. The liver is the major metabolic site.

Signs and Symptoms (Propofol Infusion Syndrome)

Respiratory failure, metabolic acidosis, rhabdomyolysis, cardiac bradyarrhythmias, hypotension and cardiac failure, anaphylaxis, hypertriglyceridemia, renal failure, hepatomegaly, hepatic steatosis, acute pancreatitis, and death.

There may be green discoloration of the urine due to the presence of phenolic chromophores.

Treatment

i. Administration of $NaHCO_3$.
ii. Extracorporeal membrane oxygenation (ECMO).
iii. Cardiac pacing.
iv. Hemodialysis.

Postmortem Findings

Pulmonary edema, visceral congestion, petechial hemorrhages on lungs, hemorrhagic pancreatitis and hepatic steatosis.

Medico-legal Aspects

- Cases of accidental overdose and suicide have been seen mostly among nurses and physicians.
- Homicides involving anesthetics have been reported for which blood and gastric fluid samples, injection sites should be preserved.
- Propofol is also coabused with other drugs, such as benzodiazepines, barbiturates and opioids.

> **NOTA BENE**
> The death of singer Michael Jackson from propofol in 2009, the identification of propofol as an anesthetic, and the coroner's ruling the death a homicide received extensive publicity.

FM 10.1
Describe general principles and basic methodologies in treatment of poisoning with regard to insulin.

INSULIN

Introduction: Insulin is a potent hypoglycemic agent and if severe lowering of the blood sugar persists for many hours, then brain damage and death will occur. In massive doses, especially intravenously, death can take place within few hours.

Signs and Symptoms

- *Sympathomimetic effect:* Nausea, vomiting, sweating, hyperventilation, tachycardia, labile BP.
- *Neuroglycopenic effects:* Abnormal behavior, altered level of consciousness, generalized tonic clonic seizure, lethargy, coma, cerebral edema, hypertonia, hyperreflexia, extensor plantar response.
The most significant complication is hypoglycemic encephalopathy. Alcohol co-administration leads to a poorer prognosis.

Diagnosis

- Blood samples are preserved (to distinguish between human, bovine and porcine insulin and detect adjuvants, such as zinc which assists in tracing the origin of the extrinsic insulin).
- Samples should be taken soon after death and the plasma immediately separated from the cells, and kept deep-frozen until analysis.
- Postmortem blood glucose levels are generally unhelpful in confirming hypoglycemia, but vitreous humor is more useful.
- Measurements of the C-peptide and insulin levels could be useful to differentiate between exogenous

and endogenous insulin, particularly in unconscious hypoglycemic patients.
- **Radioimmunoassay (RIA)** is used for measurement of insulin in the body. The method most used is *chemiluminescent immunoassay* and the measurement of blood insulin is possible even when embalming fluid had contaminated the blood.

False negative analysis may be due to:
- Prolonged interval between injection and death (if the person was comatose for many days).
- Postmortem glucose measurements since postmortem glycolysis may falsely elevate blood glucose levels.

Treatment

i. Management of hypoglycemia is with dextrose (0.5–1 g/kg bolus in unconscious patients followed by various concentrations of intravenous dextrose). Intramuscular glucagon administration is another option.
ii. Ryle's tube feeding with a mixed meal should be initiated.
iii. Intravenous lorazepam for seizures and treatment of electrolytes imbalance.

Postmortem Findings

If death from insulin is suspected (which looks like a natural death with no obvious anatomic cause of death found at autopsy), either from suicide/parasuicide (usually amongst nurses and doctors who have access to large doses), homicide or rarely from accidental overdose (usually in hospital), then a search of the body must be made for recent needle marks and the surrounding skin, subcutaneous tissue and underlying muscle excised and sent unfixed for assay (occult injection sites can be a mucosal surface or scrotum in male).

Medico-legal Aspects

- Insulin, unless suspected, is an effective homicide method.
- Oral hypoglycemic agents, such as sulfonylureas and biguanides, may be taken as an overdose, either suicidal or accidentally.

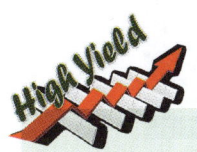

- Paracetamol (PCM) inhibits prostaglandin synthesis.
- PCM produces liver damage through toxic metabolite *N-acetyl-p-benzoquinone imine* (NAPQI).
- PCM causes renal tubular necrosis.
- Primary organ affected by PCM poisoning is liver.
- *Rumack-Matthew nomogram* can help in planning treatment of PCM poisoning.
- **Fatal dose of PCM:** 10–15 g (20–30 tablets).
- **Antidote for PCM poisoning:** N-acetyl cysteine (NAC).
- Metabolic acidosis is seen in iron toxicity.
- Treatment for iron toxicity is chelation therapy (*deferoxamine*—antidote).
- No specific antidote for acute phenothiazine poisoning.
- **Action of benzodiazepine:** Enhance inhibitory actions of GABA in brain.
- **Classic presentation of BZD overdose:** CNS depression with normal vital signs (no irregularity in respiration or BP).
- **Fatal dose of BZD:** 100–300 mg/kg body wt.
- **Screening test for BZDs:** Bratton-Marshall test.
- **Antidote for BZD poisoning:** Flumazenil.
- **Signs and symptoms of acetylsalicylic acid (aspirin) toxicity:** Nausea, vomiting, sweating, slurred speech, hypertension, tachycardia, tachypnea, ringing in ears, irritable, pulmonary edema, coma.
- **Salicylate jag:** Restlessness and mental aberrations seen in chronic salicylism—similar to alcohol intoxication.
- Aspirin causes metabolic acidosis.
- **Fatal dose:** Sodium salicylate and aspirin: 15–20 g (200 mg/kg).
- *Reye's syndrome* may develop in children <15 years on intake of aspirin. Features are acute onset of hepatic failure and encephalopathy.
- **Screening test for aspirin:** Ferric chloride test.
- **Treatment of aspirin poisoning:** Alkalization of urine and treatment of acidosis with $NaHCO_3$.

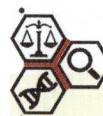

Interesting case

Benzodiazepine Poisoning (Case of a German Nurse, 2020)

On three occasions—twice in September 2017 and once in March 2019—a 54-year-old German nurse put out drugged homemade cookies and coffee in a kitchenette of the hospital for her colleagues at the Kerckhoff Clinic, Bad Nauheim **(Fig. A)**. The cookies and coffee were laced with the anti-anxiety drug oxazepam **(Fig. B)**. Several of her colleagues reported dizziness, drowsiness, confusion, slurred speech, diplopia and fainting after eating the cookies.

Police began to focus on the nurse after analyzing the clinic's duty roster, and noticing she had been on duty when each of the incidents occurred. During a search of her residence, they found empty packages of oxazepam that came from the clinic, and traces of the substances in a blender. The woman was detained in September 2019, but she denied having poisoned her colleagues. The suspect, who asserted to have brought the blender to work to whip up smoothies, argued that any co-worker could have tampered with the appliance. But the Judge did not buy that argument, stating she could have easily created the beverages at home and brought them to work. Furthermore, none of her colleagues claimed to have ever seen her consuming her own concoctions. Prosecutors could not find what could have motivated the woman to poison her colleagues.

In May 2020, the former German nurse was convicted by a court of causing dangerous bodily harm for poisoning her colleagues. She was sentenced to 3 years in prison. As one of the victims had a life-threatening reaction to the drugs, prosecutors initially charged the woman with one case of attempted murder. The charge was dropped once the court ruled there had been no intent to kill.

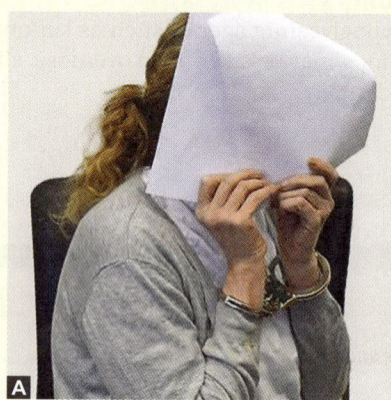
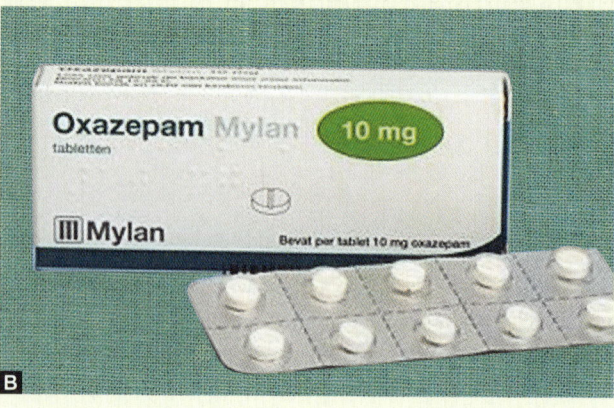

CHAPTER 59: Drug Dependence and Date Rape Drugs

LEARNING OBJECTIVES

Must know
1. Drug abuse and drug dependence
2. Drug addiction and drug habituation
3. Amphetamine and LSD intoxication
4. Hallucinogens, solvents and designer drugs
5. Withdrawal symptoms and treatment in alcohol, opioids and cocaine dependence

Desirable to know
1. Physical and psychological dependence producing substances
2. MDMA, inhalants abuse
3. Date rape drugs
4. PM findings in death due to drug abuse

Definitions

- **Drug:** Any substance, when taken into the living body, may modify one or more of its functions.
- **Hallucinogens:** Classes of drugs that involve visual, auditory, or other hallucinatory experiences and create a sensation of feeling separated from reality.
- **Designer drug:** Synthetic structural analogues/congeners of controlled substances with slightly modified chemical structures intended to mimic the pharmacological effects of known drugs of abuse so as to evade drug classification and/or detection in standard drug tests, e.g., LSD, PCP, methcathinone, GHB, MDMA etc.
- **Psychoactive drug** is one that is capable of altering the mental functioning.
- **Drug dependence** is a compulsion to take a drug to produce a desired effect or to prevent unpleasant effects when the drug is withheld, i.e., it is necessary for either physical or psychological well-being.

Drug dependence includes both 'addiction' and 'habituation' **(Diff. 59.1)**.

Nowadays, words 'addiction' and 'addict' are not used in medicine due to their derogatory implication. Instead 'abuse' or 'harmful use' or 'dependence' is used.

> **NOTA BENE**
>
> **Hard and soft drugs** are terms to distinguish between psychoactive drugs that are addictive and non-addictive.
> - *Hard drugs* lead to severe physical addiction, e.g., heroin, methamphetamine, alcohol and nicotine.
> - *Soft drugs* do not cause physical addiction but may lead to psychological dependence, e.g., cannabis, mescaline, psilocybin and LSD.
>
> The distinction between soft drugs and hard drugs is important in the drug policy of the Netherlands, where cannabis production, retailing and use come under official tolerance, subject to certain conditions.

PATTERNS OF DRUG USE DISORDERS

There are four important patterns of drug use disorders, which may overlap with each other:
i. Acute intoxication
ii. Withdrawal state

DIFFERENTIATION 59.1: Drug addiction and drug habituation

S.No.	Feature	Drug addiction	Drug habituation
1.	Compulsion	Present	Desire, but no compulsion
2.	Dependence	Psychological and physical	Psychological, but not physical
3.	Dose	Tendency to increase	No tendency to increase
4.	Withdrawal symptoms	Characteristic symptoms	None or mild
5.	Harm	Both—individual and society	Individual only

iii. Dependence syndrome
iv. Harmful use.

- **Acute intoxication** is a transient condition, resulting in disturbance of the level of consciousness, cognition, perception, behavior or other psycho-physiological functions and responses. This is usually associated with high blood levels of the psychoactive substance.

  The intensity of intoxication lessens with time, and effects gradually disappear in the absence of further use of the substance. Recovery is complete, except where tissue damage or some complication has arisen.

- **Withdrawal state** is characterized by a group of symptoms, often specific to the drug used which develop on total or partial withdrawal of a drug, usually after repeated and/or high-dose use. The duration usually is of few hours to a few days. Typically, the patient reports that withdrawal symptoms are relieved by further substance use.

- **Dependence syndrome:** Cluster of physiological, behavioral and cognitive phenomena in which the use of substances takes on a much higher priority for a given individual than other behaviors that once had greater value. It is characterized by the desire (often strong, sometimes overpowering) to take psychoactive drugs, alcohol or tobacco.

- **Harmful use:** Continued drug use despite awareness of harmful medical and/or social effect of the drug being used/or a pattern of physically hazardous use of drug (e.g., driving during intoxication). The diagnosis requires that actual damage should have been caused to the mental or physical health of the abuser. Harmful use is not diagnosed, if dependence syndrome is present.

DSM-5 Criteria for Substance Related and Addictive Disorders

The DSM-5 recognizes **substance-related disorders** resulting from the use of 10 separate classes of drugs—alcohol, caffeine, cannabis, hallucinogens (phencyclidine or similarly acting arylcyclohexylamines, and other hallucinogens, such as LSD), inhalants, opioids, sedatives, hypnotics, or anxiolytics, stimulants (including amphetamine-type substances, cocaine, and other stimulants), tobacco, and other or unknown substances.

Addictive disorders include gambling disorder and other potential behavioral addictions (internet addiction, sex addiction, exercise addiction, shopping addiction, etc.) not included due to "insufficient peer-reviewed evidence to establish the diagnostic criteria and course descriptions..."

Substance-related disorders divided into two groups:
1. **Substance-induced disorders** include conditions of intoxication or withdrawal and other induced mental disorders.
2. **Substance-use disorders** relate to pathological patterns of behaviors related to the use of a particular substance.

Criteria for Substance Use Disorders

- The essential feature is continued use despite significant substance-related problems
- Changes in brain circuits may persist, exhibited in repeated relapses and intense drug cravings
- Criteria include impaired control, social impairment, risky use, and pharmacological symptoms (withdrawal/tolerance)

a. 11 diagnostic criteria (some classes of substances have 10 criteria)
b. At least 2 or more signs and symptoms are present within a 12-month period
c. Must include a pattern of use leading to clinically significant impairment or distress

Diagnostic Criteria

1. Substance often taken in larger amounts or over a longer period of time than intended
2. A persistent desire or unsuccessful efforts to cut down or control use
3. A great deal of time spent in activities necessary to obtain the substance, use it, or recover from its effects
4. Craving, or strong desire or urge to use
5. Recurrent use resulting in failure to fulfill major role obligations at work, school or home
6. Continued use despite having persistent or recurrent social/interpersonal problems caused or exacerbated by use
7. Important social, occupational or recreational activities given up or reduced because of use
8. Recurrent use in situations which is physically hazardous
9. Use is continued despite knowledge of having a persistent or recurrent physical/psychological problem likely to have been caused or exacerbated by use
10. *Tolerance:* The need for markedly increased amounts of substance to achieve intoxication or desired effect, or a markedly diminished effect with continued use of same amount
11. *Withdrawal:* A characteristic syndrome, or use to relieve or avoid withdrawal.

PSYCHOACTIVE SUBSTANCES

The major dependence producing drugs are given in **Table 59.1**.

Alcohol

Alcohol dependence (earlier called *alcoholism*) is a psychiatric diagnosis in which an individual uses alcohol

TABLE 59.1: Dependence producing drugs

S.No.	Drug	Physical dependence	Psychological dependence	Tolerance
1.	Alcohol	Moderate	Moderate	Mild
2.	Cannabis	Little	Moderate	Mild
3.	Cocaine	Little	Moderate	None
4.	Opioids	Severe	Severe	Severe
5.	Amphetamine	Moderate	Moderate	Severe
6.	LSD	None	Mild	Mild
7.	Barbiturates	Moderate	Moderate	Severe
8.	Inhalants	Little	Moderate	Mild
9.	Nicotine	Mild	Moderate	Mild
10.	Caffeine	Mild	Moderate	Mild

despite significant areas of dysfunction, evidence of physical dependence and/or related hardship. It is more common in males and often associated with drug dependence/abuse.

Alcohol dependence has been classified into five types based on the pattern of use (not on the basis of severity):
 i. *Alpha alcoholism:* Excessive and inappropriate drinking to relieve physical and/or emotional pain with no loss of control but ability to abstain present.
 ii. *Beta alcoholism:* Excessive and inappropriate drinking with physical complications (e.g., gastritis, cirrhosis) due to cultural drinking and poor nutrition but there is no dependence.
 iii. *Gamma (malignant) alcoholism:* Physical and psychological dependence with tolerance and withdrawal symptoms with inability to control drinking.
 iv. *Delta alcoholism:* Inability to abstain, tolerance, withdrawal symptoms, amount of alcohol consumed can be controlled and social disruption is minimal.
 v. *Epsilon alcoholism:* Dipsomania and spree-drinking.

The treatment can be broadly divided into:
 i. Detoxification (detox)
 ii. Treatment of alcohol dependence.

Detoxification: Treatment of alcohol withdrawal symptoms, i.e., symptoms produced by removal of the 'toxin' alcohol. The most common withdrawal syndrome is *hangover (Refer to Chapter 47).*

Treatment of alcohol dependence: After detox is over, there are several methods for further management:
 a. Behavior therapy (aversion therapy is commonly used), psychotherapy and group therapy.
 b. *Deterrent agents* (alcohol sensitizing drugs): Disulfiram, citrated calcium carbimide, metronidazole, nitrafezole and methyltetrazolethiol can be used.
 c. *Anticraving agents:* Acamprosate, naltrexone and fluoxetine are used.

 d. *Other medications:* Benzodiazepines, antidepressants, antipsychotics, lithium, carbamazepine and even narcotics have been used.

Opioids

Addiction with opiates involves dopaminergic pathways and reward circuits that control processes, such as hunger, thirst and drug addiction.

- Most common dermatologic manifestation is the **'needle tracks'**, the hypertrophic linear scars that follow the course of large veins (concealment of intravenous marks is done by making tattoos at unusual sites).* Other manifestations include tetanus, skin infections, abscesses, hepatitis, HIV/AIDS, pneumonia, endocarditis, osteomyelitis, fat necrosis, lipodystrophy, skin atrophy and amenorrhea.
- The onset of **withdrawal symptoms** occurs within 12–24 hours (h) and symptoms subside within 7–10 days of the last dose of opioid.

Signs and symptoms: Nausea, vomiting, anorexia, sweating, diarrhea, yawning, lacrimation, rhinorrhea, tachycardia, pupillary dilatation, insomnia, muscle cramps, generalized bodyache, anxiety, piloerection (*goose skin*), and mild elevation of blood pressure, body temperature and respiratory rate. The heroin withdrawal syndrome is more severe than that of morphine.

Treatment
The treatment can be divided into:
 i. **Treatment of overdose:** Narcotic antagonists (e.g., naloxone and naltrexone) are used.
 ii. **Detoxification**
  - Methadone (25–50 mg twice daily), a substitution drug is used in the West to recover from the withdrawal symptoms.
  - Clonidine, 0.3–1.2 mg/day is used which is gradually tapered off in 10–14 days. Use of naltrexone (100 mg orally, alternate day) with clonidine is recommended.
  - *Other drugs:* Other detox agents like levo-alpha acetyl methadol (LAAM), propoxyphene, diphenoxylate, buprenorphine and lofexidine provides an alternative to methadone.
 iii. **Maintenance therapy:** Methadone is commonly used. Buprenorphine and LAAM are considered effective in long-term management. Opioid antagonist like naltrexone combined with clonidine is effective for detox and maintenance therapy.
 iv. **Other methods:** Individual psychotherapy, cognitive, family, group or motivational enhancement therapy with rehabilitation at the social and occupational levels are other methods of treatment in dependence disorder.

---

* IM or subcutaneous injection (skin popping) are associated with map shaped *'geographical ulcers'.*

> **FM 12.1**
> Describe features and management of abuse/poisoning with cannabis, and cocaine.

Cocaine

Cocaine use produces a mild physical, but a strong psychological dependence. A **triphasic withdrawal syndrome** follows an abrupt discontinuation of chronic cocaine use.

Signs and symptoms: In the early phase (*crash phase*, 9 h to 4 days), there is anorexia, depression, agitation, excessive craving, hypersomnia, fatigue and exhaustion which is followed by normal mood, anxiety and anhedonia (next 4–7 days). In third phase (*extinction phase*, after 7–10 days), there are no withdrawal symptoms, but increased vulnerability to relapse.

Treatment
a. Bromocriptine and amantadine are useful in reducing cocaine craving. Gabapentin is being used in adult addicts.
b. *Other useful drugs*—desipramine, topiramate, imipramine and trazodone (both for reducing craving and for antidepressant effect).
c. Treating underlying psychopathology—most important step. Psychosocial treatment techniques, like supportive psychotherapy and contingent behavior therapy are useful.

> **NOTA BENE**
> **Speedball** (powerballing) refers to the intravenous use of cocaine with heroin or morphine in the same syringe.

Cannabis

Cannabis produces a mild physical dependence and withdrawal syndrome. This syndrome begins within few hours of stopping cannabis use and lasts for 4–5 days. Psychological dependence ranges from mild (occasional '*trips*') to severe (compulsive use) form.

Signs and symptoms: Chronic users and abrupt cessation may experience malaise, irritability, agitation, insomnia, drug craving, depression, tremors, nausea, sweating and bodyache. Hippocampus is said to be affected which results in impairment of attention, learning, memory, retention and retrieval. Effects on the lungs are similar to nicotine.

♦ Chronic use may lead to **'amotivational' syndrome** with loss of age-appropriate behavior, like lethargy, lack of interest in day-to-day activities at home and school. Decreased sperm count and sperm motility, and morphologic abnormalities of spermatozoa following marijuana use have been reported.

Treatment: Since the withdrawal syndrome is mild, supportive and symptomatic treatment is given. Psychotherapy and family therapy are also important in dependence.

Barbiturates

Barbiturates produce marked physical and psychological dependence. Tolerance develops rapidly and is usually marked. There is also a cross-tolerance with alcohol.

Withdrawal syndrome can be very severe and usually occurs in individuals who are taking >600–800 mg/day of secobarbital equivalent for more than 1 month.

Signs and symptoms: It is characterized by marked restlessness, tremors, hypertension, seizures and in severe cases, a psychosis resembling delirium tremens. The withdrawal syndrome is at its worst in about 72 h after the last dose. Coma followed by death can occur in some cases.

Treatment: Treatment is conservative. Pentobarbital substitution can be given. Follow-up supportive treatment is important for associated depression.

> **FM 12.1**
> Describe features and management of abuse/poisoning with amphetamines.

Amphetamines

It is a CNS stimulant which can be used by snorting, smoking, ingestion and intravenously. Among common users are students and sportspersons who require to overcome the need for sleep and fatigue. Symptoms are similar to cocaine abuse.

Signs and symptoms (Acute Intoxication)
i. **CVS:** Tachycardia, hypertension, hemorrhage, cardiac failure and cardiovascular shock.
ii. **CNS:** Seizures, hyperpyrexia, tremors, ataxia, euphoria, pupillary dilatation and tetany.
iii. **Psychiatric:** Anxiety, irritability, panic, insomnia and hostility.

Acute intoxication may present as a paranoid hallucinatory syndrome which closely mimics *paranoid schizophrenia*. The distinguishing features include rapidity of onset, prominence of visual hallucinations, absence of thought disorder, appropriateness of affect, fearful emotional reaction and presence of confusion.

Chronic use leads to severe compulsive craving for the drug and a high degree of tolerance (needs 15–20 times the initial dose to obtain the same effect). Tolerance usually develops to the CNS, as well as CVS effects of amphetamines. Tactile hallucinations may occur in chronic amphetamine intoxication.

Withdrawal symptoms include depression, apathy, suicidal tendency, fatigue, hypersomnia with alternating insomnia and agitation.

Treatment: Patient should be kept in a dark room, acidification of the urine and gastric lavage is done. Acute intoxication is treated symptomatically—for hyperpyrexia (cold sponging, cooling blanket and antipyretics), hypertension (sodium nitroprusside or α-adrenergic antagonists), seizures (lorazepam or diazepam) and psychotic symptoms (haloperidol).

For withdrawal symptoms, symptomatic treatment, antidepressants and supportive psychotherapy is indicated.

> **NOTA BENE**
> - **Marquis test:** A drop or two of the reagent (mixture of formaldehyde and sulfuric acid) is placed on the sample to be tested. If amphetamines are present, the reagent turns orange-brown.
> - **Liquid gold** (slang for urine of amphetamine addicts sold on the streets): A significant proportion of ingested amphetamine is excreted unchanged in the urine, consumption of which is an economical way of amphetamine intake.
> - **Methamphetamine** (methyl homolog of amphetamine; *ice, speed, crank, glass, meth, chalk, crystal or yabba*) has developed into the stimulant of choice for adolescents as it is superior to amphetamine in CNS effects. Methamphetamine use is associated with violent criminal behavior (including sexual assault) through systemic dynamics (e.g., drug trafficking) and pharmacological effects (e.g., agitation, paranoia and psychosis). Recently, there has been a resurgence of amphetamine use with the availability of 'designer' amphetamines, like MDMA (3, 4-methylenedioxymethamphetamine street name: *ecstasy or XTC*). Combining 'ecstasy' with psilocybin mushrooms is called '**hippy flipping**'.
> - Amphetamine is one of the drugs included in the 'dope test' for athletes.

FM 12.1
Describe features and management of abuse/poisoning with following chemicals: Hallucinogens, solvent and designer drugs.

HALLUCINOGENS

Categories of Designer Drugs

1. **Synthetic cannabinoids** mimic the euphoria caused by smoking or otherwise ingesting the marijuana (cannabis) plant. They are available as:
   i. A liquid form that is typically used in e-cigarettes or other types of vaporizers.
   ii. Sprayed on dried plant material and smoked, it is called synthetic marijuana or synthetic cannabis.

> **NOTA BENE**
> - The liquid in e-cigarettes can contain multiple substances including nicotine, THC, cannabinoid oils, flavorings, and additives that are known to be carcinogenic. E-cigarette or vaping use-associated lung injury (EVALI) remains a major concern of acute lung injury. E-cigarettes work by heating a liquid, called 'vape,' that produces an aerosol, which is then inhaled into the lungs. Adolescent EVALI presents with variable symptoms which range from constitutional symptoms to GIT, respiratory, and neurologic. Dyspnea and cough are the most common respiratory complaints. In severe cases, there is acute respiratory distress syndrome leading to death.
> - In India, vaping is illegal and banned under **Prohibition of E-cigarettes Act, 2019**. Anyone involved in production, manufacturing, sale, transportation, import, export, advertisement and storage of e-cigarettes is punished with imprisonment up to a 1 year with/without fine up to ₹1 lakh (repeat offense—1–3 years with fine up to ₹5 lakh.

2. **Synthetic cathinones (stimulants):** Synthetic cathinones are a class of lab-made stimulants chemically related to substances found in the khat plant. Khat is a shrub grown in East Africa and southern Arabia that some people consume for its stimulant effects. Illicit synthetic cathinones are more commonly known as "bath salts."* Synthetic cathinones are CNS stimulants and reproduce the euphoria and hallucinations associated with cocaine, LSD and methamphetamine.
   Adverse effects include panic attacks, hallucinations, extreme agitation, paranoia, and dangerous behavior.
   Street names: Vanilla Sky, Cloud Nine, Bath salts, Ivory Wave, Mephedrone—Meph, Meow-meow, M-Cat, MMC Hammer, Bubbles, PVP—Flakka.

3. **Synthetic opioids** include morphine and the illicit drug heroin, most infamous synthetic opioids being fentanyl (most common cause of overdose deaths in the US).

> **NOTA BENE**
> **U-47700:** U-47700, nicknamed 'U4', 'pinky' or 'pink,' is a highly potent *synthetic opioid* that looks like a light pink or white powder. Often, it is either pressed into pills to look like legal pain tablets or sold in baggies. Abuse of this drug is similar to prescription and designer opioids and heroin.

Designer hallucinogens: Numerous designer hallucinogens like MDMA, Ketamine, Rohypnol, GHB etc. are available under various names. These psychoactive substances are popular due to the 'trip' one experiences within 30–45 min after taking these recreational drugs.

Lysergic Acid Diethylamide (LSD)

LSD (*acid, blotters*) is obtained from rye fungus and is rapidly absorbed from the GIT with onset of action in 30–40 minutes (min). LSD presumably produces its effects by an action on the 5-HT levels in the brain.

Although, tolerance and psychological dependence occur with LSD use, no physical dependence or withdrawal syndrome is seen. A common pattern of LSD use is *trip* (occasional use followed by a long period of abstinence).

---
* The name derives from instances in which the drugs were disguised as bath salts.

Signs and symptoms (Acute Intoxication)

a. **Somatic or physical:** Dizziness, dilated pupils, nausea, flushing, hyperthermia, paresthesia, hyperactive reflexes and tremors.
b. **Perceptual:** Altered changes in vision and hearing, like floating feeling, illusions, sensation of synesthesia, i.e., 'seeing' smells and 'hearing' colors.
c. **Psychic or changes in sensorium:** Delusional ideation, body distortion, suspiciousness to the point of toxic psychosis, depersonalization and loss of sense of time.

Treatment includes removing the patient from aggravating situation, anxiolytics and symptomatic treatment.

> **NOTA BENE**
>
> **Ehrlich's reagent test:** A rapid screening test for LSD makes use of the Ehrlich (Van Urk) reagent. When suspected sample is added to this solution, it turns bluish purple (violet) indicating positive test.

Methylenedioxymethamphetamine (MDMA)

MDMA **(ecstasy or Molly)** is similar to mescaline and also known as one of the '*club drugs*' or '*rave drug*'. It is supposed to interact with serotoninergic neurons in the CNS.

Acute symptoms include euphoria, heightened sensual awareness, and increased psychic and emotional energy. MDMA produces less amount of emotional lability, depersonalization and disturbance of thought.

Adverse effects include nausea, teeth grinding, blurred vision, anxiety, panic attacks and psychosis. MDMA has been associated with sudden death due to cardiac arrhythmia.

Treatment: No specific treatment for acute overdose, only symptomatic treatment is given.

> **NOTA BENE**
>
> **Phencyclidine (PCP)**
> PCP is a white, crystalline powder or a clear, yellowish liquid. It is used recreationally as a psychedelic and hallucinogen.
>
> **Street names:** Angel dust, super kools, dips, wack, rocket fuel, crystal, tic-tac, purple rain, zombie.
>
> **Route of administration:** Smoking, IV, snorting, ingestion and transdermal. It is well absorbed from all routes of administration.
>
> **Mechanism of action:** Dopaminergic, anticholinergic and opiate-like activities.
>
> **Signs and symptoms:** Effects are usually dose dependent, and onset is rapid when smoked or injected (1–5 min) and are delayed when snorted or ingested (30 min).
> - *Physiological*: Hypertension, tachycardia, tachypnea with shallow breathing, salivation, flushing, and diaphoresis, generalized numbness of extremities, blurred vision, grimacing facial expression, speech difficulties, ataxia, muscular in-coordination, nystagmus and anesthesia.
> - *Psychological*: Euphoria or lethargy, disorientation, invulnerability, loss of coordination, distorted sensory perceptions, impaired concentration, disordered thinking, illusions and hallucinations, agitation, combativeness, memory loss, bizarre behavior, paranoia, sedation, stupor, seizures, coma and death.
>
> **Fatal dose:** About 1 mg/kg in adults.
>
> **Diagnosis:** Blood levels peak in 1–4 h after ingestion. PCP use can be detected in urine by immunoassay up to a week.
>
> **Treatment:** Supportive treatment.
> i. GI decontamination: Activated charcoal is administered and repeated every 4 h.
> ii. Adequate hydration with NS in order to maintain urine output of 2–3 mL/kg/h.
> iii. Benzodiazepines for managing aggressive behavior and diphenhydramine for acute dystonic reactions.
> iv. Hyperthermia is treated with aggressive mechanical cooling.
> v. Acidification of urine (PCP is a weak base) to increase urinary excretion is not recommended.

Inhalants

They are commonly abused because of their easy availability, rapid action and low cost.

- The three major classes of inhalants are:
  i. *Solvents:* Paint thinners, gasoline, glues, dry-cleaning fluid and correction fluid.
  ii. *Gases:* Butane lighters, propane tanks, refrigerant gases, aerosol products—spray paints, deodorant sprays and anesthetic gases—ether, chloroform and halothane.
  iii. *Nitrites:* Cyclohexyl nitrite, amyl nitrite.

Techniques for Inhalation

- *Sniffing*: Inhaling fumes from the liquid in an open container.
- *Bagging*: Placing the chemical in a bag and then putting it over the face.
- *Huffing*: Applying the chemical to a cloth/rag and then inhaling it by covering nose and mouth with the cloth/rag.

Acute symptoms: Initially, there is mild stimulatory effect (euphoria, enhanced musical appreciation and aphrodisiac effect) which is followed by inhibition and syncope. Concentrated amount of these aerosols may cause suffocation, heart failure and death.

Adverse effects include hearing loss, peripheral neuropathies or limb spasms, CNS, liver and kidney damage, blood oxygen depletion, bone marrow damage, and Kaposi's sarcoma.

Chronic abuse cause behavioral disturbances, such as inattentiveness, lack of coordination and general disorientation.

Treatment of acute inhalant intoxication is usually supportive, like providing oxygen and phenytoin for cardiac arrhythmias, bretylium for ventricular fibrillation and checking methemoglobin or carboxyhemoglobin level.

Nicotine

Nicotine, the active ingredient in cigarettes causes intoxication, dependence, tolerance and withdrawal syndrome. Each cigarette contains 10 mg of nicotine and per cigarette delivers 1–3 mg of nicotine. Abusers tend to hide or lie about their use, and begin to develop tolerance and the pleasure associated with continued use.

Action: Nicotine affects cholinergic receptors at the nucleus accumbens. It also increases acetylcholine, serotonin and beta-endorphin release.

Smokers tend to have a significant risk of coronary artery disease, lung cancer, emphysema and laryngeal carcinoma. Smokeless tobacco can cause tooth loss, leukoplakia and oral cancer. The negative impact of passive smoking is well established.

Treatment: Nicotine replacement therapy or bupropion can be used in those who are motivated to quit. The nicotine patch method, gum and spray are the most useful form available. Medications, like clonidine and nortriptyline can be used as second line of treatment.

DATE RAPE DRUGS

- **Date rape:** Forcible sexual intercourse of a woman by a male acquaintance, during a voluntary social engagement in which the woman did not intend to submit to the sexual advances, and resisted the act by verbal refusals, denials and/or physical resistance.
- **Date rape drug (predator drug):** Any substance that is administered to lower sexual inhibition and enhances the possibility of unwanted sexual intercourse and renders the individual vulnerable to a *drug facilitated sexual assault (DFSA)* including rape.
- **Drink spiking:** The act of surreptitious administration of such drugs to drinks. Although, drink spiking is often associated with malicious acts including assault, theft and DFSA, it is also used for misguided pranks or jokes. In the UK, drink spiking with intent to commit a sexual assault or other serious criminal act is an offense that may result in imprisonment for 10 years.
- Gamma hydroxybutyrate (GHB), ketamine, and flunitrazepam (Rohypnol) are the most common date rape drugs ('club drugs'), though alcohol is the most common drug used to facilitate date rape **(Table 59.2)**. Other drugs which are also associated with date rape are marijuana, benzodiazepines, cocaine, heroin, amphetamines and choral hydrate.
- Although, these drugs differ in their effect on the body, they all act as sedatives, frequently causing unconsciousness and amnesia. The drugs often have no color, odor or taste and are easily added to flavored drinks without the victim's knowledge. Because of the effects of these drugs, victims are physically helpless, unable to refuse sex, and unable to remember what happened. Date rape drugs are particularly dangerous when mixed with alcohol and can lead to a coma or even death.
- **Chloral hydrate:** A solution of chloral hydrate and alcohol constituted the infamous '**knockout drops**' or '**Mickey Finn**' which is used in DFSA.

TABLE 59.2: Characteristics of common date rape drugs

S.No.	Feature	GHB	Flunitrazepam	Ketamine
1.	Chemical	GHB is metabolite of GABA, the inhibitory neurotransmitter	Benzodiazepine	Sympathomimetic amine similar to phencyclidine
2.	Street names	Grievous bodily harm, liquid G, liquid ecstasy, scoop	Roofies, R2, roofenol, roche, rope, forget pill	K, Ket, special K, super acid, smack K, kit-kat
3.	Properties	Powder or liquid, colorless, odorless, salty taste	Odorless and tasteless pill	Colorless and odorless liquid, or white or off-white powder
4.	Onset of action	15 min	15–20 min	20 min
5.	Duration	1.5–2 h	4–6 h	6–24 h
6.	Signs and symptoms	Initially relaxation, disinhibition, euphoria, followed by nausea, drowsiness, dizziness, amnesia, hallucinations, delirium, sedation	Lack of muscle control and motor abilities, confusion, slurring, amnesia, nausea, dizziness, sleepiness, unconsciousness	Dissociative anesthesia, confusion hallucinations, impaired motor function, nystagmus, amnesia, sedation, respiratory depression
7.	Management	Supportive, no antidote	Supportive, antidote is flumazenil	Supportive, ECG monitoring
8.	Specimens	Blood (in NaF and potassium oxalate): within 24 h of incident Urine (100 mL): within 96 h	Urine: Flunitrazepam metabolites within 12 h after ingestion	Urine: Norketamine and dehydronorketamine, using GC-MS or LC-MS analyses

This patient gave a history of heroin abuse. Identify the route of intake from the scars (arrows).

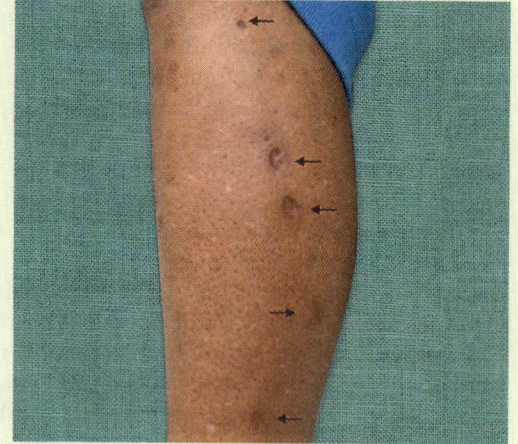

A. Mainlining B. Skin popping
C. Intramuscular D. Chasing the dragon

[*Courtesy:* Dr Sirunya Silapunt, Associate Professor of Dermatology, McGovern Medical School, Houston (Cureus 10(6): e2726)]

COMPLICATIONS OF DRUG ABUSE

The different routes of intake may produce different physical lesions.

i. **Oral:** Self-neglect, malnutrition and dental decay.
ii. **Injections:** The peripheral veins in the arms, hands, legs and sometimes, abdomen, groin or neck are damaged. Over-use of the same veins produces thrombosis and phlebitis, and pulmonary embolism. The veins become dark in color, hard and may ulcerate. When healed, there may be white or silvery linear scars in the axis of the limb.
   - Intra-arterial injection may cause vascular damage and gangrene.
   - Fragments may be injected that may lead to microemboli in the lungs and liver where they can form granulomas and even abscesses.
   - *Infection:* Cellulitis and skin abscess formation at the injection site.
   - Fat atrophy and necrosis, and chronic myositis may be seen.
   - Septicemia and subacute bacterial endocarditis may occur.
   - Shared syringes and needles can transmit hepatitis B and C, HIV, syphilis and malaria.
iii. **Inhalation:** It may precipitate asthma or bronchitis, pneumothorax and vomiting.
iv. **Other complications:** Pulmonary tuberculosis, pneumonias, accidents from traffic, falls and fires (because of impairment of alertness and behavior), theft, prostitution, personal violence and homicide.

Death from poisoning can occur from the effects of the drugs or from contaminants, such as strychnine which are used to dilute the drugs.

v. Acute and chronic liver disease.
vi. Kidney problems and amyloidosis.
vii. Psychiatric complaints.

POSTMORTEM FINDINGS

External

i. There are often signs of wasting of the body.
ii. Froth may be seen at the mouth and nose.
iii. The regional lymph nodes may be enlarged.
iv. The body may be extensively tattooed to hide scars. Linear needle track scars, often pigmented, are usually found overlying fibrosed veins of the antecubital fossae, forearms and dorsa of the hands in '*mainliners*'. Punctate areas of black discoloration (*soot tattooing*) are caused by deposition of carbonaceous materials along the track of the needle. Such tattooing is called '**turkey skin**', resembling the bird. The usual sites for subcutaneous or IM injections are upper arms and thighs.
v. Additional damage to the skin and subcutaneous tissues results from attempts by the addict to obliterate the track by overlaying it with a cigarette burn or abrading with sandpaper or using chemicals. Multiple circular sunken atrophic scars (*tissue paper scars*) suggest skin popping, followed by skin infection.
vi. Recent injection sites may show zones of inflammation surrounding or adjacent to a needle puncture site.
vii. Subcutaneous heroin users show a higher incidence of abscesses. Healing by fibrosis may produce hyperpigmented macules or retracted circumscribed scars, which resemble those from smallpox vaccinations.
viii. Chronic edema of the hands, secondary to occlusive thrombophlebitis in the forearms is seen occasionally in long-term addicts.
ix. Habitual inhalation of cocaine or heroin (snorting or sniffing) causes perforation of the nasal septum.

Internal

i. There may be phlebitis, phlebosclerosis, thrombosis, and recent and resolving perivenous hemorrhage. The vein and surrounding tissue should be preserved for chemical analysis.
ii. Typical visceral findings include *non-specific triad* of edema, bronchopneumonia and aspiration of gastric contents.
iii. Pericardial, pleural and peritoneal effusions may be found.
iv. **Stomach** may contain pills or capsules.

v. **Liver:** Most common changes from parenteral drug abuse consist of hepatic lymphadenopathy and hepatic portal triaditis. The liver may be slightly enlarged or show evidence of cirrhosis.
vi. **Spleen:** Splenomegaly and portal lymph node hyperplasia are common. The most constant finding in both spleen and portal lymph nodes is the presence of large germinal centers, but the morphological features are not specific.
vii. Hyperplastic changes in the reticuloendothelial system are common.
viii. **Lungs:** Pleura may show petechial hemorrhages, and lungs are congested and edematous.
ix. **Heart** may show valvular disease.
x. In mainliners, the crystals lodge in pulmonary capillaries and produce a foreign body granulomatous reaction. Pulmonary hypertension with right ventricular hypertrophy occurs due to extensive microcrystalline pulmonary emboli.
xi. **Brain:** It may show edema and focal areas of necrosis involving the globus pallidus and hippocampus due to hypoxia.

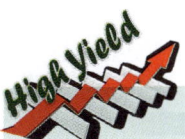

- **Drug:** Any substance, when taken into the living body, may modify one or more of its functions.
- **Psychoactive drug** is one that is capable of altering the mental functioning.
- **Drug dependence:** Compulsion to take a drug to produce a desired effect or to prevent unpleasant effects when the drug is withheld, i.e., necessary for either physical or psychological well-being.
- **Hard drugs** lead to severe physical addiction, e.g., heroin, methamphetamine, alcohol, nicotine.
- **Soft drugs** do not cause physical addiction but cause psychological dependence, e.g., cannabis, mescaline, psilocybin, LSD.
- **Speedball:** IV use of *cocaine + heroin/morphine* in same syringe.
- **Hippy flipping:** Combining 'ecstasy' + psilocybin mushrooms.
- **'Knockout drops' or 'Mickey Finn':** Solution of chloral hydrate + alcohol.

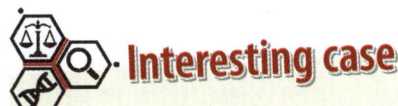

Gamma Hydroxybutyrate Toxicity

Drug facilitated sexual assaults are increasingly occurring in the past few years. Varela *et al.*, reported a case of sexual assault using gamma hydroxybutyrate (GHB) **(Fig. A)**. It was mixed in her drinks without her knowledge. Symptoms may mimic those of alcohol and not all patients are screened for GHB.

A 20-year-old woman presented herself in the emergency department suspecting that she had probably been sexually assaulted. The previous night she went to a discotheque where she had two drinks and smoked cigarettes, but denied any illegal drug use. At this point, she had a gap in her memory. Her next memory was that she woke up in bed in a strange flat with two unknown men who took her to the street, left her and disappeared.

She complained of mild proctalgia (anal pain) and vulvodynia (pain around the opening of vagina). Her medical history was irrelevant. She had been sexually active since the age of 17. Physical examination showed the presence of a red hematoma on the inside of the right thigh. The external and internal genitalia, perineum and anus were normal, and the hymen was broken and healed. Presence of spermatozoa in vaginal samples was confirmed by optic microscopy. Psychiatric evaluation uncovered no psychopathological data apart from a reactive depression. The routine screening of the urine sample for opioids, cocaine, cannabis, amphetamines, benzodiazepines and ethanol was negative. A further determination of GHB by gas chromatography-mass spectrometry came positive.

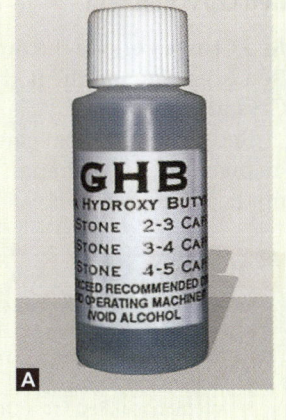

Source: Varela M, Nogué S, Orós M, et al. Gamma hydroxybutyrate use for sexual assault. Emergency Medicine Journal 2004; 21:255-256.
(*Courtesy:* Dr Maria Varela, Department of Gastroenterology, Hospital Universitario Central de Asturias, Spain)

Supplement

LEARNING OBJECTIVES

Desirable to know
1. Red cross emblem
2. Novus actus interveniens
3. The Juvenile Justice Act, 2015
4. The Sexual Harassment of Women at Workplace Act, 2013
5. The Clinical Establishments Act, 2010
6. Decompression sickness (DCS)
7. Altitude illness
8. Boric acid poisoning
9. Hydrofluoric (HF) acid poisoning
10. Methemoglobinemia inducing agents
11. Ergot poisoning
12. *Cantharides* (Spanish fly) poisoning
13. Isopropyl alcohol poisoning
14. Curare poisoning
15. *Conium maculatum* (hemlock) poisoning
16. Quinine toxicity
17. Carbon dioxide (CO_2) poisoning
18. Hydrogen sulfide (H_2S) poisoning
19. Biological weapons
20. Naphthalene poisoning
21. Kerosene oil poisoning
22. Botulism
23. *Lathyrus sativus* poisoning
24. Poisonous mushrooms
25. *Argemone mexicana* poisoning

MEDICAL JURISPRUDENCE

Red Cross Emblem

Red Cross is one of the three emblems of International Red Cross and Red Crescent Movement. The other two are the Red Crescent and the Red Crystal. The Red Crescent emblem is used in 33 Islamic countries, while Israel uses the Red Crystal emblem.

Red Cross emblem can be used only by those belonging to the Red Cross Movement and Army Medical Services involved in humanitarian work, mainly at times of armed conflicts and natural disasters, and it is not an emblem of medical professionals.

> **NOTA BENE**
> As specified by the Geneva Conventions, the emblem can be used only by:
> - Facilities for the care of injured and sick armed forces members
> - Armed forces medical personnel and equipment
> - Military chaplains
> - International Red Cross Organizations

The use of the emblem by Government medical institutions, like hospitals, clinics and blood banks, doctors, private nursing homes and also on ambulance vehicles is equivalent to abuse, and is punishable with a fine of ₹ 500 and forfeiture of the goods or vehicles on which the emblem has been used.

CHAPTER 60 : Supplement

Novus Actus Interveniens

- *Novus actus interveniens* (Latin, 'new intervening act') is an independent event which, after the accused's act has been concluded either caused or contributed to the consequence concerned.
- This new act breaks the causal chain between the accused's action and the liability that is implicated to him as a result thereof. A requirement to constitute a *novus actus* is that the secondary act was not reasonably foreseeable.
- As a *novus actus* is an 'independent' intervening act, it can be occasioned by anyone or anything other than the accused. This general category also includes the injured party himself, doctor or even an act of God.
- *Novus actus* is a defense for the accused who wish to prove that his liability is limited or non-existent and should be attributed on another party.
- This must be distinguished from *contributory negligence*. If an act or omission occurs before the incident that gives rise to the injury—contributory negligence.
- If an independent act occurs after the damage-causing incident, it is *novus actus*, e.g., when a patient is hospitalized with fracture femur due to assault, and sustains further head injury in hospital due to fall (as a result of wet floors).

> **NOTA BENE**
>
> **Volenti non fit injuria** (Latin, 'to a willing person, injury is not done') is a defense to an action in negligence. If a plaintiff (patient), with full knowledge, voluntarily consents the risk of injury, he will not recover any damages. The defendant (doctor) needs to prove not only that the plaintiff accepted the risk of injury but also accepted that if injury should happen, the plaintiff would accept the legal risk.
>
> The **eggshell skull rule (thin-skull rule)** is a legal doctrine used in both civil and criminal law that holds an individual liable for all consequences resulting from their activities leading to an injury to another person, even if the victim suffers unusual damages due to a pre-existing vulnerability or medical condition.

■ MEDICAL ACTS

The Juvenile Justice (Care and Protection of Children) Act, 2015

Introduction: This Act came into force from January 2016 and repeals the Juvenile Justice Act, 2000. The JJ Act, 2015 provides for strengthened provisions for both children in need of care, and protection, and children in conflict with law. The law intends to act as deterrent for child offenders committing heinous offenses such as rape and murder, and protect the rights of victim.

Definitions

- *Child:* A person who has not completed 18 years of age.
- *Child in conflict with law:* A child who is alleged to have committed an offense and has not completed 18 years of age on the date of commission of such offense.
- *Petty offenses:* Offenses for which the punishment is imprisonment up to 3 years under the IPC.
- *Serious offenses:* Offenses for which the punishment is imprisonment from 3 to 7 years.
- *Heinous offenses:* Offenses for which the punishment is imprisonment for 7 years or more.

Juvenile Justice Board

A Board to try child offenders should consist of a Judicial Magistrate of First Class (or Metropolitan Magistrate) with at least 3 years experience and two social workers, out of whom at least one should be a woman. They will form a Bench and have the powers of Judicial Magistrate of the First Class, and the Magistrate on the Board is designated as the Principal Magistrate.

Order that may be passed if a child is found guilty of an offense:
a. send home after advice or admonition and counseling to the parent/guardian and the juvenile.
b. participate in group counseling.
c. perform community service.
d. pay fine, either by the parent or the juvenile, if he is over 14 years of age and earns money.
e. release on probation of good conduct and placed under the care of any parent/guardian (after executing a bond, with/without surety) or any fit institution for the good behavior and wellbeing of the juvenile for any period not exceeding 3 years.
f. send to a special home (reformatory school, formerly called as Borstal) for a period of 3 years.

Several rehabilitation and social reintegration measures have been provided.
- Under the institutional care, children are provided with various services including education, health, nutrition, de-addiction, treatment of diseases, vocational training, skill development, life skill education, counseling, etc., to help them assume a constructive role in the society.
- Non-institutional options include: sponsorship and foster care including group foster care for placing children in a family environment which is other than child's biological family.

Heinous offenses committed by child above 16 years
- Children in the age group of 16–18 years may be tried as adults in cases of heinous offenses after preliminary assessment (by psychologists or psycho-social workers or other experts) with regard to his mental and physical capacity to commit such offense, ability to understand the consequences of the offense and the circumstances in which he allegedly committed the offense should be done.
- The Board can transfer such cases to a Children's Court (Court of Session).
- The provisions provide for placing children in a 'place of safety' both during and after the trial till they attain the age of 21 years after which an evaluation shall be conducted by the Children's Court. After the evaluation, the child is either released on probation, and if the child is not reformed then the child will be sent to a jail for remaining term.

Age Determination
- If it is obvious based on the appearance that the said person is a child, then the trial proceeds without waiting for further confirmation of the age.
- In case there is doubt regarding whether the person is a child or not, then age determination is done using the following evidence:
  a. Date of birth certificate from the school, or the matriculation certificate; and in its absence, birth certificate given by a corporation/municipal authority/panchayat.
  b. In the absence of any of the above, age shall be determined by an ossification test or any other latest medical age determination test.

Adoption of Orphan, Abandoned and Surrendered Children
- To streamline adoption procedures for orphan, abandoned and surrendered children, the existing Central Adoption Resource Authority (CARA) is given the status of a statutory body to enable it to perform its function more effectively.
- It provides for detailed provisions relating to adoption and punishments for not complying with the laid down procedure.
- Processes have been streamlined with timelines for both in-country and inter-country adoption including declaring a child legally free for adoption.
- As per the provisions, a single or divorced person can also adopt, but a single male cannot adopt a girl child.

Inclusion of New Offenses Committed Against Children
- Several new offenses committed against children—sale and procurement of children for any purpose including illegal adoption, corporal punishment in child care institutions, use of child by militant groups, offenses against disabled children, and kidnapping and abduction of children are included in the Act.
- Penalties for cruelty against a child, offering a narcotic substance to a child, and abduction or selling a child have been prescribed.
- The penalty for non-registration of child care institutions is imprisonment up to 1 year with/without fine of ₹ 1 lakh.
- The penalty for giving a child intoxicating liquor, narcotic or psychotropic substances is imprisonment up to 7 years with/without fine of ₹ 1 lakh.

Prohibition on Disclosure of Identity of Children
- The name, address, school, photograph or any other particular of child in conflict with law or victim or witness of a crime should not be disclosed in the newspaper, magazine or audio-visual media.
- Disclosure may be permitted, if it is in the best interest of the child.
- The police should not disclose any record of the child for the purpose of character certificate or otherwise in cases where the case has been closed or disposed of.
- Any person contravening the provisions may be punished with imprisonment for a term which may extend to 6 months with/without fine up to ₹ 2 lakh.

Delhi Anatomy Act, 1953

Introduction: This Act is meant to provide for unclaimed bodies of deceased persons to teaching medical institutions for the purpose of anatomical examination and dissection.

- **Unclaimed body:** The body of a person who dies in a hospital, prison or public place, which has not been claimed by any of his near relatives or personal friends within such time as may be prescribed.
- If the body of such person is not claimed by any of his near relatives/friends within a period of 48 h, the authorized officer shall proceed to deal with the body in the manner laid down in the Act.

Unclaimed Dead Bodies in Hospitals, Prisons and Public Places

- If a person dies in a hospital/prison and his body is not claimed by any of his near relatives or friends, the in-charge of hospital/prison should report it to the authorized officer who will hand it over to a teaching medical institution (except when cause of death is in doubt).
- If a person dies in any public place (no permanent place of residence) and the body is not claimed by any of his near relatives/friends, the authorized officer may hand it over to a teaching medical institution (except when cause of death is in doubt).
- When there is any doubt regarding the cause of death, the authorized officer should forward the unclaimed body to the Police Officer.
- Where any unclaimed body is not required by the teaching medical institution, it is disposed off as per the Act.

Duties of Hospital/Medical Institution

- When a person dies in a hospital/prison, the in-charge should immediately inform the nearest relative mentioned in the records of the patient/prisoner. If the relative/friends do not claim the body within 48 h, it is disposed off in the manner as laid down in the Act.
- In case of any dispute, the DM/Magistrate of the First Class to decide as to whether a person is or is not a near relative/friend of the deceased.
- The dead body is removed to the hospital/teaching medical institution as the case may be for preservation from decay, pending claim.
- In the Anatomy Department, the body should be washed and preserved by means of formalin or glycerin solution. Those which are not required for immediate use, should be kept in a tank containing preservation solution.
- Dead bodies not required by a teaching medical institution to be handed over to a social organization/local body concerned undertaking cremation/burial according to the rights of the community of the dead person.

Penalty: Anyone contravening the provision of the Act is punished with fine which may extend to ₹ 500.

The Factories Act, 1948

Introduction: This Act prohibits the employment of children below 14 years and 15-18 years as belonging to the adolescent group. Adolescents require fitness certificate prior to employment in a factory job.

- A child who has completed his 14th year can work in a factory as a 'child' after obtaining a certificate of fitness from certifying surgeon. A child who has completed his 15th year can work in a factory as an 'adult' after obtaining a certificate of fitness.
- The Act also prescribed a maximum 48 h/week, not exceeding 9 h/day with atleast half hour rest after 5 h continuous work. A child is not allowed to work in any factory for more than 4.5 h/day and during the night.
- A female or male adolescent who has not attained the age of 17 years and allowed to work as an adult can work only between 6 AM to 7 PM.
- This Act provides for a maximum punishment up to 2 years with/without fine up to ₹ 1 lakh.

The Sexual Harassment of Women at Workplace (Prevention, Prohibition and Redressal) Act, 2013

Introduction: This Act has been drafted to address sexual harassment at the workplace and creates a mechanism for redressal of complaints. It also provides safeguards against false or malicious charges. Under the Act, which also covers students in schools and colleges, as well as patients in hospitals, employers and local authorities will have to set up grievance committees to investigate all complaints.

Salient Features

- **Sexual harassment** includes unwelcome acts or behavior like physical contact and advances, a demand or request for sexual favors or making sexually colored remarks or showing pornography and any other unwelcome physical, verbal or non-verbal conduct of sexual nature.

- Aggrieved woman includes all women, irrespective of her age or employment status, whether in the organized or unorganized sectors, public or private and covers clients, customers and domestic workers as well.
- Workplace include organizations, department, office or branch unit in the public and private sector, organized and unorganized, hospitals, nursing homes, educational institutions, sports institutes, stadiums, sports complex and any place visited by the employee during the course of employment including transportation (*Vishaka guidelines* was confined to the traditional office set-up where there is a clear employer-employee relationship).
- Employee covers regular, temporary, ad hoc, daily wage employees and also includes volunteers.
- Employer includes the head of the government department, organization, institution, office, branch or unit, the person responsible for management, supervisions or control of the workplace, and in relation to a domestic worker, the person who benefits from that employment.
- The redressal mechanism is in the form of Internal Complaints Committee (ICC) and Local Complaints Committee (LCC). All workplaces employing ≥10 workers are mandated under the Act to constitute an ICC. The ICC will be a 4 member committee under the Chairpersonship of a senior woman employee and will include 2 members from amongst the employees preferably committed to the cause of women or has experience in social work/legal knowledge and includes a third party member (NGO, etc.) as well.
- Complaints from workplaces employing <10 workers or when the complaint is against the employer will be looked into by the LCC. A District Officer notified under the Act will constitute the LCC at the district level. LCC will also look into complaints from domestic workers.
- A complaint of sexual harassment can be filed within a time limit of 3 months. This may be extended to another 3 months if the woman can prove that grave circumstances prevented her from doing the same.
- The Complaints Committees have the powers of civil courts for gathering evidence.
- The Committee is required to provide for conciliation before initiating an inquiry, if requested by the victim.
- The Committee is required to complete the inquiry within a time period of 90 days. On completion of the inquiry, the report is sent to the employer or the District Officer, as the case may be, they are mandated to take action on the report within 60 days.
- If found guilty, then the Committee can recommend action in accordance with the provision of service rules applicable to the accused. The Committee can also recommend deduction of an appropriate amount from the salary of the accused or asked to pay the amount. In case the accused fails to pay, District Officer may be asked to recover the amount as an arrear of land revenue.
- In case the allegation is not proved, then the Committee can write to the employer/District Officer that no action needs to be taken.
- In case of malicious or false complaint, the Act provides for penalty according to the Service Rules. However, this clause has a safeguard in the form of an enquiry prior to establishing the malicious intent. Also, mere inability to prove the case will not attract penalty under this provision.
- It prohibits disclosure of the identity and addresses of the aggrieved woman, respondent and witnesses. However, information regarding the justice secured to any victim of sexual harassment under this Act wit hout disclosing the identity can be disseminated.
- Penalties have been prescribed for employers. Non-compliance with the provisions of the Act is punishable with a fine of up to ₹ 50,000. Repeated violations may lead to higher penalties and cancellation of license or registration to conduct business.

The Clinical Establishments (Registration and Regulation) Act, 2010 (CEA)

Introduction: The CEA lays down the requirement for a National and State Council for mandatory registration of clinical establishments and provides for penal consequences in case of non-registration. It is implemented in the Union Territories, and States like Arunachal Pradesh, Mizoram, Himachal Pradesh, Rajasthan, Uttarakhand, Sikkim, etc. (total of 19 States and Union Territories). Rest of the States have to adopt the CEA by passing resolutions in the Assemblies since the health is a State subject.

Salient Features

- As per Sec. 12 (2) of CEA, medical practitioners will have to provide 'facilities to stabilize the emergency medical condition of any individual who is brought to his/her clinical establishment.'
- Clinical establishment means a place established as an independent entity—a hospital, maternity or nursing home, dispensary, clinic or an institution that offers services (diagnostic or investigative) in any recognized system of medicine. It includes a clinical establishment owned or controlled by the Government, trust (public or private), corporation (including a society), local authority or a single doctor, but does not include the clinical establishments of the Armed Forces.

- Penalties
  - Any person contravening any provision of this Act, if no penalty is provided elsewhere, is fined up to ₹ 10,000 for the 1st offense, up to ₹ 50,000 for the 2nd offense and up to ₹ 5 lakh for any subsequent offense.
  - Penalty for non-registration: Fine is up to ₹ 50,000 for 1st contravention, up to ₹ 2 lakh for 2nd contravention and up to ₹ 5 lakh for any subsequent contravention.
  - Any person, who knowingly serves in a clinical establishment not registered under this Act is fined up to ₹ 25,000.

DECOMPRESSION SICKNESS (DCS)

Definitions

- **Decompression sickness (diver's or Caisson disease, 'bends')** is a disorder in which nitrogen (main inert gas) dissolved in the blood and tissues by high pressure forms bubbles as pressure decreases.
- **Dysbarism** is a term that covers all the adverse effects of pressure.
- **Barotrauma** describes the mechanical damage from gas released into the tissues.

DCS is hazardous for fliers and divers who are involved in recreational diving (e.g., scuba diving), deep-water exploration and rescue or salvage operations.

At low depths, the greatly increased pressure (e.g., at 100 feet, the pressure is four times greater than at the surface) compresses the respiratory gases into the blood and other tissues. During ascent from depths >9 meters (30 feet), gases dissolved in the blood and other tissues escape as the external pressure decreases.

Predisposing factors: Exercise, injury, right to left cardiac shunt, obesity, dehydration, alcoholic excess, hypoxia, medications (e.g., narcotics or antihistaminics) and cold.

Signs and Symptoms

The onset occurs within 30 minutes (min) to 6 hours (h).

- Symptoms are pain in the joints ('**bends**' in 60–70% cases due to gas bubble formation) with shoulder being the most common site; neurological symptoms ('**staggers**' in 10–15% cases) with headache and visual disturbances; skin manifestations (10–15% of cases) like itching, sensation of tiny insects crawling over the skin (*formication*) and pruritic rash, and pulmonary decompression sickness ('**chokes**') with pleuritic substernal pain, persistent cough and dyspnea (rare in divers).
- Other symptoms include numbness, confusion, nausea, vomiting, loss of hearing, weakness, paralysis, dizziness, vertigo, paresthesias, aphasia and coma.
- Sequelae include hemiparesis, neurologic dysfunction and bone damage.

Treatment

i. Administration of 100% oxygen.
ii. Aspirin may be given for pain, but narcotics should be used cautiously.
iii. Rapid transportation to a treatment facility for recompression, hyperbaric oxygen, hydration treatment of plasma deficits, and supportive measures is necessary.

ALTITUDE ILLNESS

Five manifestations of altitude illness are:
i. Acute mountain sickness
ii. High-altitude pulmonary edema
iii. High-altitude encephalopathy
iv. Subacute mountain sickness
v. Chronic mountain sickness (*Monge's disease*)

Lack of sufficient time for acclimatization, increased physical activity and varying degrees of health may be responsible for the acute, subacute and chronic disturbances that result from (hyperbaric) hypoxia at altitudes >2,000 meters (6,560 feet).

Acute Mountain Sickness

The severity of acute mountain sickness (AMS) correlates with altitude and rate of ascent.

- *Initial manifestations* include headache (most severe and persistent symptom), lethargy, drowsiness, dizziness, chilliness, nausea, vomiting, facial pallor, dyspnea and cyanosis.

- Later, there is facial flushing, irritability, difficulty in concentrating, vertigo, tinnitus, visual and auditory disturbances, anorexia, insomnia, dyspnea and weakness on exertion, increased headaches (due to cerebral edema), palpitations, tachycardia, Cheyne-Stokes breathing and weight loss. More severe manifestations include pulmonary edema and encephalopathy.

Voluntary periodic hyperventilation may relieve symptoms. In most individuals, symptoms clear within 24–48 h, but in some instances, if the symptoms are sufficiently persistent or severe, the patient must return to lower altitudes.

Treatment

- Definitive treatment is immediate descent, which is essential, if reduced consciousness, ataxia or pulmonary edema occurs.
- Administration of oxygen, 1–2 L/min, often relieve acute symptoms. If immediate descent is not possible, portable hyperbaric chambers can provide symptomatic relief depending on altitude and severity.
- Acetazolamide, 250 mg every 8–12 h or dexamethasone, 8 mg initially, followed by 4 mg every 6 h for as long as symptoms persist is recommended.

TOXICOLOGY

> **NOTA BENE**
>
> **Diagnostic ECG**
> - *Bradycardia and atrioventricular block*: Cholinergic agents (carbamate and OPC insecticides), cardiac glycosides and tricyclic antidepressants.
> - *Ventricular tachyarrhythmia*: Cardiac glycosides, fluorides, methylxanthines, sympathomimetics, chloral hydrate, aliphatic and halogenated hydrocarbons.
>
> **Diagnostic X-ray**
> - *Pulmonary edema (ARDS)*: CO, cyanide, opioid, paraquat, phencyclidine, sedative-hypnotic, salicylate, inhalation of irritant gases, fumes, vapors (acids and alkali, ammonia, aldehydes, chlorine, hydrogen sulfide, isocyanates, metal oxides, mercury, phosgene).
> - *Aspiration pneumonia*: Petroleum distillate ingestion.
> - *Presence of radiopaque densities on abdominal X-rays*: Calcium salts, chloral hydrate, chlorinated hydrocarbons, heavy metals, illicit drug packets, iodinated compounds, potassium salts, psychotherapeutic agents, lithium, enteric-coated tablets, or salicylates.
>
> **Response to antidotes useful for diagnostic purposes:** Resolution of altered mental status and abnormal vital signs within minutes of IV administration of dextrose, naloxone, and flumazenil is diagnostic of hypoglycemia, narcotic poisoning and benzodiazepines respectively, and of anticholinergic poisoning by physostigmine.

BORIC ACID (HYDROGEN BORATE/ORTHOBORIC ACID)

Introduction: Boric acid is a weak acid of boron which is used as an antiseptic, insecticide (especially for cockroaches), flame retardant, as a neutron absorber and as a precursor of other chemical compounds. Boric acid crystals are white, odorless, nearly tasteless and dissolves in water.

Metabolism: Boric acid is not metabolized; it is eliminated unchanged in the urine.

Signs and Symptoms

System	Signs and symptoms
GIT	Nausea, vomiting, diarrhea and occasionally crampy abdominal pain—may be confused with acute gastroenteritis. Emesis and diarrhea may be bluish-green
Dermal	Generalized erythema creating a **'boiled lobster'** appearance with massive areas of desquamation indistinguishable from toxic epidermal necrolysis or staphylococcal scaled skin syndrome in the neonate. Rash is particularly seen on the palms, soles and buttocks
CNS	Irritability, seizures, delirium and coma may occur
Renal	Oliguria, renal tubular damage and elevated serum creatinine
CVS	Tachycardia, hypotension
Other	Hepatic injury, hyperthermia

Cause of death: Death results from circulatory collapse.

Fatal dose: 15–20 g in adults; 5–6 g in children and 2–3 g for infants.

Treatment: Supportive treatment. Activated charcoal is not recommended because of its poor adsorptive capacity for boric acid. Hemodialysis and exchange transfusion may be helpful.

Medico-legal aspects: Because of the wide availability of boric acid, accidental intake by children occurs frequently. It may be taken by mistake and suicidal purposes. The abandonment of boric acid as an irritant and particularly its removal from nursery setting (for treatment of napkin dermatitis) have led to a marked decrease in the incidence of significant boric acid poisoning.

HYDROFLUORIC (HF) ACID

Introduction: Hydrofluoric acid, one of the strongest inorganic acids, is used mainly for industrial purposes (e.g., glass etching, metal cleaning, electronics manufacturing).

Action

- The two mechanisms that cause tissue damage are corrosive burn from the free hydrogen ions and chemical burn from tissue penetration of the fluoride ions.
- Systemic toxicity occurs secondary to depletion of total body stores of calcium and magnesium, resulting in enzymatic and cellular dysfunction, and ultimately cell death.

Routes of exposure: Exposures to HF occur via dermal, ocular, inhalation, oral and rectal routes.

Signs and Symptoms

System	Signs and symptoms
Skin	Pain,* blanching, white discoloration, erythema, edema, blisters, ulceration, necrosis
Ocular	Corneal erosion/opacification/scarring, decreased visual acuity, blindness
RS	Mucosal irritation/burns, laryngeal edema, airway obstruction, dyspnea, bronchospasm, chemical pneumonitis, pulmonary edema (non-cardiogenic), tracheobronchitis
GIT	Nausea, vomiting, pharyngeal erythema and edema, abdominal pain, gastritis, hematemesis, gastric necrosis and perforation, pancreatitis, colitis and perforation (rectal administration)
CVS	Ventricular dysrhythmias, cardiac arrest
Metabolic	Hypocalcemia, hypomagnesemia, hyperkalemia, metabolic acidosis
MS	Corrosion and decalcification of bone

Fatal dose: >15 mg/kg.

Treatment

The treatment of HF exposures focuses on preventing systemic absorption and correcting electrolyte abnormalities.
 i. **Decontamination**
  - *Inhalation:* Remove the patient from the exposure and administer oxygen.
  - *Skin:* The affected part is washed thoroughly with water and then massaged with calcium gluconate gel. All blisters should be removed and the underlying tissues cleaned.
  - *Eye:* Immediate copious irrigation with water or normal saline for at least 20 min is required.
  - *Ingestion:* Immediate rinsing out of the mouth with water or milk may benefit. Nasogastric aspiration, gastric lavage and whole bowel irrigation are not recommended. Activated charcoal is not indicated and emesis is contraindicated.
 ii. Calcium gluconate (10-30 mL of 10% solution diluted in 150 mL 5% dextrose administered IV over 10 min) is the antidote for hypocalcemia.
 iii. Hemodialysis is useful.
 iv. Supportive care.

Postmortem Findings

External: Greenish gray or black color chemical burns on skin, puckered skin on finger pads and toe pads.

---
* Pain is deep, burning, or throbbing, and often disproportionate to apparent skin involvement.

Internal
  i. *GIT:* Erosive cheilitis, glossitis, esophagitis and gastritis.
  ii. *RS:* Pulmonary congestion and edema.
  iii. *Liver:* Centrilobular macrovesicular steatosis.

Medico-legal aspects: Suicidal poisoning has been reported. More commonly seen as occupational exposure (hands being the commonest part injured) with some reports of unintentional poisoning. It can be used as chemical terrorism agent.

METHEMOGLOBINEMIA INDUCING AGENTS

- A large number of chemical agents are capable of oxidizing ferrous hemoglobin to its ferric state (methemoglobin), a form that cannot carry oxygen and thus inducing a functional anemia. In addition, the shape of oxygen-hemoglobin dissociation curve is altered, aggravating cellular hypoxia.
- Drugs and chemicals known to cause methemoglobinemia include benzocaine, antimalarial agents, dapsone, aniline dyes, nitrites, nitrates, nitrogen oxide gas, nitrobenzene and many others.

Signs and Symptoms

- The severity of symptoms depends on the percentage of hemoglobin oxidized to methemoglobin, severe poisoning is usually present when methemoglobin fractions are >40–50%.
- Even at low levels (15–20%), victims appear cyanotic (especially of the nails, lips and ears), because of the '**chocolate brown**' color of methemoglobin *('chocolate cyanosis')*, but they have normal PO_2 results on arterial blood gas determinations.
- It may cause dizziness, nausea, headache, dyspnea, confusion, seizures and coma.
- Severe metabolic acidosis may be present. Hemolysis may occur, especially in patients susceptible to oxidant stress (i.e., those with G-6-PD deficiency).

Diagnosis is suggested by finding of chocolate brown blood (dry a drop of blood and compare with normal blood).

Treatment
  i. Administer high-flow oxygen.
  ii. Administer activated charcoal.
  iii. Methylene blue, 1–2 mg/kg (0.1–0.2 mL/kg of 1% solution) IV enhances the conversion of methemoglobin to hemoglobin by increasing the activity of the enzyme methemoglobin reductase. Dose may be repeated once in 15–20 minutes, if necessary.

ERGOT

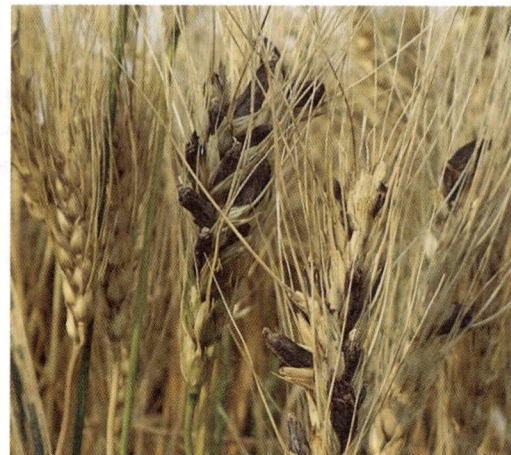

Fig. 60.1: *Claviceps purpurea* (Ergot)
(*Courtesy*: Dr Andrew Friskop, Assistant Professor and Cereal Crop Extension Plant Pathologist, North Dakota State University, US)

Introduction: Ergot is the dried sclerotinum of the fungus *Claviceps purpurea* which grows on stale grains, particularly rye, barley, maize and wheat **(Fig. 60.1)**.

Active principles: Several alkaloids are present, important ones are ergotoxin, ergotamine and ergometrine. It also contains some amount of histamine, tyramine and acetylcholine.

Action: Ergot is primarily a vasoconstricting agent. It stimulates the smooth muscles of arterioles, intestines and uterus.

Signs and Symptoms

Acute Poisoning

System	Signs and symptoms
GIT	Thirst, nausea, vomiting, diarrhea, abdominal colic
RS	Respiratory distress, feeling of tightness in the chest
MS	Tingling and numbness of hands and feet, paresthesias, cramps in muscles
Others	Dizziness, dimness of vision, feeling of coldness, hypertension, dilated pupils, bleeding from nose, unconsciousness

Fatal dose: 1–2 g.

Fatal period: Few days.

Chronic poisoning (ergotism) may either be convulsive or gangrenous in type.
- In **convulsive type**, there is twitching, tingling, numbness and pain in the muscles. There may be headache, drowsiness, giddiness, formication and convulsions.
- In **gangrenous type**, which resembles Raynaud's disease, there is a burning pain (called *St. Anthony's fire*) in the limbs with alternating heat and cold sense, numbness and tingling or anesthesia. In fingers, toes, ears, nose, hands and feet, there may be dry gangrene without swelling and ulceration.

Treatment

i. Stomach wash is done. Activated charcoal is given.
ii. Emesis (ipecac syrup) and purgation are also useful.
iii. Nitroprusside or nitroglycerin for vasospasm.
iv. Prazocin, captopril, nifedipine and cyproheptidine for limb ischemia.
v. Vitamin A is useful in convulsive variety.
vi. Phenobarbital or diazepam may be given to sedate the patient.

Postmortem Findings

Non-specific: Internal organs are congested.
- In *convulsive type*, degenerative changes may be seen in the posterior column of the spinal cord.
- In *gangrenous type*, there is degeneration of the intima of the arterioles with thrombus formation. Gangrenous change may be present in some parts of the body.

Medico-legal Aspects

- Poisoning is mostly accidental. It may occur due to consumption of bread prepared with affected rye or grain. This may cause mass poisoning in an area.
- Ergot is used as an abortifacient. Systemic poisoning may occur.
- Chronic poisoning used to occur when ergot preparation was used in the treatment of migraine or prolonged uterine hemorrhage.

CANTHARIDES (SPANISH FLY)

Introduction: The Spanish fly (*Cantharis vesicatoria*, blister beetle) is 2 × 0.6 cm in dimensions **(Fig. 60.2)**. The powder of the dried body is grayish-brown and contains shiny green particles.

Active principle: Cantharidin.

Action: It is locally irritant and nephrotoxic agent.

Absorption: Cantharidin is readily absorbed from all surfaces, including the skin.

Signs and Symptoms

Locally, on application to the skin, redness and burning pain are produced, which is followed by formation of vesicles.

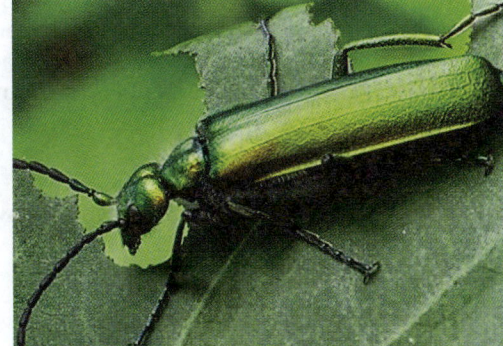

Fig. 60.2: *Cantharis vesicatoria* (Spanish fly)

On ingestion, there is burning sensation in the mouth, throat and abdomen, nausea and vomiting of blood-stained material, pain in abdomen, severe thirst, tenesmus and difficulty in swallowing and speech. Later, a dull pain is felt in the loins, desire to micturate, but urine is scanty and bloodstained. Priapism in males and abortion in pregnant females may occur. The patient becomes prostrated with convulsions, and coma preceding death.

Fatal dose: 15–30 mg of cantharidin or 1.5 g of powder.

Fatal period: 24 h.

Treatment

Gastric lavage, demulcents (but not fat) and symptomatic treatment.

Postmortem Findings

External: Inflammation and vesicles are seen in the mouth.

Internal

i. **GIT:** The mucous membrane of the esophagus and stomach is often swollen and engorged, and may show patches of ulceration and hemorrhages. Stomach may contain shiny greenish particles of the insect.
ii. **Kidneys:** Congested with hemorrhage in the pelvic calices.
iii. **Lungs:** Edematous and congested with subpleural hemorrhagic spots.

Medico-legal Aspects

- It is used as counterirritant to the skin in the blistering plaster, as aphrodisiac, and as hair oils to promote growth. So, accidental poisoning may occur.
- It is used as an abortifacient.
- Suicide/homicide is rare.

ISOPROPYL ALCOHOL

Introduction: Isopropanol is found in rubbing alcohol (70% isopropanol), antifreeze, hand sanitizers, skin lotions, mouthwashes and home cleaning products.

Physical properties: It is a colorless, volatile liquid with a faint odor of acetone, and is slightly bitter in taste.

Metabolism: It is well absorbed through the mucous membrane of the respiratory tract and GIT, and reaches a peak concentration approximately 30–120 min after ingestion. It is metabolized in the liver and converted to acetone which is excreted in the urine and breath.

Action: It is 2–3 times more potent than ethanol and more toxic than methyl alcohol. Both the CNS depressant effects and the fruity odor on the patient's breath are due to acetone.

Signs and Symptoms

i. The primary toxicity with isopropanol is CNS depression.
ii. Unlike methanol and ethylene glycol, isopropanol *does not cause* metabolic acidosis.
iii. It causes hypotension, cerebral depression and drunkenness. There is loss or sluggishness of reflexes. Pupils are constricted in coma. There are signs of renal damage.

Death from ingestion of isopropanol is uncommon.

Fatal dose: 250 mL (>100 mg/dL in blood).

Fatal period: Few hours.

Treatment: It is mainly supportive with intravenous hydration along with thiamine, folate and a multivitamin.

Postmortem Findings

- **Externally**, non-specific findings.
- **Internally**, the organs are congested. Lungs and kidneys are congested and edematous. There may be renal degeneration.

Medico-legal aspects: Poisoning is accidental, mostly by way of external medicinal use.

PERIPHERAL NERVE POISONS

Curare

Introduction: The alkaloid is a peripheral muscle relaxant and is available from the plant *Chondrodendron tomentosum* or from some species of *Strychnos* plants. It is not poisonous when swallowed.

Active principles: d-tubocurarine, dimethyl tubocurarine, syncurine and succinylcholine chloride.

Action: It blocks the postsynaptic nicotinic acetylcholine receptors in the muscles, thus causing flaccid paralysis of skeletal muscles.

Signs and Symptoms

It causes paralysis of voluntary muscles, followed by paralysis of respiratory muscles resulting in death from asphyxia. The mental faculties remain clear till the end.

Fatal dose: 30–60 mg of curarine parenterally.

Fatal period: 1–2 hour.

Treatment

i. Artificial respiration and O_2 should be given.
ii. If applied to a wound or introduced by an arrow, a ligature should be applied proximal to the site and is washed with a solution of $KMnO_4$.
iii. Atropine 0.6–1.2 mg, followed by physostigmine (1–2 mg, *physiological antidote*) or neostigmine (0.5–1 mg) subcutaneously should be given.

Postmortem findings: Those of asphyxia. Skin and tissue from the wound due to the arrow or injection should be preserved.

Medico-legal aspects: Most deaths are from its use in anesthesia. It is also used as arrow poison.

Conium maculatum (Hemlock)

Introduction: This plant is also known as *spotted hemlock,* because of the purple spots on its stem. It grows in wastelands. All parts of the plant are poisonous. The whole plant has a mousy odor which is intensified by crushing the leaves or stems.

Active principles: Coniine, methyl coniine and six other alkaloids. Coniine content is highest in the unripe fruit and seeds.

Routes of exposure: Symptoms may be caused by ingestion, injection or even inhalation of coniine (volatile alkaloid).

Action: It causes paralysis of the motor nerve terminals in the muscles, gradually spreading to the motor cells of the spinal cord and the brain.

Signs and Symptoms

- Nausea, unpleasant mousy odor in breath.
- Ingestion causes burning in the mouth and throat, gastric inflammation, vomiting, diarrhea, slow respiration and pulse, mental confusion, tremors and blindness.
- This is followed by progressive muscular paralysis due to depression of the motor nerves. The lower limbs are affected first and the paralysis ascends till the muscles of respiration are affected.
- Delirium, convulsions and coma may supervene, and the patient dies of asphyxia due to respiratory paralysis. The mind remains clear till the end.

Fatal dose: 60 mg coniine or a piece of plant about 1 cm in diameter.

Fatal period: Few hours.

Diagnosis: Coniine and other alkaloids can be measured in the urine by various methods including gas chromatography, mass spectrometry and thin layer chromatography.

Treatment

i. Gastric lavage with $KMnO_4$.
ii. Artificial respiration.
iii. Oxygen inhalation.
iv. Stimulants.
v. Symptomatic treatment.

Postmortem findings: Those of asphyxia, the remains of the roots or leaves should be looked for in the stomach contents and preserved for chemical analysis.

Medico-legal aspects: Poisoning is mostly accidental, the plant being mistaken for parsley or some harmless herb.

> **NOTA BENE**
> Hemlock was administered to Socrates, the Greek Philosopher in 399 BC as a form of execution.

CARDIAC POISONS

Cleistanthus collinus

Introduction: *Cleistanthus collinus* (common name: **oduvanthalai**) is a toxic shrub **(Fig. 60.3)**. All parts of this plant are toxic. Mechanisms of toxin-mediated injury and the pathogenesis of organ dysfunction are not clearly known.

Active principles in the leaf: Aryl-naphthalene lignan lactones Diphyllin and its glycoside derivatives cleistanthins A and B.

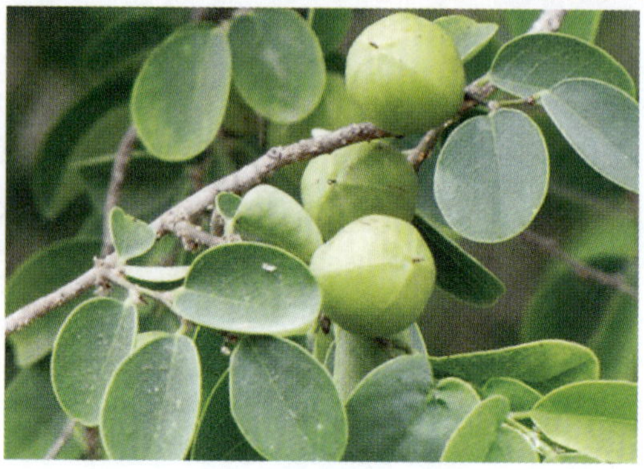

Signs and Symptoms

i. It results in renal tubular dysfunction, with resultant hypokalemia and normal anion gap metabolic acidosis. ARDS is seen in severe cases.
ii. Cardiac dysrhythmia is commonly seen.
iii. Hypokalemic metabolic acidosis and cardiotoxicity are described as the cardinal features of *oduvanthalai* poisoning.

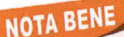

Fig. 60.3: *Cleistanthus collinus* (Oduvanthalai).

Cause of death: Mortality is due to cardiac arrhythmias, acute renal failure, shock and respiratory failure.

Detection: Enzyme-linked immunosorbent assay (ELISA) for cleistanthins A and B.

Treatment: Monitoring and correction of electrolyte imbalances and symptomatic treatment. N-acetylcysteine, L-cysteine, melatonin and thiol-containing compounds have all been suggested as possible antidotes.

Medico-legal Aspects

- The leaves are used for poisoning humans (suicide or homicide) and animals (cattle and fish) and as an abortifacient.
- The most common types of plant poisons consumed for suicidal purposes by young women in South India are *Cleistanthus collinus* and *Thevetia peruviana* (yellow oleander).

Quinine

Introduction: The bark of *Cinchona* plant contains quinine, quinidine, cinchonidine and other alkaloids. Quinine occurs as white needle-shaped, odorless, crystalline and bitter powder.

Action: It is a protoplasmic poison with anesthetic and sclerosing effect. It stimulates and then depresses the CNS. It causes circulatory failure by direct and indirect actions.

Signs and Symptoms

On ingestion, there is pain in the abdomen, vomiting, diarrhea, headache, giddiness, tinnitus, partial deafness, loss of vision, scotoma, confusion, muscular weakness, itching, tachycardia, hypotension and cyanosis.
- There may be oliguria, hemolysis, hematuria and uremia.
- Respiration is rapid and shallow, pupils are fixed and dilated, delirium and coma.

Cause of death: Death occurs from respiratory failure.

Cinchonism or quinism is caused by repeated therapeutic doses or overdose of quinine.
Symptoms are tinnitus, vertigo, deafness, diplopia, scotoma, blindness, skin rash, hypoglycemia and cardiac arrhythmias.

Fatal dose: 2–8 g.

Fatal period: About 6 h.

CHAPTER 60 : Supplement

Treatment
i. Assisted ventilation, if necessary. Continuous cardiac monitoring is needed.
ii. Gastric lavage is done and magnesium sulfate is used for purgation.
iii. Activated charcoal.
iv. For cardiac toxicity, IV bolus of sodium bicarbonate is given.
v. Ventricular tachycardia may be treated with magnesium IV or overdrive pacing.
vi. Intravenous fluids are given to promote diuresis.
vii. *Protection of vision:* Blocking of bilateral stellate ganglion is sometimes recommended.
viii. Symptomatic treatment.

Postmortem findings: Non-specific. Organs are congested, and hemolysis of red cells may be found. Renal tubules may be blocked by hemoglobin.

Medico-legal Aspects
- Accidental poisoning occurs due to medicinal overdose.
- Suicide/homicide is rare.
- It is used as an abortifacient.

CARBON DIOXIDE (CO_2)

Properties
- CO_2 is a heavy, colorless and odorless (slightly irritating) gas.
- Constituent of atmosphere air (0.4%).
- Slightly acidic in taste.

Sources
- It is formed during respiration, combustion, fermentation and putrefaction of organic matter, mine explosion, refrigerating plants and limekilns.
- Found in old wells, mine shafts and damp cellars.
- Solid form is known as *dry ice*.

Uses: CO_2 is used in the food industry in the carbonation of beverages, fire extinguishers as an 'inerting' agent and in the chemical industry.

Action: Its mode of action is as an asphyxiant (lack of O_2), although it also exerts toxic effects at cellular level. Pure CO_2 causes vagal inhibition along with glottis spasm leading to instant death.

Signs and Symptoms

Blood CO_2 (%)	Signs and symptoms
0–2	No symptoms
2–5	Increased respiration, throbbing headache
5–10	Hyperpnea, tinnitus, mental confusion, muscular tremors
10–20	Slow respiration, fall in blood pressure
20–40	Dyspnea, muscular weakness, fall in blood pressure, loss of reflexes
40–60	Dyspnea, feeling of tightness in chest, tinnitus, muscular weakness, drowsiness, unconsciousness, coma and death
60–80	Immediate unconsciousness, convulsions, death due to asphyxia (cerebral hypoxia)

Solid CO_2 may cause burns following direct contact. If it is warmed rapidly, large amounts of carbon dioxide are generated, which can be dangerous, particularly within confined areas.

Fatal concentration
- Minimum: 25–30%.
- Maximum: 60–80%.

Concentrations >10% may cause convulsions, coma and death.

Fatal period: Instant collapse and death.

Treatment

The treatment requires immediate removal from the source, administration of oxygen and appropriate supportive care including assisted ventilation.
   i. Shift to fresh atmosphere.
   ii. Maintain body warmth.
   iii. Artificial respiration with oxygen therapy.
   iv. Tham (2-amino-2 hydroxymethyl-1, 3-propanediol), an amine buffer may be given IV.
   v. Cardiac stimulants, like amphetamine sulfate can be used.
   vi. Dry ice burns are treated similarly to other cryogenic burns, requiring thawing of the tissue and suitable analgesia.

Postmortem Findings

Features of asphyxia are found.
   i. Cyanosis; pupils are dilated.
   ii. Marked capillary and venous congestion.
   iii. Petechial hemorrhages.
   iv. Froth at the nostrils and mouth.
   v. Blood is dark and fluid.
   vi. Deep congestion of the viscera.

Medico-legal Aspects

- Poisoning is mostly accidental. The gas being heavier settles at the bottom and may affect workmen associated with well sinking, well cleaning and descending in pits and ship holds.
- Blood CO_2 accumulates during postmortem. Of critical importance is analysis of air-sample collected from the scene for CO_2 content.
- Sometimes, anesthetist causes fatality by giving CO_2 in place of O_2 by mistake.

HYDROGEN SULFIDE (H_2S)

Properties
- H_2S is a colorless, transparent gas with smell of rotten eggs.
- It dissolves in water, and burns in air with a pale blue flame.
- H_2S has been referred to as the '**knock-down gas**' because inhalation of high concentrations (700–1000 ppm) can cause immediate loss of consciousness and death.
- H_2S in combination with CO_2 and methane formed in sewers is known as '*sewer gas*'. H_2S is the chief and dangerous constituent in sewer gas.

Sources
- **Natural:** Caves, volcanoes, decaying fish, sewage, manure and putrefying cadaver.
- **Industrial:** Petroleum and tanning industry, silk, rayon and paper manufacturing processes.

Action
- H_2S does not combine with hemoglobin, but does so with methemoglobin to form sulfmethemoglobin.
- It causes asphyxiation by interfering with the use of oxygen in the cytochrome oxidase system.
- Its toxicity and rapidity of action is comparable to hydrocyanic acid (HCN).

Signs and Symptoms

Significant H_2S poisoning usually occurs by inhalation. As a cellular poison, H_2S affects all organs, particularly the CNS and the respiratory system.

System	Signs and symptoms
CNS	Headache, vertigo, nystagmus, weakness, convulsions coma
RS	Rhinitis, dyspnea, cyanosis, crackles, apnea, pulmonary edema
CVS	Chest pain, bradycardia, arrhythmia, myocardial depression
Ocular	Lacrimation, photophobia, conjunctivitis ('*gas eye*')
Metabolic	Metabolic acidosis

The presence of H₂S is apparent because of the characteristic rotten egg smell. However, concentrations >150 ppm may overwhelm the olfactory nerve, so that the victim may have no warning of exposure.

Fatal dose and fatal period

H_2S concentration (ppm)	Clinical effects
>200	Anosmia, pulmonary edema
>500	Hyperpnea, apnea, rapid unconsciousness, 'knock-down' or immediate collapse
>1000	Respiratory paralysis, death

Exposure of >700–800 ppm can cause immediate cardiopulmonary arrest.

> **NOTA BENE**
> - **Detection:** H_2S, if present in significant concentration, can be tested by exposing a filter paper moistened with lead acetate. The filter paper will turn black.
> - **Spectroscopic test:** It is characterized by absorption spectrum of two bands consisting of one band in the red between C and D and a fainter band between D and E.

Differential diagnosis: Smoke inhalation, CO, cyanide and hydrocarbons.

Treatment

High-flow (100%) O_2 is the mainstay of therapy for H_2S poisoning.
 i. Remove the victim into fresh air.
 ii. Artificial respiration and 100% O_2 is given.
 iii. *Antidote:* Amyl nitrite and sodium nitrite (without thiosulfate) enhance formation of methemoglobin which in turn is spontaneously detoxified in the body.*
   - Break 0.3 mL ampoule/pearl of amyl nitrite in a gauze and hold over the patient's nose for 15–30 seconds.
   - 0.3 g of sodium nitrite in 10 mL of sterile water is given slow IV for over 2–3 min.
 iv. *Supportive measures:* Correction of electrolyte imbalance, metabolic acidosis and pulmonary edema.

Postmortem Findings

 i. Signs of asphyxia (cyanosis, frothing at the mouth and nose, and petechial hemorrhages in respiratory mucosa) are seen.
 ii. Rotten egg odor is present around the nostrils and mouth.
 iii. Greenish discoloration of viscera, gray matter of brain and bronchial secretions may be found.
 iv. Pulmonary edema and congestion of viscera are seen.
 v. **Brain:** Subcortical white matter demyelination and globus pallidus degeneration.

Medico-legal Aspects

- Poisoning is always accidental, causing number of deaths in sewer workers. The petroleum industry is responsible for most cases of H_2S toxicity in North America.
- H_2S has recently been implicated in suicides in Japan.

> **Chemical or detergent suicide:** In Japan, it is a method of committing suicide and has gained popularity in other countries from internet suicide websites. A near-instant death may occur by mixing common household chemicals—bath sulfur (5–30% calcium polysulfides) with toilet bowl cleaner (15% HCl)—to create H_2S gas in cars, closets or other enclosed spaces.

Chronic H_2S exposure causes headache, weakness, nausea, weight loss, ataxia and tremors.
- Patient can lose their ability to smell/detect the gas even though it is still present in the environment (olfactory fatigue/paralysis).
- Low-level exposure of H_2S affects the mucous membranes, and may cause conjunctivitis, pharyngitis, green-gray line on gingiva and wheezing.

---

*Based on the similarities in cyanide and H_2S toxicity, induced methemoglobinemia may be used for the treatment of H_2S toxicity. Methemoglobin acts as a scavenger, and it is more attracted to H_2S than cytochrome oxidase.

BIOLOGICAL WEAPONS

Definitions

- **Biological weapons** are microorganisms or toxins found in nature which can be used to incapacitate, kill or otherwise impede an adversary.
- **Bioterrorism** is the deliberate release of viruses, bacteria, toxins or other harmful agents causing illness or death in people, animals or plants.

Types of Biological Warfare Agents

The CDC in the US has categorized these biological warfare agents as under **(Table 60.1)**:
  i. **Category A:** These high-priority agents can be easily transmitted and disseminated, result in high mortality, have potential major public health impact, may cause public panic or require special action for public health preparedness.
  ii. **Category B:** These agents are moderately easy to disseminate and have low mortality rates.
  iii. **Category C:** These agents are emerging pathogens that might be engineered for mass dissemination because of their easy availability, ease of production and dissemination, high mortality rate or ability to cause a major health impact.

TABLE 60.1: Categories of biological warfare weapons

Category A	Category B	Category C
Anthrax	Brucellosis	Nipah virus
Botulinum toxin	Water borne threats (e.g., *Vibrio cholera*)	H1N1, a strain of influenza
Viral hemorrhagic fever	Food poisoning threats (e.g., *Salmonella, E. coli*)	SARS
Bubonic plague	Ricin and abrin	
Smallpox	Q-fever	
Tularemia	Staphylococcal enterotoxin B	
	Typhus, viral encephalitis	

Some of them are described below:

1. **Anthrax:** Anthrax is a non-contagious disease caused by the spore-forming bacterium *Bacillus anthracis*. It usually affects animals. Humans who have contact with infected animals or animal products, such as wool or hide can get the disease.
   Mode of transmission: Anthrax is propagated by terrorists in a powder form. Common method is by sending letters smeared with spores to target victims. When the letter is handled, spores enter the body by inhalation and skin contact.
   Anthrax spores are highly stable and can be dispersed by enclosing them in bombs and ammunitions. When the bombs explode, anthrax spores are liberated into the atmosphere.
   Symptoms: three types of anthrax infections depending upon the route of entry of the spores:
   a. *Cutaneous:* Symptoms are caused by skin contact with infected animal materials. Blisters and ulcers develop in the skin.
   b. *GIT:* It is caused by consumption of undercooked meat of infected animals. Symptoms are fever, nausea, hemoptysis and bloody diarrhea.
   c. *Respiratory:* It is caused by inhalation of the spores. Symptoms are fever, cough and myalgia. Later, serious respiratory symptoms may appear.
   Treatment: It can be treated with antibiotics. Anthrax vaccination is available as a prophylactic measure.
2. **Botulism** is caused by a toxin generated by bacterium *Clostridium botulinum*, and results in serious neurological symptoms. This toxin is more toxic than cyanide, and is readily available because of its widespread use in cosmetology.
   Mode of transmission: The toxin is propagated as lyophilized powder enclosed in rockets and bombs. The toxin enters the body through air, contaminated food and water.
   Symptoms: Botulism causes death by respiratory failure and paralysis.
   Treatment: Antitoxin is effective in reducing the severity of symptoms.
3. **Plague:** Plague is caused by *Yersinia pestis*, a bacterium found in rodents and their fleas. Rodents are the normal host of plague and the disease is transmitted to humans by flea bites (*bubonic plague*) and occasionally by aerosol (*pneumonic plague*).
   Mode of transmission: One of the methods is by releasing infected rat fleas in enemy country. The fleas are kept in porcelain containers attached to projectiles, like rockets and bombs before firing at targets.

Symptoms: Swollen and tender lymph nodes called *buboes*. If untreated, the bacteria spread through the bloodstream and infect lungs causing pneumonia. In *pneumonic plague*, the person has fever, weakness and rapidly developing pneumonia with dyspnea, chest pain, cough and bloodstained sputum. If untreated, death occurs due to respiratory failure and shock.

Treatment: It is treated with broad-spectrum antibiotics. There is no vaccine available to prevent plague.

4. **Smallpox:** Smallpox is caused by the virus *variola major* which is highly contagious and has a high mortality rate (20–40%). It occurs only in humans and has no external hosts or vectors.

   Mode of transmission: It is spread through aerosols and infected material. Even though smallpox has been eradicated throughout the world, virus samples are still available in laboratories of some countries (Russia and US).

   As a biological weapon, smallpox is dangerous because vaccines are no longer administered to the general population, and in the event of an outbreak most people would be unprotected.

   Symptoms: Fever, headache, fatigue, diarrhea, vomiting and a specific rash. The rash first starts as flat red spots which turn into blisters. Blisters contain a clear fluid, initially, and then pus, as the disease progresses.

   Treatment: There is no specific drug to treat smallpox.

5. **Viral hemorrhagic fever:** This includes hemorrhagic fever caused by members of the family *Filoviridae* (e.g., Ebola and Marburg virus) and by the family *Arenaviridae* (e.g., Lassa and Machupo virus). Ebola and Marburg virus have high mortality rates. It is believed that some terrorist group possesses Ebola virus culture.

   Death from Ebola virus disease is commonly due to multiple organ failure and hypovolemic shock.

   Treatment: There is no effective treatment and prophylaxis for these viral infections, although vaccines are in the process of development.

6. **Tularemia:** Tularemia or rabbit fever is caused by *Francisella tularensis* bacterium through contact with fur, inhalation or ingestion of contaminated water or by insect bites. It is a highly infectious disease and requires only a small number of organisms (10–50) to cause it.

   Mode of transmission: If it is used as a weapon, the bacteria would likely be made airborne for exposure by inhalation.

   Symptoms: On inhalation, there is severe respiratory illness, including life-threatening pneumonia, and if left untreated, systemic infection may result.

7. **Brucellosis:** Brucellosis is an infectious disease caused by *Brucella* bacteria. The bacteria affect cattle, dogs, pigs and other animals. Humans become infected by coming into contact with animals or animal products contaminated with these bacteria.

   Mode of transmission: Air, water and food articles are contaminated by terrorists. The bacteria can also enter through skin wounds. When cattle are infected, their milk contains the bacteria. Intake of unpasteurized milk can transmit the bacteria to those people who consume the milk.

   Symptoms: Fever, headache, back pain and weakness are seen. Sometimes, endocarditis and encephalitis may develop.

8. **Ricin toxin:** Ricin obtained from *Ricinus communis*, is one of the most poisonous naturally occurring substances known. Ricin is toxic by numerous exposure routes and its use by terrorists might involve poisoning of water or foodstuffs, inoculation via ricin-laced projectiles, or aerosolization of liquid ricin or distribution of powder.

9. **Nipah virus:** Nipah virus, a highly virulent zoonotic paramyxovirus, is believed to be introduced into pig farms by fruit bats through their saliva, urine and feces. It is transmitted to humans who came into close contact with infected animals.

   Mode of transmission: It is an extremely pathogenic organism with a case mortality close to 40%. It can be aerosolized with the capacity for widespread dispersal.

   Symptoms: Non-specific—severe headache, fever, vomiting, myalgia, disorientation, respiratory diseases, neurological deficits and encephalitis, and may cause coma or death.

   Treatment: Other than ribavirin, which is expensive and has undesirable side effects, there are no specific antiviral drugs and there is no vaccine.

NAPHTHALENE

Introduction: It is a solid volatile substance obtained from the middle fraction of coal-tar distillation and has chemical properties similar to benzene. It occurs as large, lustrous, white crystalline balls with a characteristic odor (*'mothballs'*) (Fig. 60.4).

Uses: Deodorant in lavatories, as a pesticide in mothballs, and in the dye industry for the manufacture of indigo and certain azo dyes.

Action: It causes hemolysis with subsequent blocking of renal tubules and hepatic necrosis. Patients with hereditary deficiency of glucose-6-phosphate dehydrogenase (G-6-PD) in the red cells are more susceptible to hemolysis.

Absorption and metabolism: Toxic effects follow from its absorption from the skin, respiratory tract and GIT. It is metabolized in the liver to α-naphthol, β-naphthol and their quinines.

Signs and Symptoms

- **On ingestion**, there is gastric irritation with nausea, vomiting, abdominal pain and fever in 1–2 days, followed by acute hemolytic crisis on 3rd to 5th day. The symptoms include pallor, mild jaundice, burning sensation in the urethra, and pain in the bladder and loins. The urine may be dark-brown or black containing albumin and hemoglobin. Severe poisoning may damage the liver and kidneys, and result in cyanosis, profuse perspiration, convulsions, coma and death.
- **On inhalation**, it causes headache, malaise, nausea, vomiting, conjunctivitis, mental confusion and visual disturbances.
- **Contact** with naphthalene dust on bedding may cause dermatitis, conjunctivitis, vomiting, headache, jaundice and hematuria.

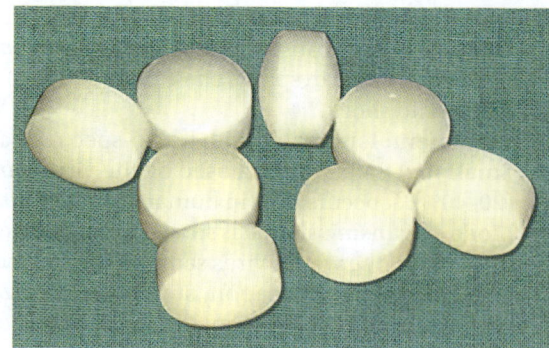

Fig. 60.4: Naphthalene balls

Complications: Acute nephritis, jaundice, hemolytic anemia and optic neuritis.

Fatal dose: Approximately 2 g.

Fatal period: Few hours to 2–3 days.

Diagnosis: Identification of 1-naphthol and 2-naphthol in urine can confirm diagnosis.

Treatment

i. The patient should be kept warm.
ii. The stomach should be washed out with warm water or saline.
iii. Ipecac syrup induced emesis is indicated, followed by activated charcoal.
iv. Milk and fatty meals should be avoided as they facilitate absorption.
v. Bowels should be cleared by magnesium sulfate or whole bowel irrigation with polyethylene glycol lavage.
vi. Sodium bicarbonate should be administered to maintain an alkaline urine so as to prevent the precipitation of acid hematin crystals and blocking of the renal tubules.
vii. If cyanosis is present, methemoglobinemia is suspected and treated with methylene blue 1–2 mg/kg IV.
viii. Blood transfusion may be necessary.
ix. Hydrocortisone is helpful in limiting naphthalene hemolysis.

Postmortem Findings

i. Skin may be yellow.
ii. The gastric mucosa may be yellow, congested or inflamed.
iii. Liver and kidneys may show severe damage.
iv. Respiratory tract may show signs of irritation.
v. Other visceral organs may be congested.

Medico-legal Aspects

- Accidental poisoning in children with poison being inhaled from clothes stored in naphthalene mothballs.
- Toxicity from ingestion of naphthalene has occurred in children mistaking mothballs for candy.
- Suicidal ingestion may also occur.

KEROSENE OIL POISONING

Introduction

- In general, among the petroleum distillates, ether, petrol, naphtha and benzine are highly poisonous when swallowed or inhaled.
- Kerosene oil is the most common amongst the hydrocarbons causing accidental poisoning in children.

Action: It causes local irritation to the mucosa of the GIT, and after absorption it has neurotoxic, nephrotoxic and respiratory depressing effects.

Signs and Symptoms

Ingestion results mainly in respiratory symptoms. Signs and symptoms usually begin within 30 minutes and may progress during the first 24–48 h and then subside in next 1–2 weeks.

System	Signs and symptoms
Local	Irritation of oral mucosa and kerosene taste
GIT	Sensation of burning in the throat, nausea, vomiting, colicky pain and diarrhea; breath, vomit and urine smells of kerosene
RS	Coughing, choking, cyanosis, bronchopneumonia, pulmonary edema, slow and shallow respiration
CNS	Giddiness, headache, lethargy/drowsiness, restlessness, weakness, muscle twitchings, seizures and coma
Others	Pyrexia, arrhythmias, hemolytic anemia, acute renal failure, hepatotoxicity and bone marrow suppression

Inhalation of fumes causes choking, cough, respiratory distress, pyrexia, headache, vertigo, nausea, vomiting and lung complications, followed by intense excitement, hallucinations and convulsions. In fatal cases, cyanosis, unconsciousness and coma precede death.

Cause of death: Death is due to respiratory failure.

Fatal dose: 10–50 mL.

Fatal period: Few hours.

Investigations

Chest radiograph shows bilateral punctuate mottled densities (fine perihilar opacities) involving multiple lobes, but particularly the lower lobes, and atelectasis.

Treatment

- In case of **cutaneous exposure**, decontamination is done by removing the clothing and thoroughly washing the skin with soap and water.
- In case of **inhalation**, the patient must be removed to the open air and artificial respiration is given.
- In case of **ingestion**, the patient needs to be observed for at least 24 h in the hospital for any signs of kerosene toxicity.
    i. *Gastric lavage and emesis are contraindicated, except*:
        - When the patient presents within 1 h of ingestion or large amount has been ingested (>1 mL/kg).
        - When the patient is in coma.
        - When kerosene is mixed with pesticides, heavy metals and other toxic substances.
        In no case, should it ever be done without intubation, as there is a risk of aspiration.
    ii. Activated charcoal is not useful as it poorly adsorbs most hydrocarbons.
    iii. Bacterial pneumonia is uncommon. Prophylactic antibiotic therapy is not recommended. Antibiotics are indicated in limited situations, like malnutrition or immunocompromised state.
    iv. Corticosteroids are not recommended, except when administered concurrently at the time of aspiration.
    v. Bronchodilators are used for chlorinated or fluorinated solvent intoxication.
    vi. Oxygen therapy is given in hypoxemia.

Complications: *Aspiration pneumonitis is the most common complication of kerosene ingestion*, followed by CNS and CVS complications.
- *Respiratory:* Aspiration and lung injury secondary to pneumonitis. Secondary effects in the lungs include pneumothorax, pyopneumothorax, pneumatocele or bronchopleural fistula.
- *CNS:* Seizures, encephalopathy and memory loss.
- *CVS:* Myocarditis and cardiomyopathy.

Postmortem Findings

i. Acute gastroenteritis and kerosene odor may be observed on opening the chest and abdominal cavity.
ii. **Stomach:** Petechial hemorrhages with congested mucosa.
iii. **Lungs:** Petechial hemorrhages, congested, edematous and bronchopneumonia.
iv. Degenerative changes in the liver and kidneys and hypoplasia of the bone marrow occur after prolonged period of inhalation.
v. Organs are congested, and other signs of asphyxia may be seen.

In case of suspected death from kerosene, the lungs, brain and other viscera should be preserved in *saturated saline* for chemical analysis.

Medico-legal Aspects

- In North India, it accounts for about 50% of infants and children brought to hospital for accidental poisoning, who have taken kerosene mistaking it for water. However, ingestion of large quantities is unusual because of its foul taste (rarely consume more than 30 mL).
- Kerosene is occasionally used for self-immolation and suicidal purpose (IV kerosene injection has also been reported).
- Homicidal attempts by pouring kerosene on clothes and igniting them are common in case of dowry deaths in India.
- Inhalation of volatile hydrocarbons is common abuse in adolescents and young adults for recreation, similar to drugs and alcohol.
- Aspiration may occur during attempt to siphon off gasoline.

FOOD POISONING

Definitions

- **Food poisoning** include all illnesses which result from ingestion of food containing bacterial or non-bacterial products including viruses, environmental toxins or toxins present within the food itself.
- **Food-borne disease outbreak** is defined by the following criteria:
  i. Similar illness, often gastrointestinal, in a minimum of two individuals
  ii. Evidence of food as the source.

Causes
  i. Poisoning due to bacteria and toxins.
  ii. *Poisons of vegetable origin (natural food poisons):* *Lathyrus sativus*, poisonous mushrooms and *Argemone mexicana*.
  iii. *Poisons of animal origin:* Poisonous fish and mussel.
  iv. *Chemical:* Intentionally or accidentally added, products of food processing and radionucleotides.

Bacterial Food Poisoning

Bacterial food poisoning results from the ingestion of contaminated food, uncooked food or imperfectly cooked food. It is divided into two groups:

  i. **Infection type** (*inflammatory diarrhea*) results from multiplication within the body of pathogenic organisms contained in the food. Organisms belong mainly to the *Salmonella* group and occasionally organisms, like *Proteus*, *E. coli*, *Bacillus cereus*, *Streptococci*, *Shigella* and paratyphoid bacilli are also involved. *Salmonella* invade and destroy the mucosa of the small intestine.
  Symptoms: Sudden onset of nausea, vomiting, abdominal pain and foul smelling watery diarrhea stained with blood and/or mucus occurs in 12 h to two days. Diarrhea in several patients after 24–48 h of eating the same meal indicates ingestion of *Salmonella*.
  ii. **Toxin type** (*non-inflammatory diarrhea*) results from ingestion of preformed toxins (*exotoxins*) from bacterial proliferation in prepared food (canned or preserved food), e.g., enterotoxin of *Staphylococci*, *Clostridium perfringens* or *Bacillus cereus*. The materials usually affected are meat, milk, fish or egg.
  Symptoms: Salivation, diarrhea, nausea, abdominal cramps and vomiting occur for a short time and the patient recovers as soon as the enterotoxins have been neutralized and metabolized, usually within 24 h of poisoning.

Acute diarrhea in food poisoning usually lasts <2 weeks. Diarrhea lasting 2–4 weeks is classified as *persistent*. Chronic diarrhea is defined by duration of >4 weeks.

> **NOTA BENE**
>
> **Organisms suspected based on presentation**
> - Upper GI symptoms (nausea and vomiting predominate) occurring in 1–6 h (*Staphylococcus aureus*), 8–16 h (*Bacillus cereus*), 6–24 h (Mycotoxins), 12–48 h (Norovirus).
> - Lower GI symptoms (abdominal cramps, diarrhea predominate) occurring in 2–36 h (*Clostridium perfringens and Bacillus cereus*), 6–96 h (*Salmonella* spp., *Shigella, E. coli*), 6 h to 5 days (*Vibrio cholerae*), 1–10 days with bloody diarrhea (*E. coli*), 3–5 days (Rotavirus), 3–7 days (*Yersinia enterocolitica*).

CHAPTER 60 : Supplement

Postmortem Findings
i. The mucosa of the GIT is swollen and often intensely congested, and there may be minute ulcers.
ii. Fatty degeneration of the liver.
iii. The causative organism can be isolated from the blood and viscera.

> **NOTA BENE**
> - **Exotoxins:** Toxin protein released from gram-positive and gram-negative bacteria. Exotoxins are antigenic, inactivated by heat, and are secreted, or similar to endotoxins, may be released during lysis of the cell, e.g., cholera, botulinum, pertussis and diphtheria toxins.
> - **Endotoxins** are heat stable lipopolysaccharide complex of the outer membrane of the cell wall of gram-negative bacteria, such as *E. coli, Salmonella, Shigella, Pseudomonas, Neisseria, Haemophilus influenzae, Bordetella pertussis* and *Vibrio cholerae.* Unlike exotoxin, it is not secreted in soluble form by live bacteria, but is a structural component in the bacteria which is released mainly when bacteria are lysed.
> - **Enterotoxin:** A toxin produced by bacteria that is specific for intestinal cells and causes the vomiting and diarrhea associated with food poisoning.

Botulism (Allantiasis)

The term 'botulism' is derived from '*botulismus*' meaning sausage.
- Botulism is an intoxication, not an infection. The causative organism *Clostridium botulinum* (gram-positive spore forming anaerobic bacilli) which multiplies in the food, e.g., sausages, tinned meat, fish and fruits, before it is consumed, and produces a powerful exotoxin—a neurotoxin.
- Botulinum toxin, also called '*miracle poison*', is one of the most poisonous biological substances known.
- Eight antigenically distinguishable exotoxins (A, B, C_1, C_2, D, E, F and G) have been identified. Type A is the most potent toxin, followed by types B and F toxin. *Types A, B and E are commonly associated with systemic botulism in humans.*

Action
- The toxin inhibits acetylcholine and paralyzes the nerve endings by blocking the nerve impulses at the myoneural junctions.
- Its action is selective, being confined to the cholinergic fibers of the autonomic nervous system.
- It affects the peripheral cholinergic nerve terminals including neuromuscular junctions, post-ganglionic parasympathetic nerve endings and peripheral ganglia without affecting the CNS.

Modes of entry
Following are the four modes of entry for botulinum toxin:
i. Food-borne botulism is caused by eating foods that contain the toxin.
ii. Wound botulism is caused by toxin produced from a wound infected with *C botulinum*.
iii. Infant botulism (intestinal botulism) is caused by consuming the spores of the botulinum bacteria (consumption of honey during the first year of life), which then grow in the intestines and release toxin.
iv. Inhalation by laboratory workers and after cosmetic use.

Signs and Symptoms
The incubation period is 12–30 h.
- **Classic triad of botulism:** Bulbar palsy and symmetric descending paralysis, lack of fever, and clear senses and mental status ('clear sensorium').
- Initial symptoms are dry/sore mouth or throat, difficulty with visual accommodation, diplopia, dysphonia, descending bilaterally symmetrical motor paralysis initiated by—abducent (VI) or oculomotor (III) nerve palsy (strabismus, blepharospasms), dysphagia, constipation, hypothermia, respiratory insufficiency and urinary retention.
- The GIT symptoms, like nausea, vomiting and abdominal pain are rare.
- The patient is conscious till death which is preceded by coma or delirium.

Fatal dose: 0.01 mg or even less.

Fatal period: 24–48 h, may extend to a week.

Differential diagnosis: Toxin type of food poisoning, poliomyelitis, myasthenia gravis, encephalitis, multiple sclerosis, Guillain-Barré syndrome, diphtheria, tetanus, and poisoning from CO, organophosphates and elapid snakebite.

Treatment
i. Maintenance of ABC.
ii. Decontamination—gastric lavage, activated charcoal, purgatives and whole bowel irrigation.

iii. Polyvalent botulinum antitoxin (types A, B and E) one vial by slow IV in normal saline and one vial IM, repeated at 2–4 h intervals IV.
iv. Botulism immune globulin (BIG), 50 mL is given IV daily, till the patient recovers.
v. Frequent dose of brandy is beneficial as alcohol precipitates toxin.

Medico-legal Aspects

- Unintentional outbreak of food-borne botulism is caused from foods that are not canned properly or improper handling during manufacture.
- Iatrogenic botulism can also occur from accidental overdose of botulinum toxin resulting in lawsuits alleging negligence (complications such as immune reaction and brain injury may occur).
- Botulinum toxin poses a major biological weapon because of its extreme potency and lethality, ease of production and transport. Dissemination of aerosols of toxin can produce mass casualties.

> **NOTA BENE**
> - **Infant botulism** is a neuroparalytic disease which affects otherwise healthy children <1 year old. Early symptoms are constipation, generalized weakness and weak cry.
> - SIDS could be attributed to *C. botulinum* intoxication.
> - *Botulinium toxin* type A (Botox) was approved by the US Food and Drug Administration (FDA) for the treatment of strabismus, blepharospasm and hemifacial spasm. It is also used for treatment of frown lines between the eyebrows (glabellar lines), spasticity and muscle pain disorders and cervical dystonia.

POISONOUS FOODS

Poisonous foods are those which contain poison derived from plants, animals and inorganic chemicals.

Lathyrus sativus ('Kesari Dhal')

Introduction: This is a variety of pulse and is the staple food for the low-income groups in some areas of Central India. Consumption of *L. sativus* seeds in quantities exceeding 30% of the total diet for more than 6 months has been known to cause paralysis. Men are more susceptible than women.
Active principle: β-N-oxalyl amino-alanine (BOAA), a neurotoxic amino acid present in the seed cotyledons.

Signs and Symptoms

The continued use of *L. sativus* produces **neurolathyrism**, which is characterized by progressive spastic paraplegia with preservation of sphincters, sensation and mental activity.
- There may be pain in the back or weakness of legs and difficulty in sitting down and getting up. The patient is unable to walk without the aid of a stick, the legs tremble and are dragged along with difficulty.
- A spastic gait develops characterized by 'walking on tiptoes' with the legs crossing scissor-wise. Later, complete paraplegia occurs.
- There is no atrophy or loss of the tone of muscles and no reaction of degeneration.
- The knee jerks are increased, ankle clonus is marked and Babinski's sign is present.

Treatment

- Rich diet with exclusion of the pulse, massage and application of electricity are useful.
- Steeping the pulse in hot water and parboiling remove 90% of toxic amino acid.

Death is very rare. At autopsy, lateral columns of the spinal cord may show sclerosis.

Mushrooms

Introduction: Some species are non-poisonous and are used as food. Common poisonous fungi are *Amanita phalloides* and *Amanita muscaria* (deadly agaric/death cap).

Active principles and action: *Amanita muscaria* contains an alkaloid muscarine which stimulates postganglionic cholinergic fibers. *Amanita phalloides* contains phalloidin, phallon, α-amanatin which are cyclopeptides and virotoxins. They are powerful inhibitors of cellular protein synthesis.

Signs and Symptoms

In some cases, irritant symptoms may be present, in others neurotic, and in some, there may be a combination of both.
- *Irritant symptoms* are delayed by 6–24 h and include constriction of the throat, burning pain in the stomach, nausea, vomiting and diarrhea, followed by cyanosis, slow pulse, labored respiration, sweating, collapse and death.
- *Neurotic symptoms* are giddiness, headache, delirium, diplopia, constriction of the pupils, cramps, twitching of the limbs, convulsions, salivation, bradycardia and coma. Icterus, hepatic and renal failure occurs in 3–6 days.

Fatal dose: 2–3 mushrooms.

Fatal period: Usually 24 h.

Diagnosis: *Meixner test* (*Wieland test*) for detection of toxins (α-amanitin) in stools and vomitus.

Treatment

i. *Supportive*: It comprises of aggressive correction of fluid and electrolyte losses, and in the advanced stages, attention to liver and renal failure.
ii. *Specific*: Decontamination is required to remove the toxin rapidly. Activated charcoal and lactulose are ideal.
iii. In *amatoxin type of poisoning*, penicillin, silybin, thioctic acid and corticosteroids have been tried for their synergistic effect in inhibiting the binding of both toxins and interrupting enterohepatic recirculation of toxins.
iv. In *muscarine poisoning*, the specific antidote is atropine sulfate, 0.01–0.02 mg/kg/dose IV repeated every 30 minutes until atropinization.
v. For convulsions, diazepam may be given.
vi. Hemodialysis may be done.
vii. Symptomatic treatment.

Postmortem Findings

- Inflammation of the mucous membrane of the GIT, and fatty degeneration of the liver, kidneys and heart may be found.
- In case of neurotic symptoms, congestion of the brain and petechial hemorrhages in serous membranes are seen.

Argemone mexicana (Prickly Poppy)

Introduction: It grows wild all over India in the cold season. All parts of the plant are poisonous. The *Argemone* or *katkar* oil causes **epidemic dropsy**. The flowers are yellow and seeds are dark-brown in color, smaller than *mustard seeds* and covered with minute, regularly arranged projections and depressions **(Fig. 60.5)**.

Active principles: The plant contains two alkaloids—berberine and protopine. The oil contains two alkaloids, sanguinarine and dihydrosanguinarine. They cause abnormal permeability of blood vessels.

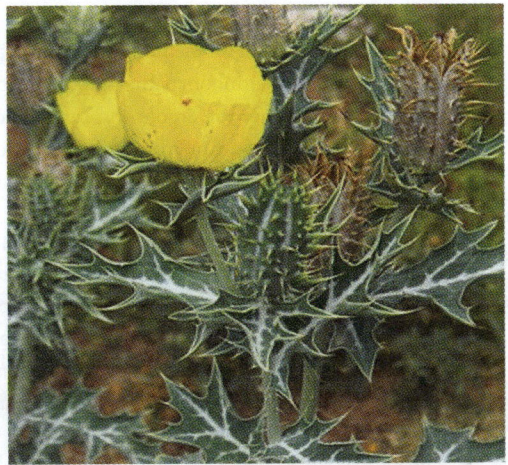

Fig. 60.5: *Argemone mexicana* (Prickly poppy).

Signs and Symptoms

Symptoms appear slowly with loss of appetite, diarrhea, marked edema of the legs, and sometimes generalized anasarca.

System	Signs and symptoms
Heart	Myocardial damage and dilatation of the heart
CVS	Hypotension, breathlessness and feeble pulse
Hepatic	Enlarged and tender liver
PNS	Tingling and hyperesthesia of skin and tenderness of the calf muscles. The jerks are feeble or absent
Ocular	Dimness of vision (in about 10% of cases) due to increased intraocular pressure
Skin	Bluish mottling of the skin due to dilation of the peripheral vessels

Cause of death: Death occurs from severe damage to the heart.

Treatment: Good diet, decontamination, withdrawal of oil, diuretics, corticosteroids and supportive treatment.

Medico-legal aspects: The oil from the seeds is sometimes used as an adulterant of mustard oil or other edible oil.

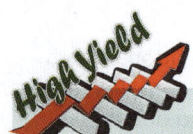

- Usage of Red Cross emblem by medical professionals is punishable offense.
- **Novus actus interveniens:** An independent event which, after the accused's act has been concluded either caused or contributed to the consequence concerned.
- Juvenile court deals with cases of children up to the age of 18 years.
- Juvenile offenders (<18 years) should not be sentenced to death or life imprisonment.
- If the dead body of an unknown person is not claimed by any of his near relatives/friends within a period of 48 h, the authorized officer shall proceed to deal with the body in the manner laid down in the Delhi Anatomy Act.
- The Factories Act, 1948 prescribes a maximum 48 h/week, not exceeding 9 h/day with at least half hour rest after 5 h continuous work. A child is not allowed to work in any factory for more than 4.5 h/day and during the night
- **Sexual harassment** includes unwelcome acts or behavior like physical contact and advances, a demand or request for sexual favors or making sexually colored remarks or showing pornography and any other unwelcome physical, verbal or non-verbal conduct of sexual nature.
- **Decompression sickness (Caisson disease):** Nitrogen dissolved in the blood and tissues by high pressure forms bubbles as pressure decreases.
- Symptoms of Caisson disease are pain in the joints ('**bends**') with shoulder being the most common site; neurological symptoms ('**staggers**') with headache and visual disturbances; skin manifestations, and pulmonary decompression sickness ('**chokes**').
- Chronic mountain sickness is known as *Monge's disease*.
- Boiled lobster appearance of skin is seen in boric acid poisoning.
- **Xenobiotics causing methemoglobinemia:** Benzocaine, antimalarial agents, dapsone, aniline dyes, nitrites, nitrates, nitrogen oxide gas, and nitrobenzene.
- Victims with methemoglobinemia have a '**chocolate brown**' *('chocolate cyanosis')*.
- Ergot is the dried sclerotinum of the fungus *Claviceps purpurea*.
- **Active principles in ergot:** Ergotoxin, ergotamine and ergometrine.
- Chronic poisoning (ergotism) may either be convulsive or gangrenous in type.
- In gangrenous type, there is a burning pain (called *St. Anthony's fire*) in the limbs with alternating heat and cold sense, numbness and tingling or anesthesia.
- Priapism occurs in males in cantharidin poisoning.
- Treatment of isopropyl alcohol poisoning is supportive.
- Hemlock was administered to Socrates as a form of execution.
- Most common plant poison used for suicidal purposes by women in South India is *Cleistanthus collinus*.
- H_2S is known as *'knock-down gas'* as it can cause immediate loss of consciousness and death.
- **Chemical or detergent suicide:** Death may occur by mixing common household chemicals—bath sulfur (5–30% calcium polysulfides) with toilet bowl cleaner (15% HCl)—to create H_2S in enclosed spaces.
- Smallpox can be a dangerous biological weapon, because vaccines are no longer administered.
- Viral hemorrhagic fever includes hemorrhagic fever caused by members of the family Filoviridae (e.g., Ebola and Marburgvirus) and by the family Arenaviridae (e.g., Lassa and Machupo virus).
- Gastric lavage and emesis are contraindicated in kerosene oil poisoning.
- Most common complication of kerosene ingestion is aspiration pneumonitis.
- Acute diarrhea in food poisoning usually lasts <2 weeks. Diarrhea lasting 2–4 weeks is classified as persistent. Chronic diarrhea is defined by duration of >4 weeks.
- **Classic triad of botulism:** Bulbar palsy and symmetric descending paralysis, lack of fever, and clear senses and mental status.
- **Active principle of Lathyrus Sativus:** b-N-oxalyl amino-alanine (BOAA), a neurotoxic amino acid.
- Use of *L. sativus* produces neurolathyrism, characterized by progressive spastic paraplegia with preservation of sphincters, sensation and mental activity.
- Argemone or katkar oil causes epidemic dropsy.
- **Active principles in Argemone mexicana:** The plant contains two alkaloids—berberine and protopine and the oil contain two alkaloids, sanguinarine and dihydrosanguinarine.

Answer Key

Chapter No.	Answers
Chapter 1	1. (a) 176 CrPC (b) 304-B IPC 2. D
Chapter 2	1. Dichotomy 2. C 3. 2nd image 4. B
Chapter 3	1. Active euthanasia
Chapter 5	1. Spreading callipers 2. Turner syndrome 3. Male skull 4. Option 1 5. (A) About 14 years (B) 20–21 years 6. (A) <21 years (B) Metopic suture, 1 year 7. Bullet scar
Chapter 6	1. (A) Arch (B) Loop (C) Whorl 2. (A) Cheiloscopy (B) Type I 3. Animal hair 4. Palatoscopy
Chapter 7	1. 1. B 2. D 3. A 4. C 2. T-shaped or 'bucket handle' incision 3. (A) Macronodular cirrhosis (B) Coronary artery atherosclerosis (blockage) (C) Polycystic kidneys (D) Stab injury of heart
Chapter 8	1. (A) Homicidal (B) Suicidal 2. Dyadic death 3. (A) Cyanosis (B) Petechial hemorrhages (C) Congestion of viscera 4. Option 2
Chapter 9	1. C 2. A 3. D; Glove and stocking PM staining 4. A 5. A 6. D
Chapter 10	1. 1. C 2. D 3. B 4. A 2. La facies sympathique; Left side 3. Hangman's fracture 4. Option 2 5. Electrical cord which is used for homicide purpose; Ligature strangulation 6. Traumatic asphyxia
Chapter 11	1. (A) Graze abrasions (B) Patterned abrasion (C) Scratch abrasion 2. D 3. C 4. 7–12 days 5. Patterned bruise, Tyre 6. Lacerated wound; Weapon with blunt round end (e.g., hammer) 7. Homicidal cut throat injury 8. Incised looking lacerated 9. Chop wound with underlying fracture of skull 10. Fabricated injury

Answer Key

Chapter No.	Answers
Chapter 12	1. Option 2 2. D 3. Wad; Smooth bored firearm (shotgun) 4. Right to left; Nearly horizontal; Tattooing can be seen 5. Contact shot; Double barrel shot gun 6. Near shot (about 2 feet) 7. Option 1 8. Shotgun; Distant shot 9. B
Chapter 13	1. (A) Depressed fracture (B) Linear fracture (C) Hinge fracture (D) Sutural fracture 2. Fracture of middle cranial fossa; Contrecoup contusion 3. (A) 4 (B) 3 (C) 2 (D) 1
Chapter 14	1. Second degree burn 2. 30% 3. Option D 4. Septicemia 5. Option A 6. Option D 7. Joule burn; Electrocution
Chapter 15	1. (A) Secondary injury (B) Primary impact injury—bumper fracture
Chapter 17	1. Grievous injury 2. A, B, C, E, F, G 3. Fat embolism
Chapter 20	1. Modified Benke's technique 2. (A) 5 months (B) Full term (C) 9 months 3. Fetus was viable 4. IUD; Spalding sign 5. Live born 6. Caput succedaneum

Chapter 23	1. 1. D 2. A 3. B 4. C
	2. (A) Probable sign—immunological test
	   (B) Presumptive—Jacquemier's or Chadwick's sign
	   (C) Positive sign—linear arrangement of vertebral column

Chapter 24	1. Smegma can be seen; Yes
Chapter 26	1. 1. D 2. A 3. B 4. C
Chapter 28	1. C 2. 1. D 2. A 3. B 4. C 3. 1. C 2. A 3. B 4. D
Chapter 29	1. 1. B Rh +ve 2. A Rh +ve 3. O Rh –ve 4. AB Rh +ve
Chapter 32	1. 1. Parrot's perch 2. Falanga 3. Water boarding 4. Dry submarine
Chapter 35	1. (A) Infant feeding tube (B) Ryle's tube (C) Intravenous set (D) Stomach wash tube
Chapter 36	1. B 2. Carbolic acid poisoning
Chapter 45	1. 1. Viper 2. Banded krait 3. Common cobra 4. Common krait
Chapter 59	1. B

Index

Page numbers followed by *b* refer to box, *f* refer to figure, *fc* refer to flowchart, and *t* refer to table.

A

ABAcard test 489*f*
   strips 500, 502
Abdomen 124, 126, 287, 350, 411, 516
   distended 172*f*
   enlargement of 405
Abdominal cavities 125*f*, 134, 386
Abdominal cramps 732
Abdominal injuries 287, 288, 329
Abdominal pain 434, 604
Abdominal viscera, vaginal herniation of 433
Abdominal wall 412
Abdominal X-rays 718
ABO blood
   group antigens 502
   types 500*t*
ABO system 490, 490*t*
Abortion 71, 380, 380*f*, 382*f*, 387
   artificial 381
   blood 493
   causes of 381
   classification of 380, 381*fc*
   complications of 387
   illegal 30
   natural 380, 385
   pills 382
   stick 382, 383, 383*f*, 386*f*, 387
   unsafe 380
Abortus 380, 387
Abralin 594
Abrasion 213, 214, 215*f*, 216, 216*f*, 221, 222, 263, 426
   age of 215, 216*t*
   collar 243, 244*f*, 261
   types of 214*f*
Abruptio placenta 359
Abrus 598
   precatorius 382, 594, 594*f*, 595
Abscess 103
Absorption 558, 564, 569, 575, 579, 582, 621, 632, 637, 642, 644, 650, 667, 684, 688, 695, 698, 730
Abuse
   perianal signs of 442*t*
   simulation of 455*f*
   types of 375
Acarophobia 475
Acceleration injury 262, 284*f*
Accident 224, 230, 402, 536
Accidental cases 674
Accidental choking 198
Accidental drowning 209
Accidental ingestions, management of 540
Accidental laceration 223
Accidental marks 116

Accidental poisoning 535
Accidental strangulation 194
Acetabulum 316
Acetaminophen 692
   test for 693
Acetic acid 136, 552
Acetone-chlor-hemin crystal test 488
Acetylcholine 678*f*
Acetylcholinesterase, inhibition of 678
Acetylsalicylic acid 697
   toxicity 701
Achlorhydria 667
Acid 540, 549
   diuresis 542, 548
   elution test 408, 414
   hydrolysis 697
   ingestion 555
   of sugar 552
   phosphatase 432, 498
      test 498, 499
Acid-base imbalance, severe 666
Acidosis 538, 609, 689
Aconite 658, 664
Aconitine, toxicity of 659
Aconitum
   ferox 658
   napellus 658
Acoustic barotrauma 325
Acquired immunodeficiency syndrome 103, 510, 518, 521
   (Prevention and Control) Act 520
Acridine-orange fluorescent stain 155
Acrophobia 475, 484
Acro-reaction test 311, 313
Act of Commission 32, 372
Act of Omission 32, 372
Activated charcoal 540, 547, 548
Acute radiation syndrome 353
Acute respiratory distress syndrome 340
Addiction 373, 376, 391, 392
Addictive behaviors 470, 478
Adipocere 175, 175*f*, 176
Adipose tissue 341, 350
Adoption 481
Adrenal cortex, cells of 580
Adrenal hyperplasia, congenital 86
Adult homosexual behavior 443*t*
Adultery 69, 395, 397, 437, 438, 491
   decriminalization of 437*t*
Advanced life support 667
Age assessment protocol 97*b*
Agglutination test 407
Agonal period 149, 157
Agonal regurgitation 356
Agonal thrombi 130
Agoraphobia 475, 484

Agrochemicals 533
Air 172
   bags, role of 320
   blast 324, 330
   current 175
   drying 295
   embolism 229, 286, 342, 384
   insufflations 383
   movement 164
   sample collected, analysis of 726
Airway 537
   edema 555
   support 638
Albumin 541
   solution 300
Albuminuria 534, 564
Alcohol 136, 159, 322, 540, 552, 620, 621, 704
   absorption of 621*t*
   bootlegged 633
   dehydrogenase method 629
   dementia 631
   hangover 623, 634
   influence of 628
   intoxication 623*b*, 672
   level, specific for 635
   smell of 626
   solution of 108
   testing 115
   withdrawal symptoms
      sign of 635
      treatment of 705
Alcoholic hallucinosis 629, 631
Alcoholic paranoia 629, 631
Alcoholic peripheral neuropathy 631
Alcoholism 154, 629, 704
   treatment of 635
Aldehyde 718
   syndrome 630
Aldrich-Mees lines 560, 560*f*
Aldrin 683
Algolagnia 446
Algophobia 475
Algor mortis 163, 177
Alkali 540, 549
   ingestion 555
   poisoning 555
Alkaline
   diuresis 542, 548, 638
   fuchsin 499
Alkalis 559
   strong 533, 554
Alkaloids 614, 618, 654
Alkalosis 149
Alkyl phosphates 678
Allantiasis 733
Allethrin 685

Index

Allograft 149
Alopecia 466f, 579
   traumatic 374
Alphos 687
Alphos poisoning 688, 691
   management of 689fc
   test for 691
Altruistic surrogacy 69
Aluminum phosphide 687, 687f
Alveolar damage, diffuse 127
Alzheimer's disease 509
Amanita
   muscaria 734
   phalloides 540, 734
Amateur tattoos 103
Ambenonium 678
Amelia 371
Ameloglyphics 118
Amenorrhea 413, 571
Amiodarone 659
Amitriptyline 696
Ammonia 549, 552, 554, 718
Ammoniacal vapor 555
Ammonium
   chloride 572
   molybdate test 500
Amnesia 566
Amnestic disorder 479
Amniotic fluid embolism 384, 387
Amotivational syndrome 706
Amphetamine 532, 614, 621, 654, 706, 709
   sulfate 726
Amussat's sign 188
Amygdalin 666
Anal canal, anatomy of 440
Anal evidence 429
Anal fissures 441
Anal hair, shaving of 441f
Anal opening 441
Anal pain 711
Anamnestic evidence 177
Anaphylaxis 154
Anatomical Russian method 524
Ancillary care 50
Androgen
   insensitivity, incomplete 85
   receptor deficiency 85
Anemia 159, 173, 570
   cause of 570, 574
Anemic anoxia 153
Anesthesia
   complications of 355
   death of 353, 354
   spinal 355
Anesthetic devices 356
Aneurysms 275, 278f
Anhidrotic heat exhaustion 297
Aniline dyes 736
Anilingus 443
Animal activity 457
Animal hair 112, 113f
Animal origin, poisons of 732
Animal red blood cells 488f
Anisocytosis 570
Ankylosis 301
Annealing 506
Anomaly, congenital 390
Anorexia 301, 554
   nervosa 477, 478f, 484

Anosmia 727
Anoxemia 159
Anoxia 153
   classification of 153fc
   types 153
Anoxic anoxia 153
Antabuse 630, 635
Antacids 689
Antecedent causes 150
Antemortem 142f
   abrasion 216
   bruise 220
   burns 306
   sign of 303, 304f, 313
   clot 128, 128f
   drowning 206, 208, 211
   sign of 204f
   hanging 190, 210
   sign of 187, 187f
   injuries 204
   thrombi 130
Anterograde amnesia 269
Anthrax 728
Anthropometry 106
Anthropophagy 447
Antibiotics 699
Antibody 376, 519
   fragments, digoxin-specific 661
Anti-cholestatic modalities 588
Anticholinergic agents 621
Anticholinergic syndrome 642
Anticholinesterase 607
Anticraving agents 705
Antidotal therapy 668
Antidote 547, 553, 559, 578, 616
   administration of 540
   pharmacological 541
   physiological 541, 580, 723
   serological 541
Antidotum arsenici 559
Antiglobulin
   consumption test 489
   inhibition test 140
Anti-human hemoglobin serum 489
Antimony 259
Antioxidant agents 583, 681, 690
Antiretroviral therapy 520
Antivenom 607
   treatment 606
Anxiety 470, 474, 474f, 566, 673, 699
Aorta 287
   rupture of 287
   wounds of 287
Aortic aneurysm 153
Aphasia 51, 467
Apnea 727
   test 148
Apoplexy 203, 273, 280
Apoptosis 411
Apostasy 395
Apparent death 159, 159b
Appeals 64
Appellate powers 22
Arachnophobia 475
Arcus senilis 99
Arenaviridae 729, 736
Argemone 735, 736
Argemone mexicana 732, 735, 735f, 736
   poisoning 712

Arguments for Consumer Protection Act 64
Arousal 477
Arrhythmia 609
Arsenic 115
   natural sources of 557
   poisoning 558, 560t, 561, 562
   postmortem imbibition of 561
   sulfide 557
   trioxide 557
Arsenious oxide 557, 557f
Arsenophagists 560
Arsine gas exposure 559
Arson 306
Arterial air emboli 133
Arterial bleeding 494, 494f
Arterial blood pH 537
Artifacts 455, 457, 459, 526
   resuscitative 356, 460
Artificial intelligence 525, 527
Aryl phosphates 678
Ashley's rule 87, 104
Aspartic acid racemization 93
Asphyxia 152, 162, 183, 185, 185fc, 191, 194, 198, 203, 300, 726
   pathophysiology of 183, 183fc
   traumatic 183, 200f, 211, 544
Asphyxial conditions 184f
Asphyxial deaths 125, 183, 184f, 186
Asphyxial torture 513
Asphyxiant 533, 671, 674, 725
Asphyxiophilia 448
Aspiration
   pneumonia 186
   pneumonitis 731
Aspirin 39, 621, 697, 699, 701
   poisoning, treatment of 701
   screening test for 701
Assault 332
   nature of 114
Assisted reproductive
   technology 398, 400
   Act 68
Asthma 680
Atavism 411, 414
Ataxia 727
Atherosclerosis 293
Atherosclerotic vessels 279
Atomic absorption
   spectroscopy 259, 547
Atria mortis 147, 157
Atrioventricular block 718
Atrium, right 286
Atropa belladonna 641, 644
Atropine 614, 641, 645, 681
   poisoning 645
Atropinization 680, 735
Attempt to murder 333
Auditory hallucination 464, 484
Auditory meatus, external 301
Autistic thinking 471
Auto-brewery syndrome 628
Autoerotic asphyxia 209-211, 448
Autograft 149
Autogynephilia 448
Automated fingerprint identification
   system 110
Automatism 269, 639
Autonomic ganglia 660
Autonomic ganglionic effects 679

Index

Autopsy 120, 133, 180, 269, 270, 271, 274, 277, 278, 281, 284
  academic 120
  appearance 275f, 276f, 279f, 281f
  clinical 120
  digital 139
  endoscopic 121
  instruments for 122, 123f
  medico-legal 120, 121, 131
  needle 121
  negative 138
  pathological 44, 121
  radiology 140
  room hazards 138
  second 139, 139b
  skin incision for 126
  viscera preserved during 135t
Avulsed laceration 222f
Axillary hair 113
Axonal injury, diffuse 269
Axonal swelling 270f
Azotemia 582

B

Baar technique 360
Baby's cry 365
Bacillariophyceae 207
Bacillus cereus 732
Back 124
  spatter 244
Baclofen 699
Bacterial contamination 563
Bacterial food poisoning 732
Bacterial meningitis 278
Bacterial phosphotriesterases 681
Bacteroides group 384
Baecchi stain 499
Baldness 99
Ball sign 368, 408
Ballataka 595
Ballistics 235
Ballottement 406
Bangarus fasciatus 599
Bansdola 191, 211
Barberio's test 498, 498f, 502
Barbiturate 159, 540, 637, 638, 639, 700, 706
  automatism 639, 640
  blisters 640
  fatal dose of 640
  poisoning 640
Baritosis 584
Barium 583
  poisoning 585, 586
  sulfate dust, inhalation of 584
  sulphide 583
Barotrauma 717
Barr body 82, 83f, 493
Bartholin cyst 392
Basilar artery, bifurcation of 278f
Bastinado 516
Battered baby syndrome 373, 374f
Battered wife syndrome 435
  symptoms of 435b
Battery and plastic industries 582
Battle's sign 267, 267f, 291
Baux score 305
Bayard's ecchymoses 184
Bayard's spots 210
Beard and moustache 113

Beating-heart donor 149
Bedside
  diagnosis 698
  tests 546t
Bee 532, 610
  management of 599
Behavior 625
Behavioral disorders 469
  classification of 470t
Behavioral syndromes 470
Belly scales 600
Beneke's technique 132, 360, 378
Benzene 654
  hexachloride 683
Benzidine test 487
Benzocaine 736
Benzodiazepine 696, 700, 709
  poisoning 702
    antidote for 701
Benzophenone 697
Benzoylecgonine 650, 653
Benzyl-isoquinoline derivatives 614
Berry aneurysms 144, 279, 279f
Bertillon system 106
Beta-alcoholism 705
Beta-amyloid precursor protein 270
Beta-blockers 651
Bicyclists, injuries to 321
Bile 564
Biliverdin reductase 219
Billiard ball ricochet effect 252f
Biochemical disturbances 138
Bioethics 46, 59
Biological functions, disturbance of 474
Biological surrogacy 69
Biological tests 406
Biological warfare weapons,
    categories of 728t
Biological weapons 712, 728
Biomedical technology 46
Bipolar disorder 474
Birth
  asphyxia 371
  trauma 370
Bisexual 443
Bite mark 116
  swab from 442
Bitten part, care of 607
Bitter almonds 66f
Bitter-sweet taste 659
Black eyes 218f, 263, 291
  causes of 264, 264f
Black powder 241
  grading of 242
Black's law dictionary 32
Blackfoot disease 561
Blackmail 413, 491
Bladder 288
  tumors of 153
Bland liniments 596
Blast injury 324, 326f, 330, 331
  classification of 325t
Blast wave 324
Bleeding 251, 428, 440f
  increased 278
  source of 292
Blister 302, 309
  beetle 721
  gases 674

Blood 134, 178, 189, 508, 545, 559, 629, 726
  alcohol concentration 621, 621f
  analysis of 486
  cherry-red coloration of 673, 673f
  donation 520
  doping 491
  during autopsy, collection of 145
  extravasation of 196f, 220, 458
  genetic markers in 490
  loss 338
  medico-legal application of 491
  non-human 489f
  pressure 350, 522
  salicylate level 698
  sample 429
  spitting of 51
  tests for 488
  transfusion 35
Blood group 490
  incompatibility 381
  typing 500
  medico-legal aspects of 491
Blood vessel 206, 264, 390
  air in 458
  changes in 368
Blood-brain barrier 563
Bloodstain 83
  analysis 486, 486fc, 495
  fluid 277
Blunt force
  injuries 217
  trauma 213
Blunt injury 285
Blunt trauma 184
Blunt weapon
  shape of 223
  trauma 286
Boat tail bullet 240
Bodily distress 478
  disorders of 470, 478
Bodily experience disorders 478
Body
  affecting rigor mortis 167t
  behavior of 315
  condition of 173
  coverings of 165
  dysmorphic disorder 476
  fate of 175
  fluids 492, 501, 518
  freezing 180
  glycogen stores 350
  hair 113
  integrity dysphoria 478
  measurement 106
  parts of 188, 192, 497
  posture of 165
  skeletonization of 173
  stuffers 617
  surface area 305
Body packer 617, 617f, 618
  syndrome 617f
Bolam test 33
Bolitho test 33
Bomb
  explosion 325f
  pulse dating 143
Bone 134, 200
  age estimation 97
  age from ossification of 94

Index

and joint 289
carpals 95
clavicle 95
contusion 221
corrosion of 719
cutter 123
decalcification of 719
detect arsenic in 562
femur 95
fibula 95
fracture of 335
fragments, depression of 265
hip 95
humerus 95
indices of long 80
marrow 83, 100
    changes in 178
pain 582
pearls 310, 313
radius 95
saw 123
scapula 95
stature from 100
sternum 95
tarsals 95
tibia 95
ulna 95
Bordetella pertussis 733
Boric acid 549, 718
    poisoning 712, 736
Botulinum toxin 728, 733, 734
Botulism 584, 712, 733
    classic triad of 733, 736
    immune globulin 734
Botulismus 733
Bowel 534
    sounds, diminished 643
Boxer's encephalopathy 269
Boyde's method 91, 93
Brachial index 81
Brachycephalic skull 80*f*
Bradycardia 156, 269, 718
Bradykinesia 673
Brain 136, 147, 171, 189, 192, 206, 270, 303, 326, 356, 360, 560, 566, 573, 580, 583, 639, 668, 690, 711
    abscess of 186
    contrecoup injury of 272*f*
    contusions, types of 270
    damage 35
    death 147, 148, 148*b*
    delivery of 130
    diffuse injury to 282
    dissection of 131
    edema 147
    examination of 131
    fingerprinting 523
    fixation of 131
    function 147, 148
    hemorrhages, types of 329
    herniation 283, 283*f*
    infarction of 186
    injury to 268
    knife 123
    mapping 523
    swelling 282, 283*f*
    tissue 263

Brain injury 268
    classification of 268*fc*
    stratification, severity of 268*t*
    traumatic 262, 268, 269
Brainstem 132
    death 147, 157
    reflexes, absence of 148
Brass chills 585
Bratton-Marshall test 697, 701
Brawner rule 483
Braxton-Hick's contractions 406, 414
Breadth 228
Breast 412, 425
    changes 411
Breath 629
    alcohol 628
    control play 448
Breathalyzer 629
Breeding program 509
Brentamine
    fast blue test 498*fc*
    test 498
Breslau's second life test 367, 378
Broken neck sign 611
Bromocriptine 696
Bronchi 354, 580
Bronchioles 206, 303
Bronchitis 301
Bronchopneumonia 301
Bronchorrhea 679*f*
Brooke formula 300
Brown recluse spiders 610
Brucella 381
Brucellosis 728, 729
Bruise 163, 213, 217, 221, 222, 327
    age of 218, 219*t*
    artificial 51, 596, 597
    factors influencing 217
    intradermal 217
    patterned 218
    true 596
Bryan-Leishman stain 499
Bubonic plague 728
Buccal coitus 444, 445
Buccal epithelial cells 82, 508
Buccal swabs 508
Bucket-handle incision 125
Buddha tree 663
Bulbar paralysis 607
Bulbocavernosus reflex test 393
Bulbouretral gland 496
Bulimia nervosa 477, 478*f*
Bulky foods 541
Bullet 238, 254, 260
    caliber of 238, 260
    close shot entry wound of 248*f*
    emboli 260
    exits 250
    handling of 254*f*
    path of 257
    preservation of 254*f*
    tumbles 250
    types of 239, 239*f*, 260
    wounds 253
Bullous lesions 672
Bumper impacts 316
Bungarus caeruleus 599
Buprenorphine 705
Buried alive 201

Burking 200, 201*f*, 211
Burn 115, 298, 300, 308*f*, 309, 341, 374, 513
    accidental 306
    age of 305*t*
    cause of death in 312
    classification of 298*f*, 298*t*, 299
    contact 298
    degree of 299, 299*f*
    effect of 298
    electric 298
    endogenous 309
    exogenous 310
    filigree 311*f*
    flash 309
    friction 215
    immersion 307
    lightning 298
    microwave 298
    postmortem findings in 302*f*
    radiant heat 298
    self-inflicted 306
    steam 307
    types of 298
Burning 247, 372
    acrid taste 660
    micturition 434
Burnt bones 306
Burtonian line 574
Butterfly bruise 217, 374

C

Cabot's rings 570
Cadaveric donation, case of 62
Cadaveric spasm 167, 168, 168*f*, 205*f*, 257, 655
Cadmium 582, 583
    dust, inhalation of 582
    poisoning, target organ in 585
    ring formation 582
Café coronary 198, 211
Caffeine 543, 621
Caffey syndrome 211, 379
Caisson disease 717, 736
    symptoms of 736
Calcined bone 140
Calcium 376
    disodium ethylenediaminetetraacetic acid 569
    disodium versenate 541
    gluconate 553, 609, 683, 719
    oxalate crystals 553
    polysulfides 727
    salts 580
Caliber 260
Calliphora vomitoria 174
Calliphoridae 653
Calomel 563
Calotropis 382, 383, 597, 597*f*, 598
    gigantea 597
    procera 597
Camel and llama, exception of 488
Cancellous bone unite faster, fractures of 290
Candida 628
Canine 92, 116
Cannabinoid hyperemesis syndrome 648
Cannabis 646, 647, 647*f*, 706
    americana 646
    driving under influence of 648
    indica 646
    mexicana 646

Index

preparations of 646, 646t
sativa 646
toxicity, management of 649
Cantharides 721
  poisoning 712
Cantharis vesicatoria 721, 721f
Capgras syndrome 462
Capital murder 333
Capital punishment 11
Capsicum
  annuum 596, 596f
  seeds 642
Caput succedaneum 365, 365f, 378
Carabelli's cusp 94
Carabelli's tubercle 94
Carbamate 677, 678f
Carbol marasmus 554
Carbolic acid 136, 543, 549, 553
  poisoning 554f
Carbolism 553
Carboluria 553
Carbon dioxide 725
  ice 180
  poisoning 712
Carbon dot powders 527
Carbon monoxide 183, 671
  poisoning 157, 680
Carbonated drinks 621
Carcinogenic effect 487
Cardiac arrest 719
Cardiac arrhythmias 156, 584
  antidote for 661
Cardiac concussion 287
Cardiac disease 69
Cardiac failure, severe 127
Cardiac glycosides 718
Cardiac poisons 533, 658, 724
Cardiac stimulants 726
Cardiac tamponade 153, 286, 287, 287f
Cardiac troponin, degradation of 179
Cardinal manifestation 284
Cardiomyopathy 153
Cardiopulmonary bypass 659
Cardiorespiratory depression 696
Cardiovascular collapse 661
Cardiovascular disease 86, 153
Cardiovascular support 638
Cardiovascular system 627
Care, degree of 33
Carotid artery, root of internal 278f
Carpal bones, ossification of 96f
Carphologia 642, 643
Cartilage 83
Carunculae hymenales 402
Cascabela thevetia 661, 662, 662f, 664
Casper's dictum 173
Catalytic color tests 487
Catamite 439
Cataplexy 480
Cataract, subcapsular 578
Catarrhal changes 560
Catatonia 470, 472
Catharsis 696
Cathartics 542
Catheterization 643
Caucasian skull 81
Causative weapon 216
Caustic agents 549
Caustic alkali 543, 554

Caustic ingestion, neutralizing agents
  for 551
Cecum 560
Celiac disease 349
Cell death proteins 179
Celphos 687
Centerfire 241, 241f
Central Adoption Resource Authority 714
Central Consumer Protection Authority 63
Central Drug Standards and Control
  Organization 51
Central nervous system 147, 153
  effects 679, 695
  infections 615
  symptoms 634
Central venous pressure 275
Cephalhematoma 365, 365f, 378
Cephalic index 80, 80f, 80t, 141
Cerbera odollam 663, 663f, 664
Cerberin 664
Cerebellar hemorrhage 632
Cerebellum 132, 283
Cerebral anoxia 191, 194
Cerebral concussion 268
Cerebral contusion 270, 274
Cerebral cortex 132, 147
Cerebral edema 282, 282f, 571, 673
  diffuse 668
  malignant 282
Cerebral hemisphere, swelling of 274
Cerebral hemorrhage 672
  non-traumatic 280
Cerebral laceration 270
Cerebral malaria 154
Cerebrospinal fluid 134, 134f, 178
Cerebrum 131, 356
Cervical
  canal 383
  cell 436
  spine 284f
  upper 284
  vertebrae, fracture of 185, 191
  zygapophysial joint 284
Cervix 411, 412, 428
  abrasion of 428
  dilation of 383
Chadwick's sign 405, 413
Chalcosis corneae 578
Chalcosis oculi 578
Charaka's oath 52
Charas 646, 649
Charcot-Bouchard aneurysms 279
Charles Bonnet syndrome 464
Chasing dragon 614, 617
Cheiloscopy 110, 119
Chelating agents 541, 542t, 565
Chelation therapy 694
Chemical
  analysis 544
  antidotes 541
  asphyxiants 671
  burns 298, 308
  castration 395
  colitis 552
  combination 534
  methods 629
  peels 103
  peritonitis 681
  pneumonitis 582

  suicide 727, 736
  thermometer 526
  warfare 593, 674
Chemiluminescence 487
Chemotherapy 392
Cherry-red color lungs 304f
Chest 127, 285, 286, 359, 516
  changes in 365
  graze abrasion on 317f
  injuries 329
  pain 659
  X-ray 342
Chevalier d'eon de beaumont 448
Cheyne-Stokes respiration 159, 679
Chilblains 294
Child abuse 116, 307f, 358, 375
Child adoption 400
Child Welfare Committee 67
Chlamydia 381
Chloasma 405
Chloral hydrate 136, 709
Chlordane 683
Chlordecone 683
Chlordiazepoxide 631
Chloride 567
Chlorinated hydrocarbons 683, 686
Chlorinated phenol 553
Chlorine 718
Chloroform 136, 356
Chlorpyriphos 678
Chlorthion 678
Chocolate cyanosis 720
Choke bore 237, 260
Cholera 558
Cholestyramine 588, 683
Choline
  and spermine test 500
  iodide crystals 498f
  periodide appear 497
Cholinergic agents 621
Cholinesterase 680t
  activity, depression of 680
Chondrocytes viability 179
Choral hydrate 709
Christmas tree stain 499, 502
Chromatin positivity 83t
Chromatography 546
Chromic acid 543
Chromodacryorrhea 679f
Chronic poisoning 391, 392, 532, 535, 554, 565,
  570, 581, 660, 684, 721, 736
  signs of 697
Chvostek sign 553
Chylothorax 286
Cinchona plant contains quinine, bark of 724
Cinchonidine 724
Cinchonism 724
Cinnabar 563
Circle of Willis 131, 133, 278, 278f, 279f
Circulatory collapse 584
Circulatory failure 355, 632
Circulatory system, effects on 571
Cirrhosis 544
Cisvestism 448
Citrated calcium carbimide 630
Civic benefit 28
Civil case 10, 12, 143
Civil court 9, 9fc
Civil law 4

Index

Civil negligence 33, 34
  cases arising 491
Civil responsibility 481
Claustrophobia 475, 484
Claviceps purpurea 720, 720*f*, 736
Clavicle, X-rays of 95
Cleistanthins 724
Cleistanthus collinus 724, 724*f*
Clinical Establishments Act 712
Clitoris 404
Clomipramine 696
Clonidine 681, 705
Clostridia 220
Clostridium
  botulinum 728
  tetani 339
Clostridium perfringens 170, 339, 384, 732
  septicemia 162
Clot organization, signs of 290
Coagulopathy 607
Coal gas 671
Cobra 600, 602, 603, 603*f*
  bite 611, 612
Cocaethylene 650
Cocaine 533, 614, 647, 650, 650*f*, 654, 706, 709
  bugs 652, 653
  fatal dose of 653
  poisoning 653
  washed-out syndrome 652
Cocainism 652
Cocainomania 652
Cocainophagia 652
Code of Ethics and Regulations 46
Code of Medical Ethics 29
Codeine 614, 615
Coercion technique 514
Coercive sexual sadism disorder 446
Coffee-ground appearance 552
Cognition 467, 469
Cognitive dysfunction 269
Cognitive impairment 673
Cognitive-behavioral therapy 434
Cognizable offense 5, 18
Cold
  application of 214, 293
  injury 293
  stiffening 167, 169
  torture 512
  water drowning 203
Colica pictorum 569
Collateral negligence 38
Colloids 300
Colonic mucous membrane 564
Colonic strictures 552
Colposcopic examination 428
Coma 152, 609, 632, 679
  cocktail 537, 547
  stage of 615, 622
Commercial surrogacy 69
Common carbamates 678, 685
Common date rape drugs 709*t*
Commotio cordis 287
Communication
  effective 55
  skills 54, 55, 55*b*
  strategies 55
  technique 514
Community health providers 21
Complete androgen insensitivity syndrome 85

Completion illusion 465
Compos mentis 13, 481
Compression fracture, anteroposterior 197
Compulsive sexual behavior disorder 478, 481
Concave lens appearance 276*f*
Concealed sex 82
Concussion 203, 269
  mercurilis 566
Conduction system anomalies 376
Condyle 292
Conflict resolution techniques 54
Congenital diseases 370
Congenital ovarian hypoplasia
      syndrome 84
Conium maculatum 723
  poisoning 712
Conjunctiva 558, 626
  congested 192*f*
Connective tissue histochemistry 344
Consciousness 469
  loss of 274
Consensual sodomy 445
Consent 25, 40, 44, 68, 69, 418
  absence of 419
  for Act 34
  presumption of 43, 420
  types of 40*fc*
  validity of 481
Constipation 540, 571
Constitution 20
Constitution of Ethics Committee 49
Consumer commissions, structure
      of 63*fc*
Consumer Protection Act 63
Contact blanching 161
Contact injury 263, 587
Contact pallor 159, 161
Contact shot head, signs of 261
Contact shotgun injury 245*f*
Contamination 475
Contraception 395
  methods of 396, 396*fc*
Contraceptives, barrier 396
Contrecoup contusion 270*f*, 271
Contrecoup lacerations 288
Contusion 213, 217, 270
  collar 244
Conversion therapy 448
Convex lens appearance 275*f*
Convulsions 537, 584, 609, 655
Cookie cutter appearance 246
Copper 382, 575
  acetoarsenite 557, 557*f*
  arsenite 557
  carbonate 575
  ions 575
  poisoning 576, 578
  subacetate 575, 575*f*
  sulfate 575, 575*f*, 591
    poisoning, acute 577*f*
Coprinus atramentarius 630
Coprophagia 451
Coprophilia 451
Coral snake 599
Cord
  knots of 371
  pressure on 371
Cord around neck 371, 371*f*
Core temperature, measurement of 164

Cornea 149, 177
  capacity 301
  erosion 719
  opacity of 160
  retrieval 77
  transplantation 77
Corneal reflexes, loss of 160
Corneal tear, partial thickness 334*f*
Coronary artery 129*f*, 154
  disease 153, 630
  extramural 128
  lumen 154
  occlusion of 157
  right 154
  spasm 155
  system 154
Coronary atherosclerosis 154
Coronary lesions, acute 128
Coronary ostia 154
Coroner's court 8
Coroner's inquest 7, 8
Corporal evidence 177
Corporate negligence 38
Corpus delicti 79
Corrosive poisons 539, 549, 551*f*
Cortex 111, 112
Cortical blindness 673
Cortical bone histology 100
Cortical sulci 269
Corticosteroid 735
  therapy 607
Cosmetic autopsy incision 515
Cosmetic tattoos 103
Cotard's syndrome 462
Councilman rib shear 123
Coup
  contusion 270
  injuries 271, 272
  mechanism of 272*f*
Court 6
Court of law 9, 28
Court ordered examination 28
Court questions 16, 17
COVID-19 outbreak 26
Cowper's glands 496
Crack baby 652
Crack dancing 652
Crack lung 652
Cramps 583
Cranial bones, reflection of 360*f*
Cranial sutures 143
Craniocerebral injury 262
  classification of 263*t*
Craniofacial reconstruction 524
Creatine phosphokinase test 500
Creche coronary 199
Crepitant lungs 366
Cribriform 402
Crime against human body 5
Crime against property 5
Crime scene 121, 216, 253, 525, 526
  investigation 525, 528
  reconstruction 492
  types of 525, 527
Criminal abortion 100, 380, 381, 385, 387, 413
  complications of 384, 384*t*
  methods for 381
  procure 383*f*
  samples collected in 387*b*

Index

Criminal cases 10, 143, 394, 467, 492, 523
Criminal causes 372
Criminal court 9, 9*fc*, 10
Criminal identification, method of 106
Criminal law 4
Criminal Law (Amendment)
    Act 417, 418
Criminal negligence 33, 34
Criminal Procedure Code 5
Criminal responsibility 482, 648
Crocodile skin lesions 310*f*
Cross-examine witness 14
Croton tiglium 593, 594*f*, 598
Cruelty 395
Crural index 81
Crush asphyxia 199
Crush syndrome 340, 348
Crystal tests 488
Crystalline 587
    calcium phosphate 91
Cul-de-sac delivery 198*f*
Cullen's sign 218
Culpable homicide 332
Cultivating opium 532
Cunnilingus 444, 445
Cupping 382, 382*f*, 387
Cuprimine 541
Curare poisoning 712
Curling's ulcer 301, 304, 313
Curren's rule 483
Custodial rape 418, 437
Custody, chain of 122, 526
Cut laceration 222, 222*f*
Cut throat injury 372
    crime scene of 526*f*
Cutaneous blood vessels, dilatation
    of 642
Cutis anserina 204, 205*f*, 211
Cyanide 540, 567, 667, 718, 727
    analysis, specimen for 670
    antidote kit 668
    in autopsy, toxic symptoms
        of 669
    kit 668
    poisoning 670
    poisoning, antidotal for 669
    presumptive test for 669
Cyanmethemoglobin 668
Cyanosis 184, 575, 609, 726
Cyberchondria 476
Cyclic antidepressants toxicity 651
Cyclodienes 683
Cyclothymic disorder 474
Cylinder bore 237, 260
Cypermethrin 685
Cytochrome
    C oxidase 575
    P450 oxidase system 692
Cytomegalovirus 48

D

Dactylography 106
Daily dairy report 515
D-allethrin 685
Danbury tremors 566
Dangerous weapon 336
Data privacy 26
Davidson body 83*f*
Davidson-Smith body 83

Dead bodies
    cooling of 163
    disposal of 373
    examination of 386
    identification of 80
    mummified 176*f*
    on water, floatation of 174
    samples collected from 508
    submerged 204*f*
Dead people 79
Dead persons, number of 327
Dead-born 364
    fetus 369
    signs of 368, 378
Deafness, permanent 334
Death 146, 148*b*
    accidental 561
    anaphylactic 156
    autoerotic 448
    case of 356
    cause of 330
    changes after 158*t*
    circumstances of 327
    clinical 157
    complications of 229
    cot 376
    crib 376
    custodial 121, 512, 515, 516*f*
    dyadic 149
    hyperventilation 209
    manner of 149, 149*fc*, 149*t*, 150*t*, 527
    mechanism of 149, 150*t*, 202*f*
    modes of 152, 152*t*, 157, 165
    moment of 147, 157
    mother 371
    natural 149
    neglect 349
    neonatal 358, 378
    operative 353, 354
    penalty 11, 418
    presumption of 181
    primary cause of 150
    proximate causes of 152
    secondary cause of 150
    signs of 158
    sudden 379
    suspected 125*t*
    time of 115, 124, 139, 142, 142*t*, 182, 376,
        492, 527
    unexpected 379
Decamethrin 685
Deceleration injury 262, 284*f*
Deciduous teeth, eruption of 92*f*, 92*t*
Decomposed bodies 140
Decompression sickness 712, 717, 736
Decubitus 216
    position, left lateral 440*f*
Defense injuries 231
Deferasirox 541
Deferiprone 541
Deferoxamine 541
Defloration 401, 413
Delhi Anatomy Act 715
Delirium 479, 642, 679
    tremens 629-631, 635
Delivery 401
    mismanagement of 35
Delta alcoholism 705
Deltamethrin 685

Delusion 461, 471, 483
    type of 462, 462*t*, 463*f*, 484
Delusional disorder 472
Delusional parasitosis 653
Dementia 293, 479
    pugilistica 269
Demirjian method 91, 93
Demonstrate venous air embolus 144
Dense fibro fatty tissues 263
Dental enamel 179
Dental identification 116, 305
Dental profiling 116
Dental pulp 179
Dental tissue 502
Dentition, period of mixed 92
Deoxyribonucleic acid 306
    amplification 506
    analyses 116, 524
    denaturing, cycle of 506
    fingerprinting 504, 506, 509*f*, 510, 511
    index system, combined 510
    methylation profiling 501
    polymerase 506
    profiling 505*f*, 507
    sequencing 510
    signature 506
    sources of 508*fc*
    storage 508
    testing 510
Dependence syndrome 704
Depersonalization-derealization
    disorder 477
Depressed mood 473
Depression 474*f*, 566, 673
    stage of 651
    symptoms of 473*f*
Depressive cognition 473
Depressive disorder 349, 474
Depressive episode 473
Depressive ideation 473
Deprivation technique 514
Derive sexual pleasure 447
Dermabrasion 103
Dermal nitrate 259
Dermatitis, cases of contact 596
Desferrioxamine 542, 694
Designer hallucinogens 707
Desipramine 696
Destocking 302
Determine maturity 361
Deterrent agents 705
Detoxification 622, 705
Deuel's halo sign 368, 408
Dextran and Hartmann's solution 300
Dextrose 537, 580
Dhat syndrome 390
Dhatura 641, 645
    alba 641
    fastuosa 641
    ferox 641
    fruit 642*f*
    poisoning 643*f*
        antidote for 645
    seeds 596, 642, 644*f*
    signs of 645
    stramonium 641
    symptoms of 645
Diabetes mellitus 51, 103
Diaphanous test 159

Diaphragm 286, 329
  position of 366
Diarrhea 534, 540
  acute 732
Diastasis 266
Diatom's test 207, 207f, 211
Diazepam 532, 630, 681, 683, 699
Diazinon 678
Dichotomy 29
Dieldrin 683
Dietary management 572
Diethylstilbestrol, use of 39
Diffusion precipitation test 489
Digital rectal thermometer 164f
Digitalis 658
  purpurea 658, 660, 661f, 664
Digitoxin 664
Digoxin-fab 661
Dille-Koppanyi test 638, 640
Dimenhydrinate 514
Dimercaptosuccinic acid 541
Dimethyl mercury 563
Diphenoxylate 705
Diphtheria 733
Diphtheroids 170
Diplopia 623, 642
Dipsomania 465
Disabled persons 25
Disagreeable odor 660
Disaster 140
Discharge 428
Discover rule 64
Disease
  classification of 150
  signs of 124
Disguise, delusion of 462
Disodium phosphate 542
Disruptive behavior 470, 479
Disseminated intravascular coagulation 340, 355
Dissociative amnesia 477
Dissociative disorders 470, 477
Dissociative fugue 477
Dissociative identity disorder 477
Distant shot rifled firearm entry wounds 249f
Disulfiram 630, 635
  ethanol reaction 630
Dithiocarbamates 583
Diuresis 696
Diver's disease 717
Divorce 389, 399, 481, 491
  grounds for 395
Doctor at crime scene 526
Doctor-patient
  communication 55
  relationship 35
Documentary evidence 12
Dolichocephalic skull 80f
Domestic violence 73
Donor insemination, indications for 400
Dopamine β-hydroxylase 575
Dothiepin 696
Double barrel shotgun 238f
Double-condom sign 617f
Dowry death 333, 347
Doxepin 696
D-penicillamine 565, 576
Dried seminal stains 497
Dried tobacco leaves 660f

Drowning 159, 201, 205f, 372
  classification of 202fc
  molecular diagnosis of 208
  near 203, 211
  primary 201
  secondary 203
Drowsiness 643
Drug 322
  abortifacient 381
  abuse, complications of 710
  addiction 703
  allergy 103
  analeptic 639
  anesthetic 356
  antipsychotic 695
  combinations 647
  cytotoxic 86
  date rape 703, 709
  dependence 703, 705t
  designer 703
  facilitated sexual assault 709
  habituation 703
  hard 703, 711
  illicit 618
  narcoanalysis 527
  narcotic 532, 547
  neuroprotective 681
  overdose 625
  psychoactive 703, 711
  soft 703, 711
  teratogenic 70
  truth 524, 527
  use of generic names of 24
Drugs and Cosmetic Rules 533
Drug-facilitated rape 418
Drunk and disorderly 30
Drunk driving 628
Drunken gait 642
Drunken person, bounding pulse of 278
Drunkenness 269, 625
Dry mouth 645
Dum-dum bullet 239
Duodenum 544
Duplex bullet 239
Dupuytren's and Wilson's classification 312
Duquenois-Levine test 649
Durham's rule 483
Dyed starch substrates 501
Dying victim, tendency of 672
Dysarthria 622, 638, 642
Dysbarism 717
Dyserythropoiesis 570
Dysmenorrhea 571
Dyspareunia 434
Dyspepsia 51
Dysphagia 642
Dysphasia 673
Dyspnea 534, 584
Dyspraxia 673
Dysrhythmia 651
  ventricular 696, 719
Dystonic drug reactions 656

E

Ear 325, 626
  bleeding from 187
  crepitance test 366, 378
  lobes, piercing of 81
  print 118

Ear-to-ear incision 360
Eating disorder 470, 477
Ebola virus 729
Ecbolics 381, 387
Ecchymoses 338, 426
Eccrines 108
  methyl ester, formation of 650
Echis carinatae 599
Echopraxia 467
Ecstasy 647
Ectopic bruise 218, 218f
Edema 148
  aquosum 206
Edgeoscopy 110
Edges stick together 290
Edrophonium 678
Egg freezing 399
Eggshell skull rule 713
Ehrlich's reagent test 708
Ejaculation, premature 389
Ekbom syndrome 462, 463f, 653
Elapid snakebite 733
Elapidae bite 603, 608
Elastic tissue 344
Elbow, X-rays of 95
Electra complex 436
Electric torture 513
Electrical injury 308, 309f
Electrical petechiae 311
Electrical stimulation 209
Electro-chemical methods 259
Electro-chemical sensor 258
Electroconvulsive therapy 76
Electrocution 308, 313
Electrolyte
  abnormalities 355
  imbalance 543
  management 698
Electronic media 31
Electronic records 12
Electronic registration 109
Electrophoretic methods 488
Electrophysiological tests 680
Elemental hallucinations 464
Elemental mercury 563, 564, 564f
Embalming artifacts 458
Embalming fluid components 180t
Emblem 712
Embolism 340
Embryo 361
Embryonic stem cell 48
Emergency cases 25
Emergency preservation 159
Emergency resuscitation 159
Emergency treatment 76
Emetics 540
Emmenagogues 382, 387
Emotional abuse 375
Emotional lability 679
Empathy 467
Emphysema 205, 582
  aquosum 205, 211
Emphysematous bulla 286
Employee's Compensation (Amendment) Act 65
Employees' State Insurance Act 65
Employees' State Insurance Corporation 65
Emprosthotonus 655
En bloc removal 126

Index

En masse 125, 494
Enamel pearls 94
Enamel protein 93
Encephalitis 680, 733
Encephalopathy 631
Endangers life 335
Endocrinal disturbances 138
Endocrine 154, 381
   disorders 390
Endometrial surface, color of 127
Endosulfan 683, 684
Endotoxins 733
Endrin 683, 684
   fatal dose of 686
   poisoning, treatment of 686
Enterotome 123
Enterotoxin 732, 733
Entomology 174
Entrance tests 21
Envenomation 606, 606b, 606t
Environmental artifacts 459
Environmental contamination 561
Environmental temperature 164, 171, 175
Enzymatic change 178
Enzyme 169, 178
   activity 343f, 498
   bioscavengers 681
   groups of 541
   histochemistry 155
   markers 492
   synthesis 687
   typing 501
Enzyme-linked immunosorbent assay 407, 608, 724
Eonism 448f, 453
Ephebophilia 450
Epidemic dropsy 735
Epidermis 103f
Epididymis 496
Epidural hematoma 273, 275f, 279f, 303, 680
   cause of 291
   diagnosis of 291
Epidural hemorrhage 279, 280
Epidural space 274
Epilepsy 51, 62, 656
   traumatic 268, 345
Epsilon alcoholism 705
Equipment failure 354
Erectile capacity 393
Erectile dysfunction 389, 393, 399
   causes of 389, 390t, 391f, 399
Ergometrine 736
Ergot 720, 736
   poisoning 712
Ergotamine 552, 736
Ergotism 721, 736
Ergotoxin 736
Erotic asphyxiation 448
Erotomania 462, 484
Erythema pernio 294
Erythroblastosis fetalis 371
Erythromycin 621
Erythrophobia 475
Erythropoietin 491
Erythroxylum coca leaves 650, 650f
Esophageal mucosa 554f
Esophageal perforation 539
Esophageal squamous epithelium 549
Esophageal tears 540

Esophagus 126, 544, 639
   carcinoma 349
   squamous epithelium of 555
Ethanol 620
Ether 136
Ethics and Medical Registration Board 22
Ethics committee 49, 49b
Ethmoid sinus 207
Ethyl alcohol 620
Ethyl mercury 563
Ethylene glycol 136, 634, 635
   poisoning 620, 635
Ethylenediaminetetraacetic acid 541
Euthanasia 30, 47, 59
Evidence
   and samples, collection of 430f
   collection of 254
   types of 13f
Evisceration techniques 126fc
Ex officio members 20
Excitement, stage of 614, 647, 651
Excretion 553, 558, 564, 569, 575, 579, 632, 642, 644, 650, 667, 684, 688, 695, 698
Exhibitionism 449, 449f, 453
Exhumation 7, 143
   artifacts 459
Exit tests 21
Exotoxins 733
Exploding bullet 240
Explosive
   classification of 325
   irritability 566
Extracampine hallucinations 464
Extracellular fluid 136
Extradural hematoma 273, 274
   causes 273
   types 273
Extragenital injury 425, 426f
Extrapyramidal signs 695
Extremity 359
Eye 124, 191, 200, 204, 374, 600f, 626
   burns 552
   changes in 160, 177
   crow feet appearance of 302f
   instilled into 597
   movement, abnormal 609
Eyeball 177
Eyebrow 113, 362f, 363f
Eyelashes 113, 363f
Eyelids 216
   muscles of 166

F

Face 124, 187, 191, 200, 203, 359
   permanent disfiguration of 335
Facet joint 284
Facial hair growth 178
Facial injuries 283
Facial lacerations 319f
Facial motor response 148
Facial pallor 159, 571
Facial recognition 111
Facial reconstruction 524, 527
Facial sensation 148
Factitious disorder 470, 479
Factories Act 715, 736
Factum probandum 6
Factum probans 6
Falanga 516

Family courts 11
Family violence 58
Fanconi's syndrome 571
Fang mark 602f
Fasciotomy wound, surgical 607f
Fat embolism 341, 384
   cause of 348
   syndrome 341, 348
Fatal airway obstruction, acute 198
Fatal blood alcohol level 634
Fatal concentration 725
Fatigue 405
Fatty degeneration 580
Fatty foods 621
Fatty liver 544
Fear-related disorders 470
Febrile illnesses 625
Fecal matter 502
Fecal stains 498
Feces 545, 590
Feeding disorder 470, 477
Feet-first impact 328f
Feigned insanity 467, 468, 484
Feigned pregnancy and delivery 413
Female genitalia 127
Femur 100, 318, 508
   fracture of 335f, 342
   lower end of 362, 363, 363f
Ferric chloride test 556, 698
Ferric hydroxide 559
Fertility 389
Fetal cells 408
Fetal death 372f
   accidental causes of 371
   diagnosis of 364
Fetal heart sounds 407
Fetal movements 407
Fetal skull, technique of opening 361
Fetal souffle 407
Fetal viability 378
Fetex paste 383
Feticide 358
Fetishism 449, 450f, 453
Fetus 361, 362t, 378
   age of 361
   compressus 409, 414
   estimate age of 364
   papyraceus 409, 410f, 414
   sex of 72
   viability of 364
Fever 534, 609, 610
Fibers 111, 112t
   artificial 112
   natural 112
Fibrin 344
Fibroblasts 344
Fibrosis 509, 544
Fibrous layer 264
Fibrous tissue 84, 290
Fibula 318
Fictitious child 410, 414
Field impairment tests 620, 627f
Filoviridae 729
Finger nose test 627
Fingernails 124
Fingerprint 106, 256
   classification 109
   development 108
      techniques for 109t

Index

powder 564
recording of 107
ridges, types of 107t
system 106
temporary loss of 107
types of 107f, 108
Firearm 235, 255t
case of 167
classification of 236
parts of 161, 260
types of 260
Firearm injury 115, 216, 235
accidental 257
types of 243
Firearm wound 213, 243, 249
characteristics of 243
Firecracker burn 299f
Fired bullet 254, 255f
Fireman's cramps 295
First information report 5
First molar 92
First permanent tooth 104
First premolar 92
First trimester abortion, cause of 387
Fixed noose 186f
Flaccid quadriplegia 583
Flail chest 286, 291
Flame burns 298
Flecainide 659
Florence test 497, 498f, 502
Fluid 539
management 698
resuscitation 300, 693
Flumazenil 697
Flunitrazepam 709
Fluorescence 487
in situ hybridization 499
technique 493
tissue spectroscopy 179
Fluoride 136
Fluoroimmunoassay 407
Focal lesions 291
Focal neurologic symptoms 271
Fodere's test 366, 378
Folate 722
therapy 633
Fomepizole 632
Fontanelle, closure of 368
Food bolus 198f
Food poisoning 533, 732
toxin type of 733
Food-borne
botulism 734
disease 732
Foot, bones of 364
Forehead 273
Foreign body 127, 383
in situ 452f
ingestion of 539
insertion 402
Foreign hair 441
Foreign objects, insertion of 451
Forensic
anthropology 140
autopsy 120
ballistics 235
entomology 174
evaluation 500t
experts 58

medicine 3, 18, 285
odontology 115
pathology 3
podiatry 110
practice, samples encountered
in 508
psychiatrist, role of 467
psychiatry 461
serology 486
specimens 510
toxicology 531, 532, 547
Forensic science
laboratory 429
uses in 525
Formaldehyde 136, 180
Formalin 137, 552
fixed brain 131f
Formic acid 136
Formicophilia 444
Forrest test 695
Fossa navicularis 401, 404, 428
Fourchette 404, 427
rupture of 411
Foxglove 664
Fracture 187, 304
abduction 196, 197
adduction 196
antemortem 290
avenue 304
avulsion 196, 289
basilar 267
blood loss in 338t
blow-out 266
boxer's 289, 292
brawler's 289, 292
bucket-handle 375
bumper 316f, 323
cervical spine 319
chance 320
classification of 290f
comminuted 266, 266f, 289
complex 290
complications of 290
compound 289
compression 289
contrecoup 266
contusion 271
cranial fossa 267, 267f
crush 289
depressed 265, 265f
direct 289
distraction 289
elevated 266
first 250f
fissure 265
focal 289
green-stick 289
gutter 266
Hangman's 190, 190f, 210
healing of 290
hinge 267, 267f, 323
hyoid bone 195, 196, 197f, 285, 458
indirect 289
inward compression 196, 196f
knob 375
LeFort's 292
linear 265, 265f
maxillary 289
mosaic 266

motorcyclists 267, 320, 323
open 289
partial 289
pelvic 290
penetrating 289
penis 391
ping-pong 266
pond 266, 266f
postmortem 290
rib 285, 286
ring 266, 266f, 329f
seat belt 320
signature 265
simple 289
spiral 289
street 304
subsequent 250f
sutural 266, 267f
tooth 335
transverse 267, 289
tug 197
type of 265
undertaker's 459, 460
Fracture-a-la-signature 265
Fragilis 384
Frangible bullet 239
Fraternal twins 409, 410, 414
Free fatty acids 350
Fregoli's phenomenon 462
Fresh blood, passage of 552
Fresh water drowning 202f, 206
Friction skin, cross section of 107f
Fronal sinus print 118
Frontal lobes 270f
Frostbite 295
Frotteurism 450, 450f, 453
Fugue 484
Full metal jacket 238, 239f
Full term baby 363f
Fulminating poisoning 532, 552, 588
Fumes 582
Fumigants 533, 677
Fundal height 405
Fundus 342
uteri, level of 406f
Fungicides 677
Funnel-shaped depression 441
Furrow 186

G

Gacyclidine 681
Gagging 199, 199f, 211
Gait 625, 673
Galea aponeurotica 263, 264
Gallbladder, distended 351f
Galton system 106
Gambling disorder 478
Gamete
intrafallopian transfer 399
storage of 69
Gaming disorder 478, 481
Gamma alcoholism 705
Gamma hexachlorobenzene 683
Gamma hydroxybutyrate 709, 711
Gamophobia 475
Gang rape 418, 437
Gangrene 103, 220, 340
Gangrenous type 721
Ganja 649

Index

Gas
  chromatography 546
  stiffening 167, 169f
Gas-liquid chromatography 546, 629
Gasoline 540
Gastric contents 545
Gastric decontamination 538
Gastric inflammation 723
Gastric lavage 538, 539, 539f, 559, 569, 584, 591, 595, 597, 634, 659, 662, 673, 680, 696, 723, 736
Gastric mucosa, bluish discoloration of 548
Gastric neoplasm, malignant 621
Gastric perforation 539
Gastric resection 621
Gastric ulcers 621
Gastritis 621
Gastroenteritis 579, 584, 680
Gastrointestinal system 153, 627
Gastrointestinal tract 126, 533, 568
Gel electrophoresis 505
Gelineau's syndrome 480
Gender dysphoria 448
Gender identity disorder 448
Gender incongruence 481
Gene editing 527
Genetic profile 504
Genital area 359
Genital evidence 429
  collection 430f
Genital injury 425, 426
Genital organs
  development of 435
  female 288
  injuries to 288
  male 289
Genitalia 209, 216, 419
  anatomy of male 496
  external 82, 124, 161
  normal female 401, 401f
Genitals, fondling of 433
Genitourinary irritants 382
Genitourinary system 153, 375
Genome
  editing 527
  modification 48
Genotype sex 82
Geographical distribution 376
Germicide 564
Gerontophilia 450
Gestation, period of 408
Gestational surrogacy 69, 399
Gettler test 206, 211
Giddiness 609
Giemsa stain 499
Gingival tissue, cellular changes in 179
Gingivostomatitis 565
Glaister-Keen globe 426, 428, 438
Gland 601
Glass blower's shakes 566
Gliding contusion 271
Gliotic scars 271
Glomerulonephritis, chronic 69
Glottis, acute edema of 300
Glucose estimation 267
Glue sniffing 134
Glutaraldehyde 552
Glutethimide 540

Glycerin 108
Glycosides 661
Gonadal agenesis 83
Gonadal biopsy 82
Gonadal dysgenesis 83, 84
Gonads, internal 82
Goodell's sign 406, 414
Goose skin 211
Gossypiboma complication 36
Gossypol 396
Gram-negative bacteria 300
Granulomatous hepatitis 544
Graphology 118
Gravedigger's tools 459
Gravindex test 407
Graze abrasion 215
Greasy substances 559
Green bullet 240
Green pigment molecule 170
Green tobacco sickness 660
Grenz rays 109
Grey turner's sign 218
Grief disorder, prolonged 477, 481
Griess test 259
Grievous hurt 42, 117, 333
  clause 334t
Grievous injury 348
Grunwald Giemsa stains 499
Guillain-Barré syndrome 733
Guillotine 11
Gun oils, test to identify 261
Gun powder 241, 260
  composition of 241t
Gunshot entrance wounds, atypical 252
Gunshot injuries 244f
Gunshot residues 258
  tests to 261
Gustafson's criteria 94t
Gustafson's method 91, 93, 94f
Gustatory hallucination 464
Gut fermentation syndrome 628
Gutzeit tests 559
Gynecological examination 402
Gynecomastia 86
Gyri, surface of 282

H

H_2-receptor antagonists 621
Haderup system 117
Haemophilus influenzae 733
Hagedorn's needle 123
Hair 80, 111, 134, 302, 502, 559, 572
  adult 113
  bulbs 222
  clipping 545
  cross section of 113f
  detect arsenic in 562
  examination of 111
  graying of 99
  loss of 580
  microscopic examination of 581
  naturally fallen 114
  parts of 112f
  plucked 508
  root 83
  shaft
    cells, destruction of 579
    single 502

  singeing of 114, 302f
  stains attached on 115t
  tip of 114f
Hair follicle 580
  cells 82
  with roots 508
Hairpin 383f
Hallucination 461, 462, 465, 484
  types of 462, 464t
Hallucinogens 703, 707
Halo sign 267
Halo vision 632
Halothane 356
Hammurabi code of medical ethics 46
Hand 124
  chopping off of 334f
  held explosive 327f
  injury 327f
  washing, repetitive 475f
Handgun 237
Handing over report 347
Handwriting 118, 626
Hanging 184, 193, 197, 209, 212
  accidental 189
  atypical 185
  autoerotic 189
  classification of 185f
  complete 185
  homicidal 190
  incomplete 185
  judicial 190
  ligature mark in 188f
  near 185
  partial 185
  postmortem 189, 190
  typical 185
Harrison and Gilroy test 259
Hash oil 646
Hashish 646, 649
Hatter's shakes 566
Haversian system 140
Head 359
  chop wound of 226f
  crush injury of 317f
  dissection of 132
  lateral convexity of 273
  permanent disfiguration of 335
  scales, large 600f
Head injury 125, 203, 262, 282, 291, 329, 371, 372, 466
  biomechanics of 263
  evaluation of 283, 291
  open 262, 291
  severe 273
  suspected 125
Headache 593, 609, 610
  causes of 727
Health, state of 534
Healthcare 68
  workers 519
Healthy hair bulb 114f
Hearing, loss of 65, 673
Hearsay evidence 15
Heart 128, 171, 206, 286, 294, 304, 329, 544, 559, 561, 565, 573, 580, 583, 589, 639, 690, 711
  at autopsy, opening of 129f
  attack 634
  auscultation of 159

beat 159
changes in 368
contrecoup contusions of 286
contusions of 286
disease
 congenital 153
 hypertensive 153
en bloc increases 367
examination of 128
hemorrhages in 589f
impaling wounds of 286
lacerations of 286
muscle 166
rate 522
rupture of 286
stab wounds of 286
Heat
 artifacts 304
 cramps 295
 edema 295
 exhaustion 296
 hematoma 303, 304f, 313
 hyperpyrexia 296
 illnesses, progression of 296f
 injury 295
 ruptures 302, 303, 313, 459f
 stiffening 167, 168f, 169
 syncope 296f, 297
Heat stroke 296, 296f, 312, 544
 victim of 297f
Heavy metal 540
 causing peripheral neuropathy 574
 causing toxicity 568
 poisoning 541, 559
Hebephilia 450
Hegar's sign 406
Heinous offenses 713, 714
Helix sign 368, 408
Helixometer 236
Hemagglutination inhibition test 489
Hemagglutinin 594
Hemangiomas 103
Hematemesis 301
 blood 493
Hematochezia 552
Hematoidin 219
Hematological disorders 275
Hematoma 265, 273, 274, 441
 delayed 273
 expanding 273
 typical 277
Hematomyelia 284
Hematorrhachis 284
Hematuria 564
Hemin crystal 488f
 test 488
Hemlock 736
Hemochromogen 488
 crystal 488f
 test 488
Hemodialysis 698, 719
Hemoglobin exhibits 492
Hemoglobinuria 559, 576
Hemolytic imbibition 206
Hemoperfusion 543
Hemophilia 509
Hemophobia 475
Hemopneumothorax 286

Hemoptysis blood 493
Hemorrhage 127, 149, 187, 222, 224, 268, 273, 292, 534, 589f
 duret 283
 external 338
 extradural 130
 flame-shaped 264
 focal 294
 internal 338
 intra-abdominal 126
 intracranial 615
 intraparenchymal 286
 intraventricular 281, 281f
 marginal 187
 meningeal 219
 primary 338
 punctate 132
 reactionary 338, 348
 risk of 539
 secondary 338, 348
 subaponeurotic 360
 subconjunctival 187, 219, 219f, 264
 traumatic 338
Hemorrhagic contusions, multiple 386f
Hemorrhagic diathesis 539
Hemorrhagic pancreatitis 294
Hemorrhagic pulmonary edema 659
Hemostatic disturbances 607
Hemothorax 127, 286
Hepatic glutathione 692
Hepatitis 384
 B 103, 138, 563
 virus 48
 C
 infection 138
 virus 48
Hepatotoxic poison 356, 544, 544t
Herbal medicines 552
Herbicides 533
Hermaphroditism, true 83, 84
Herniation contusion 271
Heroin 533, 614, 618, 647, 654, 709
Hesitation marks 328
Heteropaternal superfecundation 409
Higginson's syringe 383f
High environmental temperature 165
High tension injuries 309
Hilt-Guard abrasion 228f
Hindu Marriage Act 481
Hippocratic oath 52
Hippy flipping 707, 711
Histamine 610
Histotoxic anoxia 153, 666
Hit-and-run 314
Hoarding disorder 476
Holiday heart syndrome 620, 624
Hollow-point bullet 239
Holograph will 481
Homicidal burns 306
Homicidal drowning 209, 372f
Homicidal impulse 465
Homicidal injuries 257, 342
Homicidal laceration 223
Homicidal poison 561
Homicidal poisoning
 inform police in 547
 suspected 535
Homicidal stab wounds 230

Homicidal strangulation 194
Homicidal throttling 196
Homicidal violence, victims of 209
Homicide 6, 189, 194, 224, 230, 321, 332, 413, 536, 595, 669
Homosexuality 439
Honey comb 171
Honeymoon impotence 392
Honor killing 333
Hoppe-Seyler's test 672
Horizontal gaze nystagmus test 626f
Hormone
 replacement therapy 397
 therapy 397
Horseradish 659
Hospital records 15
Hostile witness 15, 16, 19
House fly 174
 life cycle of 174f
Household disinfectants 552
Household emetics 540
House-mite allergy 376
Human behavior 54
Human bites 223
Human blood 489, 489f
Human chorionic gonadotropin 407
Human DNA quantitation 492
Human enamel 93
Human experimentation 49
Human genome 504
Human gestation 361
Human hair 112, 112f, 113f
 ethnic differences in 113
Human immunodeficiency virus 520, 521
 (Prevention and Control) Act 520
 infection 138, 519
 medico-legal aspects of 518
 positive, sexual partner of 519
 prevent transmission of 521
 test 518, 520
Human leukocyte antigen system 492
Human organ 77
 donation of 60
 recipients of 61t
 removal of 61
 transplantation of 61
Human red blood cells 488f
Human saliva detects 501
Human spermatozoa, size of 498
Human T-lymphotropic virus 48
Humanitarian 70
Humerofemoral index 81
Humidity 164
Hunger strikers 53
Huntington's disease 509
Huperzine A 681
Husband insemination, indications for 400
Hutchinson's pupil 274
Hybridization 506
Hydrargyrism 565
Hydrocarbons 727
Hydrocephalus 371f
Hydrochloric acid 543, 549, 552
Hydrocution 203
Hydrofluoric acid 543, 552, 666, 719

Index

Hydrogen
  borate 718
  cyanide 666
  peroxide 552
  rich saline 673
  sulfide 718, 726
    poisoning 712
Hydrolases 681
Hydrophidae 599
Hydrophobia 475
Hydroquinone 553
Hydrostatic lungs 206
Hydrostatic test 366, 367, 367*t*, 378
Hydroxypatite 91
Hygroscopic oily liquid 660
Hymen 402, 404, 427
  rupture of 428*f*
  types of 402, 402*f*
Hymeneal examination 428
Hymeneal swelling 428
Hyoid bone 196*f*
Hyoscine 614, 641, 645
Hyoscyamine 641, 645
Hyoscyamus niger 641, 644
Hyperbaric oxygen, use of 673
Hypercalciuria 582
Hypercuprosis, symptoms of 576
Hyperdynamic septic shock 339
Hyperemia 301, 544
Hyperflexion injuries 284
Hypergonadotropic hypogonadism 86
Hyperkalemia 719
Hypernatremia 275
Hyperphosphorylated tau protein, deposition of 269
Hyperpnea 727
Hypersomnolence disorders 480
Hypertension 537, 609, 610
Hypertensive intracranial hemorrhage, location of 291
Hyperthermia 537, 609, 656
  malignant 355, 537, 656, 696, 699
Hypertonic solutions 300
Hypertrophy, ventricular 129
Hyperventilation 297
Hypnagogic hallucinations 480
Hypnopompic hallucinations 480
Hypocalcemia 656, 719
Hypochondriacal delusion 462, 483
Hypochondriasis 476
Hypoglycemia 680
Hypokalemia 584
Hypokalemic paralysis 584
Hypomagnesemia 719
Hypomania 473
Hypoparathyroidism 376
Hypophosphite 688
Hypotension 269, 537, 584, 607, 659, 673
Hypothermia 162, 294, 312, 376, 537, 539
  effects of 293
  mimicking sexual assault 294*f*
Hypothyroidism 293
Hypovolemic hypodynamic septic shock 339
Hypoxanthine 160
Hypoxia 35, 147
Hypoxic encephalopathy 186
Hypoxyphilia 448
Hysterectomy, complications of 35

Hysteria 656
Hysterical coma 615
Hysterical women 216
Hysterosalpingogram 394
Hysterotomy 71

I

Iatrogenic botulism 734
Iatrogenic deaths 369
Iatrogenic pneumothorax 286
Icard's test 159
Ideal homicidal poison 537, 659
  qualities of 536
Ideal infanticidal poison 372, 378
Ideal suicidal
  agent 669
  poison 536, 537, 616, 690
IIrritable mood 473
Iliac crest 221
Illegal substance 646
Illicit liquor 633
Illusion 461, 464, 465, 484
Imipramine 696
Immaturity 370
Immersion blast 324, 330
Immersion syndrome 203, 211, 294
Immunological tests 407
Immunosuppressant steroid 673
Impotence 100, 389, 399
  causes of 392, 392*f*
Imprint abrasion 215
Impulse 461, 465, 484
  control disorders 470, 478
  disorder 466*f*
  types 465
In situ dissection 126
In vitro fertilization 30, 48, 398
Incendiary bombs 324
Incendiary bullets 240
Incest 397, 436, 438
Incisors 116
Indecent assault 417, 452
Indian Evidence Act 6
Indian Medical Council (Professional Conduct, Etiquette and Ethics) Regulations 29
Indian Medical Council Act 29
Indian Penal Code 5
Indirect agglutination inhibition test 407, 407*fc*
Industrial methylated spirit 621
Inertial injuries 263
Infancy, mandibles of 99
Infant
  botulism 734
  postmortem examination of 359
  viability of 364
Infant death 370
  causes of 370*fc*
  sudden unexpected 376
Infanticide 6, 358, 378, 413
Infantile 402
  whiplash syndrome 374, 379
Infantilism 448
Infantophilia 450
Infection 268, 381
  bacterial 175, 220
  neonatal 370
  type 732
Infectious disease, acute 544

Infertility 389, 399
  delusion of 462, 463*f*, 483
Inflammatory diarrhea 732
Influenza 544
Informed consent 74, 422
  doctrine of 40
Inframammary incision 125
Infrared
  photography 217, 253
  spectrophotometry 112
Ingestion 583, 584, 662, 719
Inguinal region 360*f*
Inguinal thighs 360*f*
Inhalable submicronic atropine respiratory fluid 681
Inhalation, techniques for 708
Inhaled anesthetic, case of 356
Inhaled poisons 538
Inheritance powder 531
Inherited disorders 509
Inhibits protein 687
Injured person, neglect of 340
Injury 127, 159, 213, 263, 332, 359, 372, 391, 440, 444, 451
  accidental 342
  age of 216
  cause of 223
  classical 318
  classification of 213, 325
  compensable 33
  contrecoup 271, 272, 291, 317
  cycle 320
  dangerous 336
  dicing 319, 321, 323
  disposition of 315
  documentation 318
  duration of 347
  endangering life 336
  enlisting 327
  examination of 232
  exclusion of 625
  explosion 324
  external 124, 173, 321, 327
  fabricated 232*b*
  fatal 79
  flaying 317
  internal 321, 375*f*
  major sites of 319*f*
  manner of 214, 216, 221
  nature of 214, 216, 223, 224, 347, 526
  non-kinetic 214
  non-motion 214
  patterned 217
  patterns 328
  photographs of 425
  primary 314, 315*f*, 316, 320, 323, 330
  report 345
    contents of 346*fc*
  secondary 316, 320, 323, 326, 330
  site of 58
  status of 347
  tertiary 316, 326, 330
  triad of 379
  type of 124, 130, 285, 346
Inorganic acids 549
Inorganic irritants 382
Inorganic mercuric salts,
  ingestion of 564

Inorganic mercury 566
　compounds 565
　toxicity, chronic 566
Inorganic metallic irritants 557, 582
　copper 575
　lead 568
　mercury 563
　thallium 579
Inorganic salts 563
Inotropic therapy 659
Inquest 6
　types of 7
Insanity 51, 461
　acute attack of 630
　legal test of 482, 484
　true 467, 468
Insect
　activity 457
　tactile hallucinations of 630
Insecticide 564, 677
　classification of 685
　substance, types of 677
　types of 685
Insemination
　artificial 30, 44, 68, 397, 398, 398f
　donor, artificial 397
　homologous, artificial 397
Insomnia 566, 673
　disorders 480
Instantaneous rigor 167
Instruments 124
Insulin 700
Insurance fraud 523
Intellectual development, disorders of 469
Intention tremors 566, 673
Intercostal blood vessels, lacerations of 286
Intermediary coup contusion 271
Intermembral index 81
Intersex 67, 82, 83
Interstitial emphysema 286
Intestinal colic 51
Intestinal contents 178
Intestines 126, 294, 304, 544, 573, 589
　changes in 367
　injuries of 287
Intoxicated patient, management of 624fc
Intoxicated persons 293
Intoxication 534
　accidental 581
　acute 704, 708
　chronic 565
　diagnosis of 623
　mild 688
Intracavernosal injection 393
Intracerebral hematoma 279, 281f
Intracerebral hemorrhage, cause of 291
Intracranial hematoma 273, 274f
Intracranial hemorrhage, undiagnosed 35
Intracranial mass lesion 283
Intracytoplasmic sperm injection 48, 399
Intradural bleeding 275
Intragluteal coitus 443
Intraocular pressure, loss of 160
Intrapartum
　asphyxia 370
　death 358, 378
Intrauterine
　devices 396
　instillation 71
　life 91, 106

Intravenous marijuana syndrome 647
Intravenous potassium supplementation 584
Introitus 412
Investigation *vs.* inquiry 8
Iodide 563
Iodine 540
　poisoning 590, 591
Ionizing radiation
　burns 298
　effects, acute 353
　reactions 353
Iris muscle 147
Iron 26, 382, 693
Irritability 269
Irritant 533
　gases 671
　　inhalation of 718
　non-metallic 587
　poison 545
　torture 513
Ischemic anoxia 153
Ischemic colitis 552
Ischemic injury, diffuse 282
I-shaped incision 125
Isocyanates 718
Isoenzyme methods 489
Isograft 149
Isopropyl alcohol 712, 722
　poisoning, treatment of 736
Isotonic crystalloids 300
Istanbul protocol 514, 517
Itai-Itai disease 585

J

Jacket, advantages of 239
Jacketed bullets 238
Jacquemier's sign 413
Jaundice 384, 544
Jaw, spacing of 92
Jigai ritual 231
Joint 647f
　deformity 301
Joule burn 309, 310f
Judgment, error of 36
Judicial death sentence, execution of 412
Judicial electrocution 311
Judicial execution 669, 670
Judicial stricture 17
Juvenile court deals 736
Juvenile Justice Act 712, 713
Juvenile Justice Board 11, 713

K

Karyorrhexis 570
Kastle-Meyer test 487, 487fc
Katayama's test 672
Katkar oil 735, 736
Kayser-Fleischer ring 578
Kelocyanor 668
Keloid 301
Kennedy phenomenon 252, 261
Keratin tissues 561
Keratoconjunctivitis 597
Kernohan-Woltman notch 283
Kernohan-Woltman sign 291
Kerosene 136, 540
　ingestion 731
　oil
　　burns 301
　　poisoning 712, 730

Ketamine 681, 709
Ketoacidosis 680
Kevorkian sign 160, 160f, 181
Keyhole autopsy 121
Keyhole defect 250f
Kidney 127, 136, 178, 206, 288, 294, 304, 351, 544, 553, 558, 561, 565, 573, 577, 580, 583, 589, 608f, 639, 690
　cortical pallor in 685f
　effect on 571
　hemorrhages in 589f
　tuberculosis of 153
　tumors of 153
King cobra 599
Kleihauer-Betke test 408, 414
Kleine-levin syndrome 480
Kleptomania 465, 466f, 478, 484
Klinefelter syndrome 84, 85b, 85f
Klismaphilia 451
Knee
　capping 512
　chest position 440f
　reflexes 626
Knife wound, double-edged 228
Knitting needle 383f
Knock-down gas 726, 736
Knockout drops 709, 711
Korsakoff's psychosis 620, 629, 631, 635
Krait 599, 602, 604
Krönlein shot 253
Kuchila 654
Kunkel's test 672
Kussmaul 566

L

Labia 426
　majora 401, 404, 411
　minora 401, 404, 411
Labor
　courts 11
　prolonged 371
Lacerated wound 213, 221, 222f, 303, 346
　healing of 223t
Lactate dehydrogenase isoenzyme 500
Ladder tears 318
Lamendin method 93
Laminaria 383f
Lanugo hair 113, 361, 363f
Laryngeal spasm 198, 203, 354
Larynx 195f, 206, 285, 303, 304f
　edema of 186
　paralysis of 583
　spasm of 370
Latex test 489
Lathyrus sativus 732, 734
　poisoning 712
Lattes crust
　method 490
　test 490
Law, types of 4
Lawful homicide 332
Lax sphincter 441f
Lead 115, 382, 568
　acetate 568, 568f
　bullets 238f
　carbonate 568
　combines 568
　encephalopathy 571
　lines 572
　osteopathy 571

Index

oxides 568
palsy 571
poisoning 117, 570, 570f, 574
salts 568
snowstorm 260
sulfide 568
tetraoxide 568, 568f, 569f
Leathery skin 302f
Leathery stomach 554
Lee Jones test 667
Left coronary artery 128
Leg, avulsion injury of 317f
Legal restrictions, evasion of 24
Legitimacy 68, 69, 397, 410, 414
Lendrum's stain 387
Lenticulostriate artery 292
Leopard rosettes 155f
Leprosy 103
Lesbianism 443, 445
Lesions
   diffuse 291
   produced simulate bruises 596
Leterm mortem 13
Lethargy 584
Letulle's technique 360
Leucomalachite green 487
Leucomelanosis 560
Leukemia 570
Levallorphan 617
Levo-alpha acetyl methadol 705
Lewis system 490
Lichtenberg flowers 311, 311f, 312
Lie-detector 527
   legal 17
Life and health, dangerous to 656
Life insurance policy 27
Life support measures 588
Ligament, yellow 284
Ligase chain reaction 510
Ligature 186
   description 186
   during suspension, slipping of 189
   strangulation 191, 191f, 372f
   test 159
Ligature mark 187, 191, 372f
   appearance of 189
   description of 186
Light weapons 337
Lightning burns, characteristic of 313
Lilliputian hallucination 464
Limbs 124, 361
   movements of 365
   paralysis of 51
Linea nigra 405f
Linear abrasion 214
Linear hemorrhages 218
Lines of Zahn 341
Linseed oil 666
Lip prints 110
   types of 111f
Liquid chromatography 546, 692
Liquid fats, unsaturated 175
Lithium 540, 694
   toxicity 651
Lithopedion 410
Litigation, danger of 397
Live birth
   determinants of 368
   signs of 364, 365, 378
Live born 364, 378

Live donation, case of 62
Liver 126, 206, 288, 294, 304, 329, 351, 544, 545, 560, 561, 565, 573, 577, 580, 583, 589, 596, 690, 711
   effects on 572
   ethanol in 622fc
   failure 630
   necrosis, acute 544
   transplantation 591
   with gallbladder, part of 135f
Living cadavers 149
Living persons 79, 135t
Livor mortis 160
L-line-X-ray fluorescence 573
Local diseases 390, 392
Locard's exchange principle 108, 431
Locard's principle 108
Lochia 411
   alba 412
   order of 414
   rubra 412
   serosa 412
   significance of 411
   types of 412t
Loco parentis 42, 44
Lofexidine 705
Long-scarf syndrome 194
Loose aponeurotic tissues, account of 263
Lower limb 95, 96f
   bones of 100
   technique for 605f
Low-order explosives 325
Low-tension injuries 309
Loxosceles species 610
Lucid interval in insanity 466
Lugol's iodine 436f
   test 435, 438
Luminescent smoking vomit 590
Lung 127, 134, 189, 192, 200, 204, 229, 286, 294, 303, 325, 329, 366f, 559, 580, 583, 589, 639, 659, 690, 698, 711
   blast 325
   changes in 366
   floatation test 205, 366
   injury, acute 616
   irritants 674
   laceration of 286
   non-crepitant 366
   respired 366
   unrespired 366
Lust murder 446, 447, 453
Lymphadenopathy 610
Lynching 190
Lysergic acid diethylamide 707
Lysol 553

M

Maceration 181, 368, 369f
   earliest sign of 368, 378
Machupo virus 729, 736
Macropsia 465
Madea's formula 178
Madonna-mistress complex 392
Madonna-Whore complex 392
Magenstrasse 551
Maggots 134
Magic bullet 261
Magistrate inquest 7
Magistrate's court 8, 10
Magnan's syndrome 652, 653

Magnesium 376
   citrate 542
   sulfate 681, 690
Magnus test 159
Malaria 381
Malate dehydrogenase 155
Male genitalia, chopping off of 334f
Male's propensity 448
Maleness 621
Malformation, congenital 370
Malingering 59, 492
Malnutrition 349
Mandelin test 616
Mandible
   age estimation from 98
   fracture, site of 292
   male 88, 88f
Mandibular canines 93
Mandragora officinarum 641
Mania 473
   symptoms of 473f
Manic episode 473
Mannitol 542
Maqianzi 654
Marburg virus 729
Marchiafava-Bignami syndrome 629, 631
Marijuana 646, 649, 709
Marital rape 434
Marital status 373
Marjolin's ulcer 301
Marquis test 616, 707
Marriage 389, 399, 481
   and divorce, nullity of 394, 397, 411, 413
   cases, nullity of 491
   false promise of 419
Marshal and Hoare formula 164
Marshall and Tewari tests 259
Marshall's triad 327, 327f, 330
Martius scarlet blue stain 340
Masochism 447, 453
Masochistic asphyxial death 448
Masque ecchymotique 200
Mass destruction, weapon of 593
Mass disaster 140
Masseter muscles 130
Mastectomy 103
Master-servant rule 39
Mastoid ecchymosis 267
Mastoid process, right 125f
Masturbation 402, 450
Maternal blood 408
Maternal illness 381
Maternity
   disputed 491
   leave 413
Matted pubic hair 497
McEwan's sign 623, 634
McNaughten rule 482
Mechanical antidotes 540
Mechanical injuries 213, 214f
Meconium 361, 367
Mediation 63
Medical acts 713
Medical Advisory Council 21
Medical alert tattoos 103
Medical and surgical history 425
Medical cannabis 649
Medical care personnel 253
Medical certificates 12
Medical defense procedure 36

Index

Medical education technologies 22
Medical error 39
Medical ethics 22, 45, 46, 59
Medical etiquette 45, 59
Medical evidence 12
 types of 19
Medical examiner system 7, 9
Medical facilities, duties of 73
Medical indemnity insurance 36, 64
Medical indications 403
Medical institution, duties of 715
Medical jurisprudence 3, 18, 712
Medical maloccurrence 38
Medical malpractice 29
Medical negligence 29, 34, 35t
Medical practice
 ethical aspects of 45
 social aspects of 45
Medical practitioner 20, 430, 514
 duties of 24fc
 regarding organ transplantation, duties of 62
Medical records 536
 maintenance of 23, 24
Medical tattoos 103
Medical Termination of Pregnancy Act 49, 70
 abortion under 71t
Medical termination of pregnancy, indications for 69, 70f
Medical torture 514
Medical treatment, high cost of 47
Medical witness, deposition of 14
Medicinal poisons 692
Medico-legal
 application 109, 114, 117
 autopsy, components of 122fc
 cases, managing 54
 issues 53, 321, 359, 394, 444
 problems 35
 register 345
 report 12, 536
 work 55
Medulla 111, 112
Medullary hemorrhages 608f
Medullary index 112, 119
Medullary paralysis 657
Megaloblastic anemia 570
Meixner test 735
Melasma 405, 405f
Melena 301
Mellanby effect 634
Membranes, rupturing of 383
Membranous glomerulopathy 565
Memory 469, 625
 loss 673
Meningeal vessels 580
Meninges 668
 cross section of 262f
Meningitis 680
Menorrhagia 571
Menstrual history 424
Mental disability 423
Mental disorder 481
 classification of 469, 470t
Mental duel 17
Mental dysfunction 482
Mental function assessment, higher 469
Mental health establishment 74
 registration of 77

Mental healthcare 74
Mental Healthcare Act 73, 74fc
Mental illness 74, 76, 469
 treatment of 74
Mental retardation 74, 461, 484
Mental status
 altered 623
 examination 468
Mentally ill person 461, 483
 examination of 483
 treatment of 75fc
Meprobamate 540
Mercurial erethism 566
Mercurialentis 566
Mercurialism 564, 567
Mercuric chloride 543, 563
Mercuric cyanide 563
Mercuric sulfide 563, 564f
Mercurous chloride 563
Mercury 382, 383, 563, 718
 concentration of hair 565
 exposures 563
 toxic inorganic salt of 567
 toxicity 566
 vapor, inhalation of 565
Mercury poisoning 567
 acute 564
 chronic 565, 566
 diagnosis of 565
Mercy killing 47
Mesobuthus tamulus 609
Messenger RNA 501
Metabolic abnormalities 381
Metabolic acidosis 149, 584, 633, 688, 696, 719, 722
Metabolic conditions 615
Metabolic disorders 275, 625
Metabolism 523, 553, 582, 614, 621, 637, 655, 678, 692, 722, 730
Metabolites 533
Metal fume fever 577, 582, 585
Metal oxides 718
Metal-jacketed bullet, partial 239
Metallic arsenic 557
Metallic fouling 255
Metallic lead 568
Metallic salts 533, 540
Metallic taste 560
Metal-plating 582
Metaphyseal sclerosis 572
Methadone 614, 705
Methamphetamine 707
Methanol 180, 632
 antidote for 635
 fatal dose of 635
 metabolism of 632fc
Methemoglobin 668
Methemoglobinemia 712, 720, 736
Methyl
 alcohol 632
 isocyanate 675
 mercury 563
Methylenedioxymethamphetamine 708
Methyltetrazolethiol 630
Meticulous record keeping 36
Metoclopramide 621
Metronidazole 630
Micropsia 464, 465
Middle cranial fossa, fracture of 267, 267f

Middle ear 131, 207, 367
 test 367
Migratory bruise 218, 218f
Minamata disease 566
Mind, unsoundness of 395, 461
Mineral acids 549
Mineral stains 493
Mineralized methylated spirit 621
Miosis 548
Miracle poison 733
Misbehave 30
Missile injury 262
Mitochondrial DNA 510
Modern medicine, proficiency in 30
Moist heat 308
Molar, second 92
Molecular death 146, 147, 157, 159
Molotov cocktail 324, 330
Monday morning fever 585
Monge's disease 717, 736
Mongolian skull 81
Mongolian spots 81
Monilethrix 114
Monoclonal antibody mouse antihuman semen 500
Monovalent antivenom 607
Monozygotic twins 414
Montgomery's test 40
Montgomery's tubercles 405f, 411, 412
Mood 468
 disorders 470, 473
Morbidity statistics 151t
Morning sickness 405
Morphine 533, 597, 614, 615, 618
 poisoning 618, 619
Morphinism 618
Mortality audits 36
Mortality statistics 151t
Mosaic pattern 266
Mosaicism 84
Motor behavior, disorders of 471
Motor disturbances 673
Motor neuropathy 579
Motor vehicle collision 314
Motor Vehicles (Amendment) Act 628
Motorcycle injuries 320
Motorcyclists experience 321
Mountain sickness 717
Mouth 726
 dryness of 642
Movement disorders, sleep-related 480
Mucocutaneous junctions 216
Mucopolysaccharides 344
Mucosal irritation 719
Mucous membrane 543t, 544, 580
 inflammation of 735
Mucus secretion 376
Muddy water 206f
Mugging 191, 211
Muir and Barclay formula 300
Multiple brain petechiae, differential diagnosis of 282
Multivitamin 722
Mummification 175, 176, 369, 369f
Mumps 86
Munchausen syndrome 377, 379
Murder 332
Musca domestica 174
Muscarine poisoning 735

Index

Muscarinic symptoms 612
Muscle 269, 294
   cramps, severe generalized 610
   fibers 165
   flaccidity of 159
   involuntary 166
   primary relaxation of 170
   relaxants 699
   secondary relaxation of 169, 170
   severing of 335f
   spasm, acute 699
   stiffness of 583
   twitching 365
Muscular activity 166
Muscular disease 630
Muscular fasciculations 609
Mushrooms 734
Musket 237
Muslim marriages 481
Mustard seeds 735
Mutilated bodies 140, 145
Mutilomania 465
Muzzle
   blast 242
   flash 242
   impression 247, 255
   imprint 244, 244f, 248f, 261
   velocity 236
Myalgia 583
Myasthenia gravis 733
Mydriasis 548, 583
Myelodysplastic syndromes 570
Myocardial fiber necrosis 294
Myocardial infarction 154, 154f, 155f, 155t, 157
Myocardial ischemia, chronic 154
Myocarditis 153
Myocardium 659
   examination of 129f
Myoclonus 583
Myoglobinuric renal failure 542
Myotoxic 601
   venom 611
Myrtiformes 402

N

N-acetyl cysteine 693
N-acetyl-para-aminophenol 692
N-acetyl-P-benzoquinone imine 692
Nail 134, 502, 559, 579
   clipping 545
   detect arsenic in 562
   print 118
   scrapings 442
   scratches 426f
Nalmefene 617
Nalorphine 617
Naloxone 537
Naltrexone 617
Name, erasure of 31
Nano-medicine, application of 565
Nanotechnology 527
Naphthalene 729
   balls 730f
   poisoning 712
Narcissism 449
Narcolepsy 480, 484
   tetrad of 484
Narcosis, stage of 615, 647
Narcotic antagonist naloxone 616

Narcotic overdose 680
Narcotic poisons 613
Narcotics Drugs and Psychotropic Substances Act 532
Nasal drops 681
Nasal edema 376
Nasal shields 600f
Nation Human Rights Commission 139
National AIDS Control Organization guidelines 518
National Commission 63
National Committee on Radiation Protection 353
National Eligibility-cum-Entrance Test 21
National Guidelines for Stem Cell Research 51
National Human Rights Commission 515
National Medical Commission 20, 21, 439
National register 22
National security 523
Natural disease 138, 218, 340, 356
   history of 300
Naturally fallen hair, root of 114f
Nausea 540, 559, 609
Nauseous metallic taste 563
Near contact shot 245
Neck 124, 130, 187, 188, 191, 192, 285, 303, 360
   autopsy of 186
   dimension of 188
   fractured 285
   injuries 285, 329
   structures 130
Necklacing 306, 313
Necrophagia 447, 453
Necrophilia 447, 453, 454
Needle tracks 705
Negligence
   basic principle of 33fc
   composite 38
   concurrent 38
   defenses against 36
   gross 33
   professional 29, 32
Negroid skull 81
Neisseria 733
Neocortical death 147
Neologisms 471
Neonaticide 358, 378
Neostigmine 608, 678, 723
Nephritis, chronic 153
Nephrolithiasis 153
Nephropathy
   acute 571
   chronic 572
Nephrotoxic poisons 544, 544t
Nerin 664
Nerium odorum 383, 661, 662, 662f, 663
   active principle in 664
Nerve
   damage, peripheral 35
   poisons, peripheral 722
   trauma 390
Nervous apoplexy 156
Nervous disturbances 560
Nervous system 345, 579
Neurasthenia 51, 467
Neurocognitive disorders 470, 479
Neurodevelopmental disorders 469, 470
   classification of 470t
Neurogenic cardiovascular failure 355, 357

Neurolathyrism 734
Neuroleptic malignant syndrome 651, 656
Neurologic criteria 148b
Neurologic disorders 680
Neurological conditions 390, 625
Neurological sequelae 355, 673
Neuromuscular paralysis 537
Neuro-ophthalmological sequelae 682
Neuropathy, peripheral 579, 630
Neuropsychiatric effects 566
Neuropsychological sequelae, delayed 672
Neurosis 466, 483
Neurosurgical complication 275
Neurotic 533
   symptoms 735
Neurotoxic 601
   amino acid 736
   organophosphates 667
   venom 602, 611
Neurotoxin 602
   enzymes 610
Neutron activation analysis 259, 545
Neutrophil 83f
Newborn, normal skull of 98f
Nicotiana tabacum 658, 660
Nicotine 621, 658, 709
   patch 534
      method 709
   poisoning 665
   properties of 660
   replacement therapy 709
Nicotinic effects 679
Nightmare disorder 480
Nihilistic delusion 462, 483
Nipah virus 729
Nitrafezole 630
Nitric acid 543, 549, 550t
Nitrite 736
   test 259
Nitrobenzene 736
Nocturnal penile tumescence testing 393
Nodding face sign 292
Nomogram method 164
Non-accidental injury, sites of 373f
Non-cellular semen markers 499
Non-cognizable offense 5, 18
Non-communicating lacerations 288
Non-environmental causes 296
Non-fatal parathion poisoning 680
Non-habitual passive patient 440
Non-immune hydrops fetalis 371
Nonporous surface 109
Nontoxic shot 240
Non-traumatic causes 277
Non-venomous snakes
   belly scales of 601f
   head scales of 600f
Noonan syndrome 86
Nortriptyline 696
Nose
   bleeding from 187
   print 118
Nostril 600f, 726
   hair 113
Notifiable clauses 28
Novus actus interveniens 712, 713, 736
Nuclear sexing 82
Nuclear terrorism 354
Nucleic acid sequence 510

Nulliparous 412f
  uterus 413
Nullity of marriage, grounds for 399
Nuremberg code consisting 49
Nux vomica 654
Nymphomania 443, 445
Nystagmus 626
Nysten's law 181

O

Oath 16, 51
  administration of 53
  refusing 16
Obscure autopsy 138
Obscure syndrome 138
Obsessive-compulsive disorder 470, 475, 475f
Obstetric history 424
Obturator foramen 89f
Occupational diseases 65
Occupational hazards 639
Occupational marks 118
Ochronosis 553, 554
Ocular movement 148
Odollam 658, 664
Odor 543
Oedipus complex 436
Offense 5, 18, 34
  and penalties 61, 64, 68, 71, 72, 77
  and punishments 66
  common weapons of 336f
  types of 66fc
Oleander 658, 661, 662f
Oleic acid 175
Olfactory hallucination 464
Oliguria 564, 607
Onanism 450
One leg stand test 627
Oniomania 465
Oocyte 68
  cryopreservation 399
OPC poisoning 686
  management of 680fc
Ophitoxemia 602
Ophthalmia 51
Ophthalmoscope 160
Opiate 613, 618, 621
Opioid 356, 613, 618, 718
  overdose, earlier 617
  semi-synthetic 614, 618
Opisthotonus 655, 655f
Opium 159, 378, 615
  poisoning 618
Optic atrophy 571, 632
Optic neuritis 632
Oral contraceptive pills 396
Oral evidence 14
Oral multi-b vitamins 630
Orbicularis oculi 166
Orbital plate, fracture of 264
Organ contusion 218
Organ donation
  after death 44
  ethical issues in 62
Organic compounds 563
Organic impotence 399
Organic irritants 382
  animal 599
  plant 592

Organic mercury 564
  compounds 566
  intoxication, chronic 566
Organic residues, instrumentation for 259
Organic salts 563
Organophosphates 677, 733
Organophosphorus compounds 677
  poisoning 679f
Orifices, natural 124
Orphan, adoption of 714
Orthoboric acid 718
Osiander's sign 406
Osteogenic granulation tissue 290
Osteomalacia, fractures with 582
Othello syndrome 462, 463f
O-tolidine test 487
Ouchterlony method 489
Ovary 127
  corpus luteum in 408
Ovum donation 44, 399
Oxalic acid 543, 549, 552
Oxide 563
Oxidized hemoglobin 668
Oximes 681
Oxygen inhalation 723
Oxytocin infusion 71

P

P300 brain response 523
Pachymeningitis hemorrhagica interna chronica 276
Pack rape 418
Painful paroxysmal skeletal muscle contractions 295
Painter's colic 569
Palatoscopy 118
Palliative care 48
Palmar injuries 328
Palmer's notation 117
Palmer's sign 406, 414
Palms and soles, hyperkeratosis of 560f
Palpation 40
Paltauf's hemorrhage 205, 211
Pancreas 127, 287, 294
Pancuronium 537
Panic attacks 475
Panic disorder 475
Papanicolaou's stain 436, 499
Papaver somniferum 613, 613f
Paper chromatography 546
Paracetamol 692
  poisoning
    antidote for 701
    signs of 692t
    symptoms of 692t
Paradox guns 237, 238f, 260
Paradoxical undressing 294
Paraffin
  melted 108
  test 259
Paraldehyde 136
Paralyses, types of 682t
Paranoia 467
Paranoid schizophrenia 706
Paraoxon 678
Paraphenylene diamine 115
Paraphilia 417, 437, 446, 453
Paraphilic disorder 446, 447, 453, 470
  types of 447t

Paraquat 684, 718
  poisoning 685f
  tongue 685f
Parasitosis, delusion of 462, 463f
Parasomnia disorders 480
Parasuicide 467, 536
Parasympathomimetic agents 621
Parathyroid extracts 553
Paratyphoid bacilli 732
Paraverbal component 55
Pareidolic illusion 465
Parenchymatous degenerative changes 544
Paresthesia 579
Parkland formula 300, 312
Parotid gland, modified 601
Parous uterus 413
Parous woman 412f
Parturition 493
Paternalism 43
Paternity 410, 414
  disputed 491
  leave 413
  testing, sample collection for 492
Patient's general condition, maintenance of 543
Pedal cycle injuries 320
Pederasty 439, 444
Pedestrian accidents, cause of death in 323
Pedestrian injuries 314, 315f
Pedestrian walks 316
Pedophilia 450, 453, 454
Pellets 254
Pelvic ultrasonography 394
Pelvis 89f, 126, 318
  and long bones, fracture of 341
  female 88, 89f
  male 88, 89f
Penal erasure 43
Penicillamine 541, 542
Penicillin 39
Penile biothesiometry 393
Penis examined 435
Pentazocine 356
Perception, disorders of 471
Percussion cap 240
Perianal abrasions 440f
Pericarditis 153
Pericardium 130
Perinatal mortality 358
Perineal swab 430f
Perineum 401, 411, 412
Periodic acid-Schiff stain 155
Periorbital hematoma 263
Peritoneal effusions 351
Peritonitis 552
Perjury 16, 19
Permanent teeth 91, 92, 92t, 117
  eruption of 92f, 92t
  successional 91
Personal illusions 464
Personality changes 673
Personality disorder 470, 479, 481
  multiple 477
Perthes syndrome 199
Per-vaginum examination 428
Pesticide 533, 677
  classification of 677t
  poisoning 685, 687
  substance, types of 677
  types of 685

Index

Petechiae 282, 338
Petechial hemorrhages 726, 731
Pethidine 356, 614
Petroleum products 533
Petrous hemorrhages 207f
Petty offenses 713
Pfropf schizophrenia 472
Phadebas test 501, 502
Phantom pregnancy 409, 414
Pharaoh's serpents 567
Pharaonic incest 436
Pharyngeal reflexes 148
Phenanthrene derivatives 614
Phencyclidine 708, 718
Phenol 180, 553, 554
Phenolphthalein test 487
Phenotype sex 82
Phenyl mercury 563
Phenytoin 694
Phobia, types of 475t
Phobic disorder 474
Phosfume 687
Phosgene 671, 718
Phosphine 687
Phosphoglucomutase 492
Phosphorous poisoning 589f, 590, 591
    antidote for 591
    chronic 590, 591
Phosphorus 136, 587
    pentoxide 687
    poisoning 591
Phossy jaw 117, 591
Phostoxin 687
Physical abuse 375
Physical ailments, treatment of 74
Physical antidotes 540
Physical health consequences 434
Physical injuries 213
Physical morphology 82
Physical torture, types of 513t
Physician-patient relationship, types of 32
Physostigmine 643, 678
Phytotoxin 592, 598
Picana 516
Picrotoxin exposure 656
Piggy back bullet 239, 239f
Pill-rolling movement 642, 643, 643f
Pilocarpine 580
Pinch mark 374f
Pink disease 566
Pinpoint pupil 615f
Piskacek's sign 406
Pitiless vipers 599
Placenta 359, 385
    early separation of 370
    previa 359
Planar chromatography 546
Plant
    penicillin 683, 686
    toxic part of 618
Plaque
    hemorrhage 128
    jaune 271, 291
    rupture 128
Plasma
    cholinesterase 680
    magnesium 206
Plastic bag asphyxia 200, 201f
Plastic bullets 240

Plastic cups 246
Plastic print 108
Pleura 303
Pleurisy 286
Pleurosthotonus 655
Ploucquet's test 366, 378
Plumbago rosea 383
Plumbism 569, 573, 574
Pluripotent stem cell 48
Pneumonia 286, 294, 300, 680
Pneumonic plague 728
Pneumothorax 127, 133, 286, 356
P-nitrophenol test 680
Podography 110
Poecilotheria species 610
Poikilocytosis 570
Poison 531, 532, 543, 543t, 547, 578, 667
    agricultural 677
    apparatus 601
    bullets 240
    causing rhabdomyolysis 611
    classification of 533
    contact 538, 677
    elimination of 542
    injected 538
    medico-legal aspects of 532
    nut 654
    toxicodynamics of 534
Poisoning
    acute 532, 552, 558, 564, 569, 579, 622, 660, 720
    amatoxin type of 735
    cases 24, 535
    concomitant 648
    management of 537, 538fc
    moderate-to-severe 688
    symptoms of chronic 697
    treatment of 579, 671, 677
Poisonous foods 734
Poisonous mushrooms 712, 732
Poisonous snakes 599
Pokkuri death syndrome 138
Police inquest 7
Police intimation, informed refusal for 423
Poliomyelitis 733
Polychromatophilia 570
Polyembolokoilamania 451
Polygraph 522, 523, 527
    test 522f
Polymerase chain reaction 504-506
Polypropylene 137
Polythiol resins 565
Polyvalent antivenom 607
Polyvalent botulinum antitoxin 734
Poppy seeds 614f
Poroscopy 110, 119
Porous surface 109
Porphyrinuria 569
Post-assault activities 424
Postcoital test 394
Post-concussion syndrome 269
Posthumous births 411, 414
Post-immersion syndrome 203, 211
Post-lumbar puncture headache 355
Postmortem 142f, 594
    abrasion 216
    ant bites 457f
    artifacts 455, 455t
    blisters 456f

    bruise 220
    burns 306, 313
    caloricity 165, 181
    changes 455
    chest X-ray 133
    clot 128, 128f
    corrosion 459
    examination 154, 156, 191, 194, 200, 203, 253, 294, 301, 321, 355, 386, 543
        essential instruments for 123b
    glycogenolysis 165
    insect bites 216
    interval 176
    luminescence 171
    maceration 459
    report 536
    samples 629
    submersion 208
    suspension 189
Postmortem staining 160, 163, 181, 204, 220, 294, 302, 455
    color of 181
    development of 161
    fate of 162
Post-traumatic stress disorder 469, 476, 514
    symptoms 476f
    development of 431
Potassium
    arsenate 557
    chloride 580
    chromate 543
    ferric hexacyanoferrate 580
    ferrocyanide 576
        test 672
    hydroxide 554
    iodide 383
    permanganate 541, 552
    serum level of 584
Potency test 400
Powder tattooing 246
Powerballing 706
Prazosin therapy 609
Preauricular sulcus 87, 88
Precipitate labor 371, 372f
Precipitin
    methods 488
    test 140, 501
Preconception and Prenatal Diagnostic Techniques Act 71
Preeclamptic toxemia 370
Pre-embryo 361
Pregnancy 401, 404, 425
    and delivery, medico-legal aspects of 412
    conclusive signs of 407, 414
    diagnosis of 414
    in dead, diagnosis of 408
    length of 70
    physical sign of early 414
    positive proof of 408
    positive signs of 408
    signs of 405, 405f, 405fc, 406f, 407, 408, 408t, 414
    symptoms of 408, 408t, 413
Premolar, second 92
Prenatal diagnostic procedures 44
Prenatal Diagnostic Techniques (Regulation and Prevention of Misuse) Act 71
Pressure abrasion 215
Pressure test 159

Preternatural combustion 306
Priapism 736
Prinsloo Gordon artifact 456, 460
Print media 31
Privileges and Rights of Patients 32
Procedural law 4
Proctalgia, mild 711
Procurator fiscal 9
Professional negligence deaths, cases of 34
Prohibition of E-cigarettes Act 707
Propellant charge 241
Propofol 700
  toxicity 357
Propoxyphene 705
Prostaglandins 71
Prostate 127, 171
  gland 496
  specific antigen 499, 502
Prostatic secretions 496
Protection of Children from Sexual Offences Act 28, 66, 67fc
Protection of Women from Domestic Violence Act 73
Protein markers 492
Proteinuria 582
Proteomes 527
Proteus 170
Pseudocide 536
Pseudocyesis 409, 414
Pseudohermaphroditism 83
Pseudomonas 733
  aeruginosa 300
Psilocybin 532
Psychiatric assessment 468
Psychiatric disorder 461, 474
Psychoactive substances 704
Psychologic symptoms 425
Psychological autopsy 121
Psychological disorders 625
Psychological effects, long-term 434
Psychological maltreatment 375
Psychological torture 513
Psychomotor activity 473
Psychomotor hallucination 464
Psychophysiological detection 522
Psychosis 466, 483, 673
Psychosocial examination 393
Psychotic disorders 470, 472
Psychotropic substance 532, 547
Pterygia 99
Pubic hair 113, 426, 430f, 435, 442
Pubic symphyseal surface 97f
Pubic symphysis 97t, 143
Pubis, symphyseal surface of 97
Pugilistic attitude 167, 302
Pulmonary artery 287
Pulmonary decompression sickness 717
Pulmonary edema 583, 584, 632, 681, 718, 727
Pulmonary embolism 341, 348
Pulmonary fat embolism 220
Pulmonary functions, impairment of 584
Pulmonary thromboembolism 341f
Punch drunk syndrome 269
Punctate basophilia 570, 574
Pupil 148, 160
  bilateral fixation of 274
  constricted 548, 679f
  dilated 548, 643f
Pupillary athetosis 659

Pupillary irregularity 631
Pupillary reflexes, loss of 160
Puppe's rule 249, 250f, 261
Puppet organs 304
Purple glove syndrome 694
Pus, collection of 131
Putrefaction 169, 368, 369f, 455, 456
  artifacts of 456f
  medico-legal importance of 173
  order of 172t
  sign of external 170f
Pyloric stenosis 621
Pyothorax 127
Pyrethrins 685
Pyrethroids 685
Pyrethrum 685
Pyridine ferriprotoporphyrin 488
Pyridostigmine 678
Pyrocatechol 553
Pyrogallol solution 133
Pyromania 465, 478
Pyruvate dehydrogenase 557

Q

Q-fever 728
Quaker buttons 654
Quaternary injuries 326, 330
Quickphos 687
Quinacrine dihydrochloride 83
Quinidine 542, 724
Quinine 542, 614, 658, 724
  overdose of 724
  toxicity 712
Quinism 724

R

Rabbit punch 284
Raccoon eyes 218f, 264
Radiation
  exposure 70
  injury 214
  sickness 353
  type of 353
Radiocontrast agents 552
Radioimmunoassay 407, 608
Radioisotopes 407
Radiological examination, indications of 140b
Railway injuries 322
Railway spine 284, 285, 291
Railway track, decapitation in 322f
Raindrop pigmentation 560, 560f
Raman spectroscopy 501
Rape 69, 394, 397, 417, 420, 437
  accused, examination of 435, 436
  cases, trial of 420
  criminal breach of 413
  deflorate 432
  medico-legal aspects of 419
  punishment for 418, 418t
  survivor of 426f, 427f
  trauma syndrome 434
  trial, cross-examination in 420
  victim
    medical examination of 420
    revealing identity of 420
Rat hole 246
Rayalaseema phenomenon 253
Raygat's test 366, 378

Reaction
  allergic 355, 566
  anaphylactic 356, 610
  antivenom 607
  behavioral 695
  dystonic 696
  electrodermal 522
  fatal 610
  hypersensitivity 39
  supravital 147, 179
  systemic 353
  vital 216, 305
Reactive symptoms 477
Recent delivery
  in dead, signs of 412
  in living, signs of 411
  signs of 411f, 412
Recoil imprint 261
Rectovaginal fistulas 552
Rectum 441, 534, 560
Red blood cells 202f
  basophilic stippling of 570f
Red phosphorous 587, 588f
Red-white-blue sign 610
Refeeding syndrome 350, 352
Reflex
  cardiac arrest 156
  hallucination 464
  vagal inhibition 185
Regional injuries 262
Rehabilitation 714
Relationship management 55
Remote causes 301, 339
Remote delivery
  in dead, signs of 412
  in living, signs of 412
Renal excretion 542
Renal failure 607, 634
  acute 384
  chronic 582, 630
Renal impairment, case of 574
Renal infarcts 127
Renal parenchyma 589f
Reproductive organs 288
Reproductive system 153, 571
  male 496, 496f
Res ipsa loquitur 36, 43
Res judicata 36
Residual air 367
Respiration 158, 159, 522
  artificial 723, 726
Respirator lung 286
Respiratory complications 301
Respiratory depression 609
  classic triad of 614
Respiratory failure 354, 583, 607, 632, 659
Respiratory infection 376
Respiratory movements, cessation of 183
Respiratory paralysis 727
Respiratory system 153, 544
Respiratory tract
  irritant, severe 687
  lumen 376
  obstruction of 354
Restless legs syndrome 480
Restlessness 609
Restraints 76
Restriction enzyme digestion 505
Reticulocytosis 570

Index

Retina 160, 177
Retinal hemorrhages 631
Retinal stippling 571
Retrograde amnesia 269
Retroperitoneal organs 329
Reye's syndrome 680, 698
Rhabdomyolysis 355, 609
    causes of 340
Rhesus incompatibility 370
Rhesus system 490
Rheumatism 51
Rhinorrhea 609, 679*f*
Rhombic prism-shaped crystals 654
Rib 285
    knob fractures of 374*f*
Ricin 728
    poisoning 598
    toxin 729
Ricinus communis 592, 592*f*, 598
Ricochet bullet 252, 252*f*
Ridgeology 110
Ridges 544
Rifle 237
Rifle barrel 236*f*
Rifle cartridge, parts of 241*f*
Rifle firearm 236, 238, 250, 255, 260
    caliber of 237*f*
    injuries 249*t*
    wounds 246
Rifle weapon 236
    cartridges of 239*f*
    parts of 236*f*
Rifling, advantages of 237
Rights and Privileges of Registered Medical Practitioners 31
Rights of Children 58
Rights of Persons with Mental Illness 74
Rights of Sperm Donors 397
Rights of Transgender Persons 68
Rigor mortis 165, 165*f*, 166*f*, 166*t*, 168, 169, 177, 181, 204, 369, 455
    testing for 166
Rimfire cartridge 241*f*
Ring precipitin test 489, 489*f*
Ring sign 267
Ringed sideroblasts 570
Risus caninus 655
Risus sardonicus 655, 655*f*, 657
Road traffic accident 273, 314
Robert's sign 368
Rodenticides 533, 677
Rohypnol 709
Roll-over crash 319
Romberg test 627
Rope burns 328
Round nose soft bullet 238
Routine viscera preservation 135*f*
Rubber bullets 240
Rubber bush 597
Rule of Hasse 361, 378
Rule of Palms 299, 312
Rule of Thumb 164
Rules of Consent 41
Rum fits 631
Rupture of hymen, causes of 402
Russell's viper 599
    venom 608
Russian roulette 257
Rust stains 493
Ryle's tube 539

S

Saccharides 542
Saccharomyces families 628
Sacrum 89, 89*f*, 98
Sadism 446, 453
    reverse of 447
Sadomasochism 448
Safe kit 421, 422*f*
Salicylate 540, 718
    jag 701
Saline diuresis 542, 584
Saliva 501
    dribbling of 187, 187*f*
    swabbing of 116
Salivary gland, modified 601
Salivation 732
    signs of 626
Salmonella 732, 733
    ingestion of 732
Salt abrasion 103
Salt water drowning 206
Sandwich technique 129
Sanitary tampons 402
Sapphism 443
Saturnism 569
Satyriasis 443
Saw-scaled viper 599
Scalds 298, 307, 307*f*
    burns from 114
    characteristic of 313
    types 307
Scalp 362*f*
    contusion 263
    cross section of 262*f*
    hair 113, 363*f*, 545
    hematoma 263, 265
    reflection of 131*f*
Scalpel 123
Scandinavian method 639, 640
Scars 102, 301
    age determination of 102*t*
Scheele's acid 666
Scheele's green 557
Schizoaffective disorder 472
Schizophrenia 470, 472, 484, 485
    classification of 472
    symptoms of 471*f*
Schizotypal disorder 472
Schneider's first-rank symptoms 471
Sciatica 51
Sclera 177, 554
Sclerosis, multiple 733
Scopolamine 641, 645
Scoptophilia 449, 453
Scorpion 532, 609
    antivenom 609
    bite 612
    sting, management of 599
Sea snake 604
Sea water drowning 202, 202*f*, 202*fc*, 205
Seat belt
    abrasion 321, 322*f*
    caused by 323
    injuries 320*b*
    role of 320
    syndrome 320, 323
Seclusion 76
Second impact syndrome 269
Second trimester abortion, cause of 387

Secondary mental syndromes 470
Secondary sexual characters 98
Seeds, dust of 593
Sehrt's sign 206
Seizures 537
    alcoholic 629, 631
    control 651
Selenium, deficiency of 376
Self-poisoning 639
Self-throttling 196
Semecarpus anacardium 595, 595*f*, 598
Semen 441
    examination of 497
    test for 500
Semenogelin 500
Semi-jacketed bullet 239*f*
Semilunar hymen 427
Seminal fluid 432
Seminal identification, purpose of 497
Seminal plasma 496
Seminal stains 431, 441, 496, 497, 500, 503
Seminal vesicles 496
Semi-smokeless powder 242
Semi-solid soap mixed 383
Semisomnolence 480
Sensorium 708
Separated labia 363*f*
Sepsis 300, 680
    cause of 384
Septic abortion 384
    complication of 387
Septic inflammation 103
Septicemia 136, 149, 341
Sertraline 588
Serum 386
    ceruloplasmin 575
    sickness 607
    truth 524, 527, 639
Sessions case 5
Sex 81, 362
    chromatin 82
    chromosomes 82-84
    determination 83, 90*t*, 93
        method of 104
        tests 30
    of deceased 305
    presumptive evidence of 81
    verification tests 82
Sex-linked acts 417
Sexual abuse 375, 416
    indicators of 434
Sexual acts with animals 417
Sexual asphyxia 209, 209*f*
Sexual assault 66, 116, 216, 416, 419, 425, 426*f*, 452*f*, 497*fc*, 522, 711
    corroborative signs of 431
    evidence of 526
    forensic evidence kit 422*b*
    survivor 421, 420, 421*fc*
Sexual battery 418
Sexual development 99
    classification of 84*fc*, 84*t*
    disorders of 83, 84, 84*fc*, 84*t*
Sexual dysfunction 389, 432, 434
Sexual harassment 66, 416, 417, 715, 736
Sexual Harassment of Women at Workplace Act 712, 715
Sexual history 424
Sexual identities 67*t*
Sexual intercourse 393, 402, 427, 427*f*, 438

Index

Sexual norms 513
Sexual offense 416, 437
Sexual Offenses Act 452
Sexual paraphilia 448
Sexual potency 389
Sexual torture 514
Sexual violence 416, 417f
Sexually active woman 432
Sexually transmitted
   diseases 395, 425
   infections 434
Shaken baby syndrome 374, 379
Shaken infant syndrome 375f
Shaking palsy 566
Shallow water drowning 203
Sharp force
   injuries 217
   trauma 214
Sharp wound, characteristics of 224f
Sheehan's hemorrhage 130
Shigella 732, 733
Shock 300, 607, 632
   anaphylactic 339
   bacteremic 154
   burn 339
   cardiogenic 339, 659
   combating 689
   endotoxic 339
   hemorrhagic 384
   hypovolemic 300, 338, 348
   neurogenic 300, 339, 348
   psychogenic 339
   septic 339, 348
   surgical 354
   traumatic 339
   vasovagal 156, 339
   waves 242f
Shooting 512
Shorr stain 499
Shot, welding of 237
Shotgun 236-238, 249, 255
   and rifle, cartridge of 240
   barrel 236f, 237
   caliber of 238f
   cartridge, parts of 241f
   choking of 237f
   injury 247f, 247t
   pellets 237
   range, barrel lengths of 237
   weapons, cartridges of 239f
Shoulder
   and neck, skin of 171f
   joints 95, 303f
Sickle cell
   anemia 509
   crisis 154
Silver nitrate 103
Silybin 735
Simon's sign 189
Sims-Huhner test 394
Sin of Gomorrah 443-445
Single bullet 261
Single-edged knife, parts of 231f
Sinking fetal lungs 367f
Sinsemilla 647
Skeletal age estimation 143
Skeletal changes 99
Skeletal injuries 374
Skeletal muscle 147, 356

Skeleton 82
Skin 123, 134, 159, 543t, 551, 554, 577
   applied to 596, 597
   blackening of 302f
   burns 551
   changes in 365, 365t
   color of 218
   degloving of 302, 302f
   dry hot 642
   erosion of 551f
   grayish discoloration of 554f
   incisions 125, 125t
   pigmentation of 405
   rashes 560
   slippage 368
Skull 80, 303
   and brain 130
   and meninges 273
   bullet wounds in 250f
   cross section of 262f
   female 87, 87f
   inbending of 264f
   linear fracture of 374f
   male 87, 87f
   suture closure 97, 98f, 98t
   types of 80t
   vault 386
   X-rays 268
Skull fracture 264, 268, 290t, 292, 320
   age of 290
   compound 267
   depressed 265
   growing 267
   types of 265, 265f
Slap mark 374f
Sleep 534
   apnea, prolonged 376
   attacks 480
   deprivation 514
   disorders 480
   drunkenness 480
   paralysis 480
   talking 480
   terrors 480
   wake disorders 480
   walking 484
      disorder 480
Sleeping beauty syndrome 480
Sleeping pills 637
Sleep-related bruxism 480
Slippery elm bark 383, 383f
Slurred speech 609
Small blood vessels 269
Small bowel prolapse 384f
Small intestine 137, 206, 287, 560, 561, 577
   upper part of 135f
Smallpox 728, 729, 736
Smears 137
Smegma 435
Smelter's shakes 585
Smoke
   inhalation 727
   soiling 243
Smokeless powder 241
Smooth bore
   firearms 237
   weapons 236

Snake 532, 599, 611
   classification of 599
   non-venomous 599, 600, 601f, 608f
   venom 601, 602t
      metalloproteases 608
   ophthalmia 604, 607
Snakebite
   diagnosis of 611
   external features of 608f
   first aid in 611
   management of 599, 606fc
   poisoning 612
   treatment 611
Sneezing 365
Snorting cocaine 651f
Snowfield vision 632
Social anxiety disorder 475
Social phobia 475
Social reintegration measures 714
Socrates 736
Sodium 376, 557
   amytal 523
   bicarbonate 681
   carbonates 549
   citrate 180
   formaldehyde sulfoxylate 565
   hydroxide 549, 552, 554
   oxalate 180
   polystyrene sulfonate 580
   rhodizonate test 259
   sulfate 542
   thiosulphate 591, 668
Sodomy 394, 439, 440, 441f, 442-445
Soft tissue injury 263
Soft-point bullet 239
Solid blasts 324, 330
Somatic cell nuclear transfer 48
Somatic death 146, 157, 158
Somatic motor effects 679
Somatic neuromuscular junction 660
Somnambulism 480, 484
Somniferous poisons 613
Somniloquy 480
Somnolentia 480, 484
Sophisticated tool 259
Sorbitol 542
Southern blotting 505
Souvenir bullet 239
Spalding's sign 368, 408
Spanish fly 712, 721, 721f
Spark burns 309
Sparrow foot marks 323
Species of semen, confirmation of 502
Species origin, identification of 500
Spectacle hematoma 264
Spectroscopic examination 487
Spectroscopic test 672, 727
Speech 118, 473, 626
Speed balling 614
Sperm 68
   bank 397
   donation of 44
   motility of 499
Spermatozoa 496
   absence of 502
Spermatozoon 499f
Spermine picrate crystals 498f
Sphenoid sinus 207
Spider bites 610

Spill burns 307
Spinal cord 132, 284
    remove 144
Spinal poisons 654
Spleen 126, 206, 287, 294, 304, 307, 329, 560, 580, 711
Split laceration 221, 222*f*
Split transplants 149
Spontaneous cardiac rupture, common site of 291
Stab injury 167
Stab wound 213, 227, 228*f*, 229, 229*f*, 336*f*, 346
    classification of 227*f*
Stagnant water 174
Stains 426, 428, 497
Standardized field impairment tests 626, 627*b*
Staphylococcal enterotoxin B 728
Staphylococcus 170, 339
    aureus 300, 732
Starvation 349, 350*f*
    acute 349, 350, 352
    chronic 349, 350, 352
    deaths 349, 352
State Commission 63
State Medical Council 22, 23*fc*
Static test 366
Statutory rape 28, 417, 418, 437
Steering wheel impact abrasions 321
Steering wheel impact injury 318, 323
Stem cell
    lines, period for 49
    research 48
    therapy 49
Stenotic lesions 154
Stereotypy 471
Sterility 100, 389, 393, 399
Sterilization 395, 396, 399
    classification of 395*fc*
Sternal notch 125*f*
Sternal rib 100
Sternum 286, 361, 363
Steroid
    anti-inflammatory 673
    injectable 396
Steroidal contraception 396
Sticky mucus 559
Stillborn 358, 364, 378
    fetus 369
Stomach 126, 206, 294, 304, 544, 553, 554, 559, 561, 573, 580, 589, 596, 639, 690, 698
    barium meal X-ray of 118
    bowel test 367, 378
    changes in 367
    contents 177, 545
    corrosive agent in 551*f*
    injuries of 287
    mucosa of 562, 668
    mucous membrane of 544*t*
    perforation of 456*f*, 551*f*
    poisons 677
    washing 538
Stone baby 410
Stools 558
Strain 263
Strangulation 190, 192*f*, 193, 372
Streak gonads 84
Streptococcus 170, 339
Stress 470
    disorders 476, 481

Stretch lacerations 221
Striae gravidarum 405*f*
Stroke, lightning 311
Stroma-free methemoglobin 668
Strychnine 542, 614, 654
    poisoning 655-657
    tree 654
Strychnos nux-vomica 654, 654*f*, 657
Stud guns 237
Stupor 467
    stage of 614
Sturner's formula 178
Subarachnoid hematoma 277, 279*f*
    types 278
Subarachnoid hemorrhage 130, 279, 280
    traumatic 329
Subclavian catheters 286
Subcutaneous bruise 217
Subcutaneous tissue 189*f*, 192*f*, 196*f*
Subdural hematoma 275, 276*f*, 277*t*, 374*f*, 680
    cause of 275, 275*t*, 291
    types 276
Subdural hemorrhage 279-281, 292
Subdural hygroma 277
Subendocardial hemorrhage 130, 544
Subendocardial infarcts 154
Subfalcine herniation 274, 277
Subgaleal hematoma 374*f*
Subgaleal hemorrhage 263, 264*f*
Subpoena 11, 16
Substance
    abuse 322
    disorders 704
    use 470, 478
Succinylcholine 699
Sudden cardiac death 287
Sudden death 6, 153, 157, 286
    cause of 157, 355
Sudden infant death syndrome 139, 370, 376, 376*f*
Sudorifics 542
Suffocation 197, 300, 371
Suicidal burns 306
Suicidal cases 595
Suicidal impulse 465
Suicidal injury 257, 342
Suicidal lacerations 223
Suicidal poisoning 535, 674, 720
Suicidal strangulation 194
Suicide 6, 189, 209, 210, 224, 230, 321, 322*f*, 356, 536, 413, 561
    bomber 327
    commit 74
    complex 149
    detergent 727, 736
    physician-assisted 48
    tree 663, 664
    victims 257
Sulfate 542, 588
Sulfhemoglobin 170
Sulfonylureas 630
Sulfuric acid 543, 549, 550*t*, 552
Summons 11, 19
    case 6, 18
Sun stroke 296
Sunflower cataract 578
Supracallosal hernia 283
Suprapubic puncture 134*f*
Supravital stain 499

Surgery, legal 17
Surgical devices 356
Surgical emphysema 356
Surgical excision 607
Surgical operation 340, 402
Surgical technique 51, 356
Surrogacy Act 69
Surrogacy, types of 69
Surrogate
    characteristics of 69
    mother 399, 400
    parenting 399
Sushruta oath 52
Sveshnikov's sign 207
Swab sticks 430
Swallow tail appearance 222*f*
Sweat glands, profusion of 108
Sweating 269
Swelling 220, 426, 428
Swiss cheese 171
    appearance 309
Swyer syndrome 84
Symphysis pubis 125*f*, 414
Syncope 152
Synovial fluid 178
Synthetic cannabinoids 707
Synthetic cathinones 707
Synthetic dyes 493
Synthetic opioids 614, 618, 707
Syphilis 103
Syphilitic chancre 436
Syringe aspiration 382

T

Tachyarrhythmia, ventricular 718
Tachycardia 297, 609, 610
Tactile hallucination 464, 652
Tail wag 252
Tail wobble 252
Takayama 488
    test 488*f*
Talunex 687
Tandem bullet 239
Tannic acid 103, 541
Tap test 609
Tardieu's spot 184, 188, 194, 210
Tarsal bones 363*f*
Tattoo 103, 103*f*, 243, 244*f*, 247, 260
    classification of 103
    mark 102, 105
Taurodontism 94
Tear 221, 428, 440*f*
    gases 674
Teardrop sign 267, 292
Teeth
    charting of 116, 119
    dislocation of 335*f*
    enamel of 368
    number of 93*t*
    pink 171
    pulp 83
    two sets of 91
Teichmann test 488, 488*f*
Telemedicine
    consultation through 26
    guidelines for 26*b*
Telephone scatologia 451
Telephonicophilia 451
Temporal lobes 270*f*

Index

Temporal muscles 130
Temporal scalp contusion 274
Temporary lethargy 269
Temporary teeth 91, 92, 104
Temposil 630
Tenacious froth 205f
Tendons, severing of 335f
Tensile strain 263
Tension 699
   pneumothorax 286
Tentorial hernia 283
Test tube baby 398
Testamentary capacity 468, 481, 484
Testes, ultrasonography of 393
Testicular feminization syndrome 85
Testicular syndrome 86
Testimony 16
Testosterone levels 82
Tetanus 656, 733
Tetracycline 39
Tetraethyl lead 568
Tetramethylbenzidine 487
Tetrathiomolybdate 578
Textiloma denotes complication 36
Tezampanel 681
Thalassemia 509
Thallium 115, 580, 581
   acetate 579
   poisoning 580, 580t, 581
   stress test 581
   sulfate 579
   toxicity 580, 581
Thanatochemistry 176
Thanatology 146, 157
Thanatomicrobiome 176, 179
Thanatopraxia 180
T-handled chisel 123
Therapeutic artifacts 457
Therapeutic hazard 39
Therapeutic misadventure 39, 44
Thermal injury 293
   classification of 293fc
Thermic fever 296
Thermogenic anhidrosis 297
Thevetia peruviana 724
Thevetin 664
Thevotoxin 664
Thiamine 537, 630, 632, 722
Thigh
   avulsion injury of 317f
   bite mark on 426f
Thin-skull rule 713
Thioctic acid 735
Thiopentone sodium 523
Third labial touches eye 600f
Third molar 92
Third party artifacts 457
Thoracic blood vessels 329
Thoracic cavity 366f
Thorax 124, 125, 360
   opening 360
Thought and speech, disorders of 471
Thought blocking 471
Thromboembolism 340
   development of 348
Thrombosis 340
Throttling 194, 195, 210, 216
Thumb pressure 161

Thunderclap headache 279
   cause of 291
Thymol 383
Thyroid 580
   cancer 39
   cartilage 285
Tibia 100
   causes fractures of 318
   fracture of 315f
   upper end of 363, 363f
Ticks 118
Tiger snake 599
Time since death, estimation of 161f, 176
Tincture iodine 541
Tingling sensation 583
Tinnitus 673
Tissue
   death of 220
   deep 218
   depth method 524
   slices 155
   tags 222
   type of 217
Tobacco 660, 664
   smoke 557
Toes, frostbite of 295f
Toluidine blue 438
Tongue 191, 204, 350, 626
   falling back leading 354
   paralysis of 583
   protruding 302f
   protrusion of 187
Tonsillar hernia 283
Tonsillar herniation 277
Tooth
   dislocation 290t
   enamel, radiocarbon analysis of 93
   forceps 123
   grinding 480
   parts of 91f
Torn frenulum 374f
Tort 33
Torture 512, 516
   and Human Rights 30
   physical 512
   reasons for 512
   sequelae of 514
   types of 512
Toucherism 450
Toxalbumin 592, 598
   ricin, containing 592
Toxaphene 683
Toxemia 300
Toxic
   chlorinated insecticides 686
   compounds 557, 563, 568, 568t, 575, 579, 583
   dose 699
   manifestations 695
   part 613, 641
   peptides 610
   principles 602
Toxicity 678
   reduction of 690
   results 355
Toxicokinetics 534
Toxicological analysis 545
Toxicological artifacts 458

Toxicological examination 356
Toxicological procedures 545
Toxicological studies,
       preservative for 145
Toxicology 531, 718
   analytical 546
   clinical 531
   general 531
   history of 531
   modern 531
Toxidrome 613, 615, 615t, 618
Toxin 532
   alcohol 705
   detection of 735
   type 732
Toxinology 532
Toxoplasma 381
Tracer bullet 240
Trachea 205f, 206, 206f, 294, 303, 304f, 354, 539, 580
   mucous membrane of 285
Tracheal reflexes 148
Traité des poisons 531
Tramline bruise 455f
Trance disorder 477
Tranquilizers 695
Transcapsular laceration 288
Transgender 67, 82, 82f, 443
Transgender Persons (Protection of Rights)
      Act 67
Transient psychotic disorder 472
Transillumination test 159
Transmittable diseases 48
Transmural infarcts 154
Transplantation of Human Organs Act 30, 60
Transplants, types of 149
Transportation injuries 314
Trans-sexualism, male-to-female 448
Transtentorial herniation 277
Transvaginal sonography 408
Transvestic fetishism 448
Transvestism 82, 448, 453
Trauma 322, 332, 345, 387
   concealed 138
   concomitant 300
Traumatic cardiac rupture, common sites of 286, 291
Traumatic causes 277
Traumatic dislodgement 335f
Traumatic injuries, sequelae of 326
Traumatic lesion, disease from 340
Tremors 583, 610, 727
Tremulousness 630
Treponema pallidum 48
Tribadism 443, 445
Trichotillomania 465, 466f, 476
Tricology 111
Tricyclic antidepressants 542, 621, 696
Trimetazidine 690, 696
Triphasic withdrawal syndrome 706
Triple base powder 241
Troilism 449
Tropical anhidrotic asthenia 297
Tropical immersion foot 295
T-shaped incision 125
Tuberculosis 103, 138
Tubular necrosis, acute 294, 544
Tularemia 728, 729

Index

Tumbling bullet 252, 261
Tunnel vision 632
Turner's syndrome 82, 84, 85b, 85f
Twins 376
   identical 409, 410, 414
Twisting neck 372
Two-finger test 403, 428
Tympanic membrane, perforation of 334f
Typhus 728
Tyre sign 444
Tyre tread marks 317
Tyre treadmark over neck 317f

U

Ubiquinone 588
Ueno's sign 207, 207f
Ulcers 51, 294, 544
   pressure 216
Ulmus fulva 383
Umbilical cord 360, 365t
   blood, banking of 48
   changes in 365
Unbearable pain 47
Uncal hernia 283
Unclaimed body 715
Unconsciousness 269
Uncus, herniation of 283f
Under Hindu Adoption and Maintenance Act 481
Unethical conduct, exposure of 24
Unfavorable witness 16
Universal antidote 547
Universal system 117
Unlawful homicide 332
Unmarried woman 397
Unnatural deaths 150
Upper cervical vertebrae, spinous process of 284
Upper limb 95, 96f, 166
Upper respiratory tract 200
Uranism 451
Ureaplasma 381
Uremia 159
Ureteric ligation 35
Urethra 534
Urethral discharge 442
Urinary bladder 127, 633
   contents of 178
   distention of 642
Urinary disturbances 405
Urinary output 537
Urine 134, 134f, 136, 386, 442, 502, 545, 553, 558, 559, 564, 629
   alcohol 628
      concentration 628
   alkalization of 698
   analysis 394
   extravasation of 288
   sample 429
Urningism 443
Urobilin 502
Urolagnia 451
Ursodeoxycholic acid 588
Uterine
   cavity, shape of 412f
   perforation 384f
   souffle 406, 407
   wall 412

Uterus 171, 411
   after delivery, size of 412t
   descends 414
   midway, fundus of 414
   post-delivery, upper border of 411f

V

Vacuum aspiration 383, 383f
Vagal inhibition 156, 191, 194, 198, 203, 384
Vagal stimulation 203
Vagina 127, 402-404, 411, 412, 428, 534
Vaginal canal, perforation of 127
Vaginal cell 436
Vaginal discharge, evidence from 431
Vaginal epithelial cells 438
Vaginal examination 428
Vaginal fluid 497
Vaginal intercourse 416
Vaginal introitus 428
Vaginal mucosal barrier 404
Vaginal reconstruction 82f
Vaginal secretion 498, 502
Vaginal squamous cells, mature 436f
Vaginal swab 430f, 502
Vaginal wall, laceration of 428f
Vaginismus 393f, 399
   types of 393t
Vagitus
   uterinus 365
   vaginalis 365
Valsalva maneuver 652
Valve, examination of 129
Valvular heart disease 153
van Gogh syndrome 472
Vanishing twin syndrome 410, 414
Variot's method 103
Vascular congestion 282
Vascular injury, diffuse 282
Vasculotoxic venom 602, 611
Vecuronium 537
Vegetable origin, poisons of 732
Vegetable stains 493
Vegetative signs 467
Venereal discharge 436
Venereal disease, transmission of 431
Venom 532
   components 602
   prevention of spread of 605
Venomous snake 599, 600, 600f, 601f, 608, 608f
   classification of 599t
   common 601, 601t
Venous air embolus 133
Venous bleeding 494, 494f
Venous congestion 185
Ventricular fibrillation 203, 294, 659
Verbal autopsy 121
Verbal component 55
Vermilion 563, 569
Vernix caseosa 359, 360f, 361, 363f, 365
Vertebral bodies, fracture of 285
Vertebral column 285
Vertical compression fracture produces 289
Vertigo 51, 673
Vesicovaginal fistulae 35
Vibrating saw 123
Vibrio cholera 728, 732, 733
Vicarious liability 44
Vicious cycle 183fc

Victim
   body 58
   detect semen from 432t
   face 444
   hygiene 432
   identification of 492
   specific blood group substance 451
   survive after injury 256
Vineyard sprayer's lung 578
Violate Provisions of Drugs and Cosmetics Act 30
Violence
   direct 264
   general 382
   indirect 264
   local 382
   physical 424
Violent exercise 382
Violent head movement 269
Violent intercourse 428
Viper 600, 602, 604
   bite 611
      local signs 603f
Viperidae 599
Viperine snake bite 594, 603, 607f, 608, 608f
Viral encephalitis 728
Viral hemorrhagic fever 728, 729, 736
Viral infections 70
Viral orchitis 86
Virchow skull breaker 123
Virchow's method 126
Virgin 401, 413
   false 404, 413
   true 404
Virginity 403
   signs of 402, 413
Virulent leprosy 395
Virus 519
Viscera 189, 294, 551
   additional 135t
   blackish 551f
   bottles, contents of 137t
   deep congestion of 726
   preservation of 135, 136
Visceral damage 458
Visceral injuries 374
Viscid actomyosin, formation of 165
Vishaka guidelines 716
Visible color reaction 487
Vision
   blurred 609
   impairment of 631
   loss of 65
   mild blurring of 610
   protection of 725
Visual hallucination 464, 484
Vital reaction, evidence of 142
Vitamin
   B 376
   C 376
   D 376
   E 376
      treatment 681
   K 588
Vitreous humor 134, 134f, 137, 160, 177, 178
Vitreous potassium 160

Index

Vitriolage 551, 551f, 556, 596
Voice 118
   recognition 111
Void marriage 394
Volatile poisons 539
Voluntary breath holding 159
Vomiting 540, 559, 609
   signs of 626
Vomitus 558
Voyeurism 449, 449f, 453
Vulva 401, 401f, 419, 426
   chancre of 392
Vulvodynia 711
Vx nerve agent 676
Vx poisoning 676

W

Wad, advantages of 241
Wadcutter 238
Waddell's triad 316, 323
Wagenaar test 488
Walk and turn test 627
Walker's test 259, 498
Walking corpse syndrome 462
Wallace rule of Nines 299, 299f, 312
Wallerian degenerative sensory neuropathy 579
Wandering bullet 260
War gases 674
Warfarin 70
Warm water immersion foot 295
Warning notice 29, 43
Warrant case 6, 18
Washerwomen's hand 204, 205f
Wasp 610
   sting, management of 599
   venom 610
Wasting disease 173
Water
   borne threats 728
   current 174
   hydrolysis in 678
   quality of 174
   salinity of 174
   submerged in 162
Water-soluble glycoprotein 592
Wax drippings 310, 313
Weakness 727
Weapon
   double-edged 228
   examination of 231, 347b
   nature of 114, 224
Wedge-shaped appearance 271
Weight loss 727
Weiss sign 553
Wenzell test 656
Wernicke's encephalopathy 620, 629, 635
Wernicke-Korsakoff syndrome 631
Wet drowning 201
Wet submarine 516
Wet-vacuum sampling device 527
Whatman FTA cards 509f
Whiplash injury 284, 291
White cell antigens 492
White deaths 294
White phosphorous 587, 588, 588f
White torture 514
Whole-bowel irrigation 569
Whole-brain death 147
Widespread petechiae 282
Widmark's formula 620, 628, 634
Widow 397
Wieland test 735
Wischnewsky spots 294
Withdrawal symptoms 630
   treatment for 635
Withdrawal syndrome 706
Witness 7, 15
   box 18
   common 15
   expert 15
   torture 514
   types of 15
Wood's lamp 438
   examination with 425
Workman's Compensation Act and Poisoning 65
Wound 213, 247, 310, 432
   accidental 225, 343
   age of 343f, 344t
      incised 224
   antemortem 343, 343f
   ballistics 242
   causes of death from 338
   chop 226, 226f
   classification of 213
   close range shotgun 246, 246f
   concealed punctured 227, 372
   contact 248f
   cut throat 225f
   defense 226, 230, 231, 232, 232f
   depth of 222
   entry 227, 249, 251
   exit 227, 249, 251
   fabricated 232
   fatal stab 230
   fictitious 232
   firearm
      entry 251f
      exit 251f
   forged 232
   gunshot 217, 243
      entry 248, 458f
   gutter 249
   head of 224
   high energy transfer 242
   homicidal 225, 343
      cut-throat 225
   incised 213, 223, 224f, 224t, 263, 346
      lacerated 221
   multiple exit 256f
   number of 230
   penetrating 227, 243, 243f, 284
   perforating 227, 234, 243, 243f
   postmortem 343, 343f
   punctured 227
   scalp 263, 264
   secondary target 256
   self-inflicted 232
   self-suffered 232
   sharp 223
   shotgun 245, 247f
   single entry 256f
   slap 253, 261
   soiling of 222
   stellate 248f
   suicidal 343
      cut-throat 225
      stab 230
   superficial perforating 253
   tailing of 224
   tangential entrance 249
   tentative 230
   therapeutic 232
   track 251
   types of 232
Wreden's test 367, 378
Wreden-Wendt tympanic cavity 367
Wrist
   drop 571, 571f
   X-rays of 95
Written consent 40
Written informed consent 413
Wydler's sign 206

X

Xenobiotics 532, 736
   causing tremors 567
Xenograft 149
Xenophobia 475
X-rays, usefulness of 253

Y

Y chromosome 93, 493
Yaw 252, 252f, 261
Yellow jackets 637
Yersinia
   enterocolitica 732
   pestis 728
Yetti 654
Y-shaped incision 125, 360

Z

Ziehl-Neelsen's method 499
Zieve syndrome 620, 624
Zinc 26, 584
   chloride 543, 584
   oxide fumes 584
   phosphide 584
   shakes 584
   stearate 584
   sulfate 584
Zip guns 237
Zoophilia 444, 445
Zoophobia 475
Zygoma 221
Zygote intrafallopian transfer 399